DAVIDSON'S
Principles and Practice of
Medicine

The Editors

Christopher R.W. Edwards
Professor of Clinical Medicine, University of Edinburgh Honorary Consultant Physician, Western General Hospital, Edinburgh. Dean of the Faculty of Medicine, Provost of the Faculty Group of Medicine and Veterinary Medicine, University of Edinburgh

Ian A.D. Bouchier
Professor of Medicine, University of Edinburgh. Honorary Consultant Physician, Royal Infirmary of Edinburgh

Christopher Haslett
Professor of Respiratory Medicine, University of Edinburgh. Honorary Consultant Physician, Royal Infirmary of Edinburgh

Edwin R. Chilvers
Wellcome Senior Research Fellow in Clinical Science, University of Edinburgh. Honorary Consultant Physician, Royal Infirmary of Edinburgh

Illustrated by Robert Britton and Hard Lines Agency

For Churchill Livingstone

Commissioning Editor   Laurence Hunter
Project Editor   Alison Bowers
Assistant Copy Editor   Kathleen Orr
Project Assistants   Jane Lyness, Sarah Cunningham
Project Controllers   Kay Hunston, Nancy Arnott
Design Direction   Erik Bigland
Design Assistant   Jim Farley
Indexer   John Sampson
Marketing   Duncan Jones, Douglas McNaughton

SEVENTEENTH EDITION

DAVIDSON'S
Principles and Practice of
Medicine

Senior Editors

C.R.W. Edwards MA MD(Cantab) FRCPE FRCP FRSE

I.A.D. Bouchier *CBE* MD FRCP FRCPE FFPHM Hon FCP(SA) FI(Biol) FRSA FRSE

C. Haslett BSc(Hons) FRCPE FRCP

Assistant Editor

E.R. Chilvers PhD FRCPE

Churchill Livingstone

EDINBURGH HONG KONG LONDON MADRID MELBOURNE NEW YORK AND TOKYO 1995

CHURCHILL LIVINGSTONE

Medical Division of Pearson Professional Limited

Distributed in the United States of America by Churchill
Livingstone Inc., 650 Avenue of the Americas, New York, NY 10011,
and by associated companies, branches and representatives
throughout the world.

First edition 1952	Tenth edition 1971
Second edition 1954	Eleventh edition 1974
Third edition 1956	Twelfth edition 1977
Fourth edition 1958	Thirteenth edition 1981
Fifth edition 1960	Fourteenth edition 1984
Sixth edition 1962	Fifteenth edition 1987
Seventh edition 1964	Sixteenth edition 1991
Eighth edition 1966	Seventeenth edition 1995
Ninth edition 1968	Reprinted 1996

ISBN 0 443 04961 0

British Library Cataloguing in Publication Data
A catalogue record for this book is available from the British
Library.

Library of Congress Cataloging in Publication Data
A catalog record for this book is available from the Library of
Congress.

Printed in Great Britain by BPC Paulton Books Limited

Preface

The seventeenth edition of *Davidson's Principles and Practice of Medicine* has undergone a major metamorphosis. The introduction of full colour into the book has not only made it more appealing to the eye but, more importantly, allowed the illustrations, diagrams and text to be more readily understood by the reader. The text itself has been extensively changed and updated with new sections on AIDS and geriatrics. Information boxes have been used to highlight the core knowledge which the student (and the examiner!) requires. In the chapters on Psychiatry and Disturbances in Water, Electrolyte and Acid-base Balance, case histories have been used to make the principles and the practice easier to appreciate. Indications for further reading have been made as up-to-date as possible and inserted at appropriate places in the text rather than at the end of the chapters.

However, despite these changes, the editorial policy continues to be that stated by Sir Stanley Davidson in his preface to the First Edition published in 1952 — 'It was also decided that no attempt should be made to describe every rare disease but to devote most of the space available to those disorders more commonly encountered in practice. The selection of the rarer diseases for inclusion and the amount of space devoted to them would be based principally on their cultural interest or their educational value as examples of applied anatomy or physiology...'. Thus the textbook is aimed principally at undergraduates. However, many postgraduate students will find that it will complement and guide their more specialist reading. To ensure its relevance and appeal to undergraduates, all the chapters of the book have been reviewed by members of the junior hospital staff of the teaching hospitals associated with the authors. Many of the changes in the book have followed from their helpful criticisms and suggestions.

Since the last edition Professor Haslett has joined the Editorial Board and Dr Edwin Chilvers been appointed as Assistant Editor. There have also been a number of changes in our contributors and our thanks go to Dr A.T. Lambie, Professor A.E.H. Emery, Professor D. deBono and Dr G.P. Crean, who made valuable contributions to previous editions. At the same time we welcome new contributors including Professor K.A.A. Fox, Professor J. Shepherd, Dr B. Frier, Dr D. Mitchell, Professor W.J. MacLennan, Professor D.J.H. Brock, Dr C.P. Swainson, Dr A.D. Cumming and Dr M.J. Mackie.

In 1974 Sir Stanley published a report in the Scottish Medical Journal on 'The Making of a Successful Textbook of Medicine'. On sending this to a colleague he noted: 'This report will give you an idea of how much work and worry there is in writing a successful book of Medicine. This is a warning to you to have nothing to do with such an idea if it is ever suggested to you!'. It is appropriate in the edition that celebrates the centenary year of Sir Stanley's birth that the Editors, who were sufficiently unwise to ignore his dictum, should remember his vision and thank all those who have shared with them 'the work and the worry'. In this respect the Senior Editors would particularly like to recognise the contribution made by Edwin Chilvers.

C.R.W.E.
I.A.D.B.
C.H.

Edinburgh 1995

Sir Stanley Davidson (1894–1981)

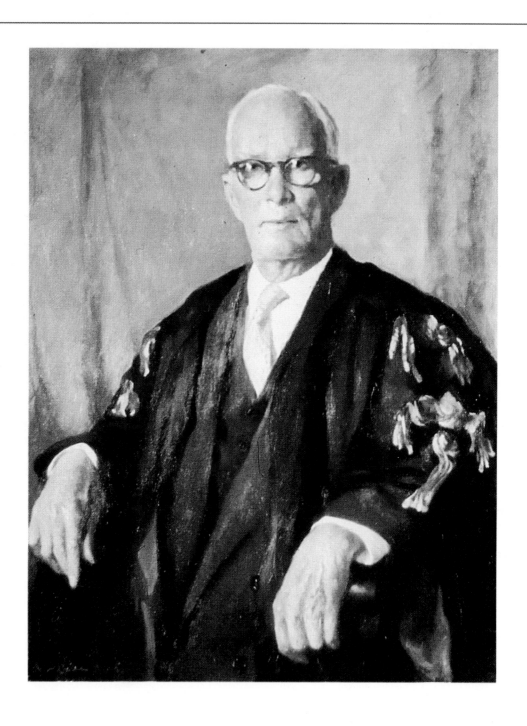

This famous textbook was inspired by one of the great Professors of Medicine of the present century. As we pass the centenary of his birth we recall some aspects of his life and times.

Stanley, as he was known by all, began his medical undergraduate training at Trinity College, Cambridge, but this was interrupted by World War I and later resumed in Edinburgh. He served in the Gordon Highlanders until he was seriously wounded in Belgium. That this period had a profound effect on his subsequent attitudes and values was clear from his emotional recollection, in later years, of the carnage and useless wastage of young life.

In the 1920s he favoured appointments in bacteriology, and this is reflected in his early interests. However, he soon decided to dedicate his life to clinical medicine and clinical research. Exciting contemporary discoveries led to an affection for haematology which he always retained and which was transmitted to many of his disciples.

In 1930 Stanley was appointed Professor of Medicine in the University of Aberdeen. This was one of the first full-time Chairs of Medicine anywhere, and the first in Scotland. The period in Aberdeen was marked by several developing qualities of academic leadership: toughness, fairness and integrity which quickly earned respect; finding and attracting young talent; recognition of the need for decent facilities and accommodation for teaching and research; and research emphasis on the needs of the community.

Appointment to the Chair of Medicine at his Alma Mater, Edinburgh, came in 1938 and he was to remain in this post until retirement in 1959. The young Derrick Dunlop was already there as Professor of Therapeutics. They were to become close friends and shared the editorship, from its first edition in 1939, of the *Textbook of Medical Treatment*, a model of common sense and lucidity.

World War II was to inhibit and delay Stanley's aspirations for the Edinburgh Medical School, but those of us who were privileged to be undergraduate students at the time have much to remember. He was a splendid educator, and a particularly gifted bedside teacher, where everything had to be questioned and explained.

He seemed to be totally at ease with everyone, and would stop and talk with students, nurses, domestic staff and frequently with a complete stranger. He had endless time to listen to and communicate with his patients, who quickly seemed to be at ease with him. His main thesis was that if you could take a good history and do a careful physical examination, the rest might not be too difficult or expensive. He gave most of the systematic lectures in Medicine himself, the substance of which was made available in typewritten notes; these were marked by an emphasis on essentials and far surpassed any textbook available at the time.

When the war ended Stanley's first priority was to develop the old municipal hospitals in the northern part of Edinburgh, to extend the teaching capacity of the Medical School and to recognise and establish units for the specialist branches of medicine that were beginning to emerge. These units were to be headed by the best physicians and teachers that could be found and were to retain commitment to general internal medicine. Within a few years Stanley's farsightedness became reality.

But Stanley will be best remembered for this textbook, *The Principles and Practice of Medicine*. He conceived the idea in the late 1940s. It was to be of modest size and price and yet sufficiently comprehensive and up-to-date to provide the good student with the main elements of sound medical practice.

The origins of the book were Stanley's lecture notes. Each of the senior members of Stanley's now extended departmental family was given a chapter to write. In the early days there was occasional annoyance when a carefully drafted manuscript was massacred by Stanley's editorial pencil; but no offence was taken because none was intended. The book was to be readable without ambiguity, uncertainty or wordiness. The result, a masterpiece of clarity and uniformity of style, is the basis from which this Seventeenth Edition has evolved. Although the format and presentation have seen many changes, Stanley's original vision and objectives remain.

It is an honour to salute the memory of a great physician and teacher and, for a fortunate few, a great mentor and friend.

Edinburgh 1995   Professor John Richmond

Acknowledgements

This book represents the combined efforts of a large number of individuals and it is my pleasure to acknowledge those concerned. The chapter authors deserve particular praise for their expert contributions and for being prepared to undertake such extensive revision and updating of their chapters. Many of the changes made in this edition arose from a series of critical reviews and I am most grateful to the following individuals for undertaking such a task: Dr L. Logie, Dr D. Cameron, Dr P. Gibson, Dr L. Plant, Dr B. Walker, Dr R. Herd, Dr O. Chapple, Dr B. McIvor, Dr J. Plevris, Dr K. Simpson, Dr J. Dillon, Dr A. Haynes, Dr D. Jenkins, Dr K. Counsell, Dr W. Wallace, Dr C. Selby, Dr G. Hayden, Dr A. Hargreaves and Dr P. Sime. I am grateful to Dr Simon Walker, Department of Clinical Biochemistry, University of Edinburgh, for his careful revision of many of the tables in the Appendices.

As this is the first full-colour edition of Davidson's, I have had to beg, borrow and steal from my colleagues many highly prized illustrations. These individuals are acknowledged on page 1157. In addition the Editors are indebted to many publishing houses and international organisations for permission to reproduce material: these too are listed on pages 1157–1158.

The Editors and publisher are also most grateful for the courteous help offered throughout the project by the staff of the Erskine Medical Library, University of Edinburgh.

Finally, I am especially grateful to the staff of Churchill Livingstone, in particular Laurence Hunter and Alison Bowers, for their advice and support and to the illustrators for the many new line illustrations.

Edinburgh 1995   E.R.C.

Contributors

Joyce D. Baird MA FRCPE
Honorary Fellow, Department of Medicine,
University of Edinburgh; Former Reader in Medicine
and Honorary Consultant Physician, Western
General Hospital, Edinburgh

N.A. Boon MA MD FRCPE
Consultant Cardiologist, Royal Infirmary of
Edinburgh; Honorary Senior Lecturer,
Department of Medicine, University of Edinburgh

Ian A.D. Bouchier *CBE* FRCP FRCPE FFPHM
FIBiol FRSA FRSE
Professor of Medicine, University of Edinburgh;
Honorary Consultant Physician, Royal Infirmary
of Edinburgh

D.J.H. Brock BA PhD FRCPath FRCPE FRSE
Professor of Human Genetics, University of
Edinburgh, Western General Hospital, Edinburgh

A.D.M. Bryceson MD FRCPE FRCP DTM&H
Senior Lecturer, London School of Hygiene and
Tropical Medicine; Consultant Physician,
Hospital for Tropical Diseases, London

Graham K. Crompton FRCPE
Consultant Physician, Respiratory Unit, Western
General Hospital; Part-time Senior Lecturer,
Departments of Medicine, Western General Hospital
and Royal Infirmary of Edinburgh

Roger E. Cull BSc PhD FRCPE
Consultant Neurologist, Royal Infirmary and
Western General Hospital, Edinburgh; Part-time
Senior Lecturer in Clinical Neurosciences, University
of Edinburgh

Allan D. Cumming BSc MD FRCPE
Senior Lecturer, Department of Medicine, University
of Edinburgh; Honorary Consultant Physician,
Department of Renal Medicine, Royal Infirmary of
Edinburgh

Alex M. Davison BSc MD FRCPE FRCP
Consultant Physician, Renal Unit, St. James's
University Hospital, Leeds; Senior Clinical
Lecturer, University of Leeds

Christopher R.W. Edwards MA MD (Cantab) FRCPE
FRCP FRSE
Professor of Clinical Medicine, University
Department of Medicine, Western General Hospital,
Edinburgh; Dean of the Faculty of Medicine, Provost
of the Faculty Group of Medicine and Veterinary
Medicine, University of Edinburgh

Anne Ferguson FRCP FRCPath FRSE
Professor of Gastroenterology, University of
Edinburgh; Honorary Consultant Physician,
Gastrointestinal Unit, Western General Hospital,
Edinburgh

Niall D.C. Finlayson PhD FRCP FRCPE
Consultant Physician, Royal Infirmary of Edinburgh;
Honorary Senior Lecturer in Medicine, University
of Edinburgh

Keith A.A. Fox BSc (Hons) FRCP FESC
Duke of Edinburgh Professor of Cardiology,
University of Edinburgh; Honorary Consultant,
Cardiology Department, Royal Infirmary of
Edinburgh

Brian M. Frier BSc (Hons) MD FRCPE FRCPG
Consultant Physician, Department of Diabetes,
Royal Infirmary of Edinburgh; Part-time Reader
in Medicine, University of Edinburgh

Alasdair M. Geddes FRCP FRCPE
Foundation Professor of Infection, School of
Medicine, University of Birmingham; Honorary
Consultant Physician, University Hospital Trust,
Birmingham

Christopher Haslett BSc(Hons) FRCPE FRCP
Professor of Respiratory Medicine, University of
Edinburgh; Honorary Consultant Physician, Royal
Infirmary of Edinburgh

John A.A. Hunter BA MD FRCPE
Professor of Dermatology, University of Edinburgh;
Honorary Consultant Dermatologist, Royal Infirmary of
Edinburgh

A.A.H. Lawson MD FRCPE
Former Consultant Physician, Queen Margaret
Hospital NHS Trust, Dunfermline; Honorary
Senior Lecturer, Department of Medicine, University
of Edinburgh

G.G. Lloyd MA MD MPhil FRCPE FRCP FRCPsych
Consultant Psychiatrist, Royal Free Hospital,
London

Christopher A. Ludlam BSc PhD FRCP FRCPath
Consultant Haematologist, Royal Infirmary of
Edinburgh; Director, Haemophilia Centre; Part-time
Senior Lecturer, Department of Medicine, University
of Edinburgh

Michael J. Mackie BMedBiol MD FRCPath FRCPE
Consultant Haematologist, Western General
Hospital, Edinburgh; Part-time Senior Lecturer,
University of Edinburgh

William J. MacLennan MD FRCP FRCPG FRCPE
Professor of Geriatric Medicine, University of
Edinburgh; Honorary Consultant Physician, Royal
Infirmary of Edinburgh

David M. Mitchell MA MD FRCP
Consultant Physician and Honorary Senior Lecturer,
Department of Medicine, St. Mary's Hospital,
Paddington, London

George Nuki FRCPE FRCP
Arthritis and Rheumatism Council Professor of
Rheumatology, University of Edinburgh;
Honorary Consultant Physician, Western General
Hospital and Royal Infirmary of Edinburgh

David J.C. Shearman PhD FRCPE FRACP
Professor of Medicine and Head, Department of
Medicine, University of Adelaide; Head,
Professorial Medical Unit and Senior Visiting
Physician, Royal Adelaide Hospital, Adelaide,
Australia

James Shepherd PhD FRCPath FRCP
Professor of Pathological Biochemistry, University of
Glasgow; Honorary Consultant Biochemist,
Glasgow Royal Infirmary

John F. Smyth MA MD(Cantab) MSc(Lon) FRCPE FRCP FRCSE
Imperial Cancer Research Fund Professor of Medical
Oncology, University of Edinburgh; Honorary
Consultant Physician, Western General Hospital,
Edinburgh; Director of the Imperial Cancer
Research Fund Medical Oncology Unit,
Edinburgh

Colin A. Soutar MD FRCPE FFOM
Director, Institute of Occupational Medicine,
Edinburgh

Charles P. Swainson FRCPE
Consultant Renal Physician, Royal Infirmary of
Edinburgh; Part-time Senior Lecturer, Department of
Medicine, University of Edinburgh

R.N. Thin MD FRCPE FRCP
Consultant Physician, Department of Genitourinary
Medicine, St. Thomas's Hospital, London

A.D. Toft CBE BSc MD FRCP FRCPE FRCPG FRCPI FRCSE
Consultant Physician, Royal Infirmary of Edinburgh;
Honorary Senior Lecturer, Department of
Medicine, University of Edinburgh

A. Stewart Truswell MD FRCP FRACP FFPHM
Boden Professor of Human Nutrition, University of
Sydney; Honorary Consultant in Nutrition, Royal
Prince Alfred Hospital, Sydney, Australia

R.G. Will MA MD FRCPE FRCP
Consultant Neurologist, Western General Hospital,
Edinburgh; Part-time Senior Lecturer,
Department of Clinical Neurosciences, University of
Edinburgh

Contents

Genetic factors in disease

Contrary to common belief, genetically-determined diseases are not rare. Between 2 and 3% of all pregnancies result in the birth of a child with a condition that can be attributed to defective or absent genes. Up to 12% of paediatric hospital admissions are the result of single-gene disorders or chromosomal abnormalities. Although the frequency of adult diseases with a strong genetic component is more difficult to estimate, it may be as high as 50%. Indeed, with a few exceptions, it is difficult to conceive of any disease that is wholly non-genetic.

At conception human beings inherit two sets of genes, one from their mother and one from their father. Apart from identical twins, each individual has a unique genetic constitution or genotype. Everything that happens from fertilisation onward, whether in health or disease, is a product of interactions between the environment and the inherited genotype. It is useful to consider human diseases as lying on a continuum; at the one end are those which are entirely genetic in origin and at the other are those where the environment is the main agent. Genetics has been more successful in dealing with the former than with the latter. However, there are reasons for believing that within the next 10 years the ways in which genes influence the patterns of common disease will be within reach.

The reason for this statement is the existence of the Human Genome Project. This international programme of research seeks to determine the sequence and structure of all 100 000 functional human genes by the turn of the century. Although driven by molecular geneticists, the Project has enormous implications for all types of human disease. By describing the genetic susceptibility factors in common disorders, it should be possible to manage and treat those at risk by sophisticated manipulation of their environments.

CATEGORIES OF GENETIC DISEASE

Diseases influenced by genetic factors may be grouped into five categories (Table 1.1). In Mendelian, chromosome and mitochondrial disorders, inherited or new mutation in the genetic material is the causative event, and these mutations may be transmitted from one generation to another. In somatic cell disorders mutation occurs after fertilisation and only in some cell types, and is not transmitted through the germ line. In multifactorial disorders the role of genetic factors is less clear-cut, and difficult to disentangle from the effects of the environment.

THE CHROMOSOMAL BASIS OF INHERITANCE

The study of genetics begins with chromosomes, which were recognised as the carriers of inherited factors well

Table 1.1 Main categories of genetic disease

Category	Description
Mendelian disorders	Caused by mutation at single locus. Can be inherited or result from new mutation. Obey simple rules of transmission.
Chromosome disorders	Usually caused by new mutation. When inherited show modified patterns of Mendelian transmission.
Multifactorial disorders	Diseases influenced rather than caused by genetic factors. No clear pattern of transmission.
Mitochondrial disorders	Caused by mutations in the mitochondrial genome. Transmitted through the maternal line.
Somatic cell disorders	Involve mutations in somatic cells. Tissue limited. Somatic mutations are not inherited or transmitted.

before the discovery of DNA. Each species has its own chromosome complement, with characteristic number and appearance; in eukaryotes like humans the chromosomes are confined within the cell nucleus and only clearly seen under the light microscope at certain stages of the cell cycle.

The chromosome number of the diploid human cell is 46, made up of 22 pairs of autosomes, with an X and a Y in males and two X chromosomes in females. The haploid female cell (the egg) has 22 autosomes and an X, and the haploid male cell (the sperm) 22 autosomes and an X or a Y. Each chromosome has a single molecule of double-stranded DNA containing the genetic information, which is coiled around basic histone proteins and then supercoiled into chromatin fibres. This extraordinarily compact structure allows as much as 2 metres of DNA to be packaged into chromosomes whose diameter may be as little as 2 microns.

CELL DIVISION

There are two types of cell division: mitosis and meiosis (Table 1.2). Mitosis occurs in dividing somatic cells, from fertilisation onward, and is the process whereby genetically identical daughter cells are generated from a parental cell.

In contrast meiosis, which occurs only in germ cells, has two different functions. One is to reduce the chromosome complement to half (the haploid state) so that the union of two germ cells at fertilisation restores the normal diploid number of 46 chromosomes. The other function is to generate diversity. This is achieved by the exchange of material between homologous chromosomes prior to the first meiotic division. This means that a child does not inherit an unchanged set of chromo-

Table 1.2 Differences between mitosis and meiosis

	Mitosis	Meiosis
Site	All somatic cells	Sperm and egg cells
Time	At all times	Post-puberty in male. Starts in utero in female, then suspended until puberty
Key feature	No pairing of homologous chromosomes	Pairing of homologous chromosomes
Result	Diploid daughter cells identical to parental cells	Haploid cells with recombinant chromosomes

somes from each parent, but rather a set from each in which some of the DNA has been scrambled.

Mitosis

Mitosis is a critical part of a carefully programmed process known as the cell cycle. This starts at a stage called G1 (gap 1), where the cell prepares its chromosomes for replication. During the **S (synthetic)** phase, DNA replication takes place and each of the 46 chromosomes is duplicated into sister chromatids held together at a central constriction called the centromere. At the end of S phase there is another gap phase (G2), which leads eventually into actual **mitosis (M)**. Thereafter the cycle is repeated for dividing cells while non-dividing cells (e.g. neurones) shift into a stationary or G0 phase.

The length of the cell cycle varies, but for cultured mammalian cells is of the order of 24 hours. Most of this time is spent in interphase, representing G1, S and G2, while actual mitosis is probably complete in under one hour. The four mitotic stages are divided for convenience into prophase, metaphase, anaphase and telophase (Fig. 1.1), although in reality mitosis takes place as a continuous process.

During the long period of **interphase** chromosomes are extended and diffuse, and cannot be clearly seen under the light microscope. The important event is DNA replication during S phase. Each chromosome has its own pattern of DNA synthesis, with some segments replicating early and others late. In female cells where only one of the two X chromosomes is genetically active (see p. 14), the other 'inactive X' is always the last to complete replication.

- **Prophase** is heralded by the onset of chromosome coiling and condensation. Each chromosome can now be seen under the light microscope as a pair of long parallel strands, or sister chromatids, held together at the centromere.
- **Metaphase** is marked by the breakdown of the nuclear envelope. The released chromosomes move to the equatorial plate of the cell. A spindle consisting

of protein microtubules attaches the centromere of each chromosome to complex structures called centrioles at opposite poles of the cell. The drug colchicine, much used in examining chromosomes, interferes with spindle formation and conveniently arrests mitosis at the metaphase stage. Homologous chromosomes do not associate in any specific way during metaphase.

- **Anaphase** starts when the centromeres divide so that each chromatid becomes a daughter chromosome. The spindles contract and pull each daughter chromosome to an opposite pole of the cell. Occasionally, both chromatids end up at the same pole, an error called mitotic non-disjunction, and this results in one daughter cell having an extra chromosome and the other a missing one (see Fig. 1.15, p. 18).
- At **telophase** a nuclear envelope forms round each set of daughter chromosomes and they begin to unwind. The cytoplasm divides (cytokinesis) to give two daughter cells, each (in the absence of errors) genetically identical to the parent cell.

Meiosis

As in mitosis, cells enter meiosis after an interphase in which the chromosomes have already replicated. The main differences which characterise meiosis are (a) that there are two successive cell divisions, meiosis I and meiosis II, without any DNA replication in between, (b) that there is exchange of genetic material between homologous chromosomes in meiosis I, and (c) that the whole process can take years instead of hours.

The stages of the two meiotic divisions are named as in mitosis. However, prophase I is long and critical to the generation of diversity. Homologous chromosomes pair to form bivalents, starting at the telomeres and moving towards the centromere in a process called synapsis. At this stage there is crossing-over or exchange of material between the chromatids of homologous chromosomes. As the homologous chromosomes are not identical the crossing-over produces new or recombinant chromosomes. The non-sister chromatids that have crossed are visible as cross-shaped connections called chiasmata. On average there are about 50 chiasmata per male cell or at least one chiasma per chromosome arm.

After the long prophase I the two successive meiotic divisions follow without further DNA replication. At metaphase I, paired homologous chromosomes line up along the equatorial plate and spindles form. At anaphase I, each member of the pair moves towards the pole of the cell, but in contrast to mitosis there is no division of centromeres. Thus after telophase I and cytokinesis there are two cells, each with a haploid set of 23 chromosomes. A reductive division has been completed.

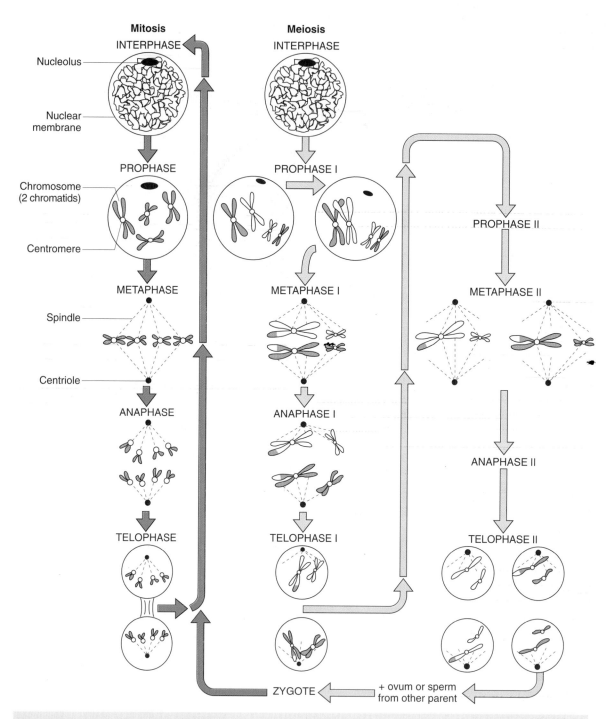

Fig. 1.1 The stages of mitosis and meiosis.

The second meiotic division is essentially identical to mitosis. There is no interphase, and after a brief prophase II sister chromatids line up along the equatorial plate in metaphase II. Centromeres divide and at anaphase II daughter chromosomes are pulled to the poles of the cell. After telophase II and cytokinesis there are now four cells, each with a haploid set of chromosomes. Some, as a result of interchange of DNA in prophase I, will be new recombinant chromosomes, while others will be identical to those that entered meiosis I.

X and Y chromosomes in meiosis

Pairing of homologous chromosomes is a key feature of meiosis I. In male germ cells there is pairing between the tips of the short arms of X and Y, in a region known as pseudoautosomal, and only here does DNA exchange take place. Obviously, in female germ cells there is normal recombination between the two X chromosomes.

Fertilisation

The union of a haploid sperm with a haploid egg restores the diploid state of 46 chromosomes in the zygote. A sperm with a Y chromosome dictates a male zygote and a sperm with an X chromosome a female. Since each chromosome assorts independently during meiosis there are at least 2^{23} different possible combinations of chromosomes in the germ cells of each parent, and indeed many more when the generation of new chromosomes by recombination is taken into account. A conservative calculation suggests that the possible combinations of chromosomes in zygotes is of the order of 6×10^{43}.

THE CHEMICAL BASIS OF INHERITANCE

Chromosomes are particulate and visible structures in the cell nucleus which carry the units of inheritance. Their behaviour during mitosis shows how genetic material can be faithfully transmitted from the one-cell zygote to all successive cells and why each one of the 5×10^{12} cells in a person is (in the absence of errors) genetically identical. Recombination of chromosomes in meiosis indicates a mechanism for producing individual differences. All this is achieved through the special chemical properties of the genetic material.

THE STRUCTURE OF GENES

The genetic material is made up of deoxyribonucleic acid or DNA. Cellular DNA is a large double-stranded molecule with chains twisted into a double helix (Fig. 1.2). Each strand is composed of varying patterns of four distinct units, the nitrogenous bases, strung in seemingly

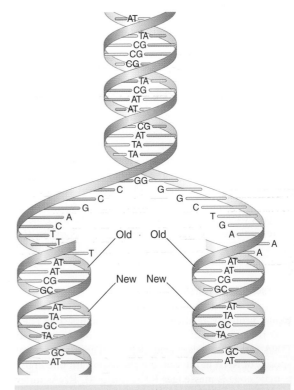

Fig. 1.2   The structure of DNA showing semi-conservative replication.

random sequence along a deoxyribose-phosphate backbone. The nitrogenous bases adenine and guanine are purines while cytosine and thymine are pyrimidines; they are referred to as A, G, C and T. In the double helix the strands are held together by specific hydrogen bonding between pairs of bases, with A always bonding with T and G always bonding with C. This means that the two strands of the double helix are complementary, so that a sequence of TAGGC in one strand is matched by ATCCG in the other.

During the S stage of mitotic interphase each chromosome replicates its DNA. The mechanism of replication is achieved by an unwinding of the double helix and the synthesis of a new daughter strand on each parental strand. Thus a TAGGC sequence in one parental strand is complemented by ATCCG in its new daughter strand and ATCCG in the other parental strand is complemented by TAGGC in its new daughter strand. The two identical DNA molecules thus produced each have one original and one new strand, a process called semi-conservative replication (see Fig. 1.2). There is evidence that each chromosome at early interphase has one huge double-stranded DNA molecule. After replication identical double-stranded DNA molecules, each representing the genetic content of a chromosome, pass to each daughter cell at mitotic cell division.

THE FUNCTION OF GENES

The function of genes is to provide exact information for the synthesis of the specific aminoacid sequence of the proteins they control. The language of this connection is called the genetic code, and it is founded on triplet codons, with three sequential nitrogenous bases specifying particular aminoacids. However, since there are 4 bases in DNA and therefore 4^3 (or 64) possible codons, while there are only 20 aminoacids, the genetic code is said to be <u>degenerate</u>. Several codons specify the same aminoacid (e.g. there are 6 for leucine), while 3 represent stop signals.

Transcription of DNA into RNA

Turning the information content of DNA into a particular protein is relatively complex. The first step (Fig. 1.3) is transcription of one strand of double-stranded DNA into ribonucleic acid (RNA). There are several species of RNA in the cell, but the important one in the genetic code is messenger RNA (mRNA). RNAs differ from DNA in that the base uracil (U) replaces thymine (T), and they are single-stranded. mRNA is exactly complementary to the DNA strand from which it is transcribed, with U (instead of T) representing the pairing partner for adenine (A).

Before mRNA migrates from the nucleus to the cyto-

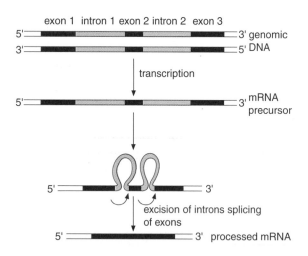

Fig. 1.3 Transcription of DNA into RNA and excision of introns.

plasm it undergoes processing. <u>In most eukaryotic genes there are stretches of DNA, called intervening sequences or introns, which lie between other sequences called exons.</u> In the precursor mRNA, sequences that are complementary to the introns are spliced out and removed. Thus <u>mature mRNA is a single-stranded complementary copy of the original exon structure of the gene.</u>

Translation of RNA into protein

In the cytoplasm each mRNA molecule becomes associated with one or more ribosomes (Fig. 1.4). It is now the template for a different species of RNA, transfer-RNA (tRNA). Each tRNA molecule carries an aminoacid and has a codon complementary to a codon in the mRNA. As the ribosome moves along the mRNA, aminoacids are added successively to a growing polypeptide chain, until a stop codon is reached. The eventual sequence of aminoacids in the polypeptide is thus dictated by the sequence of codons in mRNA, itself determined by the sequence of bases in the exon structure of the gene.

THE ANATOMY OF THE GENOME

The haploid human genome has about 3.5×10^9 <u>base pairs (bp) of DNA.</u> Scattered through the genome are about <u>100 000 functional genes</u>, usually as single copies, which are either transcribed and translated into protein or simply transcribed into RNA. However, <u>the bulk of human DNA, including the intervening sequences within genes, has no known function.</u> Much of this is <u>repetitive DNA, tracts of very similar sequences which may be repeated hundreds or even thousands of times</u> at different sites in the genome. Although the purpose of this DNA remains unclear, <u>it is stably inherited and has become of great importance in tracking functional genes as they are passed through families and populations.</u>

Normal variation

Individual uniqueness is founded on variation in the sequences of a person's DNA. Some genetic variation is sufficiently common to constitute a polymorphism in the observed phenotype, e.g. the ABO blood group or HLA systems. <u>Much of this 'expressed' variation arises from single base changes in the DNA encoding biosynthetic enzymes or structural proteins in the cell.</u>

It is now apparent that, in addition to expressed variation, <u>there is a huge amount of polymorphism in introns and in the tracts of DNA that lie between genes.</u> This is 'silent' variation which does not find its way into RNA or protein. Again some arises from single base changes in DNA. But there is also a different type of polymorphism,

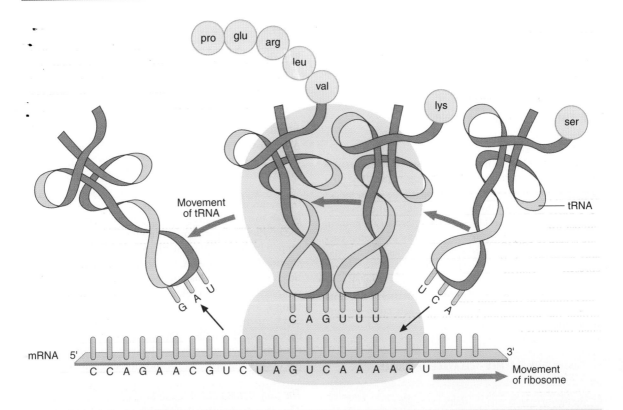

Fig. 1.4   Translation of RNA into protein. The ribosome is shown as the bell-shaped structure moving along the mRNA. A transfer-RNA (tRNA) carrying the aminoacid, serine, is seen arriving from the right and a tRNA which has discharged its aminoacid is departing at the left. The growing protein chain remains attached to the ribosome (centre).

where the number of units in a repetitive sequence varies between individuals. This type of polymorphism has been given the name 'variable number of tandem repeats' (VNTRs), and is the basis for the science of genetic fingerprinting.

Pathological variation

When a DNA change has pathological consequences it is referred to as a mutation. Many mutations are the result of single base pair changes in the exon sequence of a gene, so that there is an aminoacid substitution in the encoded protein (Table 1.3). Others are deletions, sometimes of a whole gene and sometimes of a critical part of a gene. A new type of mutation recently discovered is caused by a sudden and often gross expansion in the number of trinucleotide repeat units in a repetitive sequence. The special feature of mutation that distinguishes it from normal variation is that the function and/or quantity of encoded proteins is usually substantially disturbed.

Table 1.3   Types of mutation in human genetic disease

Type	Examples	
Point mutations	*all*	Sickle cell anaemia
	most	Cystic fibrosis
	most	β-thalassaemia
Deletions	*most*	α-thalassaemia
	most	Duchenne and Becker muscular dystrophies
Trinucleotide repeat expansions	*most*	Fragile X syndrome
		Myotonic dystrophy
		Huntington's disease
	some	Spinocerebellar ataxia

MANIPULATING AND TRACKING GENES

The ability to isolate genes, to insert them into microbial hosts where they may be grown in multiple copies, and then to rescue them for further study, is part of the science of genetic engineering. Much of the detailed technology is beyond the scope of this chapter. However, tracking genes that may cause inherited disorders is a central part of medical genetics and employs many of the same basic techniques.

THE TOOLS OF GENE TRACKING

Restriction enzymes

Cellular DNA consists of a series of large molecules which are difficult to handle in the test tube. The first step in manipulating DNA is to cut it into small pieces with a restriction endonuclease (usually called restriction enzyme). Over 1000 restriction enzymes are known; each cleaves double-stranded DNA at a specific recognition site usually made up of a four-base or six-base sequence. Cleavage may be symmetrical or asymmetrical, as shown in the information box. Any change in the recognition site as a result of mutation or normal variation abolishes the ability of the restriction enzyme to cut the DNA.

RESTRICTION ENZYMES—CLEAVAGE OF DOUBLE-STRANDED DNA

Restriction enzyme	Restriction sequence
• *Hae* III	↓ GGCC CCGG ↑
• *Taq* I	↓ TCGA AGCT ↑
• *Hpa* I	↓ GTTAAC CAATTG ↑
• *Eco* RI	↓ GAATTC CTTAAG ↑

Arrows show where restriction enzymes cleave the DNA

Hybridisation

Double-stranded DNA can be rendered single-stranded by boiling and then immobilised on filters. If a segment of exogenous single-stranded DNA ('probe DNA') has a complementary sequence to any part of the immobilised material, it will seek it out and hybridise to it. This is one of the essential keys to the analysis of DNA.

Probes

Probes are specific sequences of DNA often representing known genes, segments of genes or short synthetic oligonucleotides. To be useful in hybridisation they must be made single-stranded and tagged with a radioactive or fluorescent marker.

Southern blotting

A much-used technique for examining the genes in different people is the Southern blot (Fig. 1.5). Cellular DNA, isolated from white blood cells, amniotic fluid cells or a chorionic villus biopsy, is digested to small fragments with a suitable restriction enzyme. The DNA is then run out on an agarose gel by electrophoresis, with the smaller fragments migrating most rapidly. The gel is dipped briefly in strong alkali to render the DNA single-stranded, and the fragments are then transferred by blotting to a nitrocellulose or nylon filter. After baking to bind the DNA, the filter is immersed in a solution containing a radioactive probe which hybridizes only to complementary sequences. After washing, the filter is exposed to X-ray film. The position of dark bands on the film, known as an autoradiogram, indicates any differences in the genes of the individuals examined.

The polymerase chain reaction (PCR)

This is a technique for amplifying small segments of genomic DNA to copy numbers as high as 10^8 to 10^{10}. The amplified DNA becomes the predominant species in the mixture and so abundant that it can be seen on a gel after conventional staining with ethidium bromide. However, before a piece of DNA can be amplified by PCR, it is necessary to know its base sequence.

APPLICATIONS OF GENE TRACKING

Direct tracking

When the exact sequence change responsible for a mutation is known, it is possible to search directly for the presence or absence of mutant alleles using the PCR. An example of this is shown in Figure 1.6, where the bands from individuals heterozygous or homozygous for the common cystic fibrosis mutation, ΔF508, are shown on a polyacrylamide gel. For virtually all cloned genes this type of analysis is now possible. But it does have limitations. If a genetic disorder is made up of a large number of different mutations in the same gene, each mutation must be searched for in a separate analysis. This is cumbersome and expensive, and in practice only the more common mutant alleles are sought. Thus in cystic fibrosis, where there are over 400 mutant alleles, it is normal practice to search for the five or six that make up about 85% of cases.

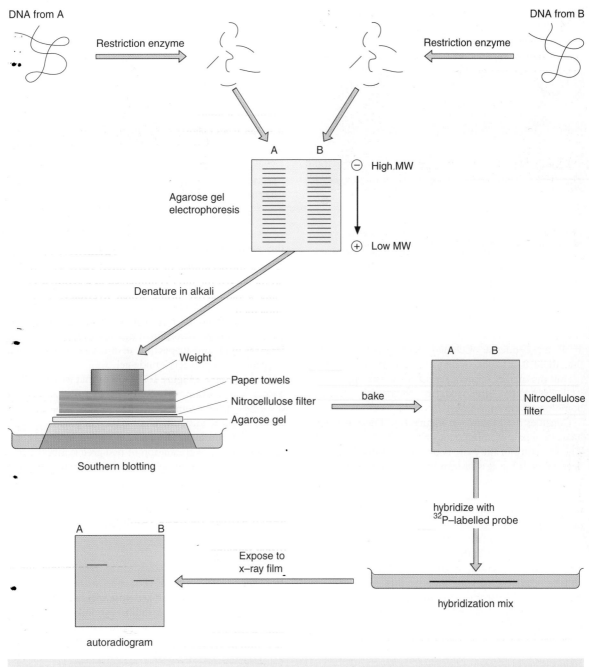

Fig. 1.5 Southern blotting.

Indirect tracking

Segments of DNA that are very close together on a chromosome tend to stay together during meiosis; in other words they do not recombine. Thus if we wish to track a gene that has not yet been cloned, we can often do this <u>by following the behaviour of a nearby gene that has been cloned, and by using the latter as a marker of the former.</u> In fact the marker does not have to be a gene

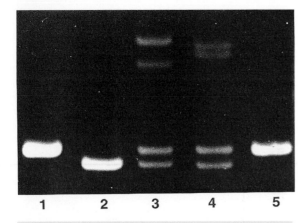

Fig. 1.6   Detection of the most prevalent mutant allele (△F508) responsible for cystic fibrosis. Because there is a 3 bp deletion in this allele, the band from an affected homozygote (2) migrates more rapidly than those from normal homozygotes (1 and 5). Heterozygotes (3 and 4) have both fast- and slow-moving bands.

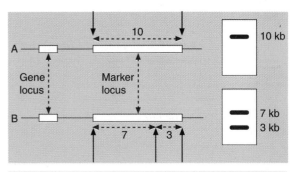

Fig. 1.7   A marker locus in which there is a restriction fragment length polymorphism (RFLP).

at all; any sequence of cloned DNA will do, provided that there is a probe available to recognise it. To be useful, the marker sequence must be polymorphic since it is generally employed to distinguish between homologous chromosomes.

Consider the example in Figure 1.7. There is a gene locus on a pair of homologous chromosomes, A and B. The structure of the gene is unknown, since it has not been cloned, but it is known that mutation in the gene causes disease. How do we discover whether the mutant gene is on chromosome A or B? Fortunately, very close to the gene locus there is a sequence of DNA that is polymorphic. Some chromosomes have a particular restriction enzyme site in the middle of the sequence while others do not. If the sequence is digested with the appropriate restriction enzyme, subjected to Southern blotting and reacted with a probe that recognises the sequence, the A chromosome will show one band on X-ray film and the B chromosome two bands. Provided that we know that the mutant gene is on the chromosome with one band, we can conclude that the same disease-causing gene will continue to be marked by a one-band pattern as it is passed to successive generations. It is now a marked gene.

The marker system in Figure 1.7 is known as a restriction fragment length polymorphism or RFLP, since the polymorphism is identified by the size of the bands seen on a Southern blot. It is not a very useful polymorphism since there are only two possibilities, defined by the presence or absence of the restriction site. There is a strong a priori chance that both chromosomes will have the same marker sequence. More valuable polymorphisms are those based on VNTRs, where there are a large number of different alleles and where the chance of two homologous chromosomes having different markers is high. Much of current gene tracking uses 'microsatellites', where the repeat unit is a CA dinucleotide. Microsatellite polymorphism is usually studied by PCR amplification and inspection of the size of the repeat sequence on a polyacrylamide gel.

The diagram in Figure 1.7 assumes that we can follow a single chromosome on a Southern blot. For autosomal disorders chromosomes come in pairs, so gene tracking is slightly more difficult. What is seen in practice, for an autosomal dominant disorder, is shown in Figure 1.8 (see Fig. 1.9 for explanation of pedigree symbols). It is immediately apparent, even without understanding the detailed behaviour of the chromosomes, that the two affected children in the pedigree have the same band pattern as the affected father, while the unaffected child has a different one.

GENETIC LINKAGE

In order to use a marker sequence to track a gene we need to know that the two are close together (linked) on the same chromosome. Establishing linkage is usually carried out by genetic methods, that is by studying the behaviour of gene and marker as they pass through the generations of large numbers of families. If gene and marker are on different chromosomes they will behave independently. If they are far apart on the same chromosome they will still behave independently, because of meiotic recombination. Only when they are quite close to each other do they begin to operate as a linked unit. Calculating the degree of genetic linkage uses sophisticated applied statistics and is beyond the scope of this chapter. It is sufficient to know that genetic linkage is measured by a reverse parameter, the recombination

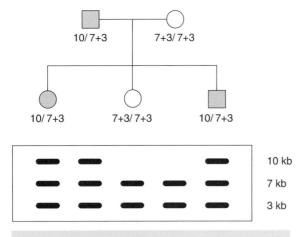

Fig. 1.8   Using an RFLP to track a disease gene from affected parent to affected children.

fraction (θ). A recombination fraction of 5% indicates that gene and marker remain as a linked unit in 95% of meioses and separate in 5%. A rough rule-of-thumb is that a 5% recombination fraction means that gene and marker are separated by about 5×10^6 bp of DNA, or 5 megabases.

SINGLE GENE DISORDERS

Single gene disorders, more accurately termed single locus disorders, refer to mutation in either one or in a pair of homologous alleles at a single locus. These disorders are inherited according to simple Mendelian laws and risks of recurrence in a family can be predicted exactly. If the locus is on one of the 22 autosomes it is called autosomal, and if on the X or Y chromosomes it is called sex-linked. Some of the more common single gene disorders are listed in Table 1.4.

AUTOSOMAL DOMINANT INHERITANCE

Disorders which are inherited as autosomal dominants show clinical symptoms in heterozygotes, that is in people who have one normal and one mutant allele at the locus involved. Pedigrees are characterised by vertical transmission, with affected individuals nearly always having one affected parent (Fig. 1.9). Because the normal and mutant alleles segregate to different gametes during meiosis (Fig. 1.10) there is a 50% chance that the child of an affected parent will also be affected. Males and females have the same chance of being affected. The unaffected children of an affected parent are free of the mutant gene and their offspring will all be unaffected.

Table 1.4   More common single gene disorders

Disorder	Frequency per 1000 births in the UK
Autosomal dominant	
Familial combined hyperlipidaemia	5.0
Familial hypercholesterolaemia	2.0
Dominant otosclerosis	1.0
Adult polycystic kidney disease	0.8
Multiple exostoses	0.5
Huntington's disease	0.5
Neurofibromatosis	0.4
Myotonic dystrophy	0.2
Congenital spherocytosis	0.2
Polyposis coli	0.1
Autosomal recessive	
Cystic fibrosis	0.4
α_1-antitrypsin deficiency	0.2
Phenylketonuria	0.1
Congenital adrenal hyperplasia	0.1
Spinal muscular atrophy	0.1
Sickle cell anaemia	0.1
β-thalassaemia	0.05
X-linked recessive	
Fragile X syndrome	0.5
Duchenne muscular dystrophy	0.3
X-linked ichthyosis	0.2
Haemophilia A	0.1
Becker muscular dystrophy	0.05
Haemophilia B	0.03

In some of the more common disorders inherited as autosomal dominants both parents may be affected. If Figure 1.10 is redrawn to show this (try on a piece of paper), it will be clear that two of the four possible gametes will carry mutant alleles. One of the four possible offspring will inherit no mutant alleles, two will inherit one mutant allele and one normal allele, and the fourth will inherit mutant alleles on each chromosome. Thus three-quarters of offspring will be affected. For a true dominant, such as Huntington's disease, people with two mutant alleles are no more severely affected than those with one mutant allele. For an incomplete dominant, such as familial hypercholesterolaemia, two mutant alleles cause more severe disease than does one.

Complicating factors

In some dominantly inherited disorders, such as achondroplasia, new mutations are relatively common. They are assumed to occur in the germ cells of unaffected parents. If the disorder is severe and affected individuals do not reproduce, the case may appear as a 'sporadic' without family history. If an affected individual reproduces, his or her offspring have a 50% chance of inheriting the condition. There is a general rule that the more severe the condition and the lower the reproductive fitness, the higher the proportion of new mutations among affected cases.

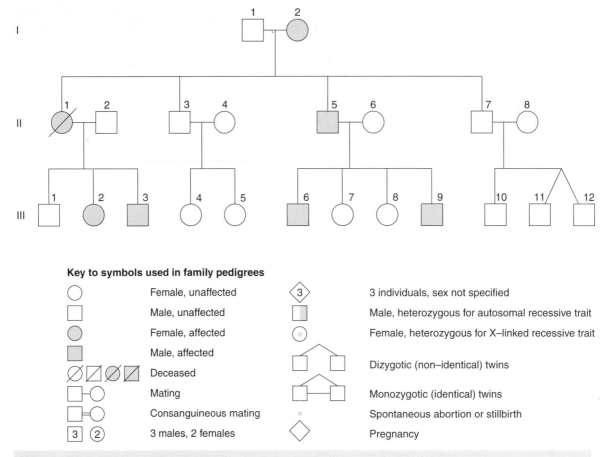

Key to symbols used in family pedigrees

○	Female, unaffected	◇3◇	3 individuals, sex not specified
□	Male, unaffected	▨	Male, heterozygous for autosomal recessive trait
●	Female, affected	⊙	Female, heterozygous for X–linked recessive trait
■	Male, affected		
⊘ ⧄ ⊘ ⧄	Deceased	Dizygotic (non–identical) twins
□—○	Mating	Monozygotic (identical) twins
□—○	Consanguineous mating	• Spontaneous abortion or stillbirth
3 ②	3 males, 2 females	◇ Pregnancy

Fig. 1.9   Pedigree showing autosomal dominant transmission of a disorder. Common pedigree symbols are shown.

In several autosomal dominants the manifestation of clinical symptoms is quite variable. For example, in Marfan syndrome the disorder may affect the skeletal system (long, thin extremities), the heart (aortic dissection) and the eyes (dislocated lenses). In some individuals all three systems are involved, in others only one system. This is called variable expressivity. Although it can occur among affected people in the same pedigree, substantial variation is more common between pedigrees and probably reflects different mutant alleles at the same locus.

In other autosomal dominants, even though the individual is known to carry the mutant gene, there is no appearance of disease at all. This is termed non-penetrance. A trivial explanation for non-penetrance is found in late-onset autosomal dominants, like Huntington's disease or myotonic dystrophy, where a mutant gene carrier may die before his or her age of onset. Such people are still capable of passing the gene and disease to their descendants.

It has been noted in disorders like myotonic dystrophy that the age of onset may become earlier and the severity of symptoms greater in successive generations. This is called anticipation. For many years the actuality of anticipation has been disputed and explained as arising from the tendency of doctors to examine more carefully younger members of families in which the disorder is segregating. Now that the myotonic dystrophy gene has been cloned, it is known that mutation causes an unstable trinucleotide repeat sequence. The size and instability of the repeat sequence can (though it does not always) increase in successive generations, and there is a rough correlation with severity. Thus anticipation now has biological reality.

AUTOSOMAL RECESSIVE INHERITANCE

Disorders inherited as autosomal recessives show clinical symptoms only in homozygotes, that is in people who have two mutant alleles, one on each of homologous chromosomes. Both sexes can be affected. Heterozygous

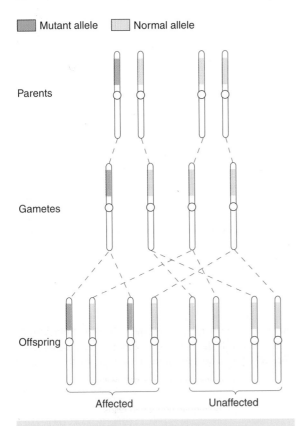

Fig. 1.10 **Autosomal dominant inheritance.**

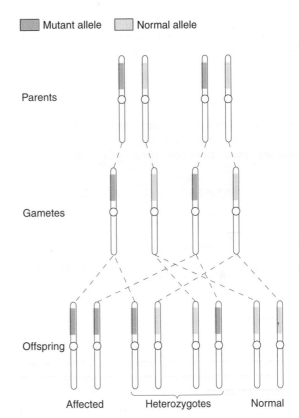

Fig. 1.11 **Autosomal recessive inheritance.**

carriers of a single mutant allele are clinically normal and thus most affected cases, arising from the mating between two heterozygotes, appear without warning. As shown in Figure 1.11, such matings have a 25% chance of producing an affected homozygote, a 50% chance of a (normal) heterozygote and a 25% chance of a normal homozygote.

People affected with autosomal recessive disorders, who reproduce, usually have clinically normal children, although all these will be heterozygotes. Occasionally, an affected individual may mate with a heterozygote for the same disease. In such cases there is a 50% chance of an affected child and a 50% chance of a heterozygous child.

Hardy–Weinberg equilibrium

Although autosomal recessive disorders are rare, the frequency of heterozygotes can be quite high. The relationship between heterozygote and homozygote frequencies in outbred populations is given by the Hardy–Weinberg equilibrium (see information box).

Compound heterozygotes

In most single locus disorders many different mutant alleles are found in the population. If someone with cystic fibrosis, for example, inherits a different mutant allele on each chromosome, he or she is termed a compound heterozygote at the molecular level but an affected homozygote at the clinical level. This is not as complicated as it sounds; the person is heterozygous for each mutant allele, while the net effect is disease-causing. The term double heterozygote is reserved for clinically normal people who are heterozygous for mutant alleles at separate loci.

SEX-LINKED INHERITANCE

Disorders determined by mutant genes carried on the X or Y chromosomes are called sex-linked. However, as there are only a few known genes on the Y chromosome, sex linkage is largely synonymous with X linkage. One exception is the SRY gene, which produces the testis-determining factor, the most important determinant of male sex. As a male passes his Y chromosome only to his sons, the SRY gene shows male-to-male transmission. A similar pattern can be expected for Y-linked genetic disorders, though none has yet been described.

X-linked recessive inheritance

A typical pedigree for a severe X-linked recessive disorder, such as Duchenne muscular dystrophy, is shown in Figure 1.12. Because females have two X chromosomes and males only one, a male who inherits a mutant gene from his symptomless heterozygous

(carrier) mother will be affected. He is called a hemizygote. It is often found that affected boys have an affected maternal uncle, a pattern known as a 'knight's move'.

As shown in Figure 1.12A, a mating between a normal father and a carrier mother has four possible outcomes, each with a 25% chance: an affected son, a normal son, a carrier daughter or a normal daughter. The father contributes only a normal X chromosome to his daughters and a normal Y chromosome to his sons, and thus it is the carrier status of the mother that is all-important. If she changes partners, the risks to her children are unchanged.

In less severe X-linked recessives, such as haemophilia, affected males may reproduce. In this case (Fig. 1.12B), all his daughters will be carriers and all his sons will be normal.

X-linked dominant inheritance

Although this is rare, it does occur, an example being vitamin D resistant rickets. If the mother is affected, there is a 50% chance of an affected child, and it can be of either sex. If the father is affected there is also a 50% chance of an affected child. However, in this case all

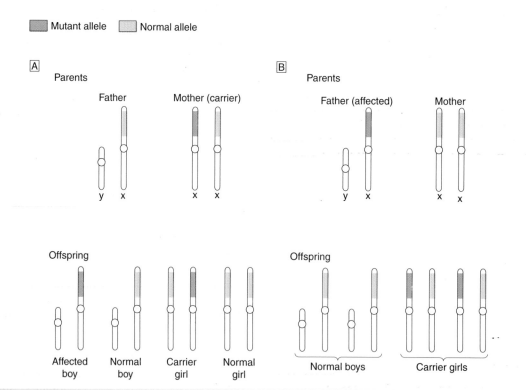

Fig. 1.12 X-linked recessive inheritance. In **A** the mother carries the mutant allele on one of her X chromosomes, while in **B** the father (who is affected) carries the mutant allele on his single X chromosome.

the daughters are affected and none of the sons. This illustrates a key feature of all X-linked inheritance—dominant and recessive—the absence of male-to-male transmission.

X inactivation

Females have two X chromosomes and males only one. At first sight one might expect there to be twice as much protein product of an X-linked gene in female compared to male cells. In fact this does not happen, because of a phenomenon first recognised by Mary Lyon in 1962, and called lyonisation or X chromosome inactivation.

At about the 16th day of life, when there are approximately 5000 cells in the embryo, one of the two X chromosomes in female cells is inactivated and appears as a dark-staining mass (Barr body) in the nucleus. Inactivation is random and can affect either the paternally or maternally derived X chromosome. However, once inactivation has occurred all the descendent cells in a particular tissue have the same X chromosome in the inactive state. By a mechanism which is poorly understood the relevant X chromosome is imprinted with the information that it is to remain inactivated in subsequent cell divisions. Inactivation is not permanent, for in the primordial germ cells of females both X chromosomes become fully active again.

Most of the genes on an inactivated X chromosome are not transcribed and therefore produce no protein product. There are some exceptions; several genes on the tip of the short arm of the X (the pseudoautosomal region where there is pairing with the tip of the short arm of the Y chromosome during meiosis) escape inactivation, and continue to be expressed in normal fashion. But for a large majority of X-linked genes the encoded proteins are found at similar levels in male and female cells, a phenomenon known as dosage compensation.

There are important clinical consequences of X inactivation, particularly for carriers of X-linked recessive disorders (Fig. 1.13). For example, in carriers of Duchenne muscular dystrophy the original inactivation of progenitor muscle cells may by chance affect mainly the normal (paternally derived) X chromosome, so that descendent cells express mainly the mutant gene. Such women may have symptoms of the disorder, and are known as manifesting heterozygotes. Conversely, if inactivation affects mainly the abnormal (maternally derived) X, it will be difficult to detect carriers by biochemical tests, such as serum creatine kinase assay. About one third of female carriers of Duchenne muscular dystrophy have creatine kinase values in the normal range. Likewise, in X-linked dominant disorders some heterozygous females may have only mild or subclinical disease, since their abnormal X has been preferentially inactivated.

MITOCHONDRIAL INHERITANCE

Although most human genes are carried on nuclear chromosomes, a small number are found in cytoplasmic organelles called mitochondria. Each mitochondrion has several copies of a circular chromosome, encoding protein components of the respiratory chain and oxidative phosphorylation system, as well as some special types of RNA.

Mitochondrial inheritance passes through the maternal line, since the sperm contributes no cytoplasm to the zygote. Thus a disorder, in which all the children of an affected mother are affected while those of an affected father are not, might arise from a mitochondrial mutation. An example of mitochondrial inheritance is the eye disease, Leigh's hereditary optic atrophy.

CHROMOSOMAL DISORDERS

Chromosomal disorders are extremely common and probably affect more than half of all conceptions. However, most spontaneously miscarry, so that the liveborn frequency is about 0.6%, of which one third are clinically serious. There are two broad types of chromosome aberration; numerical, where there is an incorrect number of chromosomes in somatic cells, and structural, where there is an alteration in the structure of one or more chromosomes. Most chromosome abnormalities are de novo events, that is they are the result of major mutations in the parental germ cells, while some are inherited according to Mendelian principles.

Karyotyping

Although human chromosomes may be visualised in any growing tissue, such as bone marrow, skin fibroblasts, amniotic fluid cells or chorionic villus, they are most conveniently studied in peripheral blood lymphocytes. Heparinised venous blood is set up in culture and phytohaemagglutinin added to stimulate T-cell division. After two to three days, cell division is arrested at metaphase by the addition of colchicine which interferes with spindle formation. A hypotonic solution swells the cells and separates the individual chromosomes. After fixation the cells are spread on microscope slides and air-dried. Chromosomes can be stained with a variety of

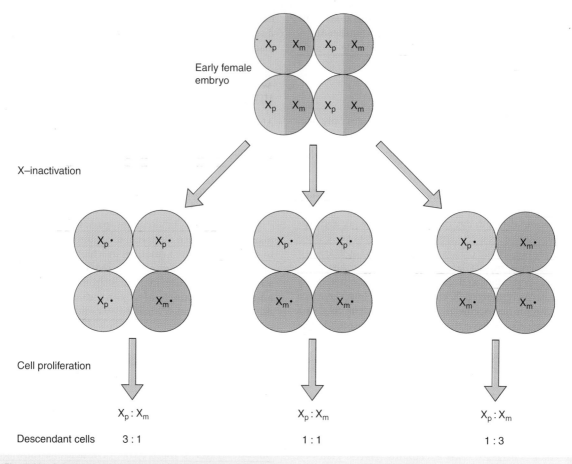

Fig. 1.13 Schematic representation of X chromosome inactivation. In cells of the early female embryo both X chromosomes (Xp, Xm) are active. X inactivation is random so that in different blocks of cells variable proportions of cells contain active Xp or active Xm. The descendent lines derived from the original inactivation events retain the same proportions of active and inactive X chromosomes.

dyes, a favourite being Giemsa. A suitable metaphase spread is photographed through a high-power microscope, the individual chromosomes cut from the photograph and arranged in homologous pairs to produce the karyotype (Fig. 1.14). A Giemsa-banded (G-banded) karyotype has 300 to 400 alternating light and dark bands, which are characteristic of each chromosome pair.

Chromosome nomenclature

In the normal human karyotype the chromosomes are arranged as 22 pairs of autosomes and the sex chromosomes (XX in females and XY in males). The position of the centromere allows division of chromosomes into three groups:

- *metacentrics*, where the centromere is approximately in the middle (1, 3, 16, 19 and 20);

- *acrocentrics*, where the centromere is close to one end (13, 14, 15, 21, 22 and Y);
- *sub-metacentrics*, where the centromere is in an intermediate position (the remainder).

Each chromosome has a short arm called *p* (petit) and a long arm called *q*. Arms are divided into regions, bands and sub-bands by a numerical system; e.g. 7q21.2 means the long arm of 7, region 2, band 1 and sub-band 2.

Karyotypes are described by a shorthand notation of symbols, which lists the total number of chromosomes, the sex chromosome constitution and any description of abnormality. Thus a normal female is 46,XX and a normal male 46,XY. A female who has lost an X chromosome (Turner syndrome) is 45,X and a male with an extra Y chromosome 47,XYY. A (+) or (−) sign is placed before an appropriate symbol to indicate an additional or missing whole chromosome, and after the

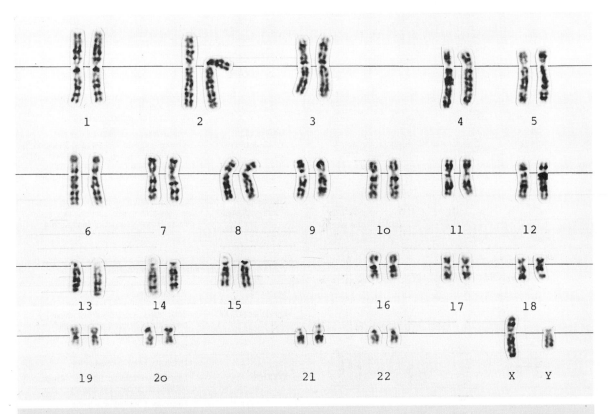

Fig. 1.14   Karyotype of a normal male on Giemsa banding (G-banding).

symbol to show only part of a chromosome. Thus a male with Down syndrome caused by an extra chromosome 21 is 47,XY,+21 and a female with part of the short arm of chromosome 5 missing is 46,XX,5p−.

NUMERICAL CHROMOSOME ABERRATIONS

The chromosome number of the normal human germ cell is 23 and of the normal somatic cell 46. A chromosome number that is an exact multiple of 23, but exceeds the diploid number of 46, is called polyploidy. Triploidy (69 chromosomes) is seen quite often in spontaneous abortions (or in early prenatal diagnosis), but is essentially incompatible with life. Tetraploidy (92 chromosomes) is also seen occasionally in spontaneous abortions but virtually never in liveborns.

The more common types of numerical chromosome aberration result from the gain or loss of one or a few chromosomes, and are called aneuploidy (Table 1.5). Aneuploidy is usually the consequence of the failure of paired homologous chromosomes to separate at meiotic anaphase, a phenomenon known as non-disjunction.

This can happen at either the first or second divisions of meiosis (Fig. 1.15), and leads to cells with an extra copy of a chromosome (trisomy) or cells with a missing copy of a chromosome (monosomy). Non-disjunction can also occur in mitotic division, resulting in a mosaic, a person with cell lines with two different chromosome complements.

Autosomal aneuploidies

The most common aneuploidy in humans is trisomy 21 which causes Down syndrome. The overall frequency is about 1 in 700 births, about 95% of which are trisomies for chromosome 21 and the remainder translocations (see below). The incidence increases sharply with advancing maternal age, particularly for mothers over 35. Two other fairly common autosomal aneuploidies are trisomy 18 and trisomy 13. Both are associated with multiple dysmorphic features at birth and only 10% of infants survive the first year (Table 1.6). The frequency of trisomy 18 is one in 3000 livebirths and of trisomy 13 one in 5000 livebirths. In both the incidence increases with advancing maternal age (Fig. 1.22, p. 24).

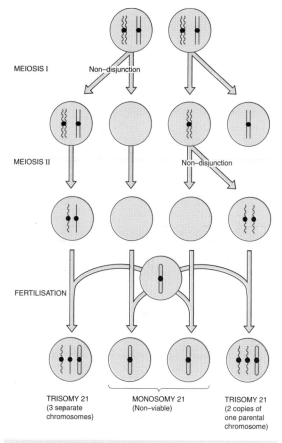

Fig. 1.15 The origin of trisomy 21 is non-disjunction of chromosomes 21 either at meiosis I or meiosis II. The homologous chromosomes 21 in the cells at the top are represented by different configurations so that their origins in the zygotes (bottom row) can be traced.

TRISOMY 21 (3 separate chromosomes)

MONOSOMY 21 (Non–viable)

TRISOMY 21 (2 copies of one parental chromosome)

Table 1.6 Common autosomal aneuploidies

Syndrome	Main features
Down syndrome (trisomy 21)	Flat profile, small nose, upward-slanting eyes, low-set ears. Single palmar (simian) crease in 50%. Floppiness in neonate. IQ usually less than 50. Congenital heart malformations and reduced life expectancy in 40%.
Trisomy 18 (Edwards syndrome)	Characteristic skull with small chin and prominent forehead, low-set ears. Clenched hands with overlapping index and fifth fingers, single palmar crease, rockerbottom feet. Frequent malformations of heart, kidney and other organs.
Trisomy 13 (Patau syndrome)	Cleft lip and palate, polydactyly, small head and close-set tiny eyes, abnormal ears, scalp defects. Frequent congenital heart disease.

Table 1.7 Sex chromosome aneuploidies

Syndrome	Main features
Klinefelter (47, XXY)	Small testes, poorly developed secondary sexual characteristics, gynaecomastia, infertility. May be mild reduction in verbal skills.
	Frequency 1 in 1000 male births.
XYY Male	Largely asymptomatic. Often tall. May be behavioural problems in later life.
	Frequency 1 in 1000 male births.
Turner (45, X)	Short stature, webbed neck, primary amenorrhoea, lack of secondary sexual characteristics, often coarctation of aorta.
	Frequency 1 in 5000 female births.
Trisomy X (47, XXX)	Largely asymptomatic, but 20% mildly mentally handicapped.
	Frequency 1 in 1000 female births.

Sex chromosome aneuploidies

With the exception of chromosome 21, aneuploidies of the X and Y chromosomes are more common than those of the autosomes. As with autosomal trisomies the origin is non-disjunction during one of the meiotic divisions.

Table 1.5 Numerical chromosome abnormalities

Description	Karyotype
Tetraploidy	92, XXYY; 92, XXXY; etc
Triploidy	69, XXY; 69, XYY; etc
Trisomy 21	47, XX, +21; 47, XY, +21
Trisomy 18	47, XX, +18; 47, XY, +18
Trisomy 13	47, XX, +13; 47, XY, +13
Klinefelter syndrome	47, XXY
Trisomy X	47, XXX
Turner syndrome	45, X
XYY male	47, XYY

However, the clinical effects are less severe (Table 1.7). Indeed, the 47,XYY male, at one time associated with criminality, is usually asymptomatic and has relatively minor and variable behavioural problems in later life. Intelligence tends to be 10 or 15 points below expectation.

STRUCTURAL CHROMOSOME ABERRATIONS

Structural abnormalities arise from chromosome breakage. When a chromosome breaks there are two unstable and sticky ends which normally rapidly rejoin. However, if a segment is lost after breakage the result is a deletion, a chromosome with an important part of the genetic material missing. If more than one break occurs, perhaps in different chromosomes, DNA repair mechanisms are unable to distinguish the sticky ends and there is the possibility of aberrant rejoining. Some of the different

Table 1.8   Types and nomenclature of structural chromosome aberrations

Type	Example	Explanation
Deletion	46, XX, del (5p) or 46, XX, 5p-	Deletion of short arm of chromosome 5. Cri-du-chat syndrome.
Ring	46, XX, r (15)	A ring chromosome 15
Duplication	46, XY, dup (2) (p13–p22)	A duplication of the short arm of chromosome 2 between p13 and p22
Isochromosome	46, X, i (Xq)	The X has split transversely with duplication of the long arm and no short arm
Inversion	46, XY, inv (11) (q13q22)	Inversion of the long arm of 11 between q13 and q22
Translocation	46, XX, t (4; 12) (p14; p13)	Reciprocal translocation between chromosomes 4 and 12, with breakpoints at p14 in 4 and p13 in 12

types of abnormal chromosome which result from breakage and incorrect reunion are listed in Table 1.8.

Translocations

Translocations are a particularly important type of abnormal chromosome. Two main types are known: Robertsonian and reciprocal translocations.

Robertsonian translocations

These are also known as centric fusions and involve breaks at or near the centromeres in two acrocentric chromosomes, leading to a cross-fusion of products (Fig. 1.16). No essential chromosomal material is lost in the discarded segments and no vital genes are damaged. The carrier of a Robertsonian translocation, although having only 45 chromosomes, is clinically normal. However, he or she has an increased chance of having chromosomally unbalanced and abnormal offspring.

This is illustrated in Figure 1.17 for the relatively common centric fusion between chromosomes 14 and

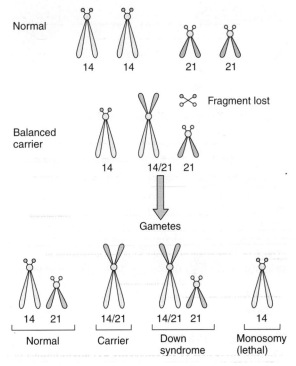

Fig. 1.17   Centric fusion between chromosomes 14 and 21. Segregation of these chromosomes into gametes is shown, together with the consequences of fertilisation by a normal gamete.

21. During meiosis the fused 14;21 chromosome may segregate along with an unchanged 21 into a gamete. If this is fertilised by a normal gamete, the resulting zygote has an extra copy of chromosome 21 and will have Down syndrome. The risk of a carrier of a balanced 14;21 translocation having a child with Down syndrome is estimated empirically (see p. 23).

Reciprocal translocations

In reciprocal translocations (Fig. 1.16) there is a two-way exchange of material between homologous or non-

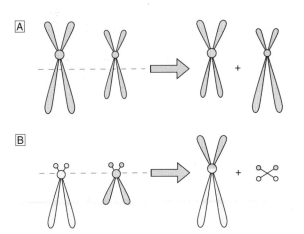

Fig. 1.16   Examples of chromosomal translocations: A, reciprocal and B, Robertsonian.

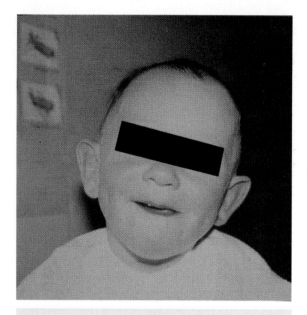

Fig. 1.18   A young boy with fragile X syndrome.

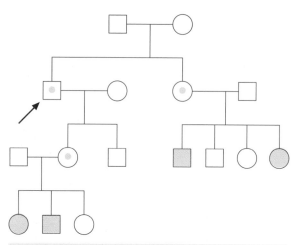

Fig. 1.19   Type of pedigree seen in the fragile X syndrome.
Symbols representing pre-mutation carriers have a central dot. The arrowed individual is a normal transmitting male. Key: p. 12.

homologous chromosomes. Autosomes or sex chromosomes may be affected, and no chromosomal material is lost. Carriers of reciprocal translocations are phenotypically normal, and as in Robertsonian translocations, the medical significance is for future generations. Theoretical calculations can be made of the proportions of offspring likely to have balanced or unbalanced constitutions, but these are not seen in practice. The actual risks depend on the chromosomes involved in the translocation and the sex of the carrier (see p. 23).

The fragile X syndrome

The most common source of inherited mental retardation is the fragile X syndrome, occurring in about 1 in 1500 males. The cytogenetic benchmark of this condition is a non-staining gap on the long arm of the X chromosome, the position being designated Xq27.3. However, the fragile site can only be visualised in culture media with folate depletion or thymidine excess, and even then cytogenetic diagnosis is unreliable. Clinically, the syndrome is characterised by moderate to severe mental retardation, a long face with large everted ears and large testes (Fig. 1.18). Some 30% of female carriers also show a degree of mental impairment.

The gene responsible for the fragile X syndrome, called FMR-1, has been cloned. An unusual feature is an unstable CGG trinucleotide repeat in exon 1 of the gene. Normal males and females have between 6 and 54 copies of this repeat, with a median value at about 30.

Affected males and carrier females have large and variable expansions of the CGG repeat, ranging from 200 to several thousand copies. A male with a large repeat is invariably mentally retarded (even when the fragile site cannot be seen under the microscope), while the intellectual capacities of carrier females are less predictable.

What makes the genetics of the fragile X syndrome so unusual is the existence of a 'premutation' genotype. Carriers of the premutation, a CGG expansion in the range of about 60 to 200 copies, are phenotypically normal. Male carriers transmit the premutation to their offspring without change in size of the repeat; they are known as normal transmitting males. However, in female premutation carriers there is a high chance of expansion to the full mutation on transmission to their children; the risk is nearly 100% if the premutation is at the top end of the range, i.e. 200 copies. The type of unusual pedigree seen in families segregating fragile X syndrome is shown in Figure 1.19.

GENOMIC IMPRINTING

One of the axioms of genetics is that a mutation has the same effect whether inherited from the father or the mother. It is now evident that this is not always true. Some genes and chromosomal segments may be differentially imprinted during male and female meioses. This means that the expression of the gene is affected by the parental origin of the chromosome.

The clearest example of genomic imprinting comes from two clinically distinct but cytogenetically indistinguishable disorders, Angelman and Prader–Willi syn-

Angelman syndrome   Prader–Willi syndrome

Deletion of 15qll–13

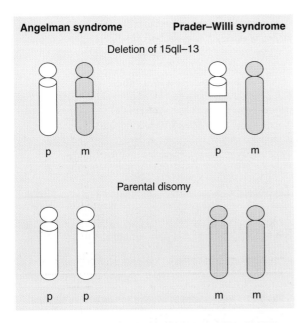

Fig. 1.20   Types of chromosome 15 found in Angelman and Prader–Willi syndromes. p = paternal; m = maternal.

MULTIFACTORIAL DISORDERS

In many of the common disorders of mankind there is evidence for genetic factors, but no clear pattern of inheritance. The disease may occur more frequently in members of a family (familial aggregation) than in the general population. It may be limited to one ethnic group in a common environment. These disorders are said to be multifactorial, meaning that they are caused by an unknown number of genes interacting with often equally unknown environmental factors. Normal traits, such as intelligence, height, weight and blood pressure, also have multifactorial origins.

Twin studies

A much used method for determining the genetic contribution to a multifactorial trait is through the study of twins. Twins occur in about 1 in 90 deliveries, with one third monozygotic and two-thirds dizygotic. Monozygotic twins are genetically identical while dizygotic twins have on average half their genes in common. If a disorder is determined by alleles at a single genetic locus, monozygotic twins should have complete concordance, with each pair either having the disorder or not having the disorder. When environmental factors are important, the concordance rate in monozygotic twins will be less than 100%.

Many comparisons have been made of disease concordance rates in monozygotic (MZ) and dizygotic (DZ) twins (Table 1.9). When the difference is large (e.g. manic depression) it is assumed that genetic factors are important, and when small (e.g. spina bifida) that environmental factors predominate. However, these comparisons give no indication of the number or nature of the genes involved. Furthermore, many named dis-

dromes. In Angelman syndrome children have severe motor and intellectual retardation, hypotonia, an ataxic gait and a wide mouth and protruding tongue. In Prader–Willi syndrome there is short stature, obesity and mild to moderate mental retardation. In each syndrome about half the patients have a deletion of the same region of the long arm of chromosome 15.

It has been shown that in Angelman syndrome the deletion arises on the chromosome 15 inherited from the mother, and in Prader–Willi on the chromosome 15 inherited from the father. This is reinforced by the finding that in some cases of Angelman syndrome there are two paternally derived chromosomes 15 and no maternal 15, while in some cases of Prader–Willi there are two maternally-derived chromosomes 15 and no paternal 15 (Fig. 1.20). This suggests that for normal development one needs a particular segment of chromosome 15 from each parent. Absence of the maternal segment due to deletion or paternal disomy gives Angelman syndrome, while absence of the paternal segment due to deletion or maternal disomy leads to Prader–Willi syndrome.

Studies of genomic imprinting in humans are still at an early stage. Evidence from mice, where controlled breeding experiments can be carried out, suggests that it may be a relatively common phenomenon in mammalian species.

Table 1.9   Twin concordance for some congenital malformations and diseases of adulthood

Disorders	Concordance (%) MZ Twins	DZ Twins
Congenital malformations		
Cleft lip + palate	35	5
Cleft palate alone	25	5
Club foot	30	2
Dislocation of hip	40	3
Pyloric stenosis	20	2
Spina bifida	6	3
Adult diseases		
Alzheimer's disease	40	10
Epilepsy	40	10
Hypertension	30	10
Manic depression	80	10
Multiple sclerosis	20	5
Schizophrenia	40	10

orders (e.g. hypertension) are so obviously heterogeneous that it makes little sense to lump them together
in a single study.

Dissecting out genes in multifactorial disorders

When it proves difficult to pinpoint the environmental
factors in a disorder, it is sometimes profitable to try
instead to identify contributing genes.

One approach is to examine whether a particular allele
occurs more frequently in affected than in unaffected
people. Clearly one needs to have some clues as to which
genetic locus to examine. In many autoimmune disorders there is prior evidence that the major histocompatibility locus (HLA) may be involved. Indeed
there are some striking associations between certain
HLA antigens and these disorders. The best-known is
between the HLA B27 antigen and ankylosing spondylitis; this antigen is found in 95% of patients and only
7% of the normal population.

Another approach is called sib-pair analysis. Sibs have
half their genes in common, and thus at any locus one
quarter of sib pairs will have two alleles in common, one
half will have one allele in common and one quarter will
have no alleles in common. If enough sib pairs can be
assembled, where both members are affected, it is possible to search for deviations from the 1:2:1 ratio in allele
sharing. For example, in insulin-dependent diabetes
mellitus, some 60% of affected sibs share alleles at the
HLA locus, considerably more than the expected 25%.
Likewise, some 80% of twins concordant for homo-
sexuality share alleles from the tip of the long arm of the
X chromosome. The conclusion in both cases is that
loci have been identified which contribute to genetic
susceptibility.

CANCER GENETICS

The genetics of cancer is complicated, and is only now
being unravelled. Most common cancers are not
inherited, but occur as sporadic events in people with
little relevant family history. Nonetheless, cancer often
shows familial aggregation. Furthermore, there are a
number of Mendelian conditions associated with
tumours, where the inheritance is as an autosomal dominant or recessive, and where it is apparent that the cancer
is the result of mutation at a single genetic locus.

Tumour-suppressor genes

The prototype disease for the study of cancer genetics is
retinoblastoma, a childhood eye tumour with an incidence of 1 in 20 000. A majority of cases are sporadic
and usually only affect one eye. Other cases are inherited

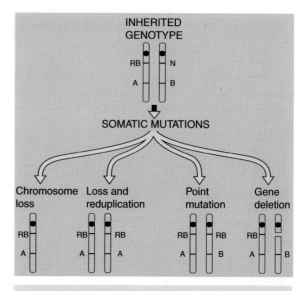

**Fig. 1.21   Mechanisms by which a person with an inherited
susceptibility to retinoblastoma (RB) develops the
cancer through a second somatic mutation.**

from an affected parent and invariably affect both eyes.
These familial forms are associated with a high risk of
other malignancies, such as osteosarcoma.

It is now known that retinoblastoma arises from
mutation in a gene called RB. In familial retinoblastoma
the mutation is inherited from an affected parent (or
arises as a new mutation in the parental germ cells). But
not all children inheriting a mutant RB gene develop
cancer. A second event is necessary, affecting the normal
gene on the homologous chromosome (Fig. 1.21). This
can be a point mutation, a deletion or the loss of the
whole normal chromosome. The important point is that
both RB genes must be affected before retinoblastoma
develops. The chance of the second event occurring in
someone who has inherited a mutant RB gene is high—
nearly 90%—so that developing retinoblasts must be
quite susceptible to mutation. In sporadic retino-
blastomas there have to be two independent mutations
of the RB genes at a very early stage of retinoblast development.

The retinoblastoma gene was the first example of a
class of tumour-suppressor gene. These are genes which
may be seen as having an in-built braking effect on cell
proliferation. Other examples are to be found in Wilms'
tumour (a childhood kidney tumour) and polyposis coli
(an inherited cancer of the bowel).

Oncogenes

In some respects oncogenes may be seen as the opposite
of tumour-suppressor genes, in that they are genes that

become activated in the development of cancer. Before activation they are normal cellular genes, called proto-oncogenes, some of which encode growth factors or growth factor receptors. Activation can occur by any mechanism that changes the genetic material. One well-known example is the Philadelphia chromosome, which is found in 95% of white cells of patients with chronic myeloid leukaemia. The Philadelphia chromosome results from a reciprocal translocation between the long arms of chromosomes 9 and 22. The *abl* proto-oncogene is translocated from its normal position on chromosome 9 to a new position on chromosome 22, where it comes under the influence of another gene that activates it. This leads to unregulated production of a specific protein and proliferation of the cells in which the translocation has occurred.

Somatic cell genetics

Although it is now clear that some cancers can be inherited as simple Mendelian traits, with clear patterns of transmission, this is the exception rather than the rule. Even though most cancers involve quite substantial changes in the genetic material, such mutations are somatic and there is no risk to future generations.

MANAGEMENT, TREATMENT AND PREVENTION OF GENETIC DISEASE

Very few genetic diseases can be successfully treated. The emphasis in clinical genetics is therefore to assist people to avoid occurrences and recurrences by genetic counselling, and, if need be, by prenatal diagnosis.

GENETIC COUNSELLING

Genetic counselling is the communication of information about disorders with a genetic component. The essential features are given in the information box.

The most important is the establishment of a correct

ESSENTIAL FEATURES OF GENETIC COUNSELLING

- **Take history** (proband and family)
  Construct pedigree
  Examine proband
  Establish diagnosis
- **Counselling**
  Risk estimation
  Options available
- **Follow-up**
  Arrange necessary procedures
  Review and support

---

diagnosis, for without this any advice given may be completely misleading. During the counselling process the consultand will be given an estimate of the risks of occurrence or recurrence of the disorder. These calculations are often more difficult than they seem and, except in simple cases, should be left to the clinical geneticist.

It must also be noted that the psychological reactions of consultands to information about genetic disorders can be complex. The initial response may be one of shock and denial, perhaps an inability to accept that a child is really affected. This can be followed by anger and hostility directed at the counsellor, as bearer of bad news. Feelings of guilt are common in parents who have produced an affected child, and accusations may be levelled against one branch of the family. Anxiety and even depression follow, and make the absorbing of information difficult. Finally, and with sensitive help from the counsellor, the consultand reaches a state of acceptance, when the options available can be realistically discussed. These discussions should be non-directive.

Exact risks

In most Mendelian conditions, provided that the diagnosis is unequivocal, an exact risk of recurrence or occurrence can be given. Straightforward situations are outlined in Figures 1.10 to 1.12.

Combined risks

It often happens that a risk calculated from Mendelian principles is modified by other factors. An obvious example is in a late-onset autosomal dominant like Huntington's disease. A person with an affected parent starts with a 50% risk of inheriting the disorder. But as he gets older and passes the typical age of onset, his probability of carrying the mutant gene obviously declines. The 'conditional' information from his age is combined with the prior risk, using Bayes' theorem, to give a final risk. For example, a 70-year old man, with no signs of the disorder but with an affected parent, has a risk of Huntington's of only 5%. Although Bayes' theorem calculations are widely used in genetic counselling, they should not be attempted by the amateur.

Empiric risks

Risks in non-Mendelian conditions are usually estimated empirically, i.e. by experience. The recurrence risk for a congenital malformation is the same as the concordance rate in dizygotic twins (see Table 1.9). Of special concern to the genetic counsellor is the risk of abnormal offspring to the carrier of a balanced translocation. Although these risks are based on small numbers and therefore imprecise (Table 1.10), they are

Table 1.10 Risk of abnormal offspring for carriers of a balanced translocation

Translocation	Risk (%) Carrier father	Carrier mother
Centric fusion 13; 14	1	1
Centric fusion 14; 21	1	15
Centric fusion 21; 22	5	10
Centric fusion 21; 21	100	100
Reciprocal (any)	10	10

usually regarded as grounds for offering prenatal diagnosis to those parents who so wish.

PRENATAL DIAGNOSIS

It is possible to diagnose a large number of chromosome disorders, single gene defects and even congenital malformations in the first or second trimester of pregnancy.

Two procedures may be employed to obtain fetal tissue. Transabdominal amniocentesis is the most widely used (see information box below), and has an excellent safety record with fetal loss rates well below 0.5%. Recently, chorionic villus sampling (CVS), by either the transcervical or transabdominal routes, has become the preferred method. The safety of CVS is yet to be satisfactorily established, and is probably associated with greater fetal loss (about 2%) than that seen with amniocentesis. However, since it may be carried out in the first trimester, any subsequent termination of pregnancy can be done before the mother has felt fetal movements.

MAIN FEATURES OF AMNIOCENTESIS

- Conventionally performed around 16 weeks of gestation, though it can be done as early as 10 weeks.
- Ultrasound is used to locate the placenta, to detect twins and to exclude major structural fetal abnormalities.
- An outpatient procedure using normal sterile techniques.
- Between 10 and 20 ml amniotic fluid is aspirated. Both the cells and the protein of amniotic fluid are fetal in origin.
- Supernatant fluid: measurement of alphafetoprotein (AFP) in the fluid allows detection of spina bifida, anencephaly, and occasional other major structural birth defects.
- Cells: Cells are cultured for 10 to 14 days and used for detection of chromosomal abnormalities. After 4 to 6 weeks' culture there is sufficient tissue for determining enzymes whose deficiency signals a Mendelian disorder.

In all forms of fetal tissue sampling, ultrasonography is used to guide biopsy. An experienced ultra-

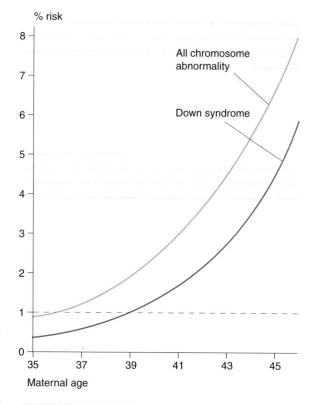

Fig. 1.22 Risk of Down syndrome and other chromosome abnormalities with advancing maternal age.

sonographer can also detect major structural malformations of the fetus.

The most common reason for prenatal diagnosis is advanced maternal age. The risk of Down syndrome (as well as that of several other chromosome aneuploidies) rises rapidly after age 35 (Fig. 1.22). Chromosome studies are carried out after 10-day culture of amniotic fluid cells, or after 48-hour culture of chorionic villus. If prenatal diagnosis is carried out by amniocentesis, it is standard practice to measure the alphafetoprotein (AFP) concentration in the amniotic fluid supernatant. This permits the diagnosis of anencephaly, spina bifida and several other congenital malformations, which are associated with elevated AFP levels.

Most of the common single gene disorders can now be diagnosed in utero. The laborious use of enzyme assay on cultured amniotic fluid cells (4 to 6 weeks of culture) is now being supplanted by direct DNA analysis of chorionic villus (see Table 1.4, p. 11).

Prenatal screening

Prenatal diagnosis is used for pregnancies where there is a known increased risk of an abnormal fetus. It is an exact procedure. Prenatal screening applies to all pregnancies, and is a crude system for detecting those with elevated risks. It must always be followed by more exact diagnosis.

Measurement of elevated maternal serum AFP to screen for increased risk of fetal spina bifida and anencephaly is widely used in the United Kingdom. Some 2 to 3% of women have raised values and ultrasonography, amniocentesis and amniotic fluid AFP determination is usually carried out to confirm or exclude the diagnosis. Low maternal serum AFP is an indicator of a risk of Down syndrome. The risk may be refined by measuring other maternal serum markers, such as chorionic gonadotrophin and unconjugated oestriol, but ultimately there is need for amniocentesis and cytogenetic evaluation of the fetus.

Alternatives to prenatal diagnosis

Because prenatal diagnosis can lead to termination of pregnancy, some people find it unacceptable. Alternative ways of avoiding the birth of an affected child are limited: forgoing reproduction or, in the case of a recessive disorder, artificial insemination by a screened donor. However, it is now possible in some situations to carry out prenatal diagnosis on a blastocyst, and if it is free of defective genes, to implant it in the mother. Pre-implantation prenatal diagnosis is still in the early stages of development.

GENE THERAPY

Attempts to treat genetic diseases have tended to focus on alleviating the metabolic or biochemical consequences of the gene defect; for example by dietary restriction of phenylalanine in children with phenylketonuria. None of these approaches has been very successful, and genetic diseases are conventionally regarded as untreatable. However, the advent of gene therapy, the introduction of normal genes into tissues expressing defective ones, promises to change this dismal conclusion.

The problems of moving gene therapy from the laboratory into the clinic remain formidable, as suggested by the information box. The most likely candidates are recessively inherited disorders, where gene supplementation rather than gene replacement is adequate. At present only somatic gene therapy is permitted, and thus there is no chance that genetic changes introduced would be transmitted to the germ line. Despite these problems clinical trials of gene therapy for several genetic (and non-genetic) disease are underway, and there is every chance of at least moderate success within the next few years.

PROBLEMS OF GENE THERAPY

- Targetting suitable cells (in vitro or in vivo)
- Designing vector for gene delivery
- Getting appropriate expression of inserted gene
- Ensuring stability of inserted gene
- Avoiding damage to other genes
- Assessing longer-term effects

THE HUMAN GENOME PROJECT

This is a loosely coordinated international effort to clone and sequence all 100 000 genes by the year 2000. Eventually it is planned to sequence all 3×10^9 base-pairs of the human genome. The consequences for all branches of medicine and biology will be enormous. Two quotations make the point: 'the genetic messages encoded within our DNA molecules will provide the ultimate answers to the chemical underpinnings of human existence' (James Watson), and 'in the 21st century all biology will be gene-based and all biologists will be geneticists' (Sydney Brenner).

FURTHER READING

Pena S D J, Chakraborty R 1994 Paternity testing in the DNA era. Trends in Genetics 10: 204–6
Plomin R, Owen M J, McGuffin P 1994 The genetic basis of complex human behaviors. Science 264: 1733–9
Poulton J 1992 Mitochondrial DNA and genetic disease. Bioessays 14: 763–8
Wilkie A 1994 The molecular basis of dominance. Journal of Medical Genetics 31: 89–98

GLOSSARY OF GENETIC TERMS

allele: alternative forms of a gene at a given locus
aneuploid: incorrect chromosome number
autosome: any chromosome other than a sex chromosome
centromere: the constricted part of a chromosome where the chromatids are joined
consultand: person seeking genetic information
crossing-over: see recombination
dominant: a trait expressed in a heterozygote
diploid: the number of chromosomes in somatic cells
eukaryote: an organism whose cells have true nucleus bounded by nuclear membrane
exon: segment of a gene containing coding sequences
expressivity: variation in severity of the same genetic disorder
genetic locus: the site of a gene on a pair of homologous chromosomes
genome: the complete genetic makeup of a species
genotype: the genetic constitution of an individual; often this refers to a single locus

(Glossary continues overleaf)

haploid: the number of chromosomes in a germ cell

haplotype: a group of closely sited alleles on a single chromosome

hemizygous: alleles on the X chromosome in males

heterozygote: a person who has different alleles at a locus on homologous chromosomes

homologous chromosomes: paired chromosomes

homozygote: a person who has identical alleles at a locus on homologous chromosomes

intron: segment of a gene that is transcribed but excised before translation

karyotype: the chromosome constitution of a person

linkage: tendency of alleles at loci which are near each other on a chromosome to be inherited as a block

lyonisation: see X inactivation

monosomy: one of homologous chromosomes is missing

mosaic: cells of different genotype in a person

non-disjunction: failure of homologous chromosomes to separate in anaphase

nucleotide: the building block of DNA and RNA, comprising a base, a pentose sugar and a phosphate group

oligonucleotide: synthetic single-stranded segment of DNA, typically 5 to 50 nucleotide bases in size

penetrance: frequency of expression of a gene

phenotype: a characteristic which is the result of inheritance of a gene or set of genes

polymorphism: alternative alleles or phenotypes found in a population

proband: the person who draws attention to the family

probe: a sequence of DNA used to identify a complementary sequence

recessive: a trait expressed only in homozygotes

recombination (crossing over): formation of new combinations of alleles during meiosis

somatic: not involved in the germ-line

X inactivation (lyonisation): random inactivation of one of the two X chromosomes in female cells

2

Immunological factors in disease

The science of immunology arose from <u>the study of</u> <u>man's resistance to infection</u>. It was appreciated that after an individual's recovery from a particular infectious disease, the same disease rarely occurred again. <u>This</u> <u>altered reactivity is what we now call specific immunity.</u> Immunology also encompasses <u>a number of entirely</u> <u>nonspecific antimicrobial protective mechanisms, innate</u> <u>in that they are not affected by prior contact with the</u> <u>infectious agent</u> although their activity can be up- and <u>down-regulated by a number of factors.</u>

Resistance to infection is not an essential feature of immunity. Bacteria may induce antibodies which have no obvious protective value, and immune responses are evoked by injection of intrinsically harmless non-living organic substances, such as serum protein from another individual or species.

<u>A distinction must be made between the induction</u> <u>phase of immunity in which, at the first encounter with</u> <u>antigen, a pattern is established of altered reactivity,</u> <u>involving T and B cells and the production of antibody,</u> <u>and expression of one or more types of immune response</u> <u>upon subsequent re-encounter with the same antigen.</u> Specific immune responses can also produce <u>hyper-</u> <u>sensitivity,</u> which has unpleasant and sometimes dangerous effects, upon subsequent exposure to the provoking antigen. There are also circumstances where antigen encounter leads to down-regulation of specific reactivity. This is called <u>tolerance,</u> and <u>occurs when antigen is fed,</u> <u>and in some species when antigen is encountered early</u> <u>in life.</u>

Thus immunology encompasses molecular and cellular biology of antigen recognition and of immune reactions, specific and nonspecific.

ORGANS, CELLS AND MOLECULES OF THE IMMUNE SYSTEM

LYMPHOID ORGANS

Cells and tissues involved in immunity comprise about 2% of the body-weight. Many of the cells migrate throughout the body but there are also organs where cells which participate in immune responses are collected together in an environment where they can perform their functions more effectively.

PRIMARY AND SECONDARY LYMPHOID ORGANS

Primary lymphoid organs
<u>The **bone marrow, thymus** and **fetal liver** are the</u> <u>major sites of **production of lymphocytes**, and the</u>

environments where lymphocytes undergo differentiation and proliferation so that they leave as functional effector cells.

Secondary lymphoid organs
Lymph nodes, spleen, tonsils and Peyer's patches provide an environment in which lymphocytes can interact with each other and with antigens because there are phagocytic macrophages, antigen presenting cells, mature T and B lymphocytes collected together.

DISPERSED IMMUNE CELLS

In addition to the organised lymphoid tissues, there are other sites, particularly the mucosae, where many immunocytes are dispersed between other cells, for example within the gut epithelium and lamina propria.

MIGRATION OF LYMPHOCYTES

Migration of cells between lymphoid organs is illustrated in Figure 2.1.

The exit route for lymphocytes from the bloodstream is through a specialised section of the post-capillary venules, the high endothelial venule. In the spleen it is via the marginal zone of the periarteriolar lymphoid sheath and there are similar specialised blood vessels in the lamina propria of the gut, and some other sites, to allow emigration of particular populations of lymphocytes into these parts of the body. Matching of receptors on lymphocytes to molecules on these specialised blood vessels explains the apparent selection of only certain types of cells for migration into the tissues.

Within the lymphoid tissues there are areas mainly populated by T cells (T-dependent areas) and B areas which also contain germinal centres.

There are also routes of return of lymphocytes, e.g. from the mucous membranes back to lymph nodes via afferent lymphatics, and via the thoracic duct into the venous system.

CLINICAL RELEVANCE OF THE ORGANISATION OF LYMPHOID TISSUES

An appreciation of the organisation of primary and secondary lymphoid organs, and movement of cells between them, has been critical to the development of specific immunotherapy for some immunodeficiency diseases; also the characteristics of a number of malignancies of the lymphoid tissues (lymphomas) relate to where, within the general developmental and migration sequences, the malignant clone has occurred.

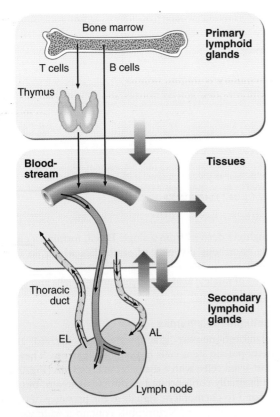

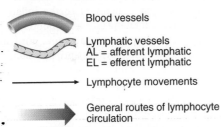

Blood vessels

Lymphatic vessels
AL = afferent lymphatic
EL = efferent lymphatic

Lymphocyte movements

General routes of lymphocyte circulation

Fig. 2.1 Organisation of the lymphoid system. There is one-way traffic of T and B cells from the primary lymphoid organs into the bloodstream, and continuous recirculation of cells between the secondary lymphoid organs, tissues and bloodstream.

Table 2.1 Lymphocyte and macrophage surface markers (cluster of differentiation, CD)

CD nomenclature	Terminology previously used	Significance of the marker
CD2	T1	All T cells are positive
CD3	T3	Present on all mature peripheral T lymphocytes, 25% of human thymocytes
CD4	T4	60% of circulating T cells, helper/inducer T cell subset
CD8	T8	Approximately 35% of circulating peripheral human T cells, suppressor/cytotoxic T cell subset
CD20	B1	Present on all human B cells from peripheral blood, lymph node, spleen, tonsil and bone marrow
CD21	B2	Similar pattern to CD20, but expression varies. This marker is useful in classifying B cell malignancies

Other markers including CD21, 19, 11, 13, 14 are used in classification of myeloid and lymphoid malignancies.

morphologically identical may be functionally very different.

Many techniques are now available to detect cell membrane molecules which indicate the stage of differentiation and activation of lymphocytes, macrophages and other cells, and thus allow subdivision of the main morphological categories. Formerly called T1, T3, etc., they have been renamed CD1, CD3, etc (CD = cluster of differentiation) (Table 2.1). Identification of CD and other surface markers on lymphocytes is valuable in clinical diagnosis (e.g. of immunodeficiency syndromes) and in the classification of lymphomas, as well as in research.

CD testing is usually done with monoclonal antibodies, and new determinants and antibodies are described each year. However, there remain some functionally distinct groups of cells and, so far, no antibody can distinguish between them, for example T suppressor and T cytotoxic cells, which can only be identified by their functional characteristics.

Antigen presenting cells

These are found mainly in the lymphoid organs and the skin, and their main role is to present antigen in a particular way to lymphocytes so as to start off the antigen specific immune responses. They include interdigitating cells in the thymus, the Langerhans cells of the skin, veiled cells in afferent lymph, interdigitating cells in the T areas of lymph nodes, and follicular dendritic cells in B areas of lymph nodes. Some macro-

CELLS INVOLVED IN IMMUNITY

A wide range of cells participate in nonspecific and specific immunity, and many of these, such as macrophages and T cells, fulfil several different functions.

Identification of cell types

There are characteristic cytological features of the various cells, but it must be appreciated that, particularly within the population of lymphocytes, cells which appear

Table 2.2   Functional classification of T cells

Cell type	Abbreviation	Marker	Properties
Immunoregulatory			
Helper	T_H	CD4	Recognise antigen in association with Class 2 HLA; provide help signals for B cells (e.g. IL-4)
Suppressor	T_S	CD8	Recognise antigen in association with Class 1 HLA; precise mode of suppression unknown
Effector			
Cytotoxic	T_C	CD8	Recognise antigen in association with Class 1 HLA; this is potentially on the surface of any nucleated cell
Mediators of delayed hypersensitivity	T_{DTH}	CD4	Recognise antigen in association with Class 2 HLA; this antigen usually will have been processed in endosomes and then presented at the surface of an antigen presenting cell. Since the tissue distribution of Class 2 is restricted, only in special circumstances are T_{DTH} cells provided with activation signals by other cells

phages probably also act as antigen presenting cells and other non-immune cells, including epithelial cells, can also perform this function.

T lymphocytes

The majority of normal human blood and recirculating T cells are small lymphocytes with a high nuclear to cytoplasmic ratio. They are derived from precursor stem cells of the bone marrow, which have matured under the influence of a hormone or factor produced by the epithelial cells of the thymus.

T cells perform important immunoregulatory functions via their secreted products, and also act as effector cells, capable of killing other cells (Table 2.2). Given appropriate stimulation they proliferate and differentiate into a range of subsets with differing functions—immunoregulatory helper (T_H), suppressor (T_S); and effector cytotoxic (T_C), capable of cell killing, and the T cells that mediate delayed-type hypersensitivity reactions (T_{DTH}), by virtue of the properties of lymphokines which they secrete. The lymphokines produce local inflammation, and attract and then activate macrophages.

Many immunological diseases, both immunodeficiency and abnormally enhanced reactivity, can ultimately be attributed to defects of T cell regulatory function. In terms of protective immunity, T cells are particularly important in defence against intracellular bacterial and protozoal pathogens, viruses and fungi.

B lymphocytes

B lymphocytes are independent of the thymus and in man probably complete their early maturation within the bone marrow. They are called B cells because they mature within the Bursa of Fabricius in birds.

When appropriately stimulated, B lymphocytes undergo proliferation, maturation and differentiation to form plasma cells, responsible for the synthesis of antibodies (immunoglobulins) in their abundant endoplasmic reticulum. Eventually there are many identical

daughters derived from a single B cell, forming a clone. The enormous diversity of antibodies which an individual can produce is explained partly by rearrangements of nucleic acid within precursor B cells and partly by random mutation.

Neutrophil polymorphs

Polymorphonuclear granulocytes are derived from haemopoietic stem cells in the bone marrow. They are short-lived cells, with a diameter of c. 5.5 μm (Fig. 2.2), are normally concentrated in the bloodstream, but can respond to chemotactic signals in the presence of tissue injury or infection. Neutrophils contain a wide variety of agents which aid their emigration to the inflamed site and promote bacterial killing (see information box). They marginate in the capillaries and move into the tissues where they can phagocytose and kill bacteria or other foreign materials which are adherent to their surface. Although they are intrinsically capable of these functions the properties of polymorphs are made much more efficient if the bacterium is coated with antibody and/or complement, and they are also influenced by a variety of cytokines released by other lymphocytes and other cells.

The importance of polymorphs is emphasised by the greatly increased susceptibility to infection found in patients with neutropenia.

Macrophages

Macrophages are derived from bone marrow precursors which differentiate to blood monocytes and finally settle in the tissues as mature, mononuclear phagocytes. Many organs contain characteristic populations of the phagocytic series, e.g. lung alveolar macrophages, liver Kupffer cells, resident and recirculating macrophages in lymph nodes, brain microglial cells, and kidney mesangial cells. Macrophages, like polymorphs, are capable of phagocytosis and killing of micro-organisms. They also secrete a number of important cytokines and are influenced

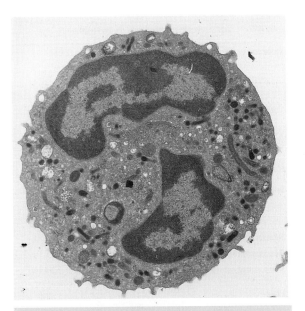

Fig. 2.2 The neutrophil granulocyte. Electron micrograph demonstrating the multi-lobed nucleus and cytoplasmic granules.

SOME RECEPTORS ON AND MOLECULES BINDING TO MACROPHAGES

- **Complement components**
  C1q, C3b, C3bi, C3d, C5a
- **Immunoglobulins**
  IgG, IgA, IgE
- **Growth factors and cytokines**
  IFN-α/β, IFNα, CSF-1, GMCSF, TNF-α
  IL-1, IL-2, IL-3, IL-4, IL-6
- **Adhesion molecules**
  e.g. LFA-1, ICAM-1
- **Phagocytic receptors**
  e.g. CR-1, CR-3, FcR
- **Glycoproteins and carbohydrates**
  e.g. mannose-6-phosphage
- **Proteins**
  e.g. fibronectin, fibrin
- **Hormones**
  e.g. calcitonin, insulin, parathormone
- **Peptides and small molecules**
  e.g. bradykinin, serotonin, substance P
- **Lipids and lipoproteins**
  Leucotrienes C, D$_4$, B$_4$, E$_2$;
  LDL; β VLDL; Modified LDL

CONSTITUENTS OF HUMAN NEUTROPHIL GRANULES

	Azurophil granules	Specific granules
• **Microbicidal enzymes**	lysozyme myeloperoxidase	lysozyme
• **Neutral proteinases**	elastase collagenases cathepsin G	collagenase
• **Acid hydrolases**	phosphatases lipases sulphatases histonase cathepsin D β glycerophosphatase esterase neuraminidase 5′nucleotidase	phosphatases
• **Others**	bactericidal/ permeability inducing protein defensins cationic proteins glycosaminoglycans chondroitin sulphate heparin sulphate	lactoferrin Vit B$_{12}$ binding protein C3bi receptor cytochrome B flavoproteins

by, and themselves influence, T lymphocytes and other important cells (see information boxes and Table 2.3).

Aggregates of macrophages, granulomas, are characteristic of many chronic infectious and idiopathic inflammatory diseases such as tuberculosis, leprosy, sarcoidosis and Crohn's disease.

Natural killer cells

Natural killer (NK) cells are large granular cells, morphologically quite similar to lymphocytes. They are thought to be important in resistance to virus infections and probably also malignancy. When a cell becomes infected by a virus or transforms into a cancerous cell its surface molecules are altered. These alterations can sometimes be recognised by NK cells which engage the infected or altered cell and kill it. NK cells bear receptors which recognise high molecular weight glycoproteins on the surface of virally infected cells, at an early stage before the virus has had a chance to reproduce. They are activated by interferons (produced by virally infected cells and sometimes by other cells such as T lymphocytes). When activated they release their granule contents into the space between the target and NK cell (Fig. 2.3), including a molecule called perforin which acts, as its name implies, by producing a hole in the cell membrane of the target cell leading to cell death.

NK cells also have receptors for immunoglobulin and thus have enhanced cell killing activity in the presence of specific antibody to virus. The antibody links host and target cell closely (Fig. 2.3). This phenomenon is called antibody dependent cell mediated cytotoxicity (ADCC), and is not confined to NK cells but can be performed by polymorphs and macrophages.

MAIN FUNCTIONS OF MACROPHAGES

- **Secretory functions** Monocytes and macrophages secrete around 100 substances whose actions range from induction of cell growth to cell death. Furthermore, single factors, such as IL-1 and tumour necrosis factor (TNF), can have many different actions.
- **Acute phase response** This is a systemic inflammatory reaction to an infection or injury comprising fever, tachycardia, shock, changes in the serum concentration of proteins such as C reactive protein and fibrinogen. IL-1, TNF and IL-6 mediate these effects.
- **Regulation of haemopoiesis** Peripheral blood leucocytes are influenced indirectly via the effects of IL-1 and TNF on T cells, and directly via factors such as macrophage colony stimulating factor which induces a peripheral blood leucocytosis.
- **Haemostasis** The host response to injury may activate the coagulation system which occasionally results in disseminated intravascular coagulation. In response to stimuli such as bacterial endotoxin and immune complexes, cells of the mononuclear phagocyte system synthesise thromboplastin, a potent activator of the coagulation pathway.
- **Lymphocyte activation** Mononuclear phagocytes are central to induction of the immune response via antigen presentation.
- **Killing of micro-organisms** Mononuclear phagocytes can migrate to and stay in the vicinity of a focus of infection and phagocytose the agents concerned. Mechanisms by which micro-organisms are recognised are ill understood. Organisms are killed by oxygen-dependent and oxygen-independent mechanisms.
- **Killing of tumour cells** Lysis of tumour cells by monocytes and macrophages is probably one of the main mechanisms of host defence against tumours, for example via TNF and gamma interferon.
- **Tissue repair and remodelling** These important functions are produced by collagenase, elastase, and substances that induce fibroblast proliferation and osteoclast bone resorption.

Eosinophils

Eosinophils are granulated blood leucocytes which can migrate into the tissues (see Fig. 2.4). They appear to be metabolically very active and among their granule mediators are the toxic protein eosinophilic major basic protein, and the anti-inflammatory histaminases and other substances which inactivate mast cell products. They are attracted by factors released by T cells, mast cells and basophils, for example eosinophilic chemotactic factor of anaphylaxis. Eosinophils have probably evolved to aid human host defences against parasites such as *Schistosoma* and worms, but they are also implicated in allergic disease such as asthma.

Their presence in the tissues, and a high count of eosinophils in the blood (eosinophilia), is therefore often a marker of allergic disease or parasitic infection.

Table 2.3 Some secretory products of macrophages

Cytokines and growth factors	IFN-$\alpha/\beta/\gamma$, IL-1, IL-6, TNF-α IL-8, gro α, MCP-1 TGFβ, PDGF, FGF, IGF, GM-CSF, G-CSF Erythropoietin, lactoferrin
Enzymes	Elastase, collagenase, lysozyme Phospholipase A$_2$, amylase Hyaluronidase, acid hydrolases β galactosidase, β-glucuronidase Nucleases, ribonucleases, acid phosphatases Sulphatases, cathepsins
Enzyme inhibitors	α_1-antiproteinase, α_2 macroglobulin Lipomodulin, α_1-antichymotrypsin Inhibitors of plasminogen and plasminogen activator
Reactive oxygen intermediates	O$_2^-$, H$_2$O$_2$, OH, Hypohalous Acid
Reactive nitrogen intermediates	NO, NO$_2$, NO$_3$
Complement components, etc.	C$_1$, C$_4$, C$_2$, C$_3$, C$_5$, Factor B, Factor D, properdin
Lipids	Leukotrienes B, C, D and E, PGE, PGF$_{2\alpha}$ PAF, prostacyclin, thromboxane A$_2$
Matrix proteins	Fibronectin, thrombospondin, proteoglycans
Coagulation factors	Factor X, factor IX, factor V, factor VII, tissue factor, prothrombin, thromboplastin

The mast cell series

These cells are bone marrow-derived and have cytoplasmic granules with particular basophilic staining characteristics. The granules contain many inflammatory and chemotactic mediators. There are several cells of this series including the basophil, the connective tissue type mast cell and mucosal mast cells. All have receptors for IgE and are degranulated when an allergen cross links two specific IgE molecules bound to the surface of the cell. Mast cells and basophils are involved in parasite immunity and IgE-mediated allergic diseases; they also participate in delayed-type hypersensitivity reactions.

MOLECULES OF THE IMMUNE SYSTEM

IMMUNOGLOBULINS

Immunoglobulin (Ig) molecules are the effector products of B cells and although they all have a broadly similar structure, minor differences within the main immunological classes (IgG, IgM, IgA, IgD and IgE) and subclasses (IgG 1, 2, 3 and 4; IgA 1 and 2) are associated with a range of important biological properties (Table 2.4). Molecules almost identical to secreted

NK Killing

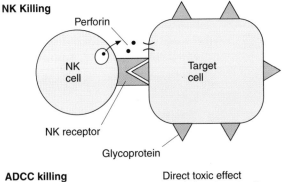

ADCC killing

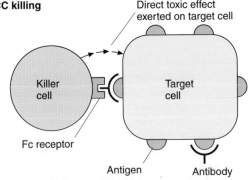

$\ddagger$ = site of cell membrane damage caused by perforin

NK = natural killer

Killer cell = may be neutrophil, monocyte or NK cell

Fc receptor = receptor for constant region of heavy chain of immunoglobulin molecule

Fig. 2.3   Direct mechanisms of cell killing. NK cells have receptors which recognise a cell membrane glycoprotein on the target cell and toxic molecules are secreted in close proximity to the target cell. In antibody-dependent cellular cytotoxicity (ADCC), a variety of types of cell can act as killer cells. They are attached to the target cell by immunoglobulin molecules. Specific antibody combines with antigen on the surface of the target cell, and the heavy chains of the immunoglobulin molecules concerned link to Fc receptors as shown.

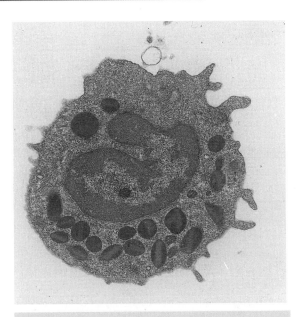

Fig. 2.4   The human eosinophil granulocyte: electron micrograph illustrating the characteristic angular granules.

immunoglobulins are incorporated in the cell membranes of B cells (surface Ig), and there are many related molecules concerned with antigen recognition and cell-cell communication.

Structure of immunoglobulin molecules

An immunoglobulin molecule is made up of distinct sub-units held together by disulphide (S-S) bonds, which can be broken by reducing agents, so that the molecule falls apart into pairs of polypeptide chains called light and heavy chains. Two types of light chain exist, kappa and lambda, of which individual immu-

noglobulin molecules have only one type, and there are several different heavy chains which confer on the Ig molecule its class-specific properties.

A typical immunoglobulin molecule such as IgG (Fig. 2.5) has two antigen-binding regions (Fab) and one Fc component which is the part of the molecule which performs the class-related functions such as complement fixation. The section of the heavy chain contained in the Fc component is responsible for the antigenic differences between the classes of immunoglobulin which enable their laboratory measurement by the use of heavy-chain-specific antisera.

The molecular basis of diversity of antigen-binding function (i.e. antibody activity) resides in the so-called variable regions of the Fab components. The antigen-combining site of an immunoglobulin molecule (the idiotype) can itself be recognised and reacted to by other immunocompetent cells, with the production of anti-idiotype antibodies which can influence the magnitude and duration of antibody production to a given antigen.

Immunoglobulin G (IgG)

In healthy adults, IgG accounts for more than 70% of the immunoglobulins in normal serum and is distributed equally between the blood and extracellular fluids. About a quarter of all the body's IgG passes out of the bloodstream each day and the same amount returns via the thoracic duct. In man, IgG is the only immunoglobulin that is transported across the placenta to reach

Table 2.4   Properties of immunoglobulins

	Sedimentation coefficient	Number of basic 4 chain units	Approximate range of concentration in normal serum	Other properties	Subclasses
IgG	7S	1	8–16 g/l	Complement fixing activity (IgG1, G3), placental transfer	IgG1, IgG2, IgG3, IgG4
IgA	7S, 10S, 11S	1 or 2	1.5–4 g/l	Present in external secretions	IgA1, IgA2
IgM	19S	5	0.5–2 g/l	Complement fixing activity, small amounts in external secretions	
IgD	7S	1	0.003–0.04 g/l		
IgE	8S	1	17–450 ng/ml	Binds to mast cells and basophils	

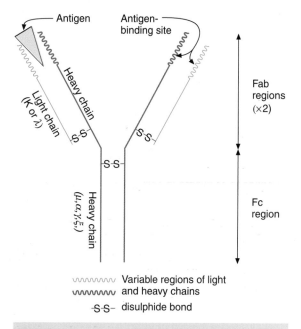

Fig. 2.5   The typical structure of an immunoglobulin molecule, illustrating the two heavy and two light chains linked by disulphide bonds; the antigen-binding sites comprise variable regions of light and heavy chains; the Fc region possesses isotype specific properties such as complement binding and the capacity to attach to mast cells.

the fetus and provide the newborn baby with passively acquired antibody during its early life.

IgG antibodies are very important in anti-bacterial immunity. They readily neutralise soluble toxins such as those responsible for many of the clinical manifestations of diphtheria or tetanus. IgG also has an opsonic effect on bacteria, coating them so that their ingestion by phagocytes is facilitated. IgG antibodies also can produce disease, e.g. by forming immune complexes, or as autoantibodies.

Immunoglobulin M (IgM)

The macro-molecular IgM is predominantly intra-vascular. It is made up of five immunoglobulin units linked with disulphide bonds to provide ten identical antigen-combining-sites, together with a J (joining) chain. IgM is especially effective in activating complement to produce immune lysis of foreign cells. IgM antibodies are also much more efficient than IgG antibodies in linking particulate antigens together for agglutination and phagocytosis, and would seem to be specially adapted for dealing with cell debris or bacteria in the bloodstream.

Immunoglobulin A (IgA)

IgA accounts for about 20% of the total serum immunoglobulins. However its function, if any, within the bloodstream and tissues is thought to be much less important than its role as a secretory antibody. The major sites of IgA synthesis are the laminae propriae underlying the respiratory tract, the gut and other mucosae. IgA is found in three main molecular forms (Fig. 2.6). In blood it is 7S, monomeric, similar in size to IgG. Dimeric 10S IgA (also containing J chain) is produced by plasma cells in the mucosae and is transported across epithelia into colostrum, saliva, intestinal juice, respiratory secretions, tears and several other body fluids. During trans-epithelial transport, another polypeptide, secretory component, is incorporated to form secretory 11S IgA, relatively resistant to digestive enzymes.

Secretory IgA confers immunity to infection by enteric bacterial and viral pathogens, and may also be involved in the regulation of the commensal gut flora. Oral immunisation is now being used to try to induce protective immunity to intestinal infections such as cholera and rotavirus.

Immunoglobulin D (IgD)

IgD is almost exclusively found on the surface of immature B lymphocytes and may be involved in their maturation and regulation.

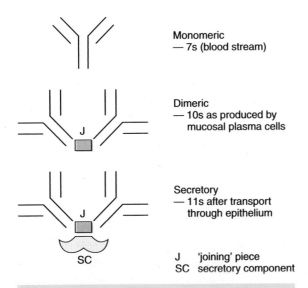

Monomeric
— 7s (blood stream)

Dimeric
— 10s as produced by
mucosal plasma cells

Secretory
— 11s after transport
through epithelium

J   'joining' piece
SC secretory component

Fig. 2.6   Forms of IgA which are present in man. J chain is synthesised by plasma cells. 10S IgA attaches to secretory component on the basolateral membrane of epithelial cells. The composite molecule is then internalised and finally expelled at the luminal surface as secretory 11S IgA, containing four light chains, four heavy chains, J chain and secretory component.

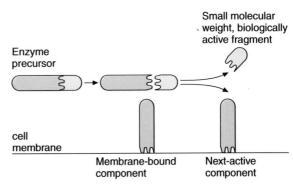

Fig. 2.7   Principles of the complement cascade. An active molecule (produced by an earlier part of the cascade and already fixed to the cell membrane) acts on an enzyme precursor breaking it into a large component which adheres to the cell membrane and is now active, and a low molecular weight fragment released into the extracellular fluid, which may have any of a variety of biological activities.

Immunoglobulin E (IgE)

IgE concentration in serum is very low. This is in part because it has a considerable affinity for cell surfaces and binds firmly to mast cells and basophils. IgE antibodies are necessary for immediate hypersensitivity reactions, such as occur in atopic individuals, e.g. in hay fever. The physiological function of IgE antibodies is obscure but appears to be important in defence against helminth parasites (worms).

COMPLEMENT

The complement system is an amplifying cascade similar to those responsible for blood clotting and fibrinolysis. Activation of this effector mechanism can be produced *either* as part of an antibody-mediated immune response (the classical pathway) *or* by bacterial or other chemical stimuli (the alternative pathway). Both of these lead to a final common sequence of events which culminates in the production of the 'membrane attack complex', in which tubules are formed which traverse the cell membrane and thus lead to cell lysis.

Complement components

There is an agreed nomenclature for the many components, e.g. C2, C3, but they do not act in the same sequence as their identification numbers. A full account of complement will be found in any textbook of immu-

nology, and this description concentrates on the general principles of the reactions and their clinical significance. Most complement components are proteins (beta globulins) made in the liver, and have proteinase activity when activated. Inhibitors are also involved at various points in the cascades and feedback loops.

Sequence of events in complement activation

Complement is usually associated with a membrane or immune complex and there is sequential activation of complement enzymes (Fig. 2.7). By virtue of its membrane effects and release of active peptides, the complement system fulfils a number of functions, including cell activation, cell lysis, inflammation and opsonisation.

An outline of the important stages of complement activation is shown in Figure 2.8. The activation of C3 by the enzyme C3 convertase is the central event of the complement sequence. The classical pathway is triggered when immune complexes combine with C1q. In the alternative pathway, a C3 convertase is generated by a process that starts with activation of complement components by materials such as bacterial cell walls and endotoxin. The alternative pathway may therefore be particularly relevant before a primary immune response has been mounted.

Biological activities and control

Some of the important biological activities of complement are listed in Table 2.5. Clinically, if the complement sequence is involved in disease, C3 may be used up in large amounts and so the finding of low blood levels of this protein is of some diagnostic value.

The complement pathway is controlled by two mechanisms. First, a number of the activated components are

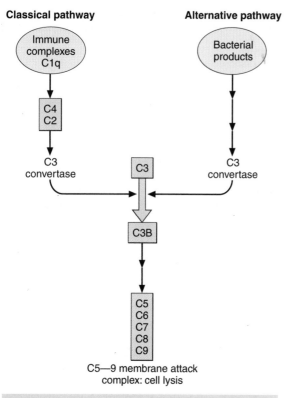

Classical pathway

Alternative pathway

C5—9 membrane attack complex: cell lysis

Fig. 2.8 Diagrammatic illustration of complement and its components. The conversion of C3 to C3B is central, and the final result is produced when the membrane attack complex causes tiny holes to appear in the cell membrane and cell death ensues.

Table 2.5 Important biologically active molecules generated during complement activation

Component	Effect
C3a	Smooth muscle contraction Vascular permeability increased Eosinophil, basophil and mast cell degranulation Platelet aggregation
C3b	Opsonisation and phagocytosis
C4a	Smooth muscle contraction Vascular permeability increased
C5a	Smooth muscle contraction Vascular permeability increased Eosinophil, basophil and mast cell degranulation Platelet aggregation Polymorph and monocyte chemotaxis Neutrophil hydrolytic enzymes released
C5a-des-arg	Neutrophil chemotaxis and hydrolytic enzymes released

able to present antigen to T cells: stimulation of T cells simultaneously with processed antigen and IL-1 is required for initiation of a specific immune response. IL-1-producing cells include circulating monocytes, macrophages, fibroblasts, B cells and epithelial cells.

Interleukin 2 (IL-2)

IL-2 is secreted by activated T cells and is responsible for amplification of the population of responding T cells and for inducing the production of other cytokines from many cell types.

inherently unstable; if the next protein in the cascade is not immediately available, the active substance decays. Secondly, there are a number of specific inhibitors, e.g. C1 inhibitor.

CYTOKINES

In the late 1960s it was recognised that lymphocyte-mediated effects were sometimes produced by soluble factors. Many such factors were described and various tests of antigen-specific cell-mediated immunity were developed, based on the presumed secretion of these factors by T cells. Now many secreted products of T and other cells have been studied in great detail, their biochemical nature is known, and even their genes have been cloned. It has become clear that many of the properties of lymphokine are possessed by only a few molecules. The main sources and targets of some well-characterised cytokines are shown in Table 2.6.

Interleukin 1 (IL-1)

IL-1 is secreted by many cell types in the presence of antigen or tissue injury. Cells that produce IL-1 are also

Table 2.6 Actions of some cytokines

Cytokine	Major source	Principal actions
IL-1	Activated macrophages and other APC	IL-1 plus antigen stimulates proliferation of antigen-specific T cells, leading to secretion of IL-2
IL-2	Activated T cell	Amplifies T cell proliferation and production of other cytokines
IL-3	Activated T cells	Stimulates proliferation of haemopoietic stem cells
IL-4	Activated T cells	Stimulates proliferation of B cells and promotes Ig isotype switch
IL-5 and IL-6	Activated T cells	Stimulate proliferation and differentiation of B cells to antibody-producing plasma cells
IFN-γ	Activated T cells	Activates macrophages and neutrophils to increase their phagocytic and bacteriocidal activity
TNF-α	Activated macrophages	Cytotoxic to bacteria and tumour cells, but also to normal tissue (but has short half-life).

Tumour necrosis factor-alpha (TNF-α)

This cytokine was so named because of its observed cytotoxicity to tumour cells. It is produced by mononuclear phagocytes in vitro when they are stimulated with bacterial endotoxin. Also known as cachectin, TNF-α has profound effects on general cellular metabolism; it causes weight loss, fever, acute phase reaction (associated with infection or tumour formation). It activates other mononuclear cells and granulocytes and increases their nonspecific killing capability.

Interferon-gamma (IFN-γ)

This is produced mainly by activated T cells following exposure to antigens or mitogens. However, it can also be secreted by activated macrophages and NK cells. It increases class II expression on epithelial cells (among other cell and tissue types). This leads to increased antigen presenting activity. It also activates macrophages for anti-tumour activity, in synergy with TNF-α.

Interleukin 8 (IL-8)

This is a member of the family of small peptides which are called chemokines. Most of these small peptides are highly chemotactic for inflammatory cells. IL-8 is emerging as an extremely important neutrophil chemotactic agent in vivo.

THE MAJOR HISTOCOMPATIBILITY COMPLEX

Although the major histocompatibility complex (MHC) was originally identified by its role in transplant rejection, it is now recognised that proteins encoded by this region of the genome are involved in many aspects of immunological recognition. These include interactions between different lymphoid cells as well as between lymphocytes and antigen presenting cells.

The MHC gene cluster is located on chromosome 6 (Fig. 2.9). It contains genes coding for the 'Human Leucocyte Antigens' (HLA), cell surface glycoproteins which are found on many cells, not only leucocytes. It also contains the genes for some important complement proteins. An individual inherits one HLA haplotype from each parent and since there are several gene loci, and a large number of different specificities at each locus, this makes for a very large number of HLA genotypes within a population.

Of the MHC encoded proteins, Class 1 antigens HLA-A and HLA-B are present on all nucleated cells and platelets. They comprise one peptide chain encoded by the MHC associated with a different polypeptide, beta-2 microglobulin, encoded elsewhere in the genome. Class 2 antigens, the HLA-D series, have more limited tissue distribution, including B lymphocytes, macrophages and activated T cells.

There are several important clinical applications of knowledge of the MHC.

ANTIGEN RECOGNITION BY T CELLS

Immunoglobulin (antibody) molecules recognise the general contour of an antigenic determinant. The T cell antigen receptor, a small chain related to the immunoglobulin family, can only 'see' its particular antigen when that antigen is held at the surface of another cell in close relationship to HLA. T cytotoxic cells only recognise antigens (such as a virus) in association with HLA class 1 molecules on the surface of a cell. It is as if HLA is a signpost, guiding the T cytotoxic cell to its target. On the other hand, T helper cells recognise antigen on macrophages and B cells (antigen presenting cells) in association with the HLA-D, class 2 antigens. This antigen will usually have been previously internalised and 'processed' by the antigen presenting cell.

DISEASES ASSOCIATED WITH HLA

There are a number of diseases associated with particular HLA types (Table 2.7). This may partly relate to

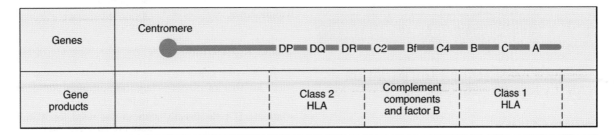

Fig. 2.9 Structure of the major histocompatibility complex on chromosome 6. HLA = human leucocyte antigens.

Table 2.7   Diseases associated with particular HLA antigens

B27	Ankylosing spondylitis
	Reiter's syndrome
B8,DR3	Addison's disease
	Thyrotoxicosis
	Myasthenia gravis
	Coeliac disease
B8, DR3, DR4	Insulin dependent diabetes mellitus
DR2	Multiple sclerosis
A3	Haemochromatosis
B13	Psoriasis

the linkage of 'immune response genes' with certain HLA genes, or to similar antigenicity of an infectious agent and the HLA gene product. Occasionally HLA status appears to be protective rather than associated with an increased frequency of a disease. These associations are of great interest scientifically but rarely of value in clinical practice.

TISSUE TYPING AND TRANSPLANTATION

In unrelated individuals, matching for HLA between donor and host improves transplant survival for some organs (e.g. kidney) but not others (e.g. liver). Tissue type details of patients awaiting transplants are collected nationally, and in difficult cases even internationally, to enable matching with suitable donors. HLA typing is also important (along with blood grouping) in the selection of live donors, e.g. of kidney or bone marrow.

FURTHER READING

Gordon S et al 1992 Macrophages in tissues and in vitro. Current Opinion in Immunology 4: 25–32
Haslett C 1993 The neutrophil. In: Holgate S T, Church M, Allergy illustrated. Gower Publications, London
MacLennan I C M 1994 Germinal centres. Annual Review of Immunology 12: 141–181
Swain S, Rest M (eds) 1994 Lymphocyte activation and effector functions. Current Opinion in Immunology 6: 355–514
Weller P 1994 Eosinophils: structure and functions. Current Opinion in Immunology 6: 85–91

IMMUNE RESPONSES AND INFLAMMATION

ANTIGEN PRESENTATION AND INITIATION OF THE IMMUNE RESPONSE

Antigen distribution

Antigen which has penetrated the tissues reaches the draining lymph nodes. If it arrives via the respiratory tract or the gut it concentrates in the organised tissues of the mucosa-associated lymphoid tissues. Antigen from the bloodstream is removed in the spleen. All of these above routes lead to the induction of a specific immune response, usually active immunity but occasionally immunological tolerance. On the other hand particulate antigen is removed from the bloodstream without induction of immunity by some macrophages in the liver and lung.

Antigen presentation

Macrophages which have phagocytosed antigen digest and process it, express it on their surface and signal B cells for activation. Antigen complexed with MHC products can switch on T cells.

The fact that T cells require antigen to be presented to them along with MHC class 1 or class 2 antigens on the surface of an antigen presenting cell means that T cells ignore antigens in the free state and are not swamped by them, for example by virus or bacteria in the bloodstream.

Antigen presenting cells in different sites appear to have slightly different properties so that the Langerhans cells of the skin seem particularly adapted towards induction of delayed type hypersensitivity. In lymph nodes, follicular dendritic cells collect antigen-antibody complexes on their surface and readily stimulate B cells whereas the T cell area dendritic cells process antigen, although without internalising it, and present it in a form readily seen by T cells at the dendritic cell surface membrane.

T CELL ACTIVATION

Activation of T helper cells (Fig. 2.10) requires two signals, antigen and IL-1. When both of these signals are received there is RNA and protein synthesis, including production of the important protein IL-2. The cell moves from G0 to G1 of the mitotic cycle.

As well as synthesis of IL-2 the activated T blast cell also expresses surface receptors for IL-2. This positive feedback loop leads to a burst of proliferative activity of cells, and they secrete a wide variety of biologically active lymphokines.

B CELL ACTIVATION

Activation of B cells can occur in two ways. There are a small number of physico-chemically unusual antigens (for example pneumococcus polysaccharide) which can stimulate B cells directly without the need for T cell involvement. Such thymus-independent antigens usually induce an IgM response with little or no memory.

Most antigens are thymus dependent. Events which

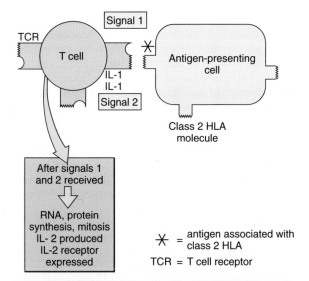

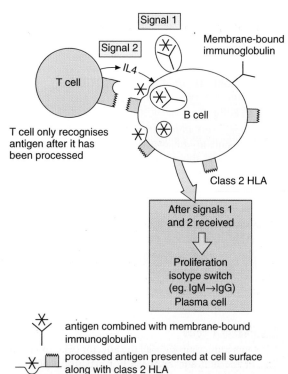

Fig. 2.10 Signals necessary for T helper cell activation.
Signal 1 is provided by the combination of antigen and Class 2 HLA on the surface of an antigen-presenting cell. Signal 2 is IL-1 which will have been released in the vicinity of the T cell by macrophages.

Fig. 2.11 B cell activation. The first signal is the simple combination of antigen with membrane-bound immunoglobulin on the surface of the B cell. The second signal requires a fairly complex series of events. Antigen is internalised by the B cell, processed and re-presented at the cell surface together with Class 2 HLA. The T cells recognise this processed antigen, and secrete a stimulatory interleukin which acts as the second signal for B cell activation.

eventually lead to antibody production by B cells require messages to be delivered by the antigen both directly to a B cell and, after intracellular processing, to a T cell (Fig. 2.11). This explains why the antigenic determinant to which antibody is being produced is not necessarily the same as the antigenic determinant recognised by T cells (in the so called hapten-carrier system). Both these determinants must be present on the same molecule for T help to be given to B cells.

B cell activation also requires two signals: first the binding of an antigenic determinant to the B cell receptor; secondly, an activating signal produced by the T cell, probably the B cell stimulatory factor IL-4, since this is capable of bringing resting B cells to the activated G1 state. Once activated the stimulated B cell acquires a number of new surface receptors for growth factors and continues to proliferate and mature. The newly active B cells express surface receptors for IL-4. Further clonal expansion of B cells is engineered by a second B cell growth factor, and other lymphokines may be synergistic.

Other signals then lead to the generation of memory B cells, final differentiation of the B cells into IgM-producing plasma cells, and also switching of the immunoglobulin produced by the stimulated cells from IgM to IgG, IgA or IgE (class switch). This is achieved by transfer of a particular gene segment for the variable segment of the heavy chain, to an alternative constant region gene so that the antibodies produced are of exactly the same specificity but of a different class.

Class switch of antibody is relevant in several clinical situations. At the first encounter with an antigen (e.g. an injected vaccine) the IgM response predominates at first, with the level of serum IgG antibody rising after 2–3 weeks. In secondary and subsequent immune responses, re-exposure to the same antigen results in a brief and transient IgM response, with rapid rise of IgG antibody, to much higher titres than in the primary response. Another application is in the serological diagnosis of infections, such as rubella. The presence of specific IgM antibody suggests recent infection, whereas antibody of the IgG class indicates only that the antigen has been encountered at some time in the past.

REGULATION OF IMMUNE RESPONSES

It is inappropriate for a specific immune response to progress and expand indefinitely, and so there have evolved several immunological factors which inhibit rather than potentiate specific immunity.

MECHANISMS OF IMMUNOREGULATION

Loss of antigen

Antigen is a very important drive to B and T cell proliferation and as the concentration of antigen in the body drops so the intensity of the drive falls off in parallel.

Presence of antibody

Antibody itself exerts negative feedback control, partly by simply neutralising the available antigen but also probably by other mechanisms. An important clinical example of this is the administration of anti-D immunoglobulin to mothers who are at risk of rhesus immunisation.

Suppressor T cells

T helpers induce virtually all the effector cells and products of the immune response but expansion of the T helpers is accompanied by the appearance of a subgroup of CD4 cells, suppressor inducer cells. These then act on a different T cell subset, the CD8 cells which actually perform the function of suppression. Although the biological activity of suppressor cells is well recognised, their cellular and molecular biology are less well studied than for helper cells. Some antigenic determinants much more readily evoke suppressor T cell responses than active immunity. If such determinants could be identified (for example in relation to allergic and hypersensitivity diseases) such diseases could be cured by the deliberate evoking of suppressive responses.

Idiotype networks

Idiotype networks may be involved in immune regulation at many stages. The principle of these is simple. It has already been explained that the antibodies produced by a clone of B cells, unique to a particular antigenic determinant, will all share the same antigen-combining site. This, composed partly of the variable regions of the light and heavy immunoglobulin chains, is called an idiotype. Since the idiotype is a protein it can itself, of course, act as an antigen and antibodies to this are called anti-idiotypes.

The antigen-combining site of the anti-idiotype antibody is often almost exactly the same in contours and other properties as the antigenic determinant originally involved. Thus anti-idiotypes have been used instead of antigen in some experimental work. One theory as to how a newborn infant can have specific antibody in cord blood (including IgE antibody) is that the stimulus is in fact IgG anti-idiotype antibody which has crossed the placenta, rather than the antigen itself.

The Fab part of an anti-idiotype molecule can itself be the target of specific antibodies, anti-anti-idiotype, and so the network continues. This may contribute to the complex immunodeficiency of old age, immunosenescence.

Anti-idiotype specificity is also expressed on T helper and suppressor cells as well as in the form of specific antibody, and can interfere and modulate what started off as an originally simple immune response to a particular antigen.

IMMUNOLOGICAL TOLERANCE

The clinical relevance of regulation of immunity is enormous. The phenomenon of tolerance, specific down-regulation of the capacity to mount an immune response to a particular antigen, has been well recognised for years. For example, potential antigens which reach the lymphoid cells of the fetus, during their immunological development, specifically suppress any future response to that antigen when the individual is immunologically mature. This is a means whereby unresponsiveness develops to the body's own constituents (self) and enables the lymphoid cells to distinguish potentially harmful non-self. Thus, immunological tolerance is what protects us against overwhelming auto (anti-self) immunity.

A state of tolerance can sometimes be induced in adult life by giving particularly large or small doses of antigen, or chemically modified antigen. Additionally, antigens which are normally encountered via the gut usually induce a state of oral tolerance. Thus food allergic diseases such as coeliac disease can be envisaged as due to a breakdown in the physiological down-regulation of immunity to dietary and other gut antigens.

Successful transplantation requires the induction of tolerance, or at least the suppression of active immunity, to the transplanted organ.

INITIATION OF THE INFLAMMATORY RESPONSE

When there is infection, injury, nonspecific inflammation or a specific immune reaction, migration of phagocytic cells and lymphocytes from the circulation into the affected tissues is central to the development of an inflammatory response.

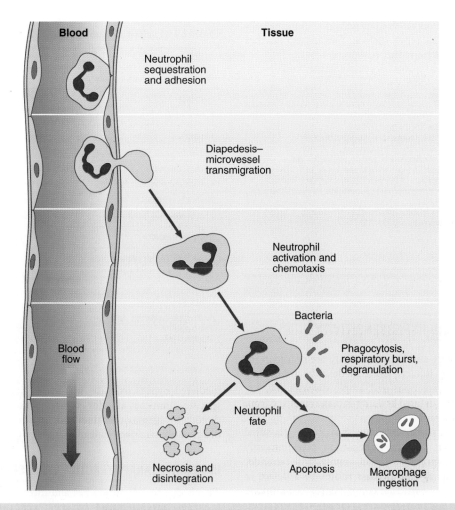

Fig. 2.12 Behaviour of the neutrophil in inflammation: the emigration of neutrophils from microvessels to the inflamed site.

Adhesion

Cells passing through the blood vessels adhere to the endothelium by the actions of inter-cellular adhesion molecules (ICAMs) of various types (e.g. selectins, integrins, addressins), which cause the leucocyte to attach to the endothelium. The density of these molecules on the leucocyte surface is higher than normal when the cells are activated, and local tissue signals such as cytokines increase the expression of the matching adhesion molecules by endothelial cells.

Transmigration

Cells move out of the bloodstream either through or between the endothelial cells.

Directed movement

Under the influence of chemotactic stimuli (such as complement components, leucotrienes, bacterial peptides, cytokines), cells move towards the site of inflammation and are retained there instead of returning into the circulation.

Local activation

With the increase in blood flow and vascular permeability, there is also accumulation of antibodies, complement components and other plasma-derived molecules. These, along with antigen, further stimulate the polymorphonuclear leucocytes, monocytes, macrophages and lymphocytes. Inflammatory and immunoregulatory mediators released by activated immune cells (and by other cell types such as fibroblasts), further potentiate the inflammatory reaction.

FURTHER READING

Bauman H, Gauldie J 1994 The acute phase response. Immunology Today 15: 74–81
Bevilacqua M P 1993 Endothelial-leukocyte adhesion molecules. Annual Review of Immunology: 767–805
Downey G P 1994 Mechanisms of leukocyte motility and chemotaxis. Current Opinion in Immunology 6: 113–125
Germain R N, Margulaies D H 1993 The biochemistry and cell biology of antigen processing and presentation. Annual Review of Immunology 403–451
Rammensec H-G, Monaco J 1994 Antigen recognition. Current Opinion in Immunology 6: 355–514

IMMUNOLOGICAL DISEASES

ALLERGY AND HYPERSENSITIVITY

The terms allergy and hypersensitivity are synonymous although allergy is often used to describe immediate hypersensitivity reactions and atopic diseases. Hypersensitivity can be defined as tissue damage resulting from an immune response.

Traditionally, hypersensitivity has been classified according to the immune mechanism predominantly involved. This remains a useful approach, a reminder that the original disease process relates to a defect in the regulation of a particular component of the immune response. This also provides a basis for rational treatment.

CAUSES OF HYPERSENSITIVITY

Hypersensitivity may result from the induction of an inappropriate pattern of immunity, for example to an environmental agent which is totally harmless. This occurs in many people who readily make IgE antibodies (atopics). Sometimes T cell mediated immunity is involved, for example in cows' milk protein sensitive enteropathy in infants.

Hypersensitivity may also occur when the immune response to an antigen such as a virus not only damages or destroys the offending agent, but incidentally produces damage to adjacent tissue. 'Innocent bystanders' are damaged by an immune response which has to be vigorous in order to kill the pathogen. A good example of this is the fibrosis and cavity formation of pulmonary tuberculosis.

There is a range of conditions in which the clinical manifestations are virtually identical to those of immune

Table 2.8   Products of mast cell degranulation

Mediator	Biological effects
Pre-formed stored within granules	
Histamine	Vasodilatation, increased capillary permeability, chemokinesis, bronchoconstriction
Heparin	Anticoagulant
Tryptase	Activates C3
β-glucosaminidase	Splits off glucosamine
Eosinophil chemotactic factor	Eosinophil chemotaxis
Neutrophil chemotactic factor	Neutrophil chemotaxis
Platelet activating factor	Mediator release
Newly synthesized	
By the lipoxygenase pathway Leucotrienes C_4 and D_4 (SRS-A)	Vasoactive, bronchoconstriction, chemotaxis and/or chemokinesis
Leucotriene B_4	
By the cyclo-oxygenase pathway Prostaglandins Thromboxanes	Affect bronchial muscle, platelet aggregation and vasodilatation

mediated hypersensitivity, but these occur when non-specific immune effector mechanisms are triggered directly by agents other than antigen, for example when drugs or physical factors lead to mast cell degranulation.

IMMEDIATE (ANAPHYLACTIC) HYPERSENSITIVITY

This is due to IgE antibodies and most if not all manifestations are produced by mast cell degranulation (Table 2.8). The pattern and severity of reaction depend on the amount and route of exposure to antigen, the density of tissue mast cells, and the amounts of IgE antibody that they bear on the surface.

Respiratory tract allergies
Relatively mild although inconvenient symptoms may occur when antigen-IgE reactions take place in the upper respiratory tract or on other epithelial surfaces. For example, reactions to pollens or animal dander may cause rhinorrhoea, sneezing, conjunctivitis. On the other hand, inhalation of the antigen can lead to intense bronchospasm in atopic asthma. Skin prick tests with common inhalant allergens can give the clinician a reasonably good indication of a patient's likely sensitivities.

Anaphylaxis
Systemic anaphylaxis consists of a group of much more severe reactions which may occur rapidly if the antigen

is injected, as in the case of a drug such as penicillin or the sting of an insect. Rarely, anaphylaxis can be produced by ingested food in a highly sensitised individual.

The features are bronchospasm, laryngeal oedema with extreme dyspnoea and cyanosis, and a marked fall in blood pressure (anaphylactic shock). There may also be nausea, vomiting and diarrhoea.

Systemic anaphylaxis is a potentially fatal condition if not treated promptly with adrenaline and an antihistamine followed, in severely ill patients, by intravenous corticosteroids.

Urticaria

Urticaria, the formation of weal and flare lesions in the skin, is an anaphylactic phenomenon which can develop as a result of absorption of antigen (some foods and food additives) from the intestinal tract. Not all urticaria is caused by immune reactions. The mediators that cause urticaria can be released by other means, especially physical agents such as trauma or cold.

Other atopic diseases

There are a number of other, less well characterised diseases in which IgE is certainly involved, although other immune effector mechanisms are also implicated. These include atopic eczema, and some acute reactions to foods, particularly in infants.

CYTOTOXIC HYPERSENSITIVITY

In this type of hypersensitivity, IgG or IgM antibodies react with antigens in the tissues or on the surface of cells; for damage to result, complement alone or complement together with various effector cells (neutrophils, eosinophils, macrophages) interacts with the antigen-antibody complex. The injury is clearly localised to a single tissue or organ, and most examples of this form of hypersensitivity are auto-immune diseases (Table 2.9).

Table 2.9 Some examples of cytotoxic hypersensitivity

Disease	Antigen to which the antibody is directed
Autoimmune haemolytic anaemia, transfusion reactions	Erythrocyte surface antigens
Idiopathic thrombocytopenic purpura	Platelet antigens
Goodpasture's syndrome (a form of glomerulonephritis)	Glomerular basement membrane
Myasthenia gravis	Acetylcholine receptor at the motor end plate on the surface of myocyte

IMMUNE COMPLEX REACTIONS

Immune complex reactions occur when IgG or IgM antibodies combine with soluble antigen; antigen-antibody complexes are deposited in blood vessel walls and in the tissues. Complement, platelets, mast cells, basophil and polymorph leucocytes are all involved in the subsequent inflammatory processes. Factors that determine the deposition of immune complexes in tissues also include the size of the immune complexes, the ratio of antigen to antibody, the nature of the antigen, and local haemodynamics. There are several types of situations in which a disease is caused by immune complex formation.

Extrinsic allergic alveolitis

Immune complexes may be formed in the lungs, in response to repeated inhalation of antigenic materials from moulds, plants or animals. In farmer's lung and bird fancier's lung there are circulating IgG antibodies to fungi which have been induced by repeated exposure to mouldy hay or to avian antigens. When antigen enters the body by inhalation, local immune complexes are formed in the alveoli and local inflammation then interferes with pulmonary function.

Arthus reactions

An Arthus reaction may occur when an antigen is injected into the skin of a subject who has previously encountered that antigen and has high titres of serum antibody. The reaction of preformed antibody with this antigen results in a high concentration of local immune complexes. The reaction develops in some 6–24 hours with oedema, haemorrhage and necrosis at the injection site.

Serum sickness

In serum sickness IgG antibody is produced in response to the injection of foreign antigen in large quantity, as when horse serum is used to confer passive immunity. The antibody reacts with remaining antigen to form circulating, soluble immune complexes. Local swelling at the injection site, urticaria, fever, enlargement of the lymph nodes, arthralgia and sometimes glomerulonephritis occur about 10 days after initial exposure to the antigen. As the immune complexes are formed, the antigen concentration is rapidly lowered. Since the process continues only as long as the antigen persists, the disease is usually self-limiting.

Persistent infection

In some cases a chronic infection (e.g. infective endocarditis, malaria or viral hepatitis) together with a weak antibody response leads to the chronic formation of immune complexes and their deposition in the tissues.

Autoimmunity

In autoimmune diseases, immune complexes may be deposited in the kidneys, joints, arteries, skin and elsewhere.

DELAYED-TYPE HYPERSENSITIVITY

In the classification of hypersensitivity suggested by Gell and Coombs in 1963 delayed-type hypersensitivity (cell-mediated or type IV) was used as a general category to describe all those hypersensitivity reactions that took more than 12 hours to develop. It is now evident that several different reactions can produce delayed hypersensitivity, and that although T_{DTH} cells are implicated they act by recruiting other cell types to the site of the reaction, particularly macrophages.

Contact hypersensitivity

Contact hypersensitivity, producing local eczema usually maximal at 48 hours, is most commonly caused by haptens such as nickel, chemicals found in rubber, and poison ivy. Contact hypersensitivity is predominantly epidermal and the antigen is presented by the Langerhans cell.

Chronic infections

Reactions effected by T_{DTH} lymphocytes are characteristically induced by infectious agents which are predominantly intracellular in the infected host, e.g. many viral infections and some bacterial infections such as tuberculosis, leprosy and syphilis. The classic example of this reaction is the tuberculin test. The normal tissues of the host, as well as infected cells, are damaged by the reaction.

Granulomatous diseases

Granulomatous hypersensitivity is an important form of delayed hypersensitivity, causing many of the pathological effects in diseases which involve T cell mediated immunity. It results from the persistence of antigen within macrophages which the cell is unable to destroy. There are many granulomatous diseases for which the precise initiating agent is still unknown, including Crohn's disease, sarcoidosis and some forms of granulomatous hepatitis.

Food-related intestinal diseases

T cell mediated hypersensitivity is also involved in some chronic forms of immune mediated food intolerance, such as cows' milk protein sensitive enteropathy with malabsorption, and coeliac disease.

Table 2.10   Types of transplantation

Type		Example
Autograft	From one part of the body to another	Pinch skin graft for burns
Isograft	Between genetically identical members of the same species	Live donor kidney graft between identical twins
Allograft	Between genetically different members of the same species	Most clinical transplantation
Xenograft	Between species	Use of pig heart valves in cardiac surgery

TRANSPLANTATION AND GRAFT REJECTION

Destructive diseases or failure of many organs can now theoretically be treated by transplantation of healthy donor tissues or organs (Table 2.10). However, unless donor and host are identical twins, the host T cells recognise the graft cells as 'non-self'. Major Histocompatibility Complex (MHC) host antigens are particularly important, and soon after transplantation, antibodies and antigen-specific T cell responses to donor MHC antigens are generated. Unless this can be prevented or suppressed, the graft will be damaged and ultimately destroyed by immune-mediated rejection processes.

Types of rejection

T cells, and the cytokines IL-2 and interferon γ, are particularly important in early, acute rejection, i.e. in the days and weeks after transplantation.

Rarely there is hyperacute rejection, which occurs almost immediately after revascularisation of the transplanted organ. This is due to pre-existing anti-donor IgG and IgM antibodies, and complement.

Chronic rejection, months or years after transplantation, is probably caused by several types of immune reaction and the mechanism varies for different organs.

AUTOIMMUNITY AND AUTOIMMUNE DISEASES

Normally an individual does not mount a significant immune response against its own body constituents because intricate controlling and suppressor mechanisms exist to prevent this happening. A defect in immunological tolerance may either occur spontaneously or be induced by some exogenous factor such as virus infection, often in a genetically predisposed individual.

In general, autoimmune reactions occur in related groups reflecting the spectrum of autoimmune disease, ranging from the organ-specific to the non-organ-specific. Thus there are a number of autoantibodies formed to different thyroid antigens in autoimmune thyroid disease, and patients with one of the diseases in the organ-specific group tend to have an increased prevalence of autoantibodies to the target organs of other diseases in the group. Some important autoimmune diseases are listed in the information box below.

IMPORTANT AUTOIMMUNE DISEASES

- **Organ specific**
  Hashimoto's thyroiditis
  Primary myxoedema
  Thyrotoxicosis
  Pernicious anaemia
  Autoimmune atrophic gastritis
  Autoimmune Addison's disease
  Type I diabetes mellitus
  Goodpasture's syndrome
  Myasthenia gravis
  Sympathetic ophthalmia
  Autoimmune haemolytic anaemia
  Idiopathic thrombocytopenic purpura
  Primary biliary cirrhosis
  Chronic active hepatitis
  Sjögren's syndrome

- **Non-organ specific**
  Rheumatoid arthritis
  Dermatomyositis
  Systemic sclerosis
  Systemic lupus erythematosus (SLE)

THEORIES OF AETIOLOGY OF AUTOIMMUNITY

It is likely that a range of different mechanisms underly the variety of autoimmune diseases; in particular, organ-specific diseases may have different aetiologies from multi-organ disorders.

Aberrant immunity

Genetic factors are important in autoimmune disease, as can be seen from experimental animal models, from family studies and from the association of many auto-immune diseases with the MHC system. In insulin-dependent diabetes, cells of the target organ express MHC class 2 antigens on their surfaces. This facilitates sensitisation and activation of the T_H cells. It may be that viruses are implicated in the abnormal expression of MHC antigens.

Loss of suppressor T cell (T_S) control of the T helper

(T_H) cells may underly the rising incidence of subclinical and clinical autoimmune disease with advancing years.

Antigen recognition

Sequestrated antigens are those that do not normally come into contact with the immunological system, so that immunological tolerance does not develop in early life and autoimmunisation may occur, for example after injury or surgery. Sperm, if extravasated following unilateral blockage of the vas deferens, may induce antibody formation and contribute to sterility. Sperm antibodies may also be produced following vasectomy in normal men.

Invading micro-organisms may have antigens that also occur in host tissues; a microbial antigen may thus induce the formation of antibodies which cross-react with these tissues. For example the sharing of antigen between some Group A haemolytic streptococci and the heart is thought to be the reason why rheumatic carditis is an occasional late complication of streptococcal tonsillitis.

Occasionally the development of autoantibodies is a side-effect of drug treatment. Some patients treated with methyldopa develop a haemolytic anaemia due to red blood cell autoantibodies; the anaemia resolves when treatment with the drug is stopped. Other drugs may be associated with the production of antinuclear antibodies.

AUTOANTIBODIES

While some antibodies may play a crucial role in the pathogenesis of autoimmune disease, others seem to have little pathological function but may be useful evidence of an autoimmune diathesis. The antibody that is most readily detectable and useful as a marker in the serum may or may not be implicated as a damaging agent.

In the organ-specific group of disorders, antibody in the serum may indicate that immunological damage of some degree is occurring even though there is at that time no clinical evidence of organ failure. This can be explained by the fact that most tissues have a substantial reserve of function that must be eroded before clinical disease is manifest (e.g. only 10% of pancreatic islets are required to maintain normal glucose homeostasis). The rate of progression of the disease process may be over many years or more rapid; so far, the genetic factors in an individual patient that determine the rate of progression have not been identified.

IMMUNODEFICIENCY DISORDERS

Virtually any component of the immune system, specific or nonspecific, can be absent or abnormal; the con-

Table 2.11 Classification of primary immunodeficiency diseases

Humoral immunodeficiences
X-linked hypogammaglobulinaemia
Transient hypogammaglobulinaemia of infancy
Common, variable, unclassifiable immunodeficiency
Selective IgA deficiency

Cellular (T-cell) immunodeficiencies
Congenital thymic aplasia (DiGeorge syndrome)

Combined immunodeficiencies
Severe combined immunodeficiency
Cellular immunodeficiency with abnormal immunoglobulin synthesis (Nezelof's syndrome)
Immunodeficiency with ataxia telangiectasia
Immunodeficiency with eczema and thrombocytopenia (Wiskott–Aldrich syndrome)
Immunodeficiency with lymphotoxins

Phagocytic deficiencies
Chronic granulomatous disease
Myeloperoxidase deficiency
Chediak–Higashi syndrome
Job's syndrome

Complement deficiencies

sequent immunodeficiency states vary in severity from trivial to fatal. There are many genetically determined conditions, but immunodeficiency can also result from acquired disease. This is well illustrated in the acquired immunodeficiency syndrome (see p. 89), but it is also part of common experience of many infections including influenza, infectious mononucleosis and measles. Acquired immunodeficiency may also be iatrogenic, for example as a result of corticosteroid treatment. In addition to causing susceptibility to infection, immunodeficiency may be associated with abnormally regulated immune reactions, as in allergy or autoimmunity. The classification of primary immunodeficiency diseases is shown in Table 2.11. Treatment is discussed in the section on immunotherapy.

Abnormalities of polymorph function, and deficiencies of complement components or antibodies, all result in susceptibility to bacterial infection. Deficiencies of the humoral and cellular components of the specific immunological system may occur separately or together. Table 2.11 indicates the probable sites of the primary defects in the immune system for a number of clinical patterns that have been recognised. The more precise analysis of these immunodeficiencies is being greatly aided by the development of monoclonal antibody markers for the different T cell subsets, for the different stages of maturity of B cells, and for monocytes.

SEVERE COMBINED IMMUNODEFICIENCY SYNDROME

This condition, which can be caused by several different gene defects, autosomal or X-linked, is characterised by a defect of stem-cells that leads to deficiency in both the T and B lymphocyte systems and therefore to impairment of cell-mediated immunity and of synthesis of humoral antibody. Stem-cell failure at an early stage of development gives the additional feature of agranulocytosis although the red cells and platelets are normal. About half the infants with the autosomal recessive form of severe combined immunodeficiency have a concomitant deficiency of adenosine deaminase which has enabled prenatal diagnosis by finding the enzyme deficiency in cultured amnion cells. The affected infants are susceptible to even the most benign viral infections, and may die from generalised chickenpox, measles, cytomegalovirus or other viral infections. When smallpox vaccination is inadvertently given to affected infants, this results in progressive, ultimately fatal vaccinia infection; similarly they are at risk of severe disease if given BCG.

DEFICIENCY OF IMMUNOGLOBULINS

Primary hypogammaglobulinaemia
Selective deficiency of the B lymphocyte system occurs in X-linked recessive hypo- or agammaglobulinaemia. The lack of immunoglobulins is not absolute but the patient fails to respond to antigenic stimuli. However, cell mediated immunity is normal. This disorder is compatible with survival for many years, though the patient is very susceptible to bacterial infections.

Common variable immunodeficiency
Most patients with immunoglobulin deficiency have 'acquired' or 'late onset' hypogammaglobulinaemia known as 'common, variable immunodeficiency'. This is associated with an unusually high incidence of autoimmune disease, such as pernicious anaemia and haemolytic anaemia. An occasional complication is a malabsorption syndrome which may be due to *Giardia lamblia* infection.

Isolated immunoglobulin deficiencies
IgM deficiency renders the patient susceptible to bloodborne infection such as that due to the meningococcus. Lack of IgA may be associated with gastrointestinal or respiratory tract infections.

Hypogammaglobulinaemia of prematurity
Maternal IgG is transferred across the placenta during the third trimester of pregnancy. Premature babies may thus have some degree of hypogammaglobulinaemia; for them, prophylactic IgG treatment may reduce the incidence of infections.

Other causes of immunoglobulin deficiency

Immunoglobulin deficiency may result from abnormal losses of serum proteins, for example in lymphangiectasia. Drugs may also depress the immune system; for example phenytoin or penicillamine may induce IgA deficiency.

DEFICIENCY OF CELLULAR IMMUNITY

Thymic aplasia

In this disease there is a selective deficiency of T lymphocytes, with severe lymphocytopenia and a predominance of reticulum cells in the lymphoid tissue. Because T cell mediated immunity is deficient, affected children do not respond in the normal way to antigens such as candida and tuberculin on skin testing. Infants with thymic aplasia are highly susceptible to viral infections, which usually prove fatal.

Secondary T cell deficiency

Secondary T cell defects may occur in Hodgkin's disease or sarcoidosis, and following infections such as leprosy, miliary tuberculosis or measles. It may also result from loss of lymphocytes from the gut in protein-losing enteropathy, or be due to thoracic duct fistula, and may be caused by treatment with cytotoxic drugs.

DISEASES OF COMPLEMENT

Deficiencies of complement components

In the inherited complement deficiencies there is usually a total absence of the complement protein, and this implies the lack of a functional gene. The association of C1, 4 and 2 deficiencies with immune complex-like or lupus-like disorders is probably due to the failure to eliminate immune complexes.

Deficiency of a complement inhibitor

The interactions between the complement system and the clotting, fibrinolytic and kinin pathways are illustrated in the condition of hereditary angioedema resulting from a deficiency of C1 inhibitor. This autosomal dominant condition causes sporadic attacks of tissue oedema often affecting the face and gut. Blood levels of C1 inhibitor are well below normal and the angioedema is probably produced by excessive action of C1 leading to high levels of an active peptide derived from C2, C2 kinin. The disease is treated either by the drug danazol which increases the level of C1 inhibitor, or by decreasing the activity of plasmin with epsilon aminocaproic acid.

Table 2.12 Factors which may lead to secondary immunodeficiency

Nutritional status	Calorie, protein or micro-nutrient deficiency
Old age	Immunosenescence, with some failure of self-tolerance leading to autoimmunity, as well as deficient T cell function
Post-operative	General anaesthesia induces a significant immunodeficiency for several days
Loss of protective commensal gut bacterial flora	Due to broad spectrum antibiotic treatment
Irradiation or cancer chemotherapy	
Use of drugs which suppress immunity	e.g. corticosteroids

THE IMMUNOSUPPRESSED PATIENT

Quite apart fom the specific immunodeficiency diseases described above and the acquired immunodeficiency syndrome (p. 89), complex partial or even profound immunodeficiency may occur in association with many clinical situations and diseases (see Table 2.12).

PRINCIPLES OF IMMUNOTHERAPY

The immune response to antigens and other extrinsic agents is mounted by B and T cells and their subsets to produce specific antibodies and T cells, and embraces many non-antigen specific humoral and cellular reactions and host tissue reactions to immune signals. Accordingly, there is enormous potential for preventive and therapeutic manipulation of immunity. There are promising indications that the clinical application of knowledge and technology in this field will develop rapidly.

IMMUNISATION

Active immunisation

Induction of protective immunity to many infectious diseases is the most successful and most widely applied example of immunotherapy. For active immunisation it is necessary to administer several doses of material which will induce a host-protective immune response in the form of serum antibodies, secretory antibodies or T cell mediated reactivity. In developing further strategies for immunisation against diseases not currently covered, knowledge of the natural history of the disease is essential. For example if some of the clinical manifestations are due to the host immune response rather than the pathogen itself, as in some parasite infections, care must be taken to induce mainly protective (e.g. IgG, IgA), rather than immunopathological (e.g. IgE, T cell) immunity.

Passive immunisation

Administration of immunoglobulin (preferably human) of known high antibacterial or antiviral titre is of proven clinical value in the prevention and treatment of specific infections. This is particularly so in immunocompromised individuals, for example when immunoglobulin of high titre anti-cytomegalovirus activity is used in bone marrow transplant recipients.

SPECIFIC TREATMENT OF IMMUNODEFICIENCY SYNDROMES

Knowledge of the precise mechanism and natural history of the condition is essential for the proper use of immunotherapy, either to cure by transplantation, or to treat by more temporary means such as giving immunoglobulin on a regular basis. Specific drugs to enhance immune responses are used in immunology research, as 'adjuvants' to stimulate immune responsiveness to an antigen when given at the same time. Immune modulatory agents are also used in some vaccines, e.g. alum salts given with diphtheria toxoid and tetanus toxoid as adjuvants.

With increasing experience of the use of interleukins and new techniques to enable their production in bulk, specific molecular immunotherapy of immunodeficiency states may become a reality.

The stem-cell deficiency in the severe combined immunodeficiency syndrome can be replaced by bone marrow transplantation, and 10-year survivals with maintenance of normal T and B cell function have been recorded in a few children. In thymic aplasia, transplantation of fragments of human fetal thymus provides the necessary educative environment for host stem-cells to develop into normal T cells, and this corrects the cellular immune deficiency.

Hypogammaglobulinaemia is treated by immunoglobulin injections (intramuscular or intravenous). These consist mainly of IgG and can provide effective protection against severe, recurrent pyogenic infections. Since the half-life of the gammaglobulin injected is approximately four weeks, patients are usually given a monthly injection of 100 mg/kg.

TREATMENT OF HYPERSENSITIVITY BY MANIPULATION OF ANTIGEN EXPOSURE

Reduction of antigen load

The classic example of this is the use of an elimination diet to treat a food allergy. For example, withdrawal of cows' milk in infants with enteropathy, colitis or eczema associated with cows' milk allergy; the use of a gluten-free diet in coeliac disease; and the strict avoidance of a food such as fish, egg, peanut, to which anaphylactic reaction has previously occurred.

Reduction of the antigen load is also important in inhalant allergies, for example the use of a mask by farmers with farmer's lung, bird breeders with bird fancier's lung; changes in bedding, curtains, etc. in children with asthma and house dust mite sensitivity.

Hyposensitisation

Anaphylactic individuals can be made less sensitive by multiple subcutaneous injections of antigen in gradually increasing dosage. The patient develops IgG antibodies against the antigen; these antibodies have a higher avidity for the antigen than do IgE antibodies and are able to compete successfully for the antigenic sites on the pollen or other allergen. These IgG antibodies are referred to as blocking antibodies. Hyposensitisation regimens may also induce other suppressor mechanisms that ultimately down-regulate IgE biosynthesis.

Specific hyposensitisation is of proven value in wasp and bee sting allergy. The value in other conditions, e.g. treatment with pollen antigens to prevent hay fever in previously badly affected individuals, is uncertain.

Dangers of hyposensitisation treatments

There have been fatal anaphylactic reactions reported from the injection of these desensitising vaccines. Patients with asthma are particularly susceptible. Thus if it is considered advisable for this treatment to be used, patients should be observed for 2 hours after treatment, and the injections must be given in a place where facilities for full cardio-respiratory resuscitation are available.

PHARMACOLOGICAL TREATMENT OF ALLERGY AND INFLAMMATION

Drugs used to treat IgE-mediated allergic reactions either act directly on the mast cell, block the effects of mast cell mediators, or have an antagonistic effect.

Sodium cromoglycate

This drug inhibits the release of the mediators from mast cells after the interaction of antigens with IgE antibodies. It is partially effective in preventing the induction of asthma by specific antigens. If inhaled by an asthmatic subject before exposure to the antigen, protection may last for several hours, but if given after exposure to the antigen it has little effect. The drug is also beneficial in exercise-induced asthma.

Antihistamines

The antihistamines occupy the same tissue receptors as histamine without providing any stimulus to the effector cells. The intravenous injection of an antihistamine quickly produces adequate tissue concentrations. The weal, the erythema and the itch of acute urticaria are reduced but there is no consistent improvement in lung function in acute bronchial asthma.

The failure of the antihistamines to relieve airway obstruction caused by an anaphylactic reaction has been attributed to high concentrations of histamine close to the smooth muscle cells. It may also be due to the presence of other mediators of the anaphylactic response. For example, bradykinin is rapidly inactivated in plasma by a kininase but its effects are not inhibited by antihistamines.

Adrenaline and related drugs

These act by producing effects which oppose the mediators and are more effective in emergencies than the antihistamines. Adrenaline, isoprenaline and aminophylline are efficient bronchodilators in bronchial asthma and in anaphylaxis (see information box). Urticaria is relieved and where oedema threatens the airway, the risk of asphyxia is lessened.

Despite their effectiveness these nonspecific antagonists have serious disadvantages. They act on receptors that differ from those occupied by the mediators, and their effects never precisely counteract those of the mediators. The dose of a sympathomimetic amine which relieves airflow obstruction may produce tachycardia and palpitations even when the amine is administered as an aerosol. Salbutamol does not have these disadvantages as it is a more selective β_2 adrenoceptor agonist.

DRUGS USED TO SUPPRESS IMMUNITY

These drugs are invaluable in the treatment of many chronic inflammatory and autoimmune diseases, and are used in combination to prevent rejection after tissue or organ transplantation.

Corticosteroids

Corticosteroids such as prednisolone interfere at many points in the immune response, affecting lymphocyte recirculation and cytotoxic effector cells. The anti-inflammatory effect of steroids is due to their inhibition of neutrophil adherence to vascular endothelium in an inflammatory area and suppression of monocyte/macrophage functions such as microbicidal activity and response to lymphokines.

ALLERGIC EMERGENCY—ANAPHYLACTIC SHOCK

Precipitated in a sensitised individual by:
- **parenteral exposure to**
  blood products
  vaccines
  many drugs
  heparin
  hypo-sensitising preparations
- **insect stings**
  bee
  wasp
- **oral exposure**
  drugs (e.g. penicillin)
  foods (e.g. peanuts, shellfish)

Clinical features:
- laryngeal oedema
- bronchospasm
- hypotension

Primary treatment:
- lay patient flat; raise legs
- adrenaline i.m. (or, cautiously, i.v. in lower dose)
  0.5–1 ml adrenaline injection 1 in 1000;
  repeat every 10 mins if necessary
- antihistamine by slow i.v. injection; continue for
  24–48 hrs

If necessary:
- emergency tracheostomy or cricopharyngotomy; i.v. fluids, oxygen, i.v. aminophylline, nebulised salbutamol, assisted respiration, i.v. corticosteroids

---

Immunosuppressive drugs

The production of immunoglobulins and the cellular immune response are dependent upon the division of lymphoid cells. Drugs that interfere with dividing cells are therefore all potentially immunosuppressive and were originally developed as anti-tumour agents. Of these, azathioprine, cyclophosphamide and methotrexate have been used for immunosuppression. Such drugs may have serious adverse effects, including bone marrow suppression and recrudescence of latent tuberculous, viral or fungal infection. A further possible hazard is an increased incidence of malignant tumours, such as lymphomas, possibly on account of the suppression of immunological surveillance of the body tissues in relation to infection with oncogenic viruses.

Cyclosporin A

This is a naturally occurring fungal metabolite. It suppresses both humoral and cell mediated immunity, and has been shown to have a direct suppressive (but non-cytotoxic) effect on B cells and T helper cells. Resting cells which carry the vital memory of immunity to microbial infections are spared, and there is little toxicity for dividing cells in the gut and bone marrow. Cyclosporin must be used at doses below those causing nephrotoxicity, so blood levels have to be monitored regularly.

NEW APPROACHES TO IMMUNOTHERAPY

Plasmapheresis
Apheresis is the generic term for removal of a component from the blood; a prefix indicates whether this is plasma, leucocytes, etc. Plasmapheresis (plasma exchange) is used in a variety of conditions, e.g. to remove acetylcholine-receptor antibodies in myasthenia gravis, glomerular basement membrane antibodies in Goodpasture's syndrome (see Table 2.13). It is sometimes used in conjunction with cytotoxic drugs and corticosteroids in order to retard the resynthesis of antibody.

Intravenous immunoglobulin
In addition to the use of immunoglobulin preparations for replacement therapy in immune deficiency syndromes, intravenous infusion of immunoglobulin preparations is beneficial in several diseases (see information box). The mode of operation is uncertain, but may be by an immunosuppressive action, e.g. anti-idiotype activity.

USE OF IMMUNOGLOBULIN THERAPY

Intramuscular

Normal human Ig
- Prevention of hepatitis A

Hyperimmune Ig
- Anti-rhesus D
- Anti-zoster
- Anti-hepatitis B
- Anti-cytomegalovirus
- Anti-rabies
- Anti-rubella
- Anti-tetanus

Intravenous

Replacement therapy
- Hypogammaglobulinaemia, paediatric AIDS

Treatment of
- Idiopathic thrombocytopenic purpura
- Neonatal allo-immune thrombocytopenia
- Kawasaki's disease
- Guillain–Barré syndrome
- Myasthenia gravis

Monoclonal antibodies
Many potentially therapeutic monoclonal antibodies are being produced by biotechnology companies and research institutes. Antibodies against lymphocyte surface molecules such as CD3 can be used to eliminate cell populations or block their functions. Antibodies to cytokines and other mediators provide an alternative approach to immunomodulation. Antibodies which neutralise bacterial endotoxin are in clinical trial in patients with sepsis syndrome and shock, and it may soon be possible to target cytotoxic drugs onto tumour cells by linking these to tumour-specific antibodies.

Table 2.13 Clinical uses of plasmapheresis

Indication	Presumed mode of action
Hyperviscosity syndromes (e.g. Waldenström's macroglobulinaemia)	Removal of large molecules (IgM, occasionally IgA)
Thrombotic thrombocytopenia (exchange with fresh, frozen plasma)	Uncertain
Rapidly progressive glomerulonephritis	Removal of autoantibodies or inflammatory mediators
Guillain–Barré syndrome	Removal of autoantibodies or inflammatory mediators
Myasthenia gravis Malignant exophthalmos Pemphigus	Removal of antibodies

---

FURTHER READING

Bochner B S, Undem B J, Lichtenstein L M 1994 Immunological basis of allergic asthma. Annual Review of Immunology 707–735

Lee R S, Auchincloss H 1994 Mechanisms of tolerance to allografts. Chemical Immunology 58: 236–258

Möller, G (ed.) 1993 Chronic graft rejection. Immunological Reviews 134: 5–116

Naparstek Y, Plotz P H 1993 The role of autoantibodies in autoimmune diseases. Annual Review of Immunology 79–105

Steinman L, Todd J A (eds) 1992 Autoimmunity. Current Opinion in Immunology 4: 699–779

A. D. M. Bryceson, C. A. Soutar

3

Climate and environmental factors in disease

Many factors affect the patterns of disease around the world. Environmental factors are important among them. Climate is the most striking factor. It affects health indirectly through its influence on plants, animals, insects and microbes, and directly by taxing the body's physiological reserves. The environment contains, for example, minerals such as fluorine and iodine that affect health through excess (fluorosis, p. 561) or deficiency (goitre, p. 561). Naturally occurring toxins such as aflatoxin (p. 533), and natural sources of radiation may cause disease. Pollution of the environment by chemical and radioactive waste is an increasingly important cause of disease and ill health.

INDIRECT EFFECTS OF CLIMATE ON HEALTH AND DISEASE

Climate chiefly determines the distribution, type and density of vegetation, including crops. It influences the range of animals that can be hunted or tended. It controls the growth and distribution of microbial organisms and of insects that may transmit them or may act as pests. Thus wealth, nutrition, education and development, and their interaction with health, depend to a large extent on climate. Some examples are given in Table 3.1.

Microclimates

Most people live in the temperate zones, which are warm and moist. The adverse effects of climate are best seen by examining the zones of extreme climate (Table 3.2). The health of people in many developing countries is poor. This is due largely to adverse climate and poverty, such that the country may not be able to educate or protect the health of its exploding population. It is important, however, not to overgeneralise. Within the broad ranges of gross climate, there are microclimates which further affect the distribution of disease. For example, mosquitoes breed on surface water and rest above ground, so the distribution of malaria is an absolute reflection of peak annual temperature, whereas phlebotomine sandflies find their very precise requirements for temperature and moisture in burrows, tree-holes, cracks and crevices where the microbes that they carry can also find vertebrate reservoirs; so they transmit disease over a wide climatic and geographic range.

Season

Within any climatic zone, season is also an important determinant of disease. In semi-arid zones food is scarce before the rains and malnutrition occurs; during the rains malaria and gastrointestinal disease increase. Very dry weather, be it hot, cold, at altitude or due to air-conditioning, damages the upper respiratory mucosa, permitting infection. In sub-Saharan Africa this leads to annual epidemics of meningococcal meningitis in March and April. Figure 3.1 illustrates some of the effects of seasonal climate on disease.

DISORDERS RELATED TO HEAT

In cool climates heat production in the body is balanced by loss from the surface chiefly by radiation and convection. When the environmental temperature approaches that of the body, evaporation of sweat becomes the most important mechanism in maintaining body temperature. A hard spell of work in a hot environment may generate 6–8 litres of sweat, each containing 2 g sodium chloride.

Acclimatisation to heat (see information box) is an essential preparation for workers exposed to excessive

Table 3.1	Indirect effects of climate on disease: some examples		
	Climate	**Effect**	**Disease in man**
	Cold/dry	Crowding, extra clothing, little washing Damage to upper respiratory mucosa	Louse-borne infections Respiratory tract infection
	Hot/dry	Cyclical drought Damage to upper respiratory mucosa Production of concentrated urine Sandflies flourish	Malnutrition Respiratory tract infection Urolithiasis Zoonotic cutaneous leishmaniasis
	Hot/moist	Sweaty skin Seasonal rivers Tse-tse fly numerous along rivers	Pyoderma Onchocerciasis, seasonal malaria Trypanosomiasis
	Hot/wet	Soil rich in microorganisms Interaction of two microorganisms Precise requirement met for vector Crowding, riverine festivals Filarial infection	Tropical and buruli ulcers Burkitt's lymphoma Loa loa infection Cholera, e.g. in Ganges delta Endomyocardial fibrosis

PHYSIOLOGICAL CHANGES OF ACCLIMATISATION TO HEAT

Increased
- circulatory volume
- cardiac output
- aldosterone production
- renal retention of sodium
- responsiveness of sweating
- fluid requirement

Decreased
- heart rate
- volume of sweating

heat in certain industries in cool climates, as well as for people who travel to the tropics. This can be achieved by progressive daily exercise under artificially produced or natural hot weather conditions for 10 to 14 days. With these adjustments the individual is able to work and remain well in a hot environment, provided an adequate intake of water and salt is maintained. The most serious disorder related to heat is heat hyperpyrexia or heatstroke. Less serious but more common disorders are listed in Table 3.3 overleaf.

HEAT HYPERPYREXIA (HEATSTROKE)

Heatstroke is a syndrome due to overheating the body. It occurs when the core, or rectal, temperature rises through 41°C. It is associated with cessation of sweating and leads to tissue injury. It occurs world-wide and carries a mortality of 10–75%, according to duration of illness and efficiency of treatment. Risk factors are listed in the information box (p. 54). Most important are high environmental temperature and humidity. Impaired or impeded sweating may be due to ectodermal dysplasia, prickly heat or unsuitable clothing. 'Leisure drugs' such as methylenedioxy methamphetamine ('speed') may cause hyperpyrexia.

In heatstroke, blood is directed to the periphery, depriving organs of oxygen, and causing brain and liver damage, rhabdomyolysis, and disseminated intravascular coagulation. Above 42°C, hypothalamic control of temperature is lost.

Clinical features

The onset is usually dramatic with no warning in a person who appears to be neither dehydrated nor deficient

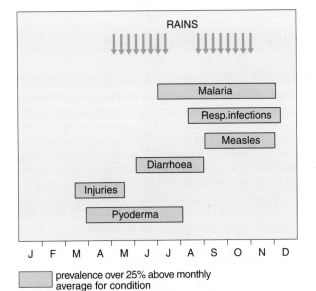

prevalence over 25% above monthly average for condition

Fig. 3.1 Seasonal variation of disease in a community in Southern Ghana (based on Parry 1984—see Further Reading).

Table 3.2   Characteristics of extreme climatic zones

Characteristic	Rain-forest	Tropical savanna	Tropical deserts	Mountains	Tundra
Climate	Hot/wet	Hot/moist	Hot/dry	Cold/moist	Cold/dry
Water	Plenty	Seasonal	Scarce/local	Variable	Variable
Leaf crops	Plenty	Seasonal	Oases only	∝ rainfall	Scarce
Grains	Scarce	Plenty	Scarce	Grown	Grown
Herds, flocks	Scarce	Plenty	Tended	Plenty	Tended
Diet	↓ protein	↓ seasonally	↓ vitamins	∝ rainfall	↓ seasonally
Insects	+++	++	+	∝ temperature	+ (summer)
Microbes	+++	++	+	∝ temperature	+
Inhabitants	Gatherers, farmers	Nomads, farmers, urban population	Nomads, settlements	Farmers, urban population	Nomads, farmers

+ Occasional
++ Common
+++ Frequent

in salt, but who may have noticed that perspiration has diminished. Loss of consciousness is rapid and may be preceded by prodromal signs of cerebral irritation. On examination a dry burning skin is found (the 'hot dry man'). When the temperature reaches 41° to 42°C the patient loses consciousness and dies, unless treated. Hyperpyrexia may be complicated by acute circulatory failure, hypokalaemia, acute renal or hepatic failure and haemorrhage.

> **RISK FACTORS FOR DEVELOPING HEAT HYPERPYREXIA (HEATSTROKE)**
>
> **Environmental**
> - Temperature ≥35°C
> - Humidity ≥75%
> - Lack of wind
>
> **Endogenous**
> - Deficient sweating
> - Obesity
> - Debility (age, cardiac failure)
> - Alcoholism
>
> **Exogenous**
> - Inappropriate clothing
> - Dehydration
> - Febrile illness
> - Exertion
> - Medication e.g. anticholinergics, phenothiazines, amphetamines

Management

The aim is to reduce the temperature as quickly as possible. In the field, the patient is moved into the shade, the clothing removed and the skin kept wet and fanned vigorously. In hospital this is done by spraying the naked patient with water or loosely wrapping the individual in a cool, wet sheet and promoting evaporation by fanning. Ideally, the water should be at 15°C and the airstream at 30–35°C. The use of iced water, or immersion in cold water, causes vasoconstriction and is less efficient. Cooling should be stopped when the rectal temperature has fallen to 39°C. The airway must be maintained and oxygen given. Potassium deficiency should be corrected and severe haemorrhage controlled by blood transfusion. Acute circulatory failure (p. 212), acute renal

failure (p. 626), hepatic failure (p. 510) or disseminated intravascular coagulation may require treatment. Parenteral antimalarial therapy (p. 152) should be given concurrently if malaria is a possibility. With energetic early treatment, 90% of patients recover.

Prevention

Acclimatisation, suitable clothing, avoidance of risk factors (see information box), and adequate water and salt intake are important. Keep cool and do not overwork in very hot, humid weather.

DISORDERS RELATED TO COLD

FROSTBITE

Dry cold, below 0°C, freezes poorly-insulated tissues such as fingers, especially in people exercising at altitudes where oxygen demand is high and availability low. The intense pain of impending frostbite progresses to loss of sensation. Superficial frostbite causes blistering of skin; in deep frostbite there is necrosis of tissue leading to gangrene. Frostbite is treated rapidly, rewarming the whole patient with good insulation and hot drinks, and by warming the affected part in water at 40°C. Warming must be continuous, to prevent refreezing.

HYPOTHERMIA

Hypothermia, which is defined as a fall in the core temperature to below 35°C, is a medical emergency which requires urgent therapy. People cannot acclimatise to cold as they can to heat.

Hypothermia occurs most commonly in the elderly, particularly when immobile and living alone, but can occur in a variety of other situations or secondarily as a complication of illness (see information box). It is a particular problem in workers in exposed conditions,

Table 3.3   Minor clinical syndromes due to heat

	Miliaria rubra (prickly heat)	Heat syncope	Heat exhaustion
At risk	Europeans in the tropics	Unacclimatised, overdressed	Those making extra effort in hot weather
Cause	Blocked sweat ducts	Relative fluid volume depletion	Fluid and salt depletion
Symptoms	Itching, scratching	Sudden onset: faintness, headache, collapse	Gradual onset: headache, giddiness, anorexia, muscle cramps, irritability, *beware* lack of thirst
Signs	Papular rash on covered skin, erythema, secondary infection	Cold, clammy, hypotensive	Tachycardia, dehydration, hypotension
Management	Reduce need to sweat Keep cool and dry Calamine lotion	Cool environment Oral fluids Allow to acclimatise	Cool environment Fluid and salt replacement (oral or intravenous) *Beware* hyperpyrexia

such as North Sea oil-rigs and fishing fleets, and for long-distance swimmers, mountaineers and hill walkers.

Clinical features

The rectal temperature is, by definition, below 35°C and may be as low as 25°C. It is important that the true core temperature is recorded using a thermocouple or a low-reading thermometer. The patient feels tired and mood and motor function are impaired. He/she feels cold, looks pale and the muscles become stiff. Heart rate and blood pressure fall. When the temperature falls below 26°C the patient becomes unconscious and may develop general oedema. Pupillary and tendon reflexes disappear.

Investigations

Haemoconcentration and metabolic acidosis are common. The electrocardiogram may show a characteristic J-wave which occurs at the junction of the QRS complex and the ST segment (Fig. 3.2). Abnormalities of cardiac rhythm occur, including ventricular fibrillation. Although the arterial oxygen tension may be normal when measured at room temperature, it should be remembered that the arterial PO_2 falls by 7% for each °C fall in core temperature. Serum aspartate aminotransferase and creatine kinase may be elevated secondary to muscle damage and the serum amylase is often high due to subclinical pancreatitis.

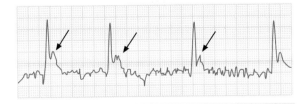

Fig. 3.2 Electrocardiogram showing J-wave (arrowed) in a hypothermic patient.

Management

The patient is kept in a warm room and allowed to rewarm gradually under blankets. If no shelter is available rewarming may be achieved by placing the patient, up to the neck, in a plastic sack or space blanket. A rise in temperature of 0.5°–1°C per hour is optimal. Particular attention must be paid to the development of arrhythmia. It is important to monitor the serum potassium and blood gases. Careful attention to the lungs is necessary as there is a high prevalence of pneumonia which should be treated with an appropriate antibiotic. Maintenance of blood pressure and volume are essential and can be achieved using glucose and saline or albumen. Drug overdose and hypothyroidism must always be excluded. Active rewarming may be too rapid and cause shock, but is needed in severe hypothermia with cardiopulmonary arrest or the development of unresponsive dangerous arrhythmia. Warmed oxygen and intravenous fluids may be used.

Prognosis

There is a particularly high mortality rate in hypothermic patients over the age of 75. Care must be exercised in pronouncing hypothermic individuals dead. No certification of death should be issued until patients have been rewarmed to 36°C and have been unresponsive at that temperature. This applies particularly to younger patients, who are capable of surviving hypothermia for surprisingly long periods.

DISORDERS RELATED TO ALTITUDE

The partial pressure of atmospheric oxygen decreases with altitude so that oxygen tension in the lungs falls from 19.9 kPa at sea level to 5.7 kPa at the top of Mount Everest (8848 m). Physiological acclimatisation starts at about 1500 m and most people feel the need to acclimatise by about 3500 m. Physically fit young people acclimatise best and do better with each ascent. Lowlanders, however, never attain the performance of highlanders. Lack of acclimatisation is shown by increased respiration, Cheyne–Stokes respiration, mild headache and irritability, easy fatiguability and sleeplessness.

Acclimatisation continues successfully up to 5330 m, above which maximal heart rate and cardiac output start to fall, pulmonary diffusion becomes impaired, arterial oxygen saturation falls and physical performance declines. Short bursts of work can be undertaken, but at the risk of producing an exaggerated lactic acidosis. Prolonged residence above this height causes anorexia, weight loss, decreasing mental and physical capacity and increasing susceptibility to infection. There are no permanent habitations above 4575 m.

ACUTE MOUNTAIN SICKNESS

This is experienced by people who go too high too quickly; some suffer at 2500 m, others reach 5500 m without trouble. The cause of the syndrome is unknown.

Clinical features

The earliest symptoms are headache, loss of appetite, nausea and vomiting, followed by lassitude, muscle weakness, breathlessness, dizziness, a rapid pulse and insomnia. Retinal haemorrhages may occur. Acute mountain sickness may herald the onset of two severe and often fatal complications: pulmonary oedema and, less commonly, cerebral oedema. Youth, speed of ascent, reascent, exertion and absolute altitude are associated factors. Cerebral oedema causes drowsiness, irritability, nightmares, confusion, fits and coma. Papilloedema is a late sign. Venous thromboses, which may lead to pulmonary embolism, may afflict the partially acclimatised; they are due to increased viscosity of blood and are prevented by adequate hydration and exercise.

Management

Acute mountain sickness may be prevented by time spent acclimatising, ascending gradually, sleeping at a level below the high point attained in a day, and adequate hydration. Alcohol avoidance is also very important and people with pre-existing cardiovascular or respiratory disorders should not go to altitude. Acetazolamide, in a dose of 500 mg at night, causes metabolic acidosis and increased drive to ventilation. It is effective in preventing acute mountain sickness, but not its complications. These are treated by descending 500–1000 m rapidly and by giving oxygen. Frusemide 40–120 mg daily and nifedipine 10 mg repeated as necessary is the treatment for pulmonary oedema, and dexamethasone for cerebral oedema. It is important to stress that these are only adjuvants to descent.

PHYSIOLOGICAL CHANGES OF ACCLIMATISATION TO ALTITUDE

Increased
- Ventilation causing respiratory alkalosis
- Urinary bicarbonate excretion
- Pulmonary diffusion
- Red blood cell mass
- Cardiac output
- Tissue capillarity

CHRONIC MOUNTAIN SICKNESS

This is due to alveolar hypoventilation and chronic hypoxia brought about by inappropriate polycythaemia, and may affect highlanders as well as acclimatised lowlanders. Clinical features include cyanosis, cardiac failure, pulmonary hypertension and neuropsychiatric symptoms. Chronic mountain sickness is treated by taking the patient down as near as possible to sea level.

Other problems at altitude

People with sickle cell disease (homozygous Hb S, p. 792) are at risk of infarction at 2000 m, which is equivalent to the pressure in a commercial airliner flying at 11 000 m. Heterozygotes can normally tolerate altitudes of 3000 m or more. Patients with myocardial disease should not ascend rapidly above 2000 m.

DISORDERS RELATED TO CHANGES IN BAROMETRIC PRESSURE (DYSBARISM)

At sea level the barometric pressure is 760 mmHg, or one atmosphere. Under water, pressure rises by one atmosphere for every 10 m of depth. Following Boyle's Law, the volume of enclosed gas varies inversely with the surrounding pressure. This pressure/volume effect accounts for most diving pathology. As the greatest *changes* in pressure happen at shallow depths, many of the problems associated with diving occur at shallow depths.

BAROTITIS ('MIDDLE-EAR SQUEEZE')

'Middle-ear squeeze' is the commonest injury of divers. Barosinusitis ('sinus squeeze') is less common.

Unless air is allowed into the middle ear to equalise pressure, the lining becomes oedematous, then haemorrhagic and the tympanic membrane may rupture at depths of 1–2 m. Rarely the round or oval window may rupture, causing severe vertigo, tinnitus and deafness. Both forms of squeeze, and reverse squeezes during decompression, also occur during air travel, especially in babies and those with upper respiratory tract disease.

Middle-ear squeeze is prevented by Valsalva manoeuvre, or by ascending in response to pain, and is treated with decongestants such as 1% ephedrine nasal drops.

SHALLOW WATER BLACKOUT

Swimmers and free divers (snorkelling without compressed air) may hyperventilate deliberately before submerging in order to drive off CO_2 and so reduce the stimulus to breathe. The raised ambient pressure maintains a high arterial O_2 tension, but this falls profoundly when the diver is eventually forced to surface. The resulting cerebral hypoxia is made worse by cerebral vasoconstriction induced by the low $PaCO_2$, and can result in unconsciousness and drowning.

PULMONARY BAROTRAUMA

This occurs in scuba divers breathing compressed air. On ascending from a depth of 10 m to the surface the lung volume doubles. Unless air is driven off by repeated exhalation, the alveoli become over-pressurised and rupture. This can happen in dives of no more than 2 m.

Clinical features
Air from ruptured alveoli may escape in one of three ways and cause:

- interstitial emphysema in the chest, neck or retroperitoneal space with pain, crepitus, impaired venous return and characteristic radiographic appearances
- pneumothorax
- air embolism. Air leaks into the pulmonary capillaries, reaches the coronary or cerebral arteries, impairs local circulation, increases capillary permeability and precipitates intravascular coagulation.

The clinical condition is usually evident within minutes of surfacing, and varies from minor changes of mood to apnoea, coma and cardiac arrhythmia.

Management
Treatment requires recompression in a recompression chamber. While transporting the patient supine to the treatment centre it is important to maintain a good airway, administer 100% oxygen, treat any dysrhythmia, treat hypotension with fluids and dopamine 2–5 μg per min by i.v. infusion and control seizures with diazepam. Air embolism is one of the commonest causes of death among divers.

DECOMPRESSION SICKNESS

This is known as 'the bends'. The amount of gas dissolved in tissue depends upon the partial pressure of that gas in a mixture of gases, the ambient pressure and the duration under pressure. Tissue metabolism removes oxygen from dissolved inhaled air. Therefore, during a long deep dive, dissolved nitrogen accumulates in tissues, especially fatty tissues, a process known as 'on-gassing'. When that tissue is saturated, bubbles form. As pressures fall during ascent, saturation levels are easily

reached. Gas bubbles are released ('off-gassing') and cause decompression sickness.

Symptoms are usually evident within an hour of surfacing and rarely start later than 4 hours after surfacing (see information box).

FEATURES OF DECOMPRESSION ILLNESS

Musculoskeletal
- Cause: gas released into muscle, skin and lymphatics
- Effects: pain in limbs, pruritus, marbled skin, painful lymph nodes, lymphoedema

Neurological
- Cause: gas released into central nervous system and other organs
- Effects: pain in head, neck and abdomen, paraesthesiae, dermatomal numbness and pain, paraplegia, bowel and bladder disturbance, other CNS changes, vestibular damage ('the staggers'), chest pain and dyspnoea ('the chokes')

Treatment of decompression sickness is by recompression. Prompt treatment usually leads to complete recovery, but delayed treatment may result in permanent disability. Those with neurologic or pulmonary signs benefit from the emergency measures described for gas embolism, plus generous intravenous fluid replacement, during transport to the treatment centre.

DISORDERS RELATED TO POLLUTION

The environment, external, at home or at work, may contribute to risks of diseases in which the environmental contribution is not easily recognised in the individual patient, for instance chronic bronchitis or cancer. Occasionally environmental factors cause a distinctive clinical illness which may suggest the cause. The emphasis in this section is on disease resulting from the general or home environment, since an adequate description of occupational diseases is not possible here.

AIR POLLUTION

The major air pollutants are particles and the gases sulphur dioxide, nitrogen dioxide, ozone and other photochemical oxidants, and carbon monoxide.

Nitrogen dioxide
The major source of man-made emissions is the combustion of fossil fuels, particularly by power stations and motor vehicles. Nitric oxide (NO), the main constituent of these emissions, reacts with atmospheric oxidants such as ozone to form nitrogen dioxide (NO_2). Emis-

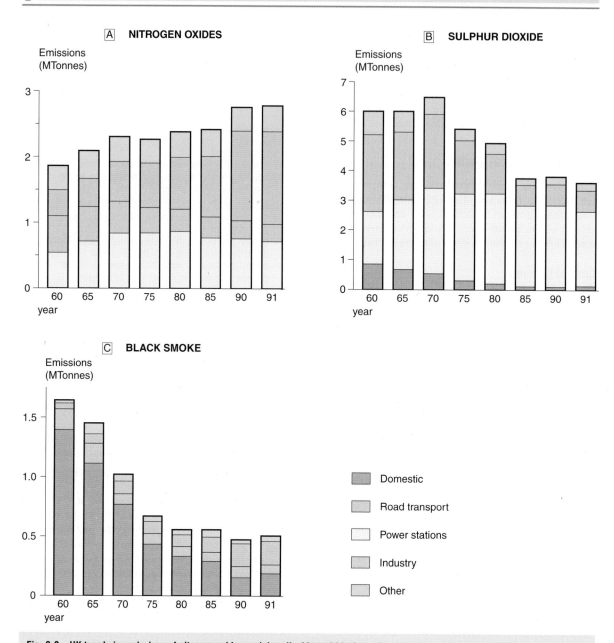

Fig. 3.3 UK trends in emissions of nitrogen oxides, sulphur dioxide and black smoke. Reproduced with permission from the Lung and Asthma Information Agency Factsheet 93/5, Trends in outdoor air pollution in the UK.

sions of nitrogen oxides (Fig. 3.3) have increased over recent decades, mainly as a consequence of increases in road transport. The introduction of catalytic converters will reduce future emissions from motor vehicles. Local generation of nitrogen oxides occurs during the manufacture of nitric acid, by explosives and by welding processes.

Sulphur dioxide and black smoke

Sulphur dioxide (SO_2) is created by burning fossil fuels containing sulphur. SO_2 may be further oxidised to SO_3 and form sulphuric acid on contact with water. Power stations are now the main source of emissions, although coal-burning industrial incinerators and other industrial processes may make local contributions. Emission levels are declining (Fig. 3.3) and this trend is likely to continue.

Diesel vehicles are now the major source of black smoke (small particles produced by incomplete combustion) following the decline in coal burning. Although overall emissions have dropped considerably (Fig. 3.3), emissions from diesel vehicles are increasing.

Ozone

Ground level ozone is a 'secondary' pollutant, being formed by atmospheric photochemical reactions and catalysed by volatile organic compounds. Ozone production may occur at considerable distances from precursor substances and it is particularly dependent on weather conditions, especially intense sunlight.

Carbon monoxide

The largest sources of carbon monoxide emissions are incomplete combustion processes, such as motor vehicles, industrial processes and incinerators. Tobacco smoking is usually the dominant contributor to carbon monoxide toxicity in those who smoke.

Although in the UK the underlying trend for toxic gaseous emissions is downwards it is important to recognise that there may be local variations. For example, levels of NO_2 and SO_2 tend to be higher in urban areas, whereas ozone concentrations tend to be higher in rural areas. Furthermore, daily pollution levels may deviate substantially from average values (Fig. 3.4).

Health effects

Temperature strongly influences daily mortality from cardiorespiratory disease, and adverse effects of some air pollutants can also be demonstrated. Winter smog comprises particulates, sulphur dioxide and sulphuric acid, and can cause an increase in mortality in subjects already suffering from chronic cardiorespiratory disease. Examples include 4,000 deaths in the London smogs of 1952 due to coal combustion, and episodes in West Germany in 1985 and 1987, where pollutants from industrial sources to the east were transported several hundred kilometres on the wind. Such high levels of pollution are now relatively rare in Europe but evidence of fluctuations in mortality in relation to lower levels of pollution are being evaluated. Non-fatal effects include temporary changes in lung function, exacerbations of symptoms of chronic bronchitis and asthma, and increases in hospital admissions for respiratory and cardiovascular conditions.

In summer smog, ozone and other oxidants may acutely cause eye, nose and throat irritation, chest discomfort, cough and headache, with small impairments of lung function. Athletic performance may be impaired.

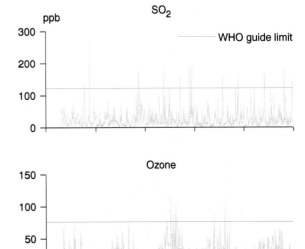

Fig. 3.4 Daily maximum hourly levels of SO_2 and ozone in central London. Reproduced with permission from the Lung and Asthma Information Agency Factsheet 93/5, Trends in outdoor air pollution in the UK. ppb = parts per billion.

Exposure to very high levels of nitrogen dioxide, as in silo-fillers' disease or through shot-firing in mines, can lead to pulmonary oedema and sometimes obliterative bronchiolitis. It is uncertain whether the concentrations found in the general environment, or in homes where gas cookers are used, influence health adversely. The level of nitrogen dioxide does influence the formation of photochemical oxidants, including ozone, in the presence of sunlight.

When exposure to carbon monoxide leads to blood carboxy haemoglobin levels in the range 3–10%, the effect will be to reduce work capacity in healthy young adults, aggravate angina symptoms during exercise, and impair mental vigilance. Higher levels additionally may cause headache, dizziness, fibrinolysis, and in pregnant women, reduced fetal birth weight and retarded postnatal development.

Prevention and management

Prevention is by long-term control of industrial pollution. Susceptible subjects may reduce their exposure to sulphur dioxide or ozone by staying at home. Indoor concentrations of fine particulates tend to be much lower than outdoor levels. Reduction of physical activity out of doors prevents excessive inhalation of pollutants due to hyperventilation. Restricting traffic may have only modest beneficial effects on ozone and other levels in the short term, and has led to the overloading of public transport systems with consequent longer exposures out of doors. Treatment is that of asthma or chronic bronchitis or carbon monoxide poisoning, as indicated.

Furthermore, patients with common respiratory illnesses, including asthma and chronic bronchitis, are particularly vulnerable to the adverse effects of pollution and need to be warned when high levels of pollution are anticipated.

At work, a variety of local sources can generate harmful airborne pollution. Numerous chemical or biological agents may be inhaled as dusts, liquid droplets or gases, and may cause acute rhinitis, pharyngitis, tracheobronchitis, pulmonary oedema, asthma, chronic airflow obstruction, pneumoconiosis, infections or cancers. In the UK employers are legally required to assess and control risks of exposure to chemical substances.

LEAD POISONING

In the general population the major source of lead is usually in food and drink. In industry, inhalation of contaminated air may be more important. The major sources of lead in the environment are fuel additives released in automobile emissions, and from various industrial sources. Lead is deposited near roads and in the vicinity of lead smelters, or where discarded battery cases are burned. Other sources include lead water pipes and tanks, and storage of food, wine or beverages in lead-soldered cans or pottery in which lead in the glaze and pigments has not been adequately stabilised; or illicit whisky made in stills improvised from discarded automobile radiators. Children are particularly at risk if they chew and eat lead-based paint from old houses or the soil around these houses.

The earliest effects of lead are interference with the enzymes responsible for manufacturing haemoglobin, with resulting anaemia.

Clinical features
Symptoms may include fatigue and lassitude, generalised aches and pains in muscles and joints, abdominal discomfort, diarrhoea or a bad taste in the mouth. Severely affected patients may have abdominal pains, colic, constipation and a motor peripheral neuropathy. In extreme cases renal tubular damage and encephalopathy occur, particularly in children. Blue lines on the gum margins and radiographic lead lines on long bones are rare, except in children.

Investigations
Laboratory investigations show an elevated blood lead (whole blood, the lead is almost all bound to red cells)

and increased urinary concentrations of aminolaevulinic acid (ALA) and coproporphyrin. Red cell concentrations of ALA dehydratase are decreased. Normal blood lead levels increase with age in children, for example, an average value of about 3 μg/100 ml is to be found in the first year of life to about 13 μg/100 ml on average for ages between 4 and 13 years. Adult levels are between 10 and 25 μg/100 ml, irrespective of age. The no-effect level for anaemia is between 50 and 100 μg/100 ml (40 μg/100 ml in iron-deficient children). For noticeable brain dysfunction the level is about 50–60 μg/100 ml in children, 60–70 μg/100 ml in adults. There is currently a debate on the influence of intermediate blood lead levels on intellectual ability in children.

Management
Treatment consists of prompt removal from exposure, and supportive measures which in severe cases may include treatment of seizures with diazepam (0.5% solution, 10–20 mg, at rate of 0.5 ml (2.5 mg) per 30 s), maintenance of fluid and electrolyte balance, and treatment of cerebral oedema with dexamethasone (10 mg intravenously followed by 4 mg intramuscularly every 6 h for 2–10 days) and mannitol (50–200 g i.v. over 24 h). Chelation therapy should be instituted in symptomatic patients or those with blood levels greater than 100 μg/100 ml. Edetate calcium sodium (up to 40 mg/kg twice daily intravenously in 0.9% NaCl infusion), and dimercaprol (2.5–3 mg/kg intramuscularly every 4 h for 2 days and then reduced dose) are used parenterally, and penicillamine orally.

As with other occupational or environmental diseases, when lead poisoning is diagnosed, the Employment Medical Adviser, or Environmental Health Officer (whichever is appropriate to the source of the poisoning) should be informed so that others may be protected against the hazard.

MERCURY POISONING

The major environmental source of mercury is the natural degassing of the earth's crust. Sources of additional production by man include burning of fossil fuels, production of steel, cement and phosphate, and the smelting of metals from their sulphide ores. Food is the main route of entry in non-occupational exposures, since methyl mercury compounds accumulate in fish, to high levels in contaminated waters. Outbreaks of chronic mercury poisoning in the general population occurred in the villages round Minamata Bay, and on the Niigata River, in Japan. In both circumstances mercury compounds from local industry had contaminated the water and fish. Over a thousand cases of chronic mercury poisoning were identified. Other epidemics have occurred due to ethyl or methyl mercury fungicides on wheat intended for planting but actually used for making bread. The largest of these was in Iraq, when over 6000 people were admitted to hospital.

Clinical features

The most common signs and symptoms of chronic mercury poisoning are paraesthesia, constriction of the visual fields, impairment of hearing and ataxia. Classical symptoms of severe poisoning include erethism (irritability, excitability, loss of memory, insomnia, excessive sweating and flushing), intention tremor and gingivitis. Renal damage may occur. The clinical effects may not reverse much even after exposure ceases. Acute mercury poisoning due to the ingestion of large amounts of any mercurial compound leads to bleeding from, and necrosis of, the gut, vomiting, circulatory collapse and renal failure. Acute pulmonary oedema may result from the inhalation of mercury vapour.

Management

Chronic inorganic mercury poisoning

This is treated with dimercaprol for high exposures or symptomatic patients, or penicillamine for lower exposures or asymptomatic patients. Haemodialysis may be required for renal failure in occasional cases.

Acute poisoning

This may require respiratory support, attention to fluid and electrolyte balance, gastric lavage, oral charcoal (5–10 g in 100–200 ml water repeated every 15–20 min) and a magnesium cathartic. Treatment of organic mercury poisoning is less effective. Penicillamine (1–2 g daily orally in divided doses before food) and an oral non-absorbable thiol resin can reduce blood concentrations of mercury, though this may not be associated with much clinical benefit. Dimercaprol is contraindicated, since it increases the mercury concentrations in the brain.

FLUOROSIS

Skeletal fluorosis occurs endemically in some tropical and sub-tropical areas with high fluoride concentrations in soil and water. In non-endemic areas it may occur as a result of occupational exposure in aluminium production, magnesium foundries, fluorspar processing and superphosphate manufacture. The bones become sclerotic, and calcification occurs in other organs.

Clinical features

In children the more severe effects include genu valgus and varum, lateral bowing of the femora, sabre shins, deformities of ribs, thorax, vertebral bodies, pelvis and joints. Milder forms include mottling of the teeth. In adults, occupational exposure may lead to increased bone density and thickening of long bones, the development of exostoses and osteophytes (e.g. calcaneal spur); calcification in ligaments, tendons and muscle insertions, polyarthralgia and arthroses. The spine may become rigid and contractures of hips and knees may occur. Occupational exposure to leaks of fluorides or hydrofluoric acid may cause severe acute illness, with skin and eye burns, acute tracheobronchitis and pulmonary oedema, and hypocalcaemia due to consumption of calcium converted to calcium fluoride.

Management

No treatment is effective for fluorosis. The effects of leaks of fluoride should be treated with calcium gluconate (gel locally, and by injection).

POLYCHLORINATED BIPHENYLS

Polychlorinated biphenyls (PCBs) are liquids, first manufactured in the 1930s, which have become widely distributed in the environment, particularly in water, fish and fish-eating birds, and in soils near sources of contamination. PCBs have been used for their electrical insulating properties in transformers, capacitors (even in some domestic equipment), heat transfer and cooling systems, hydraulic systems and vacuum pumps, and a variety of other uses. Use of PCBs has now been restricted or stopped in numerous countries, but certain occupational groups are still exposed, notably in the handling of chemical wastes, dealing with fires or accidents, working in or cleaning contaminated areas or servicing and dismantling old electrical apparatus; and the public in the vicinity of incinerators are at risk if the burning temperature is not high enough. Low levels of PCBs can be detected in many members of most industrial populations, and are concentrated in human milk. Poisoning by PCBs has been recognised as a result of occupational exposure, and in outbreaks in the general population such as occurred in Japan (Yusho disease), and in Taiwan, due to contamination of rice oil.

Clinical features

The most striking effects are hypersecretion of tears, pigmentation and acneiform eruptions of the skin (chloracne, also caused by dioxins), and persistent productive cough. Headaches and other non-specific central nervous system disturbances occur, as do paraesthesiae, liver damage and immunosuppression. Some deaths have occurred, mostly from liver disease, including hepatoma. Babies of exposed mothers are small and pigmented, and fetal deaths and abnormalities were common in the Yusho outbreak. Acute exposure irritates the eyes, skin and respiratory tract.

Management

Treatment consists of withdrawal from exposure, and general supportive measures. No specific treatment is available.

ENVIRONMENTAL RADIATION

Natural sources dominate exposure of the general population to radiation, and the variations in this contribution are much larger than the total dose from man-made sources. Radiation of natural origin includes cosmic radiation, gamma rays from the earth's crust, emissions from rock and soil of radon and thoron gases (which can accumulate in houses, particularly in granite rock areas), and other radionuclides ingested in air, food and water.

Man-made environmental radiation comprises fallout from atomic weapons testing in the atmosphere in the 1950s and 1960s (mainly carbon 14, strontium 90 and caesium 137). These levels were declining until 1986 when the reactor accident at Chernobyl nuclear power station in the Western Ukraine released substantial quantities of radionuclide to the atmosphere, eventually resulting in widespread contamination throughout the whole of the Northern Hemisphere. These radionuclides can be incorporated in the food chains. Controlled discharges from nuclear installations also make a small contribution. Radiation risks from medical procedures, or from occupational sources, can be relatively high in some individuals.

Health effects

The early effects of acute radiation exposure are summarised in Table 3.4. Survivors of high-dose radiation, for example following the Hiroshima and Nagasaki atomic bombs, are known to have a high incidence of leukaemias and solid tumours, particularly of thyroid and lung. Health effects from low-dose environmental radiation are more difficult to demonstrate. Some studies of populations downwind of nuclear weapons test sites have reported small excesses of leukaemia, though the figures are not consistent and might be the result of other factors. Some clusters of leukaemia in children living near nuclear installations making controlled discharges have been reported, but the estimates of radiation exposures are too low to explain this, on currently accepted risk estimates. Some of the clusters may be chance, others, it has been suggested, are the result of changes in exposures to infectious agents, as a result of large local influxes of workers.

The Chernobyl accident is expected to result in a detectable increase in cancer in the Commonwealth of Independent States population, and possibly a detectable increase in those evacuated from the high exposure areas. In radiation workers and people living in areas of high natural background radiation, increases in frequency of chromosomal aberrations have been noted, and excesses of lung cancer have been observed in workers in uranium and salt mines.

BUILDING SICKNESS SYNDROME

This benign syndrome occurs in workers in modern air-conditioned offices. The cause(s) are unknown, but relevant factors may include fluctuating temperatures, possibly variations in humidity, the cyclical flashing of fluorescent lights, low levels of volatile organic chemicals such as formaldehyde or solvents, and psychological factors.

There are various combinations of itching, burning and discomfort of the eyes, nasal stuffiness, discomfort in the throat, headache, dryness of the skin and lethargy.

Table 3.4 Radiation Injury

| | Radiation dose | | | |
	1–2 Gy	2–5 Gy	5–10 Gy	10–20 Gy
Mortality	0%	0–80% (2 months)	80–100% (1–2 months)	100% (2 weeks)
Critical period	—	4–6 weeks	4–6 weeks	5–15 days
Vomiting	5–50% (3 hrs)	> 3 Gy 100% (2 hrs)	100% (1 hr)	100% (30 mins)
Main organ damage	Lymphocytes	Bone marrow	Bone marrow	Bone marrow and small bowel
Symptoms and signs	Moderate leucopenia	Leucopenia, purpura, haemorrhage, hair loss	Leucopenia, purpura, haemorrhage, hair loss	Diarrhoea, fever, electrolyte imbalance
Therapy	Observation	Antibiotics	Antibiotics, blood component transfusion, bone marrow transplant	Fluid and electrolytes, possible bone marrow transplant

Symptoms are worse in the second half of the working shift, and towards the end of the week, and are more common in females. They resolve rapidly on leaving the building.

No specific treatment is required, though alterations in the office environment may be helpful.

Contamination of air-conditioning systems has also occasionally been associated with asthma, humidifier fever, extrinsic allergic alveolitis, and some infections, notably legionnaires disease. These are not generally classified as building sickness syndrome.

FURTHER READING

Delaney K A 1992 Heatstroke: underlying processes and lifesaving management. Postgraduate Medicine 91: 379–388

Honigman B, Theis M K, Kaziol-McLain J, Roach R, Yip R et al 1993 Acute mountain sickness in a general tourist population at moderate altitudes. Annals of Internal Medicine 118: 587–592

Keating W R 1991 Hypothermia: dead or alive? Some patients deserve heroic measures. Lancet 1: 3–4

Margalies A D C 1987 A short course in diving medicine. Annals of Emergency Medicine 16: 689–701

National Research Council Committee on the Biological Effects of Ionising Radiations 1990 Health Effects of exposure to low levels of ionising radiation (BEIR V). National Academy Press, Washington, DC

Parry E H O (ed) 1984 The Principles of Medicine in Africa, 2nd edn. Oxford University Press, Oxford.

Pickering C A C 1989 Building sickness syndrome. Respiratory Medicine 83: 91–92

Reeves J T, Welsh C H, Wagner P D 1994 The heart and lungs at extreme altitude. Thorax 49: 631–633

Utell M J, Samet J M 1993 Particulate air pollution and health. New evidence on an old problem. American Review of Respiratory Disease 147: 1334–1335

A. M. Geddes, A. D. M. Bryceson, R. N. Thin, D. M. Mitchell

4

Diseases due to infection

Infection can involve any organ or system of the body and thus embraces all medical disciplines. In this chapter an introduction is given to the general aspects, epidemiology, diagnosis, prevention and treatment of infection as well as descriptions of individual infectious diseases. Infections involving specific organs or systems are described in the appropriate chapters.

Infection differs from other diseases in a number of aspects. The most important is that it is caused by living microorganisms which can usually be identified, thus establishing the aetiology early in the illness. Many of these organisms, including all bacteria, are sensitive to antibiotics and most infections are potentially curable, unlike many non-infectious diseases which are degenerative and frequently become chronic. Communicability is another factor which differentiates infections from non-infectious diseases. Transmission of pathogenic organisms to other people, directly or indirectly, may lead to an epidemic. Finally, many infections are preventable by hygienic measures, by vaccines or by the judicious use of drugs (chemoprophylaxis).

PATTERNS OF INFECTION

Pattern of infection in developed countries

In the twentieth century there has been a dramatic fall in the incidence of communicable diseases in developed countries. This is due to factors such as immunisation, antimicrobial chemotherapy, improved nutrition, and better sanitation and housing. Infectious diseases which have decreased, and in some instances almost disappeared, include diphtheria, poliomyelitis and tetanus. Smallpox, a lethal virus infection, has been eradicated from the world while another lethal infection, human immunodeficiency virus infection, has emerged.

The pattern of infection in developed countries during the past two decades has been influenced by a number of factors (Table 4.1). These include the development of microbial resistance, immunosuppression, foreign travel, altered sexual behaviour, drug addiction, changes in animal husbandry and food production, the availability and uptake of vaccines, and the discovery of new microorganisms. Certain infections which had decreased or come under control are again emerging (resurgent infections), e.g. tuberculosis.

Patterns of infection in tropical countries

In less advanced countries, however, especially in the tropics, infection continues to be one of the commonest causes of disease and death, particularly in children, and determines the strength of the working man, the health of the mother and the pattern of systemic disease in the community, including neoplasia. Multiple disease

Table 4.1 Influences on patterns of infection in *developed* countries

Vaccines
Improved uptake of vaccines
New vaccines, e.g. *Haemophilus influenzae* type B and hepatitis A.

Animal husbandry and preparation of food
Salmonella and campylobacter infections originating in poultry and eggs. *Escherichia coli* type 0157 causing haemorrhagic colitis associated with beef.
Listeria infections from soft cheeses.

Microbial resistance
Increased resistance in common bacterial pathogens including *Staphylococcus aureus* (MRSA), Gram-negative bacilli, *Streptococcus pneumoniae* and *Mycobacterium tuberculosis*.

Sexual behaviour
Increase in HIV infection and other sexually transmitted diseases.

International travel
Importation of malaria (50,000 cases in Europe in 1991)
Legionnaires' disease from holiday hotels.
HIV infection.

Immunosuppression
Advances in the treatment of malignant disease and in organ transplantation leading to infections with opportunistic organisms.

Resurgence of infections
Tuberculosis—world-wide especially in association with HIV infection.
Poliomyelitis in the Netherlands (in a religious sect refusing vaccines).
Streptococcal infections in the USA (including rheumatic fever).
Measles in the USA (mainly in immigrants in inner cities).
Diphtheria in the former Soviet Union.
Hepatitis A and typhoid fever in the former Yugoslavia.

entities are the rule and the clinical patterns of illness differ in many ways from those in temperate zones. The complex interaction between chronic parasitism, respiratory and diarrhoeal diseases, tuberculosis, malnutrition and its immunosuppressive effects, and HIV infection, pose special problems for the health of children. Up to 40% of children may die before they reach 5 years of age.

Chronic infections do serious damage to important organs, such as liver and kidneys in schistosomiasis, the heart in trypanosomiasis cruzi, the lungs, bones and lymph nodes in tuberculosis, the bone marrow reserves in malaria and hookworm infections, the gut in tropical sprue and the nerves in leprosy. These organs may then fail if the demand upon them is increased through work, pregnancy or additional disease. Such diseases impose chronic ill health on millions of children and adults in the tropics.

Many of the decimating diseases of the past are controllable by vaccination (yellow fever), vector control (malaria and sleeping sickness) and general improvement in living standards (plague and relapsing fever), but control is imperfect and the diseases reappear. Other epidemic diseases such as cholera in Asia and meningococcal meningitis in Africa remain largely uncontrolled, and kill hundreds of thousands of people annually. Efficient vaccines exist for many diseases such as poliomyelitis, measles, rubella, meningitis and tetanus, but in many countries they have made little impact because of cost and the practical difficulty in delivering them.

Development, especially in the form of dams and irrigation, has often encouraged the spread of vector-borne disease such as malaria and schistosomiasis, while the exploitation of the Amazonian forests has caused mutilating outbreaks of mucocutaneous leishmaniasis. Migration to urban slums increases the risk of gastrointestinal disease and tuberculosis and of 'Western' diseases such as hypertension, and in many countries has contributed materially to the AIDS epidemic which is wreaking havoc in developing countries, especially in Africa, the Indian sub-continent and South-East Asia.

Finally, in developing countries infectious diseases are frequently associated with natural disasters such as drought, flooding and earthquakes as well as with war and revolution.

Table 4.2 illustrates patterns of infection in tropical countries.

MICROORGANISM-HOST INTERACTIONS

Effects of infection on the body

Infection has many effects on the body. These are summarised in Table 4.3 and may be acute, chronic or allergic. Chronic effects are seen especially in children in tropical countries.

Pathology of infection

Disease due to infection is the result of interaction between a microorganism and the defence mechanisms of the body. The outcome of this interaction can range from no demonstrable effect to death, and will depend on the number and virulence of the organisms, the physiological and anatomical effects that they induce and the effectiveness of the natural defences.

The mechanisms by which microorganisms cause disease are summarised in the information box and discussed in other sections of this book. Organisms act directly and/or through their toxins. Many of these effects are general, but some act at certain anatomical sites, for example poliomyelitis virus in anterior horn cells, hepatitis virus in hepatocytes, pneumococcus in the lung alveoli, and tetanus and diphtheria toxins at nerve terminals.

Shock is an especial problem in severe infections. Its aetiology is complex and results from reduced systemic vascular resistance brought about by dilated small ves-

---

Table 4.2 Patterns of infection in tropical countries

Killers of children, preventable but variably prevalent
Measles
Diphtheria
Pertussis
Poliomyelitis
Tetanus
Hepatitis B
Gastroenteritis
Malaria

Chronic disabling infections, widely prevalent
Leprosy
Tuberculosis
Trachoma
Malaria
Trypanosomiasis cruzi
Amoebiasis
Intestinal helminths
Schistosomiasis
Filarial infection

Epidemic diseases, actual* and potential
Louse-borne typhus and relapsing fever
Cholera*
Malaria
Visceral leishmaniasis*
Human immunodeficiency virus infection*
Tuberculosis*, in association with HIV epidemic
Influenza

Infections liable to focal outbreaks (zoonotic or vector-borne)
Dengue fever, e.g. Thailand
Plague, e.g. Vietnam
Cutaneous leishmaniasis, e.g. Sudan
African trypanosomiasis, e.g. Zambia
Yellow fever, e.g. Kenya, Nigeria
Anthrax

PATHOLOGY OF INFECTION

Microbe mediated	Host mediated
• Direct cell destruction, e.g. poliomyelitis, rabies, hepatitis	• Neutrophils and macrophages
• Exotoxin, e.g. tetanus, cholera, botulism, diphtheria	• Complement activation
• Endotoxin, e.g. typhoid, Gram-negative septicaemia, meningococcal infection	• Activation of clotting cascade
	• Immune mechanisms
	• Secondary autoimmune mechanisms

---

sels and leaky capillaries under the influence of several mediators, which include kinins, complement components, histamine, cytokines and endogenous opiates (see Chapter 2). The commonest cause of shock in infection is endotoxin from Gram-negative bacteria. The cycle of shock, tissue anoxia and organ failure is difficult to break and may kill the patient quickly.

Table 4.3 Clinical effects of infection on the body

Acute
Fever; anorexia, protein catabolism, nitrogen imbalance, acute phase protein response, hypoalbuminaemia, low serum iron, sequestration of iron, anaemia, neutrophilia
Inflammation; pain, dysfunction, tissue damage
Convulsions; especially in children
Shock; sustained fall in circulating blood volume associated with lowered systemic vascular resistance
Haemorrhage; haemolytic anaemia, intravascular coagulation
Organ failure; kidneys, liver, lung, heart, brain

Chronic
Weight loss and muscle wasting
Malnutrition; especially associated with diarrhoea
Retardation of growth and intellect in children
Anaemia; iron sequestration, maturation arrest in marrow, folate deficiency
Tissue destruction; e.g. lung in pneumonia or tuberculosis, nerves in leprosy, liver in hepatitis B
Post-infective syndromes; e.g. lactose intolerance, malabsorption, irritable colon, depression, post-viral fatigue syndrome

Allergic
Rash; e.g. erythema with streptococci, urticaria with helminths, maculopapular in typhoid and endocarditis, erythema nodosum in tuberculosis
Arthritis; e.g. in rheumatic fever, Reiter's syndrome
Pericarditis; e.g. in meningococcal infection
Encephalitis; e.g in measles or following vaccines
Peripheral neuropathy; e.g. in post-infective polyneuritis
Haemolytic anaemia; e.g. in infectious mononucleosis
Nephritis; e.g. in streptococcal infection.

Host response to infection

Non-specific defences

The body has a number of 'natural' antimicrobial defences, especially on the skin and at mucosal surfaces (e.g. lysozyme secretion, gastric acid, intestinal enzymes, vaginal secretions). However, these nonspecific systems are not entirely adequate and pathogenic microorganisms can breach them under conditions such as trauma and intense exposure to pathogens. The colonisation of host tissues by pathogens is then counteracted by the body's immune response. Host immunity is expressed through several different mechanisms which depend upon antigen-specific lymphocytes and their products. Polymorphs and macrophages play an important part in defence against microorganisms, especially bacteria (see pp. 29–30).

Immune response

The immune system has evolved largely to block the access of pathogenic organisms to host tissues and, where this fails, to limit their colonisation and spread. Microorganisms carry molecules which are foreign to the host, and some bacteria secrete toxins. Both antibody and cell-mediated immune mechanisms may be directed against these antigens (see p. 31). T lymphocytes can kill virus-infected cells, and they also secrete a variety of cytokines which attract and promote the antibacterial and antiviral activity of other inflammatory and immune cells (p. 30), particularly macrophages. Eosinophil granulocytes are important in host defence against parasites, e.g. worm infestations. Anti-

bodies can neutralise bacterial toxins and bind to the surface of microorganisms, where they inhibit spread and initiate complement fixation which promotes phagocytosis of microorganisms. The complement membrane attack complex may destroy certain bacteria, especially Gram-negative organisms.

Source and spread of infection

Infection may originate from the patient (autogenous), usually from skin, nasopharynx or bowel, or from outside sources (exogenous), often another person who may either be suffering from an infection or carrying a pathogenic microorganism. Carriers are usually healthy and may harbour the organism in the throat (for example diphtheria), bowel (salmonella) or blood (hepatitis B or HIV). Non-human sources of infection include water (cholera), milk (tuberculosis), food (botulism), animals (rabies), birds (psittacosis) and also the soil (Legionnaires' disease).

Microorganisms may be transmitted by several routes. Autogenous infection may develop as a result of local spread, e.g. from bowel to peritoneum, or by the bloodstream. An example of the latter is endocarditis caused by *Streptococcus sanguis* originating in the patient's mouth and entering the blood during dental procedures. Exogenous infection may be acquired directly or indirectly by one of the routes shown in Table 4.4.

Incubation period is the period between the invasion of the tissues by pathogens and the appearance of clinical features of infection. **Period of infectivity** is the time that the patient is infectious to others. Details of the

Table 4.4 Source and spread of infection

SOURCE/ROUTE OF TRANSMISSION	METHOD OF SPREAD	EXAMPLES OF INFECTION
Contact: person to person	Skin or mucous membrane contact	Impetigo, scabies, wound infection, infectious mononucleosis. Sexually transmitted diseases (including HIV & hepatitis B)
soil	Via wounds and abrasions	Tetanus, Buruli ulcer, hookworm, mycetoma
water	Penetration of skin	Schistosomiasis, leptospirosis
Airborne spread	Respiratory droplets or dust	Measles, rubella, whooping cough, scarlet fever, mumps, meningococcal infection. Upper respiratory tract infection, influenza
	Water aerosols	Legionellosis
Faecal/oral spread	Faecal contamination of food or drink	Salmonella infection, bacillary and amoebic dysentery, enteroviral infections, cholera, giardiasis, hepatitis A, campylobacter infection
Transplacental	Maternal blood	Rubella, CMV infection, toxoplasmosis, syphilis, malaria, HIV infection
Medical and nursing procedures	Needles, ventilators, infusion fluid	Hepatitis B, staphylococcal infection, pseudomonas infection
Zoonoses (Animal, fish or bird to man)	Beef or pork	Tapeworms, toxoplasmosis, trichinella infection
	Poultry or eggs	Salmonellosis
	Milk	Tuberculosis, campylobacter infection, brucellosis
	Cheese	Listeriosis, brucellosis
	Rats' or dogs' urine	Leptospirosis, Lassa fever
	Dogs' faeces	Toxocara infection, hydatid disease
	Dog bite	Rabies
	Birds	Psittacosis
	Fish	Tapeworms, mycobacterial infections
Arthropods (see Table 4.49)		

incubation periods of major infections and periods of infectivity in childhood infectious diseases are summarised in Tables 21.10 and 21.11, pp. 1154–1155.

MAJOR MANIFESTATIONS OF INFECTION

A knowledge of infections prevailing in the locality is an essential guide to diagnosis especially with imported infections, as is a knowledge of where and how to find the relevant organism. Enquiry should be made about contacts among family, friends and workmates. Persons following certain occupations may be exposed to infection, e.g. leptospirosis occurs in abattoir and farm workers and anthrax in handlers of hides and bone meal.

A recent history of laparotomy or of obscure abdominal pain should suggest subphrenic or intrahepatic abscess as a cause of unexplained fever.

Residence or travel abroad raises the possibility of malaria, amoebic abscess of the liver or other exotic disease. In many infections a diagnosis can often be made on clinical features, e.g. measles or chickenpox. In others, a diagnosis may require confirmation by microbiological, immunological, haematological, histo-

pathological or radiological investigations; see Table 4.5.

BACTERAEMIA AND SEPTICAEMIA

Bacteraemia, the presence of living organisms in the blood, can occur in healthy people without causing symptoms. For example, viridans streptococci may transiently enter the blood during dental procedures or even when teeth are cleaned vigorously. Unless there is a focus on which they can settle and multiply, e.g. an abnormal heart valve, these organisms are normally cleared rapidly from the blood by the body's defence mechanisms. Other organisms invading the bloodstream such as *Staphylococcus aureus* or *Escherichia coli* are less likely to be dealt with by the immune system and more likely to cause disease; this is referred to as septicaemia.

The organisms causing septicaemia may originate from one of the areas of the body which are normally colonised by microorganisms, such as skin, large bowel or genital tract. Alternatively, the source may be infection in a major organ such as kidney or liver.

Septicaemia can be complicated by metastatic septic lesions in organs or tissues. Examples include staphylococcal osteomyelitis, pnemococcal pneumonia and

Table 4.5   Methods used to diagnose infection

MICROBIOLOGICAL

[A]   **Recognition of causative agent**

1. In stained or fresh preparations, usually a smear*: malaria in blood slide, *Vibrio cholerae* in stool, diphtheria in throat swab, bacilli in urine, staphylococci in pus smear, entamoeba in rectal scrape, plague bacilli in buboe aspirate, schistosome ova in rectal snip, rickettsia in rash aspirate[+], fungi in skin scrapings, pneumococci in purulent sputum, spirochaetes in condylomata (dark ground microscopy), leprosy bacilli and leishmania in slit skin smear.

2. By electron microscopy: viruses in stool; herpes viruses in skin.

3. By histology of biopsy specimen: acid-fast bacilli in leprosy and tuberculosis, pneumocystis in pneumonia, hepatitis B in liver[+], rabies virus in brain[+].

[B]   **Culture of causative organism**

1. From blood: typhoid, brucellosis, Gram-negative septicaemia, pneumococcal pneumonia, HIV.

2. From bone marrow: tuberculosis, brucellosis, leishmaniasis, histoplasmosis.

3. From other body fluids, faeces or tissues: urinary tract infection, bacillary dysentery, sputum in pneumonia, liver in tuberculosis.

IMMUNOLOGICAL

[A]   **Detection of microbial antigen**
Meningococcal and pneumococcal disease (blood, CSF, sputum, urine).

[B]   **Detection of antibody of IgM class**
Toxoplasmosis, hepatitis A.

[C]   **Demonstration of antibody**

1. Rising titre: typhoid, brucellosis, HIV infection.

2. Closely linked to clinical syndrome: amoebic abscess, visceral leishmaniasis.

3. Screening for latent disease: syphilis, schistosomiasis, trypanosomiasis cruzi.

[D]   **Delayed hypersensitivity skin testing**
Tuberculosis, histoplasmosis, leishmaniasis.

NON-SPECIFIC

[A]   **Tissue biopsy**

1. Characteristic histology: hepatitis, leprosy.

2. Suggestive histology: tuberculosis, toxoplasmosis.

[B]   **Radiology**
Association of site and pattern with infection: lobar pneumonia, renal tuberculosis, muscular cysticercosis.

[C]   **Scanning**

1. Isotope: detection of abscess, osteomyelitis.

2. Ultrasound: abscess, hydatid cyst.

3. CT or MRI; intracranial infection, deep abscesses, mediastinal lymph node enlargement.

---

* Most of these are simple side room techniques which clinicians should be able to perform
[+] Usually performed using immunofluorescent staining

---

meningococcal meningitis. Figure 4.1 outlines common sources of septicaemia, the causative organisms and examples of metastatic lesions. Table 4.6 lists organisms cultured from the blood of patients during a period of one year in a large district general hospital.

Circulatory failure—the septic shock syndrome—is the most dangerous complication of septicaemia and is usually caused by the endotoxins produced by Gram-negative bacilli such as *E. coli*. It can also be associated with Gram-positive organisms, particularly pneumococci and streptococci. The clinical features and pathophysiology of septic shock are dealt with in Chapter 5.

Blood cultures are the most important initial investigation in septicaemia (Table 4.6) but if shock develops then tests of hepatic, renal and cardio-pulmonary function and of coagulation must be performed and monitored.

The treatment of septicaemia involves the prompt administration of a broad-spectrum antibiotic or a combination of antibiotics. The choice usually has to be made on an empirical basis before the results of cultures are available. Examples of initial therapy include ceftazidime alone or an aminoglycoside such as gentamicin plus a β-lactam antibiotic, e.g. azlocillin.

Shock is managed as described on page 212.

INFECTION IN IMMUNOCOMPROMISED PATIENTS

The term 'immunocompromised' refers to individuals whose resistance to infection has been reduced by disease (congenital or acquired) or by therapeutic measures such as the treatment of malignant disease or organ transplantation. Increased susceptibility to infection may result from a defect in the immune system and/or neutropenia.

The infection may be endogenous, i.e. arising from within the patient, or exogenous. Endogenous infection may be due to invasion of tissues or organs by bacteria, e.g. *E. coli*, or by fungi such as *Candida albicans* which are present in health in the patient's gastrointestinal tract, or by reactivation of organisms which have remained dormant since primary infection earlier in life. Examples of latent organisms which can cause infection in immunocompromised patients include the herpes group of viruses (varicella zoster, *Herpes simplex*, Epstein–Barr virus and cytomegalovirus), Mycobacteria, *Toxoplasma gondii* and Leishmania.

Infection is a common cause of death in immunocompromised patients, in whom it may have a fulminating onset or be refractory to therapy. Diagnosis can be difficult as the infections may present atypically, sometimes with very few signs and symptoms until well advanced. Because of the body's reduced defences

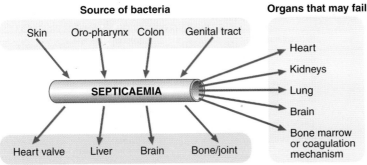

Fig. 4.1 Septicaemia: source of infection, metastatic lesions and complications.

Table 4.6 Number of clinically significant blood culture isolates in a UK district general hospital in 1992

Gram-positive bacteria	
Staphylococcus aureus	68
Streptococcus pneumoniae	59
Staphylococcus epidermidis	26
β-haemolytic streptococci	22
Enterococcus faecalis	9
Enterococcus faecium	7
Viridans streptococci	7
Other organisms	3
Gram-negative bacteria	
Escherichia coli	81
Klebsiella species	27
Proteus species	16
Enterobacter species	11
Neisseria meningitidis	8
Haemophilus influenzae	8
Bacteroides fragilis	7
Pseudomonas aeruginosa	7
Salmonella typhi	7
Xanthomonas maltophila	5
Acinetobacter species	4
Other organisms	10
Mixed cultures (2 or more organisms)	24

against infection, treatment should be started on clinical suspicion, modified according to the results of investigations.

Table 4.7 lists the important organisms causing infections in immunocompromised patients.

RASHES

Rashes are common clinical features of many systemic infectious diseases. They can be classified as maculopapular (discrete or sometimes confluent red spots which can be elevated), nodular, erythematous (a diffuse red eruption which blanches on finger pressure), haemorrhagic, vesicular (associated with blister formation), urticarial or chancres. Certain infections are associated with specific skin lesions which are characteristic of that infection. Table 4.8 gives examples of infections associated with the various types of rashes. Figure 4.2 illustrates the common types of eruption (measles, scarlet fever, chickenpox, meningococcaemia). Drugs, including antibiotics, are a common cause of rashes.

TRAVELLERS' DIARRHOEA

Pathogens which may be responsible for travellers' diarrhoea are shown in the information box. Commonly, no organism is identified.

SOME CAUSES OF TRAVELLERS' DIARRHOEA

- Enterotoxigenic Escherichia coli
- Vibrio parahaemolyticus
- Salmonellae
- Campylobacter jejuni
- Shigellae
- Giardia lamblia
- Vibrio cholerae
- Rota and Norwalk viruses

An attack of diarrhoea lasting 2–5 days commonly affects travellers, particularly when visiting developing countries. The onset is usually abrupt and the stool is watery. Abdominal cramps, anorexia and vomiting are common and there may be fever. Examination of the abdomen usually shows no abnormality but there may be diffuse tenderness.

The disorder usually resolves spontaneously. Antidiarrhoeal agents are best avoided, especially in children, as they may occasionally cause toxic dilation of the bowel. Loperamide 4 mg will stop the diarrhoea if prolonged or very severe. Antibiotics are not necessary for mild attacks, especially as they may induce antibiotic resistance. Severe attacks can be aborted in most cases with two doses of 500 mg of ciprofloxacin 12 hours apart. Dehydration should be prevented by drinking of non-alcoholic fluids and the use of oral rehydration sup-

Table 4.7 Microorganisms causing infections in immunocompromised patients

Defect in host response	Microorganism	Infections (examples)
Phagocytic abnormalities (Polymorphs, macrophages)	*Staph aureus*	Skin, soft tissue
	Strep pneumoniae	Pneumonia
	L. pneumophila	Pneumonia
	Strep pyogenes	Septicaemia
	H. influenzae	Meningitis
	Gram-neg bacilli	Septicaemia
	Candida albicans	Fungaemia
Cell-mediated defects (T cells)	Herpes viruses	Shingles
	Parvovirus	Bone marrow infection
	Candida albicans	Pneumonia
	Cryptococcus	CNS infections
	Mycobacteria	Tuberculosis
	Listeria monocytogenes	Meningitis
	Pneumocystis carinii	Pneumonia
	Toxoplasma gondii	Encephalitis
	Leishmania	Leishmaniasis
	Cryptosporidium	Enteritis
Humoral defects (Immunoglobulins)	*Strep pneumoniae*	Pneumonia
	Strep pyogenes	Septicaemia
	Ps aeruginosa	Septicaemia
	N meningitidis	Meningitis
	H influenzae	Pneumonia

Table 4.8 Patterns of rash associated with infection

Macular or maculo-papular
Measles*
Rubella
Enteroviral infections
Herpesvirus type 6 infections
Infectious mononucleosis
Toxoplasmosis
Cytomegalovirus infections
HIV seroconversion illness
Typhoid and paratyphoid fevers
Rickettsial infections
Dengue fever
Secondary syphilis
Drug rashes

Haemorrhagic
Meningococcal infection*
Viral haemorrhagic fevers
Leptospirosis
Septicaemia with DIC†
Rickettsial infections
Trypanosomiasis

Urticarial
Toxocariasis
Hydatidosis
Fascioliasis
Strongyloidiasis
Schistosomiasis

Vesicular
Chickenpox*
Shingles
Herpes simplex infections
Hand foot and mouth disease
Herpangina (mouth)
Poxviruses (monkeypox)

Nodular
Erythema nodosum
(primary TB and leprosy)

Erythematous
Scarlet fever*
Toxic shock syndrome
Lyme disease
Drug rashes
Dengue fever

Chancres (ulcerating nodules)
Syphilis
Trypanosomiasis
Typhus (tick and mite)
Anthrax
Rat-bite fever

* Rash is illustrated in Fig. 4.2
† Disseminated intravascular coagulation

plements in children, and in adults if the diarrhoea is severe.

The prevention of travellers' diarrhoea involves good hygienic practices, drinking clean water and avoiding uncooked vegetables. Doxycycline 100 mg or trimethoprim 80 mg daily will reduce the attack rate but are best reserved for susceptible individuals.

FEVER IN A PATIENT FROM THE TROPICS

Fever is a common presentation in people who have recently arrived in Britain from tropical countries. The commonest diagnoses are listed in the information box. The most important is malaria, because untreated *Plasmodium falciparum* infection in a non-immune patient (including expatriates and immigrants of over three years' duration) may become rapidly fatal. *P. falciparum* malaria usually presents within two months of arrival but occasionally up to six months, rarely longer. The clinical features of malaria are given on page 148; they may include fever, cough and diarrhoea. The pattern of fever does not distinguish malaria from other imported or domestic fevers such as influenza, but splenomegaly, thrombocytopenia and hyperbilirubinaemia strongly suggest the diagnosis. Asian immigrants are at especial risk of tuberculosis and Africans of HIV infection. Physical examination should be directed especially towards the skin (rashes in meningococcaemia, dengue, rickettsioses, typhoid), chest (bronchitis and pneumonitis are features of malaria and typhoid), lymph glands (toxoplasmosis and sero-conversion illness of infectious mononucleosis and HIV infection), spleen (malaria, typhoid, acute schistosomiasis, leishmaniasis), liver (hepatitis, amoebic abscess) and neck stiffness (meningitis).

The investigation and management of fever from the tropics is shown in the second information box.

CAUSES OF FEVER IMPORTED INTO THE UK*

Frequency	Cause	Percentage
• Common	Malaria	42
	Presumed viral	25
• Frequent	Bacterial: dysentery, upper respiratory tract including diphtheria, pneumonia; urinary tract, typhoid	16
	Proven viral: hepatitis A, HIV, EB virus, aseptic meningitis, dengue	12
• Occasional	Tuberculosis, toxo-plasmosis, rickettsial	3
• Rare	Brucellosis, amoebic abscess, visceral leishmaniasis	2

* As seen at the Hospital for Tropical Diseases, London, 1993

INVESTIGATION AND MANAGEMENT OF FEVER FROM THE TROPICS

On admission
- Thick and thin blood films for malaria; repeat if negative
- Full blood count (neutrophilia, eosinophilia, thrombocytopenia, atypical lymphocytes)
- Cultures of blood × 3 (or bone marrow × 1 if the patient has had an antibiotic), urine, throat swab and stool if diarrhoea
- Liver function tests
- Dip-stick urine for blood, protein, bile
- Store serum for possible serology later
- Consider lumbar puncture for neck stiffness
- Treat clinically diagnosed infection for which there is no rapid confirmatory test (e.g. tick-typhus) or where delay is unjustified (e.g. malaria)

Over the next three days
- Re-examine the patient and look for new signs
- Treat infection diagnosed

After three days
- Reassess: if getting better, wait; if not:
- Repeat initial tests
- Consider chest radiograph, abdominal ultrasound scan
- Consider serology for EB virus, HIV, dengue, rickettsia, toxoplasma, entamoeba, schistosoma, according to clinical and epidemiological situation
- Consider treatment on clinical grounds alone (e.g. getting worse and clinical features suggest typhoid)

After ten days
- Consider more chronic infections (e.g. tuberculosis, brucellosis, HIV, leishmaniasis)
- Consider non-infectious diseases
- Obtain a second opinion

PYREXIA OF UNKNOWN ORIGIN

Patients commonly develop transient febrile illnesses, often caused by viruses, which subside spontaneously and a definitive diagnosis is never made. Other fevers persist but a diagnosis is reached rapidly and treatment started. In a few patients fever persists and defies diagnosis.

The best definition of pyrexia or fever of unknown origin (PUO or FUO) was given by Petersdorf and Beeson in the United States in 1951 in a paper describing the results of a study which they carried out in 100 patients. They defined PUO as a temperature of 38.3°C or above persisting or recurring during a period of three weeks which included seven days' investigation in hospital. Important causes of PUO are illustrated in the information box.

IMPORTANT CAUSES OF PYREXIA OF UNKNOWN ORIGIN

Malignant disease
- Reticuloses (e.g. Hodgkin's disease)
- Hypernephroma

Diseases of connective tissue
- Polyarteritis nodosa
- Still's disease
- Lupus erythematosus

Infections
- Tuberculosis (esp. lymph gland)
- Endocarditis (e.g. Q fever)
- Abscesses (liver, paraspinal, pelvic)
- Malaria (esp. if suppressed by prophylaxis)
- Visceral leishmaniasis

Other causes
- Drug fever (esp. β-lactam antibiotics)
- Factitious fever (self-induced)
- Thrombophlebitis
- Familial Mediterranean fever
- Granulomatous diseases

Petersdorf and Beeson found that only one-third of their patients eventually proved to have an infection (the commonest being tuberculosis). Another third had malignant disease (the commonest being a reticulosis), and one-fifth diseases of connective tissue. The remainder had various less common disorders including factitious fever. This is a condition where an individual, who often has medical or nursing training, mimics pyrexia, for example by placing the thermometer on a radiator; there is usually an underlying psychiatric disorder in these cases. Table 4.9 illustrates the investigation of PUO. Repeated examination for the development of new signs is most important.

Table 4.9 Investigation of pyrexia of unknown origin

RETAKE THE HISTORY
Contact with infection (tuberculosis) or animals (brucellosis)
Sexual contacts (HIV)
Travel abroad (malaria)
Drug therapy (penicillins)
Occupation (leptospirosis)
Recent operations or dental treatment (abscess or endocarditis)

REPEAT THE EXAMINATION
Heart murmurs (endocarditis)
Splenomegaly (visceral leishmaniasis)
Lymph glands (reticulosis, HIV)
Retinal changes (tuberculosis, CMV infection and disseminated candidosis)

REVIEW RESULTS OF INVESTIGATIONS (AND REPEAT IF INDICATED)
Re-examine chest radiograph (minimal lesion)
Biochemical results abnormal (liver involvement)
Haematology results abnormal (haematological malignancy)
Microbiology results abnormal (pyuria)

CONSIDER FURTHER INVESTIGATIONS
Serological investigations (brucellosis)
CT/MRI scanning (abdominal lymph glands, tumours)
Tissue biopsies (histology and culture—TB, malignancy)

CONSIDER THERAPEUTIC TRIAL (generally as a last resort)
Antimicrobial therapy (cryptic miliary tuberculosis)
Corticosteroid therapy (connective tissue disease)
Cytotoxic therapy (lymphoma)

[Notes in parentheses indicate possible value of investigation.]

PRINCIPLES OF MANAGEMENT OF INFECTION

The management of infection depends on nonspecific and specific therapeutic measures and also on techniques of prevention of infection.

THERAPEUTIC MEASURES IN MANAGEMENT OF INFECTION

- **Non-specific management**: This includes the treatment of general symptoms such as fever, myalgia, headache and thirst, and complications such as dehydration, hypovolaemia, organ failure, haemorrhage and hyperpyrexia
- **Specific management**: This involves the use of antimicrobial agents to kill or inhibit the growth of microorganisms

The ability of one microorganism to interfere with the growth of another is called antibiosis and is due to specific diffusible metabolic products termed **antibiotics**. Since the introduction of penicillin in 1940, research has produced a wide range of antibiotics. In addition, a variety of other chemotherapeutic agents such as

metronidazole, trimethoprim, ciprofloxacin and isoniazid followed the demonstration of the therapeutic effects of sulphanilamide in 1935. A general term for all of these substances is **antimicrobial agent**. Those that kill microorganisms are referred to as bactericidal while agents that inhibit their growth are called bacteriostatic. Table 4.10 illustrates the sites and modes of action on bacteria of selected antimicrobial agents.

Effective therapy is available against all known bacteria, rickettsiae, mycoplasmas and chlamydia. Specific antiprotozoal compounds are used in the treatment of diseases such as sleeping sickness, leishmaniasis, malaria and amoebic dysentery. A number of drugs are available for the treatment of fungal infection. Antimicrobial agents active against viruses have also been discovered but few have been successful therapeutically.

ANTIBACTERIAL DRUGS

The β-lactam antibiotics

These are the **penicillins** and **cephalosporins** whose basic structure includes a 4-membered β-lactam ring (Fig. 4.3). Resistance is commonly due to bacterial enzymes called β-lactamases (penicillinases and cephalosporinases) which can cleave the ring and inactivate the antibiotic. The plasmids which code for these enzymes are transmissible between bacteria. Resistance may also be due to other mechanisms such as inability of the antibiotics to penetrate the bacterial cell wall. Penicillin-resistant pneumococci and meningococci and methicillin-resistant staphylococci (MRSA), which are also resistant to cloxacillin, are increasing problems in many countries.

The penicillins

All penicillins are bactericidal, killing bacteria by interfering with their cell synthetic processes. The range of their activity is wide as both Gram-positive and certain Gram-negative organisms are sensitive to individual penicillins (Table 4.11). Their most important adverse effect is hypersensitivity (see information box). This may take the form of urticaria and pyrexia or an acute anaphylactic reaction which may occasionally prove fatal.

ADVERSE EFFECTS OF THE PENICILLINS

Hypersensitivity	Dose-related
- Skin rash (urticaria or maculo-papular)	- Encephalopathy
- Anaphylaxis	- Neutropenia
- Drug fever	- Haemolysis
- Interstitial nephritis	

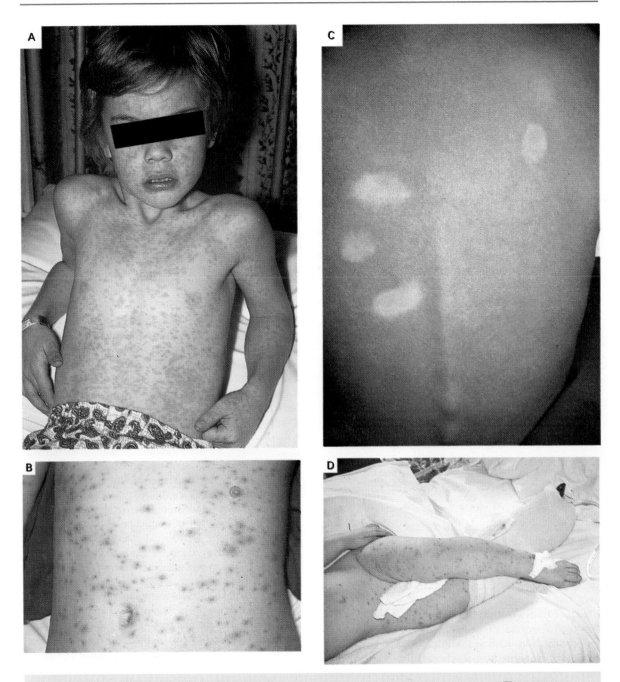

Fig. 4.2   **Childhood rashes:** skin eruptions in [A] measles, [B] chickenpox, [C] scarlet fever (note blanching on pressure) and [D] meningococcal infection.

Although penicillin is otherwise a safe antibiotic, its accumulation in patients with renal failure may lead to encephalopathy. In these patients dosage must be modified and guided by blood levels. In severe infections penicillin should be given intravenously; it should never be given intrathecally.

(i) Benzylpenicillin is rapidly absorbed following intramuscular injection and is excreted by the kidneys

Table 4.10   Mechanisms of action of antimicrobial agents

Site of action in bacteria	Mode of action	Antibiotic
Nucleic acid synthesis	Interrupts folate synthesis Inhibits DNA supercoiling Breaks DNA strands Inhibits RNA polymerase	Sulphonamides/trimethoprim 4-quinolones Nitrofurantoin Rifampicin
Protein synthesis	Binds to 30S ribosome and causes RNA code misreading Binds to 50S ribosome subunit and blocks translocation Inhibits transfer of amino acids to ribosome Binds to 30S ribosome and blocks RNA attachment	Aminoglycosides Macrolides Chloramphenicol Tetracycline
Cell membrane function	Disrupts cell membrane Inhibits sterol synthesis	Polymyxins Amphotericin
Cell wall synthesis	Inhibits carriage of subunits from cell membrane to cell wall Inhibits final cross-linkage of peptidoglycan	Vancomycin Cephalosporins/penicillins

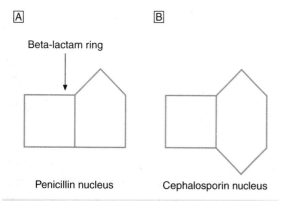

Fig. 4.3   The β-lactam antibiotics: nuclei of Ⓐ penicillin; Ⓑ cephalosporin.

within a few hours. Probenecid, 2 g daily by mouth, will raise the blood level of penicillin by delaying its excretion by the kidney and thus allow smaller doses or less frequent administration. Penicillin is also used prophylactically to prevent endocarditis, tetanus and gas gangrene.

(ii) Phenoxymethylpenicillin is incompletely absorbed from the stomach and is only used for less serious infections such as tonsillitis.

(iii) Cloxacillin and flucloxacillin are semi-synthetic penicillins which are stable to staphylococcal β-lactamases. For oral therapy flucloxacillin is superior to cloxacillin as it is almost twice as well absorbed from the gut.

(iv) Temocillin is active against penicillinase-producing Gram-negative bacilli.

(v) Ampicillin is a semi-synthetic penicillin which has a bactericidal action against both Gram-positive and certain Gram-negative organisms. It is susceptible to degradation by β-lactamases and not well absorbed with food. Maculopapular rashes occur in approximately 5% of all patients given ampicillin and in over 90% of patients given it for infectious mononucleosis; this antibiotic should not therefore be prescribed for sore throats which may be due to infectious mononucleosis. There are a number of ampicillin esters including bacampicillin and pivampicillin. These are better absorbed and produce higher blood levels of ampicillin.

(vi) Amoxycillin is an analogue of ampicillin which has a similar antibacterial spectrum but is more reliably absorbed from the gastrointestinal tract. Clavulanic acid is a β-lactam agent with only weak antibacterial activity. It is, however, a potent inhibitor of many β-lactamases and can protect β-lactamase-susceptible antibiotics, such as amoxycillin, from inactivation by these enzymes. A combination of amoxycillin plus sodium clavulanate called **co-amoxyclav** is available (Augmentin). There is also a combination of ampicillin and another beta-lactamase inhibitor called sulbactam (Unasyn).

(vii) Ticarcillin. Carbenicillin was initially the only penicillin with activity against *Pseudomonas aeruginosa*. This organism, however, is only moderately sensitive to carbenicillin, which has been replaced by its more active analogue ticarcillin. There is a preparation containing ticarcillin plus clavulanic acid (Timentin).

(viii) Mezlocillin, azlocillin and piperacillin. These acylureidopenicillins have a wider range of activity than ampicillin and are also more effective against many Gram-negative bacilli. They are used in combination with other antibiotics for the treatment of undiagnosed infections in immunocompromised patients. Azlocillin is more active than ticarcillin against *Ps. aeruginosa*, and is usually used in combination with an aminoglycoside for pseudomonas infections.

The cephalosporins

The cephalosporins have a wide range of activity against many important Gram-positive and Gram-negative bac-

Table 4.11 The penicillins

	BETA-LACTAMASE STABLE	ROUTE OF ADMINISTRATION	AVERAGE ADULT DOSE (mg given 6-hrly)	INDICATIONS
Benzylpenicillin	–	Parenteral	600–2400	Streptococcal and meningococcal infections, anthrax, diphtheria, gas gangrene, syphilis, yaws, gonorrhoea, actinomycosis
Procaine penicillin	–	Parenteral	300 (daily)	As for benzylpenicillin
Phenoxymethylpenicillin	–	Oral	500	Mild streptococcal infections
Cloxacillin/flucloxacillin	+	Parenteral/oral	500–2000	Staphylococcal infections
Ampicillin/amoxycillin	–	Parenteral/oral	250–1000	Infections caused by aerobic Gram-negative bacilli, streptococci, salmonellae and shigellae
Amoxycillin plus calvulanic acid (co-amoxyclav)	+	Parenteral/oral	250–1000 (Amox dose)	As for amoxycillin plus staphylococci and bacteroides
Ampicillin plus sulbactam (sultamicillin)	+	Oral	375 (12-hrly)	
Carbenicillin	–	Parenteral	1000–5000	Pseudomonas infections
Ticarcillin	–	Parenteral	1000–5000	Pseudomonas infections
Ticarcillin plus clavulanic acid ('Timentin')	+	Parenteral	3200 (6–8-hrly)	Pseudomonas and proteus infections
Azlocillin	–	Parenteral	1000–5000	Pseudomonas infections
Mezlocillin	–	Parenteral	1000–5000	Infections caused by aerobic Gram-negative bacilli
Piperacillin	–	Parenteral	1000–5000	Infections caused by aerobic Gram-negative bacilli
Temocillin	+	Parenteral	1000–2000 (12-hrly)	Infections caused by Gram-negative bacilli

teria and are therefore of value for the treatment of serious infections and for the initial empirical therapy of undiagnosed infections. The information box lists the

---

CEPHALOSPORINS

Injectable:

- First generation: Cephradine (also oral)
  Cephazolin
- Second generation: Cephamandole
  Cefuroxime (also oral)
- Third generation: Cefotaxime
  Ceftazidime
  Ceftizoxime
  Cefodizime
  Cefpirome
  Cefsulodin (Pseudomonas infections only)
  Ceftriaxone (long serum half-life)

Oral

- First generation: Cephalexin
  Cephradine
  Cefadroxil
- Second generation: Cefalor
  Cefixime
  Ceftibuten
  Cefuroxime axetil
- Third generation: Cefpodoxime proxetil

---

cephalosporins available in 1995. They have been developed over the past 30 years and the historical classification by 'generations', although helpful, is not ideal. The first generation agents developed in the 1960s have generally been replaced by the newer compounds. The second generation drugs are more stable to β-lactamases. The third generation agents are more active than the second against Gram-negative bacilli; however, they are less active against Gram-positive bacteria, especially *Staph aureus*. The third generation agents are very expensive.

Cefoxitin, a broad-spectrum cephamycin antibiotic, has activity against *Bacteroides fragilis*, an anaerobic bacillus which is a common cause of intra-abdominal sepsis, and is used for such infections.

The orally active cephalosporins are principally used for the treatment of lower respiratory, ear and urinary tract infections. They all have a similar spectrum but the newer agents are more resistant to beta-lactamases.

The dose of the cephalosporins ranges from 250–2000 mg 6–8-hourly depending on the weight of the patient, renal function, and severity of infection. Cefuroxime is probably the best cephalosporin for general use. Ceftazidime is the most active against Gram-negative bacilli. It is used for the treatment of septicaemia and infections in the immunocompromised. Ceftriaxone has a much longer serum half-life (10 hrs) than the other cephalosporins (1 hr) and need only be given once a day. The newer agents such as cefotaxime and ceftriaxone are now used extensively for the treatment of meningitis.

Adverse reactions are similar to those of the penicillins. A small number of penicillin-sensitive patients may also be allergic to the cephalosporins, which should be avoided if there is a history of significant hypersensitivity to the penicillins.

Other β-lactam agents

(i) Imipenem is a β-lactam antibiotic with a very broad spectrum which includes aerobic and anaerobic Gram-positive and Gram-negative organisms. It is partially inactivated by a renal enzyme and is therefore given along with an inhibitor of this enzyme called **cilastatin**. Side-effects are similar to other β-lactam antibiotics.

(ii) Aztreonam is a monocyclic β-lactam antibiotic the efficacy of which is limited to Gram-negative aerobic bacteria including *Ps. aeruginosa* and *Haemophilus influenzae*. Side-effects are similar to those of other β-lactam antibiotics.

The macrolide antibiotics

These are erythromycin, clarithromycin, azithromycin and spiramycin.

(i) Erythromycin has a similar although not identical spectrum to penicillin and is commonly used to treat infections caused by Gram-positive organisms in penicillin-allergic patients. It is also effective in whooping cough, Campylobacter enteritis and Legionnaires' disease provided it is given early enough in the course of these illnesses. It has activity against mycoplasmas and chlamydia and is an effective antibiotic for the treatment of many acute respiratory infections. Erythromycin is prescribed in a dosage of 250–500 mg by mouth every 6 hours. There is a preparation for intravenous injection. Diarrhoea, vomiting and abdominal pain are the principal side effects. Cholestatic jaundice may rarely develop if the course of treatment exceeds 10 days.

(ii) Clarithromycin has slightly greater activity than erythromycin, and achieves higher concentrations in tissues. The dose is 200–500 mg twice daily.

(iii) Azithromycin has more activity than erythromycin against certain Gram-negative organisms, including *H. influenzae*, but is less active against Gram-positive bacteria. As with clarithromycin, tissue levels are high but plasma levels are low. The serum half-life is long, allowing once-daily administration (500 mg). Because of their greater activity against *H. influenzae* and also against the organisms causing atypical pneumonia (mycoplasma, chlamydia and legionella), clarithromycin and azithromycin may replace erythromycin for the treatment of lower respiratory tract infections.

(iv) Spiramycin is a macrolide used as second-line treatment for toxoplasmosis.

The tetracycline antibiotics

Tetracycline, oxytetracycline and **chlortetracycline** are closely related bacteriostatic agents which, for practical purposes, have an identical range of activity. The adult dose is 250–500 mg 6-hourly before meals because the absorption of most tetracyclines is reduced by chelation with calcium (e.g. in milk). **Doxycycline** is an exception and also has the advantage that it is given only once daily, 200 mg on the first day and 100 mg thereafter.

The tetracyclines inhibit the growth of a wide range of Gram-positive and Gram-negative bacteria although in the context of treating lower respiratory tract infections their value is limited by the emergence of tetracycline-resistant pneumococci and *H. influenzae*. The tetracyclines are also active against rickettsiae (typhus fevers), *Coxiella burnetii* (Q fever), *Mycoplasma pneumoniae* and chlamydia (lymphogranuloma venereum, psittacosis and non-gonococcal urethritis) and are effective in brucellosis. They are also employed systemically in acne vulgaris and rosacea (see p. 955) where their beneficial effect is not due solely to their antibacterial action. Chlortetracycline is used for the local treatment of skin infections as it does not cause cutaneous sensitisation.

The tetracyclines are generally safe antibiotics, with few side-effects. The commonest is diarrhoea, which usually stops when the antibiotic is discontinued. Tetracyclines chelate with calcium and are deposited in developing bone and teeth causing a brown discoloration. They should not therefore be given to children or pregnant women. With the exception of doxycycline and minocycline, the tetracyclines can exacerbate renal failure and should not be given to patients with impaired renal function.

The aminoglycoside antibiotics

Streptomycin, kanamycin, gentamicin, tobramycin, netilmicin, amikacin and neomycin have similar chemical structures and adverse effects. They are not absorbed and for systemic treatment must be given by injection (except neomycin).

(i) Streptomycin has the important property that it is bactericidal against the tubercle bacillus (see p. 358). It is given with two other antituberculous drugs and this triple therapy prevents the emergence of resistant strains. For long-term therapy the daily dose of streptomycin should not exceed 1 g. It is also useful in the treatment of brucellosis.

(ii) Gentamicin is active against most Gram-negative bacilli, including *Ps. aeruginosa*. It is also active

Table 4.12 The aminoglycosides: dosages

Aminoglycoside	Max. daily dose(mg/kg/24 hrs)	Maximum plasma levels	
		Peak level	Pre-dose level
Gentamicin	5	10 mg/l	2 mg/l
Tobramycin	5	10 mg/l	2 mg/l
Netilmicin	6	12 mg/l	2 mg/l
Amikacin	15	30 mg/l	10 mg/l

Notes:
1. Plasma levels should be monitored in all patients if possible and MUST be measured in the elderly, in infants, and if high doses are given or if RENAL FUNCTION IMPAIRED
2. Gentamicin, tobramycin and netilmicin usually given 8- or 12-hrly if renal function normal. Single daily dosage sometimes used
3. 60–80 mg 12-hrly of gentamicin recommended for streptococcal endocarditis.

against penicillin-resistant staphylococci but inactive against anaerobes and streptococci with the exception of *Enterococcus faecalis*; in serious infections caused by this organism gentamicin is combined with ampicillin. The dose of gentamicin depends on renal function and the age and weight of the patient (see Table 4.12). 5 mg/kg body weight per 24 hours in divided doses (usually given 8-hourly) is indicated for most infections. Up to 7.5 mg/kg may be required for serious infections and in neonates. 2 mg/kg is sufficient for uncomplicated urinary tract infections and for synergistic therapy with penicillin for the treatment of streptococcal endocarditis. Serum concentrations of gentamicin must be measured during therapy to ensure efficacy and also to prevent toxicity due to unduly high levels, especially in renal failure and in the elderly. These measurements are usually carried out on 2 specimens of blood, the first taken one hour after a dose (peak) and the second just before the next dose (trough concentration). One hour levels should be between 4 and 10 mg/l and trough levels less than 2 mg/l.

(iii) Tobramycin is more active than gentamicin against *Ps. aeruginosa* but has no other advantage.

(iv) Netilmicin, a gentamicin derivative, is stable to three of nine aminoglycoside-inactivating enzymes, and should be reserved for infection caused by gentamicin-resistant organisms. Netilmicin is slightly less nephrotoxic than gentamicin, to which it is preferred in the elderly and if renal function is impaired.

(v) Amikacin has less intrinsic antibacterial activity than gentamicin, but has the advantage of being stable to 8 of the 9 aminoglycoside-inactivating enzymes, in contrast to gentamicin which is susceptible to 6 of the 9. For this reason amikacin is active against many gentamicin-resistant Gram-negative bacilli and should be

reserved for the treatment of infections caused by these organisms.

(vi) Neomycin is too toxic to be given parenterally but local applications containing neomycin are used in infections of the skin and eye. Neomycin may be used orally in hepatic encephalopathy to reduce the numbers of colonic bacteria.

The aminoglycosides are all nephrotoxic and ototoxic. The commonest adverse effect of the aminoglycosides is on the eighth cranial nerve. Aminoglycosides, especially gentamicin, should not be administered together with the diuretic frusemide, as additive ototoxicity may result from the combination.

The toxicity of the aminoglycosides is related to the age of the patient, the serum level of the antibiotic and the duration of administration. The aminoglycosides are principally excreted from the body by the kidneys and the risk of toxicity is increased when there is impairment of renal function. Serum levels of the aminoglycosides must be measured in all patients to prevent toxicity and also to ensure therapeutic blood levels.

Other antibiotics and chemotherapeutic agents

Chloramphenicol has a range of activity similar to that of the tetracyclines with the important difference that it is effective in enteric fever. It is more active than the tetracyclines against *H. influenzae* and is the antibiotic of choice in meningitis due to this organism. The daily oral dose for an adult is 1–3 g. Preparations for parenteral administration are also available. Chloramphenicol eye drops and ointment are useful for purulent conjunctivitis.

Chloramphenicol has in its chemical structure a benzene ring of the type known to cause bone marrow aplasia. Although pancytopenia due to chloramphenicol is very uncommon, it is almost invariably fatal; this antibiotic should be used systemically only if there is no adequate alternative therapy. It is inexpensive and therefore used widely in developing countries. Chloramphenicol should never be given to premature infants or to the newborn because of the risk of the development of the frequently fatal 'grey baby syndrome'. This is a state of acute circulatory failure caused by the very high blood levels of chloramphenicol due to its inadequate conjugation in the liver at this age.

Clindamycin (7-chlorolincomycin) has a similar antibacterial spectrum to penicillin against most Gram-positive organisms including penicillin-resistant staphylococci. It penetrates well into bone and is therefore useful for osteomyelitis caused by *Staph aureus*. The other principal indication is for the treatment of infections caused by *B. fragilis*. The dose is 300 mg 6-hourly, orally or by injection.

Clindamycin is the commonest cause of **antibiotic-**

associated colitis. This adverse reaction, which can also complicate treatment with other antibiotics, especially ampicillin, is due to selective overgrowth of *Clostridium difficile* which produces a toxin detectable in the faeces and is the direct cause of the disease. Treatment is with vancomycin or metronidazole, the latter being less costly.

Sodium fusidate is bactericidal against *Staph aureus* and is useful in infections caused by penicillin-resistant staphylococci. The dose is 250–500 mg 8-hourly by mouth. Nausea and vomiting are common. An intravenous preparation is available; jaundice has occasionally been associated with its use. It is expensive and is indicated only for serious infections due to staphylococci, especially osteomyelitis and endocarditis.

Spectinomycin is an aminocyclitol compound with certain structural similarity to streptomycin, although it is not an aminoglycoside. Its only clinical use is for the treatment of gonorrhoea if penicillin is contraindicated because of allergy or bacterial resistance.

Vancomycin and teicoplanin are glycopeptide bactericidal antibiotics. Indications for their use are limited to serious infections such as endocarditis (treatment and prophylaxis) or septicaemia caused by *Staph aureus* and *Staph epidermidis*, including methicillin-resistant strains (MRSA & MRSE). Oral vancomycin (125 mg 6-hourly) is used for antibiotic-associated colitis. Teicoplanin has a longer serum half-life than vancomycin and can therefore be given once a day.

Parenteral administration of vancomycin is by slow intravenous infusion of 500–1000 mg over 60 minutes every 12 hours if renal function is normal. Plasma levels must be monitored—peak (1 hr) levels should not exceed 30 mg/l and pre-dose levels must not exceed 10 mg/l. Side-effects include fever, rash and, if plasma levels exceed recommended concentrations, nephrotoxicity and ototoxicity. The daily dose must be reduced in renal failure.

Sulphonamides have largely been superseded by antibiotics although their usefulness was extended by the discovery of their synergistic action with trimethoprim, dapsone and pyrimethamine. Co-trimoxazole, a preparation containing sulphamethoxazole and trimethoprim, is active against a wide range of bacteria. Dapsone-sulphamethoxazole is used to treat malaria, and pyrimethamine-sulphamethoxazole to treat toxoplasmosis.

The sulphonamides most suitable for clinical use are short-acting preparations such sulphadimidine, which is rapidly absorbed and quickly excreted in the urine in a soluble form. One of the few remaining indications for the sulphonamides is cystitis (see p. 649) Sulphonamides have a wide range of potential hazards (see information box).

ADVERSE EFFECTS OF THE SULPHONAMIDES

- Skin rash including Stevens–Johnson syndrome (erythema multiforme and mucous membrane ulceration)
- Drug fever
- Blood dyscrasias including haemolysis in glucose-6-phosphate deficiency
- Nephritis
- Photosensitivity (topical use)
- Interaction with warfarin and sulphonylurea drugs

Co-trimoxazole consists of trimethoprim and sulphamethoxazole which act by inhibiting enzymes at two successive stages in the synthesis of para-aminobenzoic acid to folic acid and DNA. Co-trimoxazole is used for treatment of exacerbations of chronic bronchitis (p. 331) and urinary tract infections (p. 649). It is also effective in the treatment of invasive salmonella infections (p. 122). The adult dose is 2 tablets (each containing 80 mg of trimethoprim and 400 mg of sulphamethoxazole) given twice daily by mouth. There is also a preparation for injection. Double-dose co-trimoxazole is used to treat pneumonia caused by *Pneumocystis carinii* (p. 101).

The adverse effects are those of the sulphonamides (see information box above). The Stevens–Johnson syndrome has been reported in association with co-trimoxazole. In addition, haematological reactions to trimethoprim including thrombocytopenia and megaloblastic anaemia may occur due to folate deficiency. Side-effects are commonest in the elderly, in whom co-trimoxazole should be avoided.

Trimethoprim on its own is used for the treatment of urinary tract infection in a dose of 200 mg twice a day, or 100 mg each evening for long-term chemoprophylaxis. It is also used for the treatment of respiratory tract infections. Side-effects are less than with co-trimoxazole especially in the elderly.

Nalidixic acid was the first 4-quinolone to be introduced, 30 years ago. These agents are inhibitors of DNA gyrase, the enzyme responsible for supercoiling of bacterial DNA. While nalidixic acid has only modest antibacterial activity and is poorly absorbed from the gut, several new 4-quinolones have been developed with significantly greater activity and improved absorption.

Ciprofloxacin is the most important of the new 4-quinolones. It has a relatively broad spectrum with particularly high activity against aerobic Gram-negative bacilli including salmonellae, shigellae, campylobacter and pseudomonas species. It is also active against chlamydia and mycoplasmas but not against anaerobic bacteria. Although many Gram-positive organisms are sensitive to ciprofloxacin, the activity is only moderate

Table 4.13   Indications for the use of the 4-quinolone antibiotics

Treatment of gonorrhoea
Acrosoxacin (300 mg single dose)

Treatment of urinary tract infections
Nalidixic acid (1 g 6-hourly)
Norfloxacin (400 mg 12-hourly)
Cinoxacin (500 mg 12-hourly)

Broad spectrum
Ofloxacin [UTI, LRTI, STD] (200–400 mg daily)
Ciprofloxacin [UTI, LRTI, STD, GI infections, typhoid fever, septicaemia, meningococcal prophylaxis] (see text for dose)

All given orally–ciprofloxacin also available for i.v. injection
UTI: urinary tract infection
LRTI: lower respiratory tract infection but not pneumococcal
STD: sexually transmitted diseases
GI: gastrointestinal infections.

especially against pneumococci. Ciprofloxacin diffuses readily into infected tissues and cells. The oral dose is 250–750 mg 12-hourly and for intravenous infusion 200 mg 12-hourly.

Ciprofloxacin has a wide range of indications including gastrointestinal, urinary tract and lower respiratory tract infections (not pneumococcal), septicaemia and gonorrhoea.

Indications for the other available 4-quinolones are listed in Table. 4.13. With the exception of ofloxacin which has an oral and intravenous formulation, they are given orally. The adverse reactions encountered with the 4-quinolones are summarised in the information box.

SIDE-EFFECTS OF 4-QUINOLONES

- **Gastro-intestinal**:   Nausea, vomiting, diarrhoea
- **Rashes**:   Maculo-papular, photosensitivity, urticaria
- **Neurotoxicity**:   Insomnia, dizziness, headache, convulsions (rare)
- **Drug interactions**:   NSAIDs, theophylline, peptic ulcer drugs

Contraindicated in children and pregnancy
(Arthropathy in young animals)

Metronidazole. This imidazole compound has high activity against anaerobic bacteria and intestinal protozoa but none against aerobic bacteria. It is effective against infection due to *Trichomonas vaginalis*, *Giardia lamblia* and *Entamoeba histolytica* and is widely used for the treatment and prophylaxis of infections caused by anaerobic bacteria, notably *B. fragilis*. It is active against *Clostridium tetani* and *Cl. difficile*. Side-effects of metronidazole are usually limited to headache and nausea but it should not be given to women during the first trimester

of pregnancy as fetal abnormalities have been reported in animals given high doses for prolonged periods. Alcohol should be avoided during therapy with metronidazole which has a similar action to disulfiram. The oral dose varies from 200–400 mg 3 times a day. 800 mg 3 times a day is required for intestinal amoebic infections. There are preparations for intravenous infusion and rectal use.

Tinidazole is similar to metronidazole but has a longer serum half-life (12 hours as compared to 7 hours), allowing less frequent administration, and is less toxic.

Mupirocin is not related to any other antibiotic and is only indicated for application to the skin or anterior nose for the treatment of skin infection or eradication of nasal staphylococcal carriage.

Antituberculous drugs
These are discussed on page 361.

ANTIFUNGAL DRUGS

For therapeutic purposes, fungal infections are classified either as superficial (skin or mucous membranes) or systemic. The former usually respond readily to topical application of an anti-fungal agent (see Table 4.14). Systemic fungal infections usually occur in compromised hosts and can be extremely difficult to cure. Relatively high doses of antifungal agents given for prolonged periods of time may be required for these infections and expert advice should be sought for their management.

Nystatin is the most commonly prescribed agent for

Table 4.14   Antifungal drugs

	Dose
For topical application	
Nystatin	
Clotrimazole	
Econazole	
Amphotericin	
For oral administration	**Dose**
Miconazole	250 mg 6-hourly
Ketoconazole	200 mg daily
Fluconazole	50–200 mg daily (max 14 days)*
Itraconazole	100–200 mg daily
Flucytosine	200 mg daily
Griseofulvin	500 mg daily
Terbinafine (ringworm only)	250 mg daily
For intravenous infusion	
Amphotericin (also a liposomal preparation)	Initially 1 mg/kg/day (consult expert)
Miconazole	600 mg 8-hourly
Flucytozine	200 mg daily
Fluconazole	200–400 mg daily

* Up to 400 mg daily for several weeks may be necessary in severely immunocompromised patients with invasive fungal infections.
Invasive fungal infections requiring high doses and prolonged therapy should be treated by physicians with experience of these diseases.

the treatment of Candida infections of skin and mucous membranes. It is not absorbed when given by mouth and cannot be administered parenterally because of its low solubility and toxicity. A suspension, tablets and pessaries are available for the treatment of oral, intestinal and vaginal thrush.

Clotrimazole, econazole, miconazole, isoconazole, sulconazole, tioconazole and **ketoconazole** all belong to the imidazole group of antifungal agents. They are effective against a wide range of fungi. The first two agents are used for the topical therapy of superficial fungal infections. Miconazole and ketoconazole are absorbed from the gut and have been successfully used for the treatment of systemic fungal infections as well as for superficial mycoses. There is also an intravenous formulation of miconazole. Hepatotoxicity (occasionally fatal) has been reported during ketoconazole therapy. Liver function tests should be performed during long-term therapy and it should NOT be used for superficial infections.

Fluconazole is an oral triazole antifungal drug indicated for mucocutaneous and systemic candidiasis and for cryptococcal infections. **Itraconazole**, also a triazole, is indicated for oropharyngeal and genital candidiasis and for tinea infections. It is contraindicated in liver disease. It has some efficacy in aspergillus infections.

Amphotericin is the most important antibiotic for the treatment of systemic fungal infections. It is a moderately toxic drug and side-effects are relatively common. These include fever, vomiting, thrombophlebitis, anaemia and nephrotoxicity. The antibiotic is given by intravenous infusion in increasing daily doses usually commencing with 1 mg. A liposomal preparation of amphotericin (AmBisome) is more effective and less toxic, but very much more expensive; it should only be used in renal failure or in patients who have previously suffered nephrotoxicity with conventional amphotericin.

Flucytosine is well absorbed from the gut and side-effects are relatively uncommon, although bone-marrow depression can occur. It is active only against yeasts and has been used for the treatment of systemic candidiasis, sometimes in combination with amphotericin. *C. albicans* can develop resistance to flucytosine.

Griseofulvin is concentrated in keratin and is the drug of choice for widespread or chronic dermatophyte infections such as ringworm. It is well absorbed from the gut and is given in a daily dose of 250 mg (child) or 500 mg (adult). Skin lesions respond quickly but infection of the nails requires several months of therapy. Localised and minor ringworm lesions usually respond to topical application of Whitfield's ointment or miconazole. The newer agent **terbinafine**, an allylamine anti-

fungal given in an adult dose of 250 mg daily, is as effective for ringworm when given for 2–4 weeks.

ANTIVIRAL DRUGS

The challenge with antiviral chemotherapy is to find an agent which will arrest the replication of viruses without interfering with the metabolism of mammalian cells. A further problem is that by the time a viral infection has been diagnosed much of the damage has been done to the host tissues. Table 4.15 provides information on currently available antiviral drugs. Their doses are given with the descriptions of individual viral diseases.

Acyclovir is the most effective of the available antiviral agents. It is effective for herpes simplex and varicella zoster infections, particularly in the immunosuppressed. It does not, however, eradicate the viruses from the body.

ANTIPARASITIC DRUGS

Few of the antibacterial antibiotics work against protozoa or helminths.

Amphotericin inhibits the production of ergosterol, which is the major sterol of cell membranes of the yeast stages of fungi and the amastigote stages of *Leishmania*. Conventional preparations are too toxic for routine use, as a first choice. The liposomal preparations are more efficient and less toxic but extremely expensive. **Ivermectin** is an antibiotic widely used against helminths in veterinary medicine and is valuable in human filarial infections.

Many anti-parasitic drugs are derived from traditional remedies (quinine comes from chincona bark), or ancient pharmacopoeias (stibogluconate and melarsen B contain toxic heavy metals), or from random screening (mepacrine and chloroquine). Recently the pharmaceutical industry has taken a more serious interest in tropical parasitic infections and logical derivatives are being developed. Among the most useful are those based on the imidazole ring. The nitroimidazoles, metronidazole and tinidazole, are effective against intestinal protozoa, as well as anaerobic bacteria, while the benzimidaloles, such as mebendazole and albendazole, are effective against a wide range of helminthic infections. Other azoles such as ketoconazole inhibit enzymes in the ergosterol pathway and have some action against *Leishmania* as well as fungi.

The indications and dosages are given in the individual sections.

SELECTION OF ANTIMICROBIAL AGENT

Important considerations in the choice of effective chemotherapy are the nature and site of the infection,

Table 4.15 Antiviral drugs

Drug (Doses are given in text)	Routes of Administration	Indications	Side-effects
Acyclovir	Topical Oral Intravenous	Herpes zoster Chickenpox (esp. in immunosuppressed) Herpes simplex infection: encephalitis, genital tract, eye	Rash, headache, gastrointestinal toxicity, neurotoxicity (i.v. only) Increase in urea & creatinine
Famciclovir	Oral	Herpes zoster and genital *H. simplex* infection	Rash, headache
Idoxuridine	Topical	Herpes zoster *H. simplex* keratitis	Local irritation
Amantadine	Oral	Prophylaxis of influenza A	CNS symptoms Nausea
Tribavirin	Oral	Lassa fever Respiratory syncytial virus infection in infants (inhalation)	Reticulocytosis Respiratory depression
Ganciclovir	Intravenous/oral	Cytomegalovirus infection in immunosuppressed	Leukopenia, thrombocytopenia
Zidovudine	Oral	HIV infection (incl AIDS)	CNS symptoms, anaemia, neutropenia, thrombocytopenia

the known or suspected causative organism, the characteristics of the patient, the available antibiotics, their pharmacokinetic profiles, and their cost.

The nature and site of the infection

When the nature of the infection (and the likely causative organism) can be predicted from the clinical features of the illness, treatment can proceed without isolation of the causative organism, as in the prescription of penicillin for acute follicular tonsillitis or lobar pneumonia. In exacerbations of chronic bronchitis the causative organisms are almost always pneumococci and *H. influenzae* and ampicillin or co-trimoxazole is, therefore, indicated without specific laboratory diagnosis.

If the patient is seriously ill, antibiotic therapy must be started on a 'best guess' (empirical) basis. The presentation of the illness may assist in the selection of the most appropriate agent. If there are no clues as to the nature of the infection, treatment should be started with a combination of antibiotics such as gentamicin plus a penicillin, or with a cephalosporin such as cefuroxime.

The known or suspected causative organism

When there is uncertainty about the nature of the infection a bacteriological diagnosis should be made, whenever possible, so that the appropriate antibiotic can be given. If the organism is one such as *Streptococcus pyogenes*, which has a predictable susceptibility to the generally used antimicrobial agents, no further laboratory sensitivity tests are necessary.

Sensitivity tests will be required for bacteria known to vary in their susceptibility to antimicrobial agents (an increasing problem). The acquisition of resistance occurs particularly with staphylococci, Gram-negative

bacilli and mycobacteria. Once the sensitivity of the organism has been determined, it is relatively rare for this to change during the course of treatment.

The patient

The age and sex of the patient, together with a knowledge of previous adverse reactions, immune, renal and liver function must all be considered before a final selection of the antibiotic or antibiotics is made.

Children and pregnant women should not be given tetracyclines or 4-quinolones. Co-trimoxazole is also best avoided in pregnancy and the elderly, and this compound, together with other sulphonamides, must not be given to patients with glucose-6-phosphate dehydrogenase deficiency as haemolysis may be precipitated. Chloramphenicol should be prescribed only in the circumstances described on page 79 and is contraindicated in the neonate. Ampicillin must not be given to patients suffering from infectious mononucleosis and the aminoglycoside antibiotics should be used with caution in patients with renal disease and in the elderly. Clindamycin should not be used for trivial infection because of the risk of colitis.

The available antibiotics

Having considered the above factors the clinician selects an appropriate antibiotic with reference to its microbiological and pharmacological properties, adverse reactions and cost. The British National Formulary is a valuable guide.

More than one (but rarely more than two) antibiotics may be required for the initial treatment of septicaemia or for serious infections in the immunosuppressed. The use of two or more antibacterial drugs is only occasionally of proven value in other than the seriously ill. Thus, in tuberculosis, three agents are prescribed, at least initially, to reduce the emergence of resistant strains. Two drugs with different modes of action may also be used when it has been shown that the combination is synergistic.

Antimicrobial agents are often very expensive. In general, new agents are more expensive than older compounds while parenteral preparations are always much more costly than the oral formulation. Unusual or new antibiotics should not be prescribed without good reason as the difference in cost compared with other agents can be over a hundred-fold. Particularly expensive agents include vancomycin, imipenem, the newer cephalosporins, acyclovir, zidovudine and amphotericin, especially the liposomal formulation.

PREVENTION OF INFECTION

Non-specific: Non-specific methods used to prevent the spread of infection include health education, good hygiene (especially hand-washing), safe disposal of excreta, clean water supplies, the use of antiseptics, disinfectants and disposable equipment and of sterilization facilities, mosquito nets, vector control (insects and rodents), the isolation of infectious patients (source isolation) and of those especially susceptible to infection such as the immunocompromised (protective isolation).

Specific: This involves the use of prophylactic immunisation and/or chemoprophylaxis.

Immunisation against infectious disease
Immunisation may be active or passive.

Active immunisation
Vaccines are either live attenuated organisms, inactivated organisms or toxoids (inactivated toxins) (see Table 4.16). In the UK parents are advised to have their children immunised against whooping cough, diphtheria, tetanus, measles, mumps, rubella, poliomyelitis, *Haemophilus influenzae* type B and tuberculosis (see Table on Immunisation schedule recommended in Britain, in Appendix to this book). The World Health Organization (WHO) has provided guidelines for immunisation of children in developing countries: these also appear in the Appendix, p. 1155). Indications for immunisation against influenza, hepatitis A and B, typhoid fever, cholera, plague, typhus, yellow fever, Japanese encephalitis and rabies depend upon the likelihood of exposure or upon current international health regulations.

Acute demyelinating encephalomyelitis and polyneuropathy are the most important, but fortunately very rare, complications of immunisation.

General guidelines for immunisation are given in the information box.

HIV infected persons should be immunised in the same way as other individuals but must not be given BCG, live poliomyelitis or yellow fever vaccines as disseminated infection with the vaccine strain may occur.

Passive immunisation
An injection of immunoglobulin will give temporary protection (usually) for 2–6 months against certain infectious diseases (see Appendix page 1156, Table on Indications for prophylactic immunoglobulin) by providing pre-formed antibodies against those infections.

Table 4.16 Vaccines and toxoids			
	Live attenuated vaccines	**Inactivated vaccines**	**Toxoid (inactivated toxin)**
Childhood immunisation	Measles Mumps Rubella Poliomyeltis* BCG (tuberculosis)	Pertussis *H. influenzae* Type B	Diphtheria Tetanus
Travel	Yellow fever Typhoid*	Typhoid* Cholera Rabies Japanese encephalitis Hepatitis A	
Special risk groups	Influenza*	Pneumococcal Hepatitis B Influenza* Meningococcal (Types A and C only) Plague Poliomyelitis*	

* Both live and inactivated vaccines available. Vaccinated groups are not exclusive.

The immunoglobulin preparation may be pooled (prepared from blood collected from many donors) or hyperimmune (extracted from the blood of an individual recovering from an infection or from an immunised animal). Concerns about possible contamination of immunoglobulin preparations by hepatitis viruses, cytomegalovirus and HIV are often expressed. Safety procedures in donor selection and screening, together with virus inactivation during manufacture of the products, minimises this risk. Nevertheless, a slight risk remains and blood or its products should never be given unless absolutely necessary.

Chemoprophylaxis

The use of antimicrobial agents to prevent infection is known as chemoprophylaxis. The indications for this are limited, and are listed in the Appendix on p. 1156.

Notification of infectious diseases

Clinicians in Britain have a statutory obligation to notify certain infectious diseases to the appropriate Public Health Authority. This provides epidemiological information which assists in the control of infection. The notifiable infectious diseases for the UK are listed in the Appendix, Table 21.16, p. 1156.

FURTHER READING

Ayliffe G A J, Lowbury E J L, Geddes A M, Williams J D 1992 Control of Hospital Infection. Chapman and Hall Medical, London
Bradley J R, Wilks D, Rubenstein D 1994 The vascular endothelium in septic shock. Journal of Infection 28: 1–10
Campbell A G M 1992 Immunisation Against Infectious Diseases. Department of Health/HMSO, London
Fischer P R 1993 Tropical paediatrics. Paediatric Reviews 14: 95–99
Hughes J M, La Montagne J R 1994 Emerging infectious diseases. Journal of Infectious Diseases 170: 263–264
Naber S P 1994 Molecular pathology—diagnosis of infectious diseases. New England Journal of Medicine 331: 1212–1215
Rogers D J, Packer M J 1993 Vector-borne diseases, models and global change. Lancet 342: 1282–1284
Sable G A, Donowitz G R 1994 Infections in bone marrow transplant recipients. Clinical Infectious Diseases 18: 273–284
Strickland G T 1992 Fever in the returned traveller. Medical Clinics of North America 76: 1375–1392. (*The whole volume is on Travel Medicine.*)
Tomasz A 1994 Multiple-antibiotic-resistant bacteria—a report on the Rockefeller University Workshop. New England Journal of Medicine 330: 1247–1251
Tompkins L S, Tenover F, Arvin A 1994 New technology in the clinical microbiology laboratory: what you always wanted to know but were afraid to ask. Journal of Infectious Diseases 170: 1068–1074

DISEASES DUE TO VIRUSES

Viruses are the smallest micro-organisms causing human disease. They have a simple structure comprising a strand of either DNA or RNA enclosed in a protein shell. Unlike bacteria which can grow in an inanimate medium, viruses grow only within living cells. Prions are even simpler structures composed of infectious proteins without nucleic acid. Table 4.17 presents the current classification of the viruses which cause human disease. The aim of this section is to cover the major viral diseases not covered elsewhere in the book.

RNA VIRUSES

ARENAVIRUSES

LASSA FEVER

Since the first report in 1969, the disease has so far been limited to sub-Saharan West Africa where serological studies have shown that the infection is widespread. Isolated cases and small rural outbreaks are commonest, but outbreaks in hospital have also occurred (Table 4.18).

Clinical features

The disease has the general features of a viral infection, high fever, intercostal myalgia, bradycardia, low blood pressure and leucopenia. Adherent yellow exudates on the pharynx are particularly characteristic. The fever

Table 4.17   Viruses causing human disease

| RNA VIRUSES | | DNA VIRUSES | |
FAMILY	GENUS OR TYPE	FAMILY	GENUS OR TYPE
Arenaviruses	Lassa fever virus	Adenoviruses	Numerous serotypes
Bunyaviruses	Hantaviruses	Hepadnaviruses	Hepatitis B viruses
Caliciviruses	Calicivirus	Herpesviruses	Herpes simplex virus 1 and 2
Coronaviruses	Coronavirus		Epstein-Barr virus
Filoviruses	Marburg and Ebola viruses		Cytomegalovirus
			Varicella-zoster virus
			Human herpes virus 6
Orthomyxoviruses	Influenza viruses	Papovaviruses	Papilloma viruses
Paramyxoviruses	Parainfluenza viruses	Parvoviruses	B19 virus
	Mumps virus	Poxviruses	Variola, Vaccinia
	Measles virus		Molluscum contagiosum virus
	Respiratory syncytial virus		Orf
Picornaviruses	Enteroviruses		
	Poliovirus, 3 types		
	Echovirus, 31 types		
	Coxsackie A virus, 24 types		
	Coxsackie B virus, 6 types		
	Enterovirus types 68–71		
	Hepatitis A virus		
	Rhinoviruses		
Reoviruses	Rotaviruses		
Retroviruses	HIV 1 and 2		
	HTLV 1 and 2		
Rhabdoviruses	Rabies virus		
Togaviruses	Rubella virus		
	Alphaviruses		
	Flaviviruses		

Table 4.18   Common viral haemorrhagic fevers

Disease	Viral agent	Reservoir	Transmission	Geography	Case mortality
Lassa fever	Arenavirus	Multimammate rat (*Mastomys natalensis*)	Urine	West Africa	Up to 50% (responds to tribavirin)
		Patient	Body fluids		
Marburg/Ebola virus disease	Filovirus	?	Via monkeys' body fluids	Central Africa	25–90%
		Patient			
Yellow fever	Togavirus	Monkeys	Mosquitoes	Tropical Africa S. and C. America	10–60%
Dengue	Togavirus (dengue types 1–4)	Man	*Aedes aegypti* et al	Tropical and sub-tropical coasts	Nil-10%*
Omsk	Togavirus	Musk rat	Ticks	Siberia	2%
Crimean-Congo	Bunyavirus	Ixodes tick	Ixodes tick	Africa, Asia, E. Europe	15–70%
Bolivian and Argentinian	Arenavirus (Machupa and Junin)	Rodents (*Calomys* spp.)	Urine	S. America	?
Haemorrhagic fever with renal syndrome	Hantavirus	Rodents	Faeces	North Asia North Europe	30%

* Mortality of uncomplicated and haemorrhagic dengue fever, respectively.

lasts between 7 and 17 days. In severe cases liver and renal failure, electrolyte imbalance, haemorrhage and acute circulatory failure develop, hence the classification of Lassa fever as a viral haemorrhagic fever (Table 4.18).

Case mortality is high, but mild and subclinical infections also occur.

The virus may be isolated, or antigen detected, in maximum security laboratories from serum, pharynx, pleural exudate and urine, but diagnosis will usually be established from 'paired sera', the later specimen being taken 6–8 weeks after the onset of infection. The diagnosis should be considered in Britain in patients presenting with fever within 21 days of leaving West Africa.

Management

Strict isolation and general supportive measures, preferably in a special unit, are required. Tribavirin is given intravenously (100 mg/kg, then 25 mg/kg daily for 3 days and 12.5 mg/kg daily for 4 days).

Prevention

The administration of convalescent immune plasma has been followed by recovery and is therefore recommended for prophylaxis after accidental exposure to infection.

BUNYAVIRUSES

Haemorrhagic fever with renal syndrome has occurred in outbreaks in Korea (hence its alternative name, Korean haemorrhagic fever), Manchuria and Eastern Europe. The infection causes severe capillary congestion, leakage and haemorrhage, especially in the renal medulla, so that oedema and acute renal failure develop, with oliguria and the passage of cells and protein in the urine. Untreated the mortality is high, but with proper treatment for acute renal failure (p. 626) and blood transfusion if necessary, patients should recover. A less severe form of the disease, nephropathia epidemica, is found in Scandinavia.

FILOVIRUSES

MARBURG AND EBOLA VIRAL DISEASE

In 1967 a severe infectious illness broke out among laboratory workers in Marburg, West Germany, who had handled tissues from a batch of vervet monkeys imported from Uganda. In 1976 outbreaks of the disease occurred in Sudan and Zaire from a focus on the Ebola River. The viruses causing these two outbreaks were structurally identical but are antigenically distinct. Sporadic cases have occurred elsewhere in Africa. In man-to-man outbreaks the mortality is high, but successive human passage seems to reduce virulence. The incubation period is 5–9 days.

The illness presents suddenly with fever, severe myalgia and diarrhoea, followed by pharyngitis, generalised erythematous rash and lymphadenopathy. Fatal complications include haemorrhage, secondary infection, encephalitis, renal failure and pneumonia.

Management consists of supportive measures alone.

Other haemorrhagic fevers

The term haemorrhagic fevers, while increasing in popularity, covers too wide a field of medicine to be of much value. Hence, in addition to the viral causes of haemorrhagic fever covered above and listed in Table 4.18, many other infections cause bleeding—as listed in the information box.

CAUSES OF HAEMORRHAGIC FEVERS

- **Viruses:** (see Table 4.18)
- **Rickettsia:** Rocky Mountain spotted fever
- **Bacteria:** Meningococcaemia, plague Gram-negative septicaemia
- **Spirochaetes:** Relapsing fever
- **Protozoa:** African trypanosomiasis

PARAMYXOVIRUSES

MEASLES

Measles is caused by a paramyxovirus which spreads by droplet infection. One attack confers a high degree of immunity. Most people suffer from measles in childhood, and a mother who has had the disease confers passive immunity on her infant for the first 6 months of life. In tropical countries measles is very severe, with a high mortality. The incubation period is about 10 days to the commencement of the catarrhal stage.

Clinical features (see information box)
Catarrhal stage: There is a febrile onset, with nasal catarrh, sneezing, redness of the conjunctivae and watering of the eyes. In addition, cough, hoarseness of the voice and photophobia usually appear by the second day.

CLINICAL FEATURES OF MEASLES

Catarrhal stage
- Day 1–2: Fever, running nose, red, watery eyes
- Day 2+: Cough, photophobia, Koplik's spots

Exanthematous stage
- Day 3–4: Maculo-papular rash
- Day 6–7: Fever settles and rash begins to fade

At this stage, a diagnosis of measles may be made from the presence of Koplik's spots on the mucous membrane of the mouth. These are small white spots surrounded by a narrow zone of inflammation. The disease is highly infectious during the catarrhal stage and the child is miserable and irritable.

Exanthematous stage: After 3 or 4 days Koplik's spots disappear and the red macular or maculopapular rash develops first at the back of the ears and at the junction of the forehead and the hair. Within a few hours there is invasion of the whole skin and as the spots rapidly become more numerous they fuse to form the characteristic blotchy appearance of measles (Fig. 4.2, p. 75). The rash fades after several days into a faint brown staining followed by a fine desquamation. The malaise and the fever subside as the rash fades. As with most infectious diseases, measles is more severe in older children and adults.

Complications
These are listed in the information box.

COMPLICATIONS OF MEASLES

Effects of measles virus
- Stomatitis
- Enteritis
- Pneumonia
- Keratitis

Secondary bacterial infection
- Otitis media
- Bronchopneumonia
- Conjunctivitis

Neurological complications
- Post-viral encephalitis
- Subacute sclerosing panencephalitis

Nutritional
- Severe weight loss
- Kwashiorkor (tropics)
- Corneal ulceration (tropics—Vit. A deficiency)

Management
The patient should be isolated if possible and excluded from school for 10 days from the appearance of the rash. Most patients, in spite of the high temperature, remain uncomplicated and antibiotics should be prescribed only for bacterial complications.

Prevention
Active immunisation: One injection of live attenuated measles virus (in association with mumps and rubella vaccines) is given subcutaneously to children over 1 year old.

Passive immunisation: Human normal immunoglobulin, given intramuscularly, is used for the prevention or attenuation of measles in contacts under 18 months of age and for non-immune debilitated children, especially those with malignant disease. The dose is 250 mg for children under 1 year old and 500 mg for those over this age.

MUMPS

Mumps is spread by droplet infection and affects mainly children of school age and young adults. The infectivity rate is not high and there is serological evidence that 30–40% of infections are clinically unapparent. The incubation period is about 18 days.

Clinical features
Malaise, fever, trismus and pain near the angle of the jaw is soon followed by tender swelling of one or both parotid glands. Parotid swelling alone is often the first feature. The submandibular salivary glands may also be involved. The swollen glands subside in a few days, and may be succeeded by swelling of a previously unaffected gland. Orchitis occurs in about one in four males who develop mumps after puberty; it is usually on one side only, but if it is bilateral, sterility may be a sequel. Obscure abdominal pain may be due to pancreatitis or oophoritis. Acute lymphocytic meningitis is another mode of presentation. Encephalomyelitis is rare.

Investigations
Most cases of mumps can be diagnosed on clinical grounds alone, but, if in doubt, the diagnosis can be confirmed by the demonstration of specific antibodies; or the virus may be cultured from the saliva, or from the cerebrospinal fluid in meningitis. Differential diagnosis is from salivary calculus which is unilateral and sarcoidosis which causes bilateral chronic parotitis.

Management
Apart from the relief of symptoms no other treatment is necessary. Orchitis can be relieved by prednisolone (40 mg orally daily for 4 days).

Prevention
Mumps vaccine is given at the age of 15 months along with measles and rubella vaccines.

PICORNAVIRUSES

This group of viruses consists of the rhinoviruses and enteroviruses. The latter group so-called because they

INFECTIONS CAUSED BY ENTEROVIRUSES

Echoviruses (approximately 40 strains)
- Meningitis
- Encephalitis
- Conjunctivitis
- Gastroenteritis
- Pharyngitis
- Fever and rash
- Neonatal infection

Coxsackieviruses (24 type A strains, 6 type B strains)
- Myocarditis
- Pericarditis
- Meningitis
- Herpangina
- Bornholm disease
- Hand, foot and mouth disease
- Gastroenteritis
- Pharyngitis
- Neonatal infection

Polioviruses (3 strains)
- Poliomyelitis (see p. 1090)

enter the body via the intestinal tract, cause a wide spectrum of disease (see information box). They are excreted in the stool and also, if there is respiratory infection, from the nasopharynx.

Most of the infections caused by enteroviruses are described elsewhere in the book with the exception of **herpangina** which produces a vesicular rash on the soft palate, and **hand, foot and mouth disease**, a highly infectious but benign disease of childhood characterised by vesicles on hands, feet and mouth.

RETROVIRUSES

HUMAN IMMUNODEFICIENCY VIRUS INFECTION AND THE ACQUIRED HUMAN IMMUNODEFICIENCY SYNDROME

During 1981, cases of a rare neoplasm, Kaposi's sarcoma, and *Pneumocystis carinii* pneumonia (an unusual opportunistic infection only seen in severely immunosuppressed patients) were reported in the USA in previously healthy homosexual men. This was the start of an epidemic amongst homosexual men in the USA, the term acquired immunodeficiency syndrome (AIDS) being applied to these cases. In 1984 the association between infection with the human immunodeficiency virus (HIV) and the development of AIDS was established. The AIDS epidemic has stimulated an unprecedented amount of biomedical research which has led to a major expansion of knowledge in many

aspects of this infection, but many unsolved problems remain regarding the pathogenesis, management and control of the disease.

Epidemiology

Worldwide, between five and ten million people are now thought to be infected with HIV. In 1992 in the USA, it was estimated that about one million were infected with HIV and nearly 200,000 persons had AIDS. By the end of 1993, in the UK, nearly 21,000 HIV seropositive persons and 7,500 cases of AIDS had been reported, of whom nearly 5,000 had died. 87% of AIDS cases in the UK were male and sexual intercourse between men was by far the most common risk factor for HIV infection in this group (81%). Overall, the prevalence of HIV infection in the UK is continuing to rise slowly, with the most rapid increases in case numbers occurring amongst female AIDS cases and children, indicating that heterosexual spread of HIV infection in the West appears to be increasing. So far in the UK nearly 150 children have been reported with AIDS. In sub-Saharan Africa a different distribution of HIV infection is seen where males and females are affected in equal numbers, the main risk factors being multiple heterosexual contacts and infection of children from their mothers either materno-fetally or by transmission in breast milk. Very high levels of HIV seropositivity have been reported amongst prostitutes in Central Africa. The HIV epidemic continues on a global scale, with alarming increases being reported in Central Africa, South America, the Indian subcontinent and South-East Asia.

Infection with HIV essentially requires exchange of semen, vaginal secretions, milk or blood which is infected by the virus, thus explaining the high risk group categories which are listed in the information box. The

RISK FACTORS FOR HIV INFECTION IN THE UK

(Percentages refer to all cases reported in the UK to the end of 1993)

- Sex between men   61%
- Sex between men (often bisexual) and women   15%
- Intravenous drug abuse (IVDA)   12%
- IVDA and/or sex between men   1%
- Contaminated blood/blood products or tissue transfer   7%
- Other   4%

main methods of transmission for HIV are via anal or vaginal intercourse. The risk of HIV infection is higher with anal than with vaginal intercourse, greater for the recipient of penetrative sex by either route and risk is also thought to be increased if genital trauma occurs during intercourse or genital ulceration is present as a result of other sexually transmitted diseases. Intravenous drug abusers (IVDA) are at risk of HIV infection as a result of the practice of 'needle sharing' which allows transmission of HIV infected blood from one individual to another.

Studies of many thousands of health care workers exposed to AIDS patients have revealed only a few cases where occupational exposure has resulted in HIV infection. In these cases, needle stick injury with HIV-contaminated blood, or prolonged contact of abraided skin with contaminated body fluids are the risk factors. Generally, with all risk factors for HIV, by whatever method, the greater the inoculum the greater the risk. Transmission of the virus by transfusion of infected blood or blood products (coagulation factors for haemophilia) has, in many countries, largely been overcome by routine testing of blood donors.

Virology

HIV belongs to the Lentivirinae subfamily of retroviruses. Retroviruses have an RNA genome and the unique property of transcribing a DNA copy of the RNA genome following penetration of the host cell. The DNA is then used as a template to transcribe new RNA viral copies—thus the term 'retrovirus'. Lentiviruses generally evade host immune responses, and cause persistent infections in several species. HIV has a core consisting of the RNA genome and core protein surrounded by an envelope with high lipid content rendering it sensitive to organic solvents. The unique feature of the virus is that it gains entry to host cells by binding to the CD4 receptor (see below) using the viral surface membrane glycoprotein 120. This allows viral attachment and penetration of the host cell. The CD4 receptor is present predominantly on T-helper lymphocytes, which are therefore a major target for the virus. Following penetration of the host cell, the viral RNA is transcribed by the viral enzyme reverse transcriptase into a DNA copy which becomes incorporated into the host cell genomic DNA. This viral DNA may then lie dormant within the cell or undergo replication (particularly if that cell is stimulated) resulting in transcription of RNA copies and translation to viral proteins resulting in new virus formation and assembly. Viruses then bud from the cell surface (Fig. 4.4). New virus is then available to infect other cells and repeat the process.

HIV occurs in two main types.

HIV-1 is responsible for disease in Western Europe, North America and Central Africa. HIV-1 is antigenically extremely variable and indeed many different strains may be found within a single patient. Different strains of virus also vary greatly in their in-vitro cytopathicity, cell tropism and resistance to antiretroviral drugs such as zidovudine.

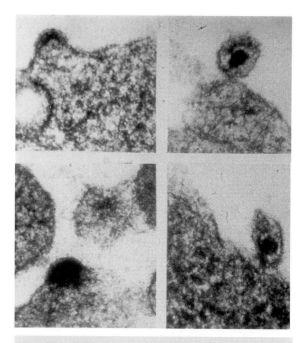

Fig. 4.4 Human immunodeficiency virus. Transmission electron micrograph of the virus budding from the surface of an infected CD4 lymphocyte.

HIV-2 is found predominantly in West Africa where it causes clinical syndromes similar to HIV-1 infection.

HIV-induced immunopathology

HIV principally affects CD4 helper T-lymphocytes (TH cells). TH cells are responsible for the initiation of nearly all immunological responses to pathogens, and following infection by HIV there is attrition of the CD4 cell population resulting in gradual and increasing failure of most aspects of immune function but particularly cell-mediated immunity. The main immunological abnormalities in HIV infection are listed in Table 4.19. The

---

Table 4.19 Immunological abnormalities in AIDS

T-helper (CD4+) lymphocytes
Decreased in number (low CD4 count in peripheral blood)
Abnormal function:
    reduced responses to antigen/mitogen
    reduced responses to interleukin-2
    reduced production of interleukin-2 and interferon gamma

B-lymphocytes
Abnormal function:
    reduced responses to specific antigen or mitogen
    polyclonal activation leading to increases in immunoglobulins

Monocytes/macrophages and dendritic cells
Defective antigen presentation
Defective cytokine secretion
Defective phagocytosis/killing

exact mechanism of the immunopathology, however, remains undetermined, since direct infection and damage by HIV to TH cells is not a sufficient explanation as it is frequently found that only 1:10 000 TH cells are actually infected by HIV. In addition to lymphocytes, HIV can infect and impair the function of many other cell types, in particular cells of the monocyte/macrophage lineage, dendritic cells and B-lymphocytes.

During the course of HIV disease there is a gradual reduction in the number of CD4 cells circulating in peripheral blood. Routine clinical measurement of the CD4 cell count is used in patients as a measure of disease progression and classification. The various complications of HIV disease correlate to an extent with the CD4 cell count which is also used to determine when anti-retroviral therapy should be instituted or when prophylactic antimicrobial agents should be used (see Table 4.20). The overwhelming abnormality of immune function caused by HIV is in cell mediated immunity which particularly protects against intracellular parasites (e.g. viruses, protozoa and mycobacteria), whereas failure of appropriate antibody responses, which also occurs with HIV infection, results in infection with capsulated bacteria.

HIV also infects cells in the central nervous system. This may be due to migration of HIV infected monocytes to the brain where they become microglial cells. This results in direct damage to the CNS, whereas most disease induced by HIV infection is a consequence of immune system failure resulting in opportunist infections and secondary neoplasms.

Testing for HIV and counselling

Although HIV infection may be suspected on clinical grounds, HIV infection is confirmed by demonstrating the presence of antibodies to HIV in the patient's serum. The current ELISA test used for detecting such antibodies is simple and cheap and has the advantage of a very low false negative rate. However, all positive results are normally confirmed by the more precise western blot test which also detects the presence of anti-HIV antibodies. Following infection, seroconversion, i.e. the detection of antibodies to HIV, may not occur for as long as three months and sometimes much longer. This means that serial testing may need to be performed on a patient following a high risk of exposure to HIV, in order to definitely exclude infection. In special circumstances where tests to detect antibody are repeatedly negative the polymerase chain reaction can be used to detect the presence of viral genomic material in peripheral blood lymphocytes to confirm that infection has occurred. However, the routine screening test remains the ELISA, which is used by centres offering a 'same day' testing service. The diagnosis of HIV infection

depends on being clinically astute, having a clear knowledge of the clinical manifestations which may occur, asking the patient for relevant risk factors, and having a high index of suspicion.

The importance of HIV testing for the patient relates to the very serious consequences, both social and medical, of having a positive test. Before a test is done it is important that adequate counselling with the patient is undertaken, including a discussion of the way in which the virus is spread, the effects the virus has, the psychological stress that a positive test will have and the effects on the individual's social, work and medical life. Issues relating to confidentiality and difficulties in obtaining life assurance and mortgages need to be discussed in the event of the test being positive. Other disadvantages of a positive test include feelings of guilt, the social stigma, and the fact that some countries will not admit HIV positive persons. The advantages of knowing that an individual is HIV seropositive include appropriate medical care and prophylactic measures, which will benefit health and the avoidance of infecting others. When the test is negative the patient should be advised to practice safe sex and abstention from other avoidable risk factors such as sharing needles for intravenous drug usage. When giving a positive result, the clinician should remember this is a disaster for the patient. Adequate time must be set aside for this without interruptions. If possible the partner, a close friend or family member should be available to provide immediate support.

Therapeutic approaches to HIV infection

Various programmes designed to prevent the spread of HIV (e.g. advice on safe sex, condoms, needles) have been in place since early in the epidemic. The overall success of these programmes is difficult to estimate accurately but the fact that currently reported numbers of AIDS cases and HIV infected inviduals in many European countries falls far short of epidemiological predictions of a few years ago must be attributed in part to these strategies. Hopes for an effective vaccine remain high but elusive at the moment despite an enormous research effort. The major therapeutic effort at present is directed to individuals already infected by HIV. There are numerous agents which interfere with HIV replication; however, the only drugs in regular clinical use are reverse transcriptase inhibitors that inhibit the spread of infectious virus into uninfected cells but do not affect replication of the HIV genome once it is integrated into the host cell.

Drugs in clinical use at the moment are zidovudine (AZT), didanosine (dideoxyinosine, DDI) and zalcitabine (dideoxycytidine, DDC). Many newer agents (e.g. protease inhibitors) are under clinical evaluation. Zidovudine is well absorbed orally and has been in general use for a number of years. It was initially shown in a large controlled study to prolong survival in patients with advanced HIV disease although toxicity was high. Lower doses have now been shown to be as effective and 500 mg or 600 mg daily is used routinely in the UK. Further studies in the USA demonstrated that early introduction of zidovudine in patients with less severe HIV disease results in a delay in the onset of AIDS. This data, however, conflicts with the findings of the large multicentre European Concorde study where zidovudine given in early HIV disease had little if any benefit with respect to delaying the onset of AIDS or improving survival. Zidovudine is known to lose its efficacy against HIV with time, so that benefits from the drug are relatively short lived and at best delay the onset of HIV related complications rather than prevent them. The current general recommendation therefore is that all HIV infected individuals with CD4 counts of greater than 500/mm^3 should not receive zidovudine. Individuals with CD4 counts between 200/mm^3 and 500/mm^3 are offered zidovudine only if there are symptoms. For patients with CD4 counts below 200/mm^3 or with AIDS, zidovudine is generally recommended. Later switching to alternative therapy with DDI or DDC may be beneficial, and the results of trials using these drugs in various combinations are awaited.

Use of zidovudine prophylactically in health care workers who have been accidentally exposed to HIV has been recommended, but disappointingly there have been several documented cases where this strategy failed to prevent infection. Side-effects of zidovudine include nausea, vomiting, headaches and myalgia, anaemia, neutropenia, and occasionally leucopenia and thrombocytopenia may occur. Macrocytosis develops in most patients.

Clinical features

Following a latent period of a few weeks, HIV infection is followed by seroconversion, which, in a third of individuals, coincides with a brief clinical illness for about two weeks, after which HIV antibodies appear in the blood. Symptoms of this illness include fever, malaise, headache, fleeting arthralgia, macular papular rash, tender lymphadenopathy and, occasionally, encephalitis. Thereafter there follows an asymptomatic phase which may last for many years. In a recent study from San Francisco, of patients infected with HIV 11 years previously, 50% had died of AIDS and of the survivors 20% had AIDS, 40% had symptoms attributable to HIV infection with 40% remaining completely symptom-free. However, it is thought that all individuals infected with HIV will eventually proceed to AIDS which is invariably fatal.

Some, but not all, HIV infected patients develop per-

Table 4.20 Classification of HIV-associated conditions

Absolute CD4 count (/mm^3)	Clinical groups		
	A	B	C
(1) > 500	A1	B1	C1
(2) 200–499	A2	B2	C2
(3) < 200	A3	B3	C3

Group A : Acute HIV infection, asymptomatic phase or persistent generalised lymphadenopathy (PGL)

Group B : Symptomatic: anything *not* included in Group C (e.g. constitutional symptoms, oral candidosis, peripheral neuropathy, idiopathic thrombocytopenic purpura, herpes zoster involving more than one dermatome, oral hairy leukoplakia)

Group C : Conditions meeting CDC/WHO case definition for AIDS (see Table 4.21).

sistent generalised lymphadenopathy (PGL) which is defined as the presence of enlarged lymph nodes greater than 1 cm in diameter in two anatomically distinct sites for greater than 3 months, in the absence of other detectable causes of lymphadenopathy. Most of these patients are asymptomatic, although a few have fever and weight loss. The diagnosis of PGL is usually made clinically; biopsy of lymph nodes shows reactive hyperplasia. The prognosis for patients who develop PGL is the same as for those who do not. Asymmetrical lymphadenopathy suggests alternative diagnoses such as lymphoma or tuberculosis.

Classification of HIV-associated conditions

Patients with acute HIV infection, or who are asymptomatic (including PGL patients who are usually asymptomatic) fall into group A of the Centers for Disease Control (CDC) classification of HIV associated conditions (Table 4.20). Group B patients have symptoms but do not have an AIDS defining condition. This group is sometimes referred to as the AIDS related complex (ARC) and is characterised by conditions not exclusively confined to immunocompromised individuals (see information box). Since these patients are relatively

---

CLINICAL FEATURES OF SYMPTOMATIC HIV DISEASE

General symptoms
- Fatigue
- Fever
- Malaise
- Weight loss
- Diarrhoea

General signs
- Lymphadenopathy
- Wasting
- Oral candida
- Oral hairy leukoplakia
- Perianal herpes
- Splenomegaly.

---

immunosuppressed they are also more prone to develop 'ordinary' infections such as herpes zoster and bacterial pneumonia. Group C includes patients who have AIDS

1. Disseminated clinical cytomegalovirus infection (not liver, spleen or lymph node)
2. Chronic (>1 month) mucocutaneous disseminated herpes simplex infection
3. Progressive multifocal leucoencephalopathy (papova (JC) virus)
4. Extra-pulmonary tuberculosis or pulmonary tuberculosis with CD4 count <200/mm^3
5. Disseminated *mycobacterium avium intracellulare* or *mycobacterium kansasii* infection
6. *Pneumocystis carinii* pneumonia
7. Candidosis of oesophagus, bronchi or pulmonary
8. Chronic (>1 month) cryptosporidiosis
9. Toxoplasmosis of brain
10. Isosporiasis
11. Disseminated histoplasmosis or coccidioidomycosis
12. Cryptococcosis
13. Extra-intestinal strongyloidiasis

Secondary neoplasms
1. Kaposi's sarcoma
2. Primary lymphoma of brain
3. Non-Hodgkin's (immunoblastic) lymphoma

Other
1. Lymphocytic interstitial pneumonia (mainly children)

* CDC: Centre for Disease Control, Atlanta, Georgia
WHO: World Health Organization

and therefore have one of the conditions meeting the CDC case definition for AIDS (Table 4.21). As demonstrated in Table 4.20, Group A, B and C patients are subdivided further according to their CD4 count. The standard classifications of HIV disease, although useful, have the disadvantage of 'pigeon-holing' patients. It is clinically more helpful to think of HIV disease as a spectrum of increasing immune deficiency which statistically increases the likelihood of opportunist infections and secondary neoplasms (see Fig. 4.5). Patients with AIDS

CD$_4$ count

Herpes Zoster
Oral Candida
Kaposi's Sarcoma
Pneumocystis pneumonia
CMV, MAI

Time

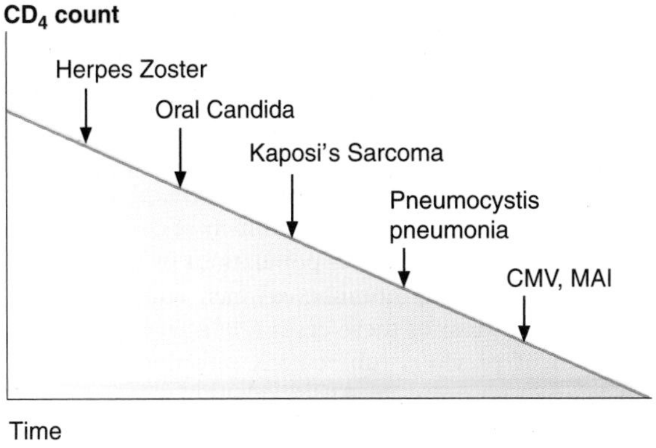

Fig. 4.5 Spectrum of diseases in HIV infection. As the CD4$^+$ lymphocyte count in the blood declines, characteristic opportunist infections and neoplasms present clinically.

have one of the major opportunist infections or one of the secondary neoplasms that characterise AIDS and these will all be described in the rest of the chapter. Survival for patients once AIDS is established is poor, with only 50% of patients still alive eighteen months beyond diagnosis. However, medical interventions have altered the course of HIV disease so that the diseases which are AIDS defining occur with more severe levels of immunosuppression than previously, thus accounting for the relatively poor outlook once AIDS is established.

Disseminated disease in AIDS

Many of the opportunist infections and secondary neoplasms seen in AIDS are disseminated at presentation. These will be described first and are listed in the information box.

DISSEMINATED DISEASE IN AIDS

Infections
- Cytomegalovirus (CMV) infection
- Bacterial septicaemia (e.g. pneumococcal, salmonella)
- *M. tuberculosis*
- *M. avium intracellulare* infection
- Toxoplasmosis
- Cryptococcosis
- Histoplasmosis

Secondary neoplasms
- Kaposi's sarcoma
- Non-Hodgkin's lymphoma

Cytomegalovirus (CMV)

CMV is a herpes virus and infection is extremely common. Approximately 50% of the general population, and 90% of homosexual men, are seropositive. Clinical disease results from reactivation of latent CMV infection in the face of severe immunosuppression, and the CD4 count is normally below 50/mm^3 when clinical disease appears. Diagnosis of CMV disease is based on the clinical picture and histology. Many organs can be involved, including the eyes, CNS, liver, gut, adrenals, mouth and lung. The most common problem is CMV choroido-retinitis (Fig. 4.6) which can lead very rapidly to blindness and is characterised by fundal perivascular haemorrhage and exudates. Overt adrenal involvement is uncommon, but can occasionally present with lassitude, postural hypotension, dehydration and hyponatraemia which responds to corticosteroid therapy. CMV encephalitis usually presents subacutely (in contrast to the more gradual progression of HIV related encephalopathy) with personality change, poor concentration, headaches and insomnia. CMV may also cause myelitis and polyradiculopathy. CMV can cause colitis presenting with diarrhoea, weight loss, anorexia and fever,

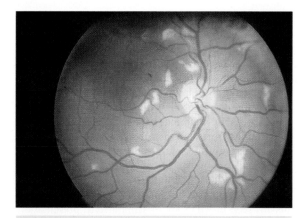

Fig. 4.6 CMV retinitis. Characteristic perivascular exudates often accompanied by haemorrhages in more severe cases.

but is a less common cause of colitis than other pathogens, which include Cryptosporidium, Giardia, Entamoeba, *Mycobacterium avium intracellulare*, Shigella and Campylobacter as well as large gut involvement by lymphoma or Kaposi's sarcoma. Sigmoidoscopy reveals diffuse submucosal haemorrhages and ulcerations. CMV may cause oesophagitis, but again oesophagitis is more frequently caused by Candida. Unlike the other sites where CMV undoubtedly does cause disease, it is a very rare cause of pneumonia although it is frequently isolated from the lung in AIDS patients. Treatment of CMV is with ganciclovir, or, alternatively, foscarnet. As both drugs have to be given intravenously, permanent venous access via a Hickman line or similar device is normally required. A favourable clinical response is normally obtained and retinal lesions may even regress. Retinitis is treated with a two-week course of induction therapy followed by maintenance therapy at a lower dose. Even with this, relapse is common but generally responds to a switch in treatment. Occasionally dual therapy with both drugs is required. The other CMV diseases require two weeks of treatment followed by careful monitoring.

Other herpes viruses
Herpes zoster infection, usually in the form of multi-dermatomal shingles, is seen in HIV infected patients belonging to Group B of the CDC classification (Table 4.20). Rarely it may cause pneumonitis or encephalitis in AIDS patients. Chronic muco-cutaneous herpes simplex infection is an AIDS defining diagnosis and infection may be very widespread, but again dissemination is unusual.

Bacterial infections in HIV
Although many of the serious opportunist infections in AIDS are due to viruses, fungi or protozoa, bacterial infections are very prevalent in these patients. This is thought to reflect the fact that cell mediated immune responses are important in certain intracellular bacterial infections such as tuberculosis, and that antibody-mediated protection and neutrophil function are also disturbed in HIV infection, allowing infection with capsulated bacteria. It is important to recognise that such infections are often not contained within a particular organ, and septicaemia causing disseminated bacterial infection is often seen in these patients. These infections will be discussed further in later sections. Neurosyphilis should be considered in the differential diagnosis of neurological disease in AIDS and, conversely, HIV infection should be considered in patients presenting with syphilis.

Mycobacterial infection
a) **Mycobacterium tuberculosis**
Although tuberculosis in HIV infected patients is not a major problem in the UK, dual infection is common in parts of the world where there is a high prevalence of both HIV and tuberculosis. This is particularly the case in developing countries such as sub-Saharan Africa where during HIV infection, tuberculosis behaves as an opportunist infection. The greater the immuno-suppression the more likely is tuberculosis to be disseminated and to present in an atypical manner. Unlike the other opportunist infections of AIDS, tuberculosis is infectious to normal individuals. On a global scale HIV is now considered the most important risk factor for the development of tuberculosis.

MAIN FEATURES OF TUBERCULOSIS IN HIV INFECTION

- Incidence reflects background prevalence in community
- Most cases due to reactivation
- TB may precede AIDS in HIV infected individual
- Extrapulmonary TB in HIV is an AIDS-defining diagnosis
- Diagnosis may be difficult
- Prognosis poor: TB may accelerate HIV disease
- Threat of multi-drug resistant TB

In the USA there had been a general decline in tuberculosis until 1986 when numbers of cases started to rise amongst certain urban populations of HIV infected individuals, mainly homosexual men and intravenous drug users. Most of these cases are in fact due to reactivation of previous tuberculous infection as a result of failing immunity. In Africa tuberculosis is the most common pulmonary complication of AIDS and one of the most important opportunist infections seen in AIDS. In the UK about 6% of AIDS patients develop tuberculosis at some stage, although this figure may change as a result of immigration to the UK of people coming from areas of the world with a high prevalence of tuberculosis who are also infected with HIV.

Tuberculosis may occur at any stage of HIV infection. When immunity is still well preserved, pulmonary disease alone is seen, often resembling post-primary disease in normal individuals, whereas when the CD4 count is low, extra-pulmonary disease involving lymph nodes, bone, pericardium, peritoneum, central nervous system, liver and marrow may occur, in addition to miliary tuberculosis. Non specific features of fever, weight loss and fatigue are also present. The diagnosis of tuberculosis classically relies on sputum examination and culture, tuberculin testing and the chest radiograph. However, in HIV infection the tuberculin test may be unhelpful as it is frequently negative because of the immune defect. As disease may be disseminated, pulmonary disease may be minimal and there may be no sputum for examination. Thirdly, the chest radiograph appearances are not always typical (Fig. 4.7). Diagnosis therefore usually relies on a high index of suspicion. Clinical response to standard treatment with isoniazid, rifampicin and pyrazinamide (see p. 361), sometimes with the addition of ethambutol, is generally excellent with rapid improvement in symptoms. However, overall survival is poor. Six to nine months of therapy is recommended but isoniazid prophylaxis should continue for life to prevent relapse. To prevent tuberculosis occurring in the first place, chemoprophylaxis is recommended for individuals who have a positive tuberculin test or individuals that come from parts of the world with a very high prevalence for tuberculosis who have almost certainly been infected in childhood. There is concern following the emergence of multi-drug resistant tuberculosis in certain groups of patients in the USA with AIDS, as the response to even second-line drugs, and hence the prognosis, is very poor and infection can be transmitted to health care workers with fatal consequences.

b) Atypical mycobacteria

Of the non-tuberculous mycobacteria, *Mycobacterium avium intracellulare* (MAI) is by far the most common mycobacterial infection seen in AIDS patients. *M. kansasii* also occurs and disseminated infection with either is an AIDS-defining diagnosis. Unlike tuberculosis, MAI is a pathogen of very low virulence and is commonly found in the environment, being present in soil, water and food. It usually causes clinical disease which is invariably disseminated only when the CD4 count is very low (less than $50/mm^3$) towards the end of the natural history of AIDS. The portal of entry is thought to be through the gut; the most common presenting features are with persistent high grade fever, night sweats, anaemia and weight loss in addition to non-specific symptoms of malaise, anorexia, diarrhoea, myalgia and occasional painful lymphadenopathy. On examination hepatomegaly is frequently present and the chest radiograph and CT scan often reveal widespread intrathoracic and intra-abdominal lymphadenopathy. The diagnosis is generally easy provided it is considered, as clinical specimens from affected organs contain numerous acid-fast bacilli. Unlike tuberculosis, MAI is universally resistant to all first line anti-tuberculous drugs. Various combinations of newer antibiotics combined with more traditional agents have been shown to produce useful clinical responses. Combination therapy is selected from ethambutol, rifabutin, clofazamine, ciprofloxacin, amikacin and azithromycin, and although some of these drugs produce troublesome toxicity, these disadvantages are outweighed by the clinical benefits in most cases.

Fungal infections

a) Candidosis

Oral candidosis is almost universal at some stage of HIV infection (Fig. 4.8), and if seen unexpectedly in the mouth of a young patient, should prompt consideration of HIV infection. Lesions in the mouth may initially respond to topical anti-fungal agents such as nystatin or amphotericin but when more advanced, systemic ther-

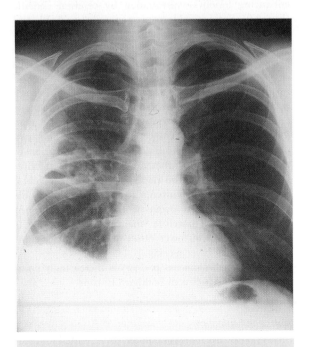

Fig. 4.7 Chest radiograph of pulmonary tuberculosis in HIV infection. Appearances are often atypical but in this case there is a typical large cavity accompanied by a pleural effusion.

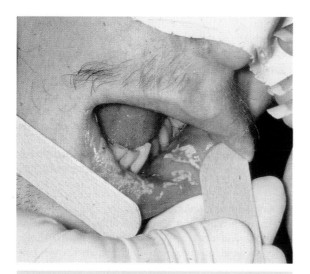

Fig. 4.8 Oral candidosis. A careful examination of the mouth is important as plaques may initially be quite small.

apy is required normally with ketoconazole or fluconazole. When Candida spreads beyond the mouth to the oesophagus or, more rarely, the lung, it becomes an AIDS-defining diagnosis. With oesophageal involvement, painful dysphagia is frequent and barium swallow may reveal a very ragged looking mucosal surface. Once Candida infection is firmly established, anti-fungal therapy has to be continuous and liver function tests should be closely monitored if ketoconazole is used. Long-term treatment with the azole drugs for prophylaxis may lead to resistance, necessitating the use of amphotericin. Widely disseminated disease is generally rare but can become a problem in patients with neutropenia, IVDA and patients with indwelling central venous lines.

b) Cryptococcal infection

Cryptococcus neoformans is the commonest cause of meningitis in AIDS patients and may also cause pulmonary involvement. Although clinically disseminated infection is relatively rare, the organism may be cultured from blood, urine, gut or bone marrow. Initial symptoms of cryptococcal meningitis are fatigue, fever and weight loss, followed by headache, nausea, vomiting and photophobia. Diagnosis may be delayed because the poor inflammatory response often masks the classical symptoms and signs of meningitis. Diagnosis is made by Indian ink staining of the CSF to identify the organism, CSF culture and measurement of cryptococcal antigen both in serum and CSF. CT scan of the brain is usually normal and CSF examination may show a monocytosis and raised protein. Standard therapy has traditionally been amphotericin with or without flucytocine.

However, because of the toxicity associated with amphotericin use, fluconazole or liposomal amphotericin are often now used with satisfactory clinical responses. Relapse is common, so long-term suppressive therapy is required with oral fluconazole.

c) Endemic fungal infection in AIDS

Disseminated infection with *Histoplasma capsulatum* and *Coccidioidomyces imitis* are seen in AIDS patients who have been exposed to these fungi in endemically restricted areas such as occur in certain parts of the United States and Africa. It is therefore vital to take a good travel history from anyone with HIV infection. Amphotericin is the treatment of choice although azole drugs such as ketoconazole may be useful.

Protozoal infection

Toxoplasma gondii infection is very common in man (see p. 162) and following severe immunosuppression with AIDS, clinical disease may emerge with fever, lymphadenopathy and headache. The brain is the most common site for lesions, which usually present with focal neurological symptoms, convulsions, cognitive impairment, confusion, lethargy or coma. Other organs including the retina may be involved. Diagnosis is usually made by cranial CT scan which shows a characteristic ring enhancing lesion(s) surrounded by cerebral oedema (Fig. 4.9). Serological tests are generally unreliable and definitive diagnosis requires demonstration of the organism in brain biopsy material. This however is rarely necessary, the diagnosis being made on clinical grounds and a satisfactory response to treatment. However, if toxoplasma serology is completely negative, a space occupying lesion in the brain of an AIDS patient is unlikely to be due to toxoplasmosis. Treatment is with folate antagonists, usually pyrimethamine and sulphadiazine given with folinic acid. A combination of clindamycin and pyrimethamine is also effective. Dexamethasone may be necessary to relieve cerebral oedema and anticonvulsants to control convulsions. Relapse is likely to occur if treatment is stopped completely and therefore maintenance therapy is recommended with lower doses of similar drug combinations taken twice weekly.

Visceral leishmaniasis (p. 156) is increasingly common in AIDS patients in Southern Europe.

Nematode infections

Strongyloides stercoralis is acquired as an endemic infection in certain parts of the world (see p. 174), normally resulting in latent infection which very rarely becomes disseminated in AIDS patients. The diagnosis is made

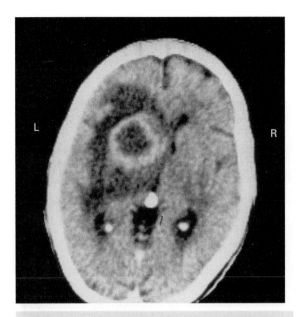

Fig. 4.9 Toxoplasma brain abscess. Characteristic ring-enhancing lesion following contrast with surrounding cerebral oedema (low attenuation area).

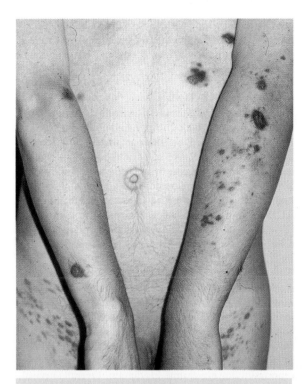

Fig. 4.10 Widespread cutaneous Kaposi's sarcoma. Lesions tend to be pleomorphic and slightly raised.

by identifying larvae in the faeces and treatment is with albendazole.

Secondary neoplasms of AIDS

Kaposi's sarcoma

Kaposi's sarcoma is the most common non-infectious AIDS-defining diagnosis in HIV disease. It is an unusual neoplastic condition which was rare before AIDS. It is unusual in that although it has many malignant features it invariably arises at multiple sites within a short space of time. The aetiology remains undetermined although novel herpesvirus-like DNA has been identified in AIDS-associated Kaposi's sarcoma. Kaposi's sarcoma is most common in homosexual male AIDS patients (about 25% of cases) and sexually transmitted HIV infection in sub-Saharan African patients, whereas it is a comparative rarity in AIDS patients with haemophilia. This suggests that a co-factor transmitted by the sexual route is required for its development. Histologically the tumour consists of spindle cells and small blood vessels. Some authorities regard it as a hyperplastic rather than a true neoplastic condition. The most common site of involvement is the skin. The mouth, the hard palate, tip of nose, penis and lower legs are also favoured sites (Fig. 4.10). Lesions are red or violatious, well circumscribed, flat or raised. In dark-skinned individuals, lesions may appear brown or even black. When multiple skin lesions are present they tend to develop along skin flexures. The prognosis for skin disease is very variable, although as the CD4 count falls, Kaposi's sarcoma tends to become more aggressive. Lymph nodes are the second most common site, and along with extranodal visceral disease indicate a poor prognosis compared to isolated skin disease. Stomach or rectal involvement may present with pain, bleeding or obstruction. Liver and spleen involvement cause hepatosplenomegaly, and pulmonary involvement may result in cough and breathlessness due to bronchial and parenchymal involvement, or the development of large pleural effusions. Patients with visceral involvement nearly all have mucocutaneous or lymph node lesions. In patients with a few skin lesions the disease may follow an indolent course whereas extensive disease tends to be more aggressive.

Skin lesions particularly on the face are unsightly and single lesions can be treated by local radiotherapy. Satisfactory palliation of disseminated disease can be achieved by combination chemotherapy with vincristine or vinblastine and bleomycin often with the addition of doxarubicin. More recently, treatment with a single agent, with liposome encapsulated daunorubicin or doxarubicin, have produced good responses comparable to combination therapy with far less drug toxicity. Treatment reduces morbidity but does not improve survival. It is noteworthy that Kaposi's sarcoma virtually never involves the brain.

Non-Hodgkin's lymphoma

This group of lymphomas arises from B lymphocytes in 80% of cases, with the remainder arising from T lymphocytes. Of the B cell tumours the majority are high grade B cell lymphomas of various histological types including immunoblastic lymphoma and Burkitt-type lymphoma. The development of one of these lymphomas in an HIV positive individual constitutes an AIDS-defining diagnosis and in contrast to their development in normal individuals, these tumours tend to arise largely at extranodal sites, most frequently the CNS, bone marrow, gastrointestinal tract and liver. They are often advanced at the time of diagnosis, producing 'B' symptoms of fever and weight loss. Diagnosis is by tissue biopsy of affected sites and histological examination. Treatment is with combination chemotherapy, and various regimens produce useful response. Primary lymphoma of the brain, however, is particularly difficult to treat, although short-term responses have been reported following cranial irradiation. Overall survival, irrespective of location or initial response to therapy, is poor and usually less than one year.

Carcinoma

There is an increased incidence of cervical dysplasia and neoplasia in HIV infected women and anal carcinoma particularly in HIV infected homosexual men. Women with HIV infection should have regular cervical smears. The association between these carcinomas and HIV is thought to be due to a greater incidence of infection by the Human Papilloma Virus in HIV-infected patients rather than a consequence of immunodeficiency.

Organ specific HIV disease

In this section organ specific disease not already covered in the previous section will be discussed.

The skin

Skin disease is extremely common in HIV infected patients. Some of these diseases are also seen in the normal population but less frequently and less severely (e.g. molluscum contagiosum (Fig. 4.11) and seborrhoeic dermatitis), whereas others are specific to HIV infection (e.g. Kaposi's sarcoma). The common skin diseases seen in HIV-infected patients are listed in the information box. In Africa, Slim disease consists of weight loss, diarrhoea (due to either HIV itself or enteric tuberculosis) and dermatitis, and is an AIDS-defining diagnosis. Management of the various skin infections observed in these

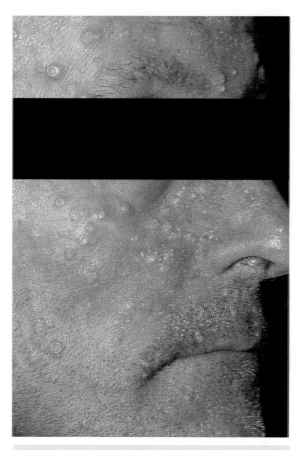

Fig. 4.11 Molluscum contagiosum. Extensive and disfiguring involvement of the face may occur.

COMMON SKIN DISEASES IN HIV INFECTION

- Seborrhoeic dermatitis
- Folliculitis/impetigo/cellulitis
- Secondary syphilis
- Herpes simplex/herpes zoster
- Molluscum contagiosum
- Fungal infections
- Kaposi's sarcoma
- Drug eruptions

---

patients is identical to the treatment given to non-HIV infected patients.

Drug eruptions

Drug induced skin eruptions are very common and more severe in HIV disease than in the general population. This is thought to be as a result of the immune dysregulation induced by HIV. Drug eruptions are a very important aspect of the care of AIDS patients as the

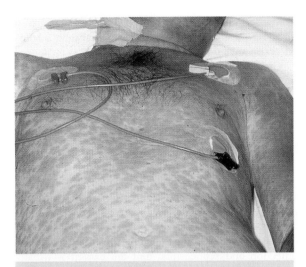

Fig. 4.12 Drug-induced skin eruption. Hypersensitivity drug reactions are common, in this case due to co-trimoxazole.

Table 4.22 Oral diseases in HIV

Disease	Treatment
Candidosis	Nystatin, amphotericin or fluconazole
Angular stomatitis	Often responds to antifungal cream or fucidic acid gel if secondary infected with *Staph aureus*
Hairy leukoplakia	Usually responds to acyclovir
Gingivitis	Metronidazole or penicillin
CMV/herpes simplex stomatitis	Appropriate antiviral therapy (ganciclovir or acyclovir)
Aphthous ulcers	Orabase triamcinalone (benzydamine mouth washes or benzocaine lozenges for pain). Thalidomide if refractory
Warts	Cryotherapy or podophyllin
Kaposi's sarcoma	Local radiotherapy if very large

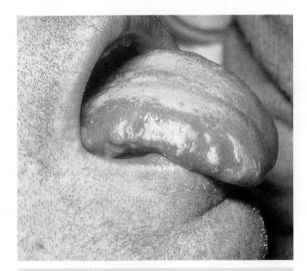

Fig. 4.13 Oral hairy leukoplakia. This tends to occur along the edge of the tongue.

majority will develop a major drug eruption at some stage. Many drugs produce these reactions but particular culprits are co-trimoxazole, which frequently induces a widespread intensely itchy maculo-papular rash (Fig. 4.12) and fansidar (pyrimethamine sulphadoxine, combination), sometimes used in prophylaxis against pneumocystis pneumonia, which may induce erythema multiforme and the Stevens–Johnson syndrome. The drugs used to treat tuberculosis may result in skin eruptions, as may dapsone. Itchy drug reactions may respond to antihistamines such as terfenadine or chlorpheniramine, although it may be necessary to stop the drug.

Oral disease

Oral disease is prominent in HIV infection (see Table 4.22), and maintenance of good dental and oral hygiene is hence very important in these patients. Because mouth lesions are so common in HIV and may be present early in HIV disease, a very careful inspection of the mouth during clinical examination is mandatory. Oral disease may cause disabling symptoms but most conditions are responsive to appropriate treatment. Oral hairy leukoplakia (Fig. 4.13) may occur in HIV infection and presents as serrated white areas normally along the sides of the tongue. These plaques are adherent and cannot be pushed off with a spatula like Candida. They are usually painless, may be caused by the Epstein–Barr virus and usually respond to acyclovir. It should be noted from Table 4.22 that for refractory aphthous ulceration thalidomide may produce useful relief but if used the dose should be kept to a minimum to prevent the development of peripheral neuropathy, and it is vital that

female patients take contraceptive measures while on thalidomide.

Gastrointestinal disease

a) **The oesophagus.** Painful dysphagia is common in HIV disease due to oesophagitis. The most common cause is, again, Candida. The majority of these patients have obvious oral candidiasis. Barium swallow appearances are characteristic but endoscopy provides definitive diagnosis. Response to fluconazole is normally excellent. Both herpes simplex and CMV are rare causes of oesophagitis and in these patients pain on swallowing and intermittent retrosternal pain are particular features. CMV characteristically causes disease in the lower third of the oesophagus. Endoscopy often reveals extremely large shallow superficial ulceration. Response to antiviral therapy is normally satisfactory but maintenance therapy for both viruses may be needed if relapse occurs. Occasionally primary lymphoma, Kaposi's sarcoma and even squamous cell carcinoma are found in HIV patients with dysphagia. Severe aphthous ulceration may spread to the oesophagus, and tablet-induced ulceration should also be considered. Finally, HIV patients are not immune from ordinary diseases and gastro-oesophageal reflux may result in oesophagitis and ulceration. In view of the wide differential diagnosis all HIV patients with dysphagia which is refractory to antifungal agents or who have low retrosternal pain should undergo endoscopy.

b) **Gastric disease.** Nausea and vomiting are very common in AIDS and are frequently the result of drug therapy, in particular high dose co-trimoxazole in the treatment of pneumocystis pneumonia. Alternatively it results from intrinsic gastric disease due to Kaposi's sarcoma, lymphoma, CMV-induced ulceration or gastric ulcer. Mallory–Weiss tears and variceal bleeding are also seen, as many AIDS patients belonging to the homosexual or IVDA risk group have high ethanol intake and hepatitis B and C are also common in this group. Nausea and vomiting in AIDS from whatever cause can be a major management problem but usually responds to either metaclopramide, domperidone, prochloperazine or ondanestron.

c) **Small bowel disease.** Weight loss, high volume diarrhoea and colicky para-umbilical pain are suggestive of specific small bowel disease which may be due to a wide range of infections (see information box). Diagnosis

---

SMALL BOWEL DISEASE IN HIV

- Cryptosporidium
- Salmonella species
- Entamoeba histolytica
- Giardia lamblia
- Campylobacter
- CMV
- Microsporidium
- Clostridium difficile
- Strongyloides stercoralis
- MAI
- Kaposi's sarcoma

---

depends on examination and appropriate culture of stools (and small bowel biopsy if necessary) to allow specific therapy with appropriate antimicrobial agents. Small bowel biopsy may also demonstrate subtotal villous atrophy, and malabsorption is a common accompaniment. HIV itself may produce mucosal changes, and autonomic neuropathy may contribute to small bowel dysfunction. High volume diarrhoea is another serious management problem in AIDS resulting in weight loss and dehydration, and requires fluid and electrolyte replacement, nutritional supplements and antidiarrhoeal agents such as loperamide, diphenoxylate and

codeine. Some patients with severe diarrhoea refractory to these measures may respond to octreotide, a somatostatin analogue.

Cryptosporidiosis, which is an AIDS-defining diagnosis if chronic, is a parasite which affects the brush border of the gastrointestinal tract and normally presents with profuse watery diarrhoea accompanied by abdominal pain, fever, anorexia, malaise, malabsorption and wasting. It may involve the biliary tract (and cause biliary tract pain), pancreatic duct and gallbladder. It is difficult to treat but spiramycin may occasionally reduce the volume of diarrhoea.

Isospora belli is related to cryptosporidium but unlike cryptosporidium normally responds well to co-trimoxazole. Bacterial infections with salmonella or shigella are often accompanied by signs of disseminated infection and septicaemia, and the patient is usually extremely ill. Response is normally good to appropriate antibiotics.

d) **Colorectal disease.** Colonic disease normally results in frequent small volume stools, left lower quadrant and suprapubic colicky pain, tenesmus and pain on defecation. A number of infectious causes are seen, two important ones being CMV and cryptosporidium. In homosexual patients a sexual history should be taken and proctoscopy performed, swabs being taken for Chlamydia and gonorrhoea. Warts and herpes simplex are common in this group and syphilis serology should be performed.

Hepatobiliary disease

Abnormal liver function tests, right upper quadrant pain and hepatomegaly are extremely common findings in AIDS patients as hepatic disease is extremely common. The main causes of hepatic disease in HIV infected patients are hepatitis A, B or C, hepatotoxic drugs and CMV and MAI infections. Investigations should include hepatitis and syphilis serology, ultrasound or CT of the upper abdomen and liver biopsy if indicated. MAI and CMV are particularly common causes of hepatitis as part of disseminated disease and CMV, Candida and Cryptosporidium are recognised causes of acalculous cholangitis. The liver may be involved in Kaposi's sarcoma and lymphoma.

Respiratory disease

Pulmonary disease is very common in AIDS and the spectrum of causes is listed in Table 4.23. The atypical fungus *Pneumocystis carinii* is the most common opportunist pathogen in AIDS in Europe and North America. Prior to the introduction of chemoprophylaxis, up to 80% of all patients with AIDS had one or more episodes of pneumocystis pneumonia. In Africa, however, pneumocystis pneumonia is unusual whereas tuberculosis is

Table 4.23 Spectrum of lung disease in AIDS

Common	Rare
Pneumocystis pneumonia	Herpes simplex/varicella zoster Adenovirus
M. tuberculosis	
M. avium intracellulare	Nocardia M. xenopi/kansasii, etc.
Strep pneumoniae	Candida/Aspergillus spp
Haemophilus influenzae	Cryptococcus/Histoplasma
Staph aureus	Strongyloides stercoralis
Moraxella catarrhalis	Toxoplasma gondii
Gram-negative bacteria	Cryptosporidia
Mycoplasma	Lymphoma
(Cytomegalovirus)	Non-specific interstitial pneumonitis Lymphocytic interstitial pneumonitis
Kaposi's sarcoma	Pulmonary drug reactions

very common. Pneumocystis infection is largely confined to the lung, where the airspaces fill with foamy exudate containing cysts and trophozoites of the organism. Pneumocystis pneumonia usually starts insidiously with an irritating dry cough and breathlessness. There is often a background of fatigue, weight loss and fever as well as other signs of HIV infection. Sputum production is unusual and audible crackles in the chest are rare. An increased respiratory rate is common with cyanosis indicative of severe disease (see information box).

PNEUMOCYSTIS CARINII PNEUMONIA

- Commonest opportunist infection in AIDS prior to chemoprophylaxis usage
- Commonly the AIDS-defining diagnosis
- 60–80% of all AIDS patients will have an episode if not taking prophylaxis
- Mortality 5–15%
- Annual incidence in AIDS (without prophylaxis) 30%
- Relapse rate (without prophylaxis) 35% by 6 months: 50–60% by 1 year

Typically, the chest radiograph shows diffuse bilateral interstitial perihilar shadowing (Fig. 4.14), although 10% of cases have a normal chest radiograph and 10% have atypical features such as focal consolidation, nodular shadows or cavities. A pleural effusion or mediastinal adenopathy are both rare in pneumocystis pneumonia and suggest alternative diagnoses such as mycobacterial infection or Kaposi's sarcoma. Non-invasive investigations, such as arterial oxygen desaturation on exercise determined by a pulse oximeter or pulmonary function testing, lack diagnostic specificity but are helpful at a stage when the chest radiograph may be normal,

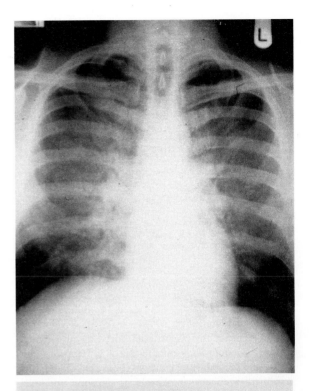

Fig. 4.14 Pneumocystis pneumonia. Typical chest radiograph appearance. Note the sparing at the apex and base of both lungs.

to confirm that organic pulmonary disease is present. As *Pneumocystis carinii* does not grow in vitro and sputum production is rare, diagnosis usually requires bronchoscopy and broncho-alveolar lavage. The lung washings reveal the cysts of *Pneumocystis carinii* with silver stain (Fig 4.15). To avoid bronchoscopy some centres induce sputum production with the use of inhaled hypertonic saline which provokes a bronchorrhoea. However, this is a difficult technique to establish and many centres still rely on bronchoscopy. Furthermore, as pneumocystis pneumonia is so common in AIDS patients, some authorities suggest empirical treatment initially without attempting to establish an aetiological diagnosis.

The treatment of choice for pneumocystis pneumonia is high dose co-trimoxazole, initially given intravenously. If a patient improves significantly a switch to oral therapy is appropriate and treatment should continue for three weeks. Alternative therapies are dapsone and trimethoprim in combination or clindamycin and primaquine in combination. Intravenous pentamidine is also effective but is not used because of toxic side effects. 80–90% of patients will respond to treatment. As a general rule, admission to intensive care units and intermittent positive pressure ventilation is avoided in these patients as the mortality is over 90%. It has been shown

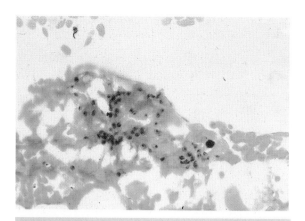

Fig. 4.15 *Pneumocystis carinii.* Bronchoalveolar lavage sample obtained at fibreoptic bronchoscopy. Methenamine-silver stain demonstrating black pneumocystis cysts.

that treatment with high dose corticosteroids at the time of admission in patients with respiratory failure reduces morbidity and mortality.

Like many of the opportunist infections already discussed, Pneumocystis pneumonia is a relapsing condition and secondary prophylaxis should be offered. Oral treatment with co-trimoxazole or dapsone and pyrimethamine provides good protection against further attacks as does nebulised pentamidine administered every four weeks. Co-trimoxazole is the most effective of these agents and primary prophylaxis (to prevent pneumocystis pneumonia developing in the first place) should be offered to all HIV seropositive patients with a CD4 count below $200/mm^3$ and all patients with AIDS. Dapsone and pyrimethamine in combination and co-trimoxazole have the added advantage of providing some protection against toxoplasmosis. Nebulised pentamidine has the disadvantage of being less effective than co-trimoxazole; relapse of pneumocystis pneumonia may be atypical affecting the upper lobes, and cases of extra-pulmonary pneumocystosis have been reported following its use.

It is important to recognise that bacterial pneumonia is also more common in HIV infected individuals than in the normal population and tends to be more severe. Response to appropriate antibiotics is usually good. Cytomegalovirus, as discussed previously, is frequently isolated from lung washings but only rarely causes pneumonitis. Tuberculosis and MAI have been previously discussed, as has Kaposi's sarcoma. Sinusitis is common in AIDS, is usually bacterial in origin, and responds to appropriate antibiotic therapy.

Neurological disease

It is now known that the HIV infects the central nervous system at an early stage in the disease. HIV seems to inflict direct damage on the central nervous system, unlike other organs, resulting in clinical disease. Indeed, in the brain this is more common than opportunist infections and secondary neoplasms. HIV can be readily isolated from brain tissue and CSF in a high proportion of patients with neurological conditions, and at postmortem pathological changes are present in the brain in about three-quarters of patients with AIDS. Neurological symptoms in HIV infection require careful investigation which often includes CT or MRI, lumbar puncture and electrophysiological studies. Very occasionally brain biopsy will be required. Causes of nervous system disease are listed in Table 4.24.

a) **Direct effects of HIV infection**. During the period of a seroconversion following HIV infection, encephalitis may occur with mood change, convulsions, or altered level of consciousness. Meningitis may also occur. During the symptomatic phase of HIV infection, HIV is present in the brain and indeed can be recovered from CSF. In late HIV disease, HIV itself can cause aseptic meningitis but more importantly causes a diffuse encephalopathy referred to as the AIDS dementia complex characterised by cognitive, motor and behavioural dysfunction. This is probably the most common neurological complication of HIV infection and probably affects the majority of AIDS patients to varying degrees. In late AIDS the majority of patients have some degree of dementia even if it is mild. Zidovudine has been shown to be effective in reducing the prevalence of AIDS dementia complex. Onset is usually insidious with increasing forgetfulness, loss of concentration and loss of cognitive skills leading to confusion, apathy, agitation

Table 4.24 Diseases of the nervous system in HIV infection and their presentation

HIV	
Seroconversion illness	Encephalitis, meningitis (uncommon)
Chronic disease	AIDS dementia complex (ADC) encephalopathy meningitis myelopathy peripheral neuropathy
Other Infections	
Toxoplasmosis	Brain abscess
Cryptococcosis	Meningitis
Papova (JC) virus infection	Progressive multifocal leucoencephalopathy
CMV	Retinitis, encephalitis
Herpes zoster	Meningitis
Tuberculosis	Brain abscess/meningitis
Syphilis	Neurosyphilis
TUMOURS	
Secondary neoplasms	Space occupying lesion
Primary lymphoma	

and social withdrawal with behavioural disturbance. Motor dysfunction normally starts with unsteadiness of gait, weakness of the legs and lack of co-ordination. A steady decline leads to global dementia with gross limb weakness and pyramidal tract signs, ataxia and incontinence. Convulsions may occur in late disease. Investigations often show cortical atrophy on CT scan and increased protein and lymphocyte count in the CSF. HIV can also cause a myelopathy contributing to the motor disturbance seen in AIDS dementia complex. A variety of peripheral neuropathies occur in HIV infection with the most common, which is probably due to HIV itself, causing a predominant sensory neuropathy.

b) **Other neurological diseases**. Apart from cryptococcal infection, other causes of meningitis include bacteria, tuberculosis, syphilis, other fungal infections and HIV itself. A diffuse encephalopathy may be caused by metabolic disturbance, Herpes zoster or simplex and CMV. Toxoplasmosis is the most common cause of a space occupying lesion in HIV disease (see p. 96). Less common causes of space-occupying lesions are primary cerebral lymphoma or lymphomatous infiltration from other sites, and tuberculosis. CMV most commonly causes choroido-retinitis presenting with blurring and then loss of vision which is often unilateral initially. Less commonly CMV causes encephalitis or radiculopathy. Progressive multifocal leuco-encephalopathy (PML) is relatively uncommon and is an opportunist infection caused by a papova virus, JC. This results in predominant damage to the white matter; the clinical course is a little more protracted than that seen in toxoplasmosis or lymphoma and definitive diagnosis can only be made on brain biopsy or at autopsy. There is no effective treatment. Peripheral neuropathies of various types in addition to those caused by HIV may occur, including ascending polyneuritis (Guillain-Barré syndrome), autonomic neuropathy, or may be secondary to Herpes zoster or CMV infection, or drug-induced—in particular as a result of the use of the antiretroviral agents dideoxyinosine and dideoxycytidine. Finally, myopathy may also occur and a polymyositis or dermatomyositis-like illness is recognised, of undetermined aetiology. Myopathy may also be caused by zidovudine.

Psychiatric problems

A positive HIV test result can result in a variety of reactions ranging from anger, guilt, anxiety with panic attacks, through to depression. Patients with HIV infection may, in fact, present with symptoms of organic brain syndromes due to HIV infection. The stress of having HIV and AIDS in terms of relationships, work and social life is likely to result in a wide range of affective disorders, with depression also common. Acute psychosis is relatively rare but does occur. More common

are mood changes, behaviour changes and cognitive disorders that herald the AIDS dementia complex.

Haematological complications

Idiopathic thrombocytopenic purpura (ITP) can complicate early HIV disease. This is thought to be related to HIV itself and is associated with anti-platelet antibodies. It is usually relatively mild and tends to resolve with the onset of AIDS. Progressive lymphopenia, in particular a progressive fall in the CD4 count, is the hallmark of HIV infection. The CD4 count is measured regularly at clinic visits in most centres and is used to predict when likely complications may be expected, when it is appropriate to start zidovudine therapy or when prophylaxis for pneumocystis should be started. Anaemia with or without other cytopenias is extremely common with the onset of AIDS. HIV itself is thought to have a suppressive effect on the marrow and anaemia may arise from a wide variety of causes relating to both the infectious and neoplastic complications of AIDS. For example, anaemia may be caused by marrow infiltration due to MAI, *M. tuberculosis* or lymphoma, chronic blood loss from Kaposi's sarcoma of the stomach or B_{12} deficiency due to malabsorption as a result of chronic gastrointestinal infections. Finally, several drugs commonly used in AIDS are myelosuppressive, in particular zidovudine, co-trimoxazole and ganciclovir.

Renal, cardiac and endocrine disease

HIV-induced nephropathy has been described, but this is rare. It is usually seen in AIDS patients who are intravenous drug users or from Afro-Caribbean ethnic groups, with intrinsic renal disease more likely due to heroin use than HIV infection. However, a large number of nephrotoxic drugs, including amphotericin B, foscarnet and pentamidine, are commonly used in AIDS patients. A variety of cardiac pathologies have been described from post mortem studies but the most consistent finding is of myocarditis. Clinical cardiac disease is relatively rare in AIDS patients and usually presents as congestive cardiomyopathy or pericardial effusion. Diffuse endocrine gland pathology has been reported from autopsy studies and clinical endocrine abnormalities have been described, but these are generally rare. CMV frequently causes adrenalitis but clinical adrenal insufficiency, although reported, is rare.

Drug interactions

It is important to remember that many of the drugs used to treat AIDS patients are toxic in their own right and this must always be considered when confronting a new clinical problem. Furthermore, many of these patients end up on large numbers of different drugs with complex interactions. For example rifampicin interacts with ketaconazole and fluconazole reducing serum levels, and ketoconazole inhibits absorption of rifampicin. This must be considered when the drugs are used in combination.

Terminal care

Despite all available treatment, AIDS remains an invariably fatal disease and good support from a partner, family and friends can be of great help during this potentially distressing time. During this phase good symptom relief is vital and attention to the control of anorexia, nausea, vomiting, dry mouth and diarrhoea are important as well as effective pain control if necessary. Many patients are anxious or depressed. Dysphagia may be a problem and many medications can be given rectally. Intramuscular injections should be avoided as in addition to being painful, they are difficult to administer: these patients are often wasted with little muscle mass. Syringe drivers for subcutaneous or intravenous delivery of antiemetics and opiates can be extremely useful.

HUMAN T-CELL LYMPHOTROPIC VIRUS (HTLV) INFECTIONS

There are two other retroviruses, HTLV1 and HTLV2, associated with disease in humans.

HTLV1 is endemic in Japan, the Caribbean and certain areas of West Africa. It is transmitted by blood transfusion, by drug abusers sharing needles and from mother to child, principally through breast-feeding. It can also be transmitted by sexual intercourse, especially from male to female.

HTLV1 is associated with adult T-cell leukaemia/lymphoma and with a degenerative neurological disease, known as tropical spastic paraplegia in the Caribbean and HTLV1-associated myelopathy in Japan. These diseases also occur in Europe and in North America in immigrants from areas of the world where HTLV1 infection is endemic.

HTLV2, a much more rarely isolated virus than HTLV1, has been isolated from Native Americans and also intravenous drug users in the United States. Its role in human disease is uncertain although it is associated with hairy cell leukaemia.

RHABDOVIRUSES

RABIES

See page 1091, Chapter 18.

ARBOVIRAL INFECTIONS

The *AR*thropod-*BO*rne viruses or **arboviruses** produce viraemia in their vertebrate hosts, and infect blood-sucking arthropod hosts during feeding. After replication in various arthropod tissues, arboviruses are transmitted in the anticoagulant saliva injected during subsequent feeding. Arbovirus vectors, in descending importance, are mosquitoes, ticks, sandflies and biting midges. Many of these viruses are zoonoses transmitted primarily between vectors and animals. Hereditary and transovarial transmission in ticks, sandflies and mosquitoes, and transstadial transmission in ticks, are probably important maintenance mechanisms. The International Catalogue lists 535 viruses (December 1990) but only 23% of all registered viruses have been associated with human disease and (by definition) only 40% are probable or proven arboviruses. Many are taxonomically unrelated but are placed into different taxonomic groups on the basis of common antigenic characteristics.

The principal groups are:

(a) **Family Togaviridae, genus Alphavirus** (former Group A arboviruses) (Type virus Sindbis). Group contains 27 viruses, all mosquito-borne. Most important viruses are Eastern, Western and Venezuelan equine encephalitis viruses that have caused epizootics in horses and human epidemics of encephalitis in the Americas, Chikungunya and O'nyong-nyong virus fevers in Africa and Ross River virus causing epidemic polyarthritis in Australia and the Pacific islands.

(b) **Family Flaviridae, genus Flavivirus** (former Group B arboviruses) (Type virus Yellow Fever). Group contains 68 members. Important tick-borne viruses are tick-borne encephalitis and Kyasanur Forest Disease. Important mosquito-borne viruses are Japanese, St Louis and Murray Valley Encephalitis viruses; yellow fever, West Nile and dengue. Uncomplicated dengue fever and the severe Dengue haemorrhagic fever/dengue shock syndrome (DHF/DSS) are the most important arbovirus diseases transmitted pan-tropically to man by peridomestic urban breeding mosquitoes.

(c) **Family Bunyaviridae, genus Bunyavirus** (Type virus Bunyamwera). Group contains 138 viruses in eighteen antigenic groups. Most important are the California Encephalitis group viruses such as LaCrosse, etc. In the Simbu antigenic group Oropouche virus is one of the few midge-transmitted viruses that cause frequent human epidemics.

(d) **Family Bunyaviridae, genus Phlebovirus.** 37 members. (Type virus Sicilian sandfly fever). Mostly associated with phlebotomine sandflies. The Uukuniemi group viruses are tick-associated. Most important phlebovirus is probably Rift Valley fever which has caused large scale epizootics and human epidemics.

Additionally there are a variety of other viruses which may cause human and animal disease. The most important are Crimean haemorrhagic fever-Congo virus (Family Bunyaviridae, genus Nairovirus); Colorado tick fever virus (Family Reoviridae, genus Coltivirus); Blue-tongue virus (Family Reoviridae, genus Orbivirus), and Vesicular stomatitis virus (Family Rhabdoviridae, genus Vesiculovirus).

Symptoms of infection are often mild, ranging from a high frequency of inapparent/mild influenza-like symptoms to more severe fevers with rash; or fever with rash, myalgia and/or arthralgia. However, a few viruses cause severe human and animal disease with encephalitis or haemmorhagic disease, with high attack rates and high morbidity and mortality. The immunity that follows is often life-long and is an important determinant of the pattern of disease in the exposed community. Normally immunity protects and prevents further epidemics, but in the case of dengue, it may also sensitise and predispose to more severe disease if the person is infected with a different, but cross-reacting, type. The incubation period is usually less than a week.

Clinical features

The presentation is with fever which may disappear after a few days, either permanently or to return accompanied by the clinical features and complications characteristic of the particular infection. In many arbovirus infections there is a maculopapular rash, conjunctival suffusion, photophobia and orbital pain. Arthralgia and myalgia are common; pain may be severe and immobilising. Lymphadenopathy is found in a few infections.

Complications

The most serious complications of arboviral infections are encephalitis and haemorrhage. The important ones causing encephalitis in man are listed above, but their distribution is wider than their names suggest. The clinical features of encephalitis are described on page 1089.

The causes of haemorrhage in arboviral infections are not fully understood. In some, such as dengue, disseminated intravascular coagulation is important; in others, notably yellow fever, haemorrhage follows severe hepatitis when deficiency of prothrombin and other coagulation factors develop. Thrombocytopenia occurs in many arboviral infections, and may contribute. Acute circulatory failure may follow haemorrhage, or occur on its own, possibly due to increased capillary permeability, as characterises dengue.

Investigations

For virological confirmation blood is transported on ice for inoculation into mice or tissue culture. It may be possible to isolate virus from CSF if there are signs of encephalitis. Serological diagnosis depends on demonstrating rising titres of antibodies, usually by complement fixation or haemagglutination-inhibition. Such antibodies are, however, usually only group specific. Neutralising antibodies may be genus specific, but are more time-consuming and expensive to assay.

Management

Treatment is supportive with attention to fluid and electrolyte balance and the circulatory state.

Prevention

This rests mainly on vector or reservoir control, but vaccines are available for some, including yellow fever, Kyasanur forest disease, European Spring-Summer encephalitis and Japanese B encephalitis.

TOGAVIRUSES

This group can be divided into the rubella virus and the former arboviruses, alphavirus and flavivirus.

YELLOW FEVER

Yellow fever, caused by a flavivirus, is normally a zoonosis of monkeys that inhabit tropical rain-forests in West and Central Africa and South and Central America, among whom it may cause devastating epidemics (Fig. 4.16). It is transmitted by mosquitoes living in tree tops (Fig. 4.17). *Aedes africanus* is the vector in Africa and the Haemagogus species in America. The infection is brought down to man either by infected mosquitoes when trees are felled, or by monkeys raiding human plantations. In the latter case *Aedes simpsoni*, which breeds in the axils of banana plants, may transmit the disease to man. In towns yellow fever may be transmitted between humans by *Aedes aegypti* which breeds efficiently in small collections of water. The distribution of this mosquito is far wider than that of yellow fever and poses a continual risk of spread.

Man is infectious during the viraemic phase which starts 3 to 6 days after the bite of the infected mosquito and lasts for 4 to 5 days. Mosquitoes become infectious 8–12 days after biting a patient and remain so for the rest of their 6–8 weeks' life span. They may pass on the virus transovarially. The incubation period is 3–6 days.

Pathology

In the liver, acute mid-zonal necrosis leads to deposits of hyalin called Councilman bodies, and intra-nuclear eosinophilic inclusions called Torres bodies; another characteristic feature is the absence of inflam-

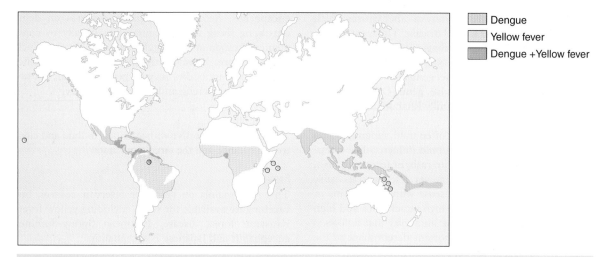

Fig. 4.16 **Endemic zones of yellow fever (gold) and dengue (green).**

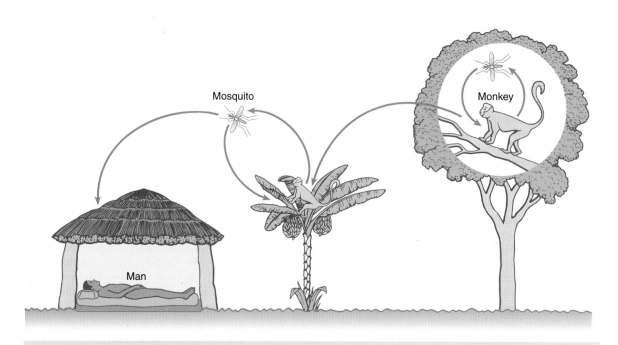

Fig. 4.17 **Transmission of yellow fever.** From tree-top cycle, via peridomestic cycle, to man.

matory infiltrate. The kidneys show tubular degeneration, which may partly be due to reduced blood flow. Widespread petechial haemorrhages are most marked in the stomach and duodenum. Haemorrhage is due to liver damage and disseminated intravascular coagulation.

Clinical features

Yellow fever is often a mild febrile illness lasting less than a week. However, the classical disease starts suddenly with rigors and high fever. Backache, headache and bone pains are severe. Nausea and vomiting start. The face is flushed and the conjunctivae infected.

Bradycardia and leucopenia are characteristic of this phase of the illness, which lasts 3 days and is followed by a remission lasting a few hours or days.

The third stage is characterised by return of fever, and the onset of jaundice, petechial haemorrhages in the mucosae, ecchymoses, haematemesis and oliguria. Patients commonly die in the third stage, often after a period of coma.

Investigations

Diagnostic procedures are listed in the information box below.

DIAGNOSIS OF YELLOW FEVER

- Clinical features in endemic area
- Virus isolation from blood in first 4 days
- Fourfold rise in antibody titre
- Postmortem liver biopsy
- Differentiate from viral hepatitis, haemorrhagic fevers, malaria, typhoid, leptospirosis, aflatoxin poisoning

---

Management

Patients should be nursed under a mosquito net until the viraemic stage has passed. Treatment is supportive, with meticulous attention to fluid and electrolyte balance, urine output and blood pressure. Blood transfusions, plasma expanders and peritoneal dialysis may be necessary.

Prevention

A single vaccination with the 17 D non-pathogenic strain of virus gives full protection for at least 10 years (Table 4.16). The vaccine does not produce appreciable side-effects, unless there is allergy to egg protein. Vaccination is not recommended in children under 9 months of age because of a slight risk of encephalitis, nor in people who are immunosuppressed. No ill-effects have been observed from vaccination during pregnancy.

Only travellers possessing valid certificates of vaccination against yellow fever are allowed to proceed from an endemic area to 'receptive areas', by which is meant countries free from the disease but in which the potential exists.

In this way the disease has been kept out of Asia. Mosquito control of airports should be maintained. The urban disease can be eradicated by the abolition of the breeding places of *Aedes aegypti* by the use of residual insecticides in houses and by mass vaccination in endemic areas. Vaccination is the only means to prevent humans being infected from forest reservoirs.

DENGUE

This disease, also caused by a flavivirus, is a risk in many tropical and subtropical countries (see Fig. 4.16), especially in coastal areas during the hot season when mosquitoes are numerous. Many large epidemics have occurred. One attack usually gives immunity for about 9 months and after several attacks a degree of permanent immunity is attained. Some cross-immunity exists between dengue and other members of the B group of arboviruses, including the virus of yellow fever. The incubation period is usually 5–6 days.

Clinical features

The disease varies in severity. The clinical features are listed in the information box. Subclinical infections are common.

CLINICAL FEATURES OF DENGUE FEVER

Prodrome
2 days malaise and headache

Acute onset
Fever, backache, generalised pains, painful red eyes, lymphadenopathy, lacrimation, anorexia, nausea, vomiting, bradycardia, prostration, depression

Fever
Continuous or 'saddle-back' with break on 4th or 5th day; usually lasts 7–8 days

Rash
Develops gradually, scarlet morbilliform on dorsa of hands and feet, spreading centripetally

Convalescence
Slow

Dengue haemorrhagic fever

This occurs in S.E. Asia, rarely elsewhere. After 3 to 4 days of fever, bleeding starts with petechiae, ecchymoses, epistaxis and melaena, and proceeds to acute circulatory failure. Even with treatment of these complications, 10% of patients die. Disseminated intravascular coagulation and complement activation which leads to vascular damage are thought to be triggered by hypersensitivity to the virus.

Investigation

This is usually easy in an endemic area when a patient has the characteristic symptoms and signs. However, the mild cases may resemble other viral disease. The virus can be recovered from the blood and antibody titres rise. Leucopenia is usual.

Management

There is no specific treatment. The severe pains can be relieved by paracetamol, but occasionally opiates are required. Aspirin should be avoided. Fluid replacement, blood transfusions and corticosteroids are indicated in the haemorrhagic varieties.

Prevention

Patients are nursed under a mosquito net. Breeding places of Aedes mosquitoes should be abolished and the adults destroyed by insecticides.

RUBELLA (GERMAN MEASLES)

Rubella is caused by a togavirus which spreads by droplet infection. One attack confers a high degree of immunity. It tends to affect older children, adolescents and young adults and spreads less readily than measles. The incubation period is usually about 18 days. The disease in children is trivial. In adults the illness may be more severe, but of short duration and of little importance except when it develops in a woman during the first 4 months of pregnancy. In such cases the child may be born with one or more congenital malformations (see information box).

RUBELLA AND THE FETUS

Risk of congenital abnormality:
- 1st four weeks of pregnancy—80%
- 16th week and onwards of pregnancy—less than 5%

Causes congenital abnormalities of:
- Heart (septal defect)
- Eye (cataract)
- Brain (mental retardation)

Clinical features

In children the constitutional symptoms are so slight that the illness is rarely suspected until the rash is seen. The spots are pink macules which appear first behind the ears and on the forehead. The rash spreads rapidly, first to the trunk and then to the limbs. Tender enlargement of the suboccipital lymph nodes is usual. In adolescents and adults the onset may be acute with fever and generalised aches, but even then the illness lasts for only 2 or 3 days. Polyarthritis is the commonest complication. Encephalomyelitis and thrombocytopenic purpura are very rare. Complete recovery from all of these complications is the rule.

The rash of rubella is very similar to that due to certain drugs, enteroviruses and also parvovirus B19 which causes **erythema infectiosum** (Fifth disease). The latter infection may be differentiated clinically by redness of the patient's cheeks ('slapped cheek' appearance). Parvovirus B19 can also cause aplastic crises in individuals with sickle-cell disease.

Serological tests are necessary for a definitive diagnosis of rubella.

Management

No treatment is available. If infection is known to have occurred during the first 16 weeks of pregnancy there is such a high chance of fetal abnormality that termination should be recommended.

Prevention

Rubella vaccine should be given to all children at the age of 15 months along with measles and mumps vaccine (MMR vaccine). A second dose of rubella vaccine alone is given to girls aged 11–13 years. Women of childbearing age who are found to be serologically negative should also be offered vaccine provided that they are not pregnant and are willing to avoid pregnancy for 12 weeks after vaccination.

DNA VIRUSES

HERPESVIRUSES

There are 6 herpesviruses which cause infection in man (Table 4.25).

Herpes simplex virus (HSV) type 1, the cytomegalovirus (CMV) and the Epstein–Barr virus (EBV) are ubiquitous agents which commonly cause asymptomatic infection in early life—hence many adults have serological evidence of past infection with these agents. Chickenpox usually causes clinical infection in childhood and 80% of adults will have antibodies to the virus in their blood. Once a herpesvirus has entered a person's body, it is there for life. The varicella/zoster virus (VSV) may reappear as shingles in later life and HSV as recurrent lesions on lip or external genitalia. CMV and EBV, however, usually only cause disease in later life if the patient has become immunosuppressed.

Human herpesvirus 6 is a recently discovered virus which is the cause of **exanthem subitum**, a benign febrile illness of children associated with a maculo-papular rash. It has also been associated with lymphadenopathy and may cause infection in the immunosuppressed.

Table 4.25 Herpesvirus infections

Virus		Infection
Herpesvirus hominis (*Herpes simplex*)	*Type 1*	*Herpes labialis* ('cold sores') Keratoconjunctivitis Finger infections ('whitlows') Encephalitis Primary stomatitis Genital infections
	Type 2	Genital infections Neonatal infection (acquired during vaginal delivery)
Cytomegalovirus (CMV)		Congenital infection Infection in immuno-compromised patients: Pneumonitis Retinitis Generalised infection
Epstein–Barr virus (EBV)		Infectious mononucleosis Burkitt's lymphoma Nasopharyngeal carcinoma Hairy leukoplakia (AIDS patients)
Varicella/zoster virus (VZV)		Chickenpox Shingles (Herpes zoster)
Human herpesvirus 6 (HHV6)		Exanthem subitum ? Cervical lymphadenopathy

---

INFECTIOUS MONONUCLEOSIS (GLANDULAR FEVER)

Infectious mononucleosis is an acute infectious disease caused by the Epstein–Barr virus which principally occurs in teenagers and young adults, although occasionally other age groups may be affected. The virus infects, and replicates in, B lymphocytes and is shed in the throat following the acute disease. Transmission is, therefore, usually by oral contact, possibly with the exchange of saliva. The incubation period is probably between 7 and 10 days.

Clinical features

The infection usually presents with malaise, tiredness, headache, abdominal discomfort, anorexia and fever. The clinical features can be variable (see the information box). The rash is especially common if ampicillin or amoxycillin has been given, occurring in around 90% of patients. Conditions to be excluded in the differential diagnosis include cytomegalovirus infection, toxoplasmosis and acute HIV infection, which can all present with lymphadenopathy, splenomegaly and fever with an atypical lymphocytosis (but not usually sore throat).

Investigations

The diagnosis is suspected by the finding of a predominance of atypical lymphocytes in the peripheral blood and confirmed by a positive Monospot or Paul–

CLINICAL FEATURES OF INFECTIOUS MONONUCLEOSIS

Acute illness
- Exudative tonsillitis
- Petechial rash on palate
- Lymphadenopathy
- Splenomegaly
- Maculo-papular rash

Abnormal laboratory test
- Atypical lymphocytosis
- Positive Monospot test
- Raised liver enzymes

Complications
- Chronic fatigue (common)
- Hepatitis (rare)
- Haemolytic anaemia (rare)
- Thrombocytopenia (rare)
- Rupture of spleen (rare)
- Meningo-encephalitis (rare)

Bunnell test. Specific virus serological tests are also available for diagnosis but are not required in most cases.

Complications

These are listed in the information box above. The chronic fatigue syndrome with prolonged debility, inability to concentrate, depression, tiredness and low-grade fever may follow infectious mononucleosis and can be associated with abnormalities of lymphocyte numbers and function. The chronic fatigue syndrome, sometimes referred to as myalgic encephalitis (ME), can, however, develop without preceding mononucleosis when it usually has an underlying psychological or stress component.

Management

This is entirely symptomatic. Rest is important during the acute illness. A 48-hour course of corticosteroids (e.g. intravenous hydrocortisone 200 mg 6-hourly or prednisolone 10 mg 6-hourly if the patient can swallow) is indicated for severe tonsillar enlargement causing dysphagia or difficulty in breathing.

CYTOMEGALOVIRUS (CMV) INFECTION

Clinical features

The various features of CMV infection are listed in the information box. Asymptomatic disease is the commonest manifestation in the immunocompetent. The cytomegalovirus is one of the most important pathogens in the immunosuppressed (especially those with AIDS), causing much morbidity and mortality in these patients. CMV (along with rubella, toxoplasmosis and syphilis) is an important, although rare, cause of congenital infection which is acquired during a pregnancy in which the mother develops symptomatic or asymptomatic CMV infection. The child may be stillborn.

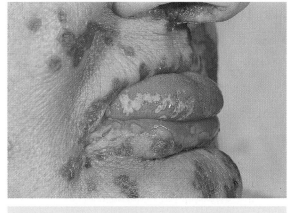

Fig. 4.18 *Herpes simplex* **virus.** Ulcerative stomatitis.

Investigations

CMV may be cultured from urine of infected patients. Diagnosis may also be confirmed by biopsy of infected tissue (e.g. lung or bowel) or by serology.

Management

The only drug which is active against CMV is ganciclovir, which is toxic and expensive and is only indicated for serious infections in the immunosuppressed. Ganciclovir is given by intravenous infusion over 1 hour, initially in a dose of 5 mg/kg every 12 hours for 14–21 days. An oral preparation has recently become available.

HERPES SIMPLEX INFECTIONS

Herpes simplex is a common virus which frequently causes nonspecific illness, often in childhood; hence many people have serum antibodies to the organism. It has assumed greater importance as a cause of serious, and sometimes fatal, infections in immunocompromised patients. There are two strains of *Herpes simplex* virus, type 1 and type 2, the latter being principally responsible for sexually transmitted anogenital infections. Infections caused by these viruses can be categorised as primary or recurrent.

Clinical features

Primary infections include ulcerative stomatitis (Fig. 4.18) (commonest in infants), keratitis (dendritic ulcer), finger infections (whitlows), vulvo-vaginitis, balanitis and encephalitis. In neonates and in the immunonosuppressed the infection may be disseminated, involving many organs and tissues, and can be fatal. The newborn may contract the infection from the mother's genital tract during birth and active genital *H. simplex*

infection is therefore an indication for Caesarean section.

Recurrent *H. simplex* infections are commonest on the lips and adjoining skin (*herpes labialis* or 'cold sore'). The lesions start as macules, become vesicular and then pustular (Fig. 4.18). Attacks of herpes labialis may be precipitated by various stimuli including sunlight, menstruation and viral and bacterial infections. Genital lesions also commonly recur.

Investigations

The virus can be cultured from lesions and infection is confirmed by rising serum antibody titres.

Management

The *H. simplex* virus is susceptible to idoxuridine and acyclovir although most infections resolve spontaneously. Drops containing idoxuridine or acyclovir are effective in eye infections. Intravenous acyclovir is indicated for disseminated infections in immunocompromised patients and also for *H. simplex* encephalitis, which has a mortality of up to 80%. The adult dose for intravenous infusion is from 5–10 mg/kg 8-hourly, the higher dose being indicated for encephalitis and the immunosuppressed. An oral preparation of acyclovir is available for infections of the skin and mucous membranes. The dose is 200–400 mg 4–5 times daily. Acyclovir will not eradicate the *H. simplex* virus from posterior root ganglia (the site of chronic asymptomatic infection), and recurrent attacks cannot therefore be prevented.

CHICKENPOX (VARICELLA)

Chickenpox (varicella) is caused by the varicella-zoster virus (VZV) which spreads by droplets from the upper respiratory tract or from the discharge from ruptured lesions on the skin or through contact with herpes zoster. Herpes zoster is due to reactivation of VZV and may be accompanied by a varicelliform rash.

Chickenpox is highly infectious and chiefly affects children under 10 years of age. Most children tolerate this disease well but, as often happens with viral infections, adults may develop a more severe illness. In patients who are immunocompromised, the disease may be severe or even fatal. The incubation period is 14–21 days.

Clinical features

Constitutional symptoms are usually brief and mild in children but can be severe in adults. Lesions are sometimes present on the palate before the characteristic rash (Fig. 4.2) appears on the trunk on the second day of the illness. Then the face and finally the limbs are involved. The spots reach their maximum density upon the trunk, and are more sparse on the periphery of the limbs. Macules appear first, and within a few hours the lesions become papular and then vesicular and, within 24 hours, pustular. Damage from scratching is frequent, since itching may be troublesome. Whether or not the pustules rupture, they dry up in a few days to form scabs. The spots appear in crops, so that lesions at all stages of development are seen in any area at the same time.

Complications

The course of the disease is usually uneventful but complications occasionally occur (see information box). Pneumonia is commonest in adults, especially in patients who smoke and the immunosuppressed.

COMPLICATIONS OF CHICKENPOX

Direct viral effects
- Pneumonia (usually adults or immunosuppressed)
- Myocarditis (usually adults or immunosuppressed)

Post-viral effects
- Encephalitis (cerebellar)
- Glomerulonephritis

Secondary bacterial infection
- Skin
- Septicaemia
- Osteomyelitis/septic arthritis

Intra-uterine infection
- Congenital limb defects (rare)

Management

No specific treatment is required in the majority of patients. Acyclovir is indicated for the immuno-compromised (10 mg/kg 8-hourly by intravenous infusion) and (orally or intravenously) for chickenpox in adults and older adolescents in whom the infection can be more severe than in children. If there is secondary infection a local antiseptic should be applied to the skin, e.g. chlorhexidine. If bacterial infection progresses, an antibiotic such as flucloxacillin 500 mg 6-hourly should be prescribed.

Prevention

Immunocompromised children in contact with chickenpox should be given an injection of human anti-varicella immunoglobulin. A vaccine is available but is not yet licensed in the UK.

PAPOVAVIRUSES

VIRAL WARTS

Most people have warts at some time of their life, usually before the age of 20. Genital warts occur during the sexually active years. Warts result from infection with the DNA human papillomavirus (HPV) of which over 60 subtypes are now recognised. Different subtypes are responsible for several clinical variants. Transmission is by contact with the virus either in living skin or in fragments of shed skin, and is encouraged by trauma and moisture (e.g. at swimming pools, amongst butchers, fishmongers, etc.). Genital warts are frequently spread by intercourse and perianal warts may reflect homosexual activity. There appears to be a close, if not causative, relationship with genital warts, especially due to HPV type 16 and 18, and carcinoma of the cervix. Other types of HPV may act as tumour promoters and, with ultraviolet radiation, cause skin cancer in immunosuppressed individuals.

Clinical features

Common warts appear initially as smooth skin-coloured papules. As they enlarge their surfaces become irregular and hyperkeratotic, producing the typical 'warty' appearance. They usually occur on the hands but may also often be seen on the face and genitalia; multiple warts are common. Plantar warts ('verrucae') are characterised by a rough surface, protruding only slightly from the skin and surrounded by a horny collar. On paring, oozing capillary loops distinguish plantar warts from corns. Often multiple, plantar warts may be painful. Other variants of warts include mosaic warts (mosaic-like plaques of tightly packed individual warts), plane warts (smooth, flat-topped papules seen most commonly on the face and backs of hands), facial warts

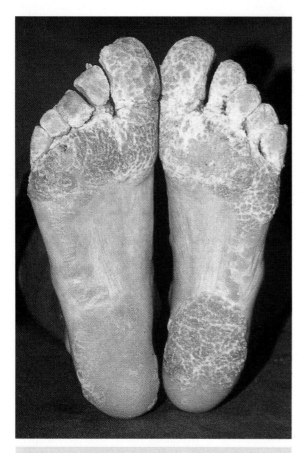

Fig. 4.19 Extensive plantar warts in a patient receiving immunosuppressive treatment.

(often filiform and hyperkeratotic) and anogenital warts (may be papillomatous and even cauliflowerlike).

Most viral warts in the healthy will eventually resolve spontaneously but this may take years. In immunocompromised patients warts persist and spread (Fig. 4.19); 70% of renal allograft recipients will have warts five years after transplantation.

Management

Warts may be treated in many different ways. Common warts in children should be managed with wart paints containing salicylic acid. Stubborn lesions should be treated with liquid nitrogen cryotherapy or removed by curettage. Anogenital warts are treated with either cryotherapy or podophyllin paint (applied initially for only 2 hours and avoided in pregnancy). Facial warts are most easily treated with cryotherapy or electrodesiccation. Plane warts are best left alone.

POXVIRUSES

SMALLPOX (VARIOLA)

As a result of the WHO programme of case detection and vaccination, it is confidently believed that smallpox has been eradicated world-wide. Apart from two laboratory-acquired infections in 1978, the last known case occurred in Somalia in 1977.

Major smallpox produces a severe constitutional illness associated with a peripherally distributed rash with lesions which, in any one area, progress in unison from macules through papules, and vesicles, to pustules. The mortality rate may be as high as 40%.

A similar virus causes **monkeypox** in primates in jungle areas of Central Africa, with lesions resembling those of smallpox. Some human cases have occurred in those in contact with infected primates but inter-human spread is exceptional.

The virus of smallpox is maintained in two designated laboratories, one in the USA and the other in Russia, in order to be able to differentiate such diseases as monkeypox from smallpox. Only staff employed in these designated laboratories or those working with the vaccinia virus now require to be vaccinated against smallpox. Limited stocks of smallpox vaccine are available for this purpose, and in case the disease should reappear.

MOLLUSCUM CONTAGIOSUM ('WATER WARTS')

This common and easily recognised poxvirus infection usually affects children and atopic or immunocompromised adults. Spread is by direct contact or by infected towelling, clothing, etc. The incubation period is 2–6 weeks.

Clinical features

Individual lesions are shiny, white and hemispherical and grow slowly up to about 0.5 cm in diameter. Their characteristic umbilicated look is due to a central punctum which may contain a cheesy core. Multiple lesions are common (Fig. 4.11). Like warts many lesions will clear spontaneously, often after brief local inflammation.

Management

No treatment may be best in some children but cryotherapy or rapid expression is tolerated well by others, especially if performed by an experienced operator.

FURTHER READING

Berkelman R L 1994 Emerging infectious diseases in the United States 1993. Journal of Infectious Diseases 170: 272–277

Halstead S B 1992 Dengue fever, viral haemorrhagic fever and rabies. Current Opinions in Infectious Diseases 5: 319–325

McKendrick M W, Balfour H H Jr 1995 Controversies in management: acyclovir for childhood chickenpox. British Medical Journal 310: 108–110

Tsoukas C M, Bernard N F 1994 Markers predicting progression of human immunodeficiency virus-related disease. Clinical Microbiology Reviews 7: 14–28

DISEASES DUE TO CHLAMYDIAE

Chlamydia are small Gram-negative organisms which, like viruses, only grow inside cells. However, they differ from viruses in that they have both RNA and DNA in their structure. They also have a cell wall and divide by binary fission. There are three species of chlamydia:

(a) *Chlamydia trachomatis* which causes trachoma, non-gonococcal urethritis and cervicitis (leading to pelvic inflammatory disease)
(b) *Chlamydia psittaci* which causes psittacosis
(c) *Chlamydia pneumoniae* which causes atypical pneumonia.

TRACHOMA

Trachoma is a specific communicable keratoconjunctivitis caused by *Chlamydia trachomatis*, and is the commonest cause of avoidable blindness in the world. Transmission is usually by contact or from fomites in unhygienic surroundings. Some infections occur during birth from infected genital passages.

Vast numbers of people suffer from trachoma in the hot, dry, dusty areas of the subtropics and tropics but it is also present in Southern Europe, and among immigrants in Britain. The disease varies markedly in incidence and in severity in different geographical regions. In endemic areas the disease is commonest in children.

Pathology

The infection lasts for years, may be latent over long periods and may recrudesce. The conjunctiva of the upper lid is first affected with vascularisation and cellular infiltration. Scarring causes inversion of the lids (entropion) so that the lashes rub against the cornea (trichasis). The cornea becomes vascularised and opaque.

Clinical features

The onset is usually insidious and infection may not be apparent to the patient. Early symptoms include conjunctival irritation and blepharospasm, but the problem may not be detected until vision begins to fail. Trachoma may also present as an acute ophthalmia neonatorum.

The early follicles of trachoma are characteristic (Fig.

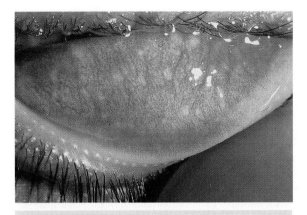

Fig. 4.20 Trachoma. Characterised by hyperaemia and numerous pale follicles.

4.20), but clinical differentiation from conjunctivitis due to other viruses may be difficult.

Investigations

Intracellular inclusions may be demonstrated in conjunctival scrapings by staining with iodine or immunofluorescence. Chlamydia may be isolated in chick embryo or cell culture.

Management

Ophthalmic ointment or oily drops of 1–3% tetracycline should be applied twice daily for 3 months. In mass therapy in endemic areas topical application twice daily for 3–6 consecutive days each month for 6 months has given good results. Oral tetracycline (15 mg/kg daily), doxycycline (15 mg/kg daily) or sulphonamide (30 mg/kg daily) given for 2 weeks is just as effective. Deformity and scarring of the lids, corneal opacities, ulceration and scarring require surgical treatment, after control of local infection.

Prevention

Personal and family cleanliness should be improved. Proper care of the eyes of newborn and young children is essential. Family contacts should be examined. Population surveys lead to discovery and treatment of asymptomatic infections. Trachoma clinics are required in areas of high endemicity.

FURTHER READING

Centers for Disease Control and Prevention (CDC) 1993 Morbidity and Mortality Weekly Report: Recommendations for the prevention and management of *Chlamydia trachomatis* infections. MMWR 42 (RR-12): 1–39

DISEASES DUE TO RICKETTSIAE

Rickettsia are rod-shaped, spherical or pleomorphic Gram-negative organisms which are smaller than the true bacteria but still visible using the light microscope. Most are intracellular pathogens which grow only in living cells.

These organisms are natural parasites of the cells of the intestinal canal of arthropods, although some species may parasitise higher mammals including man. Infection is usually conveyed to man through the skin from excreta of arthropods but the saliva of some biting vectors is infected. Essential features of rickettsial infections are compared in Table 4.26. Transovarian infection to the next generation occurs in ticks and mites, which serve as reservoirs as well as vectors of infection.

Pathology

In man rickettsiae multiply in vascular endothelial cells especially of capillaries, producing lesions in the skin, central nervous system, heart, lungs, kidneys and skeletal muscles. Endothelial proliferation, associated with a perivascular reaction (nodules of Fraenkel) may cause thromboses and small haemorrhages. In epidemic typhus the brain and in scrub typhus the cardiovascular system and lungs are particularly attacked.

The common clinical findings are fever, severe prostration, mental disturbance and often a rash.

An eschar is often found in tick and mite borne typhus. An eschar is a necrotic sore, often scabbed, at the site of the bite and is due to vasculitis following immunological recognition of the inoculated organism. Regional lymph nodes often enlarge. There are epidemic, endemic, tick and scrub typhus fevers.

The investigation, management and prevention of rickettsial infections are discussed on page 116.

EPIDEMIC TYPHUS FEVER

Louse-borne or epidemic typhus is caused by *R. prowazeki* and is transmitted by infected faeces of the human body louse, *Pediculus humanus*, usually through scratching the skin, or sometimes by inhalation. Patients suffering from epidemic typhus infect the lice, which leave when the patient is febrile. In conditions of overcrowding the disease spreads rapidly. During interepidemic periods the disease may be maintained by inapparent or latent cases or perhaps by infected fleas and rats. The disease is prevalent in parts of Africa, especially Ethiopia and Rwanda, the South American Andes and Afghanistan. Large epidemics have occurred in Europe, usually as a sequel to war. The incubation period is usually 12–14 days.

There may be a few days of malaise but the onset is more often sudden with rigors, fever, frontal headaches, pains in the back and limbs, constipation and bronchitis. The face is flushed and cyanotic, eyes congested, and the patient soon becomes dull and confused.

The rash appears on the fourth to the sixth day and often resembles measles. In its early stages it disappears on pressure but soon becomes petechial with subcutaneous mottling. It appears first on the anterior folds of the axillae, sides of the abdomen or back of hands, then on the trunk and forearms. The neck and face are seldom affected.

During the second week symptoms increase in severity. Sores collect on the lips. The tongue becomes dry, brown, shrunken and tremulous. The spleen is palpable,

Table 4.26 Essential features of rickettsial infections

Disease	Reservoir	Vector	Primary-Complex[1]	Rash	Gangrene	Target organs	Mortality
Epidemic typhus	Man	Louse	—	Morbilliform Haemorrhagic	Often	Brain, skin, bronchi, myocardium	Up to 40%
Endemic typhus	Rat	Flea	—	Slight	—		Rare[2]
Rocky Mountain spotted fever	Rodents, dogs, ticks	*Ixodid* ticks	Often	Morbilliform Haemorrhagic	Often	Bronchi, myocardium, brain, skin	2–12%[3]
Other tick-borne typhus	Rodents, dogs, ticks	*Ixodid* ticks	Usual	Maculopapular	—	Skin, meninges	Rare[2]
Scrub typhus	Rodents, mites	*Trombiculid* mites	Often	Maculopapular	Unusual	Bronchi, myocardium, brain, skin	Rare[2]
Rickettsialpox	Domestic mouse	Mite	Usual	Maculopapular	—	—	Rare[2]
Trench fever	Man	Louse	—	Maculopapular	—	—	Rare[2]

[1] Eschar at bite site and local lymphadenopathy. [2] Except in infants, elderly and debilitated. [3] Highest in adult males.

the pulse feeble and the patient stuporous and delirious. The temperature falls rapidly at the end of the second week and the patient recovers gradually. In fatal cases the patient usually dies in the second week from toxaemia, cardiac or renal failure or pneumonia.

Common complications are listed in the information box below.

COMPLICATIONS OF LOUSE-BORNE TYPHUS

- **Vascular**: Venous thrombosis, gangrene of fingers, toes, nose and genitalia
- **Infective**: Parotitis, bronchopneumonia
- **Brill's disease**: A mild relapse many years later

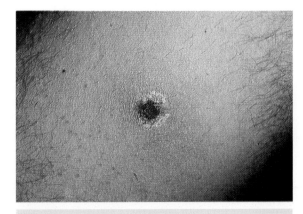

Fig. 4.21   Tick-borne typhus fever: eschar at the site of the tick-bite.

ENDEMIC TYPHUS FEVER

Flea-borne or 'endemic' typhus caused by *R. mooseri* is endemic world-wide. Man is infected when, by scratching, he introduces the faeces or contents of a crushed flea which has fed on an infected rat. The incubation period is 8–14 days. The symptoms resemble those of a mild louse-borne typhus. The rash may be scanty and transient. Laboratory aids to diagnosis are discussed on page 116, together with treatment.

ROCKY MOUNTAIN SPOTTED FEVER

The casual organism *R. rickettsii* is transmitted by the bite of hard (*Ixodid*) ticks which carry the infection to rodents and dogs and on occasion to man. It is widely distributed and increasing in western and south-eastern states of the USA and also in South America. The pathological changes are similar to those in epidemic typhus. The incubation period is about 7 days.

There may be an eschar at the site of the bite (Fig. 4.21) with enlargement of the regional lymph nodes. Symptoms closely resemble those of louse-borne typhus. The rash appears on about the third or fourth day, at first like measles, but in a few hours the typical maculopapular eruption develops. Each day it becomes more distinct and papular and finally petechial. The rash first appears on the wrists, forearms and ankles, spreads in 24–48 hours to the back, limbs and chest and lastly to the abdomen where it is least pronounced. The fully developed rash often affects also the palms, soles and face. Petechiae may appear in crops. Larger cutaneous and subcutaneous haemorrhages may appear in severe cases. The liver and spleen become palpable. Complications are as in louse-borne typhus, but gangrene is more common. Untreated, the course of the disease may be mild or rapidly fatal.

Other forms of tick-borne typhus fever

The causal agents of African tick-borne typhus in South and East Africa are *R. conori* and a substrain *R. conori pijperi*, the reservoir hosts being dogs and rodents. 'Fièvre boutonneuse' of the Mediterranean is similar, as is also the infection *R. australis* in Queensland. Infected hard ticks may be picked up by walking on grasslands, or dogs may bring the ticks into the house. Tourists often acquire tick typhus and import it into Britain. A careful search is needed to find the tell-tale eschar, and maculopapular rash on the trunk, limbs, palms and soles. There may be delirium and meningeal signs in severe infections but recovery is the rule.

SCRUB TYPHUS FEVER

Mite-borne or 'scrub' typhus is caused by *R. tsutsugamushi* transmitted by the bite of infective larval trombiculid mites. It occurs in the Far East, Burma, Pakistan, Bangladesh, India, Indonesia, S. Pacific Islands and Queensland, particularly where patches of forest have been cleared for plantations, that have attracted rats and attendant mites.

The pathology is similar to that of louse-borne typhus, but lesions in the lungs are more prominent. In many patients one or more eschars develop, surrounded by an area of cellulitis and enlargement of regional lymph nodes. The incubation period is about 9 days.

Mild or subclinical cases are common. The onset of symptoms is usually sudden with headache, often retro-orbital, fever, malaise, weakness and cough. In severe illness the general symptoms increase with apathy and prostration. An erythematous maculopapular rash often appears on about the fifth to the seventh day and spreads to the trunk, face and limbs including the palms and soles, with generalised painless lymphadenopathy. The rash fades by the fourteenth day. The temperature rises rapidly and continues as a remittent fever with sweating until it falls by lysis about the twelfth to the eighteenth day. In severe infection the patient is prostrate with cough, pneumonia, confusion and deafness. Cardiac failure, renal failure and haemorrhage may develop. Convalescence is often slow and tachycardia may persist for some weeks.

RICKETTSIALPOX

This is due to *R. akari*, transmitted from the domestic mouse by a mite. It appears to be restricted to New York and Philadelphia where mice are now adapted to live in communal rubbish chutes of apartment houses.

The illness starts with a papule, which develops into an eschar, and is followed a week later by the sudden onset of fever, sweating, backache and a rash, maculopapular at first but which soon vesiculates and crusts, healing without scarring.

TRENCH FEVER

This is caused by *R. quintana* and is spread to man by louse faeces. It was prevalent in the First World War in Europe among troops in the trenches and again in the Second World War in the USSR. The disease is otherwise rare. The incubation period is 10–20 days.

The onset is sudden with headache, and severe pains in trunk and limbs. The temperature rises sharply and remains raised for 5–7 days. The initial illness is like a mild case of typhus fever but febrile relapses are common, usually at intervals of 5–6 days, and may be debilitating.

Investigation of rickettsial infections

The Weil–Felix reaction is the nonspecific agglutination of the somatic antigens of non-motile *Proteus* species by the patient's serum. A four-fold rise in titre is diagnostic.

Species-specific antibodies may be detected by complement fixation, microagglutination and fluorescence in specialised laboratories. Rickettsiae may be isolated from the blood in the first week of illness by intraperitoneal inoculation into male guinea-pigs or mice.

Management of the rickettsial diseases

The various fevers due to rickettsiae vary greatly in severity but all respond to tetracycline or chloramphenicol. Tetracycline is administered in a dose of 500 mg 4 times daily. The fever usually settles within 2 or 3 days. Tetracycline should be continued for 2–3 days after the patient

is afebrile as there is a tendency otherwise to relapse. In endemic areas good results have been obtained in louse-borne typhus and scrub typhus by a single dose of 100 mg doxycycline.

Nursing care is important, especially in epidemic typhus. Sedation may be required for delirium and blood transfusion for haemorrhage. Relapsing fever and typhoid are common intercurrent infections in epidemic typhus, and pneumonia in scrub typhus. They must be sought and treated. Convalescence is usually protracted, especially in older people.

Prevention of rickettsial infections

Vector and reservoir control
See the information box.

Active immunisation
Vaccines can be prepared from killed *R. prowazeki*, *R. mooseri* or *R. rickettsii* cultured in eggs, but they are not generally available.

Chemoprophylaxis
It is likely that doxycycline 100 mg/weekly will protect those at risk.

Q FEVER

Q (Query) fever is caused by *Coxiella burnetii*, a rickettsia-like organism, which is widespread in nature and

---

VECTOR AND RESERVOIR CONTROL OF RICKETTSIAL INFECTIONS

Louse control
- Insufflate 5% carboryl or 0.5% malathion powder into clothing of population at risk
- Delouse patient's clothing by insecticide or heat (e.g. domestic tumble drier)

Flea control
- Vacuum clean floors. Treat floors and rodent burrows with residual insecticide powder
- Control rodents

Tick control
- Remove ticks from dogs, mechanically or with insecticide shampoo
- Inspect oneself twice daily for ticks and remove them before they have fed
- Creosote floors of log cabins in USA

Mite control
- Impregnate trousers and socks with insect repellent (e.g. 2% dimethyl phthallate) and use insect repellent creams on skin
- Clear campsites of all vegetation and spray ground with oily residual insecticide

---

highly resistant to drying. It is carried by ticks among animals, including cattle and sheep. Transmission to humans is air-borne through aerosols from animal birth products and contaminated dust. Unpasteurised milk is another source of infection. The incubation period of Q fever is from 7 to 14 days.

Clinical features

The clinical features of the illness are protean, ranging from subclinical infection to fatal encephalitis or endocarditis (p. 295). Acute Q fever usually starts like influenza with pyrexia followed by myalgia, headache and sweating. Many cases resolve without specific therapy. Some patients have a cough, and radiological examination may reveal a pneumonitis. Less common features of Q fever include hepatitis, myocarditis, epididymo-orchitis, iritis and osteomyelitis.

Investigations

The diagnosis of Q fever should be considered in patients living in rural areas, especially if there is occupational contact work with livestock. *C. burnetii* does not grow in the media used for routine blood cultures and it is therefore important to consider Q fever as a possible cause in patients with clinical evidence of endocarditis who have sterile blood cultures. The diagnosis of Q fever is confirmed by the detection of serum antibodies to the two polysaccharide antigens of *C. burnetii*; acute infection is confirmed by a four-fold rise in phase II antibody titre in paired specimens of blood taken at intervals of between 10 and 14 days. Phase I antibody titres rise more slowly than phase II and the persistence of both suggests chronic infection.

Management

C. burnetii is sensitive to the tetracyclines, clindamycin, chloramphenicol and rifampicin. Acute infections respond within a few days to tetracycline in a dose of 500 mg 6-hourly for 2 weeks, or doxycycline 200 mg daily for 2 weeks. The treatment of chronic infections, especially if there is endocarditis, requires prolonged therapy with tetracycline plus clindamycin or rifampicin.

FURTHER READING

Kirkland K B, Marcom P K, Sexton D J 1993 Rocky Mountain spotted fever complicated by gangrene: report of six cases and review. Clinical Infectious Diseases 16: 629–634

DISEASES DUE TO BACTERIA

Bacteria are classified according to several properties: these include their shape, growth requirements and reaction to Gram staining. Most are either round (cocci) or elongated (bacilli). Vibrios and Campylobacters are comma-shaped, spirochaetes are thin spiral filaments, and all three are motile when seen under the light microscope.

The main growth characteristic used in classification is their ability to grow in either aerobic or anaerobic environments. Some bacteria possess toxins which are responsible for producing pathological changes in tissues and organs. Examples include endotoxins produced by Gram-negative organisms such as *Escherichia coli* and exotoxins by *Corynebacterium diphtheriae*.

Certain bacteria exist in the environment in durable vegetative forms called spores.

STREPTOCOCCAL INFECTIONS

Streptococci produce a wide variety of infections (see the information box). All species can cause septicaemia.

STREPTOCOCCAL INFECTIONS

Streptococcus pyogenes
- Skin and soft tissue infection (incl. erysipelas, impetigo, necrotising fasciitis)
- Bone and joint infection
- Tonsillitis
- Scarlet fever
- Glomerulonephritis
- Rheumatic fever
- Puerperal sepsis

Enterococcus faecalis
- Endocarditis
- Urinary tract infection

Viridans streptococci (*Strep mitior, sanguis, mutans, salivarius*)
- Endocarditis
- Septicaemia in immunosuppressed

Group B streptococci
- Neonatal infections
- Female pelvic infections

Anaerobic streptococci
- Peritonitis
- Dental infections
- Liver abscess
- Pelvic inflammatory disease

NB—all streptococci can cause septicaemia

STREPTOCOCCUS PYOGENES INFECTIONS

Infections caused by *Strep pyogenes* result in features which vary with the invasiveness of the organism, its capacity to produce toxins, the site involved and the reaction of the host. If resistance is low and the invasive properties of the streptococcus are high, a rapidly spreading erysipelas, cellulitis, lymphangitis or bacteraemia may result. The organism may produce a specific exotoxin causing a widespread punctate erythema. When the infection is associated with such a rash the syndrome is known as scarlet fever. The same type of streptococcus may produce in one person acute tonsillitis, in another scarlet fever and in a third erysipelas. **Necrotising fasciitis** caused by *Strep pyogenes* causes great tissue destruction and has a high mortality.

SCARLET FEVER

Although scarlet fever is at present a mild disease, it may not necessarily remain so, as fluctuations in its severity have been recorded for the past 300 years. The primary site of infection in scarlet fever is usually the pharynx or tonsils but the disease can be associated with streptococcal infection in other sites, e.g. in the genital tract after childbirth or in wounds. It is transmitted by airborne infection, or more rarely by milk or ice-cream contaminated by streptococci. The incubation period is 2–4 days.

Clinical features

Scarlet fever occurs most commonly in children. It has a sudden onset and the more severe cases present with a sore throat, shivering, pyrexia, headache and vomiting. There is inflammation of the fauces; the tonsils are enlarged and may be covered with a follicular exudate. The exudate can be distinguished from the membrane seen in diphtheria by its yellow appearance and by being more easily wiped off. There is tender enlargement of the tonsillar lymph nodes. The rash, which usually appears first behind the ears on the second day, rapidly becomes a generalised punctate erythema (see Fig. 4.2 p. 75). It is most intense in the flexures of the arms and legs. The face is not affected by the rash, though it is usually flushed due to fever, and the region round the mouth is pale. The tongue is initially furred but shows prominent red papillae. The rash fades in about 1 week and is succeeded by desquamation. A profuse growth of *Strep pyogenes* can usually be obtained from a throat swab.

Complications

The complications are less common than formerly because of the mild form of the disease and effective chemotherapy. Otitis media, cervical adenitis and sinusitis may occur. Rheumatic fever and glomerulonephritis are rare sequelae which develop 2 or 3 weeks after the onset of any haemolytic streptococcal infection.

Management

The treatment of scarlet fever is the same as for streptococcal sore throat. Most patients respond rapidly to phenoxymethylpenicillin (250 mg for children and 500 mg for adults 6-hourly for 7 days).

ERYSIPELAS

Erysipelas is an acute streptococcal infection of the skin, commoner in the elderly.

Clinical features

The onset is abrupt with heat and pain in the infected skin and systemic upset. There is a rapidly spreading red patch of inflamed skin with underlying oedema of the subcutaneous tissues (Fig. 4.22). The edge of the patch is palpably raised and clearly defined and the lymph nodes draining the area become enlarged and tender. As the oedema subsides, vesicles and bullae appear in the central part of the affected area. The face is involved in at least 80% of all cases of erysipelas from the spread of streptococci from the nose.

Management

Erysipelas is usually brought under control within 48 hours with penicillin; hence the prognosis is excellent for a disease which used to be very serious. Recurrent infections are common.

STAPHYLOCOCCAL INFECTIONS

Staph aureus is responsible for a wide variety of suppurative conditions (Fig. 4.23). Many infections, particularly boils, carbuncles and abscesses, are due to autogenous infection as the organisms can be grown from nasopharynx and skin of up to 30% of healthy persons. The staphylococcus is readily spread from these sites and from clothing to contaminate the dust in which it survives in the dry state for weeks or months. In hospital this organism is an important cause of wound infection, pneumonia and neonatal sepsis. Under suitable conditions it multiplies freely in food and milk to produce a heat-stable toxin which is a cause of food poisoning.

Staphylococcal endocarditis (see p. 296)

This condition occurs in drug addicts, in whom it usually causes right-sided heart valve lesions, and as a complication of septic thrombophlebitis associated with intravenous cannulae and lines.

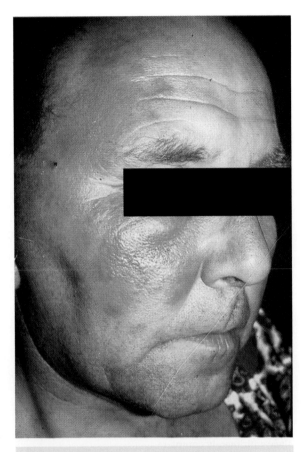

Fig. 4.22 Erysipelas. Area of clearly defined erythema with oedema of the subcutaneous tissues causing an 'orange-skin' appearance.

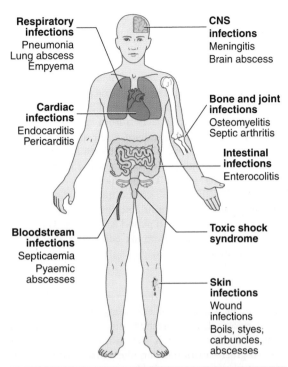

Fig. 4.23 Infections caused by _Staphylococcus aureus_.

The diagram labels the following:

- **Respiratory infections** — Pneumonia, Lung abscess, Empyema
- **Cardiac infections** — Endocarditis, Pericarditis
- **Bloodstream infections** — Septicaemia, Pyaemic abscesses
- **CNS infections** — Meningitis, Brain abscess
- **Bone and joint infections** — Osteomyelitis, Septic arthritis
- **Intestinal infections** — Enterocolitis
- **Toxic shock syndrome**
- **Skin infections** — Wound infections, Boils, styes, carbuncles, abscesses

Toxic shock syndrome

This is caused by the toxins of certain _Staph aureus_ strains and occurs in women using some types of tampon, the infection originating in the vagina and presenting with fever, rash and shock. The syndrome has also been described in men and women as a complication of staphylococcal infections of the skin, lungs and breasts. Onset is with fever followed by the development of a punctate erythematous rash as in scarlet fever. There is hypotension with shock. Renal failure may develop and death can occur if treatment is not started immediately.

Management

90% of _Staph aureus_ strains are now resistant to penicillin, which should be used only if the organism is shown to be sensitive. If the illness is severe, treatment should be commenced with flucloxacillin 500 mg 6-hourly, unless the patient is known to be allergic to the penicillins when erythromycin 500 mg 6-hourly, fusidic acid 500 mg 6-hourly or clindamycin 300 mg 6-hourly should be given. Nasal carriage of staphylococci can be eradicated by topical application of neomycin plus chlorhexidine or mupirocin.

Staph aureus strains resistant to all antibiotics except vancomycin are causing outbreaks of hospital infection in many countries. Known as methicillin- (or multiply) resistant _Staph aureus_ (MRSA), these organisms can cause serious and often fatal infections. Patients colonised by MRSA must be placed in isolation.

Staph epidermidis is a skin commensal organism which can cause serious infections in the immunosuppressed and in those with prosthetic heart valves and joint implants. Endocarditis due to this organism is particularly difficult to cure.

Methicillin-resistant _Staph epidermidis_ strains (MRSE) have now emerged as pathogens.

CORYNEBACTERIAL INFECTION

DIPHTHERIA

In many parts of the developing world diphtheria is an important cause of illness. Recent outbreaks have occurred in the former Soviet Union. It is now very rare in Britain.

Pathology

Infection with *Corynebacterium diphtheriae* occurs most commonly in the upper respiratory tract, and sore throat is frequently the presenting feature. The disease is usually spread by droplet infection from cases or carriers. The organisms remain localised at the site of infection and the serious consequences result from the absorption of a soluble exotoxin which damages the heart muscle and the nervous system. The infection may occur rarely on the conjunctiva or the genital tract, or it may complicate wounds, abrasions or diseases of the skin.

The average incubation period is 2–4 days. Cases are isolated until cultures from six daily nose and throat swabs are negative.

Clinical features

These are summarised in the information box. The disease begins insidiously. The temperature is seldom much raised although tachycardia is usually marked. The diagnostic feature is the 'wash-leather' elevated greyish-green membrane on the tonsils with a well-defined edge and surrounded by a zone of inflammation. The membrane is firm and adherent. There may be swelling of the neck ('bull-neck') and tender enlargement of the lymph nodes. In the mildest infections, especially in the presence of a high degree of immunity, a membrane may never appear and the throat is merely slightly injected.

CLINICAL FEATURES OF DIPHTHERIA

Acute infection
- Membranous tonsillitis
- *or* Nasal infection
- *or* Laryngeal infection
- *or* Skin/wound/conjunctival infection (rare)

Complications
- Laryngeal obstruction or paralysis
- Myocarditis
- Peripheral neuropathy

With anterior nasal infection there is nasal discharge, often tinged with blood. In laryngeal diphtheria there is a husky voice, a high-pitched cough, and a danger of respiratory obstruction which can be fatal if tracheostomy is not carried out. When the infection spreads towards the uvula, to the fauces and then to the nasopharynx, the patient is often gravely ill. The pulse is rapid and of poor volume and the blood pressure low. Death from acute circulatory failure may occur within the first ten days. Those who survive the earlier toxaemia

---

MANAGEMENT OF DIPHTHERIA

- Admit to isolation facility
- Administer antitoxin (4000 to 32 000 units i.m.—test dose first)
- Give benzylpenicillin 600 mg 6-hourly i.v. for 7 days
- Notify public health authorities
- Treat complications:
  Tracheostomy for respiratory obstruction.
  Monitor for, and treat, arrhythmias due to myocarditis
- Protect close contacts:
  Erythromycin prophylaxis
  Immunisation

---

may later develop arrhythmias or cardiac failure. ECG changes are common due to myocarditis. These are reversible and there is no permanent damage to the heart in those who survive.

Involvement of the nervous system sometimes occurs, and after tonsillar or pharyngeal diphtheria it usually commences with palatal palsy on about the tenth day of the illness. Paralysis of accommodation often follows and may be inferred from difficulty in reading small print. A week or two later, though somewhat rarely, weakness and paraesthesia in the limbs due to polyneuritis may develop. Recovery from such neuritis is always ultimately complete.

Management

Upon making a clinical diagnosis of diphtheria, the case should be notified to the public health authorities and sent urgently to a hospital for infectious diseases. If the clinician considers that diphtheria is likely to be the cause of the illness (see information box) antitoxin must be injected intramuscularly without awaiting the result of a throat swab. Delay increases the danger to the patient, because toxin, once fixed to the tissues, can no longer be neutralised by antitoxin. However, horse serum, in which antitoxin is contained, is liable to cause undesirable reactions as it is a foreign protein. There may be an immediate anaphylactic reaction with dyspnoea, pallor and collapse or even death. Serum sickness, with fever, urticaria and joint pains may occur 7–12 days later. If there is a previous history of inoculation of horse serum, the symptoms commonly appear in 3–4 days. As anaphylaxis is potentially lethal, all patients must be asked whether they have ever had antiserum before and whether they suffer from any allergic disorder. A small test injection of serum should be given half an hour before the full dose in every patient. 1/1000 adrenaline solution must be available to deal with any immediate type of reaction (0.5–1.0 ml intramuscularly). An antihistamine is also given.

In a severely ill patient the risk of anaphylactic shock is outweighed by the mortal danger of diphtheritic toxaemia and up to 100 000 units of antitoxin is injected intravenously if the test dose has not given rise to symptoms. For disease of moderate severity 16 000–32 000 units i.m. will suffice, and for mild cases 4000–8000 units.

Penicillin, 1200 mg 6-hourly intravenously, or amoxycillin 500 mg 8-hourly, should be administered for 1 week to eliminate *C. diphtheriae*. Patients allergic to penicillin can be given erythromycin.

Prevention

Active immunisation should be given to all children.

If diphtheria occurs in a closed community, contacts should be given erythromycin, which is more effective than penicillin in eradicating the organism in carriers. All contacts should also be immunised or given a booster dose of toxoid. Adults should be given a dilute preparation of vaccine to avoid severe reactions.

BACILLUS INFECTIONS

ANTHRAX

Anthrax is a disease of domestic animals which become infected by inhaling or ingesting spores of *Bacillus anthracis* passed in faeces. Grazing lands remain infective for years. In man anthrax is an occupational disease of farmers, butchers and dealers in hides, hair, wool and bone meal from endemic areas. Anthrax is endemic in communities where skins are used as sleeping mats, for clothing or for carrying water, and where diseased cattle are eaten. Inoculation of spores subcutaneously is more common than their spread by inhalation or ingestion. The incubation period is usually 1–3 days.

Clinical features

A cutaneous lesion begins as an itching papule which enlarges and forms a vesicle filled with serosanguineous fluid surrounded by gross oedema—the 'malignant pustule'. The lesion is relatively painless and accompanied by slight enlargement of regional lymph nodes. The vesicle dries to form a thick black eschar surrounded by blebs. Occasionally there are multiple lesions. In endemic areas patients may exhibit only slight constitutional symptoms and little oedema but in non-immune persons high fever, toxaemia and fatal septicaemia may develop.

When infected meat has been eaten an ulcer with surrounding oedema may develop in the pharynx or, more commonly, the infection causes a severe, fatal gastroenteritis.

Those who acquire the infection by inhalation may develop an acute laryngitis or a virulent haemorrhagic bronchopneumonia (wool-sorters' disease). Anthrax may also present as meningitis.

Investigations

A stained smear of fluid taken from the edge of a lesion demonstrates the organism, which can be confirmed by culture. *B. anthracis* is also recoverable from laryngeal and pulmonary anthrax and from the CSF in meningitis. Anthrax should be suspected if a group of people who have feasted on an animal which has sickened and died are taken abruptly ill with fulminating gastroenteritis. *B. anthracis* may be cultured from the faeces.

Management

Treatment is with penicillin 1200 mg 6-hourly. The organism is also sensitive to erythromycin, tetracycline, chloramphenicol and streptomycin.

Prevention

The disease is controlled in cattle by slaughter and deep burial of the diseased animal and by vaccination of healthy animals at risk. Potentially infected imports from endemic areas must be subject to strict control. Persons at risk through their occupation should be vaccinated.

BORDETELLA INFECTIONS

WHOOPING COUGH

Whooping cough (pertussis) is a highly infectious disease caused by *Bordetella pertussis*. It is spread by droplet infection and while it occurs at all ages, approximately 90% of cases are in children under 5 years of age. The incubation period is 7–14 days.

Clinical features

The first stage consists of a highly infectious upper respiratory infection lasting about 1 week during which conjunctivitis, rhinitis and an unproductive cough are present. The distinctive paroxysmal stage follows and is characterised by severe bouts of coughing. The number of such paroxysms in 24 hours varies from an occasional attack to 40 or 50 and they are more severe at night. Each paroxysm consists of a succession of short sharp coughs, gathering in speed and duration and ending in a deep inspiration during which the characteristic whoop may be heard. It may be absent in older children and in adults because the air passages are so much wider. The last paroxysm of a series frequently ends with vomiting. The paroxysmal stage lasts from 1 to several weeks.

Complications

The complications of whooping cough are listed in the information box.

COMPLICATIONS OF WHOOPING COUGH

Respiratory
- Bronchopneumonia
- Atelectasis
- Bronchiectasis

Other
- Convulsions
- Conjunctival haemorrhage
- Ulceration of frenum
- Prolapse of rectum

Investigations

Diagnosis can be difficult in the catarrhal stage when the disease is most infectious. It can be confirmed in the laboratory by the isolation of *B. pertussis* taken from the posterior wall of the nasopharynx on small swabs passed along the floor of the nose. Examination of the blood shows a lymphocytosis which, however, may not develop until the disease is well established. The diagnosis is easy in the paroxysmal stage when the whoop has developed.

Management

Erythromycin 125–250 mg 6-hourly may reduce the severity of the infection if given during the initial stage. A cough suppressant such as methadone may be helpful in controlling the severity of paroxysms. When the illness is of long duration and vomiting is frequent, skilled nursing will be required to maintain nutrition, especially in infants and young children. Feeds are usually accepted and retained if they are given immediately after the vomiting which frequently follows a paroxysm of coughing.

Prevention

Active immunisation should be given to all children except where there is a history of severe local or general reaction to a preceding dose or where there is evidence of an evolving neurological abnormality. Personal or family history of febrile convulsions or epilepsy, or a stable neurological condition, are not contraindications to immunisation. Seizures or neurological damage resulting from active immunisation are exceedingly rare (1:310 000 injections). Neurological complications after whooping cough itself are considerably more common than after the vaccine. Infants of less than three months (who are too young to be immunised) can develop severe

and occasionally fatal attacks; those who are exposed should be given prophylactic erythromycin.

SALMONELLA INFECTIONS

There are approaching 2000 salmonella serotypes, most of which originate in animals, especially poultry, and are transmitted to man either directly or in food. The exception is *S. typhi* which invariably has a human source. There are 6 clinical syndromes caused by salmonellae (see the information box).

SALMONELLA INFECTIONS

- **Typhoid and paratyphoid fever** (Enteric fever)
- **Gastroenteritis** (food poisoning)
- **Enterocolitis**
- **Septicaemia**
- **Metastatic lesions** (complicating septicaemia):
  Osteomyelitis/septic arthritis
  Liver abscess
  Brain abscess
- **Asymptomatic carrier state**

TYPHOID AND PARATYPHOID (ENTERIC) FEVERS

In many countries where sanitation is primitive, typhoid and paratyphoid fevers, which are transmitted by the faecal-oral route, are an important cause of illness. Elsewhere they are relatively rare. Nevertheless, outbreaks occur from time to time in developed countries and the infection may be contracted from returned travellers, especially if they are symptomless carriers of the infecting organism.

Aetiology

The enteric fevers are caused by infection with *S. typhi* and *S. paratyphi A* and *B*. In Britain spread is usually by carriers, often food handlers, through the contamination of food, milk or water; infected shellfish are occasionally responsible for an outbreak. The bacilli may live in the gallbladder of carriers for months or years after clinical recovery and pass intermittently in the stool and less commonly in the urine. The incubation period of typhoid fever is about 10–14 days; that of paratyphoid is somewhat shorter.

Pathology

After a few days of bacteraemia, the bacilli localise mainly in the lymphoid tissue of the small intestine. The typical lesion is in the Peyer's patches and follicles.

These swell at first, then ulcerate and ultimately heal, but during this sequence they may perforate or bleed.

Clinical features
These are outlined in the information box.

Typhoid fever: The onset may be insidious. The temperature rises in a stepladder fashion for 4 or 5 days. There is malaise, with increasing headache, drowsiness and aching in the limbs. Cough and epistaxis occur. Constipation may be present although in children diarrhoea and vomiting may be prominent early in the illness. The pulse is often slower than would be expected from the height of the temperature.

CLINICAL FEATURES OF TYPHOID FEVER

- **First week** Fever, headache, myalgia, bradycardia, constipation (diarrhoea and vomiting)
- **End of first week** Rose spots on trunk, splenomegaly, cough, abdominal distension, diarrhoea
- **End of second week** Delirium, complications, then coma and death (if untreated).

At the end of the first week a rash may appear on the upper abdomen and on the back as sparse, slightly raised, rose-red spots which fade on pressure. It is usually visible only on white skin. Around the seventh to tenth day the spleen becomes palpable. Constipation is then succeeded by diarrhoea and abdominal distension with tenderness. Bronchitis and delirium may develop. By the end of the second week the patient may be profoundly ill unless the disease is modified by antibiotic treatment. In the third week toxaemia increases and the patient may pass into coma and die. Such extreme cases are rare in countries with developed health services.

Following recovery up to 5% of patients become chronic carriers of *S. typhi*.

Paratyphoid fever: The most common variety in Britain is due to *S. paratyphi B*. The course tends to be shorter and milder than that of typhoid fever and the onset is often more abrupt with acute enteritis. The rash may be more abundant and the intestinal complications less frequent.

Complications
These are given in the information box. Haemorrhage from, or a perforation of, the ulcerated Peyer's patches may occur at the end of the second week or during the third week of the illness. Additional complications may involve almost any viscus or system because of the sep-

ticaemia present during the first week; these include cholecystitis, pneumonia, myocarditis, arthritis, osteomyelitis and meningitis. Bone and joint infection is seen, especially in children with sickle-cell disease.

COMPLICATIONS OF TYPHOID FEVER

- **Bowel** Perforation, haemorrhage
- **Septicaemic foci** Bone and joint infection, meningitis, cholecystitis
- **Toxic phenomena** Myocarditis, nephritis

Investigations
In the first week the diagnosis may be difficult because in this invasive stage with bacteraemia the symptoms are those of a generalised infection without localising features. A white blood count may be helpful as there is typically a leucopenia. Blood culture is the most important diagnostic method in a suspected case. The faeces will contain the organism more frequently during the second and third weeks. The Widal reaction detects antibodies to the causative organisms. However, it is not a reliable diagnostic test and should be interpreted with caution.

Management
Several antibiotics are effective in enteric fever. Ciprofloxacin in a dose of 500 mg 12-hourly is the drug of choice. Alternatives include co-trimoxazole (2 tablets or intravenous equivalent 12-hourly), amoxycillin (750 mg 6-hourly) and chloramphenicol (500 mg 6-hourly). However, an increasing number of salmonellae, including *S. typhi*, are now resistant to many antibiotics and some are only sensitive to ciprofloxacin. Treatment should be continued for 14 days. Pyrexia may persist for up to 5 days after the start of specific therapy. Even with effective chemotherapy there is still a danger of complications, of recrudescence of the disease and of the development of a carrier state. The chronic carrier should be treated for 4 weeks with ciprofloxacin; cholecystectomy may be necessary in some cases.

Prevention
Those who propose to travel to or live in countries where enteric infections are endemic should be inoculated with one of the three available typhoid vaccines (two inactivated injectable and one oral live attenuated).

FOOD POISONING

Food poisoning (gastroenteritis) can be due to many causes, infective and non-infective (see the information box). It presents with vomiting, diarrhoea, or both, usually between 1 and 48 hours of consumption of the contaminated food or drink. Outbreaks are common, especially in institutions and restaurants. Non-infective causes and bacterial toxins, which are pre-formed in the infected food, produce symptoms within minutes or hours of a meal, whereas the other infections may not produce illness for up to 48 hours. Infective gastroenteritis can be classified as **non-toxin type** and **toxin type**.

CAUSES OF FOOD POISONING

Infective
Non-toxin mediated
- Salmonella species
- *Campylobacter jejuni*
- *Bacillus cereus*
- Viruses, e.g. Norwalk viruses
- *Listeria monocytogenes* (causing meningitis)
- *Bacillus anthracis* (anthrax)

Toxin mediated
- *Staphylococcus aureus*
- *Clostridium perfringens*
- *Clostridium botulinum* (botulism)
- *Esch coli* 0157 (verocytotoxin-producing)

Non-infective
Allergic
- Shellfish, strawberries

Non-allergic
- Scrombotoxin (fish)
- Ciguatoxin (tropical fish)
- Fungi (e.g. *Amanita phalloides*)
- Chemicals, metals (e.g. in cooking pots)

Non-toxin-mediated food poisoning

Salmonella species (other than *S. typhi*) are very common causes of food poisoning. *S. typhimurium* and *S. enteritidis* are the most frequently isolated in Britain at present. The domestic fowl is the commonest source of infection, which may be contracted from inadequately defrosted and undercooked chicken or from undercooked or raw eggs. Intensive rearing, infected poultry food and deep freezing of carcases all contribute to the high level of human salmonella infection. Symptomless faecal carriers of salmonella who are food-handlers are also a source of infection. The size of the infecting dose of bacteria bears a close relationship to the speed of onset of symptoms and to the severity of the illness. This indicates the dangers of bacterial multiplication which may take place when food is contaminated and thereafter remains warm for many hours or days.

Campylobacter jejuni is now the commonest bacterial cause of food poisoning in Britain. Sources of infection include poultry, dogs, water and unpasteurised milk.

Bacillus cereus infection is a hazard of eating rice which has been cooked and then reheated and consumed at a later date.

Listeria monocytogenes is an environmental bacterium which can contaminate food, including poultry and cheese. It does not usually cause intestinal symptoms but is a cause of septicaemia and meningitis especially in pregnancy, the neonate, the immunosuppressed, diabetics and alcoholics.

Certain viruses (commonly referred to as small round structured viruses because of their morphology) such as Norwalk viruses, coronaviruses and rotaviruses, which can be identified only by electron microscopy of stool and are not yet culturable, commonly cause outbreaks of food poisoning, especially in institutions and catering establishments.

The protozoal organisms *Giardia lamblia* and cryptosporidium species can also cause food poisoning or waterborne outbreaks of diarrhoeal disease (p. 155).

Toxin-mediated food poisoning

Such poisoning is most commonly caused by the enterotoxin of *Staph aureus*, frequently from a food handler with a septic lesion on the hand. Incubation at a suitable temperature leads to growth of the organism and production of toxin which is relatively heat resistant and may not be destroyed by cooking.

Strains of clostridia, many of them relatively resistant to heat, can also contaminate certain foods, particularly meat. Pre-cooking of stews and pies may not destroy all the spores, and the keeping of such food will lead to the formation of heat-stable toxins which can give rise to gastroenteritis, sometimes severe.

A verocytotoxin produced by a strain of *Esch coli* (enterohaemorrhagic *Esch coli* type 0157) has recently been found to cause food poisoning, usually originating in meat, which may present as a haemorrhagic colitis. It is also a cause of the haemolytic/uraemic syndrome.

Botulism is a rare form of bacterial food poisoning due to the ingestion of the toxin produced by *Cl. botulinum* in imperfectly treated tinned food or preserved fish contaminated with the organism. The clinical features differ from all other types of bacterial food poisoning and consist chiefly of vomiting and pareses of skeletal, ocular, pharyngeal and respiratory muscles. Mortality can be high.

Clinical features

The simultaneous occurrence of symptoms in more than one member of a household or institution simplifies diagnosis. However, isolated cases are very common.

Table 4.27 Initial clinical features of food poisoning

Aetiology	Incubation	Symptoms
Chemical poison	30 minutes	Vomiting
Staphylococcal or clostridial toxin	2–6 hours	Vomiting initially—may be diarrhoea and abdominal pain later
Salmonella or campylobacter infection	12–48 hours	Diarrhoea (bloody with campylobacter), abdominal pain, vomiting. Septicaemia can occur with salmonella infection
Haemorrhagic colitis (E. coli 0157)	12–48 hours	Bloody diarrhoea predominates—may be abdominal pain.

The incubation period is a useful pointer to the aetiology (see Table 4.27).

In severe cases there may be prostration, collapse and dehydration. In the chemical and toxin types of food poisoning the onset tends to be sudden and severe and the patient may rapidly become shocked. Recovery, however, usually occurs within 24 hours. In the infective type, symptoms develop more slowly and there is usually pyrexia and toxicity. The stools are watery and offensive, and may contain blood and some mucus, in contrast to bacillary dysentery where there is also pus. Salmonella septicaemia may be associated with osteomyelitis, septic arthritis, endocarditis or meningitis.

Severe abdominal pain and blood in the stool are common in Campylobacter infections. Rarely, septicaemia may complicate Campylobacter gastroenteritis, and endocarditis has been reported. Campylobacter enteritis may be confused with ulcerative colitis and rectal biopsies can appear similar in both diseases. Bloody diarrhoea should suggest the possibility of haemorrhagic colitis due to *Esch coli* 0157.

Investigations
A specimen of the patient's stool or vomit together with the suspected food, if available, should be sent for culture. Campylobacter and organisms of the salmonella group can usually be readily isolated. In more severe cases blood should be sent for culture. Notification of salmonella infection and other types of food poisoning is compulsory in Britain.

Management
This is summarised in the information box. Most cases are mild and symptoms subside in a few days. Solid food should be withheld and the patient instructed to take fluids only. Fluid and electrolytes can usually be replaced orally. Patients who are ill or dehydrated require intravenous fluid therapy. When acute symptoms cease, a semi-fluid low-roughage diet may be taken. Codeine phosphate or loperamide is useful in controlling diarrhoea.

MANAGEMENT OF FOOD POISONING

Supportive
- Fluid and electrolyte replacement—oral or i.v.
- Bowel sedation—not for mild cases or until at least 24 hours after onset of diarrhoea. Not in children. Codeine phosphate or loperamide useful
- If chemical or poisonous food known or suspected—wash out stomach

Specific
- Majority of cases—none required
- Salmonella infections, suspected septicaemia or severe or prolonged symptoms—ciprofloxacin or trimethoprim
- Campylobacter infections—erythromycin or ciprofloxacin (although efficacy not fully proven)

Antibiotics should not be given routinely for acute diarrhoea and vomiting as they are usually ineffective and frequently exacerbate symptoms. If salmonella bacteraemia is suspected or confirmed or if diarrhoea is severe or prolonged, ciprofloxacin 500 mg 12-hourly or trimethoprim 200 mg 12-hourly should be given. Campylobacter enteritis is treated with erythromycin 500 mg 6-hourly or ciprofloxacin 500 mg 12-hourly. *Listeria monocytogenes* is susceptible to amoxycillin; gentamicin is given in addition in the immunosuppressed and for the treatment of meningitis.

If the poisoning is thought to be due to a chemical or a poisonous food, the patient's stomach should be washed out with tepid water, using the technique described on page 1132 and the stomach contents kept for analysis.

Prevention
A reduction in the high incidence of food poisoning can best be achieved by improving the standards of personal hygiene, especially in those handling food, and by stressing the importance of **hand washing** after using the lavatory. Low temperature storage is required for food which has to be kept for some hours or days before being consumed. It is essential to keep frozen poultry at room temperature for at least 12 hours before cooking or pathogens at the centre may survive unharmed. Improvements in poultry-rearing methods are urgently required.

DYSENTERY

Dysentery is an acute inflammation of the large intestine characterised by diarrhoea with blood and mucus in the stools. Its causes are bacillary or amoebic infection. The latter condition is described on page 154.

BACILLARY DYSENTERY (SHIGELLOSIS)

The bacilli belong to the genus **Shigella** of which there are four main pathogenic groups, **dysenteriae, flexneri, boydii** and **sonnei**, the first two having numerous serotypes. In Britain the majority of cases of bacillary dysentery are caused by *Sh. sonnei* although in recent years there has been a significant increase in imported infections caused by *Sh. flexneri* while indigenous sonnei dysentery has decreased. Shigella strains, especially in tropical countries, are now commonly resistant to many antibiotics. These multi-resistant organisms have been responsible for epidemics of bacillary dysentery in Bangladesh and other tropical countries.

Epidemiology

Bacillary dysentery is endemic all over the world. It occurs in epidemic form wherever there is a crowded population with poor sanitation, and has been a constant accompaniment of wars and natural catastrophes. Spread may occur by contaminated food or by flies, but contact through unwashed hands after defecation is by far the most important factor. Outbreaks occur in mental hospitals, residential schools and other closed institutions.

Pathology

There is inflammation of the large bowel which may involve the lower part of the small intestine. Sigmoidoscopy shows that the mucosa is red and swollen, the submucous veins are obscured and mucopus is seen on the surface. Bleeding points appear readily at the touch of the endoscope. Ulcers may form.

Clinical features

There is great variation in disease severity. *Sh. sonnei* infections may be so mild as to escape detection and the patient remains ambulant with a few loose stools and perhaps some colic, fever and headache. *Sh. flexneri* infections are usually more severe while those due to *Sh. dysenteriae* may be fulminating and cause death within 48 hours.

In a moderately severe illness, the patient complains of diarrhoea, colicky abdominal pain and tenesmus. The stools are usually small, and after the first few evacuations, contain blood and purulent exudate with little

BACILLARY DYSENTERY—CLINICAL FEATURES

- *Shigella sonnei* — Usually mild diarrhoea in children. Commonest type in UK
- *Shigella flexneri* — More severe diarrhoea, often blood in stool. Second commonest type in UK
- *Shigella boydii* — Rarest type. Similar clinical features to *Sh. flexneri*
- *Shigella dysenteriae* — Causes severe infections with profuse bloody diarrhoea and prostration. Haemolytic uraemic syndrome may cause renal failure. Can be fatal. Multi-resistant strains common in South-East Asia

faecal material. There is frequently fever, with dehydration and weakness if the diarrhoea persists. There is usually tenderness over the colon. Arthritis or iritis may occasionally complicate bacillary dysentery (Reiter's syndrome, p. 907).

Investigations

Diagnosis depends on faecal culture.

Management

Diarrhoea in adults may be controlled by codeine (30 mg 8-hourly), or loperamide (2–4 mg 6–8-hourly). A fluid or semi-fluid low roughage diet should be given depending on the severity of the symptoms but if diarrhoea is severe, intravenous replacement of water and electrolyte loss will be necessary (p. 130). Sonnei dysentery is usually a self-limiting disease and antibiotics are not indicated in most cases. In infections caused by dysenteriae or flexneri strains, trimethoprim (200 mg 12-hourly) or ciprofloxacin (500 mg 12-hourly) should be given.

Prevention

The prevention of faecal contamination of food and milk and the isolation of patients are methods which are theoretically important but may be difficult to apply except in limited outbreaks. Hand washing is very important.

OTHER TRUE BACTERIAL INFECTIONS

BRUCELLOSIS

Brucellosis (undulant fever, Malta fever, abortus fever) is caused in Northern Europe by infection with *Brucella abortus* which is usually spread to man by the ingestion of raw milk from infected cattle. It is an occupational hazard of veterinary surgeons, laboratory personnel and slaughterhouse workers. The infection has now been virtually eradicated from cattle in Britain. In Malta and other Mediterranean and Middle East countries the disease is frequently due to *B. melitensis* and is transmitted by infected goats or sheep. In the USA and the Far East *B. suis* acquired from pigs may be the causative organism. The incubation period is about 3 weeks. Subclinical infections are common in farmers and veterinarians.

Clinical features

The disease has features both of a bloodstream infection, and an intracellular infection. These are listed in the information box below. Untreated, the disease may last for a few days or for many months. Neutropenia and lymphocytosis occur in the more severely affected.

CLINICAL FEATURES OF BRUCELLOSIS

Onset
Acute with high continuous fever *or* insidious with fever undulating over 7–10 day periods

Symptoms
Fever, sweating, weakness, headache, anorexia, pain in limbs and back, rigors, joint pains

Signs
Fever and splenomegaly

Complications
- Relapse within 2 years of recovery
- Localised disease causing suppurative or granulomatous lesions including arthritis, spondylitis, bursitis, osteomyelitis, meningoencephalitis, endocarditis, epididymo-orchitis, pneumonia, hepatitis
- Chronic brucellosis: low-grade fever and neuropsychiatric symptoms

---

Investigations

Blood, and especially bone marrow, cultured under special conditions usually yields the organism in acutely ill patients. Brucella serology is unreliable: a four-fold rise in titre of agglutinating antibody, which detects IgM antibody, may be diagnostic but cross reactions are common. Complement fixation and anti-human globulin tests are more useful in chronic infections.

Management

Tetracycline 500 mg 6-hourly, plus rifampicin 600 mg daily for 4 weeks is curative and relapses are unusual. Streptomycin 1 g daily may be used instead of rifampicin. Tetracycline alone or co-trimoxazole, 2 tablets twice daily, are usually effective, but the disease may relapse.

Prevention

Infected herds of cattle can be identified and destroyed. The spread of brucellosis by milk is prevented by pasteurisation or boiling. Veterinary surgeons and others handling infected animals need to exercise scrupulous hygiene.

PLAGUE

Epidemics of plague, such as the 'Black Death', have attacked man since ancient times. Now, the disease is limited to rodents in the wild with occasional sporadic human cases or local outbreaks, predominantly in Vietnam and East Africa with sporadic cases in the USA and elsewhere (Fig. 4.24). The causative organism, *Yersinia pestis*, is a small Gram-negative bacillus. It is spread between rodents by their fleas. If domestic rats become infected, infected fleas may bite man. In the late stages of human plague *Y. pestis* may be expectorated and spread between humans by droplets. 'Pneumonic plague' may follow. Hunters and trappers can get plague from handling rodents.

Pathology

Organisms inoculated through the skin are taken rapidly to the draining lymph nodes where they elicit a severe inflammatory response that may be haemorrhagic. If the infection is not contained, septicaemia ensues and necrotic, purulent or haemorrhagic lesions develop in many organs. Oliguria and shock follow, and disseminated intravascular coagulation may result in widespread haemorrhage. Inhalation of *Y. pestis* causes alveolitis. The incubation period is 3–6 days, but less in pneumonic plague.

Bubonic plague

In this, the commonest form of the disease, the onset is usually sudden with a rigor, high fever, dry skin and severe headache. Soon aching and swelling at the site of the affected lymph nodes begin. The most common site of the bubo, made up of the swollen lymph nodes and surrounding tissue, is one groin. Some infections are relatively mild but in the majority of patients toxaemia quickly increases with a rapid pulse, hypotension and mental confusion. The spleen is usually palpable.

Septicaemic plague

Those not exhibiting a bubo usually deteriorate rapidly. Meningitis and pneumonia and expectoration of blood-stained sputum containing *Y. pestis* may complicate bubonic or septicaemic plague.

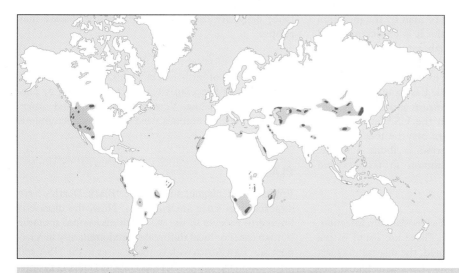

Fig. 4.24 Foci of the transmission of plague. Frequent transmission is shaded dark red, infrequent or suspected transmission pink. Adapted by permission of the World Health Organization.

Frequent transmission

Infrequent or suspected transmission

Pneumonic plague

The onset is very sudden with cough and dyspnoea. The patient soon expectorates copious blood-stained, frothy, highly infective sputum, becomes cyanosed and dies. Radiographs of the lung show a lobar opacity.

Investigations

Reports of death among rats should alert suspicion of an outbreak. Early diagnosis is urgent. An aspirate from a bubo, sputum, or the buffy coat (leucocyte fraction) of blood is used to show the characteristic organism by staining with methylene blue, or by immuno-fluorescence. Blood, sputum and aspirate should be cultured. Plague is notifiable under the International Health Regulations.

Management

If the diagnosis is suspected on clinical and epidemiological grounds, treatment must be started as soon as, or even before, samples have been collected for laboratory diagnosis. Streptomycin is given by intramuscular injection every 6 or 12 hours, at a daily dose of 30 mg/kg for 10 days, or tetracycline, 10 mg/kg 6-hourly orally or intravenously, for 10 days. Treatment may also be needed for acute circulatory failure, disseminated intravascular coagulation or hypoxia.

Prevention

Rats and fleas should be controlled (see information box p. 116). In endemic areas people should avoid handling and skinning wild animals.

A formalin-killed vaccine is available for those at occu-pational risk. Patients are isolated and attendants must wear gowns, masks and gloves. Contacts should be protected by tetracycline 2 g daily, or co-trimoxazole 1 tablet daily for a week. Postmortem examination is dangerous.

TULARAEMIA

Tularaemia is an infection due to *Francisella tularensis* transmitted to mammals and birds by the bites of infected blood-sucking flies and ticks. Man may be infected by ticks or while skinning infected wild rabbits or hares. The microorganisms enter through dermal abrasions, the conjunctiva or mouth. The disease is found in the Americas, Japan, the USSR, and most European countries excluding Britain.

Pathology

Focal areas of necrosis occur, especially in lymph nodes, spleen, liver, kidneys and lungs. There may be cutaneous, oral or ophthalmic lesions when infection is by these routes.

Clinical features

The commonest presentation is of a skin ulcer, with painful regional lymphadenopathy. There may be a systemic illness with fever, often prolonged. Sometimes the conjunctiva or throat is the site of entry, and is inflamed. Occasionally the presentation is only with lympha-denopathy.

Septicaemia is the rarest but most severe form of the disease. There is a sudden onset of high fever, prostration, aching limbs, vomiting, diarrhoea and mental confusion. Pneumonia, pleurisy and pericarditis are serious complications.

Investigations

The organism may be isolated with difficulty and danger by culture or guinea-pig inoculation. Agglutination and complement-fixation tests become positive after 10–12 days.

Management

Streptomycin, as for plague (p. 127), or gentamicin is the treatment of choice. Tetracycline (500 mg 6-hourly for 2 weeks) is less effective.

Prevention

Masks should be worn in the laboratory and gloves are used when skinning rabbits and hares in endemic areas. Adequate cooking renders infected meat safe for eating.

MELIOIDOSIS

Melioidosis is caused by *Pseudomonas pseudomallei*, which is a saphrophyte found in puddles following recent rain. Infection is through abrasions of the skin. Diabetics and patients with severe burns are particularly susceptible. The disease is commonest in the Far East, S.E. Asia and Australia, and occurs rarely in India, Africa and the USA.

Pathology

A bacteraemia is followed by the formation of abscesses in the lungs, liver and spleen.

Clinical features

There is high fever, prostration and sometimes diarrhoea with signs of pneumonia and enlargement of the liver and spleen. A chest radiograph resembles that of acute caseous tuberculosis. In more chronic forms multiple abscesses recur in subcutaneous tissue and bone.

Investigations

Culture of blood, sputum or pus may yield *P. pseudomallei*. Except in fulminating infections, antibodies may be detected by indirect haemoagglutination, direct agglutination, and complement-fixation tests.

Management

In acute illness prompt treatment, without waiting for cultural confirmation, may be life-saving. Ceftazidime 120 mg/kg plus tetracycline 3 g daily are given in divided doses for about 2–3 weeks, followed by doxycycline 200 mg daily for 2–3 months, until pulmonary cavities have healed. Abscesses should be drained surgically.

CHOLERA

Cholera is a severe acute gastrointestinal infection, caused by *Vibrio cholerae* serotype 01. Its home is in the valleys of the Ganges and other great rivers of the Far East where high humidity and population density have maintained the disease. In these valleys devastating epidemics have occurred, often following large religious festivals, and pandemics have spread throughout Asia and Europe and even to North America. The seventh pandemic began in 1961. Good hygiene has prevented its spread to Europe, but cholera is present in the Near East and Africa, where it has for the first time become endemic. In 1990 it reached Peru and has spread throughout South and Central America. The biotype of *V. cholerae*, El Tor, that is responsible for the pandemic, is more resistant than the classical vibrio, and amenable to more prolonged carriage following infection. In 1982 the classical vibrio began to re-establish itself in Bangladesh where, in 1992, a new pandemic began, with a new serotype 0139.

The organism is passed in stools, or vomit, of patients with cholera and the very much larger number of subclinical cases, who excrete it for a few days. Chronic carriage is rare. The organism survives up to 2 weeks in fresh water and 8 weeks in salt water. Transmission is normally through infected drinking water. Shellfish, and food contaminated by flies or hands, also transmit the infection.

Pathology

Cholera vibrios multiply in the lumen of the small bowel and are noninvasive. They adhere to the mucosal surface and secrete a powerful exotoxin (enterotoxin) which stimulates the adenyl cyclase-adenosine monophosphate pathway of the mucosa, resulting in an outpouring of normal alkaline, small bowel fluid. Severe dehydration follows rapidly even though absorption of fluid by the bowel is hardly impaired.

There may be acidosis and depletion of sodium and potassium with attendant complications, of which renal failure is the most important. The incubation period is a few hours to 5 days.

Clinical features

Severe diarrhoea without pain or colic, followed by vomiting, begins suddenly. After the faecal contents of the gut have been evacuated the typical 'rice-water' material is passed which consists of clear fluid with flecks of mucus. The enormous loss of fluid and electrolytes leads to intense dehydration with muscular cramps. The skin becomes cold, clammy and wrinkled and the eyes sunken. The blood pressure falls, the pulse becomes imperceptible, and the urine output diminishes. The patient usually remains mentally clear. Death from acute circulatory failure may occur within a few hours unless fluid and electrolytes are replaced. Improvement is rapid, however, with proper treatment.

Although this is the classical picture of cholera the majority of infections cause only mild illness with slight diarrhoea. Occasionally, a very intense illness, 'cholera sicca', occurs in which the loss of fluid into the dilated bowel kills the patient before typical gastrointestinal symptoms appear. The disease is more dangerous in children. The complications are listed in the information box above.

Investigations

Clinical diagnosis is usually easy during an epidemic but in other situations it is important to confirm the diagnosis bacteriologically so that an outbreak may be brought rapidly under control. *V. cholerae* has a characteristic movement that can be seen under the microscope. Culture of the stool or a rectal swab is used to isolate the organism. Other diseases such as acute bacillary dysentery, viral enteritis, *P. falciparum* malaria, food poisoning, including *Vibrio parahaemolyticus* infections from eating infected shellfish, and certain chemical poisons may produce symptoms like those of cholera. Cholera is notifiable under the International Health Regulations.

Management

The chief aim is to maintain the circulation by replacement of water and electrolytes; the earlier this is started, the better the prognosis. A quick clinical assessment of the state of dehydration is made from the appearance of the patient, the pulse, blood pressure and skin turgor. Fluids are given intravenously in severe cases or when there is vomiting. A large needle is inserted into a large vein (the femoral for example) and fluid is run in as fast as possible until pulse and blood pressure return. The rest of the estimated deficit is replaced more slowly. If intravenous fluids or drip apparatus are unavailable, fluid is administered via a nasogastric tube.

Vomiting usually stops once the patient is rehydrated and fluid should then be given orally every hour. Patients are made to drink up to 500 ml hourly. The quantity of

Table 4.28 Recommended fluid replacement for treatment of cholera

Intravenous	g/l	mmol/l		Oral	g/l
Sodium chloride	5	Na	133	Commercial salt (NaCl)	3.5
		Cl	98		
Potassium chloride	1	K	13	Potassium chloride	1.5
				or citrate	2.7
Sodium bicarbonate	4	HCO$_3$	48	Sodium bicarbonate	2.5
or acetate	6.5			Glucose*	20

* Rice flour (50 g) is more effective and cheaper than glucose.

fluid required is calculated every 8 hours from the output of urine, stool, vomit, and estimated insensible loss, which may be as much as 5 litres in 24 hours in a hot humid climate.

Total fluid requirements can be in excess of 50 litres over a period of 2–5 days. Accurate records are essential and are greatly facilitated by the use of a 'cholera cot' which has a reinforced hole under the patient's buttocks beneath which a graded bucket is placed.

The ideal fluid replacements are shown in Table 4.28. Other satisfactory fluids include Ringer lactate (BP) or Hartman's solution or Darrow's solution, in which event supplements of potassium are given as 10 mmol/l of intravenous fluid or 2–4 g potassium chloride or citrate 3 times daily by mouth. Isotonic saline is better than nothing but every 2 litres should be alternated with 1 litre of isotonic sodium lactate (18.7 g/l) or bicarbonate (14 g/l) and added potassium. Acetate is a satisfactory substitute for bicarbonate, and more stable. The presence of glucose or rice flour in the oral fluid has been shown to promote electrolyte absorption. Chlorpromazine, 50 mg 6-hourly, reduces intestinal secretion and fluid loss.

The use of correct fluids for replacement has eliminated the need for the estimation of plasma electrolytes. In children, the elderly, the anaemic and those with underlying heart disease, overvigorous intravenous rehydration may cause pulmonary oedema. Children require most careful attention to fluid balance. Ringer lactate is the fluid of choice. They are prone to hypoglycaemia. Any deterioration despite adequate rehydration is an indication for a bolus infusion of 25% glucose, 4 ml/kg and maintenance with 10 mg/kg per hour. The management of renal failure is given on page 626.

Three days' treatment with tetracycline 250 mg 6-hourly or co-trimoxazole one tablet daily reduces the duration of excretion of vibrios and the total volume of fluid needed for replacement.

Prevention

Personal prophylaxis means strict personal hygiene. Water for drinking should come from a clean piped supply or be boiled. Flies must not be allowed access to food. Vaccination with a killed suspension of *V. cholerae* may provide limited protection.

Control of water sources and of population movement and public education are most important in an epidemic. Mass vaccination with a single dose of vaccine and mass treatment with tetracycline are valuable. Disinfection of infective discharges and soiled clothing, and scrupulous hand washing by medical attendants reduces the danger of spread from treatment centres.

MYCOBACTERIAL INFECTIONS

TUBERCULOSIS (see p. 358)

LEPROSY

Leprosy is the commonest cause of peripheral neuritis in the world. It is a chronic granulomatous disease caused by *Mycobacterium leprae,* an acid and alcohol fast bacillus that has a very slow multiplication time of 12–14 days. Leprosy is one of the most seriously disabling and economically important diseases of the world and it is estimated that 20 million people are affected. *M. leprae* will grow in mice and the armadillo, but not in artificial media. Local multiplication of the organism in the foot-pads of mice is a useful technique for demonstrating the identity and viability of *M. leprae,* and the existence of drug-resistant strains for the screening of drugs, and for studying vaccines. The most important mode of spread of *M. leprae* is by droplets from the sneezes of lepromatous patients whose nasal mucosa is heavily infected. The organism may enter the body through the nasal mucosa or by inoculation through the skin.

The disease is common in tropical Asia, the Far East, tropical Africa, Central and South America, and in some Pacific islands. It is still endemic in Southern Europe, North Africa and the Middle East.

Pathology

The organisms show a predilection for peripheral nerves, skin and mucosa of the upper respiratory tract. The pathology is determined by, and reflects, the balance between the patient's cell-mediated immune response and bacillary multiplication, thus creating a spectrum of disease (Fig. 4.25).

Tuberculoid leprosy

In tuberculoid leprosy disease is confined to a few sites in skin or peripheral nerves. In skin lesions a vigorous cell-mediated immune response surrounds nerves, sweat glands and hair follicles, which are quickly destroyed. In

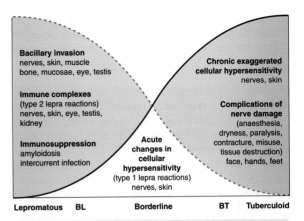

Fig. 4.25 Leprosy: mechanisms of damage and tissue affected. Mechanisms under the broken line are characteristic of disease near the lepromatous end of the spectrum and those under the solid line of the tuberculoid end. They overlap in the centre where, in addition, instability predisposes to type 1 lepra reactions. At the peak in the centre neither bacillary growth nor cell-mediated immunity has the upper hand. BL = borderline lepromatous; BT = borderline tuberculoid.

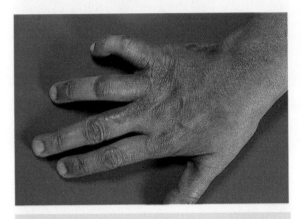

Fig. 4.26 Tuberculoid leprosy: skin lesions.

peripheral nerves, lesions are restricted to one or more of the 'sites of predilection' (Fig. 4.26) but the presence of the sheath permits the inflammation to create lethal pressure on the axons. Caseation is rare. Organisms are scanty and difficult to demonstrate.

Lepromatous leprosy

In the infective form of this disease, there is no cell-mediated immune response to *M. leprae*. Organisms are present in great abundance in the dermis, in histocytes, Schwann cells, erectores pilorum muscles and endo-thelial cells of blood vessels. Organisms are carried in the bloodstream to the peripheral nerves, eye and mucosa of the nose and upper respiratory tract, the testes and small

131

muscles and bones of the hands, feet and face, in which they multiply. Tissue damage is slow but widespread. Nephritis and amyloidosis are common late complications.

Borderline or dimorphous leprosy

Between these two 'polar' types of leprosy, there is a spectrum of manifestations grouped under the terms 'borderline' or 'dimorphous'. The host reaction varies from the near-lepromatous (Fig. 4.27) to the near-tuberculoid. *M. leprae* are demonstrable in varying numbers. In the centre of the spectrum the disease is unstable. Immunity may diminish (downgrading) in untreated patients, especially in pregnancy or other times of stress, and the disease becomes more lepromatous. Alternatively immunity may increase (upgrading or reversal), especially in response to successful chemotherapy, and the disease becomes more tuberculoid.

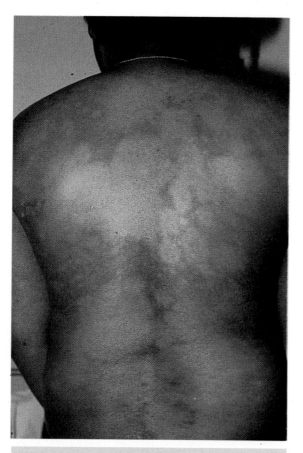

Fig. 4.27 'Borderline' or 'dimorphous' leprosy. Host reaction in this case is near-lepromatous.

Lepra reactions

Any form of leprosy may undergo an acute exacerbation or reaction which is caused by an episode of acute allergic inflammation. In lepromatous disease the reaction, lepra reaction type 2, is due to immune complex-mediated vasculitis. In borderline and tuberculoid disease the reaction, lepra reaction type 1, is due to sudden increase in cellular hypersensitivity. Borderline reactions are often associated with upgrading or downgrading. Lepra reactions may be insidious or rapid, sometimes destroying affected tissues overnight (Table 4.30).

Leprosy damages the body in three main ways:

- **Peripheral neuritis.** This leads to loss of sensory, motor and autonomic functions. Sensory loss permits trauma from pressure, friction, burns and cuts, the effects of which are intensified if there are abnormal pressures from the contractures following muscular paralysis. Autonomic nerve damage causes dry skin which cracks easily and heals slowly. Secondary bacterial infection in an anaesthetic, unprotected limb leads to cellulitis, osteomyelitis and gross tissue destruction which produces the deformities with which the disease is still, so unnecessarily, associated. Paralyses result in claw hand and dropped foot from damage respectively to the ulnar and peroneal nerves. A combination of fifth and seventh cranial nerve damage exposes an anaesthetic cornea to trauma and sepsis, so the eye is easily blinded.
- **Bacillary infiltration.** In lepromatous leprosy bacillary growth insidiously damages the infiltrated organs and renders them liable to type 2 lepra reactions.
- **Acute lepra reactions.** In children, the incubation period is 2–5 years, but post primary disease is common in young adults, as in tuberculosis (p. 358). The disease may also appear in old people, as immunity declines.

Clinical features

The onset is usually gradual. The most common first symptom is a small but persistent area of impaired sensation or numbness. In other patients the first noticeable feature may be macules, which are usually hypopigmented and erythematous. The disease may also present acutely, in a lepra reaction, with neuritis, iritis or erythema nodosum leprosum (Table 4.29).

Often the first and only lesion is the inconspicuous macule of *indeterminate leprosy*. It is situated anywhere on the body, exhibiting slight pigmentary and sensory changes. It usually heals spontaneously.

Tuberculoid leprosy

This is characterised by one or a few solitary lesions in skin and peripheral nerves. Skin lesions are macular or raised as plaques or as rings whose flat centres indicate central healing. The lesion is hypopigmented in dark skins, coppery in pale skins, with a well-defined margin. Its surface is dry, often scaly, and usually anaesthetic unless the lesion is on the face. Lesions are of almost any size and occur anywhere on the body (Fig. 4.26). The nerve twig supplying the skin lesion or a large peripheral nerve at one of the sites of predilection may be enlarged—for example, the ulnar nerve above the elbow, the median above the elbow or at the wrist, radical at the wrist, common peroneal in the popliteal fossa, posterior tibial around the medial malleolus, and great auricular across the sternomastoid muscle.

Tuberculoid leprosy tends spontaneously to heal slowly, often without residual disability. Sometimes its course is punctuated by a reaction and occasionally it downgrades into the borderline part of the spectrum.

Lepromatous leprosy

Early skin lesions are macular (Table 4.29). They are numerous, hypopigmented and erythematous. They differ from tuberculoid macules in that they are small, inconspicuous, widely scattered on the body, usually symmetrically, and with margins that merge imperceptibly with normal skin. Overlying sensation is not impaired. As the disease advances, the macular lesions become infiltrated and succulent; in advanced lepromatous leprosy nodular lesions appear, especially on the ears and face, and eyebrows are lost. Diffuse sym-

metrical thickening of the skin causes thickened brow and lobes of the ear, producing the 'leonine facies'.

Clinical evidence of nerve damage appears relatively late in lepromatous leprosy. Anaesthesia and anhidrosis are first detected in the distal aspects of the forearms and lower legs, later in a 'glove and stocking' distribution and eventually over the trunk and face, although the palms, soles, axillae and groins may be spared. The effects on other organs are summarised in the information box (above). Untreated lepromatous leprosy gradually gets worse.

THE EFFECTS OF BACILLARY INFILTRATION IN LEPROMATOUS LEPROSY

- **Skin and nerves:** see text
- **Muscles of hands, feet and face:** weakness and wasting
- **Testes:** atrophy, impotence, gynaecomastia
- **Mucosa of nose, mouth, pharynx and larynx:** rhinitis, hoarseness, perforation of nasal septum and palate, laryngeal obstruction
- **Bones of hands, feet and face:** cystic lesions of phalanges permitting fractures, loss of upper incisor teeth and nasal spine leading to nasal collapse
- **Eye:** keratitis iridocyclitis, corneal anaesthesia leading to blindness

---

Table 4.29 Clinical characteristics of the polar forms of leprosy

	Lepromatous	Tuberculoid
Skin and nerves		
Number and distribution	Widely disseminated	One or a few sites, asymmetrical
Skin lesions		
Definition		
Clarity of margin	Poor	Good
Elevation of margin	Never	Common
Colour		
Dark skin	Slight hypopigmentation	Marked hypopigmentation
Light skin	Slight erythema	Coppery or red
Surface	Smooth, shiny	Dry, scaly
Central healing	None	Common
Sweat and hair growth	Impaired late	Impaired early
Loss of sensation	Late	Early and marked
Nerve enlargement and damage	Late	Early and marked
Bacilli (Bacterial Index)	Many (5 or 6 +)	Absent (0)
Natural outcome	Progression	Healing
Other tissues	Upper respiratory mucosa, eye, testes, bones, muscle	None
Reactions	Immune complexes	Cell-mediated

Borderline or dimorphous leprosy

This may present with lesions intermediate in character between lepromatous and tuberculoid or as a mixture of them. Skin lesions are often bizarre. The eyes and nose are spared. Nerve lesions are more numerous than in tuberculoid disease. In Asia, the majority of patients have borderline lepromatous leprosy. In Africa the majority have borderline tuberculoid leprosy. If the disease upgrades, nerve damage may increase with severe residual disability. If it downgrades the complications of extensive bacillary multiplication are added to those of widespread nerve damage. In either event the patient is liable to undergo reactions.

Lepra reactions

These may be defined as episodes of inflammation in pre-existing lesions of leprosy (Table 4.30). Sometimes a reaction is the first clinical manifestation of the disease. One half of patients with lepromatous leprosy and one quarter with borderline lepromatous disease will suffer *type 2 lepra reactions* at some time during the course of their disease, most commonly in their second year of treatment. These reactions are characterised by fever and the appearance of crops of painful red papules or nodules, called *erythema nodosum leprosum*, which may necrose and discharge sterile pus, before subsiding.

Type 1 lepra reactions are especially common in borderline tuberculoid patients. They occur spontaneously or may be precipitated by treatment. Nerve function is rapidly lost, irretrievably so unless the reaction is promptly treated.

Investigations

Lepromatous and borderline lepromatous disease ('multibacillary leprosy') is diagnosed by demonstration of *M. leprae* in material obtained by a slit skin smear.

The skin is pinched between finger and thumb to expel blood, incised with the point of a scalpel and the exposed dermis scraped with the flat of the blade. The tissue juice obtained is smeared on a microscope slide and stained by a modified Ziehl–Neelsen method. Smears are made from skin lesions, earlobes and dorsum of the ring or middle finger—sites in which bacilli multiply readily and persist. Nasal mucus may also contain the organisms in lepromatous leprosy and this is a good indication of infectivity. *M. leprae* are less readily demonstrable in skin smears in borderline disease and are undetectable in tuberculoid disease.

In borderline, and especially tuberculoid disease ('paucibacillary leprosy'), the cardinal signs of leprosy are enlarged nerves and anaesthesia. Nerves are usually enlarged at sites of predilection asymmetrically and irregularly; they may be tender.

Loss or diminution of sensation, or misreference (the inability to locate accurately the site stimulated) may be detected in a skin lesion or in the distribution of a large peripheral nerve. Biopsy of skin or nerve is seldom necessary except for accurate classification.

The lepromin test

Lepromin is a suspension of dead *M. leprae*. The test is performed like the tuberculin test, but is read after 4 weeks. The result indicates the degree of cellular immunity that an individual can mount against the organism. This test is of no value in establishing the diagnosis of leprosy, but it is useful in helping to classify the disease, and so determine treatment and prognosis.

Management

Treatment of leprosy is long and often complicated. The patient must understand the disease and its complications, comply and persevere in the treatment and learn

Table 4.30 Reactions in leprosy

Lepra reaction	Type 1	Type 2
Mechanism	Cell mediated hypersensitivity	Immune complexes Arthus phenomenon
Clinical features	Painful tender nerves, loss of function Swollen skin lesions New skin lesions Rarely fever	Tender roseolar papules, may ulcerate Painful tender nerves, loss of function Iritis, orchitis, myositis, lymphadenitis Fever, oedema
Management	Mild: aspirin 600 mg 6-hourly Severe[1]: prednisolone 40–80 mg, reducing over 3–9 months	Mild: aspirin 600 mg 6-hourly Severe[1]: Thalidomide[2] or prednisolone 20–40 mg reducing over 1–6 months Local if eye involved[3]

[1] Includes any threat to nerve or eye function.
[2] See text for details.
[3] 1% hydrocortisone drops or ointment and 1% atropine drops.

Table 4.31 Main features of drugs available to treat leprosy

Drugs	Dose (mg)	Peak serum level/MIC*	Duration of MIC: days	Bactericidal activity
Dapsone	100	100–500	4–12	+
Rifampicin	600	30	1	+++
Clofazimine	100	(Stored in M.P. cells, possible depot)		?
Minocycline	100	10–20	1	++
Ofloxacin	400	—	1	++

* MIC minimum inhibitory concentration.

to look after anaesthetic limbs, control fear and cope with any stigma that exists in the community. Admission to hospital for a few days is useful to establish rapport and start education.

Specific chemotherapy

The essential features of the available drugs are given in Table 4.31.

- **Patients with multi-bacillary disease** (lepromatous and borderline lepromatous). These are preferably isolated until they are rendered non-infectious, which takes only a few days with rifampicin. Ideally treatment should be with three drugs, rifampicin, clofazimine and dapsone, to prevent the emergence of drug resistance. Rifampicin, the most expensive but most efficient bactericidal drug, need only be given monthly, because of the long generation time of *M. leprae*. It is most effective if given for two consecutive days in a daily dose of 600 mg, or 450 mg for patients under 35 kg in weight. Clofazimine is given in a dose of 50 mg daily, or 100 mg 3 times in the week (totalling 6 mg/kg per week for children). Dapsone is given in a dose of 2 mg/kg daily, not exceeding 100 mg. For mass treatment campaigns when compliance is often poor, WHO recommends that rifampicin be given in a single supervised monthly dose of 600 mg, and that a supervised monthly dose of clofazimine 300 mg be given in addition to the self-administered daily dose of clofazimine and dapsone. Patients are treated for 2 years and followed for a further 5 years.
- **Patients with paucibacillary disease** (intermediate, tuberculoid and borderline tuberculoid). These are treated with rifampicin once monthly and dapsone daily for 1 year, and are followed for a further 2 years.

  Side-effects of dapsone are rare. They include psychosis, dermatitis and haemolytic anaemia. Minocycline and ofloxacin are the most useful second-line

PROBLEMS WITH THE CHEMOTHERAPY OF LEPROSY

Compliance

Side effects of drugs
- Dapsone: dermatitis, psychosis, haemolytic anaemia
- Clofazimine: red, brown or blue-black discoloration, abdominal pain
- Ethionamide: hepatitis, especially in Asians, notably Chinese
- Rifampicin: 'flu-like syndrome after each dose

Drug resistance
- Dapsone: secondary resistance common, when given alone for lepromatous leprosy
- Rifampicin: rapid onset if given alone
- Thiacetazone: rapid onset if given alone, cross-resistance with ethionamide

drugs, less toxic but more expensive than ethionamide and thiacetazone (Table 4.31).

Treatment of lepra reactions

Chemotherapy for leprosy is maintained and appropriate anti-inflammatory drugs used. Reactional neuritis is a medical emergency as irreversible paralysis may occur overnight.

Type 2 reactions in lepromatous patients respond rapidly to thalidomide in a dose of 100 mg 6-hourly. The dose is reduced slowly over weeks or months. This drug must never be given to premenopausal women because of its disastrous teratogenic effects. If thalidomide is contraindicated or unavailable prednisolone is used. Increasing the dose of clofazimine to 200 mg or 300 mg daily for a few weeks will help control the reaction and permit prednisolone to be reduced or withdrawn. Iritis is a dangerous complication but can usually be managed by local measures.

Type 1 reactions in borderline patients are controlled with corticosteroids. Prednisolone is given in a dose of 40–60 mg daily and reduced gradually over 2–6 months for patients with borderline-tuberculoid disease, and 6–9 months for patients with borderline lepromatous disease.

Management of nerve damage

In the event of acute paralysis complicating reactional neuritis, the affected limb is splinted and exercised passively each day until function begins to return, when active exercises can be added. A patient with an anaesthetic limb must be taught to accept the limitations it imposes, to adjust life accordingly, to inspect the limb daily for trauma or infection and to learn how not to damage it.

Tarsorrhaphy helps protect an exposed anaesthetic

cornea. Secondary sepsis is treated with appropriate antibiotics, and osteomyelitis and its sequelae are managed in the most conservative manner possible. Patients with plantar ulcers are confined to bed, or given crutches or a walking plaster until healing is complete. Shoes must fit and protect anaesthetic feet against trauma and must be made specially if there is added deformity.

Prevention

In endemic areas the disease is commonest among intimate contacts of patients, and children and young adults are especially susceptible. *M. leprae* is easily spread and two-thirds of contacts undergo sub-clinical immunising infections within 2 years of regular exposure. Of the small proportion of contacts (about 1%) that develop clinical disease only about 2% will be lepromatous. Identification of this small group at risk, and logical prophylaxis, are at present impossible. No specific vaccine is available. Bacille Calmette-Guérin (BCG) is of some value, especially in Africa, and should be given to all child contacts of lepromatous patients. Dapsone and rifampicin may be given as for paucibacillary disease (above) for 6 months to child contacts of lepromatous patients. Neither measure is a substitute for 6-monthly examination of contacts.

Mass prophylaxis is impossible, but treatment and follow-up of all cases identified during a population survey reduces deformity and lowers the incidence of leprosy. With improvement of socio-economic conditions the disease tends to disappear. The rapid spread of dapsone resistance poses a great problem to existing control schemes.

FURTHER READING

Bryceson A D M, Pfaltzgraff R E 1990 Leprosy, 3rd edn. Churchill Livingstone, Edinburgh
Butler T 1994 Yersinia infections: centennial of the discovery of the plague bacillus. Clinical Infectious Diseases 19: 655–663
Crook L D, Tempest B 1992 Plague. A Clinical review of 27 cases. Archives of Internal Medicine 152: 1253–1256
Dance D A B 1991 Melioidosis: the tip of the iceberg. Clinical Microbiology Reviews 4: 52–60
Drason B S 1992 Pathogenesis and ecology: the case of cholera. Journal of Tropical Medicine and Hygiene 95: 365–372
Lienhardt C, Fine P E M 1992 Controlling leprosy: multidrug treatment is not enough alone. Lancet 305: 206–207

DISEASES DUE TO SPIROCHAETES

The classification of spirochaetal infections is outlined in the information box.

SPIROCHAETAL INFECTIONS: CLASSIFICATION

Leptospira infections
- Leptospirosis (*L. icterohaemorrhagiae*, *L. hardjo*, *L. canicola*)

Borrelia infections
- Lyme disease (*B. burgdorferi*)
- Louse-borne relapsing fever (*B. recurrentis*)
- Tick-borne relapsing fever (*B. duttoni*)
- Tropical ulcer (*B. vincenti*)
- Cancrum oris (*B. vincenti*)

Treponema infections
- Syphilis (*T. pallidum*)
- Yaws (*T. pertenue*)
- Pinta (*T. carateum*)
- Bejel (*T. pallidum*)

LEPTOSPIRA INFECTIONS

LEPTOSPIROSIS

Although over 100 serotypes of leptospiras have been identified only *L. icterohaemorrhagiae*, *L. hardjo* and *L. canicola* have been shown to cause human disease in Britain (Table 4.32).

The natural host of **Weil's disease**, caused by *L. icterohaemorrhagiae*, is the rat and other rodents. Infected urine contains spirochaetes which can penetrate the skin or mucosa of man. Abattoir and farm workers and water sports enthusiasts are most at risk.

L. canicola infection, which is contracted from dogs and pigs, usually presents as aseptic meningitis. It is not often associated with jaundice and is less severe than Weil's disease.

Table 4.32 Leptospiral infections in the UK

Organism	Source
Leptospira icterohaemorrhagiae (Weil's disease) Hepatitis Renal tubular necrosis Myocarditis Purpura Haemorrhagic conjunctivitis	Water contaminated by rats' urine
Leptospira canicola Non-specific febrile illness Aseptic meningitis	Dogs
Leptospira hardjo Non-specific febrile illness Chronic ill health Aseptic meningitis	Cattle

L. hardjo infection occurs in farm workers in contact with cattle, in whom it can cause ill-health resembling chronic brucellosis. It can also cause aseptic meningitis.

The average incubation period of leptospirosis is 10 days, the range being 4 to 21 days.

Clinical features of Weil's disease

Weil's disease usually begins abruptly with headache, severe myalgia, pyrexia, conjunctival suffusion, anorexia and vomiting. A rash may develop with petechiae, and enlargement of the liver and spleen occurs.

The temperature falls by lysis and is usually normal for 2 or 3 days. In the majority of patients, there is further pyrexia for a few days and transient meningism followed by recovery. In severe infections hepatitis, renal tubular necrosis, myocarditis and meningitis may occur during this phase. The condition may progress to acute liver necrosis. Renal tubular necrosis may lead to acute renal failure. Myocarditis is suggested by tachycardia, fall in blood pressure, arrhythmias and cardiac failure.

The majority of patients enter the convalescent phase by the third and fourth week of the illness. When there has been serious involvement of the liver, kidneys and heart, mortality in Weil's disease is in the region of 15 to 20%. Those who recover do so completely.

Investigations

A rising titre of specific leptospiral antibodies is found from the second week onwards. When there is liver involvement, liver function tests indicate hepatocellular damage with an intrahepatic obstructive element. The urine contains protein, red blood cells and cellular and granular casts in patients with renal failure; in severe cases the rise in blood urea is progressive.

BORRELIA INFECTIONS

The worldwide distribution of the major diseases caused by borrelia infection is shown in Figure 4.28.

LYME DISEASE

Lyme disease is caused by *Borrelia burgdorferi*, a spirochaetal organism transmitted by the Ixodes tick. The disease was first identified in the New England county of Lyme where a cluster of cases of arthritis of unknown aetiology occurred in the early 1980s.

Epidemiology

In the United Kingdom the vector for *B. burgdorferi* is *Ixodes ricinus*, a tick which infests dogs, sheep and deer. It is probable that deer are the principal source of infec-

tion for man and in the New Forest area of southern England approximately one-quarter of forestry workers are sero-positive for the organism.

The infection is particularly common in the eastern states of North America, especially in New England, but also occurs in Europe, particularly Sweden, and countries of Eastern Europe.

Clinical features

The information box below lists the clinical features of Lyme disease. The primary infection, which occurs two to three weeks after the initial tick bite, is often asymptomatic although it may present with influenza-like symptoms and a characteristic rash known as erythema chronicum migrans, an annular red lesion surrounding a paler area of skin. Neurological and cardiac manifestations usually occur within three to six weeks of the primary infection. Large joint arthritis is a later manifestation, while the chronic skin lesion, acrodermatitis chronica atrophica, can occur several years after the primary infection. Arthritis and cardiac involvement are seen more often in the United States whereas neurological illness and acrodermatitis are commoner in Europe.

CLINICAL FEATURES OF LYME DISEASE

Early clinical manifestations
- Rash (Erythema chronicum migrans) with or without febrile illness

Early complications
- Neurological—cranial nerve palsies, meningitis or radiculopathy
- Cardiac—conduction disorders (commonest), myocarditis, pericarditis or cardiomyopathy

Late complications
- Large joint arthritis
- Acrodermatitis chronica atrophica
- Chronic neurological—polyneuropathy, encephalopathy

Investigations

The diagnosis of Lyme disease is made on the clinical history together with a positive serum antibody test. This is usually an ELISA test confirmed by immunoblot. However, serological tests are unreliable. 30% of acute cases are seronegative; positive tests may reflect past rather than current infection. More sophisticated immunological tests are being developed.

Management

B. burgdorferi is sensitive to the β-lactam antibiotics (penicillins and cephalosporins) and to the tetracyclines.

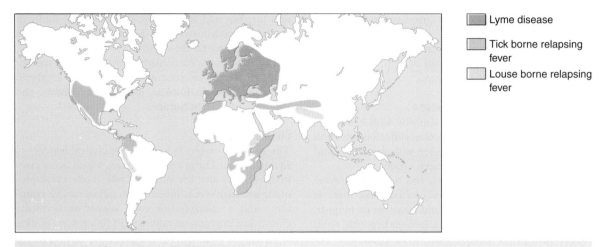

Fig. 4.28 Distribution of diseases due to Borrelia: tick-borne relapsing fever (shaded green), louse-borne relapsing fever (orange) and Lyme disease (purple).

Therapeutic options include oral doxycycline or amoxycillin given for 3 weeks. For more severe cases, intravenous benzylpenicillin or ceftriaxone is indicated. Relapses may occur, especially if treatment is delayed.

TROPICAL ULCER

Tropical ulcer is a specific infection with *Borrelia vincenti* and anaerobic bacteria. Minor injury in the presence of undernourishment, poor hygiene and debilitating disease are predisposing factors. It is most common in adolescent males, on the lower third of the leg.

Clinical features

The initial lesion is a bleb filled with sanguineous fluid. The bleb ruptures and a green-grey slough is exposed which spreads, rapidly and painfully, in the skin and subcutaneous tissue up to a diameter of 5 cm or more. In a few days these tissues slough and liquefy releasing an offensive discharge. After about a week there is usually no further spread and the necrotic tissue separates, exposing an ulcer.

In a chronic ulcer the edges are raised and slope sharply. The damage may be limited to the skin and superficial fascia, but in severe cases deep structures, including tendons and periosteum, may be invaded. The ulcer is usually solitary and heals slowly with a tissue-paper-like scar which breaks down easily. Big ulcers fail to heal and may develop malignant changes after many years.

Management

Local treatment consists in thorough cleaning of the ulcer with hypertonic saline or magnesium sulphate. Acute ulcers heal in response to procaine penicillin 300 mg intramuscularly, metronidazole 400 mg 8-hourly, or tetracycline 2 g daily for 7 days. Ulcers over 5 cm diameter need grafting. Chronic ulcers are excised and grafted.

Prevention

Where tropical ulcers are a risk, abrasions should be cleaned and covered. The provision of a good diet, washing facilities and a first-aid service have abolished tropical ulcers from labour forces on well-run estates.

CANCRUM ORIS

Cancrum oris is rare except in poorly nourished children in the tropics. It is characteristically preceded by an infective illness, especially measles. The manifestation is that of a rapidly developing gangrene, beginning inside of the mouth and penetrating through the lips and cheek. Gangrene becomes demarcated and ulceration follows resulting in severe disfigurement. Untreated it frequently causes death. *B. vincenti* and an anaerobic bacterium are frequently found in the ulcer. Penicillin (Table 4.11) arrests the infection but does not prevent gangrene of already diseased tissue. Coexistent malnutrition, anaemia or dehydration should be corrected. Subsequently skilled plastic surgery may do much to overcome the hideous defects.

Prevention depends on improved nutrition and

Table 4.33 Comparative features of the 'relapsing fevers' due to Borrelia and Spirillum

	LBRF[1]	TBRF[2]	Sodoku	Haverhill	Lyme disease
Incubation	2–12 days	2–12 days	5–21 days	1–5 days	4 days–months
Fever	4–10 days	3–5 days	7 days	3 days	Weeks
Remission	7 days	3–5 days	3–5 days	—	No consistent pattern
Relapses	0–3 days	Up to 10	Numerous	None	
JHR[3]	Severe	Mild	Mild/none	None	None
Mortality	Up to 40%	Under 10%	None	None	Rare
Major complications	Hepatitis Carditis Meningitis Shock Bleeding	Similar to LBRF but less severe Neurological in relapses	Chancre Adenitis Rash	Arthritis	Rash Arthritis Carditis Meningitis

[1] Louse-borne relapsing fever.
[2] Tick-borne relapsing fever.
[3] Jarisch-Herxheimer reaction.

hygiene in the community and on control of acute infectious diseases.

THE RELAPSING FEVERS

The relapsing fevers are a group of diseases due to infections by spirochaetes of the genus *Borrelia* transmitted by body lice or soft (Argasid) ticks. Sodoku, due to *Spirillum minus*, also relapses (Table 4.33). The louse-borne *Borrelia recurrentis* infects only man and is not transmitted from a louse to its progeny. This disease appears in epidemics particularly during wars or famine when refugees are crowded together in conditions under which infestation with the human body louse *Pediculus humanus* is frequent. It may accompany louse-borne typhus. The disease is endemic in Ethiopia from where recently recorded epidemics have probably arisen.

Species of Borrelia that cause tick-borne relapsing fever, are transmitted by various species of the genus *Ornithodoros*. Ticks live for years and once infected remain so for life and may convey the infection to the offspring. Tick-borne relapsing fever is thus an endemic disease.

LOUSE-BORNE RELAPSING FEVER

Lice cause itching. Borreliae are liberated from the infected louse when it is crushed during scratching, which also inoculates the borreliae into the skin.

Pathology

The borreliae multiply in the blood, where they are abundant in the febrile phases, and invade most tissues, especially the liver, spleen and meninges. Hepatitis causing jaundice is frequent in severe infections and there may be petechial haemorrhages in the skin, mucous membranes and serous surfaces of internal organs. Thrombocytopenia is marked.

Clinical features

Onset is sudden with fever. The temperature rises to 39.5–40.5°C and is accompanied by a rapid pulse, headache, generalised aching, injected conjunctivae and frequently a petechial rash (Fig. 4.29), epistaxis and herpes labialis. As the disease progresses, the liver and spleen frequently become tender and palpable and jaundice is common. There may be severe serosal and intestinal haemorrhage. Mental confusion and meningism may occur. The fever ends by crisis between the fourth and tenth day, often associated with profuse sweating, hypotension, circulatory and cardiac failure (see Table 4.33). There may be no further fever but, in a proportion of patients, after an afebrile period of about 7 days there may be one or more relapses which are usually milder and less prolonged. In the absence of specific treatment the mortality rate may be as high as 40%, especially among the elderly and malnourished.

Investigations

The organisms are demonstrated in the blood during fever either by dark ground illumination of a wet film or by staining thick and thin films.

Management

The problems of treatment are to eradicate the infection and to minimise the severe Jarisch–Herxheimer reaction (p. 140) which inevitably follows successful chemotherapy and to prevent relapses. The safest treatment is procaine penicillin 300 mg intramuscularly followed the next day by 0.5 g tetracycline. Tetracycline alone is

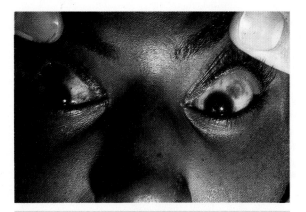

Fig. 4.29 Louse-borne relapsing fever: injected conjunctivae.

effective and prevents relapse, but gives rise to a worse reaction. Doxycycline, 200 mg once by mouth, as an alternative to tetracycline, has the advantage of being curative also for typhus, which often accompanies epidemics of relapsing fever.

Treatment is followed within a half to 3 hours by a chill or rigor, a brisk rise of temperature to 40–42°C, tachypnoea, tachycardia and often cough, confusion, distress, delirium and, occasionally, convulsions and coma. This phase is rapidly followed by profound hypotension and vasodilatation which may last from 8–12 hours and may be complicated by cardiac failure. The patient must be confined strictly to bed for 48 hours after treatment, carefully observed and managed as complications demand. Tepid sponging for fever over 41°C, careful attention to hydration, preferably by oral fluids, and prompt treatment of cardiac failure are required.

Prevention
The patient, clothing and all contacts must be freed from lice as in epidemic typhus (p. 116).

TICK-BORNE RELAPSING FEVER

This disease is conveyed by a variety of soft ticks and its endemicity is governed by the presence of the vector. In the Mediterranean area *Ornithodoros tholozani* is responsible; in the Middle East, Iran, Afghanistan and India and in the New World there are other vectors. These ticks can become infected from rodents or bats as well as by congenital transmission, and man is only an incidental host. In Central and East Africa, however, where *O. moubata* is the vector of *Borrelia duttoni*, man is probably the only important mammalian host. The disease in these areas is thus confined to old campsites, old houses and their surroundings, where *O. moubata* lives in dried mud floors and walls.

The pathological changes resemble those of louse-borne relapsing fever but with late neurological lesions.

Clinical features
These are similar to those of louse-borne relapsing fever (Table 4.33). The febrile bouts, although severe, last usually only for 3–5 days, and the apyrexial periods may also be shorter. Relapses are, however, more frequent. Iritis and neurological complications, including cranial nerve palsies, optic atrophy, localised palsies and spastic paraplegia, may develop during these later relapses.

Investigations
The methods used in diagnosis are similar to those for louse-borne relapsing fever. *B. duttoni* are, however, scantier in the peripheral blood but young mice are readily infected.

Management
Because many strains are resistant to penicillin, tetracycline 1 g daily for 7 days is given and the course repeated after an interval of a week. Good results may follow a single dose of 200 mg doxycycline.

Prevention
Ticks can be killed by lindane applied to the inside of the walls, floors and across the entrance to houses.

RAT-BITE FEVERS

There are two rat-bite fevers, one caused by *Spirillum minus*, the other by *Streptobacillus moniliformis*. The latter, in addition to being transmitted by a rat-bite, has also occurred as an epidemic due to infected milk (Haverhill fever); in other cases there has been no known contact with rats or mice. Both infections are worldwide. The incubation period of Streptobacillus fever is 1–5 days, and if *S. minus* 1–4 weeks.

The main features are summarised in Table 4.36 above. Diagnosis is by demonstration of spirochaete in fluid from chancre, lymphnode, or joint effusion, by dark ground microscopy or mouse inoculation. *S. minus* infections cross-react serologically with syphilis. The infections are cured by penicillin or tetracycline.

TREPONEMA INFECTIONS

SYPHILIS
See page 183.

YAWS

Yaws is a granulomatous disease mainly involving the skin and bones and caused by *Treponema pertenue*, mor-

Table 4.34 Comparison of the major treponemal diseases

| Disease | Organism | Source | Transmission | At risk | Lesions | | |
					Primary	Early*	Late*
Yaws	*T. pertenue*	Skin	Contact	Children	Ulcero nodule	Skin Bones	Skin, bones, palms and soles
Pinta	*T. carateum*	Skin	Contact	Family	Papule	Skin	Skin
Bejel	*T. pallidum*	Mouth utensils	Contact	Family	Rare	Skin, mucosae, bones	Skin, mucosae, bones, palms and soles
Venereal syphilis	*T. pallidum*	Genital sores, mouth	Sexual, placenta	Sexual partners, foetus	Genital ulcer, lymphadenopathy	Skin Mucosae, bones, meninges	Cardiovascular CNS, bones, etc.

* Early and late correspond with secondary and tertiary lesions.

phologically indistinguishable from the causative organisms of syphilis and pinta (Table 4.34). The three infections induce similar serological changes and possibly some degree of cross immunity. Organisms are transmitted by bodily contact from a patient with infectious yaws through minor abrasions of the skin of another patient, usually a child. The mass campaigns by WHO between 1950 and 1960 treated over 60 million people and eradicated yaws from many areas, but the disease has persisted patchily throughout the tropics and there has been a resurgence in the 1980s and 1990s in West and Central Africa and the South Pacific.

Pathology

A proliferative granuloma containing numerous treponemes develops at the site of the inoculation. This primary lesion is followed by secondary eruptions. In addition there may be hypertrophic periosteal lesions of many bones, with underlying cortical rarefaction. Lesions of late yaws are characterised by destructive changes which closely resemble the osteitis and gummas of tertiary syphilis and which heal with much scarring and deformity. The incubation period is 3–4 weeks.

Clinical features

Early yaws

The primary lesion or 'mother yaw' is usually on the leg or buttocks. The secondary eruption usually follows a few weeks or months later, as crops of papillomas covered with a whitish-yellow exudate, especially in the flexures and around the mouth. Sometimes a lesion erupts through the palm or sole, when walking becomes painful ('wet crab yaws'). Phalanges, nasal bones and tibiae swell and become distorted. Most of the lesions of early yaws will eventually subside, even if untreated.

Latent yaws

Following the spontaneous resolution of 'early yaws' serological changes may persist to be followed by further manifestations of 'early yaws', or, after an interval of as much as 5–10 years, by the tertiary lesions or 'late yaws'.

Late yaws

Solitary or multiple lesions appear as nodules or ulcers in the skin, hyperkeratotic lesions of palms or soles ('dry crab yaws') and gummatous lesions of bone. They heal with scarring. Lesions of the facial and palatal bones cause terrible disfigurement (gangosa).

Investigations and management

See the information box.

Prevention

The disease disappears with improved housing and cleanliness. In few fields of medicine have chemotherapy and improved hygiene achieved such dramatic success as in the control of yaws.

PINTA AND BEJEL

These two treponemal infections occur in poor rural populations with low standards of domestic hygiene but in separate parts of the world. They have features in common, notably that they are transmitted by contact, usually within the family and not sexually; and in the case of bejel, through common eating and drinking utensils. (Table 4.34). Their diagnosis and management is as for yaws (see the information box).

Pinta

Pinta is probably the oldest of the treponemal infections of man and *T. carateum* the parent of the organism that came to Europe with the return of Christopher Col-

DIAGNOSIS AND TREATMENT OF YAWS, PINTA & BEJEL

Diagnosis of early stages
- Detection of spirochaetes in exudate of lesions by dark ground microscopy

Diagnosis of latent and early stages
- Positive serological tests, as for syphilis (p. 183)

Treatment of all stages
- Single intramuscular injection of 1.2 g long-acting (e.g. benzathine) penicillin G

umbus' sailors in 1493, starting the epidemic of venereal syphilis known as the Great Pox. It is found only in South and Central America, where its incidence is declining. The early lesions are scaly papules or dyschromic patches on the skin. The late lesions are often depigmented and disfiguring. The infection is confined to the skin.

Bejel

Bejel is the Middle Eastern name for non-venereal syphilis, which has a patchy distribution across sub-Saharan Africa, the Middle East, Central Asia and Australia. It has been eradicated from Eastern Europe. Transmission is most commonly from the mouth of the mother or child and the primary mucosal lesion is seldom seen. The early and late lesions resemble those of secondary and tertiary syphilis (p. 184) but cardiovascular and neurological disease is rare.

FURTHER READING

Barclay A J G, Coulter J B S 1990. Tick borne relapsing fever in Central Tanzania. Transactions of the Royal Society of Tropical Medicine and Hygiene 84: 852–856

Mehens A, Antal G M 1992 The endemic treponematoses not yet eradicated. World Health Statistics Quarterly 45: 228–237

Steere A C 1989 Lyme Disease. New England Journal of Medicine 321: 586–596

DISEASES DUE TO FUNGI (MYCOSES)

There are three groups of fungi which cause human disease—multi-nucleate branched filamentous forms (moulds), round or ovoid single cells known as yeasts, and dimorphic fungi which have certain of the growth characteristics of both. Trichophyton, a fungus which causes foot infections, is an example of a filamentous fungus while *Cryptococcus neoformans*, which causes meningitis, is a yeast. *Candida albicans*, the cause of thrush, is a dimorphic fungus.

Certain fungi cause only superficial infections while others can cause invasive disease. Candida can cause both superficial and deep infections. Fungal infections are often referred to as mycoses. These diseases are listed in the information box. Pathogenic fungi are ubiquitous; their importance varies between different parts of the world. Some fungi are opportunistic and will not normally invade unless the defence mechanisms are impaired, as in the immunocompromised host. Fungal infections are transmitted by spores or hyphae, and normally enter the body through the lungs or skin, where they may cause disease, or from where they may disseminate to other parts of the body. Fungal infections tend to be chronic, and often require prolonged chemotherapy. For some infections there is still no effective treatment. Fungi also cause disease through allergy (Chapter 2) and from toxins such as ergot, muscarine and aflatoxin.

Fungal infections commonly present as skin disease, as subcutaneous swellings or as systemic infections.

FUNGAL DISEASE IN MAN

Cutaneous infections
- Dermatophytes
- Candidosis
- Pityriasis versicolor

Subcutaneous infections
- Mycetoma (Table 4.35)
- Other soft tissue infections (Table 4.36)

Systemic infections
- Histoplasmosis
- Aspergillosis
- Coccidioidomycosis
- Paracoccidioidomycosis
- Blastomycosis
- Cryptococcosis
- Candidosis

CUTANEOUS FUNGAL INFECTIONS

An intact healthy skin is especially important in the tropics, where fungal infections are common. Extensive infections may impair sweating and heat loss, and cause distress through irritation. Scratching leads to secondary pyogenic infection.

RINGWORM (tinea infections)

Ringworm is due to infection by dermatophyte fungi. There are three main genera: *Trichophyton* (skin, hair and nail infections), *Microsporum* (skin and hair), *Epidermophyton* (skin and nails).

Dermatophytes invade keratin only and in general zoophilic fungi (those transmitted to man from animals) cause a more severe but short-lived inflammatory response than anthropophilic ones (spread from person to person).

Clinical features

These depend upon the site and the species of fungus involved.

Tinea pedis ('athlete's foot')

This is the most common type of fungal infection in man. It is encouraged by the sharing of wash places and swimming pools. Infrequent washing of socks and the use of occlusive footwear encourage relapses. It may present in three main ways: soggy interdigital scaling, diffuse powdery scaling of the soles (which is often unilateral and which picks out skin creases), and recurrent bouts of vesiculation of the soles. The organisms involved are usually *T. rubrum*, *T. mentagrophytes var. interdigitale* and *E. floccosum*).

Tinea unguium (tinea of the nails)

Toe nail infection is more common than finger nail infection and is often accompanied by tinea pedis. Usually only a few nails are infected. The first changes occur at the free edge of the nail which becomes yellow and crumbly. Thickening of the nail and separation of the nail from the nail bed may follow. *T. rubrum* is a frequent cause.

Tinea manuum (tinea of the hands)

This is usually asymmetrical and involves the palms (dry powdery scaling picking out the creases) more often than the backs of the hands.

Tinea cruris (tinea of the groin)

This affects men more than women and causes well demarcated redness and peripheral scaling of the groins and upper thighs. A few vesicles or pustules are usually seen within the lesions. The eruption is often unilateral or asymmetrical, and itchy.

Tinea corporis (tinea of the trunk)

This is the archetypal 'ringworm' eruption. Erythematous scaly plaques expand slowly and clear in the centre leaving a ring-like pattern (Fig. 4.30). Peripheral scaling, a few vesicles and pustules are characteristic.

Tinea imbricata (due to *T. concentricum*), common in southern Asia, islands of the South Pacific and in some South American countries, is characterised by multiple concentric scaly rings. If untreated the eruption becomes widespread and is often intensely itchy.

Tinea capitis (tinea of the scalp)

The causative organism varies from country to country. Adults rarely develop scalp infections with anthropophilic fungi.

Anthropophilic species cause bald, slightly scaly patches with the hairs broken off a few millimetres from the

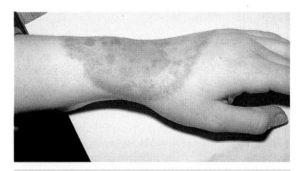

Fig. 4.30 Tinea infection of the arm and wrist.

scalp; inflammation is minimal. Some species, especially microsporum, fluoresce green under Wood's ultraviolet light, so school children may be screened in epidemics. Better hygiene and more effective therapy has made such outbreaks rare in the UK. Favus due to *T. schoenleinii* is characterised by foul-smelling, shield-like crusts and may cause permanent scarring with hair loss.

Zoophilic species (e.g. those causing cattle ringworm) induce considerable inflammation with boggy swelling and pustulation ('kerion' reaction) leading to scarring. Tinea of the beard, usually due to a zoophilic organism, shows the same features.

Complications

These include permanent alopecia due to scarring and an allergic vesicular reaction on the sides of the fingers and palms from which no fungus can be isolated (the 'ide' eruption). Atypical presentations of tinea occur in the immunosuppressed and when the rash is mistreated with topical steroids ('tinea incognito').

Investigations

Microscopic examination of skin scrapings, nail clippings or hair pluckings, cleared in potassium hydroxide, is the easiest way to check for fungi. Cultures may be carried out if facilities are available. Wood's ultraviolet light examination of the scalp is useful for screening those in institutions where outbreaks of tinea capitis occur, but some fungi do not fluoresce.

Management

Mild infections are treated with topical ointments ranging from the time-honoured but cheap Whitfield's ointment to modern preparations containing imidazoles or terbinafine. Stubborn, extensive scalp and nail infections should be treated with systemic drugs such as griseofulvin (fine particle) 500 mg daily or terbinafine 250 mg daily, the duration of treatment depending on the nature of the infection.

CANDIDOSIS (MONILIASIS)

A yeast, *Candida albicans*, is the commonest fungus of medical importance. It is ubiquitous in the environment but it may also be transmitted between people directly.

Pathology

Candidosis is usually a superficial infection of skin, nails or mucous membrane with the yeast form of the fungus, causing mild inflammation. However, these tissues are rarely affected if they are entirely healthy. Factors that predispose to candidosis are listed in the information box. A congenital immune deficiency of T lymphocytes predisposes to the syndrome of chronic mucocutaneous candidosis, while more severe, often iatrogenic, forms of immune suppression may permit systemic infection in which mycelia, as well as yeasts, invade tissue and form micro-abscesses.

FACTORS THAT PREDISPOSE TO CANDIDOSIS

Loss of integrity of skin and mucosae
- Maceration of skin due to climate or obesity
- Eczema
- Dentures

Encouragement of local multiplication of Candida
- Alteration of mucosal flora: antibiotic treatment
- Hormonal: diabetes, pregnancy

Suppression of inflammatory and immune responses
- Specific congenital T lymphocyte defect
- Leucopenia of any cause
- Immunosuppressive drugs, including topical corticosteroids
- Malignancy
- Human immunodeficiency virus infection

Clinical features

Infections of the skin may resemble those caused by other dermatophytes but are commonest where the skin is moist and in contact with itself, e.g. groins, perineum, breasts, axillae. Nail infections start at the base, forming ridges, often accompanied by paronychia. In the mouth, white curd-like patches are seen, which can be scraped away leaving a bleeding base. Atrophy of the gums and angular stomatitis are common in the elderly. Vaginitis causes intense pruritus and a thick creamy discharge. In children affected by mucocutaneous candidosis, there is widespread involvement of skin, nails, hair and mucosae, which is troublesome, disfiguring and responds poorly to treatment. Systemic candidosis may present as septicaemia or with the features of an infection of oesophagus, gastrointestinal tract, heart, lungs, urinary tract or brain meninges.

Investigation

The yeast may be identified microscopically or by culture from swabs or scrapings from the lesions and be cultured from the blood in systemic disease. Underlying local or systemic defects should be sought.

Management

Most important is to correct or control the underlying predisposition. Cutaneous candidosis is treated with a topical azole ointment (Table 4.14). Mucosal infection usually responds well to lozenges or suspension of nystatin or amphotericin. Persistent infections and nail infections require oral ketoconazole or itraconazole 100 mg daily, which may need to be maintained for some months. Systemic infections should be treated with intravenous miconazole or amphotericin and maintained on oral ketoconazole.

PITYRIASIS VERSICOLOR

This trivial but often unsightly condition is due to an overgrowth of the normally commensal yeast, *Pityrosporum orbiculare*. It is especially prevalent in hot humid climates.

Clinical features

Pityriasis versicolor mainly affects young adults. The term 'versicolor' refers to the process whereby asymptomatic fawn, scaly and slightly wrinkled macules become depigmented and non-scaly after sun exposure. The rash is most common on the upper trunk. The depigmented lesions should not be mistaken for patches of vitiligo (p. 716).

Investigation

The diagnosis can be confirmed by microscopic examination of skin scrapings cleared with potassium hydroxide.

Management

2.5% selenium sulphide in a detergent base (Selsun shampoo) is useful and relatively cheap. It is lathered on to affected areas, allowed to dry and left overnight before washing off the next morning. Applications once weekly for a month are usually adequate. Topical imidazole preparations are an effective alternative, though treatment for one month is usually required. Stubborn or widespread infections are best treated with a short course of itraconazole (200 mg daily for 7 days), or ketoconazole (200 mg daily for 2 days).

SUBCUTANEOUS FUNGAL INFECTIONS

MYCETOMA (MADURA FOOT)

Mycetoma, in this restricted sense, is a chronic fungal infection of the deep soft tissues and bones, most commonly of the limbs, but also of the abdominal or chest wall or head. It is produced by members of two groups of organisms classified as *Eumycetes* and aerobic *Actinomycetes*. A feature common to both groups is the formation of grains which are colonies of matted organisms with characteristic colours, ranging from 60 microns to 3 mm in diameter. The incidence appears to be related to climate, being especially high when an arid hot season ends in rains. The more common species of fungi causing mycetoma are shown in Table 4.35.

Pathology

The histology is that of a chronic granuloma with a fibrous stroma and cyst-like spaces in which lie the characteristic grains.

Clinical features

The fungus is usually introduced by a thorn and the infection is most common in the foot. The mycetoma begins as a painless swelling at the site of implantation which grows and spreads steadily within the soft tissues causing swelling, and eventually penetrates bones. Nodules develop under the epidermis and these rupture revealing sinuses through which grains are discharged. Some sinuses may heal with scarring while fresh sinuses appear elsewhere.

There is little pain and usually no fever, nor lymphadenopathy, but progressive disability. When the lesion is in the scalp, the skull may be affected but the dura mater appears to be an effective barrier. *Norcardia braziliensis* often affects the skin of the back. It is seldom localised and may spread widely.

Table 4.35 Fungi causing mycetoma

Species	Type of grains
Eumycetoma	
Madurella mycetomatis	Brown or black (big)
Madurella grisea	Black or brown (big)
Exophiala jeanselmei	Black
Pseudallescheria boydii	White or yellow (big)
Acremonium spp.	White or yellow
Actinomycetoma	
Actinomadura madurae	White, yellow, red (big)
Actinomadura pelletieri	Red (small)
Streptomyces somaliensis	White or yellow (big)
Norcardia brasiliensis	White, yellow (microscopic)

Investigations

Diagnosis is confirmed by demonstration of fungal grains in pus or tissue biopsy. Culture is usually necessary for species identification. Specific antibodies can usually be detected by precipitation.

Management

The difference between *Eumycetes* and *Actinomycetes* is crucial because there is no drug of proven efficacy for the former. Sporadic successes against *Eumycetes* have been reported with griseofulvin and ketoconazole, but the results have been mostly disappointing and eumycetoma requires to be excised. It has a tendency to recur.

The treatment of actinomycetoma is more helpful. It consists of rifampicin (4 mg/kg daily by mouth) or streptomycin (14 mg/kg/daily intramuscularly) for 3 months plus oral dapsone (1.5 mg/kg 12-hourly) or oral cotrimoxazole for 4–24 months. *Norcardia* infection may respond to dapsone alone. Precipitating antibodies disappear if treatment is successful.

OTHER SUBCUTANEOUS MYCOSES

These are summarised in Table 4.36.

Table 4.36 Subcutaneous fungal infections, other than mycetoma

	Zygomycosis	Chromoblastomycosis	Rhinospodidiosis	Sporothrichosis
Agent	Several	Several	*Rhinosporidium seeberi*	*Sporothrix schnekii*
Geography	Tropics	Tropics	S. America, India, etc. E. Africa	C. and S. Africa
Site	Face, limbs, systemic in immunocompromised or diabetic	Feet, others	Nose, cheeks	Limbs, rarely systemic
Presentation	Subcutaneous swellings	Mossy foot	Nasal polyps, subcutaneous nodules	Subcutaneous swellings, ulcer, lymphatic spread
Management	Potassium iodide 1.5–3.5 g daily or amphotericin B	Flucytosine and/or itraconazole	Surgery	Potassium iodide 10 g daily, itraconazole

SYSTEMIC FUNGAL INFECTIONS

HISTOPLASMOSIS

Histoplasmosis is caused by *Histoplasma capsulatum* (Darling) which is a yeast in its parasitic phase but is a filamentous fungus of soil at other times. A variant, *Histoplasma duboisii*, is found in parts of tropical Africa.

Histoplasma capsulatum multiplies in soil enriched by the droppings of birds and bats, and the spores remain viable for years. Natural infections are found in several species of small mammals, including bats. Infection is by inhalation of infected dust. The infection is an especial hazard for explorers of caves, and people who clear out bird (including chicken) roosts.

Histoplasma capsulatum is found in all parts of the USA, especially in the east central states, and less commonly in Latin America from Mexico to Argentina, in Europe, North, South and East Africa, Nigeria, Malaysia, Indonesia and Australia.

Pathology

The parasite in its yeast phase multiplies mainly in monocytes and macrophages and produces areas of necrosis in which the parasites may abound. From these foci the blood-stream may be invaded producing metastatic lesions in the liver, spleen and lymph nodes. Pulmonary histoplasmosis may cause pathological changes similar to those of tuberculosis, including the production of a primary complex with enlarged regional lymph nodes, multiple small discrete lesions and occasionally cavitation. Healed lesions may calcify.

Clinical features

These are listed in the information box below.

Investigations

In an area where the disease occurs histoplasmosis should be suspected in every obscure infection in which there are pulmonary signs or where there are enlarged lymph nodes or hepatosplenomegaly. Tissue is obtained by biopsy for an impression smear, histology, and culture. Radiological examination in long-standing cases may show calcified lesions in the lungs, spleen or other organs. In the more acute phases of the disease single or multiple soft pulmonary shadows with enlarged tracheo-bronchial nodes are seen.

Delayed hypersensitivity to the intradermal injection of histoplasmin develops in patients with either active or healed infections but is usually negative in acute disseminated disease. Complement-fixing antibodies are detected within 3 weeks of the onset of an acute primary

---

CLINICAL SYNDROMES ASSOCIATED WITH INFECTIONS WITH *HISTOPLASMA CAPSULATUM*

Infection by inhalation
- Subclinical disease: the majority of infections
- Self limiting fever, chills, cough, chest pain, fatigue, dysphoea. Occasionally fatal pulmonary insufficiency due to heavy infection causing severe alveolitis

Inoculation
- Solitary lesion of skin or mucosa

Disseminated histoplasmosis
Pattern depends on age and immunity
- **Acute** in children: severe, with fever, hepatosplenomegaly, cough, pancytopenia
- **Subacute** in the majority: fever, lymphadenopathy, hepatosplenomegaly, focal lesions of oropharynx, gut, adrenals, endocardium, meninges, brain
- **Chronic** in adults: low grade fever with fatigue. Various focal lesions possible

Chronic localised infection
- Notably pulmonary bullae resembling cavitating tuberculosis

---

infection and increase in titre as the disease progresses. Precipitating antibodies may also be detected.

Management

Specific treatment with amphotericin is indicated only in severe infections, the dosage (0.5 mg/kg, in 500 ml of 5% glucose) is given intravenously over a 6-hour period, gradually increasing to a maximum of 1.0 mg/kg. Treatment is given on alternate days to a total adult dose of 2 g. If badly tolerated, the dose may have to be reduced. Side-effects are anorexia, nausea, fever, headache, and venous thrombosis which may be controlled by the addition of 10 mg prednisolone to the intravenous solution. Plasma urea rises and haemoglobin falls during treatment but later they return to normal. Amphotericin may have to be continued for up to 3 months or longer, depending on the clinical response. Severe dyspnoea in histoplasmosis should be treated with prednisolone 20–40 mg daily for a few days.

Histoplasma duboisii

Histoplasma duboisii, the fungus of African histoplasmosis, is larger than the classical *H. capsulatum*. It is found throughout East, Central and West Africa.

This disease differs in several ways from *H. capsulatum* infection. The bones, skin, lymph nodes and liver develop granulomatous lesions or cold abscesses resembling tuberculosis, but the lungs are seldom involved. The visceral form with liver and splenic invasion is often fatal, while ulcerative skin lesions and bone abscesses follow a more benign course.

Radiological examination may show rounded foci of bone destruction sometimes associated with abscess formation. Multiple lesions of the ribs are common and the bones of the limbs may be involved. Systemic disease is treated in the same way as *H. capsulatum* infections. A solitary lesion in bone may require only local surgical treatment.

ASPERGILLOSIS

This is the most common respiratory mycosis in Britain and is discussed on page 367.

COCCIDIOIDOMYCOSIS

This is caused by *Coccidioides immitis* and found in the Southern United States, and Central and South America. The disease is acquired by inhalation. The infection behaves like tuberculosis or histoplasmosis. In 60% of cases it is asymptomatic. In 40% of cases it affects the lungs, lymph nodes and skin. Rarely it may be carried by the blood-stream to the bones, adrenals, meninges and other organs. Pulmonary coccidioidomycosis has two forms: primary and progressive. Primary coccidioidomycosis behaves like primary tuberculosis or histoplasmosis and is often asymptomatic. The progressive form of the disease is associated with marked systemic upset and features of lobar pneumonia. In more chronic cases it may resemble chronic tuberculosis. Infections, including subclinical attacks, are followed by immunity.

The fungi grow readily on culture media but as they are highly infective, diagnostic investigations are usually limited to intradermal, complement fixation and precipitin tests.

Amphotericin (as for histoplasmosis) or ketoconazole (200–400 mg daily for 1 year) may be helpful, but relapse is common. Some localised pulmonary lesions can be treated by surgery.

PARACOCCIDIOIDOMYCOSIS

This is caused by *Paracoccidioides brasiliensis* and occurs in South America. Mucocutaneous lesions occur early. Involvement of lymphatic nodes and the lungs is prominent and the gastrointestinal tract may also be attacked. Most patients respond to ketoconazole, 200 mg/day for at least 6 months; liver function must be monitored; but for those who do not, amphotericin (as for histoplasmosis) may be used.

BLASTOMYCOSIS

North American blastomycosis is caused by *Blastomyces dermatitidis*. It also occurs in Africa. Systemic infection begins in the lungs and mediastinal lymph nodes and resembles pulmonary tuberculosis. Bones, skin and the genitourinary tract may also be affected. Treatment is with amphotericin (p. 146).

CRYPTOCOCCOSIS

This is caused by *Cryptococcus neoformans*. Its distribution is world-wide. It causes local gummatous-like tumours and granulomatous lesions of the lung, bones, brain and meninges. The CSF often contains the fungus when the nervous system is affected. Immunocompromised individuals are at special risk, including those with human immunodeficiency virus infection.

The diagnosis is made by culture or recognition of spores in the CSF biopsy and serological detection of antigen.

Amphotericin should be given intravenously (p. 146) and flucytosine orally (p. 81). Surgical removal of local pulmonary lesions may be necessary. Recovery may be monitored by fall in antigen titre.

CANDIDOSIS

C. albicans is a cause of systemic fungal infection in the immunosuppressed (pp. 144, 95).

FURTHER READING

Armstrong D 1993 Treatment of opportunistic fungal infections. Clinical Infectious Diseases 16: 1–9

Burchard K W 1992 Fungal sepsis. Infectious Disease Clinics of North America 6: 677–692

Einstein H E, Johnson R H 1993 Coccidioidomycosis: new aspects of epidemiology and therapy. Clinical Infectious Diseases 16: 349–354

Hay R J, Mahgoub E S, Leon G 1992 Mycetoma. Journal of Medical and Veterinary Mycology 30. Supplement: 41–49

DISEASES DUE TO PROTOZOA

Protozoa are unicellular organisms, larger than bacteria, more complex and often motile. Many are free-living and do not infect man or other animals. Others have become specialised and have acquired precise biological niches as parasites of animals, including man. In the well-defined anatomical and biochemical microclimate of each niche, from which they seldom stray, the protozoa can multiply freely, until contained by the immune response. In order to survive transmission to another host, they must either transform into strong-walled cysts that can resist harsh external conditions (e.g. *Entamoeba*, *Giardia*), or be passaged through an insect or bug (e.g. *Plasmodium, Trypanosoma*), in which a second cycle of multiplication takes place. The vector also acts as a reservoir of infection, of variable efficiency. Some protozoa have acquired an intermediate host, in which the organism may persist dormant for many years (e.g. *Toxoplasma* in the muscles of herbivores) and man may only be an incidental host.

Protozoal diseases are of especial importance among livestock in the tropics. Epidemics of Ngama (cattle trypanosomiasis) and East Coast Fever (tyleriosis) have given rise to famine. The important human diseases due to protozoa are listed in the information box.

PROTOZOAL DISEASES OF MAN

- **In the blood:** Malaria, trypanosomiasis
- **In the gut:** Giardiasis, amoebiasis, balantidiasis
- **In the tissues:** Toxoplasmosis, leishmaniasis

MALARIA

Human malaria is caused by *Plasmodium falciparum, P. vivax, P. ovale, and P. malariae.* It is transmitted by the bite of anopheline mosquitoes, in which the parasite undergoes a cycle of development which is temperature-dependent. Malaria is therefore predominantly a disease of hot wet climates, but it used to occur in Europe as far north as England and Denmark. Malaria may also be transmitted by blood transfusion or inoculation. Trans-placental infection may occur in the child of a non-immune mother.

Malaria is endemic or sporadic throughout most of the tropics and subtropics below an altitude of 1500 m, excluding the Mediterranean littoral, the USA and Australia (Fig. 4.31). One hundred million people are attacked annually, of whom 1% die, mainly children. Following WHO-sponsored campaigns of prevention and more effective treatment, the incidence of malaria was greatly reduced in 1950–60 but since 1970 there has been a resurgence. In the 1980s *P. falciparum* became resistant to chloroquine over a steadily increasing area (Table 4.38). Most serious is the emergence of resistance in East Africa, which has spread through Central Africa and in 1989 reached most parts of West Africa. Malaria due to this parasite is more severe than that due to the sensitive parasites.

Because of increased travel and neglect of chemo-prophylaxis over 2000 cases are imported annually into Britain. Most are due to *P. vivax* from Asia. One in five, usually from Africa, is due to *P. falciparum* and of these 1% die because of late diagnosis. A few people living near airports in Europe have acquired malaria from accidentally imported mosquitoes.

Pathogenesis

Life cycle of parasite (Figs. 4.32 and 4.33)
The female anopheline mosquito becomes infected when it feeds on human blood containing gametocytes, the sexual forms of the malarial parasite. The development in the mosquito takes from 7–20 days. Sporozoites inoculated by an infected mosquito disappear from human blood within half an hour and enter the

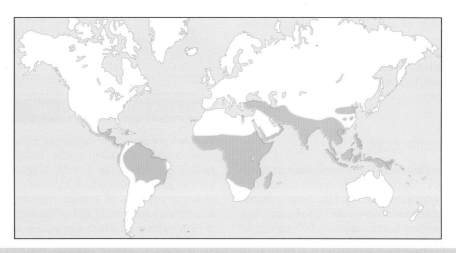

Fig. 4.31 Distribution of malaria.

Table 4.37   Relationships between life cycle of parasite and clinical features of malaria

Cycle/feature	P. vivax, P. ovale	P. malariae	P. falciparum
Pre patent period (minimum incubation)	8–25 days	15–30 days	8–25 days
Asexual cycle	48 hrs synchronous	72 hrs synchronous	<48 hrs asynchronous
Periodicity of fever	'Tertian'	'Quartan'	Aperiodic
Exoerythrocytic cycle	Persistent as hypnozoites	Pre-erythrocytic only	Pre-erythrocytic only
Delayed onset	Common	Rare	Rare
Relapses	Common up to 2 years	Recrudescence many years	Recrudescence up to 1 year

liver. After some days (Table 4.37) merozoites leave the liver and invade red blood cells where further asexual cycles of multiplication take place, producing schizonts. Rupture of the schizont releases more merozoites into the blood and causes fever, whose periodicity depends on the species of parasite.

P. vivax and P. ovale may persist in liver cells as dormant forms, hypnozoites, that are capable of developing into merozoites months or years later. Thus the first attack of clinical malaria may occur long after the patient has left the endemic area, and the disease may relapse after treatment with drugs that kill only the erythrocytic stage of the parasite.

P. falciparum and P. malariae have no persistent exo-erythrocytic phase but recrudescences of fever may result from multiplication in the red cells of parasites which have not been eliminated by treatment and immune processes.

Effects on red blood cells and capillaries

Malaria is always accompanied by haemolysis and in a severe or prolonged attack anaemia may be profound. The causes of anaemia are listed in the information box.

CAUSES OF ANAEMIA IN MALARIA

- Haemolysis of infected erythrocytes
- Haemolysis of uninfected erythrocytes
- Dyserythropoiesis
- Splenomegaly causing erythrocyte sequestration and haemodilution
- Depletion of folate stores

Haemolysis is most severe with P. falciparum which invades red cells of all ages, but especially young cells. P. vivax and P. ovale invade reticulocytes, and P. malariae normoblasts, so that infections remain lighter.

In P. falciparum malaria, red cells containing schizonts adhere to the lining of capillaries in brain, kidney, liver, lungs and gut. The vessels become congested and the organs anoxic. Rupture of schizonts liberates toxic and

antigenic substances which may cause further damage. Thus the main effects of malaria are haemolytic anaemia and, with P. falciparum, widespread organ damage.

P. falciparum does not grow well in red cells that contain haemoglobin F, C or especially S. Haemoglobin S heterozygotes (AS) are protected against the lethal complications of malaria. P. vivax cannot enter red cells that lack the Duffy blood group. West African and American Black people are protected.

Clinical features

Malaria in the non-immune

This is the pattern in children in an endemic area once they have lost the protection conferred by maternal antibodies, or in visitors of any age from a non-endemic area. The incubation period is often longer than the pre-erythrocytic cycle and may be up to several weeks for P. falciparum or months for P. vivax.

P. vivax and P. ovale malaria

In many cases the illness starts with a period of several days of continued fever before the development of classical bouts of fever on alternate days. Fever starts with a rigor. The patient feels cold and the temperature rises to about 40°C. After half to 1 hour the hot or flush phase begins. It lasts several hours and gives way to profuse perspiration and gradual fall in temperature. The cycle is repeated 48 hours later. Gradually the spleen and liver enlarge and may become tender. Anaemia develops slowly. Herpes simplex is common. Relapses are common in the first two years of leaving the malarious area.

P. malariae infection

This is usually associated with mild symptoms and bouts of fever every third day. Parasitaemia may persist for many years with the occasional recondescence of fever, or without producing any symptoms. P. malariae causes glomerulonephritis and the nephrotic syndrome, in children.

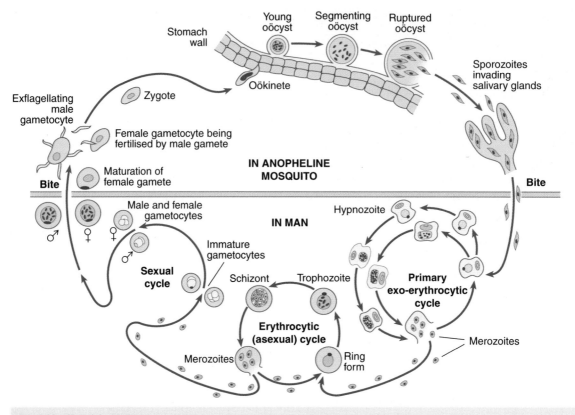

Fig. 4.32 Malarial parasites. Life cycle.

P. falciparum infections

These are more dangerous than other forms of malaria. The onset, especially of primary attacks, is often insidious with malaise, headache and vomiting. Cough and mild diarrhoea are common, suggesting influenza. The fever has no particular pattern and does not usually rise quite so high as in the other forms. The cold, hot and sweating stages are seldom found. Jaundice is common due to hepatitis and haemolysis. The liver and spleen enlarge and become tender. Anaemia develops rapidly.

A patient with falciparum malaria, apparently not seriously ill, may develop serious complications. Children die rapidly without any special symptoms other than fever. Immunity is impaired in pregnancy, and abortion from parasitisation of the maternal side of the placenta is frequent. Splenectomy increases the risk of severe malaria.

Mixed infections with more than one species of malaria parasite may occur.

The complications of falciparum malaria are listed in the information box (right).

COMPLICATIONS OF MALARIA DUE TO *PLASMODIUM FALCIPARUM*

- **Severe anaemia**

- **Organ damage due to anoxia**
  Brain: confusion, coma
  Kidneys: oliguria, uraemia (acute tubular necrosis)
  Lungs: cough, pulmonary oedema
  Intestine: diarrhoea, congestion, possibly leaky to bacteria
  Liver: jaundice, encephalopathy (rare)

- **Intravascular haemolysis**
  Blackwater fever

- **Hypoglycaemia, especially with quinine treatment**

- **Septicaemia secondary to shock**

- **Hypotensive shock**

- **Metabolic acidosis**

- **Splenic rupture**

- **In pregnancy**
  Maternal death, abortion, stillbirth, low birth weight

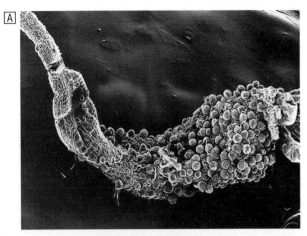

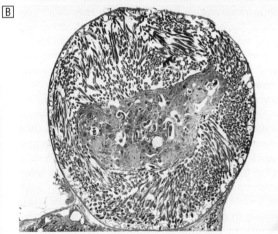

Fig. 4.33 A **Oöcysts of Plasmodium lining the stomach of an anopheline mosquito** (scanning electron micrograph); B **Sporozoites of Plasmodium within an oöcyst** (transmission electron micrograph).

Cerebral malaria

This is the most urgent complication and is manifested either by confusion or coma, usually without localising signs.

Blackwater fever

This is associated with chronic falciparum malaria, most commonly in those who have taken antimalarial treatment irregularly, or are deficient in glucose-6-phosphate dehydrogenase. Haemolysis is unpredictable and severe, destroying uninfected as well as parasitised red cells. The urine is dark or black.

Endemic malaria

The manifestations of malaria in people who grow up in an endemic area vary with the degree of endemicity, the age of the patient and the development of immunity.

In hypoendemic areas little immunity is acquired, epidemics of malaria are liable to occur and the disease does not differ materially from that in non-immunes.

In mesoendemic areas malaria is frequent but only seasonal. Repeated infections lead to anaemia, considerable enlargement of the spleen, which is in danger of rupture, and chronic ill-health with bouts of fever. The growth and development of children may be retarded.

In hyperendemic areas malaria transmission takes place throughout the year but with seasonal increases. Adults develop considerable immunity; although affected individuals may have palpable spleens and parasitaemia, malaria causes only occasional short bouts of fever.

In holoendemic areas malarial transmission is intense throughout the year and adults do not suffer from the infection although they support a low parasitaemia and the spleen becomes impalpable.

In hyperendemic and in holoendemic areas malaria may kill up to 15–20% of children below the age of 5 years. The regular taking of anti-malarial drugs prevents the manifestations of chronic malaria but may impair the development of immunity. Pregnancy lowers resistance to malaria. The associated risks are greatest in the first pregnancy (see information box p. 150).

Tropical splenomegaly syndrome

In some hyperendemic areas gross splenomegaly is associated with an exaggerated immune response to malaria and is seen, unexpectedly, in adults who have high antibody titres to malaria and low parasitaemias. The condition, which is commoner in females and in certain racial and family groups, is characterised by enormous overproduction of IgM, levels reaching 3–20 times the local mean value. Much of the IgM is aggregated with other immunoglobulin or complement and precipitates in the cold, in vitro. IgM aggregates are phagocytosed by reticuloendothelial cells in the spleen and liver, and the demonstration of this by immunofluorescence in a liver biopsy section is diagnostic. Light microscopy of the liver usually shows sinusoidal lymphocytosis. Anaemia and lymphocytosis can be confused with leukaemia. Portal hypertension may develop.

Investigations

Malaria should be considered if a febrile patient is in, or has recently left, a malarious locality. Besides malaria there are many causes for acute febrile splenomegaly in the tropics. Gross enlargement of the spleen may also result from tuberculosis, visceral leishmaniasis, schistosomiasis and chronic brucellosis as well as leukaemia and lymphoma. Well-stained blood films, thick and thin, should be repeated if necessary. *P. falciparum* parasites may be very scanty, especially in patients who have been partially treated. With *P. falciparum* only ring forms are normally seen in the early stages. With the other species all stages of the erythrocytic cycle may be found. Gametocytes appear after about 2 weeks. They persist despite treatment and are harmless. Malaria may coexist with other diseases and not be the cause of the illness in semi-immune persons in endemic areas.

Management

Chemotherapy of the acute attack

For infections with *P. falciparum* from a chloroquine-sensitive area, and for all infections with *P. vivax*, *P. ovale* and *P. malariae*, the drug of choice is chloroquine. The usual course of treatment is 600 mg of the effective *base* followed by 300 mg *base* in 6 hours then 150 mg *base* twice daily for 3–7 more days. The initial dose for children is 5–15 mg/kg. For semi-immune individuals a single dose, 600 mg for an adult, is usually adequate.

Infections with *P. falciparum* from a chloroquine-resistant area (Table 4.38) should be treated with quinine dihydrochloride or sulphate 600 mg *salt* (10 mg/kg) 3 times daily by mouth till better, and the blood is free of parasites (usually 3–5 days). This regime should be followed by a single dose of sulfadoxine 1.5 g combined with pyrimethamine 75 mg, i.e. 3 tablets of Fansidar. The dose is reduced to twice daily if quinine toxicity develops. In pregnancy a 7-day course of quinine alone should be given. Quinidine may be used in the same dosage as quinine. If sulphonamide sensitivity is suspected, quinine may be followed by tetracycline 250 mg, 6-hourly for 7 days. Alternatives to quinine plus Fansidar are mefloquine 500 mg 8-hourly for three doses or halofantrine 500 mg every 8 hours for three doses. Mefloquine may occasionally cause alarming neuro-psychiatric side effects which can persist for several days due to its plasma half-life of 14 days. Halofantrine should be avoided if the electrocardiogram is abnormal. Both drugs are expensive but are especially useful for self-medication by travellers. They should be avoided in pregnancy.

Management of complicated P. falciparum malaria

Patients with 'cerebral malaria' or other severe manifestations, or non-immune with more than 1% of red cells infected, are medical emergencies. Quinine or chloroquine is given as an intravenous infusion over 2–4 hours to avoid acute circulatory failure or acute encephalopathy. Quinine is indicated if a chloroquine-resistant infection is at all likely (Table 4.38). The dose of chloroquine is 5 mg/kg and of quinine 10 mg/kg. The dose should be repeated at intervals of 12 hours until the patient can take drugs orally. The drugs may instead be given intramuscularly but chloroquine may cause convulsions (especially in undernourished children) and quinine may cause necrosis of muscle; the hydrochloride is less irritant than the dihydrochloride. In a comatose patient lumbar puncture may be indicated to exclude coexisting bacterial meningitis.

Severe anaemia requires transfusion with packed red cells. If oliguria develops, frusemide or an infusion of mannitol may forestall renal failure. Intravenous fluid, if necessary, should be monitored by the central venous pressure because pulmonary oedema is more likely to develop if the patient is over-infused. Exchange blood transfusion is life-saving in complicated very heavy infections (over 10% of red cells infected). Hypoglycaemia, especially in children, or septicaemia may be the cause of failure to respond to treatment. Dialysis may be needed if renal failure develops.

Management of tropical splenomegaly syndrome

Splenomegaly and anaemia usually resolve over a period of months of continuous treatment with proguanil 100 mg daily, which should be continued for life to

Table 4.38 Chemoprophylaxis of malaria			
Area	**Antimalarial tablets**	**Adult prophylactic dose**	
Chloroquine resistance present[1]	Chloroquine[2]	150 mg base	Two tablets weekly
	PLUS Proguanil	100 mg	Two tablets daily
	OR Mefloquine[3]	250 mg	One tablet weekly
Chloroquine resistance absent	Chloroquine	150 mg base	Two tablets weekly
	OR Proguanil	100 mg	One or two tablets daily

[1] South America, S.E. Asia including Southern China, Indonesia, Malaysia, Philippines, Papua New Guinea, Bangladesh, India, Nepal, East, Central and West Africa.
[2] British preparations of chloroquine usually contain 150 mg base, French preparations 100 mg base and American preparations 300 mg base.
[3] Contraindicated with pregnancy, lactation, under 5 years of age, cardiotropic drugs, epilepsy, psychiatric disorders. May cause dizziness, insomnia.

prevent relapse. Complicating folate deficiency is treated with folic acid 5 mg daily.

Radical cure of malaria due to P. vivax and P. ovale

Relapses can be prevented by taking one of the antimalarial drugs in suppressive doses. Radical cure is achieved in most patients by a course of primaquine (15 mg/d for 14 days) which destroys the hyponozoite phase in the liver. Haemolysis may develop in those who are glucose-6-phosphate dehydrogenase (G6PD) deficient. Cyanosis due to the formation of methaemoglobin in the red cells is more common but not dangerous.

Chemoprophylaxis

Clinical attacks of malaria may be preventable by drugs such as proguanil which attack the pre-erythrocytic form ('causal prophylaxis'), or by drugs such as chloroquine or mefloquine after it has entered the erythrocyte ('suppression'). Tables 4.38 and 4.39 give the recommended doses for protection of the non-immune. Maloprim (pyrimethamine 12.5 mg and dapsone 100 mg) contains two compounds which block two successive enzymes in the parasite's folate pathway. It may be used to substitute for proguanil or chloroquine if either is not well tolerated. Chemoprophylaxis is begun 1 week before entering the malarious area and is continued until 4 weeks after leaving it. Resistance to the cheap and well-tolerated drugs proguanil and pyrimethamine is increasing, and frequently coincides with the much more serious spread of chloroquine resistance. Chloroquine should not be taken continuously as prophylactic for over 5 years without regular ophthalmic examination, as it may cause irreversible retinopathy. Infants under 8 weeks of age should not be given maloprim. Pregnant and lactating women may take proguanil or chloroquine safely. Fansidar should be avoided for chemoprophylaxis, as deaths have occurred from agranulocytosis or Stevens–Johnson syndrome. Mefloquine is useful in areas of multiple drug resistance, such as East and Central Africa and Papua New Guinea. Experience shows it to be safe for at least two years. There are several contraindications to its use (Table 4.38).

Table 4.39 Doses of antimalarials for children

Dose in relation to adult dose	Weight range	Age range
One-quarter	Under 5 kg	Under 1 year
One-half	5–20 kg	1–4 years
Three-quarters	20–40 kg	6–12 years
Adult dose	Over 40 kg	Over 12 years

Note: Doses according to weight are preferable to age.

Prevention

Control of anopheline mosquitoes, especially by the spraying of houses with residual insecticides, has greatly reduced or abolished the risk of malaria in many areas. However, unless eradication is complete, all visitors should take regular prophylactic drugs. *Chemoprophylaxis alone may not be sufficient to prevent malaria.* It is also important to avoid anopheline mosquitoes, which bite at night. Long sleeves and trousers should be worn outside the house. Repellent creams and sprays can be used. Screened windows, the use of a mosquito net and burning repellent coils or tablets also reduce the risk.

AMOEBIASIS

Amoebiasis is usually caused by *Entamoeba histolytica*, a potentially pathogenic intestinal amoeba that is spread between humans by its cysts. It is common throughout the tropics and occasionally acquired in Britain. *E. histolytica* must be distinguished from other species which are non-pathogenic, notably *E. hartmanni* and *E. coli*. In addition two amoebae of genera *Naegleria* and *Acanthamoeba* which inhabit polluted surface water and swimming pools all over the world are causes respectively of fulminating meningitis and granulomatous encephalitis.

Pathology

Cysts of *E. histolytica* survive well outside the body and are ingested in water or uncooked food which has been contaminated by human faeces. Lettuce is a common vehicle of infection.

In the colon the vegetative trophozoite forms emerge from the cysts (Fig. 4.34). While these remain free in the colon the condition is symptomless but some genetic strains, that can be distinguished enzymatically, may invade the mucous membrane of the large bowel. The lesions, which are usually maximal in the caecum but may be found as far down as the anal canal, are flask-shaped ulcers varying greatly in size and surrounded by healthy mucosa. A localised granuloma (amoeboma), presenting as a palpable mass in the rectum or causing a filling defect in the colon on radiography, is a rare complication. Because an amoeboma responds well to antiamoebic treatment it is important that it is not mistaken for a colonic carcinoma.

Amoebae may enter a portal venous radicle and be carried to the liver where they multiply rapidly and destroy the parenchyma, causing an amoebic abscess. The liquid contents at first have a characteristic pinkish colour which later may change to chocolate brown.

Amoebic ulcers may cause severe haemorrhage but rarely perforate the bowel wall. Cutaneous amoebiasis

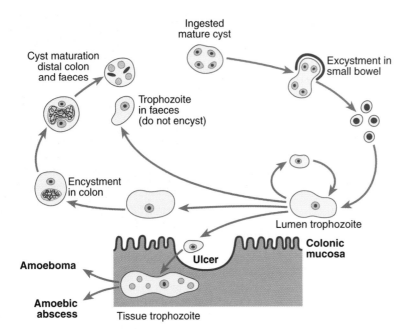

Cyst maturation distal colon and faeces

Ingested mature cyst

Excystment in small bowel

Trophozoite in faeces (do not encyst)

Encystment in colon

Lumen trophozoite

Colonic mucosa

Ulcer

Amoeboma

Amoebic abscess

Tissue trophozoite

Fig. 4.34 Amoebiasis. Life cycle of *Entamoeba histolytica.*

presents as progressive genital or perianal ulceration, usually in homosexuals, or around abdominal surgical wounds. The incubation period of amoebiasis ranges from 2 weeks to many years.

Clinical features

Intestinal amoebiasis, or amoebic dysentery
This usually runs a chronic course with grumbling abdominal pains and two or more unformed stools a day. Periods of diarrhoea alternating with constipation are common. Mucus is usually passed, sometimes with streaks of blood, and the stools often have an offensive odour. There may be tenderness along the line of the colon, usually more marked over the caecum and pelvic colon. The right iliac pain may simulate acute appendicitis. There may be more acute bowel symptoms, with very frequent motions and the passage of much blood and mucus, simulating bacillary dysentery or ulcerative colitis. This occurs particularly in the aged, in the puerperium and with superadded pyogenic infection of the ulcers.

Hepatic amoebiasis
This often occurs without a history of recent diarrhoea. It is common in the tropics and an important cause of imported fever in Britain. The abscess is usually found in the right hepatic lobe. Early symptoms may be local discomfort only and malaise; later a swinging temperature and sweating. An enlarged, tender liver, cough, and pain in the right shoulder are characteristic, but

symptoms may remain vague and signs minimal. In particular, the less common abscess in the left lobe is difficult to diagnose. There is usually neutrophil leucocytosis and a raised diaphragm with diminished movement on the right side. A large abscess may penetrate the diaphragm and rupture into the lung from where its contents may be coughed up. Rupture into the pleural cavity, the peritoneal cavity or pericardial sac is less common but more serious.

Investigations
A careful naked-eye inspection of a freshly passed stool should be made. Any exudate is examined at once under the microscope for motile trophozoites, which are about 30 microns in diameter with a clear ectoplasm and a granular endoplasm, and usually contain red blood cells. Movements cease rapidly as the stool preparation cools. Sigmoidoscopy may reveal typical flask-shaped ulcers, and a scraping should be examined immediately for *E. histolytica*. Several stools may need to be examined in chronic amoebiasis before cysts are found. The presence of cysts in the faeces does not equate with invasive amoebiasis: in endemic areas one-third of the population are symptomless passers of amoebic cysts.

An amoebic abscess of the liver is suspected from the clinical and radiographic appearances and confirmed by radionuclide or ultrasonic scanning. Aspirated pus from an amoebic abscess has the characteristic appearance described above but only rarely contains free amoebae.

Antibodies are detectable by immunofluorescence in

over 95% of patients with hepatic amoebiasis and intestinal amoeboma but in only about 60% of dysenteric amoebiasis. Tests for precipitating antibodies are less sensitive but become negative within a few months of cure.

Management

Invasive intestinal amoebiasis responds quickly to oral metronidazole (800 mg 8-hourly for 5 days), or tinidazole (single doses of 2 g daily for 3 days). Furamide 500 mg should be given orally 8-hourly for 10 days after treatment to eliminate luminal cysts. Stools are re-examined 4 weeks later.

Early hepatic amoebiasis responds promptly to treatment with metronidazole or tinidazole as above, or to chloroquine 300 mg base 12-hourly for 2 days, followed by 150 mg 12-hourly for 14 days. Furamide is given to eliminate the intestinal infection. Aspiration is also required and repeated if necessary if the abscess is large or threatens to burst, or if the response to chemotherapy is not prompt. Rupture of an abscess into the pleural cavity, pericardial sac or peritoneal cavity necessitates immediate aspiration or surgical drainage. Small serous effusions resolve without drainage.

Prevention

Personal precautions against contracting amoebiasis in the tropics and subtropics consist of not eating fresh uncooked vegetables nor drinking unboiled water.

GIARDIASIS

Infection with the flagellate *Giardia intestinalis*, known also as *G. lamblia*, is worldwide but common in the tropics. It particularly affects children in endemic areas, tourists and immunosuppressed individuals and may be a commensal in some individuals. It is the parasite most commonly imported into Britain. The cysts remain viable in water for up to 3 months and infection usually occurs by ingesting contaminated water. The flagellates attach to the mucosa of the duodenum and jejunum and cause inflammation (Fig. 4.35).

Clinical features

After an incubation period of 1–3 weeks, there is diarrhoea, abdominal pain, weakness, anorexia, nausea and vomiting. On examination there may be abdominal distension and tenderness. These features usually last for only a few days but in some individuals they continue for weeks or months. Such patients become lethargic and flatulent and lose weight. Investigation may reveal steatorrhoea, malabsorption of xylose and vitamin B_{12}, lactose intolerance and partial villous atrophy. Thus in persons returning from the tropics with diarrhoea, giar-

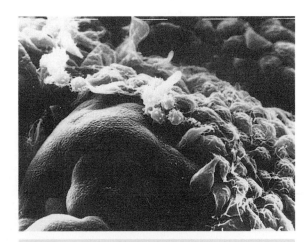

Fig. 4.35 **Trophozooites of *Giardia lamblia*** swarming over jejunal mucosa. Electron micrograph.

diasis may be confused with tropical sprue, and in residents of Western communities it must be considered in the differential diagnosis of other causes of malabsorption such as coeliac disease or Crohn's disease of the small intestine.

Investigations

Stools are obtained at 2–3 day intervals on three separate occasions and examined for cysts. The diagnostic yield is improved by examination of duodenal or jejunal fluid. Thus if endoscopy is being performed for upper gastrointestinal symptoms, it is important to remember the possibility of giardiasis and to aspirate juice for microscopic examination. If a jejunal biopsy is obtained, the mucus should be examined fresh. Histology shows giardia on the surface of the epithelium. Jejunal mucus may be obtained with a string test (Enterotest capsule).

Management

Treatment is with a single dose of tinidazole 40 mg/kg in the range 0.5–2 g, repeated after 1 week. Less effective regimens are metronidazole 2 g once daily for 3 days or 200 mg 8-hourly for 7 days, or quinacrine hydrochloride 100 mg 8-hourly for 7 days.

LEISHMANIASIS

This group of diseases is caused by protozoa of the genus *Leishmania*, conveyed to man by female phlebotomine sandflies in which the flagellate (promastigote) forms of leishmania develop. In man the leishmania are found in cells of the monocyte-macrophage system as oval forms known as amastigotes or Leishman–Donovan bodies (Fig. 4.36). Leishmaniasis may take the form of a gen-

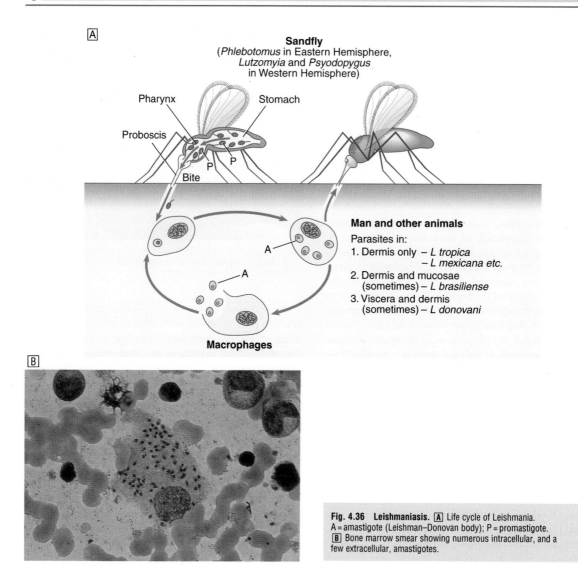

Fig. 4.36 **Leishmaniasis.** Ⓐ Life cycle of Leishmania.
A = amastigote (Leishman–Donovan body); P = promastigote.
Ⓑ Bone marrow smear showing numerous intracellular, and a
few extracellular, amastigotes.

eralised visceral infection, kala-azar, or of a purely cutaneous infection, known in the Old World as oriental sore. In South America cutaneous leishmaniasis may remain confined to the skin or metastasise to the nose and mouth.

VISCERAL LEISHMANIASIS (KALA-AZAR)

Visceral leishmaniasis is caused by *Leishmania donovani* and is prevalent in the Mediterranean and Red Sea littorals, Sudan, parts of East Africa, Asia Minor, mountainous regions of Southern Arabia, eastern parts of India, China and South America. In India, where the disease is epidemic, man appears to be the chief host. In most other areas, including the Mediterranean, dogs

and foxes are the main reservoirs of infection. Here the disease is endemic and occurs chiefly in young children or tourists. In Africa various wild rodents provide the reservoir, and the disease is rural, occurring in older children and visiting hunters and soldiers. Transmission has also been reported to follow blood transfusion in Northern Europe. The disease has presented unexpectedly in immunosuppressed patients, for example after renal transplantation and in AIDS.

Pathology

Multiplication, by simple fission, of leishmania takes place in monocytes and macrophages in various organs, especially in the liver and spleen which become greatly enlarged, the bone marrow, lymphoid tissue and the small intestinal submucosa. The disease is accompanied by malnutrition and immunosuppression which is both specific to leishmania and non-specific. Acute intercurrent pneumococcal infection or tuberculosis are common complications. Granulocytopenia and thrombocytopenia occur. Anaemia is due to haemolysis, hypersplenism and ineffective erythropoiesis. Serum albumin is low and globulin, mainly IgG, high. Hepatocellular damage and bleeding are late complications.

Clinical features

The incubation period is usually about 1 or 2 months but may be up to 10 years. The onset is usually insidious with a low-grade fever, the patient remaining ambulant, or it may be abrupt with sweating and high intermittent fever, sometimes showing a double rise of temperature in 24 hours. The spleen soon becomes enlarged, often massively; hepatomegaly is less marked. If not treated, the patient will become anaemic and wasted, frequently with increased pigmentation especially on the face. Cough and diarrhoea develop. In Africa lymphadenopathy is common, and rarely the only clinical finding.

After recovery post kala-azar dermal leishmaniasis sometimes develops. It may present first as hypopigmented or erythematous macules on any part of the body or as a nodular eruption especially on the face. Amastigotes are scanty.

Investigations

Diagnosis is established by demonstrating the parasite in stained smears of aspirates of bone marrow, lymph node, spleen or liver, or by culture of these aspirates. Antibody is detected by immunofluorescence or enzyme-linked immunosorbent assay early in the disease. The **leishmanin skin test** is negative; it is performed and read in the same way as the tuberculin test using a suspension of killed promastigotes as antigen.

Management

The response to treatment varies with the geographic area in which the disease has been acquired. In Europe and Asia the disease is readily cured, but in the Sudan and East Africa it is more resistant. Pentavalent antimonials are the drugs of choice. Sodium stibogluconate contains 100 mg Sb/ml, meglumine antimoniate contains 85 mg Sb/ml. The dose is 20 mg Sb/kg intravenously or intramuscularly daily for 20–30 days. It may be reduced progressively by 2 mg Sb/kg if not well tolerated.

, Intercurrent infection is sought and treated. Rarely blood transfusion is needed for anaemia or bleeding. Measurement of spleen size, haemoglobin and serum albumin are useful in assessing progress. A small pro-

portion of patients relapse, and should be re-treated for 2 months with a full 20 mg Sb/kg daily. Second-line drugs for patients who fail to respond to antimonials include pentamidine 3–4 mg/kg 1 or 2 times per week and liposomal or conventional amphotericin (p. 146).

Prevention

Infected or stray dogs should be destroyed in an endemic area, where they are the reservoir. Sandflies should be combated. They are extremely sensitive to insecticides. Mosquito nets treated with permethrin will keep out the tiny sandfly. Insect-repellent creams may be helpful.

Early diagnosis and treatment of human infections reduces the reservoir and controls epidemic kala-azar in India. Serology is useful for case detection in the field. There is no vaccine.

CUTANEOUS LEISHMANIASIS OF THE OLD WORLD (ORIENTAL SORE)

Cutaneous leishmaniasis is found around the Mediterranean littoral, throughout the Middle East and Central Asia as far as Pakistan, and in sub-Saharan West Africa and Sudan. It is caused either by zoonotic *L. major*, a parasite of gerbils and other desert rodents, or by the arthroponotic *L. tropica* in towns. In the highlands of Ethiopia and Kenya a third parasite, of hyraxes, *L. aethiopica*, is the cause. The disease is commonly imported into Britain. On inoculation the parasites are taken up by dermal histiocytes, in which they multiply and around which lymphocytes and plasma cells accumulate. With time, the histological appearance becomes more tuberculoid and the overlying epidermis crusts and may ulcerate centrally. Healing is accompanied by subepidermal fibrosis. The incubation period is from 2 weeks to 5 years or more but usually is from 2 to 3 months.

Clinical features

Lesions, single or multiple, on exposed parts of the body, start as small red papules which increase gradually in size, reaching 2–10 cm in diameter. A crust forms, overlying an ulcer with a granular base (Fig. 4.37). Tiny satellite papules are characteristic. Untreated, the lesion heals in 3 months to 3 years, rarely longer. Healing produces a depressed mottled scar which may be disfiguring or disabling.

Two forms of cutaneous leishmaniasis occur which do not heal spontaneously: diffuse cutaneous leishmaniasis (*L. aethiopica*) in which an immune defect permits the disease to spread all over the skin, and recidivans

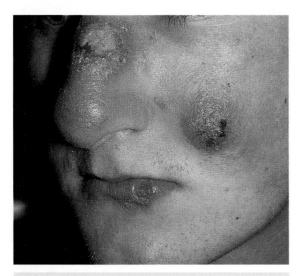

Fig. 4.37 Cutaneous leishmaniasis.

(lupoid) leishmaniasis (*L. tropica*) in which apparently healed sores relapse persistently.

Investigations
The appearance of a typical lesion in a patient from an endemic area suggests the diagnosis. Amastigotes can be demonstrated by making a slit skin smear (p. 134) and staining the material obtained with Giemsa stain or culturing it. Cultured parasites may be speciated by isoenzyme or DNA studies. The leishmanin skin is positive except in diffuse cutaneous leishmaniasis. Serology is unhelpful.

Management
Small lesions may be treated by freezing with liquid carbon dioxide, curettage or infiltration with 1–2 ml sodium stibogluconate. When the lesions are multiple or in a disfiguring site it is better to treat the patient by parenteral injections of pentavalent antimonials as outlined under visceral leishmaniasis above, but *L. aethiopica* is not sensitive to antimonials. Diffuse cutaneous leishmaniasis is treated with pentamidine once weekly.

Prevention
In addition to those prophylactic measures described under visceral leishmaniasis against animals and sandflies, a lasting immunity can be achieved by deliberate inoculation of a living culture of *L. major* on the upper arm, which produces a typical sore but protects against a subsequent, possibly disfiguring, lesion with the same species of parasite.

CUTANEOUS AND MUCOSAL LEISHMANIASIS OF THE NEW WORLD

In South and Central America, cutaneous leishmaniasis is endemic and mostly caused by *L. mexicana*, *L. amazonensis* and *L. brasiliensis*, which occur in hot, moist forest regions and are conveyed to man from a variety of animals by several species of sandflies (Fig. 4.36A). *L. mexicana* is responsible for chiclero's ulcer, the self-healing sores of Mexico, Guatemala and Honduras, and for some of the sores in the north of South America, including diffuse cutaneous leishmaniasis (*L. amazonensis*). *L. brasiliensis* extends widely from the Amazon basin as far as Paraguay and Costa Rica and is responsible for self-healing sores and for mucosal leishmaniasis. A third variety of the disease occurring in the Peruvian Andes is known as 'uta' and is caused by *L. peruviana*, dogs providing the reservoir.

Pathology
The microscopic appearances of the skin lesions may be similar to oriental sore. Mucosal lesions begin as a perivascular infiltration; later endarteritis may cause destruction of the surrounding tissues.

Clinical features
Clinically, lesions of *L. mexicana* and *L. peruviana* closely resemble those seen in the Old World but lesions on the pinna of the ear are common and are chronic and destructive. The primary lesions of *L. brasiliensis* are similar but in some areas up to 80% of infected persons develop 'espundia', metastatic lesions in the mucosa of the nose or mouth. Mucosal lesions usually occur 1–2 years after the skin lesions but may appear many years later. The nasal mucosa becomes congested and ulcerates; later all soft tissues of the nose may be destroyed. The lips, soft palate, fauces and larynx may also be invaded and destroyed leading to considerable suffering and deformity. Secondary bacterial infection is common. Two related species, *L. guyanensis* and *L. panamensis*, rarely cause espundia.

Investigations
Diagnosis depends on the history and clinical appearance, confirmed by demonstration of the parasites in smears, culture or histological section. As parasites are not easily found, the leishmanin test is of value. Serology may be useful in mucosal leishmaniasis.

Management
Purely cutaneous disease may be successfully treated by sodium stibogluconate given as recommended for visceral leishmaniasis above but in established espundia amphotericin is sometimes necessary.

AFRICAN TRYPANOSOMIASIS (SLEEPING SICKNESS)

African sleeping sickness is caused by trypanosomes conveyed to man by the bites of infected tsetse flies of either sex. The disease is naturally acquired only in Africa between 12°N and 25°S. Two trypanosomes affect man, *Trypanosoma brucei gambiense* conveyed by *Glossina palpalis* and *G. tachinoides* and *T. rhodesiense* transmitted by *G. morsitans*, *G. pallidipes*, *G. swynnertoni* and *G. palpalis*.

Gambiense trypaosomiasis has a wide distribution in West and Central Africa reaching to Uganda and Kenya; rhodesiense trypanosomiasis is found in parts of East and Central Africa where it is currently on the increase. In West Africa transmission is mainly at the riverside, where the fly rests in the shade of trees. Animal reservoirs of *T. gambiense* have not been identified, although pigs may carry it. *T. rhodesiense* has a large reservoir in numerous wild animals and transmission takes place in the shade of woods bordering grasslands. Devastating epidemics of both types have occurred. Trypanosomiasis of cattle, caused mainly by *T. brucei*, is also widespread and seriously limits grazing land and the production of meat and milk. Only a low percentage of tsetse flies are infected.

Clinical features

A bite by a tsetse fly is painful and commonly becomes inflamed, but if trypanosomes are introduced, the site may again become painful and swollen about 10 days later ('trypanosomal chancre'), and the regional lymph nodes enlarge. Within 2–3 weeks of infection the trypanosomes invade the blood stream (Table 4.40).

Gambiense infections

In these infections the disease usually runs a slow course over months or years with irregular bouts of fever and enlargement of lymph nodes. These are characteristically firm, discrete, rubbery and painless and are particularly prominent in the posterior triangle of the neck. The spleen and liver may become palpable. After some months, in the absence of treatment, the central nervous system is invaded. This is shown clinically by headache and changed behaviour, insomnia by night and sleepiness by day, mental confusion and eventually tremors, pareses, wasting, coma and death. The histological changes in the brain are similar to those found in viral encephalitis but trypanosomes are scattered in the substance of the brain and large mononuclear (morula) cells are found whose cytoplasm contains globules of IgM.

Rhodesiense infections

In these infections the disease is altogether more acute and severe than in gambiense infections, so that within days or a few weeks the patient is usually severely ill and may have developed pleural effusions and signs of myocarditis or hepatitis. There may be a petechial rash. The patient may die before there are signs of involvement of the central nervous system. If the illness is less acute, drowsiness, tremors and coma develop.

Investigations

Trypanosomiasis should be considered in any febrile patient from an endemic area. In rhodesiense infections thick and thin blood films, stained as for the detection of malaria, will reveal trypanosomes. The trypanosomes may be seen in the blood or from puncture of the primary lesion in the earliest stages of gambiense infections, but it is usually easier to demonstrate them by puncture of a lymph node. Concentration methods include buffy coat microscopy and miniature anion exchange chromatography. Animal inoculation is sometimes used for

Table 4.40 Comparison of the clinical and laboratory features of trypanosomiasis due to *T. rhodesiense* and *T. gambiense*

Feature	T. rhodesiense	T. gambiense
Incubation	7–14 days	Weeks–months
Onset	Abrupt	Insidious
Primary complex	Usual	Rare
Fever	High, swinging	Low grade
Early features	Effusions, hepatitis, myocarditis	Lymphadenopathy
Rash	Macular, petechial	Erythematous, circinate
Late features	Drowsiness, tremors, coma, death	Headache, insomnia, behavioural, tremors, paresis, wasting, coma
Duration of illness	Weeks or months	Months or years
Trypanosomes	Numerous in blood	Numerous in lymph node aspirate
Cerebrospinal fluid	Protein, cells, Trypanosomes	Protein, cells, Trypanosomes

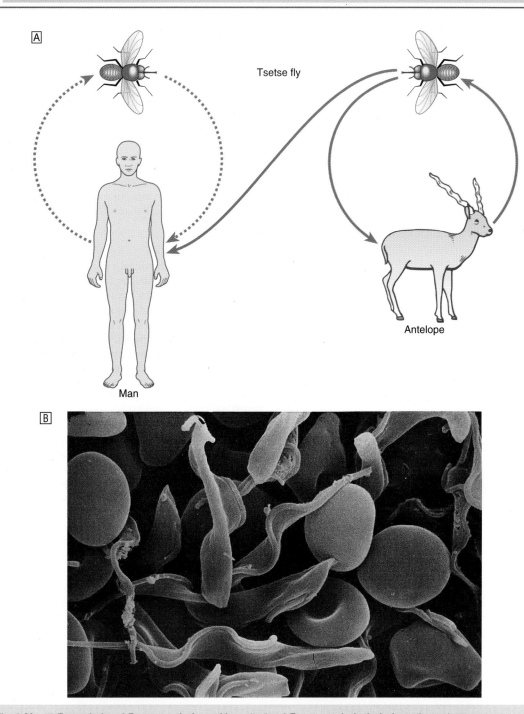

Fig. 4.38 Ⓐ **Transmission of *Trypanosomiasis gambiense*** (top) and ***Trypanosomiasis rhodesiense*** (bottom); Ⓑ **Scanning electron micrograph** showing trypanosomes swimming among erythrocytes.

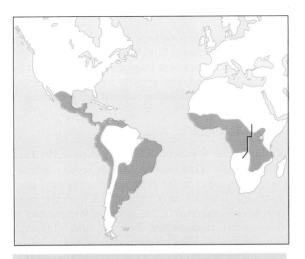

Fig 4.39 Endemic zones of American and African trypanosomiasis. Within these zones, the actual distribution may be patchy and variable. The vertical line in central Africa separates the distribution of *T. gambiense* (left) from *T. rhodesiense* (right).

the detection of rhodesiense infections. Serological tests are employed in field work.

If the central nervous system is affected the cell count and protein content of the CSF are increased and the glucose diminished. Sometimes trypanosomes may be found by centrifugation. Very high levels of serum IgM or the presence of IgM in the CSF are suggestive of trypanosomiasis.

Management

The prognosis is good if treatment is begun early before the brain has been invaded. At this stage either suramin

or pentamidine may be used, the latter being employed only for gambiense infections. After the nervous system is affected an arsenical or difluoromethyl ornithine will be required. Details are given in Table 4.41.

Prevention

A single intramuscular injection of 250 mg pentamidine gives protection against *T. gambiense* for 6 months because of the slow excretion of the drug. As the protection against *T. rhodesiense* is less sure and shorter in duration, chemoprophylaxis is not advised in rhodesiense areas. In endemic gambiense areas various measures may be taken against tsetse flies and field teams detect and treat early human infection. In rhodesiense areas control is difficult.

AMERICAN TRYPANOSOMIASIS (CHAGAS' DISEASE)

Chagas' disease occurs widely in South and Central America. The cause is *Trypanosoma cruzi* transmitted to man from the faeces of a reduviid bug in which the trypanosomes have a cycle of development before becoming infective to man. Bugs live in the mud and wattle walls and thatch roofs of simple rural houses, and emerge at night to feed on the sleeping occupants. While feeding they defecate. Infected faeces are rubbed in through the conjunctiva, mucosa of mouth or nose or abrasions of the skin. Over 100 species of mammals, domestic, peridomestic and wild, may serve as reservoirs of infection. In some areas blood transfusion accounts for about 5% of cases. Congenital transmission occurs occasionally.

Table 4.41 Chemotherapy of trypanosomiasis

Drug/route of administration	Dosage	Toxicity	Indications
Suramin, intravenous	Test dose 200 mg then 1 g in 10 ml water every 5 days, to total dose 5–6 g	Mild: proteinuria, arthralgia Severe: dermatitis, diarrhoea, nephritis (red cells and casts)	Rhodesiense and gambiense infection before CNS involvement
Pentamidine as base intramuscular	4 mg/kg, max 250 mg/dose alternate days for 10 doses	Collapse if injected intravenously, hypoglycaemia, nephritis, diabetes mellitus, injection abscess	As for suramin
Melarsoprol (Mel B) 3.6% in propylene glycol, intravenous	Three consecutive days/week for 4 weeks wk 1: 0.5 ml, 1 ml, 1 ml wk 2: 2.5 ml × 3 wk 3: 3.5 ml × 3 wk 4: 5 ml × 3	Jarisch–Herxheimer reaction, arsenical encephalopathy, mortality up to 10%*	Rhodesiense and gambiense disease after CNS involvement
Difluoromethyl ornithine intravenously	200–400 mg/kg daily × 4 wk	Diarrhoea, abdominal pain	Cerebral gambiense infections
Nitrofurazone orally	10 mg/kg 8-hourly × 10 days	Haemolysis, neuropathy	Resistance to arsenicals

* Toxicity is greatly reduced if the blood has been cleared of trypanosomes with suramin (test dose plus 1 g) a few days previously.

Pathology

The trypanosomes migrate via the blood-stream and develop into amastigote forms in the tissues. These multiply in many sites, especially in the myocardium causing pseudocysts, in smooth muscle fibres, and also in the ganglion cells of the autonomic nervous system.

Clinical features

The entrance of *T. cruzi* through an abrasion produces a dusky-red firm swelling and enlargement of regional lymph nodes. A conjunctival lesion, though less common, is more characteristic; the unilateral firm reddish swelling of the lids may close the eye and constitutes 'Romaña's sign'. Young children are most commonly affected. In a few patients an acute generalised infection soon appears, with fever, lymphadenopathy and enlargement of the spleen and liver. Neurological features include personality changes and signs of meningoencephalitis. The acute infection may be fatal to infants. In most patients the early infection is silent.

After a latent period of many years features of the chronic infection appear, notably damage to Auerbach's plexus with resulting dilatation of various parts of the alimentary canal, especially the colon and oesophagus, 'mega' disease. Dilatation of the bile ducts and bronchi are also recognised sequelae. Chronic low-grade myocarditis and damage to conducting fibres cause a cardiomyopathy characterised by cardiac dilatation, arrhythmias, partial or complete heart block and sudden death. Autoimmune processes may be responsible for much of the damage. There are geographical variations of the basic pattern of disease.

Investigations

T. cruzi may be seen in a blood film in the acute illness. In chronic disease it may be recovered by xenodiagnosis in which infection-free, laboratory-bred reduviid bugs are fed on the patient; subsequently the hind gut or faeces of the bug is examined for parasites. Complement fixation, direct agglutination and fluorescent antibody tests are positive in 95% of cases.

Management

Nifurtimox is given orally. The dose, which has to be carefully supervised to minimise toxicity while preserving parasiticidal activity, is as follows: for those under 10 years, 15–20 mg/kg; 10–17 years, 12.5–15 mg/kg; over 17 years, 8–10 mg/kg, for 90 days. Cure rates of 80% in acute disease and 90% of chronic disease are obtained, but established tissue damage is not reversed. Side-effects include anorexia, vomiting and epigastric pain; insomnia, headache, vertigo and excitability; myalgia and arthralgia; peripheral neuropathy. Surgery may be needed for 'mega' disease.

Prevention

Preventive measures include improving housing and destruction of reduviid bugs by spraying of houses with chlorinated hydrocarbon insecticides. Blood taken for transfusion in endemic areas is treated with gentian violet. Long-term resolution requires better housing.

TOXOPLASMOSIS

Toxoplasmosis is a world-wide infection caused by *Toxoplasma gondii*. Transmission from a mother infected during pregnancy to the fetus causes congenital toxoplasmosis. Infection after birth occurs from the ingestion of cysts excreted in the faeces of infected cats or from eating undercooked beef or lamb. Immunocompromised patients are particularly at risk.

Pathology

In the congenital form of the disease the organism is widespread in the central nervous system, eyes, heart, lungs and adrenals. If the infant survives, the parasite soon disappears from most organs except the central nervous system and retina. The brain shows areas of necrosis with cyst formation and patchy calcification; the spinal cord may be similarly affected. The organism commonly invades lymph nodes and spleen in the acquired disease, and less commonly liver and myocardium.

Clinical features

The manifestations in congenital infections are mainly cerebral. There may be hydrocephalus or microcephaly associated with convulsions, tremors or paralysis. Radiological examination may show patches of calcification in the brain. Microphthalmos, nystagmus and choroidoretinitis are common. The CSF is often xanthochromic with increased protein and mononuclear cells. An enlarged liver, jaundice, thrombocytopenia and purpura may also occur. Congenital infections are usually fatal, and if the child survives it is frequently disabled and blind.

Many acquired infections are symptomless. In the acute form there may be pneumonia with fever, cough, generalised aches and pains, profound malaise, a maculopapular rash and rarely jaundice and myocarditis. More chronic infections are often afebrile and there may be only enlargement of the lymph nodes with a lymphocytosis showing atypical mononuclear cells similar to those present in infectious mononucleosis. Toxoplasmosis is a cause of choroidoretinitis and uveitis in adults.

Latent toxoplasmosis may reactivate and cause encephalitis and necrosis of brain in immunocompromised patients especially in AIDS (p. 96).

Seronegative recipients of organ grafts may acquire the disease from seropositive donors.

Investigations

Serological tests are of value. Antibodies detectable by fluorescence or the dye test appear early in the disease and persist for years. Complement-fixing antibodies appear and decline more quickly. A rise in the titre of IgM antibodies indicates acute infection. Antibodies may not be detectable in adult ocular toxoplasmosis. Antibodies persisting in an infant beyond 6 months of age imply congenital toxoplasmosis. Biopsy material from a lymph node may be inoculated into mice, or show characteristic histological changes. Toxoplasma may be found in the CSF of immunocompromised patients.

Management

Most patients with acquired toxoplasmosis do not require specific therapy as the infection usually resolves spontaneously. Patients for whom treatment is essential include infants, the immunosuppressed and those with eye involvement. A combination of sulphadimidine 1 g 6-hourly and pyrimethamine in a single loading dose of 75 mg followed by 25 mg daily, both for 4 weeks, is given together with folic acid 10 mg daily. Blood count is monitored weekly.

Toxoplasmosis and pregnancy

A seronegative woman who acquires toxoplasmosis during pregnancy, is at risk of producing a damaged fetus, especially if infection takes place in the first trimester; termination should be considered. Those who are seropositive before becoming pregnant do not risk fetal damage.

FURTHER READING

Ahmed M, McAdam K P W J, Sturm A W et al 1992 Systemic manifestations of invasive amoebiosis. Clinical Infectious Diseases 15: 974–982

Bradley D 1995 Prophylaxis against malaria for travellers from the United Kingdom. British Medical Journal 310: 709–714

Farthing M J 1992 Giardia comes of age: progress in epidemiology, immunology and chemotherapy. Journal of Antimicrobial Chemotherapy 30: 563–566

Hall S M 1992 Congenital toxoplasmosis. British Medical Journal 305: 291–297

Hoffman S 1992 Diagnosis, treatment and prevention of malaria. Medical Clinics of North America 76: 1327–1355

Olliaro P L, Bryceson A D M 1993 Practical progress and new drugs for changing patterns of leishmaniasis. Parasitology Today 9: 323–328

Pépin J, Milord F 1994 The treatment of human African trypanosomiasis. Advances in Parasitology 33: 1–47

Tanowitz H B, Kirkhoff C V, Simon D 1992 Chagas' disease. Clinical Microbiological Reviews 5: 400–419

White N J, Ho M 1992 The pathophysiology of malaria. Advances in Parasitology 31: 83–173

DISEASES DUE TO HELMINTHS

Helminths cause much disease among man and domestic animals in the tropics and are a common cause of imported disease in temperate countries. Infections caused by the commoner helminths or worms are listed in the information box.

ZOOLOGICAL CLASSES OF HELMINTHS WHICH PARASITISE MAN

Trematodes or flukes
- Blood flukes: *Schistosoma haematobium, S. mansoni, S. japonicum*
- Lung flukes: *Paragonimus* species
- Hepatobiliary flukes: *Clonorchis sinensis, Opisthorcis felineus, Fasciola hepatica*
- Intestinal flukes: *Fasciolopsis buski*

Cestodes or tapeworms
- Intestinal tapeworms (adult stages): *Taenia saginata, Taenia solium, Diphyllobothrium latum, Didylidium caninum, Hymenolepis nana*
- Tissue-dwelling cysts or worms (larval stages): *Taenia solium* (cysticercosis), *Echinococcus granulosus* (hydatid disease), *Multiceps multiceps* (coenurus), *Diphyllobothrium mansoni* (sparganosis)

Nematodes or roundworms
- Intestinal human nematodes: *Enterobius vermicularis, Ascaris lumbricoides, Trichuris trichiura, Necator americanus, Ancylostoma duodenale, Strongyloides stercoralis, Capillaria philippinensis*
- Tissue-dwelling human nematodes: *Wuchereria bancrofti, Brugia malayi, Loa loa, Onchocerca volvulus* (all filarial worms), *Dracunculus medinensis* (guinea worm)
- Zoonotic nematodes: *Toxocara canis, Ancylostoma brasiliensis, Oesophagostomum* species, *Angiostrongylus cantonensis, Trichinella spiralis, Gnathostoma spinigerum, Anisakis marina*

The commonest parasitic helminth of humans in Britain is the nematode *Enterobius (Oxyuris) vermicularis* or threadworm. Other worms which may be acquired in Britain include the roundworms *Ascaris lumbricoides, Toxocara canis, Trichuris trichiura* (whipworm) *Trichinella spiralis, Taenia saginata* (beef tapeworm), *Echinococcus granulosus* causing hydatid disease, and *Fasciola hepatica*, the endemic fluke of sheep.

Helminths are the largest of human parasites. Inside a chitinous exoskeleton, they contain an efficient reproductive system that generates millions of eggs and may occupy most of the adult female or hermaphroditic worm. Nematodes and trematodes also have a mouth and intestinal tract but cestodes absorb food through the cuticle. Worms that live in the gut often have suckers or hooklets at the head end for attachment to the mucosa. They are all motile and this is essential for certain phases of their developmental cycle: e.g. the migration on grass of segments of *Taenia*, the emigration of threadworms through the anus to lay eggs, the penetration of human skin by infective hookworm larvae and the initial migratory phase of many helminths in man. But once established in their definitive site, adult worms are usually sedentary. All this is regulated by nervous and hormonal systems. A given species of helminth will only parasitise one genus or a small range of genera of higher animal hosts. It is not known what determines this selectivity, nor the worm's ability to migrate to its correct definitive site. Worms may be longlived, *Onchocerca* up to 15 years and *Schistosoma* over 30 years.

Many helminths have a complicated life cycle, often involving one or more intermediate host. Only *Strongyloides stercoralis* can complete its life cycle within man. Disease may be caused by invasive larval stages (e.g. Loeffler's syndrome), adult worms (e.g. hookworms) or their progeny, either eggs (e.g. schistosomiasis) or microfilariae (e.g. onchocerciasis). Adult worms may be present in the body for many years before, or without, producing disease. Sometimes larval stages that normally develop in intermediate hosts cause cystic disease in man (e.g. cysticercosis). Man may also suffer from invasion by larval stages of worms that normally only infect other animals (e.g. hydatid disease).

Eosinophilia is a characteristic feature of helmintic infections. The eosinophilic syndromes associated with them are summarised in the information box on page 180.

TREMATODE (FLUKE) INFECTIONS

Flukes are flat, usually oval-shaped worms, like a small thick leaf, although schistosomes are elongated. They attach with suckers. Adult worms live in pairs and produce eggs that are passed from the body in faeces, urine or sputum, according to the site of infection, which depends upon the species of fluke. The life cycles are complex and involve fresh water snails and sometimes an intermediate host that man must eat. Disease is caused by the inflammatory response, either to worms or to eggs in tissues.

SCHISTOSOMIASIS

Schistosomiasis (Bilharziasis) is one of the most important causes of morbidity in the tropics and is being spread by irrigation schemes. Schistosome eggs have been found in Egyptian mummies dated 1250 BC.

There are three species of the genus *Schistosoma* which commonly cause disease in man: *S. haematobium*, *S. mansoni* and *S. japonicum*. *S. haematobium* was discovered by Theodor Bilharz in Cairo in 1861 and the genus is sometimes called *Bilharzia* and the disease bilharziasis. The ovum is passed in the urine or faeces of infected individuals and gains access to fresh water where the ciliated miracidium inside it is liberated and enters its intermediate host, a species of fresh water snail, in which it multiplies. Large numbers of forktailed cercarie are then liberated into the water, where they may survive for 2 to 3 days. Cercariae can penetrate the skin or the mucous membrane of the mouth of their definitive host, man. They transform into schistosomulae and moult as they pass through the lungs and are carried by the blood stream to the liver and so to the portal vein where they mature (Fig. 4.40). The male worm is up to 20 mm in length and the more slender cylindrical female, usually enfolded longitudinally by the male, is rather longer. Within 4–6 weeks of infection they migrate to the venules draining the pelvic viscera where the females deposit ova.

Pathology

The pathological changes and symptoms depend on species and stage of infection (Table 4.42). Penetration of the skin by schistosomes not pathogenic in man in, for example, Scotland can produce a similar rash. Most of the disease is due to the passage of eggs through mucosa and to the granulomatous reaction to eggs deposited in tissues. The eggs of *S. haematobium* pass mainly through the wall of the bladder, but may also involve rectum, seminal vesicles, vagina, cervix and fallopian tubes. *S. mansoni* and *S. japonicum* eggs pass mainly through the wall of the lower bowel, or are carried to the liver. The most serious consequence, though rare, of the ectopic deposition of eggs is transverse myelitis and paraplegia. Granulomas are composed of macrophages, eosinophils, epithelioid and giant cells around an ovum. Later there is fibrosis and eggs calcify, often in sufficient numbers to become radiologically visible. Eggs of *S. haematobium*, and of the other two species after the development of portal hypertension, may reach the lungs.

Clinical features

During the early stages of infection there may be itching at the site of cercarial penetration lasting 1–2 days. After

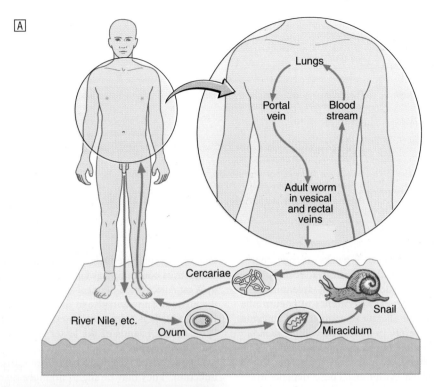

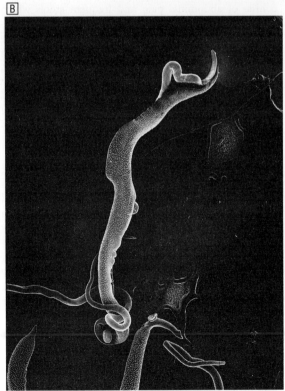

Fig. 4.40 Schistosoma. [A] Life cycle; [B] Scanning electron micrograph of adult schistosome worms showing the larger male worm embracing the thinner female.

Table 4.42 Pathogenesis of schistosomiasis

Stage	Time	S. haematobium	S. mansoni and S. japonicum
Cercarial penetration	Days	Papular dermatitis at site of penetration	As for S. haematobium
Larval migration and maturation	Weeks	Pneumonitis, myositis, hepatitis, fever, 'serum sickness', eosinophilia, seroconversion	As for S. haematobium
Early egg deposition	Months	Cystitis, haematuria	Colitis, granulomatous hepatitis, acute portal hypertension
		Ectopic granulomatous lesions: skin, CNS, etc. Immune complex glomerulonephritis	As for S. haematobium
Late egg deposition	Years	Fibrosis and calcification of ureters, bladder; bacterial infection, calculi, hydronephrosis, carcinoma	Colonic polyposis and strictures, periportal fibrosis, portal hypertension
		Pulmonary granulomas and pulmonary hypertension	As for S. haematobium

a symptom-free period of 3–5 weeks allergic manifestations may develop such as urticaria, eosinophilia, fever, muscle aches, abdominal pain, splenomegaly, headaches, cough and sweating. Patches of pneumonia may be present. These allergic phenomena (Katayama syndrome) may be severe in infections with *S. mansoni* and *S. japonicum* but are rare with *S. haematobium*. The features subside after 1–2 weeks and it may be 2 or 3 months before further symptoms. These depend upon the deposition of eggs, the intensity of infection, and the species of infecting schistosome.

Schistosomiasis haematobium

Man is the only natural host of *S. haematobium* which is highly endemic in Egypt, the east coast of Africa and the adjacent islands and occurs throughout most of Africa and in Iran, Iraq, Syria, Yemen, Lebanon and Israel. It also occurs in Turkey, Cyprus and in solitary foci in Portugal and the Maharashtra State of India (Fig. 4.41).

Painless terminal haematuria is usually the first and commonest symptom. Frequency of micturition follows, due to the contracted fibrosed or calcified bladder. Pain is often felt in the iliac fossa or in the loin and radiates to the groin. In advanced disease, pyelonephritis, hydronephrosis or pyonephrosis may lead to hypertension or uraemia. Disease of the seminal vesicles may lead to haemospermia. Females may be sterile and schistosomal lesions of the cervix may be mistaken for cancer. Intestinal symptoms may follow involvement of the bowel wall. Ectopic worms cause skin or cord lesions. The severity of *S. haematobium* infection varies greatly, and many with a light infection suffer little. However, as adult worms can live for 20 years or more and lesions may progress, these patients should always be treated.

Schistosomiasis mansoni

Man is the only natural host of importance, although the infection is also found in baboons. *S. mansoni* is endemic in the Nile Delta and Libya, Southern Sudan, East Africa continuing as far south as the Transvaal and in West Africa from Senegal and Gambia to Cameroun, throughout Zaire and also in the Arabian peninsula (see Fig. 4.41). It is found in Venezuela, Brazil and in the West Indian Islands of the lesser Antilles, Puerto Rico and Dominica.

Characteristic symptoms begin 2 months or later after infection. They may be slight, no more than malaise, or consist of abdominal pain and frequent stools which contain blood-stained mucus. With severe advanced disease increased discomfort from rectal polypi may be experienced. The early hepatomegaly is reversible but portal hypertension may cause massive splenomegaly, fatal haematemesis from oesophageal varices, or progressive ascites. Jaundice and hepatic failure are uncommon. *S. mansoni* infections predispose to the carriage of Salmonella.

Schistosomiasis japonicum

The adult worm infects, in addition to man, the dog, rat, field mouse, water buffalo, ox, cat, pig, horse and sheep. *S. japonicum* is prevalent in the Yellow River and Yangste-Kiang basins in China where the infection is a major public health problem. It also has a focal distribution in Japan, the Philippines, Celebes, and Vietnam. A related parasite, *S. mekongi*, occurs in Laos, Thailand and the Shan States of Myanmar, formerly Burma. The pathology of *S. japonicum* is similar to that of *S. mansoni* but as this worm produces more eggs the lesions tend to be more extensive and widespread. The clinical features resemble those of severe infection with *S. mansoni*, with added neurological features. The small bowel as well as the large may be affected, and hepatic fibrosis with splenic enlargement is usual. Deposition of eggs or worms in the central nervous system, especially in the brain, causes symptoms in about 5% of infections, notably epilepsy, hemiplegia, blindness and paraplegia.

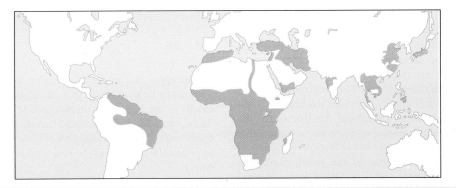

Fig. 4.41 Geographical distribution of schistosomiasis.

Investigations

A history of residence in an endemic area, with characteristic symptoms, will indicate the need for investigation. In *S. haematobium* infection dip-stick urine testing shows blood and albumin. The terminal spined eggs can usually be found by microscopic examination of the centrifuged deposit of terminal stream urine, especially after exercise. The eggs may also be found by a microscopic examination of the stools or of a 'rectal snip', taken by snipping a piece of rectal mucosa with a small curette against the proctoscope. The snip is examined fresh; live and dead ova are easily identified. A radiograph may indicate calcification of the wall of the bladder while intravenous urography or ultrasound scanning may show stenosis or dilatation of the ureters, reduction in capacity of the bladder, or hydronephrosis. Cystoscopy reveals 'sandy' patches, bleeding mucosa and later distortion.

In a heavy infection with *S. mansoni* or *S. japonicum* the characteristic egg with its lateral spine can usually be found in the stool. When the infection is light, or of long duration, a rectal snip can be examined. Sigmoidoscopy may show inflammation or bleeding. Biopsies should be examined for ova. Serological tests (enzyme-linked immunosorbent assay or immuno-fluorescence) are useful as screening tests but the diagnosis rests on demonstration of ova. The bowel symptoms and barium enema appearances of *S. mansoni* and *S. japonicum* infection may resemble those of amoebiasis or a neoplasm of the large bowel.

Management

The object of specific treatment is to kill the adult schistosomes and so stop egg laying. It may not be possible or desirable to kill all adult worms by mass treatment campaigns in communities where reinfection is likely, but a reduction in egg output of around 90% is often achieved which significantly reduces morbidity, and pos-

sibly transmission, without impairing what little acquired immunity there may be. Details of the drugs used are given in Table 4.43.

- **Praziquantel**. This is normally the drug of choice for all forms of schistosomiasis. Side-effects are uncommon and mild, and include nausea, headache, giddiness and drowsiness.
- **Oxamniquine**. This is safe in the chronic hepatic forms of the disease though it may cause fever for a few days.
- **Metrifonate**. This is an organophosphorus inhibitor of cholinesterase, and paralyses the worm. Higher or more frequent doses than those given in the Table cause abdominal pain, nausea or vomiting.

Surgery may be required to deal with residual lesions but large vesical granulomas usually respond well to chemotherapy. Ureteric stricture and the small fibrotic urinary bladder may require plastic procedures. Removal of rectal papillomas by diathermy or by other means may provide relief. Granulomatous masses in the brain or spinal cord may require neurosurgery if the manifestations do not respond to chemotherapy and corticosteroids.

Table 4.43 Drugs used in the treatment of schistosomiasis

Infection	Praziquantel*	Oxamniquine	Metrifonate
S. mansoni	30 mg/kg twice in one day	15 mg/kg 12-hourly for 2 days	Not useful
S. japonicum	40 mg/kg once	Not useful	Not useful
S. haematobium	40 mg/kg once	Not useful	7.5 mg/kg every 2 wks × 3

* Doses quoted give cure rates of about 90% and reduce egg excretion by over 99%, and are used in mass campaigns and in primary health care centres. A dose of 10 mg/kg 8-hourly × 3 days gives a cure rate of virtually 100% for all three species.

Prevention

This presents great difficulties and so far no satisfactory single means of controlling schistosomiasis has been established. The life-cycle is terminated if the ova in urine or faeces are not allowed to contaminate fresh water containing the snail host. The provision of latrines and of a safe water supply, however, remains a major problem in rural areas throughout the tropics. In the case of *S. japonicum*, moreover, there are so many hosts besides man that the proper use of latrines would be of little avail. Mass treatment of the population helps against *S. haematobium* and *S. mansoni* but this method has so far had little success with *S. japonicum*. Attack on the intermediate host, the snail, presents many difficulties and has not on its own proved successful on any scale. For personal protection, contact with infected water must be avoided. Accidental immersion or contact should be followed by a shower and vigorous towelling. Storage of water for three days will usually kill cercariae.

PARAGONIMIASIS (ENDEMIC HAEMOPTYSIS)

There are several species of the flukes of the genus *Paragonimus* which may affect man, the commonest being *P. westermani*. The adult flukes measuring 10×6 mm live in small 'nests' in the lung and elsewhere. The sputum contains ova, which may be expectorated or swallowed and passed in the faeces. Myracidia emerge in water from these eggs and seek the first intermediate host, a freshwater snail. Larvae emerging from the snail encyst as metacercariae in freshwater crabs or crayfish. Man or certain other mammals become infected if they eat these crustacea raw or inadequately cooked. Human infec-

tions are most frequent in the Far East but there are also endemic foci in South America, West Africa, Somalia and India.

Pathology

The adults lie in cysts up to 1 cm in diameter, situated chiefly in the lung and containing reddish-brown fluid. There are seldom more than 20 such cysts present. In heavy infections, cysts may also be present in the pleural or peritoneal cavities, in the brain, muscles, skin or elsewhere.

Clinical features

The first symptoms are slight fever, cough and the expectoration of brown or black sputum. Occasionally there are bouts of frank haemoptysis with severe pain in the chest. Increasing clinical signs in the chest may simulate pneumonia or pulmonary tuberculosis which may coexist. When the parasites lodge in the abdomen there may be symptoms of enteritis or hepatitis. If they settle in the abdominal wall they may produce sinuses which discharge through the skin. Cysts in the central nervous system may cause signs of cerebral irritation, encephalitis or myelitis. The disease may be extremely chronic as the adult worms may survive for 20 years.

Investigations

Ova may be found on microscopic examination of the faeces, sputum or a discharge. The radiological appearances of affected lungs are variable but the lesions are usually situated close to the pleural surfaces. Extrapulmonary lesions are diagnosed by biopsy.

Table 4.44 Diseases caused by flukes in the bile duct

Disease	Clonorchiasis	Opisthorciasis	Fascioliasis
Parasite	*Clonorchis sinensis*	*Opisthorcis felineus*	*Fasciola hepatica*
Other mammalian hosts	Dogs, cats, pigs	Dogs, cats, foxes, pigs	Sheep, cattle
Mode of spread	Ova in faeces, water	As for *C. sinensis*	Ova in faeces onto wet pasture
1st intermediate host	Snails	Snails	Snails
2nd intermediate host	Freshwater fish	Freshwater fish	Encysts on vegetation
Geographical distribution	Far East, esp. S. China	Far East, esp. N.E. Thailand	Cosmopolitan, incl. UK
Pathology	*E. coli* cholangitis, abscesses, biliary carcinoma	As for *C. sinensis*	Toxaemia, cholangitis, eosinophilia
Symptoms	Often symptom-free, recurrent jaundice	As for *C. sinensis*	Obscure fever, tender liver, may be ectopic, e.g. subcut fluke
Diagnosis	Ova in stool or duodenal aspirate	As for *C. sinensis*	As for *C. sinensis*; also immunofluorescence
Prevention	Cook fish	Cook fish	Avoid contaminated watercress
Treatment	Praziquantel 25 mg/kg 8-hourly for 2 days	As for *C. sinensis* but 1 day only	Triclabendazole 12 mg/kg. Two single doses 2 days apart*

* In UK available from the Hospital for Tropical Diseases, London..

Management

Praziquantel is given in a dose of 25 mg/kg twice daily for 2 days orally. Lesions localised to or maximal in one lobe of a lung may be treated surgically.

Prevention

In an endemic area crab or crayfish should not be eaten unless adequately cooked. Immersion of crustaceans in wine, vinegar or brine does not kill the parasites.

LIVER FLUKES

Table 4.44 sets out the main features of the diseases caused by flukes which infect the bile ducts of man. In the Far East and S.E. Asia, liver flukes are an important cause of ill-health.

CESTODE (TAPEWORM) INFECTIONS

Cestodes are ribbon-shaped worms which inhabit the intestinal tract. They have no alimentary system and absorb nutrients through the segmental surface. The anterior end, or scolex, is provided with suckers for attachment to the host. From the scolex arises a series of progressively developing segments, the proglottides, which when shed may continue to show active movements. Cross-fertilisation takes place between segments. Ova, present in large numbers in mature proglottides, remain viable for weeks and during this period they may be consumed by the intermediate host. Larvae liberated from the ingested ova pass into the tissues.

Man acquires tapeworm by eating undercooked beef infected with *Cysticercus bovis*, the larval stage of *Taenia saginata* (beef tapeworm), undercooked pork containing *Cysticercus cellulosae*, the larval stage of *T. solium* (pork tapeworm), or undercooked freshwater fish containing larvae of *Diphyllobothrium latum* (fish tapeworm). Usually only one adult tapeworm is present in the gut but up to 10 have been reported. The life-cycles of *Diphyllobothrium mansoni*, *Dipylidium caninum* and *Hymenolepsis nana* are different (Table 4.45). *Echinococcus granulosus* is a tapeworm of dogs.

TAENIA SAGINATA

This worm may be several metres long. The scolex, the size of a pin head, has four suckers; mature segments, 1.3 cm × 1 cm, contain a central stemmed uterus with lateral branches which are easily seen if the segments are left in water for 24 hours. The ova of both *T. saginata* and *T. solium* are indistinguishable microscopically. Infection with *T. saginata* occurs in all parts of the world. The adult worm produces little or no intestinal upset in human beings, but knowledge of its presence, by noting segments in the faeces or on underclothing, may distress the patient. Ova may be found in the stool.

Praziquantel is the drug of choice (Table 4.45), and prevention depends on efficient meat inspection and the thorough cooking of beef.

TAENIA SOLIUM AND CYSTICERCOSIS

T. solium, the pork tapeworm, is common in Central Europe, South Africa, South America and in parts of Asia. It is not so large as *T. saginata*. The scolex has, in addition to suckers, two circular rows of hooklets anterior to the suckers. The adult worm is found only in man following the eating of undercooked pork containing cysticerci.

Human cysticercosis

This results from ova being swallowed or gaining access to the human stomach by regurgitation from the person's own adult worm (Fig. 4.42). The larvae are liberated from eggs in the stomach, penetrate the intestinal

---

Table 4.45 Essential features of the less common tapeworm infections of man

Species	Geography	Definitive host	Intermediate host(s)	Stage and site in man	Clinical features
Multiceps multiceps	E. + S. Africa	Dog	Sheep	Larval cysts/brain	CNS
Diphyllobothrium latum	Scandinavia Asia	Fish-eating mammals	*Cyclops* Fish *Diaptomus*	Adult worm/gut	Nil *or* megaloblastic anaemia
Diphyllothrium mansoni	Africa Far East	Cats and dogs	*Cyclops*, frogs, snakes	Sparaganum/various	Subcutaneous swellings
Dipylidium caninum	World-wide	Dogs and cats	Flea	Adult worm/gut	Ova in faeces
Hymenolepsis nana	World-wide	Man	None	Adult worm/gut	Ova in faeces

Treatment of intestinal tapeworms is with praziquantel 20 mg/kg once, or niclosamide (1 g repeated after 2 h). Treatment of larval cysts and sparganosis is surgical.

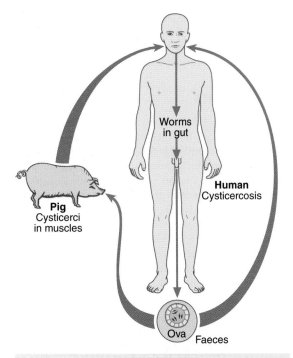

Fig. 4.42 **Cysticercosis.** Life cycle of *Taenia solium*.

mucosa and are carried to many parts of the body where they develop and form cysticerci, 0.5–1 cm cysts that contain the head of a young worm. They do not grow further or migrate. Common locations are the subcutaneous tissue, skeletal muscles and brain.

Clinical features

When superficially placed, cysts can be palpated under the skin or mucosa as pea-like ovoid bodies. Here they cause few or no symptoms, and will eventually die and become calcified.

Heavy brain infections, especially in children, may cause features of encephalitis. More commonly, however, cerebral signs do not occur until the larvae die, 5–20 years later. Epilepsy, personality changes, staggering gait or signs of internal hydrocephalus are the most common features.

Investigations

Calcified cysts in muscles can be recognised radiologically. In the brain, however, less calcification takes place and larvae are only occasionally demonstrated radiologically but usually by computed tomography. Epileptic fits starting in adult life should suggest the possibility of cysticercosis if the patient has lived or travelled in an endemic area. The subcutaneous tissue should be palpated and any nodule excised for histology.

Radiological examination of the skeletal muscles may be helpful. A fluorescent antibody test is usually positive, but is only genus-specific.

Management

Praziquantel is the drug of choice (Table 4.45). It improves the prognosis of cerebral cysticercosis; the dose is 50 mg/kg in 3 divided doses daily for 10 days. Prednisolone, 10 mg every 8 hours, is also given for 14 days, starting one day before the praziquantel. In addition, antiepileptic drugs should be given until the reaction in the brain has subsided. Operative intervention is indicated for hydrocephalus.

Prevention

Prevention of *T. solium* infection consists in cooking pork well. Cysticercosis is avoided if food is not contaminated by ova or segments. Patients with pork tapeworm probably acquire cysticercosis by ingesting ova from contaminated fingers, rather than from regurgitation of segments. Great care must be taken by nurses and other adults while attending a patient harbouring an adult worm.

ECHINOCOCCUS GRANULOSUS (TAENIA ECHINOCOCCUS) AND HYDATID DISEASE

The dog and certain wild canines are the definitive host of the tiny tapeworm *E. granulosus*. The larval stage, a hydatid cyst, normally occurs in sheep, cattle, camels and other animals that are infected from contaminated pastures or water. Man, by handling a dog or drinking contaminated water, may ingest eggs (Fig. 4.43). The embryo is liberated from the ovum in the small intestine and gains access to the blood stream and thus to the liver. The resultant cyst grows very slowly, sometimes intermittently, and may outlive the patient. It may calcify or may rupture giving rise to multiple cysts. The disease is common in the Middle East and North and East Africa, Australia and Argentina. Foci of infection persist in rural Wales and Scotland. A variant, *E. multilocularis*, which has a cycle between foxes and voles, causes a similar but more severe infection, 'alveococcosis' which invades the liver like cancer.

Clinical features

A hydatid cyst is typically acquired in childhood and it may, after growing for some years, cause pressure symptoms. These vary, depending on the organ or tissue involved. In nearly 75% of patients with hydatid disease the right lobe of the liver is invaded and contains a single cyst. In others a cyst may be found in lung, bone, brain or elsewhere.

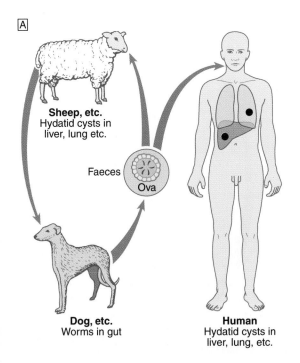

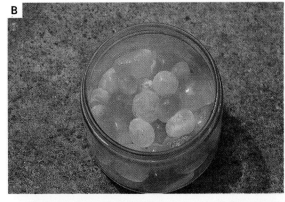

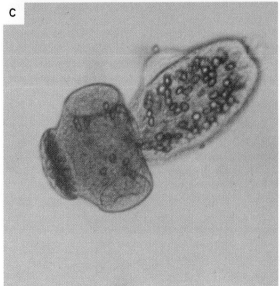

Fig. 4.43 Hydatid disease. A Life cycle of *Echinococcus granulosus*. B Daughter cysts removed at surgery. Within them are the protoscolices shown in C.

Investigations

The diagnosis depends on the clinical, radiological and ultrasound findings in a patient who has lived in close contact with dogs in an endemic area. Complement-fixation, immunofluorescent tests and enzyme-linked immunosorbent assay are positive in 70–90% of patients.

Management

Hydatid cysts should be excised wherever possible. Great care is taken to avoid spillage and cavities are sterilised with 0.5% silver nitrate or 2.7% sodium chloride. Albendazole (400 mg 12-hourly for 1–3 months) has been used for inoperable disease, and to reduce the infectivity of cysts preoperatively. Praziquantel 10 mg/kg 8-hourly for 2 weeks kills protoscolices peri-operatively.

Prevention

Prevention is difficult in situations where there is a close association with dogs and sheep. Personal hygiene, sat- isfactory disposal of carcases, meat inspection and de-worming of dogs can greatly reduce the prevalence of disease.

OTHER TAPEWORMS

There are many other cestodes whose adult or larval stages may infect man, the commonest of which are summarised in Table 4.45. Sparganosis is a condition in which an immature worm develops in man, usually subcutaneously, as a result of eating or applying to the skin the secondary or tertiary intermediate host.

NEMATODE (ROUNDWORM) INFECTIONS

Nematode infections of man may be divided into three groups: see the information box on page 163.

171

Intestinal nematodes

The commonest that cause disease are listed in the information box.

Adult male and female worms live in the lumen of the gut and do not normally invade tissues. They often have complex life cycles and may cause a syndrome of fever, cough and eosinophilia during the stage of larval invasion. Eggs or larvae are passed in the faeces and the worm does not normally complete its life-cycle in man. Strongyloides, however, behaves differently and is potentially dangerous.

Tissue-dwelling human nematodes

These are the filarial worms and the guinea worm *Dracunculus medinensis*.

These worms have complex life-cycles, with an intermediate host that is also a vector. Disease may be due to the presence of the adult worms or to their progeny, the microfilariae, which migrate in the blood or tissues, provoking a massive eosinophilia; but often the infection is long lived and well tolerated.

Zoonotic nematodes

Nematodes that normally infect other animals may cause serious incidental infections in man.

The infective larvae of these worms are unable to 'home' to their normal site for development into adults, in their abnormal host. They may wander or may become trapped in a particular organ. They tend to provoke severe inflammatory reactions characterised by eosinophilic granulomas.

ENTEROBIUS VERMICULARIS (THREADWORM)

This helminth is common throughout the world. It affects children especially. The male worm is 2–5 mm long and the female 8–13 mm. After the ova are swallowed, development takes place in the small intestine, but the adult worms are found chiefly in the colon.

Clinical features

The gravid female worm lays ova around the anus, and causes intense itching, especially at night. The ova are often carried to the mouth on the fingers and so reinfection takes place (Fig. 4.44). In females the genitalia may be involved. The adult worms may be seen moving on the buttocks or in the stool.

Investigations

Ova are detected by applying the adhesive surface of cellophane tape to the perianal skin in the morning. This is then examined on a glass slide under the microscope.

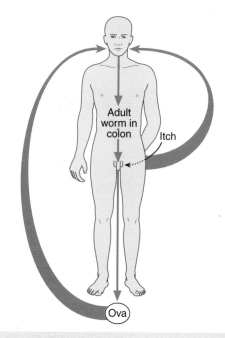

Fig. 4.44 **Threadworm.** Life cycle of *Enterobius vermicularis.*

Management

A single dose of one of the drugs in Table 4.46 is given and repeated after 2 weeks to control auto-reinfection. Where infection constantly recurs in a family, each member should be treated with mebendazole 100 mg twice daily for 3 days repeated after 10 days. During this period all night clothes and bed linen are laundered and finger nails must be scrubbed before meals.

ASCARIS LUMBRICOIDES (ROUNDWORM)

This pale yellow worm is 20–35 cm long. Man is infected by eating food contaminated with mature ova. These hatch in the duodenum and the larvae migrate through the lungs, where they moult, ascend the bronchial tree and are swallowed. They mature in the small intestine. In heavy infections, larvae in the lung may cause pneumonitis and eosinophilia.

Clinical features

Adult worms commonly cause abdominal discomfort or colic and may be vomited or passed per rectum. A tangled mass of worms may cause intestinal obstruction and heavy infestation will compete for nourishment and contribute to malnutrition. Other complications include blockage of the bile or pancreatic duct and obstruction of the appendix by adult worms.

Table 4.46   Relative activity of drugs used for the common gut nematodes

	Ascaris	Hookworm	Enterobius	Trichuris	Strongyloides
Piperazine salts 100 mg/kg	+++	+	+++	−	−
Pyrantel pamoate 10 mg/kg	+++	++	+++	−	−
Oxantel pamoate 10 mg/kg	−	−	−	+++	−
Mebendazole 100 mg (any age)	++	++	+++	++	+
Albendazole 400 mg	++	++	+	+	++
Thiabendazole 25 mg/kg	(++)	(++)	(++)	(+)	+++
Levamisole 5 mg/kg	+++	+	+	−	−
Pyrvinium 5 mg/kg	+	−	+++	−	−

Size of a single dose is given. + = quite effective, ++ = effective, +++ = very effective therapy; − = ineffective. Activities given in parenthesis indicate that the drug is not used for that species. Piperazine is cheap and safe, but with a limited range. Mebendazole given twice daily for 3 days is completely safe and eradicates most infections. Thiabendazole has a wide spectrum: it is absorbed and effective against many tissue-dwelling nematodes, but toxic, causing dizziness, headaches, anorexia, vomiting and drowsiness. A single dose antihelmintic is ideal for mass treatment and control schemes. Levamisole is the first choice for roundworms, and has a useful action against hookworms. A single dose of pyrantel pamoate and oxantel pamoate or of albendazole is used for multiple infections. (Adapted from Knight R 1982 Parasitic disease in man. Churchill Livingstone, Edinburgh.)

Investigations

The diagnosis is made microscopically by finding ova in the faeces or by observing an adult worm. A solely male infection is usually revealed only after the giving of an antihelmintic to a patient with an unexplained eosinophilia. Occasionally the worms are demonstrated radiographically by a barium examination.

Management

The appropriate drugs are listed in Table 4.46. Surgery is required if obstruction occurs and fails to respond to nasogastric suction and sedation.

TRICHURIS TRICHIURA (WHIPWORM)

Infections with whipworm are common all over the world under unhygienic conditions. Infection takes place by the ingestion of earth or food contaminated with ova which have become infective after lying for 3 weeks or more in moist soil. The adult worm is 3–5 cm long and has a coiled anterior end resembling a whip. Whipworms inhabit the caecum, lower ileum, appendix, colon and anal canal. There are usually no symptoms, but intense infections in children may cause persistent diarrhoea or rectal prolapse, and stunting. The diagnosis is readily made by identifying ova in faeces. Treatment is with mebendazole in doses of 100 mg twice daily for 3–5 days or a single dose of oxantel (Table 4.46).

ANCYLOSTOMIASIS (HOOKWORM)

Ancylostomiasis is caused by parasitisation of the small intestine with *Ancylostoma duodenale* or *Necator americanus*. It is one of the main causes of anaemia in the tropics. The adult hookworm is a greyish-white nematode about 1 cm long which lives, often in large numbers, in the duodenum and upper jejunum. Eggs are passed in the faeces. In warm, moist, shady soil the larvae develop and reach the filariform infective stage which penetrate human skin and are carried to the lungs (Fig. 4.45). After entering the alveoli they ascend the bronchi, are swallowed and develop in the small intestine, reaching maturity 4–7 weeks after infection.

Hookworm infection is widespread under insanitary conditions in the tropics and subtropics and used to be common in mines in Europe. *A. duodenale* is endemic in the Far East and Mediterranean coastal regions and is also present in Africa while *N. americanus* is endemic in West, East and Central Africa and Central and South America as well as in the Far East.

Pathology

The larvae may cause allergic inflammation at the site of entry through the skin. When infection is heavy, the passage through the lungs may cause pulmonary eosinophilia. The worms attach themselves to the mucosa of the small intestine by their buccal capsule (Fig 4.46) and withdraw blood. The mean daily loss of blood from one *A. duodenale* is 0.15 ml and for *N. americanus* 0.03 ml. The degree of iron and protein deficiency which develops depends not only on the load of worms but also on the nutrition of the patient and especially on the iron stores. Thus in a light infection there may be no anaemia. In the early stages of infection eosinophilia is common.

Clinical features

Dermatitis usually on the feet (ground itch) may be experienced at the time of infection. The passage of the

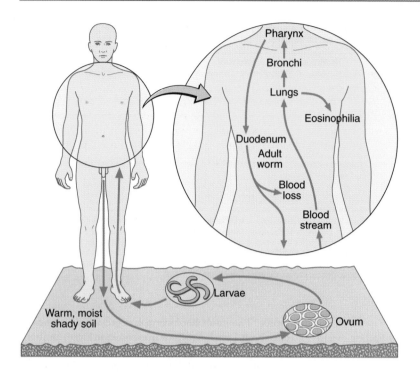

Fig. 4.45 Ancylostomiasis.
Life cycle.

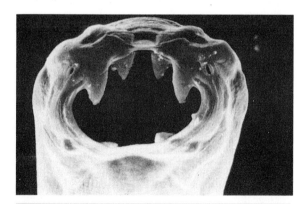

Fig. 4.46 *Ancylostoma duodenale:* electron micrograph
showing the ventral teeth.

larvae through the lungs in a heavy infection causes a
paroxysmal cough with blood-stained sputum, associated with patchy pulmonary consolidation. When the
worms have reached the small intestine, vomiting and
epigastric pain resembling peptic ulcer disease may
ensue. Sometimes frequent loose stools are passed, the
condition then resembling early sprue or giardiasis. Anaemia and hypoproteinaemia may develop in the undernourished. The mental and physical development of

children may be retarded. There may be no symptoms
in a well-nourished person with a light infection.

Investigations
The characteristic ovum can be recognised in the stool.
If hookworms are present in numbers sufficient to cause
anaemia, tests of the stool for occult blood will be positive and ova will be present in large numbers.

Management
This is listed in Table 4.46. Mebendazole twice daily for
3 days is preferred, but for single dose treatment pyrantel
is the best choice. Anaemia associated with hookworm
infection responds well to oral iron. When anaemia is
severe enough to cause heart failure, blood should be
transfused slowly, adding frusemide 20 mg to each unit.

STRONGYLOIDIASIS

Strongyloides stercoralis is a very small nematode (2
mm × 0.4 mm) which parasitises the mucosa of the
upper part of the small intestine, often in large numbers.
The eggs hatch in the bowel but only larvae are passed
in the faeces. In moist soil they moult and become the
infective filariform larvae. After penetrating human skin

they undergo a development cycle similar to that of hookworms but the female worms burrow into the mucosa and submucosa. Some larvae in the intestine may develop into filariform larvae which may then penetrate the mucosa or the perianal skin and lead to autoinfection and a very persistent infection. Man is the natural host but dogs may also be infected. Strongyloidiasis occurs in the tropics and subtropics and is especially prevalent in the Far East.

Pathology

There may be a dermatitis at the time of entry of the larval worms. In the intestine female worms burrow into the mucosa and induce an inflammatory reaction; with heavy infections the mucosa may be severely damaged leading to malabsorption. Granulomatous changes, necrosis, and even perforation and peritonitis may occur. Eosinophilia commonly persists. Actively motile larvae are passed in the faeces. Immunosuppression may cause fatal systemic strongyloidiasis.

Clinical features

These are shown in the information box below.

Systemic strongyloidiasis occurs in association with immune suppression (intercurrent disease, HTLV1 infection, corticosteroid treatment) and is rapidly fatal unless diagnosed and promptly treated.

CLINICAL FEATURES OF STRONGYLOIDIASIS

- **Penetration of skin by infective larvae**
  Itchy rash
- **Presence of worms in gut**
  Abdominal pain, diarrhoea, steatorrhoea, weight loss
- **Allergic phenomena**
  Urticarial plaques and papules, wheezing, arthralgia
- **Auto-infection**
  Transient itchy linear urticarial wheals across abdomen and buttocks (larva currens)
- **Systemic (super-) infection**
  Diarrhoea, pneumonia, meningoencephalitis, death

Investigations

Motile larvae can be seen on microscopic examination of the faeces and occasionally in the sputum. Excretion is intermittent so repeated examinations or jejunal aspiration or a string test (p. 155) may be necessary. Filarial serology is positive in 15% of patients.

Management

Albendazole is given orally in a dose of 15 mg/kg body weight twice daily for 3 days. A second course may be required. For systemic strongyloidiasis the drug is administered by nasogastric tube for a longer period.

Prevention of intestinal nematode infections

Most of these worms are transmitted through contaminated soil or unwashed hands. Safe disposal of faeces, the provision of clean drinking water and strict personal hygiene form the basis of control. Mass treatment at yearly intervals is also useful (Table 4.46). Capillariasis is prevented by cooking fish.

FILARIASES

Several nematodes of the family *Filarioidea* infect man. Larval stages are inoculated by biting flies, each specific to a particular filarial species. The larvae develop into adult worms (2–50 cm long) which, after mating, produce millions of microfilariae (170–320 microns long) that migrate in blood or skin. The life cycle is completed when the flies take up microfilariae while feeding on man. Man is normally the only host.

Disease is due to the host's immune response to the worms, particularly dying worms, and its pattern and severity vary with the site and stage of each species (Table 4.47). The worms are long-lived; microfilariae survive 2–3 years and adult worms 10–15 years. The infections are chronic and worst in individuals constantly exposed to reinfection. Filarial infections cause the highest eosinophilia of all helmintic infections, and are normally diagnosed by the morphology of the microfilariae.

LYMPHATIC FILARIASIS

Wuchereria bancrofti is conveyed to man by the bites of infected mosquitoes of a number of different species, the most common being *Culex fatigans*. The adult worms, 4–10 cm in length, live in the lymphatics, and the females produce microfilariae which at night circulate in large

---

Table 4.47 Pathology of filarial infections depends upon the site and stage of worms

Worm species	Adult worm	Microfilariae	
Wuchereria bancrofti and *Brugia malayi*	Lymphatic vessels[+++]	Blood[−]	Pulmonary capillaries[++]
Loa Loa	Subcutaneous[+]	Blood[+]	
Onchocerca volvulus	Subcutaneous[+]	Skin[+++]	Eye[+++]
Mansonella perstans	Retroperitoneal[−]	Blood[−]	
Mansonella streptocerca	Skin[+]	Skin[++]	

[+++] = severe, [++] = moderate, [+] = mild, [−] = rarely pathogenic.

numbers in the peripheral blood. In the mosquito, ingested microfilariae develop into infective larvae. As *Culex fatigans* bites at night the nocturnal periodicity of the microfilariae facilitates the spread of the infection. There is a non-periodic strain of *W. bancrofti* in some of the Pacific Islands, maintained by mosquitoes which bite in the daytime. The microfilariae are chiefly in the capillaries in the lungs when not circulating in the peripheral blood. The infection is widespread in tropical Africa, the North African coast, coastal areas of Asia, Indonesia and Northern Australia, South Pacific Islands, the West Indies and also in North and South America.

Brugia malayi resembles *W. bancrofti* closely. The microfilariae usually exhibit nocturnal periodicity. The vectors are mosquitoes mostly belonging to the genus *Mansonioides*. *B. malayi* is found in Indonesia, Borneo, Malaysia, Vietnam, South China, South India and Sri Lanka. A distinct, closely related species, *B. timori* occurs in Timor.

Pathology

The presence of adult worms in the lymphatics causes allergic lymphangitis (Table 4.47). Recurrent episodes may lead to intermittent lymphatic obstruction and transient lymphoedema, which may later become permanent in the leg, arm, genitalia or breast; and hydrocoele. Obstructed lymphatics become dilated and tortuous and may rupture. Rupture into tissues leads to cellulitis, fibrosis and elephantiasis. Increased lymphatic pressure may cause retrograde flow or rupture, in turn causing chyluria, chylous ascites and chylous pleural effusions (Fig. 4.47). The incubation period is not less than 3 months.

Clinical features

There are bouts of fever accompanied by pain, tenderness and erythema along the course of inflamed lymphatic vessels. Inflammation of the spermatic cord, epididymitis and orchitis is common. The fever abates after a few days and the symptoms and signs subside.

Further attacks follow, temporary oedema becomes more persistent, and regional lymph nodes enlarge. Progressive enlargement, coarsening, corrugation and fissuring of the skin and subcutaneous tissue with warty superficial excrescences develops gradually, causing irreversible 'elephantiasis'. The scrotum may reach an enormous size. Chyluria and chylous effusions are milky and opalescent; on standing, fat globules rise to the top. Eventually the adult worms may die but the lymphatics remain obstructed. The interval between infection and the onset of elephantiasis is usually not less than 10 years and elephantiasis develops only in association with repeated infections in highly endemic areas.

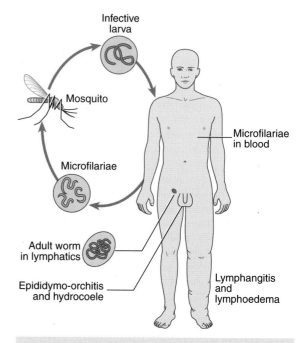

Fig. 4.47 ***Wuchereria bancrofti* and *Brugia malayi*.** Life cycle and pathogenesis of lymphatic filariasis.

Tropical pulmonary eosinophilia

Occasionally, and especially in Indians, microfilariae become trapped in the pulmonary capillaries and destroyed by allergic inflammation. The resulting pneumonitis causes persistent cough, fever, weight loss and radiological changes suggestive of miliary tuberculosis.

Non-filarial elephantiasis

Usually affecting one or both legs, this occurs in certain geographical areas which are free from filariasis. It is attributable to damage to lymphatics by silicates absorbed from soil derived from volcanic rocks.

Investigations

In the earliest stages of lymphangitis the diagnosis is made on clinical grounds, supported by eosinophilia and sometimes by positive serology. Microfilariae appear in the blood at night after about a year from the time of infection and can be seen moving in a wet blood film or by microfiltration of a sample of lysed blood. They are usually present in hydrocoele fluid which may occasionally yield an adult filaria. By the time elephantiasis develops microfilariae become difficult to find. Calcified filariae may sometimes be demonstrable by radiography. An initial exaggeration of symptoms following the administration of diethylcarbamazine suggests a filarial infection.

Immunodiagnosis

Indirect fluorescence and enzyme-linked immuno-sorbent assay detect antibodies in over 95% of active cases and 70% of established elephantiasis. Cross-reactions occur in 15% of cases of strongyloides and 5% of other intestinal nematodes. The test becomes negative 1–2 years after cure. None of these tests distinguishes between the different filarial infections. In tropical pulmonary eosinophilia, serology is strongly positive but circulating microfilariae are not found.

Management

Diethylcarbamazine kills microfilariae and adult worms. The dose is 9–12 mg/kg daily orally in 3 divided doses for 14 days. The full dose must be reached slowly, starting with 50 mg (one tablet) and doubling daily unless serious allergic reactions ensue. This course may be repeated twice at intervals of 4–6 weeks. Antihistamines or corticosteroids may be required to control allergic phenomena. Plastic surgery may be indicated in established elephantiasis. Great relief can be obtained by removal of excess tissue but recurrences are probable unless new lymphatic drainage is established. Tight bandaging, or bed-rest with suspension or raising of the affected part, or the nightly use of pneumatic stockings may control the swelling to some extent.

Prevention

Treatment of the whole population in endemic areas with diethylcarbamazine, 100 mg for adults (50 mg for children) 3 times daily for 7 days has reduced but not eliminated the infection. Children are given such a course on starting and before leaving school. This mass treatment should be combined with control of the vector by insecticides. Early chemotherapy prevents later elephantiasis. Individuals should avoid being bitten by mosquitoes (p. 153).

LOIASIS

Loiasis is caused by infection with the filaria *Loa loa*. The adults, 3–7 cm × 4 mm, parasitise chiefly the subcutaneous tissue of man. The larval microfilariae circulate harmlessly in the peripheral blood in the daytime. The vector is *Chrysops*, a forest-dwelling fly which bites by day.

Pathology

The adult worms move harmlessly about in the subcutaneous tissues and other interstitial planes (Table 4.47). From time to time a short-lived, inflammatory, oedematous swelling (a *Calabar swelling*) is produced, presumably around an adult worm. Heavy infections, especially when treated, may cause encephalitis. The incubation period is commonly over a year but may be as short as 3 months.

Clinical features

The infection is often symptomless. The first sign is usually a Calabar swelling which is an irritating, tense, localised swelling that may be painful especially if it is near a joint. The swelling is generally on a limb; it measures a few centimetres in diameter but sometimes is more diffuse and extensive. It usually disappears after a few days but may persist for 2 or 3 weeks. A succession of such swellings may appear at irregular intervals, often in adjacent sites. Sometimes there is urticaria and pruritus elsewhere. Occasionally a worm may be seen wriggling under the skin, especially of an eyelid, and may cross the eye under the conjunctiva, taking many minutes to do so. Severe unilateral headaches resembling migraine may be experienced when an adult worm moves in the retro-orbital tissues.

Investigations

The diagnosis is made by demonstrating microfilariae in the blood, but they may not always be found in patients with Calabar swellings. Antifilarial antibodies are positive in 95% of patients and there is massive eosinophilia. Occasionally a calcified worm may be seen on a radiograph.

Management

Diethylcarbamazine (see above) is curative, gradually increased to a dose of 9–12 mg/kg daily which is continued for 21 days. Treatment may precipitate a severe reaction in patients with a heavy microfilaraemia characterised by fever, joint and muscle pain and encephalitis; these patients should be given steroid cover (p. 179).

Prevention

Protection is afforded by siting houses away from trees and by having dwellings wire-screened against the fly. Protective clothing and repellents are also useful. Diethylcarbamazine in a dose of 5 mg/kg daily for 3 days each month is partially protective.

ONCHOCERCIASIS (RIVER BLINDNESS)

Onchocerciasis is the result of infection by *Onchocerca volvulus*. Although only about 0.3 mm in diameter, the adult female may be as long as 50 cm; the male is 13 cm. The infection is conveyed by flies of the genus Simulium which inflict a painful bite. In West Africa the vector is *S. damnosum*, in Northern Nigeria also *S. bovis* and in East Africa and Zaire *S. neavei*. The flies breed in rapidly flowing well-aerated water, the larvae being attached to submerged vegetation, rocks or crabs. Adult flies bite

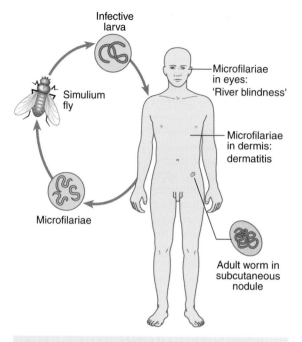

Infective
larva

Simulium
fly

Microfilariae

Microfilariae
in eyes:
'River blindness'

Microfilariae
in dermis:
dermatitis

Adult worm in
subcutaneous
nodule

Fig. 4.48 *Onchocerca volvulus.* Life cycle and pathogenesis of onchocerciasis.

during the daytime both inside and outside houses. Man is the only known definitive host.

Onchocerciasis is endemic in well-defined areas throughout tropical Africa, in Southern Arabia and Yemen and also in South Mexico, Guatemala, Colombia, Venezuela and Brazil. It is estimated that over 20 million people are infected. In parts of West and Central Africa it affects the whole adult population and blindness rates of 10% are common, reaching 35% in some parts of Ghana. Because of onchocerciasis huge tracts of fertile land lie virtually untilled, and individuals and communities are impoverished.

Pathology

Infective larvae of *O. volvulus* are introduced into the skin by the bite of an infected Simulium (Fig. 4.48). The worms mature in 2–4 months and live for up to 17 years in small colonies in subcutaneous and connective tissues (Table 4.47). At sites of trauma, over bony prominences and around joints, fibrosis may form nodules around adult worms which otherwise cause no direct damage. Innumerable microfilariae, discharged by the female *O. volvulus*, move actively in these nodules, in the adjacent tissues and widely distributed in the skin, and may invade the eye.

Live microfilariae elicit little tissue reaction, but dead microfilariae may cause severe allergic inflammation

leading to hyaline necrosis and loss of collagen and elastin. Death of microfilariae in the eye causes conjunctivitis, sclerosing keratitis with pannus formation, uveitis which may lead to glaucoma and cataract and, less commonly, choroidoretinitis and optic neuritis.

Clinical features

The infection may remain symptomless for months or years. The first symptom is usually itching, localised to one quadrant of the body and later becoming generalised and involving the eyes. Evanescent oedema of part or all of a limb in Europeans is an early sign, followed by papular urticaria spreading gradually from the site of infection. This is difficult to see on dark skins in which the commonest signs are papules excoriated by scratching, spotty hyperpigmentation from resolving inflammation and more chronic changes of a rough, thickened skin or inelastic wrinkled skin. Superficial lymph nodes enlarge and may hang down in folds of loose skin at the groins. Hydrocoele, femoral hernias and scrotal elephantiasis occur. Firm subcutaneous nodules occur in chronic infection (onchocercomas), which are palpable, 1 cm or more in diameter.

Eye disease is commonest in highly endemic areas and is associated with chronic heavy infections and nodules on the head. Early manifestations include itching, lacrimation, conjunctival injection and evidence of the features listed under pathology. Classically, 'snow flake' deposits are seen in the edges of the cornea.

Investigations

The finding of nodules or characteristic lesions of the skin or eyes, in a patient from an endemic area, associated with eosinophilia, is suggestive. Skin snips or shavings, taken with a corneoscleral punch or scalpel blade from calf, buttock and shoulder are placed in saline under a cover slip on a microscope slide and examined after 4 hours. If negative, a test dose of diethylcarbamazine is given to see if it aggravates the rash. Microfilariae are seen wriggling free in all but the lightest infections. Slit-lamp examination of the eye may reveal microfilariae moving in the anterior chamber of the eye, or trapped in the cornea. A nodule may be removed and incised, showing the coiled threadlike adult worm. Filarial antibodies may be detected in 95% of patients.

Management

Ivermectin, in a single dose of 100–200 μg/kg, kills microfilariae and prevents their return for 9 months. It is non-toxic and does not trigger severe reactions, in contrast to diethylcarbamazine which is no longer used for this infection.

In the rare event of a severe reaction, causing oedema

or postural hypotension, prednisolone 20–30 mg may be given daily for 2 or 3 days.

Adult worms are killed by suramin (1 g intravenously, weekly for 5–6 doses). But a repeated dose of ivermectin every 6–12 months is preferred to the potential toxicity of suramin (Table 4.41). Palpable nodules should be excised.

Prevention

Mass treatment with ivermectin is under trial. It reduces morbidity in the community and prevents eye disease from getting worse. Simulium can be destroyed in its larval stage by the application of insecticide to streams. Dimethylphthalate applied to skin or clothing will repel the fly for several hours. Long trousers, skirts and sleeves discourage the fly from biting.

OTHER FILARIASES

Mansonella perstans

This filarial worm is transmitted by the midges *Culicoides austeni* and *C. grahami*. It is common throughout equatorial Africa as far south as Zambia, and also in Trinidad and parts of northern and eastern South America.

M. perstans has never been shown to cause disease but it may be responsible for a persistent eosinophilia and occasional allergic manifestations (Table 4.47). *M. perstans* is resistant to ivermectin and diethylcarbamazine and the infection may persist for many years.

Mansonella ozzardi

This is non-pathogenic and is found in the West Indies and South America.

DRACONTIASIS (GUINEA WORM)

The female *Dracunculus medinensis*, which measures over a metre in length and 0.9–1.7 mm in diameter, lives in the interstitial and subcutaneous tissues of man. The male worm, which is rarely seen, is only 2.5 cm long. Man is infected by ingesting a small crustacean, *Cyclops*, which inhabits wells and ponds and which contains the infective larval stage of the worm.

Pathology

Ingested larvae mature and penetrate the intestinal wall and migrate through the connective tissues of the host. After 9–18 months the fully mature female surfaces under the skin, usually on the leg, where a vesicle is raised, ruptures and exposes the anterior end of the worm. The worm's distended uterus ruptures and dis-

charges its larvae externally. The worm is attracted to the surface by cooling, hence the larvae are likely to be expelled into water and complete the life cycle.

The disease can be extremely disabling and is especially liable to affect those who collect water at water-holes, or farmers at the beginning of the rains, and thus seriously interfere with planting. It is found in sub-Saharan Africa, Egypt, the Arabian peninsula, Iran, Afghanistan and in parts of Pakistan and India.

Clinical features

The adult worm may sometimes be felt beneath the skin. Some hours before the head of the worm emerges from the skin there is painful, hot, local inflammation which vesiculates. It takes 3–4 weeks for the larvae to be discharged during which time the ulcer persists and there is a pain and cellulitis, especially if it is close to an ankle or knee. There will be a marked allergic inflammation if the worm dies or is broken during extraction. Secondary infection is common and may cause cellulitis, arthritis or septicaemia. Tetanus is a well-recognised complication. Multiple infections may occur and reactions around aberrant worms may cause serious lesions.

Diagnosis

This is usually clinical. Discharge fluid may contain microfilariae. A radiograph may show calcified worms.

Management

Traditionally the protruding worm is extracted by winding it out gently over several days on a match stick. *The worm must never be broken.* Niridazole 25 mg/kg daily in 2 divided doses for 10 days, or mebendazole 100 mg 12-hourly for 7 days, may reduce inflammation and aid the extraction of the worm. Antibiotics for secondary infection and prophylaxis of tetanus are also required.

Prevention

The provision of a satisfactory water supply will eradicate the infection. Where this is impracticable, wells and ponds may be protected or treated chemically to kill *Cyclops*.

ZOONOTIC HELMINTH INFECTIONS

TRICHINELLA SPIRALIS

This is the most important zoonotic nematode to cause disease in man. Others are given in Table 4.48, and in the information box on page 113.

Table 4.48 **Zoonotic helminths that commonly cause incidental infections in man**

	Toxocara canis	Ancylostoma brasiliense	Angiostrongylus cantonensis	Gnathostoma spinigerum
Distribution	Worldwide	Tropics and subtropics	Far East, Pacific	Bangladesh, S.E. Asia, Far East
Vector/reservoir	Adult roundworms in dog intestine. Ova on contaminated fur and soil	Adult hookworms in dog intestine. Infective larvae on soil	Adults in lungs of rodents. Larvae in snails, slugs, crustacea	Adults in dog and cat intestine. Larvae in Cyclops, fish, frogs and snakes
Transmission	Geophagia; handling dogs, especially puppies	Larvae penetrate skin on contact with soil	Eating undercooked snails, etc.	Drinking Cyclops in water, eating undercooked frogs etc.
Site of parasite in man	Larval worms migrate and die in tissues	Larval worms migrate in skin	Larval worms in brain, meninges	Larval worms migrate subcutaneously
Clinical features	Visceral larva migrans. Febrile hepatomegaly, rarely blindness	Cutaneous larva migrans. Slowing moving inflamed irritating tracts on buttocks, feet	Eosinophilic meningitis	Recurrent migratory subcutaneous swellings
Laboratory diagnosis	Eosinophilia, serology	May be eosinophilia	Eosinophilia in CSF and blood, serology	Eosinophilia, serology
Treatment	Albendazole 400 mg daily for 7 days	Topical 10% thiabendazole; oral albendazole 400 mg daily for 2 days	Albendazole 400 mg 12-hourly for 14 days Prednisolone	Albendazole 400 mg 12-hourly for 14 days

Trichinella spiralis is a parasite of rats and pigs and is transmitted to man by eating partially cooked infected pork, usually as sausage or ham. Symptoms result from invasion of intestinal submucosa by ingested larvae, which develop into adult worms, and the secondary invasion of tissues by fresh larvae produced by these adult worms. The main tissue invaded is striated muscle, in which the larvae encyst. Outbreaks have occurred in Britain as well as in other countries where pork is eaten. Bear meat is another source.

Clinical features

The clinical features of trichinosis depend largely on the number of larvae. There may be no symptoms if there are only a few worms present, but many worms may cause nausea and diarrhoea 24–48 hours after the infected meal. A few days later, these symptoms are overshadowed by those associated with the larval invasion, namely fever and oedema of the face, eyelids and conjunctivae. Invasion of the diaphragm may cause pain, cough and dyspnoea; involvement of the muscles of the limbs, chest and mouth causes stiffness, pain and tenderness in the affected muscle groups. Fever may reach 40°C with daily remissions. Larval migration may cause acute myocarditis and encephalitis. An eosinophilia is usually found after the second week. An intense infection may prove fatal but those who survive recover completely.

Investigations

Commonly, a group of people who have eaten infected pork from a common source develop symptoms about

EOSINOPHILIC SYNDROMES ASSOCIATED WITH HELMINTIC INFECTIONS

- **Urticarial rashes**: strongyloidiasis, onchocerciasis, fascioliasis, hydatid disease, trichinosis
- **Cutaneous larva migrans**: ancylostoma brasiliense
- **Dermatitis**: onchocerciasis
- **Migratory subcutaneous swellings**: loiasis, gnathostomiasis
- **Lymphangitis, orchitis**: lymphatic filariasis
- **Myositis**: trichinosis, cysticercosis
- **Febrile hepatosplenomegaly**: schistosomiasis, toxocariasis
- **Pneumonitis**: migratory stage of larval helminths (Loeffler's syndrome), lymphatic filariasis (tropical pulmonary eosinophilia), systemic strongyloidiasis
- **Enteritis and colitis**: strongyloidiasis, capillariasis, trichinosis, rarely other intestinal worms.
- **Meningitis**: angiostrongyloidiasis, strongyloidiasis

the same time. Biopsy from the deltoid or gastrocnemius after the third week of symptoms in suspected cases may reveal encysted larvae. Serological tests are also helpful.

Management

Albendazole 400 mg daily for 6 days may relieve muscle pain. Given early in the infection it may kill newly-formed adult worms in the submucosa. Corticosteroids are necessary to control the serious effects of acute inflammation.

Table 4.49   Infections conveyed by arthropods

Name	Genus	Disease
House fly	*Musca*	Dysenteries, enteric fevers, salmonelloses; and possibly cholera, trachoma, tropical ulcer
House fly	*Tabanida*	Tularaemia, ?anthrax
Oscinid fly	*Hippelates*	Streptococcal dermatitis, conjunctivitis, ?yaws
Tsetse fly	*Glossina*	African trypanosomiasis
Mosquito	*Anopheles*	Malaria, some arboviruses, Bancroftian and Brugia filarias
	Aedes	Yellow fever, dengue and other arboviruses
	Culex	Bancroftian and Brugia filariasis, Japanese encephalitis and other arboviruses
Black fly	*Simulium*	Onchocerciasis
Midges	*Culicoides*	*Mansonella perstans, M. streptocerca, M. ozzardi*
Soft ticks	*Ornithodoros*	Tick-borne relapsing fever, Lyme disease
Hard tick	*(Ixodidae)* *Rhipicephalus,* etc.	Some typhus fevers, Kyasanur Forest disease, tularaemia, ?Q fever
Sandflies	*Phlebotomus,* etc.	Leishmaniasis, sandfly fever, bartonellosis
Lice	*Pediculus*	Epidemic typhus fever, louse-borne relapsing fever, trench fever, *Dipylidium caninum*
Mites	*Leptotrombidium*	Scrub typhus fever
	Allodermanyssus	Rickettsialpox
Winged bug	*Triatoma*	Chagas' disease
Fleas	*Xenopsylla* *Ctenocephalides*	Plague, endemic typhus fever *Dipylidium caninum*

FURTHER READING

Crompton D W, 1992 Ascaris and childhood malnutrition. Transactions of the Royal Society of Tropical Medicine and Hygiene 86: 577–579

Gryseels B, 1992 Morbidity due to infection with *Schistosoma mansoni*: an update. Tropical and Geographical Medicine 44: 189–200

Hopkins D R, Ruiz-Tiben E, Kaiser R L 1993 Dracunculiasis eradication: beginning of the end. American Journal of Tropical Medicine and Hygiene 49: 281–289

Lessnan K D, Can S, Talavera W, 1993 Disseminated *Strongyloides stercoralis* in human immunodeficiency virus-infected patients. Treatment failure and a review of the literature. Chest 104: 119–122

Malatt A E, Taylor H R 1992 Onchocerciasis. Infectious Disease Clinics of North America 6: 963–977

Pawlowski Z S 1992 Echinococcosis and cysticercosis. Current Opinions in Infectious Diseases 5: 319–325

Wen H, New R R, Craig P S 1993 Diagnosis and treatment of human hydatidosis. British Journal of Clinical Pharmacology 35: 565–74

Wolfe M S 1992 Eosinophilia in the returning traveller. Infectious Disease Clinics of North America 6: 489–502

DISEASES DUE TO ARTHROPODS

Arthropods may be responsible for disease in four ways. They may act as vectors of infectious agents (Table 4.49); they may envenomate through stings or bites; they may infest or even infect the human body directly; and they may cause allergic dermatitis.

LICE

As well as transmitting serious disease, the body louse *Pediculus humanus* causes dermatitis and sleeplessness through itching, especially in poor crowded communities in cold countries (for control see p. 116).

The head louse, *Pediculus capitis*, is cosmopolitan and increasing in prevalence in British schools. It makes the child itch and alarms parents and teachers. Tiny white oval eggs, 'nits', are seen attached to the base of hairs on the scalp. The crab louse is transmitted in shared beds. A single treatment with gammabenzene hexachloride (BHC) shampoo or lotion is usually curative. In countries, such as Britain, where resistance is developing to BHC, malathion or carbaryl is preferred (see information box p. 116).

SCABIES

This disease is due to the mite *Sarcoptes scabei*; it is common all over the world. There is itching, initially between the fingers or on the buttocks or genitals where the mite burrows, and later all over the body (Fig. 4.49). Secondary streptococcal infection is an important cause of glomerulonephritis in the tropics. Severe widespread ('Norwegian') scabies occurs in the debilitated or immunosuppressed. The diagnosis of scabies is confirmed by scraping the mite out of a burrow. Scabies is treated by

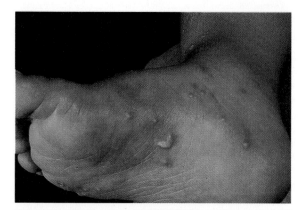

Fig. 4.49 Scabies. Tracks and papules on the soft foot skin of a child.

a single application of gammabenzene hexachloride 1% to the whole body below the neck or by 3 daily applications of benzyl benzoate 25%.

JIGGERS (TUNGIASIS)

This is due to infestation with *Tunga penetrans* (the chigoe or jigger flea). It is widespread in tropical America and Africa. Man and pigs are important hosts. The pregnant female flea burrows into the skin about the toes and soles and grows as large as a pea, packed with eggs which are subsequently discharged onto the surface. The burrows irritate and become inflamed but the chief danger is from secondary pyogenic infection or tetanus.

The chigoe or egg sac should be removed with a sterile needle and a mild antiseptic ointment applied. Massive infestations, such as may be seen in neglected children and in senile persons, may be treated by immersing the feet in an aqueous solution containing benzene hexachloride 5% and cetrimide 0.8%.

MYIASIS

This is an infestation of various tissues of man by the larvae of flies.

Cutaneous myiasis

A common cause of cutaneous myiasis is *Cordylobia anthropophaga* (Tumbu fly) which lays its eggs on laundry spread on grass. The larvae penetrate the skin and produce lesions like boils with central orifices through which the larvae breathe. On reaching maturity they emerge. A drop of thick oil or petroleum jelly usually brings a larva out in search of air and facilitates its removal. Occasionally the common warble-fly *Hypoderma bovis* may infest man.

Myiasis of wounds, sores and cavities

The larvae of many flies may infest necrotic tissues in open wounds or ulcers and occasionally invade living tissue. *Chrysomya bezziana* is found in Africa, India and South Vietnam. It may penetrate the nasal sinuses and cause great destruction. The application of 10% chloroform in a light vegetable oil is the treatment of choice for infested wounds.

Intestinal myiasis

In the tropics especially, vague digestive disturbances or abdominal cramps with diarrhoea and vomiting may be caused by fly larvae in the intestinal canal, the eggs having been ingested with food.

FURTHER READING

Estes S A, Estes J 1993 Therapy of scabies: nursing homes, hospitals and the homeless. Seminars in Dermatology 12: 26–33

SEXUALLY TRANSMITTED DISEASES

Most sexually transmitted diseases (STDs) are increasing. They include syphilis, gonorrhoea, human immunodeficiency virus (HIV) infection, genital *Herpes simplex* virus (HSV) infection, genital warts, chlamydial infection, trichomoniasis, and genital candidosis.

The approach to the patient with suspected STD

Patients who suspect an STD are anxious; staff must be friendly, sympathetic and reassuring, and doctors must put patients at ease and explain that everything is confidential. The history focuses on genital symptoms. In both sexes this covers genital ulceration, rash, itch, pain or swelling and urinary symptoms, especially burning on micturition. In men the clinician should ask about urethral discharge and in women vaginal discharge. General health must be recorded including menstruation, recent medication, especially with antimicrobial or antiviral agents. The sexual history should cover number of sexual partners, dates, casual or regular relationship, symptoms, and genital to genital, anogenital and orogenital contact. Contraception should be recorded, especially condom use. Past history should include treatment for STD, and the family and obstetric history should be recorded.

The genitals must always be examined and in females this includes passing a bivalve vaginal speculum. The history will indicate other systems requiring examination; ideally all patients should have a complete examination.

Several infections may be present at the same time;

Table 4.50 Investigations in sexually transmitted disease

Patient and focus	Investigation
FEMALES	
Cervical os	Gram stain and culture for gonococci. Chlamydia culture or antigen detection. Smear for cytological examination
Urethral meatus	Gram stain and culture for gonococci
Vagina	Gram stain and culture for candidal elements Saline mount (for microscopy) and culture for *T. vaginalis* Microscopy for bacteria causing anaerobic/bacterial vaginosis. (Culture for *Gardenerella vaginalis*)
MALES	
Urethra	Gram stain and culture for gonococci. Saline mount and culture for *T. vaginalis*. Chlamydia culture or antigen detection
ALL PATIENTS	Blood for VDRL and TPHA serum antibody tests Urine for analysis for sugar and protein when indicated
Genital ulcers	Scraping for herpes simplex virus culture. Scraping for dark ground microscopy for *T. pallidum* Swab for bacterial culture if secondarily infected
Contacts of gonorrhoea	Rectal Gram stain and culture for gonococci Throat culture for gonococci
Drug abusers and homosexual or bisexual men plus others at risk	Blood for serum markers for Hepatitis B and C for drug abusers. Blood for HIV antibodies (after counselling)

all patients should therefore have the investigations in Table 4.50 at their first visit. Positive investigations must be repeated after treatment to ensure cure.

Spread and control of STDs

Spread

The fundamental factors in spread are the acquisition of infection from one partner and its transmission to another. These depend on the availability of partners, which increases with population movement including migration from rural to urban areas and world-wide travel. Social factors which promote spread include affluence, alcohol, leisure, personal freedom, prostitution and ignorance. Additional factors are asymptomatic infection, antimicrobial resistance, and contraception. Unlike condoms and to a lesser extent the cap, oral contraceptives and the intrauterine device provide no barrier to infection. All socio-economic groups acquire STDs; people at special risk are shown in the information box.

Control

Good control of STD is based on a number of important principles:

THOSE AT PARTICULAR RISK OF STDs

- Men aged 18–34 years
- Women aged 16–24 years
- Frequent travellers
- Prostitutes
- Armed services personnel
- Merchant seamen
- Entertainers

- Good clinical practice, including accurate diagnosis, effective treatment and close follow-up to ensure cure
- Partner notification—the identification of potentially infected partners and their treatment
- Education on STD
- Screening—certain groups of at-risk patients (see the information box above) should be screened, and routine blood donor and antenatal serological testing should continue.

SEXUALLY TRANSMITTED BACTERIAL DISEASES

SYPHILIS

Syphilis is due to infection with *Treponema pallidum*. It is systemic from the beginning, infectious and chronic. There are florid features at some times but there may be long periods of latency at others. It can be transmitted to the fetus, but it responds to penicillin, which is the drug of choice.

The classification of syphilis is shown in the information box.

The division between early and late syphilis is 2 years. The course is variable, may be latent throughout, but clinical features may develop at any time, so all cases must be treated (Table 4.51).

Acquired syphilis

Early stage

The incubation period is commonly 14–28 days with extremes of 9–90 days.

Primary syphilis. The primary lesion or chancre develops at the site of infection, usually on the genitals. A small pink macule appears, becomes papular and ulcerates. The regional lymph nodes are moderately enlarged, mobile, discrete, rubbery, painless, and non-tender. Primary syphilis must be included in the differential diagnosis of all genital ulcers—see the information box.

Table 4.51 Management of syphilis

Stage	Medication	Regimen
Primary	Procaine penicillin	600–1200 mg i.m. once daily for 12 days
	Oxytetracycline	500 mg orally 6-hourly for 15 days
	Doxycycline	100 mg orally 8-hourly for 15 days
Secondary	Procaine penicillin	600–1200 mg i.m. once daily for 15 days
Tertiary	Oxytetracycline	500 mg orally 6-hourly for 15 days
Latent	Doxycycline	100 mg orally 8-hourly for 15 days
Cardiovascular and	Procaine penicillin	900–1200 mg i.m. once daily for 21 days
Central Nervous	Oxytetracycline	500 mg orally 6-hourly for 28 days
System	Doxycycline	100 mg orally 8-hourly for 28 days

CLASSIFICATION OF SYPHILIS

Acquired
- **Early**
  Primary
  Secondary
  Latent
- **Late**
  Latent
  Tertiary (benign gummatous)
  Quarternary (cardiovascular, neurosyphilis)

Congenital
- **Early**
  Clinical and latent
- **Late**
  Clinical and latent, stigmata (or scars)

Secondary syphilis. This starts 6–8 weeks after the chancre with mild fever, malaise and headache. The features are shown in Table 4.52 and Figure 4.50.

CAUSES OF GENITAL ULCERS, NON-SYPHILITIC

Common
- *Herpes simplex* (pp. 110, 188)
- Erosive balanitis (p. 188)
- Trauma with secondary infection

Uncommon
- Secondary syphilis
- Scabies (p. 181)
- Reiter's disease (p. 907)
- Stevens–Johnson syndrome (p. 973)
- Behçet's syndrome (p. 908)

The rash starts with faint macules on the trunk and proximal limbs, becomes generalised, papular, is characteristically dull red, polymorphic and symmetrical, does not itch and turns scaly. Characteristically the palms and soles are affected. Condylomata lata are flat papules in warm moist areas such as at the anus. Lymphadenopathy may be generalised with nodes like those in primary syphilis. Mucosal ulcers affect the genitals,

mouth, pharynx and larynx. Early lesions are superficial; later they develop a white base, a red margin, and coalesce to form 'snail track ulcers'.

After several months without treatment, resolution occurs and the disease enters the latent phase.

Many cases are identified in this stage following serological testing. Modern antimicrobial therapy (Table 4.51) gives cure rates over 95%.

The differential diagnosis of secondary syphilis is summarised in Table 4.52. Syphilis must be distinguished clinically from yaws (p. 140), endemic (non-venereal) syphilis and pinta (p. 141). These diseases are caused by treponemes morphologically indistinguishable from *T. pallidum* of syphilis.

Late stage
Latency may persist for many years.

Tertiary stage. (rare). This takes at least two years to develop and affects skin, mucosa and bones. The charactertistic feature is a granuloma called a gumma.
Quaternary stage. Cardiovascular syphilis and neurosyphilis take longer to develop and may lead to the patient's death.

Congenital syphilis
The fetus may contract syphilis from a mother with early acquired syphilis. With severe disease the child is born

Table 4.52 Differential diagnosis of secondary syphilis

Macular rash	Papular rash	Condylomata lata
Drug eruption	Drug eruption	Viral warts
Rubella	Scabies	
Pityriasis rosea	Acne vulgaris	
Mouth ulcers	**Genital ulcers**	**Lymphadenopathy**
Herpes simplex	Herpes simplex	Infectious mononucleosis
Aphthous ulcers	Erosive balanitis	Lymphoma
Ulcerative stomatitis		HIV infection
Agranulocytosis		

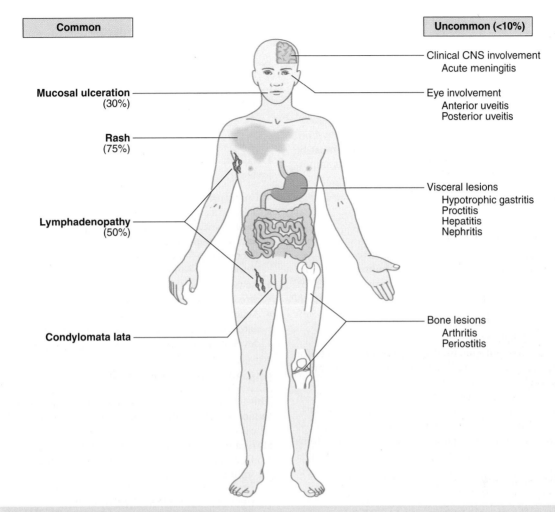

| Common | | Uncommon (<10%) |

Clinical CNS involvement
Acute meningitis

Mucosal ulceration
(30%)

Eye involvement
Anterior uveitis
Posterior uveitis

Rash
(75%)

Visceral lesions
Hypotrophic gastritis
Proctitis
Hepatitis
Nephritis

Lymphadenopathy
(50%)

Condylomata lata

Bone lesions
Arthritis
Periostitis

Fig. 4.50 Features of secondary acquired syphilis.

dead. A less severely affected baby has vesicles, bullae and mucosal ulcers at birth and disease of bones, joints, liver, kidneys and other organs. In a third group the disease remains latent for years. Congenital syphilis is rare where antenatal serological screening is practised. Treatment during pregnancy usually produces a healthy baby.

Investigations

T. pallidum is found in early acquired and congenital syphilis (Table 4.50). Serological tests for syphilis are listed in the information box.

Serological tests are positive from the fourth week of acquired syphilis and at birth in congenital syphilis. False positive results occur occasionally to the VDRL and RPR tests in other infections and also in connective tissue diseases; therefore results must be confirmed with

---

SEROLOGICAL TESTS FOR SYPHILIS

Nonspecific or lipoidal antigen tests
- Venereal Disease Research Laboratory (VDRL) test
- Rapid Plasma Reagin (RPR)
- Treponemal enzyme assay (ELISA)

Specific treponemal antigen tests
- Treponema pallidum haemagglutination assay (TPHA)
- Fluorescent treponemal antibody absorbed (FTA-abs) test
- Treponemal enzyme-linked immunosorbent assay (ELISA)

---

specific tests. When syphilis is suspected lipoidal antigen and specific tests are used together.

In the latent stages the CSF is examined to exclude or confirm neurological disease and chest radiographs

185

are taken for calcification of the ascending aorta, which indicates cardiovascular disease.

Management

Antimicrobial treatment for syphilis is summarised in Table 4.51. Tetracyclines are indicated for patients hypersensitive to penicillin, except pregnant women are given erythromycin stearate in the same dosage; erythromycin crosses the placenta poorly so the new-born baby needs careful management. All patients must be followed to ensure cure; partner notification is important.

NEUROSYPHILIS—see p. 1097.

GONORRHOEA

Gonorrhoea is caused by the Gram-negative diplococcus *Neisseria gonorrhoeae* which infects columnar epithelium in the lower genital tract, rectum, pharynx and eyes. The incubation period in men with gonococcal urethritis is 2–10 days.

Clinical features

In males the anterior urethra is the common site for infection. Anterior urethritis causes dysuria and purulent discharge but these may be mild or absent in 5–10%. The lower cervical canal is infected in 80% of women, with the urethra and rectum involved in 50%. There may be vaginal discharge and dysuria, but 60% of women with uncomplicated infection are symptom-free. Homosexual men may have asymptomatic rectal infection. Symptomless pharyngeal gonorrhoea occasionally affects males and females.

Differential diagnosis in uncomplicated gonorrhoea is given in the information box.

Investigations

Gram-negative intracellular diplococci may be seen on microscopy of infected secretions but must be confirmed by culture (Table 4.50).

Management

Uncomplicated gonorrhoea responds to a single adequate dose of a suitable antimicrobial. In Britain infections are usually sensitive to penicillin. Elsewhere, such as the Far East and West Africa, up to 50% of infections are totally resistant to penicillin. Occasional strains of *N. gonorrhoeae* isolated in Europe and more in the Far East have diminished sensitivity to ciprofloxacin. Antimicrobial regimens are shown in Table 4.53. Partners should be notified as soon as possible.

Prognosis

Symptoms gradually resolve without treatment but it is not known how long the patient remains infectious.

DIFFERENTIAL DIAGNOSIS OF UNCOMPLICATED GONORRHOEA

- **Males:** Nongonococcal urethritis
- **Females:** Urinary infection, trichomoniasis, candidosis, bacterial vaginosis
- **Both sexes:** Proctitis, pharyngitis

Delay in treatment leads to complications, which include:

- Epididymo-orchitis
- Salpingitis and pelvic infection
- Perihepatitis—characterised by right hypochondrial pain and tenderness
- Bacteraemia—rare and causes fever, joint pains and sparse peripheral pustular rash
- Acute gonococcal arthritis (p. 910) and septicaemia—rare in developed countries
- Acute purulent conjunctivitis (ophthalmia neonatorum) in infants born to infected mothers—rare in developed countries.

NON-GONOCOCCAL INFECTION

This clinically resembles gonorrhoea, but gonococci cannot be identified; a cause is recognised in only 50% (about half may be due to *Chlamydia trachomatis*, which also causes lymphogranuloma venereum—see Table 4.54), and the aetiology is obscure in the remainder (see the information box).

Non-gonococcal urethritis (NGU) in men

Urethritis in men is much more commonly non-gonococcal than gonococcal in origin. NGU also occurs in Reiter's disease (p. 907). Clinically NGU resembles gonococcal urethritis but is milder. The incubation period varies from a few days to a few weeks. Urethritis is confirmed by finding polymorphonuclear leucocytes in a Gram stain of urethral secretions; gonorrhoea is excluded by absence of organisms on Gram stain and culture. An additional urethral swab should be taken for chlamydiae. A wet preparation will show *T. vaginalis*.

Untreated NGU runs a prolonged low grade course and may be complicated by epididymo-orchitis. In Britain and some other countries epididymo-orchitis is more common with NGU than with gonorrhoea.

A satisfactory response to a single course of therapy is achieved in up to 80%. Non-responders should be retreated with an alternative regimen. Epididymo-orchitis should be treated with oxytetracycline or erythromycin 500 mg 6-hourly for 14 days (see information box). Whether or not a causative agent is identified,

Table 4.53   Treatment of uncomplicated anogenital gonorrhoea

	Drug	Route	Regimen
Penicillin sensitive	Ampicillin and	Oral	2 – 3.5 g
	Probenecid	Oral	1 g single dose
	Co-trimoxazole dispersible tablets	Oral	8 × 480 mg single dose **OR** 5 × 480 mg 12 hourly × 3 doses
Penicillin resistant	Ciprofloxacin	Oral	250 – 500 mg single dose
	Cefotaxime	i.m.	0.5 – 1.0 g single dose
	Spectinomycin	i.m.	2 – 4 g single dose
Pharyngeal gonorrhoea	Co-trimoxazole dispersible tablets	Oral	5 × 480 mg 12 hourly × 3 doses
	Ciprofloxacin	Oral	500 mg single dose

Table 4.54   Salient features of lymphogranuloma venereum (LGV), chancroid and granuloma inguinale (Donovanosis)

Condition and distribution	Organism	Incubation period	Genital lesion	Lymph nodes	Diagnosis	Management
LGV Worldwide especially E. and W. Africa, India, S.E. Asia, S. America, Caribbean	*Chlamydia trachomatis* Types L1, II, III (intracellular inclusions)	1–5 weeks	Small transient, often not recognised	Tender, unilateral, matted, adherent, suppurative, multilocular	Culture or antigen identification. Circulating (micro IF) antibodies	Oxytetracycline 500 mg 6-hourly for 14 days; increase and prolong if severe
CHANCROID Africa, S.E. Asia	*Haemophilus ducreyii* (small Gram-negative rod)	1–8 days	Multiple, irregular, tender ulcers	Tender, unilateral, matted, adherent, suppurative	Microscopy & culture of scrapings	Erythromycin 500 mg 6-hourly for 7 days or co-trimoxazole 2 (80/400 mg) 12-hourly for 7 days
GRANULOMA INGUINALE S. India, S.E. Asia, Central and W. Africa, Caribbean, S. America, Central Australia among Aborigines	*Donovania granulomatis* (Bipolar rods)	Few days—3 months	Spreading granulomas, pink & red velvety appearance	Only if secondary infected	Microscopy of scrapings	Streptomycin 1 g 12-hourly i.m. for 10–20 days or Oxytetracycline 500 mg 6-hourly for 14–21 days

CAUSES OF NON-GONOCOCCAL URETHRITIS (NGU) IN MEN

- Common approx. 50%   *Chlamydia trachomatis*
  Ureaplasma urealyticum
- Rare   *Trichomonas vaginalis*
  Herpes simplex virus
  Upper urinary tract infection
  Trauma
- Remainder   Obscure

partner notification is important because untreated female partners may develop pelvic inflammatory disease.

Non-gonococcal infection in women

This is due to *C. trachomatis* in 50% of cases and no other cause has yet been identified. *C. trachomatis* infects the lower cervical canal and rarely the urethra. Many women have additional infections; therefore all require full investigation (Table 4.50).

Uncomplicated lower genital tract chlamydia-positive or negative infection may cause no symptoms or signs, but it may also progress to pelvic inflammatory disease which may recur, become chronic, and lead to tubal pregnancy or infertility. A woman with cervical infection may infect her baby's eyes at birth. Investigations for NGU in women are outlined in Table 4.50.

The antimicrobial treatment of uncomplicated and complicated chlamydia-positive and -negative infection is the same as that for men (see the information box).

SEXUALLY TRANSMITTED VIRAL DISEASES

Viral diseases are in general more serious than bacterial diseases, because viruses are more difficult to eradicate and serious complications may occur. This is par-

---

TREATMENT OF NON-GONOCOCCAL URETHRITIS (NGU)

(All regimens for 14 days by mouth. Presence or absence of chlamydia on culture does not influence antibiotic choice)

- Oxytetracycline 250 mg 6-hourly or 500 mg 12-hourly
- Doxycycline 100 mg 12-hourly
- Erythromycin 250 mg 6-hourly or 500 mg 12-hourly
- Azithromycin 1 g as a single dose

---

ticularly true for human immunodeficiency virus (HIV) infection, which is covered in detail on pp. 89–104.

Anogenital Herpes simplex

This is due to *Herpes simplex* virus (see p. 110) spread by sexual contact. There is a severe first attack followed by milder recurrences which resemble labial herpes simplex (cold sores).

First attack

This starts with malaise, fever and local irritation followed by widespread painful tender vesicles affecting the genitals and rarely the anorectum. The vesicles rupture leaving painful tender erosions followed by further crops of lesions. Regional lymph nodes swell. There may be nerve root pains in the second and third sacral dermatomes and, rarely, retention of urine. First attacks heal in 2–4 weeks and are followed by recurrence.

Recurrent attacks

These resemble first attacks but there is one cluster of lesions covering an area of about 1 cm^2 which heals in 7–10 days.

The virus is identified by electron microscopy in vesicular fluid or scrapings from fresh erosions. Lesions always heal and local saline bathing may be all that is necessary. Acyclovir, 200 mg 5 times daily for 5 days by mouth, inhibits viral replication so if given early shortens first attacks. Acyclovir is not prescribed for mild or infrequent recurrences. A few patients suffer frequent recurrence, which may be suppressed by continuous oral acyclovir 400 mg twice daily.

Genital warts

Warts are due to the human papilloma virus (HPV—see p. 111) and are common on the genitals and anus. HPV infection predisposes to carcinoma of the cervix.

Exophytic warts can be recognised from their appearance. Flat warts are more difficult to diagnose. Atypical and persistent lesions should be biopsied. Treatment is with 10–25% podophyllin applied weekly, or 0.5% podophyllotoxin applied twice daily for three con-

secutive days per week for a maximum of 5 weeks. Alternative methods are destruction by cryotherapy, electrocautery or laser. Warts tend to recur so all patients must be followed to ensure cure. Partners must be notified.

Molluscum contagiosum

Molluscum contagiosum virus (p. 112) produces small, shiny, pink papules, with a central depression which allows differentiation from warts. Treatment is by destruction with cryotherapy or electrocautery.

Hepatitis

Hepatitis B (p. 514) is transmitted readily between homosexual men but rarely between heterosexuals. This is in contrast to Hepatitis A and C, as these are rarely sexually transmitted.

MISCELLANEOUS CONDITIONS

BALANITIS AND BALANOPOSTHITIS

Balanitis is inflammation of the glans penis; balanoposthitis involves the glans and undersurface of the prepuce. They are common in men with a long tight prepuce and poor hygiene. Causal agents include: Candida species, *T. vaginalis*, some streptococci and anaerobes, but sometimes no cause is identified. Immune deficiency, diabetes mellitus (p. 724), broad spectrum antimicrobials, corticosteroids and antimitotic drugs predispose to candidosis.

Clinical features

There is general or patchy erythema with erosions when severe and a white or purulent exudate. Circinate balanitis occurs in Reiter's disease (p. 907) with round erosions which coalesce. Balanitis xerotica obliterans (BXO) is the genital manifestation of lichen sclerosis et atrophicus; initial patchy erythema progresses to atrophy with a white appearance, meatal stenosis and phimosis. Diagnosis is from the clinical appearance. Swabs are taken to identify possible causes.

Management

Specific treatment should be given as in Table 4.55. Local saline bathing is always advised and is sufficient when no cause is found. Saline may suffice for circinate balanitis and BXO but hydrocortisone cream 1% is recommended in severe cases. Partner notification is indicated in candidosis, and trichomoniasis.

Table 4.55   Treatment of balanitis and vulvovaginal conditions

Cause	Vulvovaginal condition	Balanitis
Candidosis	Clotrimazole 500 mg pessary once **OR** Clotrimazole 200 mg pessary at night × 3 **AND** Clotrimazole cream twice daily	Clotrimazole cream twice daily
Trichomoniasis, bacterial vaginosis and anaerobic infection	Metronidazole 200 mg 8-hourly for 7 days **OR** 400 mg 12-hourly for 5 days	Metronidazole 200 mg 8-hourly for 7 days **OR** 400 mg 12-hourly for 5 days
Streptococcal infection	Amoxycillin 250 mg 8-hourly for 5 days	Amoxycillin 250 mg 8-hourly for 5 days

Table 4.56   Causes and features of vulvovaginal conditions

Condition	Cause	Features
Non infective vulvovaginitis	Chemicals e.g. antiseptics; trauma	Soreness, redness and variable discharge
Senile vaginitis	Oestrogen deficiency	Soreness, itch and pale atrophic appearance
Infective candidosis	Candida albicans	Itch, vulval oedema, thick white discharge
Trichomoniasis	T. vaginalis	Painful irritation, smell, erythema, thin yellow discharge
Bacterial vaginosis	Gardenerella vaginalis and anaerobes	Smell and off-white discharge

VULVOVAGINAL CONDITIONS

Vaginal discharge is common, may be associated with vulval inflammation, and is due to a variety of causes summarised with the clinical features in Table 4.56. All of the infections may occur without symptoms but treatment is indicated as clinical disease may develop. Investigate as in Table 4.50. Saline bathing is indicated for vulval involvement and specific treatment prescribed as in Table 4.55. Partner notification is required in trichomoniasis and recurrent candidosis.

Scabies (p. 181) and pediculosis (p. 181) can be sex- ually transmitted and this must be considered in their management.

FURTHER READING

Corcoran G D, Ridgway G L 1994 Antibiotic treatment of bacterial sexually transmitted diseases in adults: a review. International Journal of Sexually Transmitted Diseases and AIDS 5: 165–171
Holmes K K, Mardh P-A, Sparling P F, Wiesner P J 1989 Sexually Transmitted Diseases, 2nd edn. McGraw-Hill, New York
Young H 1992 Syphilis: new diagnostic directions. International Journal of STD and AIDS 3: 391–413

Diseases of the cardiovascular system

Cardiovascular disease is the most frequent cause of death in adult life in industrialised societies, and is increasingly important in developing countries. In early life minor congenital abnormalities affect 1 in 100 live births and more serious abnormalities approximately 1 in 500.

Since the 1960s, mortality from cardiac disease has steadily declined in the United States of America, and more recently in Australia, Europe and certain other countries. It is not yet clear whether this reflects changing lifestyles, improved diagnosis and management, or other factors as yet unrecognised.

Prompt recognition of the development of heart disease is limited by two key factors. Firstly, it is very commonly latent. For example, disease of the coronary arteries can proceed to an advanced stage before the patient notices any symptoms, unlike disease of other organs. Secondly, the diversity of symptoms attributable to heart disease is limited and it is common for many different pathologies to present through a common symptomatic pathway.

APPLIED ANATOMY, PHYSIOLOGY AND INVESTIGATIONS

ANATOMY

Orientation of the heart

The position of the heart in the mediastinum is such that two-thirds of its mass extends to the left of the mediastinum, with the long axis oriented towards the 'apex' of the two ventricles. The 'base' of this triangle is formed by the plane of the atrioventricular groove.

The only significant structure situated anterior to the heart, in the upper mediastinum, is the thymus gland. Posteriorly, the oesophagus lies behind the left atrium, with the descending aorta nearby, in the posterior mediastinum. Thus these structures may be visualised using transoesophageal echocardiography.

In the frontal plane, as seen on a chest radiograph, the normal heart occupies less than 50% of the transthoracic diameter. On the patient's left, the cardiac silhouette is formed by the aortic arch, the pulmonary trunk, the left atrial appendage and left ventricle. On the right, the right atrium is joined by superior and inferior venae cavae, and the lower right border is made up by the right ventricle (see Fig. 5.1A and B). In disease states, or congenital cardiac abnormalities, the silhouette changes according to the cavity dimensions.

The coronary circulation

The left main and right coronary arteries arise from the left and right coronary sinuses, just distal to the aortic valve (Fig. 5.1C). Within 2.5 cms of its origin the left main coronary divides into the left anterior descending artery (LAD), which runs in the anterior interventricular groove, and the circumflex artery (LCX) which runs posteriorly in the atrioventricular groove. The LAD gives branches to supply the anterior left ventricle, the apex, and the anterior part of the septum. The LCX gives marginal branches to supply the posterior left ventricle and inferior surface. The right coronary artery (RCA) runs in the right atrioventricular groove, giving branches to supply the right atrium, right ventricle and inferio-posterior aspects of the left ventricle (as the posterior descending vessel, in the posterior interventricular groove). In most individuals (approx. 90%) the RCA supplies the posterior descending vessel, but in the remainder there is a left dominant system which supplies this vessel from the LCX.

The sinoatrial (SA) node is supplied by the right coronary artery in about 60% of individuals and the atrioventricular (AV) node in 90%. Proximal occlusion of the right coronary artery often results in sinus bradycardia, and may also cause electrical conduction block of the AV node. Abrupt occlusions in the RCA, due to coronary thrombosis, result in infarction of the inferior part of the left ventricle and often the right ventricle. Abrupt occlusion in the LAD or LCX causes infarction in the corresponding territory, but occlusion of the left main coronary artery is usually fatal.

The venous system mainly follows the coronary arteries, but drains to the coronary sinus in the inferior atrioventricular groove, and then to the right atrium where its orifice is protected from backflow by the Thebesian valve. Small (Eustachian) veins also drain directly into the right atrium. An extensive lymphatic system drains into vessels which travel with the coronary vessels and then into the thoracic duct.

Nerve supply of the heart

The heart is innervated by both sympathetic and parasympathetic supply. Adrenergic nerves supply muscle fibres in the atria and ventricles and the electrical conducting system. Positive inotropic and chronotropic effects are mediated predominantly by β_1-adrenoceptors (β_2-adrenoceptors predominate in vascular smooth muscle). Parasympathetic pre-ganglionic fibres and sensory fibres reach the heart through the vagus nerve. Cholinergic nerves supply the AV and SA nodes via muscarinic (M2) receptors. Under resting conditions the predominant effect is due to vagal inhibitory fibres, rather than sympathetic fibres. The roles of parasympathetic and sympathetic function in disease states are still emerging, but they may exert profound influences on control of heart rate and arrhythmia generation.

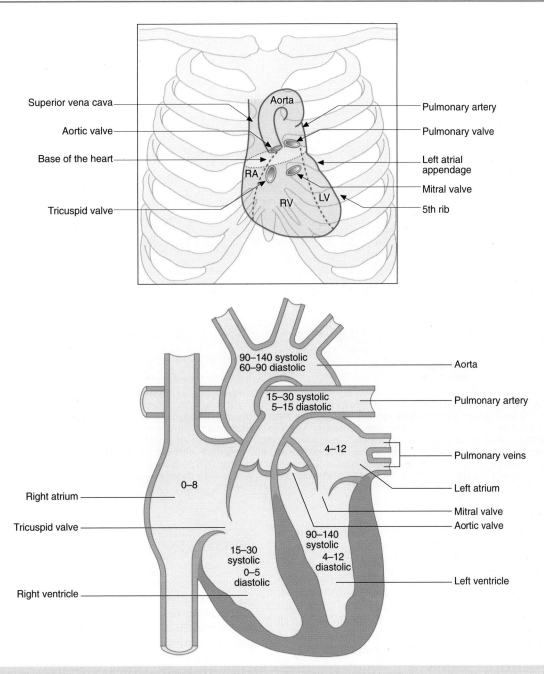

Fig. 5.1 Top: **Radiological outline of the heart** showing the positions of the major cardiac chambers and heart valves. Bottom: **Schematic diagram of the major cardiac structures** (left anterior oblique projection), with Normal Resting Pressures in mmHg. Oxygen consumption index 110–150 ml/min/m^2; cardiac output index 2.5–4.2 l/min/m^2.

The electrical conduction system

The sinoatrial node is situated at the junction of the superior vena cava and right atrium and is the origin of the impulses responsible for heart rhythm under normal conditions ('sinus rhythm'). Depolarisation of the sinus node triggers a wave front of depolarisation which travels through the atrium. Conduction directly to the ventricles is prevented by the annulus fibrosus, which insulates the atria from the ventricles. The atrioventricular (AV) node is situated beneath the right atrial endo-

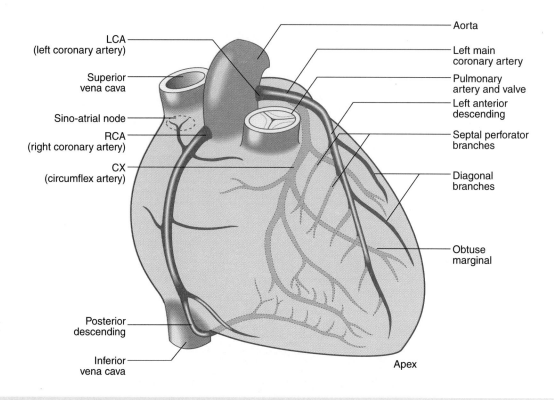

Fig. 5.1—*continued.* **Diagram of the coronary arteries of the heart** (anterior view). The left (LCA) and right (RCA) coronary arteries arise in the respective sinuses just distal to the aortic valve. The left main coronary artery divides into a left anterior descending branch which supplies the front wall and apex of the heart, and a circumflex (CX) branch which supplies the posterior wall of the heart and a variable proportion of the inferior wall. The right coronary artery gives off right ventricular branches and may give rise to the posterior descending vessel which runs in the posterior interventricular groove. The sinoatrial node (sinus node) is situated at the junction of the superior vena cava and right atrium and the atrioventricular node (AV node) is situated beneath the right atrial endocardium at the lower end of the interatrial septum.

cardium at the lower end of the interatrial septum. It conducts slowly and regulates the frequency of conduction to the ventricles. From the AV node the His bundle passes through the annulus fibrosus and divides into right and left bundles which pass down the respective sides of the ventricular septum. The left is subdivided into anterior and posterior hemibundles, and all His fibres radiate out as the Purkinje network. Injury to the right or left His bundle is evident on the electrocardiogram as the respective right or left bundle branch block, and injury to a hemibundle as a deviation in electrical axis.

The valves of the heart

The structure and function of the atrioventricular valves (mitral and tricuspid) and ventricular outflow valves (aortic and pulmonary) are considered in relation to cardiac investigations (p. 201) and to disorders of the valves (p. 280).

PHYSIOLOGY

Myocardial contraction

Myocardial cells (myocytes) are about 100 μm long and each cell branches and interdigitates with adjacent cells. An intercalated disc permits electrical conduction (via gap junctions) and force conduction (via the fascia adherens) to adjacent cells. The basic unit of contraction is the sarcomere (2 μm length), which is aligned to those of adjacent myofibrils, giving a striated appearance due to the Z-lines (Fig. 5.2). Actin filaments (molecular weight 47,000) are attached at right angles to the Z-lines, and interdigitate with thicker parallel myosin filaments (molecular weight 500,000). The cross-links between actin and myosin molecules contain myofibrillar ATPase, which breaks down ATP to provide the energy for contraction. Two chains of actin molecules form a helical structure, with a second molecule, tropomyosin,

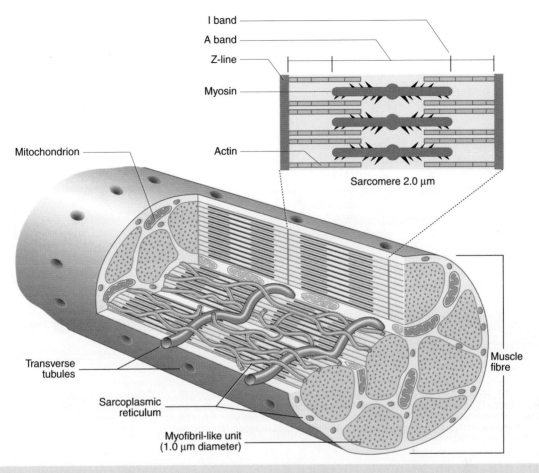

I band

A band

Z-line

Myosin

Mitochondrion

Actin

Sarcomere 2.0 μm

Muscle fibre

Transverse tubules

Sarcoplasmic reticulum

Myofibril-like unit (1.0 μm diameter)

Fig. 5.2   Schematic of a muscle fibre showing the arrangement of myofibrils, and longitudinal and transverse tubules extending from the sarcoplasmic reticulum. Expanded section shows schematic of an individual sarcomere with thick filaments composed of myosin and thin filaments composed primarily of actin.

in the grooves of the actin helix, with a further molecule, troponin, attached to every seventh actin molecule (Fig. 5.3).

During contraction, shortening of the sarcomere results from the actin and myosin molecules interdigitating, without altering the length of either molecule. Contraction is initiated when calcium is made available during the plateau phase of the action potential by calcium ions entering the cell and being mobilised from the sarcolemma. As its concentration rises calcium binds to troponin C, precipitating contraction. The force of cardiac muscle contraction, or inotropic state, is regulated by the influx of calcium ions through 'slow calcium channels'. The extent to which the sarcomere can shorten determines stroke volume of the ventricle. It is maximally shortened in response to powerful inotropic drugs or severe exercise. However, the enlargement of the heart seen in heart failure is due to slippage of the myofibrils and adjacent cells, rather than lengthening of the sarcomere.

Factors influencing cardiac output

Cardiac output is determined by the product of stroke volume and heart rate. Stroke volume is dependent upon end-diastolic pressure (preload) and peripheral vascular resistance (afterload).

Stretch of cardiac muscle (as indicated by an increment in end-diastolic volume) results in increased force of contraction (measured as increased stroke volume). This relationship is known as Starling's Law of the heart. Afterload falls as blood pressure is reduced and this allows greater shortening of the muscle fibres and hence increased stroke volume.

The contractile state of the myocardium is controlled, in part, by the neuro-endocrine system, including for

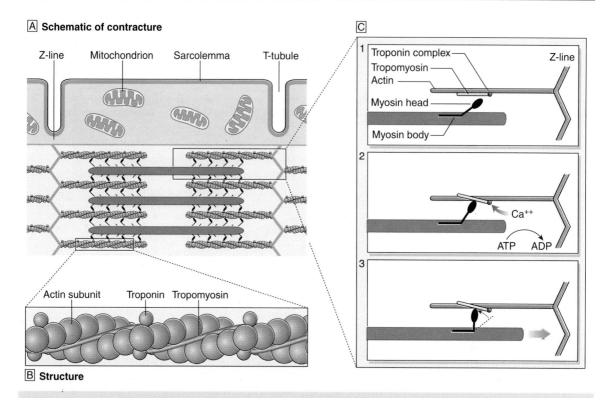

A Schematic of contracture

Z-line · Mitochondrion · Sarcolemma · T-tubule

Actin subunit · Troponin · Tropomyosin

B Structure

C

1. Troponin complex · Tropomyosin · Actin · Myosin head · Myosin body · Z-line
2. Ca^{++} · ATP · ADP
3.

Fig. 5.3 **A**, top left: Schematic of a sarcomere showing overlapping of actin and myosin filaments. **B**, below left: Enlarged diagram of the structure of an actin filament. **C**, right: Diagram of three stages of contraction resulting in shortening of the sarcomere. *Top*: The actin binding site is blocked by tropomyosin. *Centre*: ATP-dependent release of calcium ions which bind to troponin C, displacing tropomyosin. The binding site is exposed. *Bottom*: Tilting of the angle of attachment of the myosin head, resulting in fibre shortening.

example sympathetic tone and reflexes. It is influenced by various inotropic drugs and their antagonists.

Determination of the response to a physiological change, or a drug, can be predicted on the basis of the combined influence on preload, afterload and contractility.

Factors influencing resistance to coronary blood flow
Coronary blood vessels receive sympathetic and parasympathetic innervation. Stimulation of alpha receptors causes vasoconstriction and β_2-adrenoceptors vasodilatation, but the predominant effect of sympathetic stimulation in coronary arteries is vasodilatation. Parasympathetic stimulation also causes a modest dilatation of normal coronary arteries. Intracoronary acetylcholine stimulates the local release of nitric oxide ('Endothelial-Derived Relaxing Factor', EDRF) and this causes vasodilatation. In the presence of endothelial damage or atheroma acetylcholine acts directly on vascular smooth muscle, causing constriction. Other locally derived factors (for example endothelins), systemic hormones and neuropeptides all influence arterial tone and hence blood pressure (see hypertension section, p. 266).

Factors influencing resistance to systemic blood flow
Systemic blood flow is critically dependent upon vascular resistance, which varies with the fourth power of the radius of the resistance vessel. Thus small changes in calibre have a marked influence on blood flow. Metabolic and mechanical factors control arteriolar tone. Neurogenic constriction operates via alpha adrenergic receptors on vascular smooth muscle, and dilatation via muscarinic and β_2-adrenoceptors. In addition, systemic and locally released vasoactive substances influence tone (constrictors like noradrenaline, angiotensin and endothelin, dilators like adenosine, bradykinin, prostaglandins and nitric oxide). See also hypertension section, page 266.

PHYSIOLOGICAL BASIS OF PHYSICAL SIGNS

Investigation of the cardiovascular system begins with physical examination, and then proceeds to bedside and specific laboratory investigations, depending upon the clues elicited. The choice of further investigation is determined by the clinical history and physical examination. A detailed description of the techniques of physical examination is beyond the scope of this textbook, but the physiological basis of the most important physical signs will be considered (recommendations for further reading are found at the end of this section).

The arterial pulse

The arterial pulse is conveniently assessed by palpation of the radial artery, but the volume and character of the pulse are better judged in a larger vessel like the brachial or carotid artery. The following information box describes common terms in relation to the arterial pulse, and a summary of their underlying mechanisms.

THE ARTERIAL PULSE

PULSE VOLUME
Depends on cardiac stroke volume and arterial compliance.

- **Small pulse volume** (pulsus parvus) occurs in cardiac failure, hypovolaemia, vasoconstriction and any cause of reduced cardiac output
- **Large pulse volume** occurs in vasodilatation, pyrexia, anaemia, aortic regurgitation and arteriovenous shunting
- **Pulsus alternans** describes an alternating pattern of large and small volume beats, despite a regular rhythm, and is seen in cardiac failure. Uncommon and must be distinguished from coupled ectopics
- **Pulsus paradoxus**: a misleading term because it is an exaggeration of the normal variation in systolic arterial pressure seen with respiration. (Normally falls by <10 mm of Hg on inspiration). Seen in airways obstruction, pericardial tamponade and massive pulmonary embolism
- **Pulsus bisferiens**: 'double peak'. May be seen in combined aortic stenosis and regurgitation, and occasionally in hypertrophic cardiomyopathy. First component due to the percussion wave of a large volume of blood ejected in systole; second component due to elastic recoil in the arteries

PULSE RHYTHM
Regular in periodicity with sinus rhythm with the exception of the variation induced by respiration.

- **Sinus arrhythmia**: acceleration of heart rate on inspiration (in response to reduced intrathoracic pressure and reduced return to the left heart)
- **Atrial fibrillation**: totally irregular in time and volume (distinguish from sinus rhythm with multiple ectopics)
- **Ectopic beats**: usually occur before the end of diastole, hence don't produce a palpable pulse. Sensation of a 'dropped beat' followed by a beat with increased volume

---

The jugular venous pulse

The jugular venous pulse provides a convenient bedside means of measuring right atrial pressure. The internal jugular vein is in direct continuity with the right atrium, whereas the external jugular may be obstructed by muscular or fascial tissue or valves. The patient should be inclined so that the top of the venous wave may be seen (often about 45°, but this may need to be steeper or shallower according to the height of venous pulse). *The jugular venous pressure is the vertical height between the manubriosternal angle and the top of the venous wave* (normally 3–4 cms). The mid right atrium lies approximately 5 cms below the manubriosternal angle, with an average diastolic pressure of less than 8 mmHg.

THE JUGULAR VENOUS PULSE IS DISTINGUISHED FROM THE CAROTID ARTERIAL PULSE BY THE FOLLOWING CHARACTERISTICS:

- Venous pulse visible but not palpable
- Two peaks in each cycle of the venous pulse, one in the arterial
- Venous pulse obliterated by gentle pressure at the root of the neck; arterial pulse not
- Venous pulse rises and falls with respiration and position of the patient
- Abdominal compression causes the venous pulse to rise—'hepato-jugular reflux'

Abnormally low venous pressure occurs in hypovolaemia (e.g. haemorrhage). Elevated jugular venous pressure occurs in any form of cardiac failure involving the right heart; pericardial constriction or tamponade; expanded circulating volume or obstruction of the superior vena cava.

The jugular venous pressure wave is illustrated in Figure 5.4. The *a* wave is produced by atrial systole and the *v* wave by venous filling during ventricular systole. The *x* descent is produced by atrial relaxation and downward displacement of the tricuspid valve ring in ventricular systole, and the *y* descent by the fall in pressure as the tricuspid valve opens. After the *a* wave there is a small positive pressure wave during early atrial relaxation, the *c* wave, possibly due to recoil or transmission from the carotid pulse. The *c* wave can seldom be distinguished at the bedside.

The *a* wave is abolished in atrial fibrillation. Large *a* waves occur in pulmonary hypertension, right ventricular hypertrophy and tricuspid stenosis (unless the patient is in atrial fibrillation). In the presence of atrial-ventricular dissociation the atrium sometimes contracts against a closed tricuspid valve (for example in complete heart block or ventricular tachycardia), and the blood regurgitates into the venae cavae giving rise to a very large *a* wave, the *cannon wave*. Cannon waves are almost

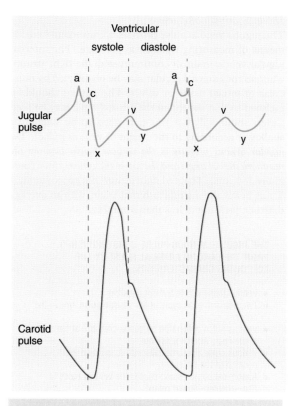

Fig. 5.4 Carotid and jugular pulses. Simultaneous central arterial and venous pulses to demonstrate carotid and jugular pulse waveform. *a* = atrial contraction; *c* = onset of ventricular contraction; *v* = pressure peak immediately prior to opening of the tricuspid valve; *c* to *x* = the x descent; *v* to *y* = the y descent.

always intermittent. In junctional rhythms regular cannon waves may occasionally be produced due to simultaneous atrial and ventricular contractions.

Tricuspid regurgitation produces giant *v* waves with each ventricular contraction, and hence the waves are visible in time with systole and with every beat.

Steep *y* descent due to an abrupt fall in diastolic pressure occurs in constrictive pericarditis, tricuspid regurgitation, and to a lesser extent in right ventricular failure.

The praecordium

Deformities of the chest wall may produce malposition of the heart and can give rise to murmurs. Pectus excavatum, visible as an indented sternum, may produce a 'benign' systolic murmur, as may kyphoscoliosis. Abnormal pulsations may be visible as a result of right or left ventricular hypertrophy, or aneurysm formation in the aorta or left ventricle. The latter produces a paradoxical bulge as the aneurysm expands in systole.

The **apex beat** is defined as the most inferior and lateral point of cardiac pulsation, and is normally in the 4th or 5th intercostal space just lateral to the mid-clavicular line. It may be visible or palpable and its position gives a guide to cardiac enlargement. Left ventricular dilatation displaces the apex towards the axilla and inferiorly. The character of the apex beat may be a guide to certain conditions, but the recording of the apex cardiogram has been superseded by echocardiography. A displaced and thrusting apex may be evident in conditions of volume overload of the ventricle (e.g. aortic or mitral regurgitation) and a sustained apical impulse with ventricular hypertrophy occurs when there is pressure of the left ventricle (e.g. aortic stenosis). A 'tapping' apex may be evident in mitral stenosis, with a brief impulse and no ventricular enlargement. In chronic obstructive airways disease, emphysema or obesity the apex may be impalpable.

A parasternal heave may be palpable at the left sternal edge in the presence of right ventricular hypertrophy, or rarely, left atrial enlargement. A systolic impulse in the 2nd left interspace is usually due to pulmonary hypertension. Very loud heart sounds may also be palpable (sometimes a 3rd or 4th heart sound in heart failure), or clicks (for example an aortic ejection click).

Palpable vibrations, 'thrills' produced by murmurs, may also be present, including the systolic thrill of aortic stenosis, or the diastolic thrill of mitral stenosis. These are palpable in areas which correspond with the murmurs and they are not produced by benign conditions.

Heart sounds

The **first heart sound** results from closure of the mitral, and to a lesser extent tricuspid, valve, and is best heard at the apex. The sound is usually appreciated as single, but may be narrowly split on account of the two components. This benign phenomenon must be distinguished from an ejection click due to aortic or pulmonary valve stenosis, or a 4th heart sound due to heart failure. The first heart sound is loud in the presence of a hyperdynamic circulation (anaemia, pregnancy, thyrotoxicosis) and soft in heart failure or if the leaflets do not close properly in mitral regurgitation or severe calcific mitral stenosis. Usually however, mitral stenosis produces a loud first sound. The intensity of the first sound will vary when the PR interval is variable (as in atrio-ventricular dissociation), depending upon the changing contribution of the atrium to diastolic filling of the ventricle.

The **second heart sound** is produced by closure of the aortic and pulmonary valves and is best heard at the base of the heart. The aortic component is loud in arterial hypertension and soft in the presence of diminished cardiac output. Similarly, the pulmonary component is loud in pulmonary hypertension and soft in pulmonary stenosis. The pulmonary valve closes shortly after the aortic valve as right ventricular emptying is more prolonged than that of the left ventricle. The pulmonary component (P2) is further delayed on inspiration as increased venous return delays right ventricular emptying. This gives rise to the physiological splitting of the second sound on inspiration. Reversed splitting (i.e. on expiration) occurs when left heart emptying is delayed, as in left bundle branch block, left ventricular failure or aortic stenosis (S2 is soft in aortic stenosis). The pulmonary component is delayed on inspiration, bringing the sounds together. Conversely, wide but variable splitting of S2 occurs with delayed emptying of the right ventricle as in right bundle branch block or pulmonary stenosis.

Wide *fixed* splitting of the second heart sound occurs in atrial septal defect on account of the balanced pressures in the atria but volume overload of the right heart and concomitant right bundle branch block. Because of the atrial connection respiration no longer produces differential effects on emptying of the two sides of the heart. In contrast, wide but variable splitting of S2 may occur with pulmonary embolism on account of raised pulmonary artery pressure.

Added heart sounds

Additional sounds are produced as a result of ventricular filling under conditions of altered loading of the ventricle. They are low pitched and occur either early (third sound) or late (fourth sound) in diastole. In sinus tachycardia the individual sounds may be difficult to distinguish, and a cadence described as a 'gallop' rhythm may result (similar to the hoof beats of a galloping horse).

The third sound (Fig. 5.5) is generated in the ventricular wall due to the vibrations caused by the abrupt cessation of rapid ventricular filling. It is common in the young, in pregnancy, and other hyperdynamic states (e.g. thyrotoxicosis). It also occurs in pathological conditions like heart failure, cardiomyopathy or volume overload of the ventricle, and may be heard best at the left sternal edge or apex.

A fourth sound (Fig. 5.5) occurs in the presence of an abnormally stiff ventricle and augmented atrial contraction. It is low pitched and occurs just before the first heart sound, in time with atrial contraction. It is indicative of a pathological state, but does not occur in atrial fibrillation, or other conditions without co-ordinated atrial contraction. It is frequently heard following myocardial infarction, heart failure, or conditions in which hypertrophy of the ventricle increases stiffness.

Early systolic or midsystolic clicks are due to abnormal valves and may be associated with a murmur of valve

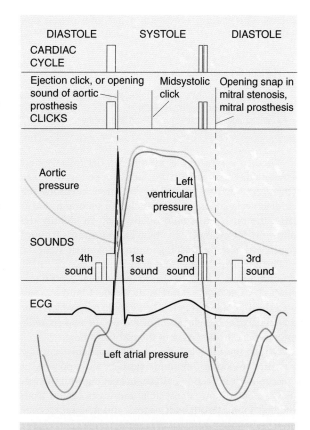

Fig. 5.5 Diagram to show the relationship of the cardiac cycle to the electrocardiogram, the left ventricular pressure wave and the position of heart sounds.

stenosis (aortic or pulmonary), or valve regurgitation (floppy mitral valve respectively). The presence of an ejection click indicates that outflow tract obstruction is likely to be valvular, rather than supra- or infra-valvular.

Prosthetic heart sounds are produced by the opening and closing of normally functioning mechanical valves, and heard as loud clicks. When a valve is obstructed by thrombus or vegetation these sounds may be lost.

Cardiac murmurs

Murmurs are associated with turbulent blood flow. When cardiac output is greatly increased, as with exercise, pregnancy or severe anaemia, blood flow through a normal aortic or pulmonary valve may become turbulent, and give rise to a systolic murmur usually best heard at the sternal border in the second left intercostal space. Murmurs also arise when blood is projected through, or leaks back across, abnormal valves, or through an abnormal channel such as a ventricular septal defect. The features are listed in the information box below.

FEATURES OF MURMURS

- Systolic or diastolic?
- Where is it heard best?
- Where does it radiate to?
- Intensity and thrill?
- Duration?
- Pitch and quality?

Whether a murmur is systolic or diastolic is best assessed by timing it with the apex beat or carotid pulse (Fig. 5.6). Changes in a murmur's intensity during the cardiac cycle are an important clue to its origin. Similarly, the pitch and sound quality help to identify the murmur; for example the 'blowing' murmur of mitral regurgitation or the 'rasping' murmur of aortic stenosis.

The intensity (loudness) is graded on a scale of 1 to 6. A grade 1 murmur is only heard under ideal conditions, grade 2 is soft, grade 3 moderate, grade 4 loud (associated thrill), grade 5 very loud and grade 6 heard without a stethoscope. The location of a murmur and its radiation reflect the direction of the turbulent flow.

Systolic murmurs associated with ventricular outflow obstruction occur in mid systole and possess a crescendo-decrescendo pattern, in keeping with the velocity of blood flow. Pansystolic murmurs extend from the first sound throughout systole, and maintain a constant intensity. Regurgitation into a low pressure chamber continues with similar velocity throughout systole, and hence the murmur is pansystolic, and of similar intensity throughout its duration. Late systolic murmurs similarly reflect the velocity of flow (for example, the dynamic obstruction of hypertrophic cardiomyopathy which occurs late in systole).

Diastolic murmurs are indicative of abnormal pathology, and do not occur under physiological conditions. Mid-diastolic murmurs occur due to flow across the mitral or tricuspid valves, in keeping with the velocity of blood flow. Early diastolic murmurs occur with regurgitation across the aortic or pulmonary valves. They begin in early diastole, decrescendo in character and blowing in quality.

Continuous murmurs result from a combination of systolic and diastolic flow (as in a persistent ductus arteriosus). They should be distinguished from sounds produced by flow in arterial shunts or occasionally by high rates of venous flow in children ('venous hum'). Extra-cardiac sounds like that of pericardial friction (see p.

Table 5.1 Murmurs and their location

SYSTOLIC MURMURS	
Mid-systolic (crescendo-decrescendo) murmurs	
Aortic stenosis	Aortic area (radiating towards neck) and/or left sternal edge
Pulmonary stenosis	
Hypertrophic cardiomyopathy	
Fallot's tetralogy	
Atrial septal defect (pulmonary flow)	
Pan-systolic murmurs	
Mitral regurgitation	Apex (radiating towards axilla)
Tricuspid regurgitation	Left sternal edge: (low pitched)
Ventricular septal defect	(harsh, rasping)
Late-systolic murmurs	
Mitral valve prolapse	Apex
Hypertrophic cardiomyopathy	
DIASTOLIC MURMURS	
Early-diastolic murmurs	
Aortic regurgitation	Left sternal edge
Pulmonary regurgitation, Graham Steell: (pulmonary regurgitation due to pulmonary hypertension and mitral stenosis)	
Mid-diastolic murmurs	
Mitral stenosis	Apex
Austin Flint: (aortic regurgitation impairing mitral diastolic flow)	Left sternal edge
Tricuspid stenosis	
CONTINUOUS MURMURS	
Persistent ductus arteriosus	Upper left sternal edge
Venous hum (positional)	Anterior chest wall/elsewhere
Arteriovenous shunts	

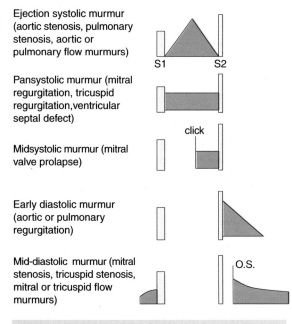

Ejection systolic murmur (aortic stenosis, pulmonary stenosis, aortic or pulmonary flow murmurs)

S1   S2

Pansystolic murmur (mitral regurgitation, tricuspid regurgitation, ventricular septal defect)

Midsystolic murmur (mitral valve prolapse)

click

Early diastolic murmur (aortic or pulmonary regurgitation)

Mid-diastolic murmur (mitral stenosis, tricuspid stenosis, mitral or tricuspid flow murmurs)

O.S.

Fig. 5.6 Diagram to show the timing and pattern of cardiac murmurs.

309) extend variably through systole and diastole, and do not have a constant relationship to the cardiac sounds. Pericardial friction is described as scratching or crunching in character.

More detailed consideration of specific murmurs and associated clinical features is given in the later sections which deal with valvular and congenital defects.

INVESTIGATIONS

Investigations can be considered in two categories: non-invasive tests conveniently performed at the bedside (e.g. ECG, echocardiography), and more complex procedures usually performed in a specialised facility (cardiac catheterisation, nuclear scanning, CT, MRI).

ELECTROCARDIOGRAPHY (ECG)

Electrocardiography is used to elucidate cardiac arrhythmias and conduction defects, and to diagnose and localise myocardial hypertrophy, ischaemia or infarction. It may also give information about electrolyte imbalance and the toxicity of certain drugs.

The fundamental basis for electrocardiography is that the electrical activation of a heart muscle cell causes a depolarisation of its membrane. The depolarisation is propagated along the length of a cell or fibre, and transmitted to adjoining cells. The result is a moving wavefront of depolarisation which passes through the heart and sets up electrical currents which are detected by surface electrodes, and amplified and displayed as the electrocardiograms. For each lead of the ECG the electrocardiogram represents summation of depolarisation and repolarisation, as seen from that position in the vertical or frontal plane. Electrocardiographic symbols and abbreviations are given in the information box.

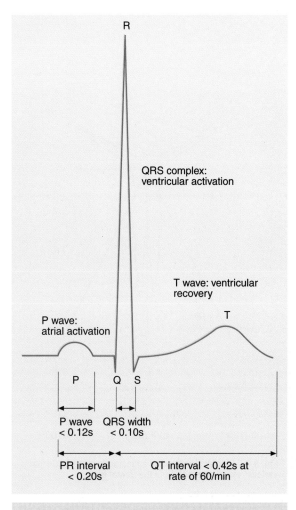

Fig. 5.7 Diagram to show the components of an ECG complex.

ELECTROCARDIOGRAPHIC SYMBOLS AND ABBREVIATIONS

I, II, III, aVR, aVL, aVF   'limb leads' (Fig. 5.8)

These reflect depolarisation of the heart from various positions in the frontal plane.

VI-V6   'chest leads' (Fig. 5.9)

These reflect electrical activation of the heart from various positions in the horizontal plane.

SA node	sinoatrial node
P wave	atrial depolarisation
QRS complex	ventricular activation
QT interval	repolarisation of the heart
R-R interval	Interval between successive R waves in the ECG

The standard 12-lead ECG

Components of the ECG complex are illustrated in Figure 5.7. Leads I, II, III, aVR, aVL and aVF are orientated in the frontal plane and are referred to as limb leads (Fig. 5.8). Leads V1 to V6 are orientated in the horizontal plane and called chest leads (Fig. 5.9). V1-V2 mainly reflect the right ventricle, V3-V4 the interventricular septum, and V5-V6 the left ventricle.

Normally, cardiac activation starts in the sinoatrial (SA) node, but this cannot be detected on the ECG. The depolarisation then spreads through the atria, producing an upright P wave in all leads except aVR (the net vector is towards all leads except aVR). The only point at which the impulse can be transmitted to the ventricles is via the atrioventricular (AV) node, through which conduction is relatively slow (the PR interval). It

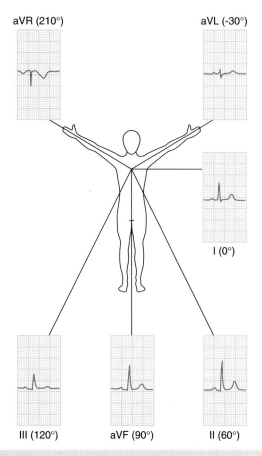

aVR (210°) aVL (-30°)

I (0°)

III (120°) aVF (90°) II (60°)

Fig. 5.8 Diagram to show the appearance of the ECG from various recording positions in the frontal plane.

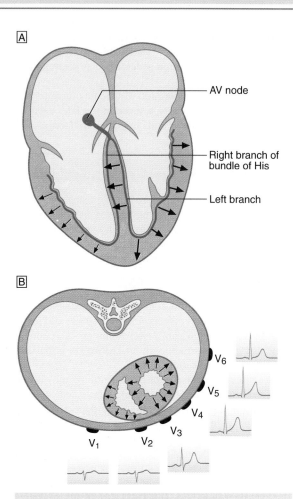

AV node

Right branch of bundle of His

Left branch

V6
V5
V4
V3
V1 V2

Fig. 5.9 Activation of the septum is from left to right followed by spreading of the impulse through both ventricles [A]. Electrocardiographic complexes from various positions in the horizontal plane and the sequence of activation from the atrium to ventricles [B].

then goes rapidly through the left and right branches of the bundle of His to ventricular muscle, triggering ventricular activation. The QRS complex represents ventricular activation, and in most leads this is dominated by the upright R wave from the left ventricle (as the depolarisation spreads towards the leads it produces a positive deflection). In lateral leads such as lead I and V6 the R wave is preceded by a small negative deflection (a Q wave) caused by activation from left to right of the interventricular septum. Septal activation is not normally detected in leads V4-V6, II, III and aVF as these are at right angles to septal depolarisation. In leads aVR and V1 the main direction of left ventricular activation is away from the electrode, giving a dominant S wave. The QRS axis is the mean frontal plane vector of the QRS complex, and can be estimated roughly by seeing which limb lead has the biggest R wave (Fig. 5.10). Normally it lies between 0° (largest R, smallest S in lead 1) and 90° (largest R, smallest S in aVF).

ECG CONVENTIONS AND HEART RATE

- Depolarisation towards electrode: positive deflection
- Depolarisation away from electrode: negative deflection
- Sensitivity: 10 mm = 1 mV
- Paper speed: 25 mm per second
- Each large (5 mm) square = 0.2 s
- Each small (1 mm) square = 0.04 s
- Heart rate = 1500/R-R interval (mm)
- If R-R interval = 5 mm, heart rate = 300/min
- If R-R interval = 25 mm, heart rate = 60/min

Exercise (stress) ECG

By performing an ECG during progressively increasing exercise (usually on a treadmill) it is possible to detect

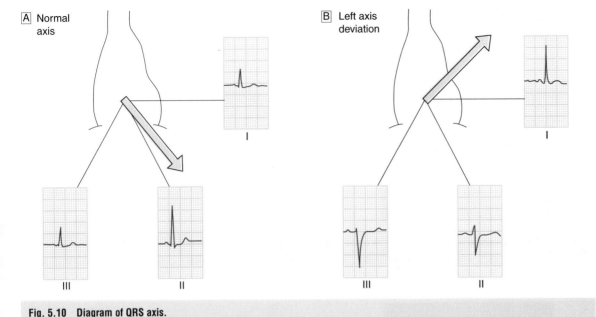

A Normal axis

B Left axis deviation

Fig. 5.10 Diagram of QRS axis.

stress-provoked arrhythmias, or evidence of ischaemia. Blood pressure recording and assessment of symptoms are performed regularly during the test. Horizontal or downsloping ST segment depression of > 1 mm suggests ischaemia. Failure to achieve an increase in blood pressure, or the occurrence of a fall in pressure during exertion, is evidence of ventricular decompensation and is usually indicative of extensive ischaemia. The inability to achieve the predicted heart rate target renders the test inconclusive, rather than negative. An exercise ECG is necessary to confirm the clinical diagnosis of ischaemic heart disease and is useful in guiding further management, or evaluating the management of arrhythmia. High risk patients may be identified on the basis of a low exercise threshold to provoke ischaemia, or functional decompensation during exercise. Following myocardial infarction an exercise test may be used in risk assessment, but sensitivity of the test is reduced (see nuclear imaging). Stress tests are *contraindicated* in the presence of unstable angina, decompensated heart failure, severe hypertension or severe outflow obstruction (e.g. aortic stenosis).

Ambulatory ECG (Holter monitoring)
Continuous recordings of one or more ECG leads may be obtained by attaching them to a small portable solid state or tape recorder. This technique is useful in detecting transient episodes of arrhythmia or ischaemia, which seldom occur fortuitously during the short time taken for routine 12-lead ECG recordings. Infrequent arrhythmias may be detected with a device which is placed over the chest during the symptomatic episode. This records the ECG for subsequent trans-telephonic transmission to a cardiac centre.

RADIOLOGY

A chest radiograph is useful for determining the size and shape of the heart, and the state of the pulmonary blood vessels and lung fields. Most information is given by a postero-anterior (PA) projection taken in full inspiration. Antero-posterior (AP) projections are convenient when the patient is confined to bed (intensive care units) but result in magnification of the cardiac shadow because of the divergence of the radiograph beam.

An estimate of overall heart size can be made by comparing the maximum width of the cardiac outline with the maximum internal transverse diameter of the thoracic cavity. This 'cardiothoracic ratio' should be less than 0.5 and the transverse cardiac diameter less than 15.5 cms. Enlargement of the cardiac silhouette occurs with pericardial effusion, and apparent enlargement may be mimicked by mediastinal masses.

Dilatation of individual cardiac chambers can be recognised by the characteristic alterations they cause to

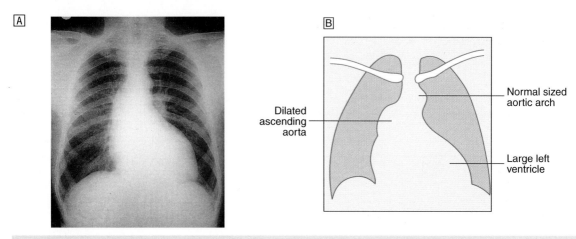

Fig. 5.11   Chest radiograph Ⓐ **from a patient with aortic regurgitation, left ventricular enlargement and dilatation of the ascending aorta.** Line diagram Ⓑ to illustrate the position of major structures.

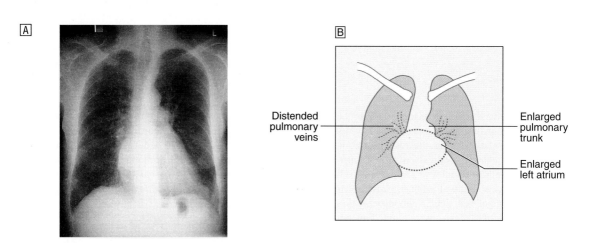

Fig. 5.12   Chest radiograph Ⓐ **of a patient with mitral stenosis and regurgitation** indicating enlargement of the left atrium and prominence of the pulmonary artery trunk. Line diagram Ⓑ to illustrate major structures.

the cardiac silhouette (see Figs. 5.11 and 5.12, and also the sections on valvular heart disease).

- Left atrial dilatation results in prominence of the left atrial appendage, a double cardiac shadow to the right of the sternum and widening of the angle of the carina as the left main bronchus is pushed upward.
- Right atrial enlargement projects from the right heart border towards the right lower lung field.
- Left ventricular dilatation causes prominence of the left lower heart border and enlargement of the cardiac silhouette. LV hypertrophy does not cause overall cardiac enlargement unless heart failure ensues.
- Right ventricular dilatation increases heart size and

displaces the apex upward. Differentiation from LV dilatation may be difficult on chest radiograph.

Lateral or oblique projections may be useful in detecting aortic or mitral valve calcification, which may be obscured by the spine on the PA view. However, echocardiography is more sensitive.

The chest radiograph in heart failure

A rise in pulmonary venous pressure from left-sided cardiac failure first shows on the chest radiograph as an abnormal distension of the upper lobe pulmonary veins (with the patient in the erect position). The vascularity of the lung fields becomes more prominent and the pulmonary artery dilated (the right lower pulmonary artery should measure less than 16 mmHg). Subsequently, interstitial oedema causes thickened interlobular septa and dilated lymphatics (when pulmonary venous pressure is in the range 20–30 mmHg. Normal is 5–14 mmHg). These are evident as horizontal lines in the costophrenic angles (Kerley 'B' lines). More advanced changes due to alveolar oedema cause a hazy opacification spreading from the hilar regions, and pleural effusions (pulmonary venous pressure > 30 mmHg).

An increased pulmonary blood flow, as in congenital heart disease with a left-to-right shunt, causes enlargement of the pulmonary artery and a generalised increase in pulmonary vascular markings. Pulmonary arterial hypertension also causes an enlargement of the main pulmonary artery and of the proximal pulmonary arteries, but the peripheral lung vascular markings tend to be diminished.

ECHOCARDIOGRAPHY (ECHO)

This uses reflected ultrasound to study blood flow, the structure of the heart and the movement of valves and cardiac muscle. Ultrasound is reflected at interfaces, between blood and more solid tissues, because the velocity of sound is almost constant in body tissues and hence anatomic dimensions can be measured.

M-mode echocardiography
The ECG is recorded simultaneously and permits accurate measurements of the timing of cardiac events including the opening and closing of valves. The ultrasound is focused into a narrow beam, and the information is presented graphically with respect to time and depicts the structures through which the beam passes. Characteristic patterns of valve movement are produced in, for example, mitral stenosis, and pericardial effusions are easily recognised.

Two-dimensional (or cross-sectional) real-time echocardiography
Using a mechanical probe with rotating crystals, or an electronic equivalent, the ultrasound beam is swung rapidly back and forth over an arc or sector. The resulting information is synthesised into a two-dimensional map or picture of the position of the reflecting structures and presented on a television screen (Fig. 5.13). The picture is the equivalent of a 'slice' through the heart, in a par-

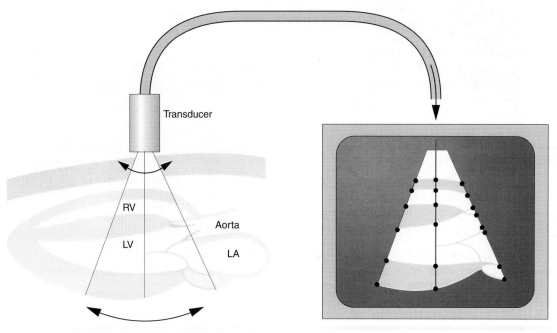

Narrow ultrasound beam rapidly oscillated through 60° or 90°

TV display builds up composite ultrasound image; image is produced and renewed fast enough to follow 'real time' movement of the heart

Fig. 5.13 Principles of 2-dimensional (2D) echocardiography. A moving 2-dimensional image of echoes detected from a 'slice' of heart can be reconstructed to show movement of the cardiac structures.

ticular plane, and the structures shown will depend on the position and orientation of the ultrasound probe. Because the beam oscillates very rapidly, the ultrasound image accurately reproduces the movement of structures in the living heart (hence 'real time') (Fig. 5.14). This type of echocardiography is particularly valuable for detecting intracardiac masses, such as thrombi or tumours, or endocarditic vegetations. It is also very useful in defining complex structural abnormalities in congenital heart disease.

Doppler cardiography

This technique depends on the fundamental principle that sound waves reflected from moving objects, such as intracardiac red blood cells, undergo a frequency shift. The speed and direction of movement of the red cells, and thus of blood, can be detected in the heart chambers and great vessels. The greater the frequency shift, the faster the blood is moving. The derived information can be presented either as a plot of blood velocity against time for a particular point in the heart (Fig. 5.15) or as a colour overlay on a two-dimensional real-time echo picture (colour flow doppler). Doppler cardiography is valuable in detecting abnormal directions of blood flow, e.g. aortic or mitral reflux, and in estimating pressure gradients, for example the gradient across a stenosed aortic valve (Fig. 5.16). Normal velocities are in the order of 1 m/sec, but in the presence of a stenosis flow velocity is increased (for example in severe aortic stenosis the peak aortic velocity may be increased to 5 m/sec). An estimate of the pressure gradient across a valve or lesion is given by the Bernoulli equation:

$$\text{Pressure gradient} = 4 \times (\text{velocity})^2$$

CARDIAC CATHETERISATION AND ANGIOCARDIOGRAPHY

In contrast to the preceding investigations, these techniques require a catheter to be inserted into a vein or artery and manipulated to the heart under radiographic fluoroscopic guidance. For example, a catheter from the femoral or brachial fossa vein can be advanced into the right atrium, and then manipulated into the right ventricle and pulmonary artery. In the presence of an atrial septal defect or patent foramen ovale, venous catheters can also enter the left atrium and left ventricle. If the atrial septum is intact, access to the left ventricle is usually obtained by retrograde passage of a catheter across the aortic valve. Left atrial pressure can be measured directly by puncturing the interatrial septum with a special catheter containing a short needle, advanced via the femoral vein and right atrium. For many purposes, however, a satisfactory approximation to left atrial pres-

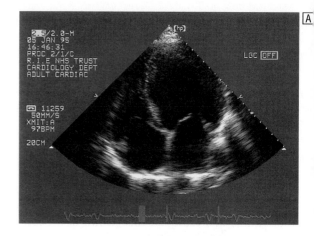

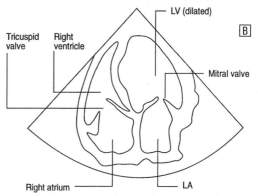

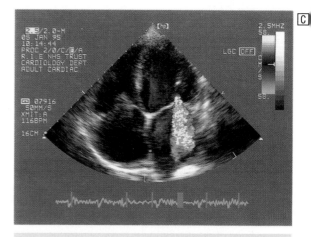

Fig. 5.14 Echocardiographic illustration of the principal cardiac structures in the '4 chamber' view. [A] Late diastole. [B] Line diagram of major features. [C] Mitral regurgitation showing flame-shaped (yellow/blue) turbulent jet into left atrium (colour-flow Doppler).

sure can be recorded by 'wedging' an end-hole venous catheter in a branch of the pulmonary artery.

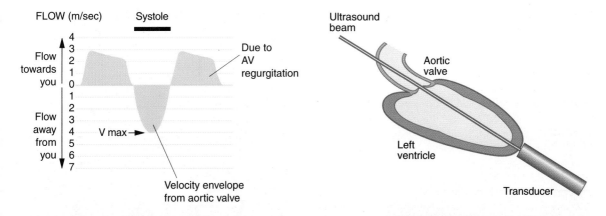

Fig. 5.15 Left: **Doppler ultrasound graph** showing spectrum of blood flow velocities in order to determine the maximum systolic blood-flow velocity through the aortic valve. Blood flow velocities are presented graphically with positive deflection indicating flow towards the transducer. The relationship between pressure drop and velocity can be used to derive an aortic outflow gradient. Peak gradient = 4(V max)^2. Right: **The Doppler ultrasound transducer**, applied to the apex of the heart and aligned with the left ventricular outflow tract.

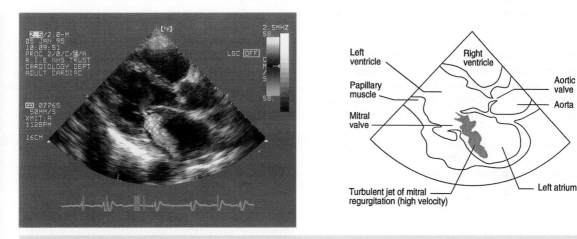

Fig. 5.16 Left: **Echocardiogram (systole).** Real time image of the heart (parasternal long axis view) showing turbulent jet (yellow/blue) of mitral regurgitation. Right: Line diagram of major features.

Cardiac catheters are usually manipulated under radiographic control, but specially designed pulmonary artery balloon catheters can be manipulated into the right atrium by monitoring the lumen pressure. The balloon is then inflated and the blood stream helps guide the catheter through the right ventricle and into the pulmonary artery. Swan-Ganz catheters are used in intensive and coronary care units to monitor pulmonary 'wedge' pressure as a guide to left heart filling pressure. A detailed diagram explaining their use is given under cardiogenic shock (Fig. 5.21, p. 216).

Pressure measurements obtained through cardiac catheters can be used to assess the severity of valvular stenoses, and measurement of ventricular end-diastolic pressure gives an indication of ventricular compliance, and indirectly of ventricular function. Measurement of oxygen saturation in samples withdrawn via the catheters at different sites in the heart allows the detection of intracardiac left-to-right or right-to-left shunts, and also allows calculation of pulmonary and systemic blood flow and the respective resistances. For example, a step up in oxygen saturation from 65% in right atrium to 80% in pulmonary artery is indicative of a large left-to-right shunt which may be due to a ventricular septal defect. Cardiac output can also be measured by dye-dilution or thermodilution techniques.

Intracardiac catheters also allow the injection of radio-opaque contrast medium into individual chambers of the

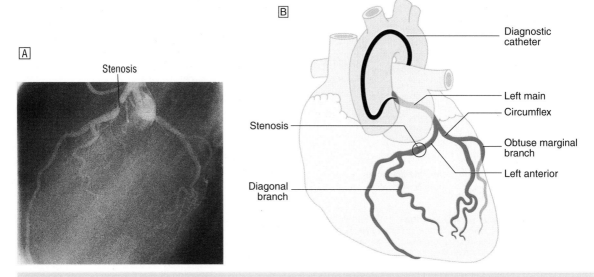

Fig. 5.17 Left: **Coronary artery angiogram** showing the left anterior descending and circumflex coronary arteries with a stenosis in the left anterior descending vessel. Right: Line diagram to illustrate vessels and branches.

heart, the aorta or pulmonary artery, or, using specially shaped catheters, into either coronary artery (Fig. 5.17). Coronary angiography to detect coronary stenoses and guide revascularisation constitutes by far the commonest indication for cardiac catheterisation in most countries.

RADIONUCLIDE SCANNING

The availability of gamma-emitting radionuclides with a short half-life has made it possible to use radionuclides for studying cardiac function non-invasively. The gamma rays are detected by means of a planar or tomographic camera and permit images of the heart to be reconstructed. Two techniques are available:

Blood pool scanning

The isotope is injected intravenously and mixes with the circulating blood. The gamma camera detects the amount of isotope-emitting blood in the heart at different phases of the cardiac cycle, and also the size and 'shape' of the cardiac chambers. By linking the gamma camera to the ECG it is possible to collect information over multiple cardiac cycles, allowing 'gating' to the systolic or diastolic phases of the cardiac cycle. Blood pool scanning provides an accurate and reproducible measure of left ventricular function, and is useful for detecting left ventricular aneurysms.

Myocardial scanning

This technique also uses gamma camera scintigraphy, but the object is usually to distinguish between ischaemic and non-ischaemic myocardium (using radioactive thallium or other tracers—see p. 251) or between normal and infarcted myocardium (using radioactive pyrophosphate). More sophisticated quantitative information is available with positron emission tomography (PET), but this is largely a research tool and is only available in a few centres.

FURTHER READING

Feigenbaum H 1993 Echocardiography. Lea and Febiger, Philadelphia. *An authoritative reference source on echocardiography*
Hampton J 1992 ECG made easy. Churchill Livingstone, Edinburgh
Hampton J 1992 The ECG in practice. Churchill Livingstone, Edinburgh
Levick J R 1991 An introduction to cardiovascular physiology. Butterworths, London. *The physiological basis of cardiac signs and investigations*
Munro J, Edwards C R W 1994 Macleod's clinical examination, 9th edn. Churchill Livingstone, Edinburgh. *A clear, concise guide to the techniques of clinical examination. Davidson's Principles and Practice of Medicine does not set out to describe these*

MAJOR MANIFESTATIONS OF HEART DISEASE

Heart disease gives rise to a relatively limited range of symptoms. Differentiation of disease conditions therefore requires emphasis on factors which provoke the

DIFFERENTIAL DIAGNOSIS OF CHEST PAIN

CENTRAL

- **Cardiac**
  Myocardial ischaemia
  (angina)
  Myocardial infarction
  Pericarditis
  Mitral valve prolapse
- **Aortic**
  Dissecting aneurysm
  Dilating aneurysm
  Aortitis (rare)
- **Pulmonary/mediastinum**
  Massive embolus
  Tracheitis
  Mediastinal malignancy
- **Oesophageal**
  Oesophagitis
  Oesophageal spasm
  Mallory–Weiss syndrome
- **Psychogenic**
  Anxiety/cardiac neurosis
- **Neurologic/skeletal**
  Herniated intervertebral
  disc
  Osteoarthritis
  Trauma (impact injuries)

PERIPHERAL

- **Lungs/pleura**
  Lobar pneumonia
  Pneumothorax
  Pulmonary infarction
  Malignancy
  Tuberculosis
  Connective tissue
  disorders (rare)
- **Chest wall disorders
  (simulating pleural pain)**
  Rib fracture/injury
  Intercostal muscle injury
  Epidemic myalgia
  (Bornholm disease)
  Costocondritis (Tietze's
  syndrome)
- **Psychogenic**
  Anxiety
- **Neurologic/skeletal**
  Herniated intervertebral
  disc
  Herpes zoster
  Thoracic outlet syndrome

symptoms and subtle differences in the way in which they are described by the patient.

CHEST PAIN

DIAGNOSTIC APPROACH TO THE PATIENT WITH CENTRAL CHEST PAIN

Chest pain is a common presentation of cardiac disease, but it can also signify disease of the lungs, the musculoskeletal system or less commonly, the gastrointestinal system. It is useful to discriminate between central and peripheral or 'pleural type' pain (see information box) and then to consider diagnostic approaches to patients presenting with these symptoms.

History

A number of key characteristics help to distinguish cardiac pain from that of other causes.

- **Location**: cardiac pain is typically centrally located

in the chest, on account of the derivation of the nerve supply to the heart and mediastinum. Pain only experienced at a peripheral site in the chest is rarely of cardiac origin (see information box above).

- **Radiation**: ischaemic pain, especially when severe, may radiate to the neck, jaw and upper or even lower arms. Pain situated over the left anterior chest, and radiating laterally, may have various other causes including pleural or lung pain, chest wall injury and anxiety.
- **Provocation**: anginal pain is precipitated by exertion (not after exertion) and is relieved by resting. With deteriorating or unstable angina, similar pain may be brought on by minimal exertion and may also occur at rest. In contrast, pain associated with a specific movement (bending, stretching, turning) is likely to be musculoskeletal in origin.
- **Character of the pain**: cardiac pain is typically described as dull, constricting or 'heavy'. It may not be appreciated as pain but as discomfort, and the constricting sensation can be described as breathlessness. Pleural pain is 'sharp' or 'catching' in quality and interrupts breathing, coughing or movement. It may originate from lung pleura or pericardium.
- **Pattern of onset**: The pain of aortic dissection, massive pulmonary embolism or of pneumothorax is usually very sudden in onset (seconds). Myocardial infarction pain usually takes several minutes, or even longer, to develop, and angina builds up gradually in proportion to the intensity of exertion.
- **Associated features**: the severe pain of myocardial infarction, or massive pulmonary embolus, or aortic dissection is often accompanied by autonomic disturbance including sweating, nausea and vomiting. Breathlessness is associated with raised pulmonary capillary pressure or pulmonary oedema in myocardial infarction, and may accompany any of the respiratory causes of chest pain. Cough is characteristically associated with tracheitis or pneumonia. Associated gastrointestinal symptoms may provide the clue to the source of non-cardiac chest pain (oesophageal reflux, oesophagitis, peptic ulceration or biliary disease).

Differential diagnosis of central chest pain

Angina

This is a choking or constricting chest pain which comes on with exertion, is relieved by rest, and is due to myocardial ischaemia. It is commonly felt retrosternally and may radiate to the left or more rarely the right arm, to the throat, jaws and teeth, or through to the back. The pain may be described as squeezing, crushing, burning or aching, but seldom stabbing. Patients may describe a choking sensation simulating breathlessness.

The pain may be brought on or exacerbated by emotion, and is frequently made worse by large meals or a cold wind. It is relieved by nitrates (see Ischaemic heart disease, p. 250). 'Unstable angina' describes a pattern of severe angina which may be precipitated by minimal exertion, or may occur spontaneously, and may culminate in infarction.

Myocardial infarction

The pain is similar in nature and distribution to angina but is more severe, persists at rest, and does not respond to nitrates. There are usually features of sympathetic nervous system activation, and vomiting is common. There may be anxiety and a frightening feeling of impending death (see myocardial infarction, p. 256). In some patients, and especially the elderly, the symptoms are atypical and may simulate other conditions.

Dissecting aortic aneurysm

The pain is severe, sharp and tearing, often felt in or penetrating through to the back. The pulse may be disproportionately slow for the severity of the pain, owing to stimulation of aortic baroreceptors (p. 275).

Pericarditic pain

This is felt retrosternally, to the left of the sternum, or in the left or right shoulder. It characteristically varies in intensity with movement and the phase of respiration (p. 308). It is described as 'Sharp' and may catch the patient during inspiration or coughing.

Musculo-skeletal chest pain

This is very variable in site and intensity but does not usually fall into the patterns described above. It may vary with posture or movement, can be brought on by exertion but often does not cease instantly on rest, and is very commonly accompanied by local tenderness over a rib or costal cartilage.

Oesophageal pain

The pain can mimic that of angina very closely, is sometimes precipitated by exercise and may be relieved by nitrates. It is usually possible to elicit a history relating chest pain to food or drink intake or oesophageal reflux. It may coexist with angina.

Examination

In uncomplicated new onset angina, physical examination is often normal. However, underlying risk factors may be evident, including hypertension and hyperlipidaemia (see p. 245). The physical features of myocardial infarction are those of the accompanying auto-

---

CHEST PAIN—SUMMARY OF DIFFERENTIAL DIAGNOSIS

Cardiac
- Angina (pain on exertion, remits at rest)
- Myocardial infarction (severe, persists at rest, other associated symptoms)
- Pericarditis (varies with breathing and posture, audible rub)

Aortic
- Dissecting aneurysm (abrupt onset, 'tearing' pain in back, asymmetric pulses, bradycardia)

Lung/Pleura
- Pneumothorax (sudden onset, asymmetric air entry, percussion note)
- Pleurisy (varies with breathing, pleural rub)

Musculoskeletal
- Local tenderness common (related to posture, not exercise duration)

Oesophageal
- May be food-related (but not invariably)

---

nomic disturbance (sweating, pallor) or those of cardiac failure (fourth heart sound, pulmonary crepitations or florid oedema), or diminished output (cyanosis, peripherally poor perfusion). The patient looks systemically 'ill'. *However, the absence of such signs does not exclude the diagnosis.*

Similar autonomic disturbance may accompany any cause of severe pain. Signs of pleural involvement (see below) provide important clues to the diagnosis, and it must be remembered that the inflammation may affect the pericardium, and/or the lung pleura. Tachypnoea or dyspnoea and cyanosis may accompany pulmonary embolism, but more commonly there are no abnormal physical signs. *Thus, proceeding to examination without a careful history may be unhelpful.*

Investigations

It must be recognised that although cardiac investigations may be specific when abnormal, lack of sensitivity means that a normal or nonspecific result does not exclude the diagnosis. For example, the first ECG in patients presenting with infarction may not show characteristic changes in up to one-third of cases. On the other hand, where typical ECG signs of acute infarction are present, the diagnosis is made and no other investigation should delay the start of treatment. The chest radiograph is not diagnostic in infarction, but may reveal pulmonary oedema. It should be performed in suspected aortic dissection or suspected pulmonary causes of chest pain. Although rapid analysis cardiac enzymes are now available, insufficient enzyme (creatine kinase, troponin, myoglobin) is released in the first 1–2 hrs of onset to be certain of the diagnosis. Thus the enzymes provide retrospective confirmation of infarction rather than a guide to immediate treatment (analgesia, aspirin, thrombolysis).

Similarly, the resting ECG and chest radiograph are often normal in angina, even when caused by severe left main or 3 vessel coronary disease. Exercise or stress provoked tests are discussed later (p. 249).

Arterial blood gases may help to guide therapy when the patient exhibits hypoxaemia or cyanosis (pulmonary embolus, extensive pneumonia) but should *not* be performed if the patient requires thrombolysis (bleeding complications).

Echocardiography should be performed when cardiac failure is associated with valvular dysfunction or muscle impairment, but need not delay the start of treatment.

Patients with acute cardiac failure and diminished cardiac output require intensive monitoring (ECG, blood pressure, urinary output, oxygen saturation), and may even require haemodynamic monitoring (pulmonary artery, pulmonary capillary pressure, cardiac output and vascular resistance) in order to titrate inotropic drug support and monitor the need for further invasive treatment or ventilation.

Thus the sequence of investigations is guided by the history, the clinical signs, and the suspected diagnosis.

DIAGNOSTIC APPROACH TO THE PATIENT WITH PERIPHERAL CHEST PAIN

History
Pleural pain is usually sharp, and worsens during the inspiratory phase of the ventilatory cycle (pleurisy). However, it can be dull and persistent, as exemplified by mesothelioma (p. 388) and other malignant tumours involving the pleura. Sudden onset of pleural pain in the absence of preceding ill health should suggest pneumothorax or pulmonary infarction; a short history of ill health is suggestive of pneumonia, tuberculosis or viral myalgia, whereas a long history of ill health should arouse suspicion of malignant disease, tuberculosis or pneumonia in an immunocompromised patient. Similarly, significant weight loss is suggestive of malignancy or tuberculosis. There may be a history of conditions favouring development of a deep venous thrombosis (p. 275) in pulmonary infarction, and arthralgia or rashes may suggest an underlying connective tissue disorder (p. 912).

Examination
On general examination there may be pyrexia (in pneumonia, but also in established pulmonary infarction), cachexia suggestive of malignancy, signs of deep venous thrombosis, or stigmata of connective tissue diseases. On examination of the chest a pleural rub may be heard on auscultation, and it is important to determine whether a pleural effusion is present. Localised chest wall tenderness or pain on 'springing' the ribs is common in chest wall disorders but rare in pleural disease.

Investigations
The chest radiograph is nearly always abnormal in cases of pleural disease, and it may be diagnostic in pneumothorax (p. 400). There may be pleural effusions which require further investigation (see below), and bilateral lower zone abnormalities are common in pulmonary infarction. Diffuse pulmonary shadowing is a common feature of infections in immunocompromised individuals, and bilateral upper zone abnormalities may be present in tuberculosis (but not in all cases).

Where pulmonary infarction is suspected, a ventilation/perfusion scan (p. 319) or pulmonary angiography may be necessary to confirm the diagnosis and ascending venography can be used to identify the site and extent of deep venous thrombosis. In bacterial pneumonia, sputum should be examined and cultured for pathogens and blood taken for white cell count and blood cultures. In cases of suspected tuberculosis sputum should be stained and cultured for mycobacteria and a tuberculin test performed, but in the absence of sputum it is often necessary to obtain bronchial washings by bronchoscopy. The sputum can be examined for malignant cells, but in suspected pleural malignancy transthoracic needle biopsy or thoracoscopy is usually necessary to obtain a histological diagnosis.

If pleural effusion is present, in the case of a small, or loculated, effusion ultrasonography may be necessary to identify the most favourable site where aspiration and biopsy can be performed. In large pleural effusions the investigation of choice is aspiration and pleural biopsy using an Abram's needle (p. 321). The fluid should be examined for bacterial pathogens, tubercle bacilli, malignant cells and a differential white cell count. It is also useful to determine pleural fluid protein, glucose and LDH levels. High titres of rheumatoid factor, anti-DNA antibodies, etc., may be found in pleural effusions complicating connective tissue diseases (p. 390). Multiple pleural biopsies should be fixed and examined histologically. If a diagnosis is not established by pleural aspiration and biopsy, thoracoscopy may be necessary to permit direct visualisation and biopsy of abnormal tissue.

BREATHLESSNESS (DYSPNOEA)

See page 323, Respiratory chapter.

ACUTE CIRCULATORY FAILURE (SHOCK)

Shock is a loosely defined term used to describe the clinical syndrome that develops when there is critical impairment of tissue perfusion due to some form of acute circulatory failure.

There are numerous causes of shock. They can be broadly classified into three major groups (see Table 5.2).

Pathophysiology

The syndrome of shock is characterised by widespread failure of the capillary system caused by a complex interaction of haemodynamic and toxic factors. Loss of capillary integrity reduces oxygen delivery to the tissues, disturbs local metabolism, and allows fluid to extravasate into the interstitial space. Generalised but patchy cell death and further capillary damage occur due to the combined effects of ischaemia, acidosis, and the release of toxic metabolites including catecholamines, angiotensin II, and cytokines such as the interleukins and tumour necrosis factor. The condition therefore often leads to multi-organ failure and death.

Many of the potential complications of shock (see Fig. 5.18) will cause additional tissue damage. For example, declining myocardial contractility may set up a vicious cycle of falling cardiac output and deteriorating tissue perfusion. Similarly, alveolar oedema and progressive lung damage (Adult Respiratory Distress Syndrome) may cause increasing hypoxia and generalised ischaemia. Secondary infections often occur because destruction of the intestinal mucosa allows commensal organisms to enter the circulation; Gram-negative septicaemia is common and may cause further damage due to endotoxic shock (see below).

Systemic activation of the clotting cascade, platelet aggregation, and reduced flow through the micro-circulation may all cause clot formation within the capillary bed (disseminated intravascular coagulation) leading to further ischaemia and cell death. Paradoxically, a generalised coagulation defect may develop as the clotting factors and platelets are consumed in the capillary bed (consumption coagulopathy) and this may lead to generalised bleeding.

Clinical features

Although the clinical features of shock depend to some extent on the underlying cause, a range of clinical features and complications are common to most cases (see information box and Fig. 5.18).

ACUTE CIRCULATORY FAILURE: GENERAL FEATURES

- Hypotension (systolic BP <100 mmHg)
- Tachycardia (>100/min)
- Cold clammy skin
- Rapid shallow respiration
- Drowsiness, confusion, irritability
- Oliguria (urine output <30 ml/hour)
- Elevated or reduced central venous pressure
- Multi-organ failure (see Fig. 5.18)

The central venous pressure (JVP) is reduced in hypovolaemic and normovolaemic shock but elevated in cardiogenic shock. This is an important distinction and direct measurement of the central venous pressure or pulmonary artery wedge pressure (see below) may be very helpful if the physical signs are difficult to interpret.

The aetiology is usually obvious in hypovolaemic shock, but intra-abdominal haemorrhage from a leaking aortic aneurysm, a ruptured spleen or an ectopic pregnancy may be difficult to diagnose.

Septic shock is usually caused by Gram-negative septicaemia and is partly due to capillary damage and increased nitric oxide production caused by the release of bacterial endotoxins. The patient is often pyrexial and there may be a history of rigors. Although there is critical impairment of cardiac output and vital organ perfusion the skin is often warm due to cutaneous vasodilatation.

In **anaphylactic shock** there may be a history of exposure to a known allergen, and the release of histamine and other mediators that may cause characteristic features such as urticaria, stridor (laryngeal oedema), wheeze and facial oedema.

The features of the major causes of cardiogenic shock are described below.

CARDIOGENIC SHOCK

The common causes are illustrated in Figure 5.19. Echocardiography is very helpful when the diagnosis is in doubt.

Table 5.2 Acute circulatory failure

Type	Examples
Hypovolaemic shock —secondary to any condition provoking a major reduction in blood volume	Internal/external haemorrhage Severe burns Acute pancreatitis Dehydration (e.g. diabetic ketoacidosis)
Normovolaemic shock —secondary to capillary damage, arteriovenous shunting and inappropriate vasodilatation	Septic shock (usually Gram-negative septicaemia) Anaphylactic shock
Cardiogenic shock —caused by any form of severe heart failure	Myocardial infarction Acute massive pulmonary embolism Pericardial tamponade

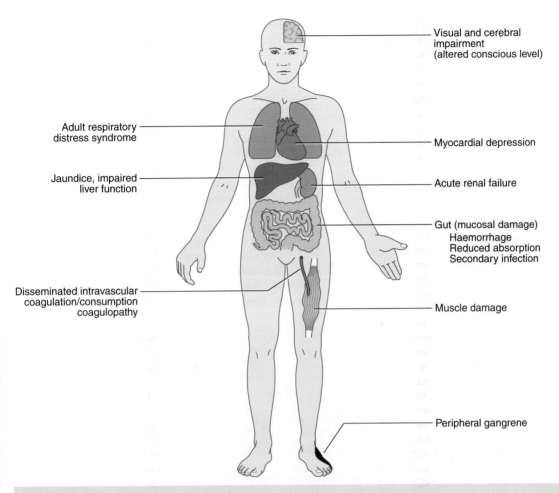

Visual and cerebral
impairment
(altered conscious level)

Adult respiratory
distress syndrome

Myocardial depression

Jaundice, impaired
liver function

Acute renal failure

Gut (mucosal damage)
Haemorrhage
Reduced absorption
Secondary infection

Disseminated intravascular
coagulation/consumption
coagulopathy

Muscle damage

Peripheral gangrene

Fig. 5.18   Some systemic complications of shock.

Myocardial infarction

Although heart failure complicating myocardial infarction can be due to mechanical problems such as mitral regurgitation or a ventricular septal defect (see p. 263) it is usually due to left ventricular dysfunction.

Hypotension, oliguria, confusion and cold, clammy peripheries are the manifestations of a low cardiac output, whereas breathlessness, hypoxia, cyanosis and inspiratory crackles at the lung bases are features of pulmonary oedema. A chest radiograph (Fig. 5.20) may reveal signs of pulmonary congestion when clinical examination is normal. If necessary a Swan–Ganz catheter can be used to measure the pulmonary artery wedge (PAW) pressure (see Fig. 5.21).

These findings can be used to divide patients with acute myocardial infarction into four haemodynamic subsets (see box).

The viable myocardium surrounding a fresh infarct may contract poorly for a few days. This phenomenon is known as **myocardial stunning** and means that, in this setting, it is often worth treating acute heart failure energetically in the hope and expectation that overall cardiac function will improve.

Acute massive pulmonary embolism

This may complicate leg or pelvic vein thrombosis and usually presents with sudden collapse. The clinical features are discussed on page 277.

Bedside echocardiography may be very helpful and usually demonstrates a small vigorous left ventricle with a dilated right ventricle; it is sometimes possible to see thrombus in the right ventricular outflow tract or main pulmonary artery. Pulmonary angiography is the definitive diagnostic procedure but may be hazardous and is often unnecessary.

Treatment (p. 279) may utilise high flow oxygen,

ACUTE MYOCARDIAL INFARCTION: PATIENT SUBSETS

- **Normal cardiac output. No pulmonary oedema**
  The normal state of affairs; carries a good outlook and requires no treatment for heart failure

- **Normal cardiac output. Pulmonary oedema**
  Usually due to moderate left ventricular dysfunction; should be treated with diuretics and vasodilators

- **Low cardiac output. No pulmonary oedema**
  Often due to a combination of right ventricular infarction and hypovolaemia due to a reduced oral intake of fluids, vomiting and inappropriate diuretic therapy. Such patients have a poor prognosis and are difficult to manage and it is usually advisable to insert a Swan–Ganz catheter and give i.v. fluids or plasma to raise the PAW pressure to between 14 and 16 mmHg

- **Low cardiac output. Pulmonary oedema**
  Usually due to extensive left ventricular damage and carries a very poor prognosis. The patient may benefit from treatment with diuretics, vasodilators and inotropes (see p. 217)

anticoagulation, thrombolytic therapy and sometimes surgical embolectomy.

Pericardial tamponade

This condition is due to a collection of fluid or blood in the pericardial sac compressing the heart; the effusion may be small and is sometimes less than 100 ml. Sudden deterioration is frequently due to bleeding into the pericardial space.

Tamponade may complicate any form of pericarditis and is often due to malignant disease. Other causes include trauma and rupture of the free wall of the myocardium following myocardial infarction.

The important clinical features of the condition are listed in the information box.

An ECG may show features of the underlying disease, e.g. pericarditis or acute myocardial infarction. When there is a large pericardial effusion the ECG complexes are small and there may be electrical alternans (a

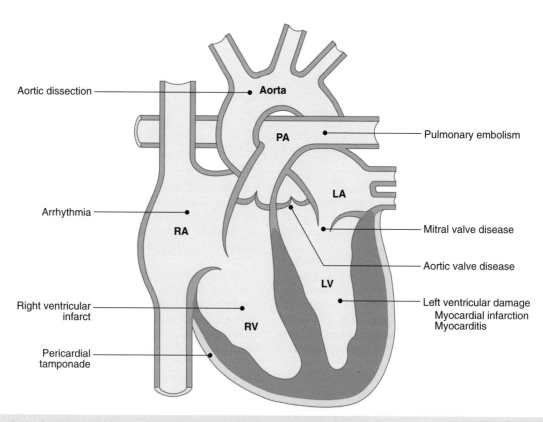

Fig. 5.19 Some causes of cardiogenic shock.

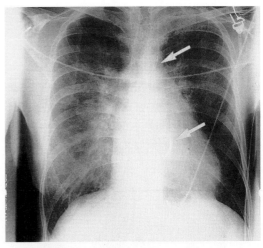

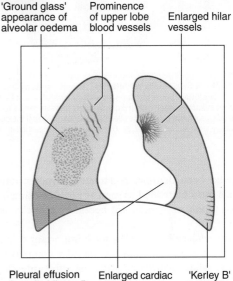

'Ground glass' appearance of alveolar oedema   Prominence of upper lobe blood vessels   Enlarged hilar vessels

Pleural effusion (usually bilateral)   Enlarged cardiac silhouette   'Kerley B' septal lines

Fig. 5.20 Chest radiograph demonstrating pulmonary oedema in a patient with a prosthetic mitral valve (arrow). This was due to fracture of one of the valve struts; the disc had fallen out of the valve and lodged in the aortic arch (arrow). **The line diagram illustrates the appearance of the chest radiograph in heart failure.**

changing axis caused by the heart moving in the bag of fluid). A chest radiograph may show an enlarged globular heart but can look normal when there is a small pericardial effusion. Echocardiography, which may be done at the bedside, is the best way of confirming the diagnosis, and helps to identify the optimum site for paracentesis.

Prompt recognition of tamponade is important because the patient usually responds dramatically to percutaneous pericardiocentesis (p. 311) or surgical drainage.

Valvular heart disease

Acute left ventricular failure may be due to the sudden onset of aortic regurgitation, mitral regurgitation or prosthetic valve dysfunction (Fig 5.20). Some of the common causes of these problems are listed in the information box.

The clinical diagnosis of acute valvular dysfunction is sometimes difficult. Murmurs are often unimpressive because there is usually a tachycardia with a low cardiac output. Transthoracic echocardiography will establish the diagnosis in most cases; however, transoesophageal echocardiography is sometimes required to identify prosthetic mitral valve regurgitation.

Patients with acute valve failure usually require cardiac surgery and should be referred for urgent assessment in a cardiac centre.

Management

General principles

The immediate objective is to restore and then maintain adequate tissue perfusion until the cause of circulatory

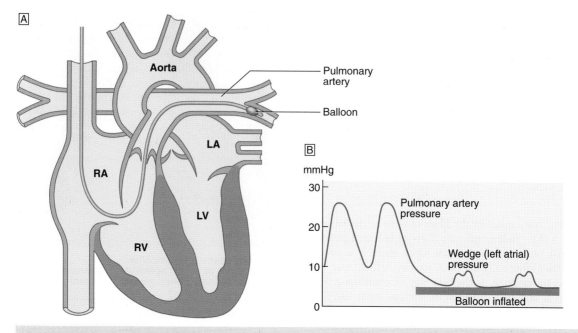

Fig. 5.21 A Swan–Ganz catheter. A There is a small balloon at the tip of the catheter and pressure can be measured through the central lumen. The catheter is inserted via a subclavian or femoral vein and advanced through the right heart until its tip lies in the pulmonary artery. When the balloon is deflated the pulmonary artery pressure can be recorded. Advancing the catheter while inflating the balloon will 'wedge' the catheter in the pulmonary artery. In this position blood cannot flow past the balloon so the tip of the catheter will now record the pressure transmitted from the pulmonary veins and left atrium B. This is known as the pulmonary artery wedge pressure and provides an indirect measure of the left atrial pressure.

failure has been identified and treated. Hypotension and hypoxia must be treated as soon as possible using intravenous fluids, oxygen, and if necessary artificial ventilation.

In hypovolaemic shock the most important step is to replace the fluid lost from the vascular compartment. Isotonic saline, plasma or a plasma substitute can be used at first, but thereafter the type of fluid lost should determine the nature of its replacement. The infusion rate should be adjusted according to estimates of the volume of fluid that has been lost, the clinical state of the patient, and measurements of the central venous pressure or pulmonary artery wedge pressure. When large transfusions are given rapidly it is important to use fluids that have been warmed to body temperature.

Even stable patients require careful monitoring to ensure that any complications are detected and treated early.

Monitoring

Although regular clinical evaluation is essential, progress can also be assessed by monitoring certain parameters at the bedside. These include:

- ECG—a standard monitor will record rate and rhythm while more sophisticated machines can moni-

tor ST segment shift, which may be useful in patients with ischaemic heart disease.

- Blood pressure—can be measured intermittently using an automatic sphygmomanometer but in critically-ill patients continuous intra-arterial monitoring using a line placed in the radial artery may be preferable. It is important to remember that cardiac output and tissue perfusion may be reduced in spite of a normal blood pressure if there is vasoconstriction and a high peripheral vascular resistance.

- Skin temperature—this reflects cutaneous blood flow and is therefore a useful indirect measure of peripheral perfusion.

- Oxygen saturation—this can be monitored easily using a finger or ear lobe probe. In general, oxygenation is satisfactory if the saturation is greater than 90%.

- Urinary flow—this is a sensitive measure of renal perfusion and can easily be monitored if a urinary catheter is in place.

- Central venous pressure (CVP)—using a catheter to measure the right atrial pressure (directly or through a manometer system) is a useful means of assessing the circulating blood volume and therefore the appropriate rate of intravenous fluid replacement. In severe hypovolaemia the right atrial pressure may be sustained by peripheral venoconstriction and at first transfusion may produce little or no change in the CVP.

- Pulmonary artery wedge (PAW) pressure—in most situations the central venous pressure is an adequate guide to the filling pressures of both sides of the heart; however, this may not be the case in critically ill patients and those with pulmonary vascular disease or right ventricular dysfunction. In these situations it may be advisable to monitor the PAW pressure using a Swan–Ganz catheter (see Figure 5.21). These catheters can also be used to measure cardiac output and other haemodynamic variables such as the systemic vascular resistance. The mean PAW or 'wedge' pressure normally lies between 6 and 12 mmHg but in left heart failure it may be as high as 35 mmHg. The optimum PAW pressure in acute circulatory failure usually lies around 15 mmHg; this is high enough to ensure good left ventricular filling but carries a low risk of pulmonary oedema.

Management of acute pulmonary oedema

This is a feature of acute left heart failure and needs urgent treatment:

- sit the patient up in order to reduce pulmonary congestion
- give oxygen (high flow, high concentration) to breathe
- use morphine (10 mg intravenous, intramuscular or subcutaneous) to alleviate breathlessness and reverse reflex peripheral vasoconstriction
- administer a powerful diuretic such as frusemide (40–80 mg intravenously); these drugs provide rapid relief because they are also vasodilators.

If these immediate measures prove inadequate, one may try to stimulate the heart using inotropic agents, or to reduce left ventricular load by using more powerful vasodilators.

Controlled vasodilatation

This is an important concept in the management of pulmonary oedema and left-heart failure. Venodilatation reduces central venous pressure and right ventricular output, and therefore slows the accumulation of pulmonary oedema, while arteriolar dilatation improves left ventricular function by reducing afterload.

Sublingual nitrate (see p. 250), given as a tablet, spray or buccal preparation, is a useful 'first aid' vasodilator. However, in severe heart failure a controlled intravenous infusion of nitrates is preferable; the dose must be adjusted according to the clinical response but most patients respond to nitroglycerine 0.6–1.2 mg/hour or isosorbide dinitrate 2–4 mg/hour. In severe heart failure

nitrates tend to act both as venous and arteriolar dilators. The main complication of vasodilator therapy is hypotension and it is seldom wise to let the systolic pressure fall below 90 mmHg. Other problems include pharmacological tolerance and adsorption and degradation of nitrate within the intravenous giving set.

Many patients treated with intravenous nitrates will benefit from long-term oral therapy with angiotensin-converting enzyme inhibitors, nitrates or other vasodilators (p. 223).

Inotropic agents

These drugs can increase cardiac output and therefore improve tissue perfusion, but often do so at the expense of increasing myocardial oxygen demand, thereby aggravating any myocardial ischaemia. In some settings it may be desirable to minimise the cardiac workload by using a combination of inotropes and vasodilators.

Inotropic drugs are usually used to reverse the effects of cardiac depressant drugs (including anaesthetics), or to stabilise a patient until a metabolic disturbance can be corrected or a mechanical defect repaired. These drugs are usually infused through a central venous catheter because local extravasation may cause tissue necrosis.

- **Dopamine.** At low doses (< 4 μg/kg per minute) this drug increases renal blood flow, glomerular filtration rate and sodium excretion by stimulating specific dopaminergic receptors; it is therefore a useful adjunct to diuretic therapy and may help to preserve renal function in shock states. At doses between 4 and 10 μg/kg per minute dopamine stimulates cardiac β_1-adrenoceptors and therefore increases the heart rate and myocardial contractility. At even higher doses it causes vasoconstriction by stimulating peripheral alpha receptors; this will increase blood pressure but may reduce tissue perfusion.
- **Dobutamine.** This is a synthetic catecholamine with marked β_1 and weak β_2 effects; it therefore increases myocardial contractility, cardiac output, heart rate and coronary blood flow. Most patients will respond to an infusion of between 2.5 and 10 μg/kg per minute. If tachycardia can be avoided the increase in myocardial oxygen supply usually outweighs the increase in oxygen demand.
- **Other catecholamines.** Adrenaline is a very potent alpha and beta agonist and is sometimes used in patients who do not respond to dopamine and dobutamine. Noradrenaline increases myocardial contractility but also produces a substantial rise in peripheral vascular resistance; it is therefore used in settings where the importance of increasing blood

pressure outweighs the disadvantages of causing peripheral vasoconstriction.

- **Cyclic nucleotide phosphodiesterase inhibitors.** These drugs are sometimes called 'inodilators' because they act as inotropes and vasodilators. Enoximone and milrinone are the most commonly used agents in this group and will increase cardiac output; they do not cause a tachycardia and may also have favourable effects on myocardial oxygen consumption and pulmonary vascular resistance. Unfortunately, the development of these drugs has been blighted by the results of clinical trials which have shown that long-term oral administration may increase mortality in patients with chronic heart failure.

Circulatory assist devices

A variety of devices can be used to provide temporary mechanical assistance to the circulation. They are often used to support the circulation while the myocardium recovers following cardiac surgery and can also be used to help patients with a cardiac problem that is amenable to surgical correction (including transplantation) while the operation is being arranged.

Intra-aortic balloon counterpulsation is the most widely used system. A balloon is inserted through the femoral artery, positioned in the descending aorta just distal to the left subclavian artery, and pumped up and down with 50 ml of carbon dioxide or helium in time with the pulse. Rapid inflation at the onset of diastole will enhance the flow of blood in the proximal and distal aorta and increase coronary, cerebral and renal perfusion. Moreover, rapid deflation of the balloon just before systole helps to unload the left ventricle and augment left ventricular ejection. Unfortunately, vascular complications may occur and the device can seldom be used for more than a few days.

Ventricular assist devices. A variety of partial heart-lung bypass machines can be used to provide short-term support to the circulation in critically-ill patients but it is only appropriate to use these devices if the patient has a treatable condition with a reasonable prospect of recovery.

Care of other systems

Acute renal failure (p. 626) is a common complication of shock because severe hypotension causes reflex renal arteriolar vasoconstriction leading to a reduction in total renal blood flow and a redistribution of blood from the cortex to the medulla of the kidney. Prolonged hypotension therefore causes a marked reduction in cortical perfusion and may lead to acute tubular necrosis or even acute cortical necrosis.

Inducing a diuresis with frusemide or the osmotic diuretic mannitol may help protect the kidney from vaso-

constriction, but the most effective antidote to renal vasoconstriction is low-dose dopamine (2–4 μg/kg per minute). Once tubular necrosis has occurred it is important to restrict fluid intake, otherwise fluid overload and pulmonary oedema will develop. In most cases renal function will recover but a period of peritoneal or haemodialysis is sometimes necessary.

Hypoxia is common in acute circulatory failure, particularly when there is pulmonary oedema. If it does not respond rapidly to oxygen and diuretic therapy, consideration should be given to endotracheal intubation and positive-pressure ventilation. Sometimes oxygenation can be further improved by using positive end-expiratory pressure (PEEP) or continuous positive airway pressure (CPAP).

Prognosis

The prognosis of acute circulatory failure is determined by the underlying cause. No amount of medication can compensate for massive and irretrievable myocardial damage, and the prognosis for circulatory failure complicating extensive myocardial infarction is poor. In contrast, the outcome following drainage of a pericardial effusion, replacement of a diseased valve, or dissolution of a pulmonary embolus may be excellent.

HEART FAILURE

Heart failure is an imprecise term used to describe the state that develops when the heart cannot maintain an adequate cardiac output or can do so only at the expense of an elevated filling pressure. In the mildest forms of heart failure cardiac output is adequate at rest and becomes inadequate only when the metabolic demand increases during exercise or some other form of stress.

In practice heart failure may be diagnosed whenever a patient with significant heart disease develops the signs or symptoms of a low cardiac output, pulmonary congestion, or systemic venous congestion.

Almost all forms of heart disease may lead to heart failure and it is important to appreciate that, like anaemia, the term refers to a clinical syndrome rather than a specific diagnosis. Good management depends on an accurate aetiological diagnosis, partly because in some situations a specific remedy may be available, but mainly because a clear understanding of the pathophysiology is essential to logical drug therapy.

Heart failure is frequently due to coronary artery disease, tends to affect elderly subjects and often leads to prolonged disability. In the United Kingdom most patients admitted to hospital with heart failure are more

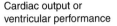

Cardiac output or
ventricular performance

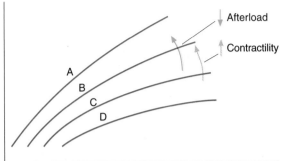

Preload

Fig. 5.22   Starling's Law. Ⓐ normal; Ⓑ mild; Ⓒ moderate; Ⓓ severe heart failure. Ventricular performance is related to the degree of myocardial stretching. An increase in preload (end-diastolic volume, end-diastolic pressure, filling pressure or atrial pressure) will therefore enhance function; however, overstretching causes marked deterioration. In heart failure the curve moves to the right and becomes flatter. An increase in myocardial contractility or a reduction in afterload (arterial resistance/blood pressure) will shift the curve upwards and to the left.

than 65 years old and the average hospital stay is around 20 days.

Although the outlook depends to some extent on the underlying cause of the problem, heart failure carries a very poor prognosis; approximately 50% of patients with severe heart failure will die within two years. Many patients die suddenly, often due to malignant ventricular arrhythmias or myocardial infarction.

Pathophysiology

The cardiac output is a function of the preload (the volume and pressure of blood in the ventricle at the end of diastole), the afterload (the arterial resistance) and myocardial contractility. The interaction of these variables is shown in Figure 5.22 which is based on Starling's Law of the heart.

Heart failure is associated with complex neurohormonal changes including activation of the renin-angiotensin-aldosterone axis and the sympathetic nervous system. At first these changes may help to optimise cardiac function by altering the afterload or preload and by increasing myocardial contractility (Fig. 5.23). However, ultimately they become counterproductive and often reduce cardiac output by causing an inappropriate and excessive increase in peripheral vascular resistance. A vicious cycle may be established because a fall in cardiac output will cause further neurohormonal activation and increasing peripheral vascular resistance.

The onset of pulmonary and/or peripheral oedema is due to high atrial pressures compounded by salt and water retention caused by impaired renal perfusion and secondary aldosteronism.

Types of heart failure

Heart failure can be described or classified in several ways:

Acute and chronic heart failure

Heart failure may develop suddenly, as in myocardial infarction, or gradually, as in progressive valvular heart disease. When there is gradual impairment of cardiac function a variety of compensatory changes (see information box) may take place. Although initially these changes may improve overall cardiac function, as the disease progresses they often become counterproductive.

COMPENSATORY CHANGES IN HEART FAILURE

Local changes
- Chamber enlargement
- Myocardial hypertrophy
- Increased heart rate

Systemic changes
- Activation of the sympathetic nervous system
- Activation of the renin-angiotensin-aldosterone system (Fig. 5.23)
- Release of antidiuretic hormone
- Release of atrial natriuretic peptide

The term *compensated* heart failure is sometimes used to describe a patient with impaired cardiac function in whom adaptive changes have prevented the development of overt heart failure. A minor event, such as an intercurrent infection, may precipitate overt heart failure in this type of patient (see information box).

FACTORS THAT MAY PRECIPITATE OR AGGRAVATE HEART FAILURE

- Inappropriate reduction of therapy
- Administration of a drug with negative inotropic (e.g. β-adrenoceptor antagonist) or fluid retaining properties (e.g. NSAIDs, corticosteroids)
- Arrhythmia
- Myocardial ischaemia or infarction
- Intercurrent illness (e.g. infection)
- Pulmonary embolism
- Conditions associated with increased metabolic demand (e.g. pregnancy, thyrotoxicosis, anaemia)

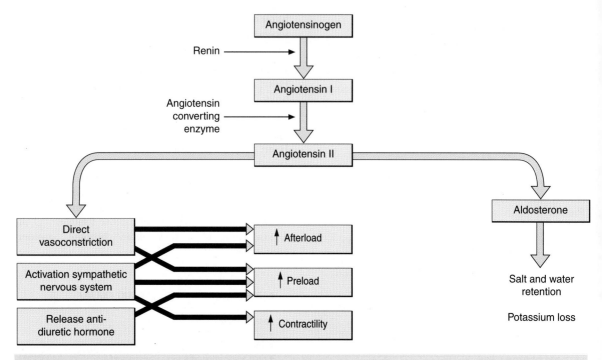

Fig. 5.23 The renin-angiotensin-aldosterone system in heart failure. Impaired renal perfusion and diuretic therapy lead to the release of renin with secondary changes in the afterload, preload and myocardial contractility.

Left, right and biventricular heart failure

The left side of the heart is a term for the functional unit of the left atrium and left ventricle together with the mitral and aortic valves, whereas the right heart comprises the right atrium, right ventricle, tricuspid and pulmonary valves.

- **Left-sided heart failure**. In this condition there is a reduction in the left ventricular output and/or an increase in the left atrial or pulmonary venous pressure. An acute increase in left atrial pressure may cause pulmonary congestion or pulmonary oedema; but a more gradual increase in the left atrial pressure may lead to reflex pulmonary vasoconstriction, which protects the patient from pulmonary oedema at the cost of increasing pulmonary hypertension.
- **Right-sided heart failure**. In this condition there is a reduction in right ventricular output for any given right atrial pressure. Causes of isolated right heart failure include chronic lung disease (cor pulmonale, p. 335), multiple pulmonary emboli, and pulmonary valvular stenosis.
- **Biventricular heart failure**. Failure of the left and right heart may develop because the disease process (e.g. dilated cardiomyopathy or ischaemic heart disease) affects both ventricles, or because disease of the left heart leads to chronic elevation of the left atrial

pressure, pulmonary hypertension and subsequent right heart failure.

Forward and backward heart failure

In some patients with heart failure the predominant problem is an inadequate cardiac output (**forward failure**) whilst other patients may have a normal or near normal cardiac output with marked salt and water retention causing pulmonary and systemic venous congestion (**backward failure**).

Diastolic and systolic dysfunction

Heart failure may develop as a result of impaired myocardial contraction (**systolic dysfunction**) but can also be due to poor ventricular filling and high filling pressures caused by abnormal ventricular relaxation (**diastolic dysfunction**). The latter is commonly found in patients with left ventricular hypertrophy and occurs in many forms of heart disease, notably hypertension and ischaemic heart disease. Systolic and diastolic dysfunction often coexist, particularly in patients with coronary artery disease.

High output failure

Conditions that are associated with a very high cardiac output (e.g. a large AV shunt, severe anaemia or thyro-

Table 5.3 Causes of heart failure

Cause	Features	Examples
Ventricular outflow obstruction (pressure overload)	Initially concentric ventricular hypertrophy allows the ventricle to maintain a normal output by generating a high systolic pressure. However, secondary changes in the myocardium and increasing obstruction eventually lead to failure with ventricular dilatation and rapid clinical deterioration	Hypertension, aortic stenosis (left heart failure) Pulmonary hypertension, pulmonary valve stenosis (right heart failure)
Ventricular inflow obstruction	Small vigorous ventricle Dilated hypertrophied atrium Atrial fibrillation is common and often causes marked deterioration because ventricular filling depends heavily on atrial contraction	Mitral stenosis Tricuspid stenosis Endomyocardial fibrosis and other disorders that cause a stiff myocardium, e.g. left ventricular hypertrophy Constrictive pericarditis
Ventricular volume overload	Dilatation and hypertrophy allow the ventricle to generate a high stroke volume and help to maintain a normal cardiac output. However, secondary changes in the myocardium eventually lead to impaired contractility and worsening heart failure	Mitral regurgitation (LV volume overload) Aortic regurgitation (LV volume overload) Atrial septal defect (RV volume overload) Ventricular septal defect Increased metabolic demand (high output)
Reduced ventricular contractility	Progressive ventricular dilatation In coronary artery disease 'akinetic' or 'dyskinetic' segments contract poorly and may impede the function of the normal segments by distorting their contraction and relaxation patterns	Myocarditis/cardiomyopathy (global dysfunction) Myocardial infarction (segmental dysfunction)

toxicosis) can occasionally cause heart failure. In such cases additional causes of heart failure are often present.

Clinical features

The clinical picture depends on the nature of the underlying heart disease, the type of heart failure that it has evoked and the neural and endocrine changes that have developed.

A low cardiac output causes fatigue, listlessness and a poor effort tolerance. The peripheries are cold and the blood pressure is low. Poor renal perfusion may lead to oliguria and uraemia.

Pulmonary oedema due to left heart failure may present with breathlessness, orthopnoea, paroxysmal nocturnal dyspnoea and inspiratory crepitations over the lung bases. The chest radiograph shows characteristic abnormalities (p. 215) and is usually a more sensitive indicator of pulmonary venous congestion than the physical signs.

In contrast, right heart failure produces a high jugular venous pressure, with hepatic congestion and dependent peripheral oedema. In ambulant patients the oedema affects the ankles whereas in bed-bound patients it col-

lects around the thighs and sacrum. Massive accumulation of fluid may cause ascites or pleural effusion.

Chronic heart failure is sometimes associated with marked weight loss (**cardiac cachexia**) caused by a combination of anorexia and impaired absorption due to gastrointestinal congestion, poor tissue perfusion due to a low cardiac output, and skeletal muscle atrophy due to immobility.

Complications

In advanced heart failure a number of nonspecific complications may occur:

- **Uraemia** reflects poor renal perfusion due to the effects of diuretic therapy and a low cardiac output. Treatment with vasodilators or dopamine may improve renal perfusion.
- **Hypokalaemia** may be the result of treatment with potassium-losing diuretics or hyperaldosteronism caused by activation of the renin-angiotensin system and impaired aldosterone metabolism due to hepatic congestion. Most of the body's potassium is intracellular, and there may be substantial depletion of

potassium stores even when the plasma potassium concentration is in the normal range.

- **Hyponatraemia** is a feature of severe heart failure and may be caused by diuretic therapy, inappropriate water retention, or failure of the cell membrane ion pump.
- **Impaired liver function**. Hepatic venous congestion and poor arterial perfusion frequently cause mild jaundice and abnormal liver function tests; reduced synthesis of clotting factors may make anticoagulant control difficult.
- **Thromboembolism**. Deep vein thrombosis and pulmonary embolism may occur due to the effects of a low cardiac output and enforced immobility, whereas systemic emboli may be related to arrhythmias, particularly atrial fibrillation, or intracardiac thrombus complicating conditions such as mitral stenosis or LV aneurysm.
- **Arrhythmias**. Atrial and ventricular arrhythmias are very common and may be related to electrolyte changes (e.g. hypokalaemia, hypomagnesaemia), the underlying structural heart disease, and the pro-arrhythmic effects of increased circulating catecholamines and some drugs (e.g. digoxin). Sudden death occurs in up to 50% of patients with heart failure and is often due to a ventricular arrhythmia. Frequent ventricular ectopic beats and runs of non-sustained ventricular tachycardia are common findings in patients with heart failure and are associated with an adverse prognosis; unfortunately, the outlook appears to be no better when antiarrhythmic drugs are used to suppress these arrhythmias.

Investigations

Simple tests (e.g. urea, electrolytes, ECG, chest radiograph) may help to establish the nature and severity of the underlying heart disease and detect any complications (see below).

Echocardiography is a very useful investigation and should be considered in all patients with significant heart failure in order to:

- confirm the diagnosis
- detect hitherto unsuspected valvular heart disease (e.g. occult mitral stenosis) and other conditions that may be amenable to specific remedies
- identify patients who will benefit from long-term therapy with an angiotensin-converting enzyme inhibitor (see below).

Management of heart failure

General measures

Bed-rest increases renal blood flow and may help to initiate a diuresis in a patient with severe heart failure.

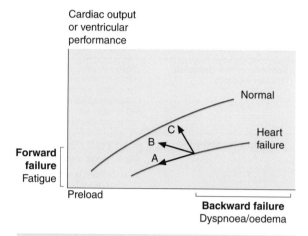

Fig. 5.24   The effect of treatment on ventricular performance curves in heart failure. A. Diuretics and venodilators, B. Angiotensin-converting enzyme inhibitors and mixed vasodilators, C. Positive inotropic agents.

However, regular stamina-building exercise (e.g. brisk walking or swimming) has been shown to improve the outlook in patients with chronic heart failure.

Patients with heart failure should be advised to avoid a high dietary salt intake, excess alcohol, and salt- or fluid-retaining drugs (e.g. NSAIDs).

Drug therapy

Cardiac function can be improved by increasing contractility, optimising preload or decreasing afterload. The effects of these measures are illustrated in Figure 5.24. Drugs that reduce preload are most appropriate in patients with high end-diastolic filling pressures and evidence of pulmonary or systemic venous congestion (backward failure); drugs that reduce afterload or increase myocardial contractility are particularly valuable in patients with signs and symptoms of a low cardiac output (forward failure).

Diuretics. These are usually the first line of treatment. The main types, mode of action, and side-effects of these drugs are described on page 602. In heart failure diuretics produce an increase in urinary sodium excretion, leading to a reduction in blood and plasma volume, and may also cause a small but significant degree of arterial and venous dilatation. Diuretic therapy will, therefore, reduce preload and improve pulmonary and systemic venous congestion; it may also cause a small reduction in afterload and ventricular volume leading to a fall in wall tension and increased cardiac efficiency.

Although a fall in preload (ventricular filling pressure) tends to reduce cardiac output, the 'Starling curve' in heart failure is flat so there may be a substantial and beneficial fall in filling pressure with little change in cardiac output (Fig. 5.24). Nevertheless, excessive diuretic therapy may cause an undesirable fall in cardiac output with a rising blood urea, hypotension and increasing lethargy.

In severe heart failure treatment with combinations of diuretics from different classes (loop, thiazide, and potassium-sparing) may increase the diuretic effect and may help to prevent hypokalaemia.

Vasodilators. The use of vasodilators in acute circulatory failure is described on page 217. These drugs are also valuable in chronic heart failure; venodilators (e.g. organic nitrates) reduce preload, and arterial dilators (e.g. hydralazine) reduce afterload (Fig. 5.24). However, their use is limited by pharmacological tolerance and hypotension, and treatment with angiotensin-converting enzyme inhibitors is usually preferable.

Angiotensin-converting enzyme inhibitors. The advent of these drugs has been a major advance in the treatment of heart failure. They act to prevent the conversion of angiotensin I to angiotensin II, thereby counteracting salt and water retention, peripheral arterial and venous vasoconstriction, and activation of the sympathetic nervous system (Fig. 5.23). They will, therefore, interrupt the vicious circle of neurohumoral activation that is characteristic of moderate and severe heart failure and will also prevent the undesirable activation of the renin-angiotensin system caused by diuretic therapy.

The major benefit of ACE inhibitor therapy in heart failure is a reduction in afterload; however, there may also be an advantageous reduction in preload and a modest increase in the plasma potassium concentration. Treating heart failure with a combination of a potassium-losing diuretic and an ACE inhibitor therefore has many potential advantages.

Clinical trials have shown that in moderate and severe heart failure ACE inhibitors can produce a substantial improvement in effort tolerance and in mortality. Using data from the SOLVD (studies of left ventricular dysfunction) trial it has been calculated that treating 1000 heart failure patients with an ACE inhibitor for 3 years would prevent about 50 premature deaths and 350 hospital admissions. Recent trials have also established that ACE inhibitors can improve outcome and prevent the onset of overt heart failure in patients with poor residual left ventricular function following myocardial infarction (see page 264).

Unfortunately these drugs can cause profound hypotension with postural symptoms and a deterioration in renal function (especially in patients with bilateral renal artery stenosis or pre-existing renal disease). Moreover, there may be a potentially catastrophic fall in blood pressure following the first dose of an ACE inhibitor, particularly if the drug is started in the presence of hypovolaemia or hyponatraemia due to prior diuretic therapy. Accordingly, it is usually advisable to withhold diuretics for 24 hours before starting treatment with a low dose, while the patient is supine and under observation. If hypotension occurs this can be counteracted by elevating the foot of the bed, intravenous saline or, in extreme circumstances, intravenous angiotensin II. Renal function must be monitored and should be checked a month after starting therapy.

- **Captopril** (average dose 25 mg 8-hourly) is a short-acting agent with an elimination half life of 6–8 hours. Unwanted effects include hypotension, hyperkalaemia, deterioration in renal function, cough, skin rash, altered taste and neutropenia.
- **Enalapril** (average dose 20 mg daily) is a long-acting agent that is only active after conversion, in the liver, to the active metabolite enalaprilat. Unwanted effects are similar to those caused by captopril.
- **Lisinopril** (average dose 10 mg daily) is a new agent that has a long half life and a similar range of side-effects.

Digoxin. This should be used as first-line therapy in patients with heart failure and atrial fibrillation when it will usually provide adequate control of the ventricular rate together with a small positive inotropic effect. The dosage and side-effects are discussed on page 239.

The role of digoxin in the treatment of patients with heart failure and sinus rhythm is less certain. There is no doubt that it can produce substantial haemodynamic and symptomatic benefit in some patients. However, it has a narrow therapeutic index and there is evidence that some of its beneficial effects are subject to tolerance. Many physicians therefore only use digoxin to treat patients with heart failure and sinus rhythm if treatment with a diuretic and an ACE inhibitor fails.

Other drugs. A variety of potentially useful oral positive inotropic agents have been developed but have been shown to *increase* mortality in clinical trials.

Anticoagulants are used to treat or prevent thromboembolism complicating atrial fibrillation.

Although not firmly established, there is growing interest in the prospect of using antiarrhythmic drugs to prevent potentially fatal arrhythmias.

HEART TRANSPLANTATION

Cardiac transplantation is an established and very successful form of treatment for patients with intractable heart failure. Coronary artery disease and dilated cardiomyopathy are the commonest reasons for transplantation. The introduction of cyclosporin for immunosuppression has improved survival, which now exceeds 90% at 1 year. The use of transplantation is limited by the availability of donor hearts so it is generally reserved for young patients with severe symptoms.

Heart transplantation is contraindicated in patients with pulmonary vascular disease due to long-standing left heart failure, complex congenital heart disease (e.g. Eisenmenger's syndrome) or primary pulmonary hypertension, because the right ventricle of the donor heart may fail in the face of increased pulmonary vascular resistance. However, heart-lung transplantation is now an option for such patients and has also been used in the treatment of terminal respiratory disease such as cystic fibrosis.

Although cardiac transplantation usually produces a dramatic improvement in the recipient's quality of life, serious complications may occur:

- *Rejection.* In spite of routine therapy with cyclosporin A, azathioprine and corticosteroids, episodes of rejection are common and may present with heart failure, arrhythmias, or subtle ECG changes; cardiac biopsy is often used to confirm the diagnosis before starting treatment with high dose steroids.
- *Accelerated atherosclerosis.* Recurrent heart failure is often due to progressive atherosclerosis in the coronary arteries of the donor heart. This is not confined to patients who were transplanted for coronary artery disease and is probably a manifestation of chronic rejection. Angina is rare because the heart has been denervated.
- *Infection.* Opportunistic infection with organisms such as cytomegalovirus or aspergillus remains a major cause of death in transplant recipients.

OTHER SYMPTOMATIC MANIFESTATIONS OF CARDIOVASCULAR DISEASE

OEDEMA

Oedema of heart failure

This is a feature of chronic heart failure and is due to excessive salt and water retention with activation of the sympathetic and renin-angiotensin systems. In ambulant or sedentary patients it usually affects the ankles, legs, thighs and lower abdomen, in that order. In a patient who is largely bed bound it is most apparent over the sacrum. The oedema of heart failure is usually accompanied by at least some other symptoms of heart

failure, and by a raised jugular venous pressure (see heart failure, p. 218).

Unless it is long-standing and the skin is very tense the oedema pits easily on pressure. Ascites may be present. A differential diagnosis is given in the information box below.

DIFFERENTIAL DIAGNOSIS OF PERIPHERAL OEDEMA

- **Cardiac failure** (right or combined left and right heart failure, pericardial constriction, cardiomyopathy)
- **Chronic venous insufficiency**
- **Hypoalbuminaemia** (nephrotic syndrome, liver disease, protein-losing enteropathy)
- **Drugs**
  Retaining sodium (fludrocortisone, non-steroidal anti-inflammatory agents)
  Increasing capillary permeability (nifedipine)
- **Idiopathic** (women > men)
- **Chronic lymphatic obstruction**

Oedema of chronic venous insufficiency

This is very common in the elderly and usually affects the lower legs only. The oedema pits readily and redistributes after a night's sleep. However, there are no other features of cardiac failure.

Oedema is a relatively late and unreliable feature of deep venous thrombosis. However ilio-femoral vein thrombosis or inferior vena cava obstruction can cause severe venous congestion and oedema.

Oedema of nephrotic syndrome

This tends to be more severe and more widely distributed than the oedema of heart failure, and often affects the face and arms. This is because patients with a nephrotic syndrome have normal cardiac output and normal or reduced circulating blood volume. The presence of proteinuria confirms the diagnosis. Hypoproteinaemic oedema may also occur in liver disease and in protein-losing enteropathy.

PALPITATIONS

Palpitations describe an abnormal subjective awareness of the heart beat. Patients can usually distinguish between sporadic and continuous palpitations (for example extrasystoles or a sustained tachycardia) and between an irregular and a regular pulse. It may be helpful to ask the patient to tap out the heart rhythm on the table. Palpitation with a regular rhythm and a normal heart rate may be due to sudden vasodilatation (e.g. following vasodilator drugs or during perimenopausal flushing).

SYNCOPE

Syncope is loss of consciousness resulting from an inadequate blood supply to the brain. This may be due to sudden vasodilatation, to a sudden fall in cardiac output, or both. Postural syncope when due to vasodilator or antihypertensive drugs is an example of the former, and diminished cardiac output from complete heart block or a very rapid tachycardia of the latter. Exertional syncope may occur under conditions of severe LV outflow obstruction (aortic stenosis).

Vasovagal fainting

This involves both a reflex cardiac slowing mediated by the vagus and a sudden withdrawal of peripheral sympathetic tone. It is a complex centrally mediated reflex which tends to be initiated when pain or a powerful emotional stimulus is inflicted against a background of intense sympathetic stimulation. A very similar reflex can also be triggered by mechano-receptors from the endocardium of the left ventricle. This accounts for the fainting reflex which occurs in patients with pulmonary embolism or aortic stenosis (pp. 277, 290).

SUDDEN CARDIAC DEATH

Cessation of the heart's activities leads rapidly to irreversible brain death and together they constitute the definition of death. Collapse with cardiac arrest is associated with three forms of cardiac rhythm:

- **Asystole** is a lack of electrical activation of the ventricle.
- **Electromechanical dissociation** occurs when the ventricle is activated but is unable to contract or to expel blood.
- **Ventricular fibrillation** is due to very rapid and incoordinate activation of ventricular muscle with consequent lack of ventricular contraction. Prolonged ventricular fibrillation leads to asystole. The cardiac arrest which can occur in the early phase of myocardial infarction is due to ventricular fibrillation in most cases (initially). (See p. 233).

OTHER CARDIOVASCULAR SYMPTOMS

Tiredness is a common complaint with severe heart failure and with ischaemic heart disease. Sometimes it is the consequence of treatment rather than the disease itself, e.g. β-adrenoceptor antagonist therapy or hypokalaemia from diuretics. In those with valvular disease without heart failure it should lead to a suspicion of infective endocarditis.

Nocturia, or a reversal of the usual diurnal rhythm of

FACTORS PRECIPITATING CARDIAC ARREST

Asystole
- Myocardial infarction (may follow VF or heart block)
- Hypoxia/poisoning
- Electrocution

Ventricular fibrillation (VF)
- Myocardial infarction, or ischaemia without infarction
- Myocarditis, cardiomyopathy, RV dysplasia
- Electrolyte disturbances: (low or high K^+, low Ca^{++} or Mg^{++})
- Electric shock
- WPW (see p. 229), long QT syndromes

Electromechanical dissociation
- Cardiac rupture
- Cardiac tamponade
- Cardiac depressant drugs, low Ca^{++}

---

diuresis, sometimes occurs in ambulant patients with cardiac failure. This probably reflects improved renal perfusion during bed-rest rather than a simple mobilisation of oedema fluid from the ankles. Reversal of the normal pattern of daytime diuresis occurs following cardiac transplantation.

Cough may be a feature of pulmonary oedema and is also a recognised side-effect of ACE inhibitors.

Anorexia, nausea and vomiting are all common in severe protracted heart failure; they may also be manifestations of digitalis toxicity (p. 239).

FURTHER READING

Barnard M J, Linter S P K, 1993 Acute circulatory support. British Medical Journal 307: 35–41
Dargie H J, McMurray J J V 1994 Diagnosis and management of heart failure. British Medical Journal 308: 321–328
Levick J R 1991 An introduction to cardiovascular physiology. Butterworths, London

DISORDERS OF HEART RATE, RHYTHM AND CONDUCTION

The heart beat is normally initiated by an electrical discharge from the sinoatrial (sinus) node. The atria and ventricles then depolarise sequentially as electricity passes through the specialised conducting tissue (Fig. 5.25). The sinus node acts as a pacemaker and has its own intrinsic rate that is regulated by the autonomic nervous system; vagal activity slows the heart rate and sympathetic activity accelerates it.

If the sinus rate becomes unduly slow a lower centre may assume the role of pacemaker. This is known as an escape rhythm and may arise in the AV node (nodal rhythm) or the ventricles (idioventricular rhythm).

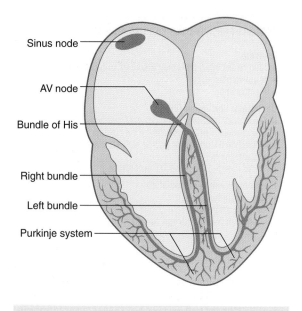

Sinus node

AV node

Bundle of His

Right bundle

Left bundle

Purkinje system

Fig. 5.25 The specialised conducting tissue of the heart.

An arrhythmia is a disturbance in the electrical activity of the heart and may be paroxysmal or continuous. Bradycardia is defined as a rate of < 60/minute, whereas tachycardia is the term used when the rate exceeds 100/min.

There are two underlying mechanisms for tachycardia:

- increased automaticity—when the tachycardia is sustained by repeated spontaneous depolarisation of an ectopic focus or single cell.
- re-entry—when the tachycardia is initiated by an ectopic beat but sustained by a closed loop or re-entry circuit (Fig. 5.26).

Most tachyarrhythmias are due to re-entry.

An arrhythmia may be supraventricular (sinus, atrial or junctional) or ventricular. Supraventricular rhythms usually produce narrow QRS complexes because the ventricles are depolarised normally through the AV node and bundle of His. In contrast, ventricular rhythms produce broad bizarre QRS complexes because the ventricles are activated through an abnormal pathway.

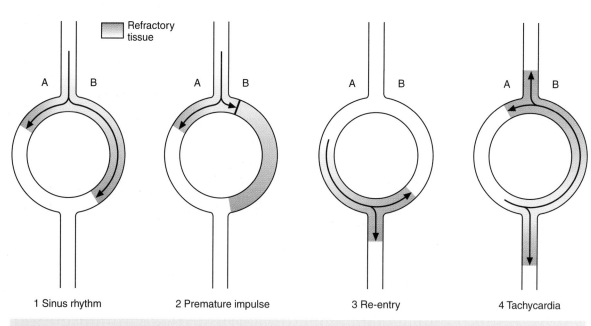

Refractory tissue

A B   A B   A B   A B

1 Sinus rhythm   2 Premature impulse   3 Re-entry   4 Tachycardia

Fig. 5.26 The mechanism of re-entry. Re-entry can occur when there are two alternative pathways with different conducting properties (e.g. the AV node and an accessory pathway, or an area of normal tissue and an area of ischaemic tissue). In this example pathway A conducts slowly and recovers quickly while pathway B conducts rapidly and recovers slowly. **(1) In sinus rhythm** each impulse passes down both pathways before entering a common distal pathway. **(2)** Because the pathways recover at different rates a **premature impulse** may find pathway A open and B closed. **(3)** Pathway B may recover while the premature impulse travels selectively down pathway A. The impulse may then travel retrogradely up pathway B, setting up a closed loop or **re-entry** circuit. **(4)** This may initiate a **tachycardia** that will continue until the circuit is interrupted by a change in conduction rates or electrical depolarisation.

However, occasionally a supraventricular rhythm can produce broad or wide QRS complexes due to coexisting bundle branch block, or the presence of accessory conducting tissue (see below).

SINUS RHYTHMS

Sinus arrhythmia

Phasic alteration of the heart rate during respiration (the sinus rate increases during inspiration and slows during expiration) is a manifestation of normal autonomic nervous activity, and is often particularly pronounced in children. A complete absence of this normal variation in heart rate with breathing or with changes in posture may be a feature of autonomic neuropathy.

Sinus bradycardia

A sinus rate of less than 60 per minute may occur in normal people during sleep and is a common finding in athletes. Some pathological causes are listed in the information box. Acute symptomatic sinus bradycardia usually responds to intravenous atropine 0.6 mg.

Sinus tachycardia

This is defined as a sinus rate of more than 100/min and is usually due to an increase in sympathetic activity associated with exercise, emotion or a variety of pathologies (see information box). The rate seldom exceeds 160/min, except in infants.

SOME PATHOLOGICAL CAUSES OF SINUS BRADYCARDIA

- Myocardial infarction
- Sinus node disease (sick sinus syndrome)
- Hypothermia
- Hypothyroidism
- Cholestatic jaundice
- Raised intracranial pressure
- Drugs, e.g. β-adrenoceptor antagonist, digoxin, verapamil

SOME PATHOLOGICAL CAUSES OF SINUS TACHYCARDIA

- Anxiety
- Fever
- Pregnancy
- Anaemia
- Heart failure
- Thyrotoxicosis
- Phaeochromocytoma
- Drugs, e.g. β-adrenoceptor agonists (bronchodilators)

ATRIAL TACHYARRHYTHMIAS

ATRIAL ECTOPIC BEATS (EXTRASYSTOLES, PREMATURE BEATS)

These usually cause no symptoms but can give the sensation of a missed beat or an abnormally strong beat. The ECG (Fig. 5.27) shows a premature but otherwise normal QRS complex; if visible the preceding P wave has a different configuration because the impulse starts at an abnormal site.

ATRIAL TACHYCARDIA

An ectopic atrial tachycardia due to increased automaticity is rare but is sometimes a manifestation of digitalis toxicity. The ECG shows an atrial rate of 140–220 per minute with abnormal P waves often accompanied by atrioventricular block (e.g. 2:1, 3:1, or variable). Management is similar to that for atrial flutter (see below).

ATRIAL FLUTTER

In this condition a rapid atrial rate of around 300/min is associated with 2:1, 3:1, 4:1 or variable atrioventricular block. The ECG shows characteristic saw-toothed flutter waves (Fig. 5.28). When there is regular 2:1 AV block it may be difficult to distinguish atrial flutter from supraventricular or sinus tachycardia because alternate flutter waves are buried in the QRS complexes; carotid sinus pressure or intravenous adenosine may help to establish the diagnosis by temporarily increasing the degree of AV block and revealing the flutter waves (Fig. 5.29).

Management

Digoxin, β-adrenoceptor antagonists or verapamil can be used to control the ventricular rate (for details see pp. 234–239). However, in many cases it may be pref-

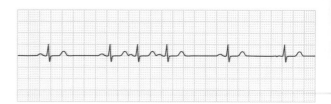

Fig. 5.27 Atrial ectopic beats. The first, second and fifth complexes are normal sinus beats. The third, fourth and sixth complexes are atrial ectopic beats with identical QRS complexes and abnormal (sometimes barely visible) p waves.

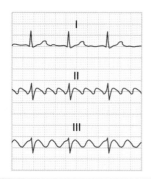

Fig. 5.28 Atrial flutter. Simultaneous recording showing atrial flutter with 3:1 block; flutter waves are only visible in leads II and III.

erable to try and restore sinus rhythm by means of atrial overdrive pacing, DC (direct current) cardioversion or drug therapy. Amiodarone, disopyramide, propafenone, flecainide or quinidine may be effective and can also be used to prevent recurrent episodes of atrial flutter (see pp. 234–239).

ATRIAL FIBRILLATION

In this arrhythmia the atria beat rapidly, chaotically and ineffectively; the ventricles respond at irregular intervals giving the characteristic 'irregularly irregular' pulse. The ECG (Fig. 5.30) shows normal but irregular QRS complexes; there are no P waves but the baseline may show irregular fibrillation waves.

Atrial fibrillation is the most common sustained cardiac arrhythmia with an overall prevalence of approximately 0.5% in the adult population, rising to 10% or more in those over 75 years old. The common causes are listed in the information box.

The onset of atrial fibrillation can cause palpitation and may precipitate or aggravate cardiac failure in patients with an abnormal heart, especially those with mitral stenosis or poor left ventricular function. Nevertheless, atrial fibrillation is often asymptomatic, particularly in the elderly.

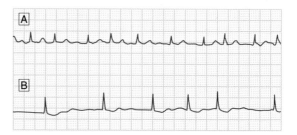

Fig. 5.30 Two examples of atrial fibrillation. The QRS complexes are irregular and there are no p waves. There is usually a fast ventricular rate, often around 180/min, at the onset of atrial fibrillation A. However, in chronic atrial fibrillation the ventricular rate may be much slower due to the effects of medication and AV nodal fatigue B.

Ineffective atrial contraction coupled with left atrial dilatation predisposes to stasis and may lead to thrombosis and systemic embolism. The risk of thromboembolism depends on the underlying cause (see below), and increases with the size of the left atrium and the age of the patient.

Management

Digoxin, β-adrenoceptor antagonists ('β-blockers') or verapamil (pp. 234–239) will reduce the ventricular rate by increasing the degree of AV block, and this alone may produce a striking improvement in overall cardiac function, particularly in patients with mitral stenosis.

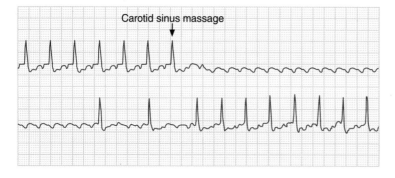

Carotid sinus massage

Fig. 5.29 Carotid sinus massage in atrial flutter: continuous trace. In this example the diagnosis of atrial flutter with 2:1 block was established when carotid sinus massage produced temporary AV block revealing the flutter waves.

Treatment of the underlying cause (e.g. thyrotoxicosis, post-operative chest infection) may restore sinus rhythm; if not, elective DC cardioversion (p. 243) should be considered. In patients with paroxysmal atrial fibrillation and those who have undergone successful cardioversion, beta-blockers, quinidine, disopyramide or amiodarone, but not digoxin, may help to preserve sinus rhythm (see pp. 234–239).

In exceptional cases refractory atrial tachyarrhythmias can be treated by deliberately inducing complete heart block using surgery or transvenous catheter radiofrequency ablation; a permanent pacemaker must be implanted at the same time.

Anticoagulation with warfarin reduces the risk of stroke or systemic embolism in patients with atrial fibrillation but can precipitate serious bleeding complications. The potential benefits of anticoagulant therapy must therefore be weighed against the possible hazards in each case. The risk of thromboembolism is greatest in patients with atrial fibrillation associated with mitral valve disease or thyrotoxicosis and those undergoing DC cardioversion, who therefore have most to gain from full anticoagulation. In contrast, patients below the age of 60 with atrial fibrillation and an otherwise normal heart are at low risk of embolism and should not be anticoagulated. In other forms of chronic atrial fibrillation the annual risk of stroke is approximately 5%; treatment with warfarin reduces this to about 1.5% per year with an annual risk of important bleeding of around 0.5%. In these patients low intensity anticoagulation (target INR 1.5–2.7) seems to offer the best risk/benefit ratio. Aspirin is less effective than warfarin in this situation, particularly in elderly patients, but is worth considering if the risks of anticoagulation are high.

Full or low dose anticoagulation should therefore be considered in all patients with chronic atrial fibrillation who have evidence of structural heart disease or are over 65 years old.

JUNCTIONAL TACHYARRHYTHMIAS (SVT)

AV NODAL RE-ENTRY TACHYCARDIA

This rhythm is due to re-entry within the AV node and produces a regular tachycardia with a rate of between 140 and 220; it tends to occur in hearts that are otherwise normal and may last from a few seconds to many hours. The patient is usually aware of a fast heart beat and may feel faint or breathless. Polyuria, due to the release of atrial natriuretic peptide, is sometimes a feature and cardiac pain or heart failure may occur if there is coexisting structural heart disease.

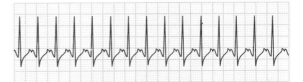

Fig. 5.31 Supraventricular tachycardia. The rate is 180/min and the QRS complexes are normal.

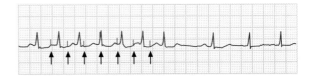

Fig. 5.32 Anti-tachycardia pacemaker. A supraventricular tachycardia is detected by the pacemaker, which terminates the arrhythmia by delivering a series of critically timed impulses (arrows) to the right atrium.

The ECG (Fig. 5.31) usually shows a tachycardia with normal QRS complexes but occasionally there may be rate-dependent bundle branch block.

Management

Treatment is not always necessary. However, an attack may be terminated by carotid sinus massage or other measures that increase vagal tone (e.g. self-induced vomiting, valsalva manoeuvre). Intravenous adenosine or verapamil will restore sinus rhythm in most cases. Suitable alternative drugs include β-adrenoceptor antagonists, disopyramide and digoxin. In an emergency the tachycardia should be terminated by DC cardioversion (p. 243).

If attacks are frequent or otherwise disabling, prophylactic oral therapy with any of the above drugs may be indicated. Further information on antiarrhythmic drugs is given on pages 234–239. In refractory cases catheter radiofrequency ablation of the re-entry circuit or an anti-tachycardia pacemaker may be helpful. Anti-tachycardia pacemakers are able to detect the onset of an abnormal rhythm and to respond by emitting appropriately timed impulses which block the re-entry circuit (Fig. 5.32).

THE WOLFF–PARKINSON–WHITE (WPW) SYNDROME

In this condition there is an abnormal band of atrial tissue which connects the atria and ventricles and can electrically bypass the AV node. In normal sinus rhythm conduction takes place partly through the AV node and partly through the more rapidly conducting bypass tract.

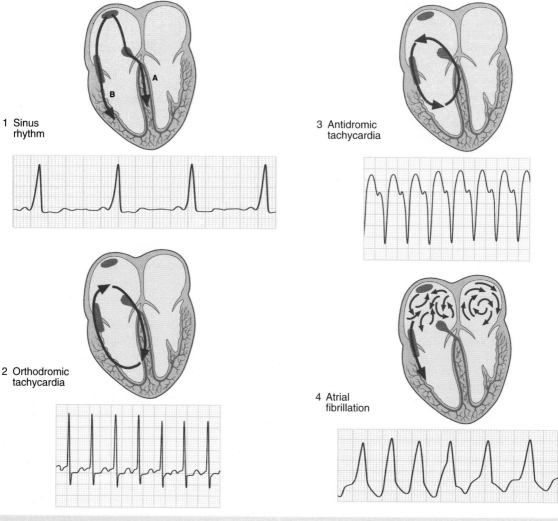

Fig. 5.33 Wolff–Parkinson–White syndrome. In this condition there is a strip of accessory conducting tissue that allows electricity to bypass the AV node and spread from the atria to the ventricles rapidly and without delay. When the ventricles are depolarised through the AV node the ECG is normal (**A**) but when the ventricles are depolarised through the accessory conducting tissue the ECG shows a very short PR interval and a broad QRS complex (**B**).
(1) Sinus rhythm. In sinus rhythm the ventricles are partly depolarised through the AV node, and partly through the accessory pathway, producing an ECG with a short PR interval and broadened QRS complexes; the characteristic slurring of the upstroke of the QRS complex is known as a delta wave. The degree of pre-excitation (the proportion of electricity passing down the accessory pathway) and therefore the ECG appearances may vary a lot and at times the ECG can look normal.
(2) Orthodromic tachycardia. This is the commonest form of tachycardia in WPW. The re-entry circuit passes antegradely through the AV node and retrogradely through the accessory pathway. The ventricles are therefore depolarised in the normal way producing a narrow complex tachycardia that is indistinguishable from other forms of SVT.
(3) Antidromic tachycardia. Occasionally the re-entry circuit passes antegradely through the accessory pathway and retrogradely through the AV node. The ventricles are then depolarised through the accessory pathway producing a broad complex tachycardia.
(4) Atrial fibrillation. In this rhythm the ventricles are largely depolarised through the accessory pathway producing a very rapid irregular broad complex tachycardia.

The ECG shows shortening of the PR interval and a 'slurring' of the QRS complex called a delta wave (Fig. 5.33A). Because the AV node and bypass tract have different conduction speeds and refractory periods, a re-entry circuit (Fig. 5.26) can develop, causing paroxysms of tachycardia (Fig. 5.33B,C). The onset of atrial fib-

rillation may produce very rapid ventricular rates because the bypass pathway lacks the rate-limiting properties of the normal AV node (Fig. 5.33D). Atrial fibrillation is therefore a potentially dangerous arrhythmia in these patients and may cause collapse, syncope and even death.

Drug treatment is only indicated in symptomatic pa-

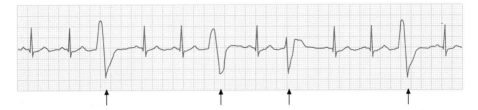

Fig. 5.34   Ventricular ectopic beats. There are broad bizarre QRS complexes with no preceding p wave in between normal sinus beats. Their configuration varies so these are multifocal ectopics.

tients and is aimed at slowing the conduction rate and prolonging the refractory period of the bypass tract, using agents such as disopyramide or amiodarone (pp. 234–239); digoxin and verapamil increase conduction in the bypass tract and should be avoided. Transvenous catheter radiofrequency ablation of the bypass tract offers a cure and is the treatment of choice for most patients.

VENTRICULAR TACHYARRHYTHMIAS

VENTRICULAR ECTOPIC BEATS (EXTRASYSTOLES, PREMATURE BEATS)

The ECG shows premature broad bizarre QRS complexes which may be unifocal, when there is a single ectopic focus, or multifocal (varying morphology with multiple foci—Fig. 5.34). 'Couplet' and 'triplet' are terms used to describe two or three successive ectopic beats, whereas a run of alternate sinus and ectopic beats is known as 'bigeminy'. Ectopic beats produce a low stroke volume because left ventricular contraction is premature and ineffective. The pulse is therefore irregular with weak or missed beats. Patients are often asymptomatic but may complain of an irregular heart beat, missed beats or abnormally strong beats (due to the increased output of the post-ectopic sinus beat). The significance of ventricular ectopic beats (VEBs) depends on the nature of any underlying heart disease.

Ventricular ectopic beats in otherwise healthy subjects

VEBs are frequently found in normal people, and their prevalence increases with age. Ectopic beats in patients with otherwise normal hearts are often more prominent at rest, and tend to disappear with exercise. The outlook is excellent and treatment is unnecessary although low dose β-adrenoceptor antagonist treatment is sometimes used to suppress anxiety and palpitation.

VEBs are sometimes a manifestation of otherwise subclinical heart disease, particularly coronary artery disease. There is no evidence that antiarrhythmic therapy is merited in such patients but the discovery of frequent ventricular ectopic beats might reasonably prompt some general cardiac investigations.

Ventricular ectopic beats associated with heart disease

Frequent VEBs are often observed during acute myocardial infarction but are of no prognostic significance and require no treatment. However, persistent frequent (> 10/hour) ventricular ectopic activity in patients who have survived the acute phase of myocardial infarction is indicative of a poor long-term outcome. Unfortunately, antiarrhythmic therapy does not improve, and may even worsen, the prognosis in these patients.

VEBs are common in patients with heart failure, when they are associated with an adverse prognosis; but again the outlook is no better if they are suppressed with antiarrhythmic drugs. Effective treatment of the heart failure may suppress the ectopic beats.

VEBs are also a feature of digoxin toxicity, are sometimes found in mitral valve prolapse, and may occur as 'escape beats' in the presence of an underlying bradycardia. Treatment should always be directed at the underlying condition.

VENTRICULAR TACHYCARDIA (Fig. 5.35)

This is a grave arrhythmia because it is nearly always associated with serious heart disease and may degenerate into ventricular fibrillation. Patients may complain of palpitation or the symptoms of a low cardiac output such as dizziness, dyspnoea or even loss of consciousness (syncope). The ECG shows broad, abnormal QRS complexes with a rate of between 140 and 220 per minute and may be difficult to distinguish from supraventricular tachycardia with bundle branch block or pre-excitation (Wolff–Parkinson–White syndrome). Features in favour of ventricular tachycardia are listed in the information box. A 12-lead (Fig. 5.36), intracardiac (Fig. 5.37) or oesophageal ECG may help to establish the diagnosis. When there is doubt, it is safer to treat for ventricular

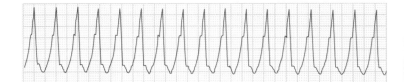

Fig. 5.35 Ventricular tachycardia—rhythm strip. Typical broad bizarre QRS complexes with a rate of 160/min.

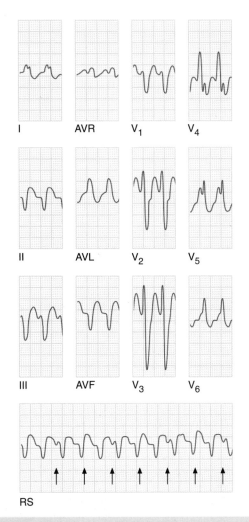

Fig. 5.36 Ventricular tachycardia—12-lead ECG. The morphology of this tachycardia is typical of VT with very broad QRS complexes and marked left axis deviation. In addition there is AV dissociation; some p waves (arrowed) are visible and others are buried in the QRS complexes.

FEATURES IN FAVOUR OF VENTRICULAR TACHYCARDIA IN THE DIFFERENTIAL DIAGNOSIS OF BROAD COMPLEX TACHYCARDIA

- A history of myocardial infarction
- AV dissociation (pathognomonic)
- Capture/fusion beats (pathognomonic—see Fig. 5.38)
- Extreme left axis deviation
- Very broad QRS complexes (>140 ms)
- No response to carotid sinus massage or i.v. adenosine

aneurysm or poor left ventricular function. In some cases ventricular tachycardia is associated with abnormal prolongation of the QT interval which may be hereditary but can also be due to hypokalaemia, hypomagnesaemia, or drugs such as quinidine, sotalol or amiodarone.

Patients recovering from myocardial infarction sometimes have periods of idioventricular rhythm ('slow' ventricular tachycardia) at a rate only slightly above the preceding sinus rate. These episodes are usually self-limiting, asymptomatic, and do not require treatment. Other forms of ventricular tachycardia, if they last for more than a few beats, will require treatment, often as an emergency.

Management

Prompt action to restore sinus rhythm is required and in most cases should be followed by prophylactic therapy. DC cardioversion is often the initial treatment of choice but if this is not available or the arrhythmia is well tolerated intravenous lignocaine may be given as a bolus followed by an intravenous infusion (see Table 5.4). Mexilitine, flecainide, disopyramide and amiodarone are suitable alternatives (see pp. 234–239). Hypokalaemia, hypomagnesaemia and acidosis must be corrected.

Oral prophylactic therapy with mexilitine, disopyramide, propafenone or amiodarone (pp. 234–239) is often necessary. The efficacy of such drug therapy should always be assessed by ambulatory ECG monitoring, exercise testing or invasive electrophysiological studies. If drug therapy fails, alternative treatments include the use of an automatic implantable cardioverter-defibrillator (see p. 243) or surgery to identify and resect the area of diseased myocardium responsible for the arrhythmia.

tachycardia which is by far the commonest cause of a broad complex tachycardia.

The common causes of ventricular tachycardia include acute myocardial infarction, myocarditis, cardiomyopathy, and chronic ischaemic heart disease, particularly when it is associated with a ventricular

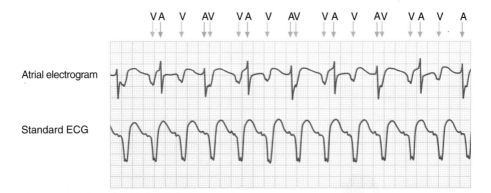

VA V AV VA V AV VA V AV VA V A

Atrial electrogram

Standard ECG

Fig. 5.37   Ventricular tachycardia—intracardiac ECG. A simultaneous recording of an atrial electrogram, obtained by placing a pacing lead in the right atrium, and an ordinary rhythm strip illustrating ventricular tachycardia with AV dissociation. Although the standard ECG shows a broad complex tachycardia with no visible p waves, dissociated atrial activity is clearly visible in the atrial electrogram. A = atrial depolarization, V = ventricular depolarization.

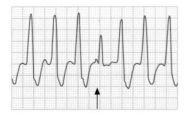

Fig. 5.38   Ventricular tachycardia—fusion beat. In ventricular tachycardia there is independent atrial and ventricular activity. Occasionally a p wave is conducted to the ventricles through the AV node. This may produce a normal sinus beat in the middle of the tachycardia (a capture beat); however, more commonly the conducted impulse fuses with an impulse from the tachycardia (a fusion beat). This phenomenon can only occur when there is AV dissociation and is therefore diagnostic of ventricular tachycardia.

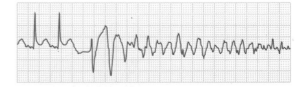

Fig. 5.39   Ventricular fibrillation. A bizarre chaotic rhythm initiated in this case by two ectopic beats in rapid succession.

CARDIAC ARREST

This describes the sudden and complete loss of cardiac function. There is no pulse, the patient loses consciousness, and respiration ceases almost immediately; death is virtually inevitable unless effective treatment is given promptly. Cardiac arrest may be due to ventricular fibrillation, asystole, or electromechanical dissociation.

Aetiology of cardiac arrest

Ventricular fibrillation

This is the commonest and the most easily treatable cause of sudden death. It may be due to myocardial infarction, ischaemia or electrocution. The presence of structural heart disease, electrolyte disturbance such as hypokalaemia, or inappropriate medication may increase susceptibility to ventricular fibrillation. The

arrhythmia produces rapid ineffective uncoordinated movement of the ventricles, which therefore produce no pulse. The ECG (Fig 5.39) shows chaotic, bizarre, irregular complexes.

Ventricular asystole

This occurs when there is no electrical activity of the ventricles and may be due to failure of the conducting tissue or massive ventricular damage complicating myocardial infarction. Cardiac massage or a blow to the chest can sometimes restore cardiac activity, although an artificial pacemaker may be needed to prevent further attacks.

Electromechanical dissociation

This occurs when there is no effective cardiac output despite the presence of normal or near normal electrical activity; it is often due to cardiac rupture or massive pulmonary embolism and is seldom amenable to treatment.

Management of cardiac arrest

Prompt treatment is essential because irreversible brain damage will occur unless some circulation of oxygenated blood can be achieved within two or three minutes.

A   Airway
Clear the airway of vomitus or debris, extend the neck and raise the chin

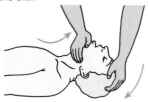

B   Breathing
   1. Direct mouth-to-mouth
      breathing

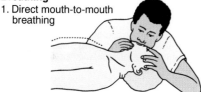

   2. Indirect mouth-to-mouth
      breathing

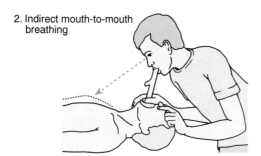

C   Circulation
Cardiac massage
(see text)

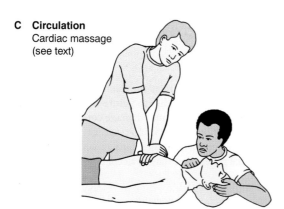

Fig. 5.40   Emergency resuscitation. The ABC of basic life support.
A. Airway.   Clear the airway of vomitus or debris, extend the neck and raise the chin.
B. Breathing.   1. Direct mouth to mouth breathing;
                    2. Indirect mouth to mouth breathing.
C. Circulation. Cardiac massage.

First, confirm the diagnosis (unconscious, death-like appearance, no pulse) and send for help. Next, deliver a sharp blow to the centre of the chest. If the heart does not start immediately, as indicated by the return of the carotid or femoral pulse, start basic life-support (Fig. 5.40). The patient should be placed on his back, on the floor or on some other firm surface, and his legs should be elevated. Mouth to mouth, mouth to nose, or mouth to airway ventilation should be used until a facemask and bag become available. Cardiac massage should be given by placing both hands on the lower sternum and applying short, sharp, forceful compressions at a rate of 60 to 100 per minute (practice with a dummy or mannikin is very helpful).

Obtain an ECG as soon as possible (many defibrillators have a facility for reading the ECG through the paddles). This will identify the underlying rhythm and allow further treatment according to the advanced life support algorithms for ventricular fibrillation or pulseless ventricular tachycardia (Fig. 5.41), asystole (Fig. 5.42) and electromechanical dissociation (Fig. 5.43).

Resuscitation is most likely to succeed when cardiac arrest is due to ventricular fibrillation, particularly if this occurs as a result of an accident or an otherwise uncomplicated myocardial infarct.

ANTIARRHYTHMIC DRUGS—PRINCIPLES OF USE

The drugs used to treat arrhythmias are potentially toxic and should be used carefully according to the following principles:
- Many arrhythmias are benign and do not require specific treatment
- Precipitating or causal factors should be corrected if possible. These may include excess alcohol or caffeine consumption, myocardial ischaemia, hyperthyroidism, acidosis, hypokalaemia and hypomagnesaemia
- If drug therapy is required it is best to use as few drugs as possible
- In difficult cases programmed electrical stimulation (electrophysiological study) may help to identify the optimum therapy
- When dealing with life-threatening arrhythmias it is essential to ensure that prophylactic treatment is effective. Ambulatory monitoring, exercise testing, and programmed electrical stimulation may be of value
- Patients on long-term antiarrhythmic drugs should be reviewed regularly and attempts made to withdraw therapy if the factors which precipitated the arrhythmias are no longer operative
- Patients who do not respond to drug therapy may benefit from other forms of therapy such as anti-tachycardia pacing, radiofrequency ablation or arrhythmia surgery

ANTIARRHYTHMIC DRUGS

The classification of antiarrhythmic drugs

Some of the drugs used to treat individual arrhythmias have already been mentioned. These agents may be classified according to their mode of action or their main site of action (see information boxes). The main uses, dosages and side-effects of the most widely used drugs are summarised in Table 5.4.

CLASSIFICATION OF ANTIARRHYTHMIC DRUGS ACCORDING TO THEIR MAIN SITE OF ACTION

- **AV node**: *adenosine, β-adrenoceptor antagonists, verapamil, digoxin*
- **Ventricles**: *lignocaine, mexilitine*
- **Atria, ventricles and accessory conducting tissue**: *quinidine, disopyramide, flecainide, propafenone, amiodarone*

CLASSIFICATION OF ANTIARRHYTHMIC DRUGS ACCORDING TO THEIR EFFECT ON THE INTRACELLULAR ACTION POTENTIAL

Class I—membrane stabilising agents (fast sodium channel blockers)
(**a**) block Na^+ channel and prolong action potential
   quinidine, disopyramide
(**b**) block Na^+ channel and shorten action potential
   lignocaine, mexilitine
(**c**) block Na^+ channel with no effect on action potential
   flecainide, propafenone

Class II—β-adrenoceptor antagonists
- *propranolol, metoprolol, atenolol, l-sotalol*

Class III—drugs whose main effect is to prolong the action potential
- *amiodarone, d-sotalol*

Class IV—slow calcium channel blockers
- *verapamil, diltiazem*

NB. Some drugs (e.g. digoxin and adenosine) have no place in this classification while others have properties in more than one class (e.g. amiodarone which has actions in all four classes).

Class I drugs

Class I drugs act principally by suppressing excitability and slowing conduction in atrial or ventricular muscle.

Quinidine. This is excreted in the urine and accumulates in renal failure. Gastrointestinal side-effects (abdominal discomfort, nausea and diarrhoea) are common; more serious side-effects include myocardial depression, ventricular tachycardia (often heralded by prolongation of the QT interval) and idiosyncratic auto-immune thrombocytopenia or haemolytic anaemia. Quinidine potentiates digoxin, by increasing plasma digoxin concentrations, and is subject to many other important drug interactions. In view of these problems it is usually used as a second or third line agent.

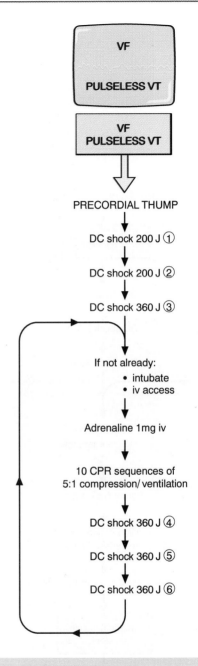

Fig. 5.41 Advanced cardiac life support. Algorithm for ventricular fibrillation or pulseless ventricular tachycardia. Reproduced with permission: copyright European Resuscitation Council; Resuscitation 22 (1992), 111–121.

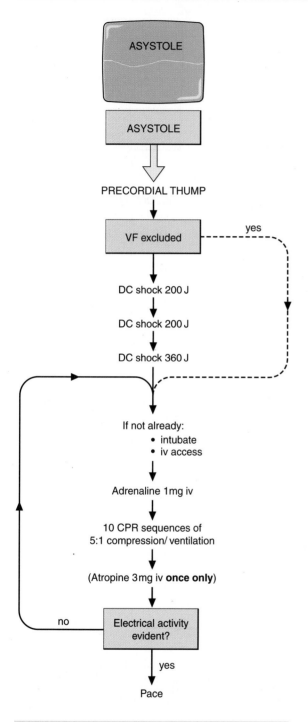

Fig. 5.42 **Advanced cardiac life support. Algorithm for asystole.** Reproduced with permission: copyright European Resuscitation Council; Resuscitation 22 (1992), 111–121.

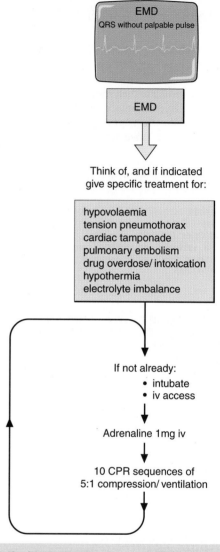

Fig. 5.43 **Advanced cardiac life support. Algorithm for electromechanical dissociation.** Reproduced with permission: copyright European Resuscitation Council; Resuscitation 22 (1992), 111–121.

Disopyramide. This has weak atropine-like effects and may cause urinary retention or precipitate glaucoma. It has a depressant effect on ventricular function and should be avoided in cardiac failure. The drug is cleared through the kidneys and liver. If it is used in patients with atrial flutter and AV block, there is a risk of a paradoxical increase in heart rate as the atria slow and 2:1 block changes to 1:1 conduction; this can be prevented by pretreatment with digoxin.

Lignocaine. This must be given parenterally, and has

Table 5.4   The main uses, dosages and side-effects of the most widely used antiarrhythmic drugs

Drug	Main uses		Dose (adult)	Important side-effects
CLASS I **Quinidine**	Prevention of VEs and AF	oral	Test dose: 250 mg Maintenance: 500 mg 12-hourly as quinidine bisulphate SR	GI upset, myocardial depression, ventricular tachycardia, haemolytic anaemia, potentiates digoxin and warfarin
Disopyramide	Prevention and treatment of all tachyarrhythmias	i.v. oral	2 mg/kg at 30 mg/min then 0.4 mg/kg per hour (max 800 mg/d) 100–150 mg 6-hourly or 250–375 mg 12-hourly SR	Myocardial depression Hypotension Dry mouth Urinary retention
Lignocaine	Treatment and short-term prevention of VT and VF	i.v.	Bolus 1.5 mg/kg 4 mg/min for 2–4 hours, then 2 mg/min	Confusion Convulsions
Mexiletine	Prevention and treatment of ventricular tachyarrhythmias	i.v. oral	Loading dose 100–250 mg at 25 mg/min then 250 mg in 1 hour then 250 mg in 2 hours Maintenance therapy 0.5 mg/min 250 mg 8-hourly	GI irritation, confusion, dizziness, tremor, nystagmus ataxia
Propafenone	Prevention and treatment of ventricular arrhythmias	oral	150–300 mg 8-hourly	Myocardial depression, dizziness
Flecainide	Prevention and treatment of all tachyarrhythmias	i.v. oral	2 mg/kg over 10 min then 1.5 mg/kg/h for 1 hour then 0.1 mg/kg/h 50–100 mg 12-hourly	Myocardial depression, dizziness
CLASS II **Propranolol**		i.v. oral	1 mg over 1 min to a maximum of 10 mg 10–160 mg 6- or 8-hourly	
Metroprolol	Treatment and prevention of SVT and AF Prevention of VEs and exercise-induced VT	i.v. oral	5 mg over 2 min to a maximum of 15 mg 50–100 mg 8- or 12-hourly	Myocardial depression, bradycardia, bronchospasm, fatigue, depression, nightmares, cold peripheries
Atenolol		i.v. oral	2.5 mg at 1 mg/min repeated at 5-min intervals (max 10 mg) 50–100 mg daily	
Sotalol		i.v. oral	10–20 mg slowly 40–160 mg 12-hourly	
CLASS III **Amiodarone**	Serious atrial and ventricular tachyarrhythmias, particularly in the WPW syndrome	i.v. oral	5 mg/kg over 20–120 min then up to 15 mg/kg/24 h Initially 600 mg/day then 1–200 mg daily	Photosensitivity, skin discolouration, corneal deposits, thyroid dysfunction, alveolitis, nausea and vomiting, hepatotoxicity, peripheral neuropathy, potentiates digoxin and warfarin
CLASS IV **Verapamil**	Treatment of SVT, control of AF	i.v. oral	5–10 mg over 30 s 40–120 mg 8-hourly or 240 mg SR daily	Myocardial depression, hypotension, bradycardia, constipation
OTHER **Digoxin**	Treatment and prevention SVT, control AF	i.v. oral	Loading dose: 0.02 mg/kg 0.5 mg over 30 min 6-hourly then 0.125–0.25 mg daily 0.5 mg 6-hourly then 0.125–0.25 mg daily	GI disturbance, xanthopsia Arrhythmias (see p. 225)
Adenosine	Treatment of SVT, aid to diagnosis in unidentified tachycardia	i.v.	3 mg over 2 s followed if necessary by 6 mg then 12 mg at intervals of 1–2 min	Flushing, dyspnoea, chest pain

SVT Supraventricular tachycardia
AF Atrial fibrillation
VE Ventricular ectopic
VT Ventricular tachycardia
VF Ventricular fibrillation
SR Sustained release formulation

a very short plasma half-life, so plasma concentration will depend on the rate of infusion. It is mainly used for the urgent treatment or prophylaxis of ventricular tachycardia or fibrillation.

Mexilitine. This can be given intravenously or orally and is used for the treatment or prophylaxis of ventricular arrhythmias. Side-effects include nausea, vomiting, confusion, dizziness, tremor, nystagmus and ataxia. Metabolism is mainly hepatic and the drug may accumulate in liver disease.

Flecainide. This can be given intravenously or orally for the treatment or prophylaxis of supraventricular or ventricular arrhythmias and may be useful in the management of Wolff–Parkinson–White syndrome. Unfortunately it is a potent myocardial depressant and cannot, therefore, be used safely in patients with poor left ventricular function. Like all antiarrhythmic drugs it can in some circumstances be proarrhythmic and has been found to be hazardous in patients with a history of myocardial infarction. Flecainide is therefore contraindicated in ischaemic heart disease except in patients with life-threatening ventricular arrhythmias who have been assessed by invasive electrophysiological studies.

Propafenone. This is indicated for the treatment or prophylaxis of ventricular arrhythmias and can also be used in the Wolff–Parkinson–White syndrome. Propafenone is a class Ic drug but also has some β-adrenoceptor antagonist (class II) properties and may precipitate heart failure or heart block in susceptible patients. Important interactions with digoxin, warfarin and cimetidine have been described.

Class II drugs

This group comprises the β-adrenoceptor antagonists (β-blockers). The agents used most commonly are:

Propranolol. This is not cardioselective and is subject to extensive first pass metabolism in the liver. The effective oral dose is therefore unpredictable and must be titrated after starting treatment with a small dose. For the same reason intravenous propranolol is very potent. CNS side-effects (e.g. nightmares, sedation) are common because the drug readily crosses the blood–brain barrier.

Metoprolol. This is a cardioselective β-adrenoceptor antagonist and may therefore have fewer side-effects than propranolol. However, it is also lipid soluble and therefore crosses the blood–brain barrier.

Atenolol. This is a cardioselective β-adrenoceptor antagonist with a long duration of action; it is largely excreted unchanged through the kidneys. CNS side-effects are rare because it is water soluble.

Sotalol. This is a racemic mixture of two isomers with non-selective β-adrenoceptor antagonist (mainly l-

sotalol) and class III (mainly d-sotalol) activity; it has a long half-life.

Class III drugs

Class III drugs act by prolonging the plateau phase of the action potential, thus lengthening the refractory period.

Amiodarone. This is the principal drug in this class although both disopyramide and sotalol have class III activity. Amiodarone has unusual pharmacokinetics and is effective against a wide variety of atrial and ventricular arrhythmias. It is probably the most effective drug currently available for controlling paroxysmal atrial fibrillation and the arrhythmias associated with the Wolff–Parkinson–White syndrome. Furthermore, it is very useful in preventing episodes of recurrent ventricular tachycardia, particularly in patients with poor left ventricular function. Amiodarone has an extraordinarily long tissue half-life (25–110 days). This means that the onset of action after oral and intravenous therapy is delayed; indeed it may take several months to reach steady state. For the same reason the drug's effects may last for weeks or months after treatment has been stopped. Side-effects are numerous and potentially serious (see Table 5.4); they include photosensitisation, corneal deposits, gastrointestinal problems, thyroid dysfunction, liver disease and pulmonary fibrosis. Drug interactions are also common; for example, the effects of digoxin and warfarin are potentiated by amiodarone.

Class IV drugs

These block the 'slow calcium channel' which is particularly important for impulse generation and conduction in atrial and nodal tissue, although it is also present in ventricular muscle.

Verapamil. This is the most widely used antiarrhythmic drug in this class; nifedipine (p. 251) has no significant antiarrhythmic effect in man. Intravenous verapamil may cause profound bradycardia and/or hypotension and should not be used in conjunction with oral or intravenous β-adrenoceptor antagonists.

Other antiarrhythmic drugs

Adenosine. Adenosine must be given intravenously and like carotid sinus massage produces transient AV block lasting a few seconds. Accordingly, it may be used to

RESPONSE TO INTRAVENOUS ADENOSINE

Arrhythmia	Response
• Supraventricular tachycardia	Termination
• Atrial fibrillation, atrial flutter	Transient AV block
• Ventricular tachycardia	No effect

terminate junctional tachycardias when the AV node is part of the re-entry circuit or to help establish the diagnosis in difficult arrhythmias such as atrial flutter with 2:1 AV block or broad complex tachycardia (see Table 5.4).

Adenosine is given as an intravenous bolus according to an ascending dosage schedule. The initial dose is 3 mg given over 2 seconds. If there is no response after 1–2 minutes 6 mg should be given and if necessary the physician should wait another 1–2 minutes before administering the maximum dose of 12 mg. Unwanted effects are shortlived and include flushing, breathlessness and chest pain. The effects of adenosine are greatly potentiated by dipyridamole and inhibited by theophylline and other xanthines.

Digoxin. This is a purified glycoside from the European foxglove, *Digitalis lanata*, which slows conduction and prolongs the refractory period in the AV node. This effect helps to control the ventricular rate in atrial fibrillation and will often interrupt re-entry tachycardias involving the AV node. On the other hand digoxin tends to shorten refractory periods and enhance excitability and conduction in other parts of the heart (including accessory conduction pathways); it may therefore increase atrial and ventricular ectopic activity and can lead to more complex atrial and ventricular tachyarrhythmias.

DIGOXIN TOXICITY

Extracardiac manifestations
- Anorexia, nausea, vomiting
- Diarrhoea
- Altered colour vision (xanthopsia)

Cardiac manifestations
- Bradycardia
- Multiple ventricular ectopics
- Ventricular bigeminy (alternate ventricular ectopics)
- Paroxysmal atrial tachycardia
- Ventricular tachycardia
- Ventricular fibrillation

Management
- Stop digoxin
- Check urea, electrolytes and plasma digoxin level
- Correct hypokalaemia and/or dehydration
- Correct bradycardia using atropine (0.6 mg i.v.) and/or temporary pacing
- Treat atrial tachycardia with β-adrenoceptor antagonists
- Treat ventricular tachycardia with lignocaine
- In overdose, specific anti-digoxin antibodies may be of value

N.B. Cardioversion carries an increased risk of provoking ventricular fibrillation

---

Digoxin is largely excreted by the kidneys, and the maintenance dose (see Table 5.4) should be reduced in children, the elderly and those with renal impairement. It is widely distributed and has a long tissue half-life so that effects may persist 24–36 hours after the last dose. Measurements of plasma digoxin concentration are useful in demonstrating that the dose being used is inadequate and in confirming a clinical impression of toxicity (see information box).

SINOATRIAL DISEASE (THE SICK SINUS SYNDROME)

Sinoatrial disease can occur at any age, but is most common in the elderly. The underlying pathology is not understood but may involve fibrosis, degenerative changes and/or ischaemia of the sinus node. The condition is characterised by a variety of arrhythmias (see

---

COMMON FEATURES OF SINOATRIAL DISEASE

- Sinus bradycardia
- Sinoatrial block (sinus arrest)
- Paroxysmal supraventricular tachycardia
- Paroxysmal atrial fibrillation
- Atrioventricular block

---

information box) and may present with palpitation, dizzy spells, or syncope due to intermittent tachycardia, bradycardia, or pauses (sinoatrial block or sinus arrest) with no atrial or ventricular activity (Fig. 5.44).

A permanent pacemaker may benefit patients with troublesome symptoms due to spontaneous bradycardias, or those with symptomatic bradycardias induced by drugs required to prevent tachyarrhythmias. Pacing the atrium may help to prevent episodes of atrial fibrillation; however, permanent pacing does not improve prognosis and is not indicated in patients who are asymptomatic.

ATRIOVENTRICULAR AND BUNDLE BRANCH BLOCK

ATRIOVENTRICULAR (AV) BLOCK

Atrioventricular conduction is influenced by autonomic activity; AV block can therefore be intermittent and may only be evident when the conducting tissue is stressed

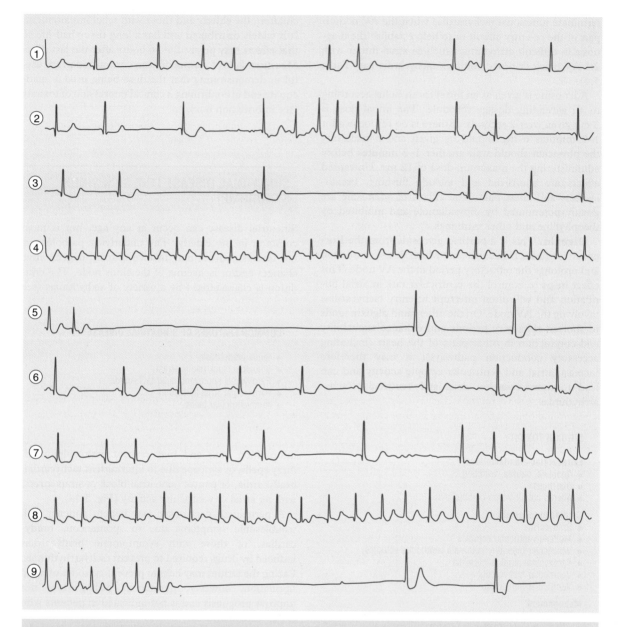

Fig. 5.44 Sinoatrial disease (the sick sinus syndrome). A continuous rhythm strip from a 24-hour ECG tape recording illustrating periods of sinus rhythm, atrial ectopics, sinus bradycardia, sinus arrest and paroxysmal supraventricular tachycardia.

by a rapid atrial rate. Accordingly, atrial tachyarrhythmias are often associated with AV block (Fig. 5.28).

First degree AV block

In this condition AV conduction is delayed so the PR interval is prolonged beyond the upper limit of normal (0.20 second). There are no symptoms and the diagnosis can only be made from the ECG (Fig. 5.45).

Second degree AV block

In this condition dropped beats occur because some impulses from the atria fail to get through to the ventricles.

In **Mobitz type I second degree AV block** (Fig. 5.46) there is progressive lengthening of successive PR intervals culminating in a dropped beat. The cycle then repeats itself. This is known as Wenckebach's phenom-

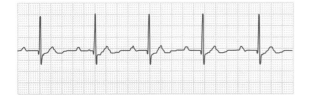

Fig. 5.45   First degree heart block. The PR interval is prolonged and measures 0.26 seconds.

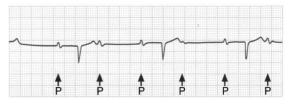

Fig. 5.48   Second degree heart block with fixed 2:1 block. Alternate p waves are not conducted. This may be due to Mobitz type I or II block.

enon and is usually due to impaired conduction proximal to the bundle of His. The phenomenon may be physiological and is sometimes observed at rest or during sleep in athletic young adults with high vagal tone.

In **Mobitz type 2 second degree AV block** (Fig. 5.47) the PR interval of the conducted impulses remains constant but some P waves are not conducted. This is usually caused by disease below the bundle of His and is more serious than Mobitz type I.

In **2:1 AV block** (Fig. 5.48) alternate P waves are conducted so it is impossible to distinguish between Mobitz type I and type II block.

Third degree (complete) AV block (Fig. 5.49)
When AV conduction fails completely the atria and ventricles beat independently (AV dissociation). Ventricular activity is maintained by an escape rhythm arising in the bundle of His (narrow QRS complexes) or the distal conducting tissues (broad QRS complexes). Distal escape rhythms tend to be slower and less reliable.

THE AETIOLOGY OF COMPLETE HEART BLOCK

Congenital

Acquired
- Idiopathic fibrosis
- Myocardial infarction/ischaemia
- Inflammation:
  acute (e.g. aortic root abscess in infective endocarditis)
  chronic (e.g. sarcoidosis, Chagas' disease)
- Trauma (e.g. cardiac surgery)
- Drugs (e.g. digoxin, β-adrenoceptor antagonist)

The aetiology is shown in the information box above.

Complete heart block produces a slow (25–50/min) regular pulse that, except in the case of congenital complete heart block, does not vary with exercise. There is usually a compensatory increase in stroke volume with a large volume pulse and systolic flow murmurs. Cannon

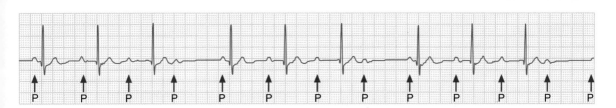

Fig. 5.46   Second degree heart block (Mobitz type I—Wenckebach's phenomenon). The PR interval progressively increases until a p wave is not conducted. The cycle then repeats itself.

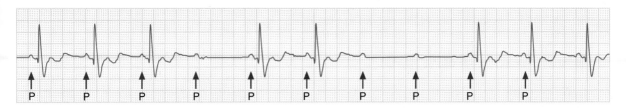

Fig. 5.47   Second degree heart block (Mobitz type II). The PR interval of conducted beats is normal but some p waves are not conducted.

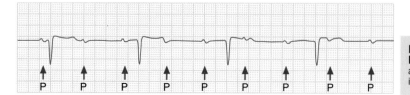

Fig. 5.49 Complete (third degree) AV block. There is complete dissociation of atrial and ventricular complexes. The atrial rate is 80/min and the ventricular rate is 38/min.

waves may be visible in the neck and the intensity of the first heart sound varies due to the loss of AV synchrony.

Adams–Stokes attacks

Episodes of ventricular asystole may complicate complete heart block or Mobitz type II second degree AV block and can also occur in patients with sinoatrial disease. This may cause recurrent syncope or 'Adams–Stokes' attacks.

A typical episode is characterised by a sudden loss of consciousness which frequently occurs without warning and may result in a fall. Convulsions (due to cerebral ischaemia) can occur if there is prolonged asystole. There is pallor and a deathlike appearance during the attack but when the heart starts beating again there is a characteristic flush. In contrast to epilepsy, recovery is rapid.

Management

AV block complicating acute myocardial infarction

Acute *inferior* myocardial infarction is often complicated by transient AV block because the right coronary artery supplies the junctional tissues and bundle of His. However, there is usually a reliable escape rhythm and if the patient remains well no treatment is required. Clinical deterioration due to second degree or complete heart block may respond to atropine (0.6 mg intravenously, repeated as necessary) or, if this fails, a temporary pacemaker. In the vast majority of cases the AV block will resolve within 7–10 days.

Second degree or complete heart block complicating acute *anterior* myocardial infarction is usually a sign of extensive myocardial damage and therefore carries a poor prognosis. Asystole may ensue and a temporary pacemaker should be inserted as soon as possible. If the patient presents with asystole, atropine (0.6 mg intravenously, repeated if necessary) and isoprenaline (1–5 mg in 500 ml 5% dextrose, infused intravenously at the minimum rate needed to produce a satisfactory heart rhythm) may help to maintain the circulation until a temporary pacing electrode can be inserted.

Chronic AV block

Patients with symptomatic bradyarrhythmias associated with AV block should receive a permanent pacemaker (see below).

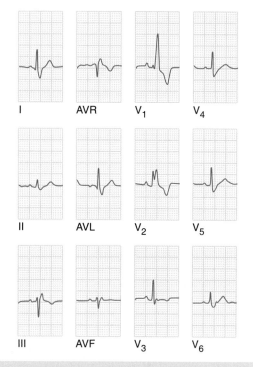

Fig. 5.50 Right Bundle Branch Block. Note the wide QRS complexes with 'M'-shaped configuration in leads V1 and V2 and a wide S wave in lead I.

Asymptomatic first degree or Mobitz type I second degree AV block does not require treatment but may be an indication of serious underlying heart disease.

A permanent pacemaker is usually indicated in patients with asymptomatic Mobitz type II second degree or complete heart block because there is evidence that pacing can improve their prognosis. An exception may be made in young asymptomatic patients with congenital complete heart block who have a mean day-time heart rate of more than 50 per minute.

BUNDLE BRANCH BLOCK AND HEMIBLOCK

Interruption of the right or left branch of the bundle of His delays activation of the appropriate ventricle, broadens the QRS complex (0.12 seconds or more) and produces the characteristic alterations in QRS morphology shown in Figures 5.50 and 5.51.

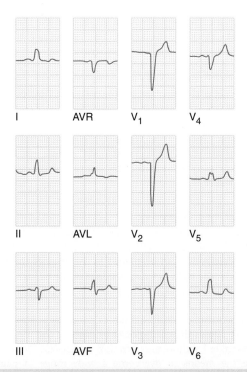

Fig. 5.51   Left Bundle Branch Block. Note the wide QRS complexes with the loss of the Q wave or septal vector in lead I and 'M'-shaped QRS complexes in V5 and V6.

Right bundle branch block is a common normal variant but left bundle branch block usually signifies important underlying heart disease. Both forms of bundle branch block may be due to conducting tissue disease but are also features of other types of heart disease (see information box).

THE COMMON CAUSES OF BUNDLE BRANCH BLOCK

LBBB
- Coronary artery disease
- Hypertension
- Aortic value disease
- Cardiomyopathy

RBBB
- Normal variant
- Right ventricular hypertrophy or strain, e.g. pulmonary embolism
- Congenital heart disease, e.g. ASD
- Coronary artery disease

The left branch of the bundle of His divides into an anterior and posterior fascicle. Damage of the conducting tissue at this point (hemiblock) does not broaden the QRS complex, but alters the mean direction of ventricular depolarisation (mean QRS axis) causing left axis deviation in left anterior hemiblock and right axis deviation in left posterior hemiblock. The com-

bination of right bundle branch and left anterior or posterior hemiblock is known as bifascicular block.

ELECTRICAL TREATMENT OF ARRHYTHMIAS

EXTERNAL DEFIBRILLATION AND CARDIOVERSION

The heart can be completely depolarised by passing a sufficiently large electrical current through it from an external source. This will interrupt any arrhythmia and produce a brief period of asystole which is usually followed by the resumption of normal sinus rhythm. Modern defibrillators deliver a direct current (DC), high energy, short duration shock via two electrodes coated with conducting jelly, positioned over the sternum and the left axilla or scapula.

Energy applied during a critical period around the peak of the T wave may provoke ventricular fibrillation so when this technique is used to treat organised rhythms such as atrial fibrillation or ventricular tachycardia the shock should be synchronised with the ECG and is normally given 0.02 sec after the peak of the R wave. The precise timing of the discharge is not important in ventricular fibrillation.

In ventricular fibrillation and other emergencies the energy of the first shock should be 200 Joules; there is no need for an anaesthetic if the patient is unconscious. Elective cardioversion requires a general anaesthetic. High energy shocks may cause myocardial damage so if there is no urgency it is appropriate to begin with a low amplitude shock, going on to larger shocks if necessary. In atrial fibrillation a synchronised shock of 100 Joules may restore sinus rhythm and in more organised rhythms such as atrial flutter or supraventricular tachycardia energies of 50 Joules or less may suffice.

Digoxin toxicity increases the risk of untoward arrhythmias after cardioversion, and ideally digitalis therapy should be withdrawn 36 hours before elective cardioversion. Patients with long-standing atrial arrhythmias are at risk of systemic embolism during cardioversion, so it is wise to delay the procedure until the patient has been adequately anticoagulated for at least 6 weeks.

Automatic implantable cardioverter-defibrillator
These devices, which are usually implanted in the abdomen, can detect and then correct episodes of ventricular tachycardia or fibrillation by delivering a low energy shock (10–20 Joules) via epicardial or endocardial electrodes. They are extremely expensive and should be reserved for patients with life-threatening arrhythmias that are not amenable to other forms of therapy.

Radiofrequency catheter ablation

The aim of this new technique is to interrupt a re-entry circuit by selectively damaging endocardial tissue with radiofrequency energy delivered through a transvenous catheter. Radiofrequency ablation has become the treatment of choice for symptomatic Wolff–Parkinson–White syndrome and is a promising treatment for other atrial and junctional tachycardias. The procedure is often time-consuming but does not require an anaesthetic and can produce a lifetime cure.

ARTIFICIAL PACEMAKERS

Temporary pacemakers

In an emergency it is sometimes possible to pace the heart by passing an electric current through electrodes placed on the chest wall, passed down the oesophagus, or inserted directly through the chest wall into the myocardium. None of these methods is satisfactory for more than a few minutes, if at all, and the most effective technique for temporary artificial pacemaking is to insert a bipolar pacing electrode via an antecubital, subclavian or femoral vein and position it under fluoroscopic control in the apex of the right ventricle. The electrode is then connected to an external pulse generator which can be adjusted to alter the energy output or pacing rate. The threshold is the lowest output that will reliably pace the heart and should be less than one volt at implantation. The generator should be set to deliver an output that is at least twice this figure and may require daily adjustment because the threshold tends to rise, due to inflammation and oedema around the tip of the electrode.

Temporary pacing may be indicated in the management of transient heart block and other arrhythmias complicating acute myocardial infarction, as a safety measure in patients with heart block or sinoatrial disease (that does not require permanent pacing) undergoing a general anaesthetic, or as a prelude to permanent pacing. Complications include pneumothorax and other forms of trauma related to the insertion of the wire, local infection or septicaemia (usually *Staph. aureus*), and pericarditis. Failure of the system may be due to lead displacement or a progressive increase in the threshold (exit block). The complication and failure rate increase with time and it is seldom wise to use a temporary pacing system for more than 10–14 days.

The ECG of a patient whose rhythm is controlled by an artificial ventricular pacemaker placed in the right ventricle shows regular broad QRS complexes with a left bundle branch block pattern. Each complex is immediately preceded by a 'pacing spike'. Nearly all pulse generators are used in the 'demand' mode so that a spontaneously generated QRS complex will inhibit the pacemaker.

Permanent pacemakers

Permanent artificial pacemakers utilise the same principles, but the pulse generator is implanted under the skin. Electrodes can be placed in the apex of the right ventricle, the right atrial appendage or both (Fig. 5.52).

Most permanent pacemakers are programmable so the rate, output, etc. can be altered by an external programmer using radiofrequency or magnetic signals. This facility allows the cardiologist to prolong the life of the pacemaker by choosing optimum settings and may provide the means to overcome a wide range of pacing problems. For example, programming can be used to increase output in the face of an unexpected increase in threshold, or to alter sensitivity if the pacemaker is inappropriately inhibited by electrical potentials generated in the pectoral muscles (myopotential inhibition).

Atrial pacing may be appropriate for patients with sinoatrial disease without AV block, and ventricular pacing is the only suitable mode for patients with continuous atrial fibrillation. In dual (atrial and ventricular) chamber pacing the atrial electrode can be used to detect spontaneous atrial activity and trigger ventricular pacing, thereby preserving atrioventricular synchrony and allowing the ventricular rate to increase together with the atrial rate during exercise and other forms of stress. Dual chamber pacing is expensive but has many advantages when compared to simple ventricular pacing; these include superior haemodynamics leading to a better effort tolerance, a lower prevalence of atrial arrhythmias in patients with sinoatrial disease and the ability to

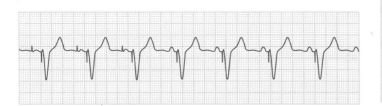

Fig. 5.52 Dual chamber pacing. The first 3 beats show atrial and ventricular pacing with narrow pacing spikes in front of each P wave and QRS complex. The last 4 beats show spontaneous p waves with a different morphology and no pacing spike; the pacemaker senses or tracks these P waves and maintains AV synchrony by pacing the ventricle after an appropriate interval.

prevent or cure the 'pacemaker syndrome' (a fall in the blood pressure and dizziness precipitated by the start of ventricular pacing).

There are also 'rate-responsive' pacemakers which react (by changing the pacing rate) to parameters such as the QT interval (an index of sympathetic activity), respiration, or physical movement. This type of pacemaker helps to maintain an optimum heart rate and can be used in patients who are not suitable for atrial triggered pacing, e.g. patients with atrial fibrillation.

FURTHER READING

Arrhythmia Octet 1993. Lancet 341: 1189–1193, 1254–1258, 1317–1322, 1386–1391, 1454–1458, 1512–1519, 1578–1582, 1641–1647. *A series of eight articles that provide a comprehensive and up-to-date review of all aspects of arrhythmias*
Bennett D H 1993 Cardiac arrhythmias. Practical notes on interpretation and treatment, 4th edn. Butterworth-Heinemann, London

ISCHAEMIC (CORONARY) HEART DISEASE

Coronary heart disease is the commonest form of heart disease and the single most important cause of premature death in the developed world. In the UK one in three men and one in four women die from this disease; an estimated 330 000 people have a myocardial infarct each year and approximately 1.9 million people have angina. The death rates from coronary heart disease in the UK are among the highest in the world (nearly 170 000 people died from coronary heart disease in the UK in 1992) but are falling slowly; unfortunately, the incidence of the condition is increasing rapidly in Eastern Europe and many developing countries.

PATHOPHYSIOLOGY, RISK FACTORS AND PREVENTION

Disease of the coronary arteries is almost always due to atheroma and its complications, particularly thrombosis. However, occasionally the coronary arteries are involved in other disorders such as congenital anomalies (e.g. anomalous origin, fistula or malformation of a major coronary artery), aortitis, polyarteritis and other connective tissue disorders.

ATHEROMA

Atheroma or atherosclerosis is a patchy focal disease of the arterial intima. Some arteries such as the radial artery and the internal mammary artery are largely spared, while others, notably the coronary arteries, are at high risk. Coronary artery, cerebral and peripheral vascular disease often coexist but seldom develop at the same rate.

In western countries atheromatous plaques begin to appear in the second and third decade of life. The nature and composition of these plaques change as they evolve (see Fig. 5.53).

Fatty streaks develop as circulating monocytes migrate into the intima, take up oxidised low density lipoprotein (LDL) from the plasma, and become lipid-laden foam cells. As these foam cells die and release their contents, extracellular lipid pools appear. Smooth muscle cells then migrate into and proliferate within the plaque. As the lesion grows it encroaches into the lumen of the vessel and erodes the media.

A mature fibrolipid plaque has a core of extracellular lipid, surrounded by smooth muscle cells, and is separated from the lumen by a thick cap of collagen-rich fibrous tissue. Such plaques may rupture or fissure allowing blood to enter and disrupt the arterial wall; this may compromise the lumen of the vessel and often precipitates thrombosis and local vasospasm. Plaque rupture may lead to rapid growth of the lesion or occlusion of the vessel and is thought to be the cause of most acute coronary syndromes.

The number and state of evolution of plaques both increase with age, but the rate of progression of individual plaques, even in the same patient, is very variable.

Clinical features

The clinical manifestations and pathological correlates of coronary artery disease are shown in Table 5.5.

Risk factors

The causes of coronary disease can be studied either in animal models or by looking for associations between clinical coronary disease and variables such as smoking and plasma cholesterol. Animal models do not accurately reproduce human pathology, and epidemiological studies are often unable to distinguish between risk factors, which bear a causative relation to the disease, and risk markers, where the variable measured is not itself the cause, but is linked to something which is.

Some risk factors for coronary disease are listed in the information box below. There is increasing evidence that there may be different risk factors for angina (development of plaque) and myocardial infarction (development of plaques, plaque rupture and thrombosis).

The excess risk multiplies when there is more than one risk factor; people with a combination of risk factors (e.g. smoking, hypertension and diabetes) therefore have the greatest risk of developing coronary heart disease. It is important to distinguish between *relative* risk (the

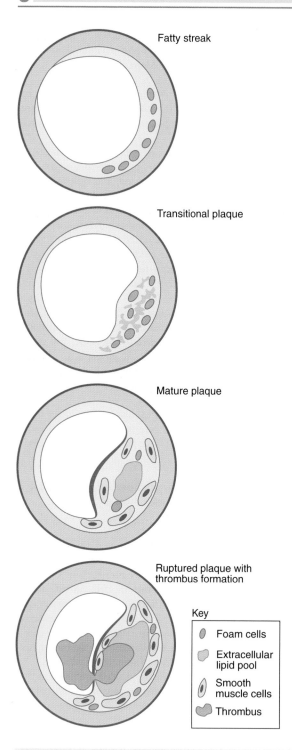

Fatty streak

Transitional plaque

Mature plaque

Ruptured plaque with thrombus formation

Key

Foam cells	
Extracellular lipid pool	
Smooth muscle cells	
Thrombus	

Fig. 5.53 The evolution of an atheromatous plaque.

Table 5.5 Coronary artery disease: clinical manifestations and pathology

Clinical problem	Pathology
Stable angina	Fixed atheromatous stenosis of one or more coronary arteries
Unstable angina	Dynamic obstruction due to plaque rupture with superimposed spasm and thrombosis
Myocardial infarction	Acute occlusion due to coronary thrombosis
Heart failure	Myocardial dysfunction due to infarction or ischaemia
Arrhythmias	Altered conduction due to ischaemia or infarction
Sudden death	Ventricular arrhythmia or acute myocardial infarction

proportional increase in risk) and *absolute* risk (the actual chance of an event). Thus a man of 35 with a plasma cholesterol of 10 mmol/litre who smokes 40 cigarettes a day is many times more likely to die from coronary disease within the next decade than a non-smoking woman of the same age with a normal cholesterol, but the likelihood of his dying during this time is still small (high relative risk, low absolute risk).

The risk of suffering a coronary event is analogous to the risk of being involved in a road accident. An inexperienced driver in an old car with poor brakes, bald tyres and defective steering is much more likely to have an accident than an experienced driver in a new car. However, accidents are rare and there is a random element which means that occasionally the good driver will have an accident a few minutes after leaving home.

SOME IMPORTANT RISK FACTORS FOR CORONARY ARTERY DISEASE

Fixed	**Modifiable**
• age	• smoking
• male sex	• hypertension
• family history	• lipid disorders
	• diabetes mellitus
	• haemostatic variables
	• sedentary lifestyle
	• obesity
	• polyunsaturated fatty acid deficiencies

- **Age and male sex.** Obviously these risk factors cannot be corrected; however, there is good evidence that hormone replacement therapy reduces the risk of ischaemic heart disease in post-menopausal women.
- **Family history.** Coronary artery disease often runs in families. This may be due to genetic factors or the effects of a shared environment (similar diet, smoking

habits, etc). At present it is estimated that about 40% of the risk of developing ischaemic heart disease is controlled by genetic factors, and 60% by environmental factors. Hyperlipidaemia, hyperfibrinogenaemia and abnormalities of other coagulation factors are often genetically determined. Recent studies have identified a common deletion polymorphism of the angiotensin-converting enzyme (ACE) gene which is associated with increased levels of circulating ACE and an excess risk of coronary artery disease.

- **Smoking.** Tobacco is probably the most important *avoidable* cause of coronary disease. There is a strong, consistent and dose-linked relationship between cigarette smoking and ischaemic heart disease. The relative risk is highest in young people and becomes significantly lower within 6 months of quitting.
- **Hypertension.** The incidence of coronary artery disease increases as blood pressure rises and the excess risk is related to both systolic and diastolic blood pressure. Antihypertensive drugs have been shown to reduce coronary mortality but by less than might have been anticipated, possibly because many of these agents have potentially adverse effects on lipid and glucose metabolism (see pp.270–271).
- **Hypercholesterolaemia** (see pp.765–767). Patients with familial hyperlipidaemia have a high incidence of premature coronary disease and many epidemiological studies have demonstrated a positive correlation between mean population plasma cholesterol concentration and morbidity and death from coronary disease. The excess risk is closely related to the plasma concentration of LDL cholesterol and is inversely related to the plasma HDL cholesterol concentration. There is also a weak correlation between plasma triglyceride concentration and the incidence of coronary artery disease. Moreover, numerous clinical trials have shown that lowering high cholesterol concentrations by diet or drugs can reduce the risk of cardiac events (though sometimes at the cost of other morbidity).
- **Haemostatic factors.** High levels of fibrinogen and factor VII are associated with an increased risk of myocardial infarction (coronary thrombosis).
- **Physical activity.** Regular exercise (brisk walking, cycling or swimming for 20 minutes two or three times a week) appears to have a protective effect which may be related to its ability to increase HDL cholesterol, lower blood pressure, reduce blood clotting, and promote collateral vessel development.
- **Diabetes mellitus** is associated with an increased incidence of ischaemic heart disease and with a tendency to diffuse coronary atheroma. Insulin resistance (normal glucose homeostasis with high levels of insulin) is associated with obesity and physical inactivity

and is also a potent risk factor for coronary heart disease. These factors are thought to account for the high incidence of ischaemic heart disease in some Asian communities.

- **Obesity** is probably an independent risk factor although it is often associated with other adverse factors such as hypertension, diabetes and physical inactivity.
- **Alcohol.** A moderate intake of alcohol (2–4 units a day) appears to offer some protection from coronary disease; however, heavy drinking is associated with hypertension and an excess of cardiac events.
- **Other dietary factors.** Diets deficient in polyunsaturated fatty acids are associated with an increased risk of coronary disease. This may be independent of the tendency of diets with a high polyunsaturated/saturated ratio to lower cholesterol. Low levels of vitamin C, vitamin E and other antioxidants may enhance the production of oxidised LDL (see Fig. 5.53) and are important independent risk factors for coronary disease.
- **Mental stress.** There is very little evidence to support the popular view that stress causes coronary heart disease; however, there is no doubt that stress can aggravate the symptoms of established heart disease.

Strategies for the prevention of coronary disease

Primary prevention

There has been controversy over whether efforts to prevent coronary disease among the healthy population (primary prevention) should concentrate on identifying and treating those individuals who are thought to be at high risk or should aim to modify the lifestyle of the whole population. The two approaches are not incompatible and both should be pursued. High risk individuals usually have a combination of risk factors and can be identified using composite scoring systems; however, they are relatively few in number and constitute only a small proportion of those who will ultimately develop coronary disease.

Some reasonable public health advice is summarised in the information box below.

POPULATION ADVICE TO PREVENT CORONARY DISEASE

- Do not smoke
- Take regular exercise
- Maintain 'ideal' bodyweight
- Eat a mixed diet with fruit and vegetables as well as meat and dairy products
- Aim to get no more than 30% of energy intake from fat

Secondary prevention

There is strong and compelling evidence that the correction of risk factors, particularly smoking and hypercholesterolaemia, will improve the outlook for most patients with established coronary or vascular disease (secondary prevention). For example, giving up smoking after a heart attack halves the risk of recurrence (see page 265).

Many clinical events offer an unrivalled opportunity to introduce effective secondary preventive measures. For example, patients who have just survived a myocardial infarction or undergone a major procedure such as coronary artery bypass grafting are usually keen to help themselves and may be particularly receptive to appropriate lifestyle advice.

ANGINA PECTORIS

Angina pectoris is the term used to describe discomfort due to transient myocardial ischaemia and constitutes a clinical syndrome rather than a disease; it may occur whenever there is an imbalance between myocardial oxygen supply and demand (see information box).

FACTORS INFLUENCING MYOCARDIAL OXYGEN SUPPLY AND DEMAND

Oxygen demand	Oxygen supply
Cardiac work	*Coronary blood flow**
• Heart rate	• Duration of diastole
• Blood pressure	• Coronary perfusion
• Myocardial contractility	pressure (aortic diastolic-
	right atrial diastolic
	pressure)
	• Coronary vasomotor tone
	Oxygenation
	• Haemoglobin
	• Oxygen saturation

* **N.B.** coronary blood flow is confined to diastole

Coronary atheroma is by far the most common cause but angina is also a feature of aortic valve disease, hypertrophic cardiomyopathy and some other forms of heart disease.

Clinical features

The history is by far the most important factor in making the diagnosis. Stable angina is characterised by left-sided or central chest pain that is precipitated by exertion and promptly relieved by rest.

Most patients describe a sense of oppression or tightness in the chest—'like a band round the chest'; 'pain' may be denied. When describing angina the victim often closes a hand around the throat, puts a hand or clenched fist on the sternum, or places both hands across the lower chest. The term 'angina' is derived from the Greek word for strangulation and many patients report a 'choking' sensation. Breathlessness is sometimes a prominent feature.

The pain may radiate to the neck or jaw and is often accompanied by discomfort in the arms, particularly the left, the wrists and sometimes the hands; the patient may also describe a feeling of heaviness or uselessness in the arms. Occasionally the pain is epigastric or interscapular. Angina may occur at any of these places of reference without *chest* discomfort but a history of precipitation by effort, and relief by rest or sublingual nitrate, should still allow the condition to be recognised.

Symptoms tend to be worse after a meal, in the cold, and when walking uphill or into a strong wind. Some patients find that the pain comes when they start walking and that later it does not return despite greater effort ('start-up angina'). Some experience the pain when lying flat (decubitus angina), and some are awakened by it (nocturnal angina).

Angina may also occur capriciously as a result of coronary arterial spasm; occasionally this is accompanied by transient ST elevation on the ECG (Prinzmetal's or variant angina).

CLINICAL SITUATIONS PRECIPITATING ANGINA

• Physical exertion
• Cold exposure
• Heavy meals
• Intense emotion
• Lying flat (decubitus angina)
• Vivid dreams (nocturnal angina)

Physical examination is frequently negative, but should include a careful search for evidence of:

• **important risk factors**
  e.g. nicotine stains, hypertension, hyperlipidaemia (tendon xanthomas, thickening of the achilles tendons, arcus lipidis, etc.), diabetes, myxoedema
• **contributory disease**
  e.g. obesity, anaemia, thyrotoxicosis, aortic valve disease
• **left ventricular dysfunction**
  e.g. gallop rhythm, cardiomegaly, basal crackles, elevated venous pressure
• **generalised arterial disease**
  e.g. carotid bruits, peripheral vascular disease.

Differential diagnosis

This includes musculoskeletal, pericardial and oesophageal pain. Musculoskeletal pains are provoked by specific movement rather than by walking, and background pain often persists at rest; there may be associated chest wall tenderness. The pain of pericarditis is occasionally provoked by exercise, but its other characteristics (p.309) should help to establish the diagnosis. Angina occurring at rest may be confused with oesophagitis, with or without a hiatus hernia, but pain due to oesophagitis usually has a burning quality and is relieved by antacids. Oesophageal spasm, however, causes a different type of pain which may be difficult to distinguish from variant angina.

Investigation

Resting ECG

The ECG may show evidence of previous myocardial infarction but is normal in most patients. Occasionally there is T wave flattening or inversion in some leads providing non-specific evidence of myocardial ischaemia or damage.

The most convincing ECG evidence of myocardial ischaemia is obtained by demonstrating reversible ST segment depression or elevation, with or without T wave inversion, at the time the patient is experiencing symptoms (whether spontaneous or induced by exercise testing).

Exercise ECG

A formal exercise tolerance test is usually performed using a standard treadmill or bicycle ergometer protocol to ensure a progressive and reproducible increase in work load while monitoring the patient's ECG (preferably all 12 leads), blood pressure and general condition. Resuscitation facilities must be available and the test should be stopped if the patient develops significant chest pain or discomfort, a serious arrhythmia, a fall in blood pressure or marked ST segment changes. Planar or downsloping ST segment depression of 1 mm or more is indicative of ischaemia (Fig. 5.54); upsloping ST depression is less specific and often occurs in normal individuals.

Exercise testing can be used to confirm or refute a diagnosis of angina and is also a useful means of assessing the severity of coronary disease. The amount of exercise which can be tolerated and the extent and degree of any ST segment change (see Fig. 5.55) provide a useful guide to the likely extent of coronary disease.

Unfortunately, exercise testing is not infallible and may produce false positive results (see information box).

SOME CAUSES OF EXERCISE-INDUCED ECG CHANGES THAT MAY LEAD TO A FALSE POSITIVE EXERCISE TEST

- Digoxin therapy
- Left ventricular hypertrophy
- Left bundle branch block
- Wolff–Parkinson–White syndrome

Isotope scanning

Myocardial perfusion scanning may be helpful in the evaluation of patients with an equivocal or uninterpretable exercise test and those who are unable to exercise. The technique involves obtaining scintiscans of the myocardium at rest and during stress after the administration of an intravenous radioactive isotope such as thallium 201 (^{201}Tl); it may be used in conjunction with conventional exercise testing or some form of pharmacological stress such as a controlled infusion of dobutamine. Thallium is an analogue of potassium and is taken up by viable perfused myocardium. A perfusion defect present during stress but not rest provides evidence of reversible myocardial ischaemia (Fig. 5.56), whereas a persistent perfusion defect seen during both phases of the study is usually indicative of previous myocardial infarction.

Measurement of the ejection fraction by radionuclide blood-pool scanning can provide relevant information about ventricular function.

Coronary arteriography

This provides detailed information about the extent and nature of coronary artery disease (Fig. 5.57) and is usually performed with a view to coronary bypass grafting or angioplasty (p. 253). In some patients diagnostic coronary angiography may be indicated when non-invasive tests have failed to elucidate the cause of atypical chest pain.

Management

The management of angina pectoris involves:

- a careful assessment of the likely extent and severity of arterial disease and any contributory factors
- the identification and control of significant risk factors

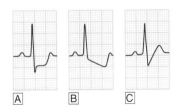

Fig. 5.54 Forms of exercise-induced ST depression. Planar A or downsloping B ST depression is usually indicative of myocardial ischaemia but upsloping C depression may be a normal finding.

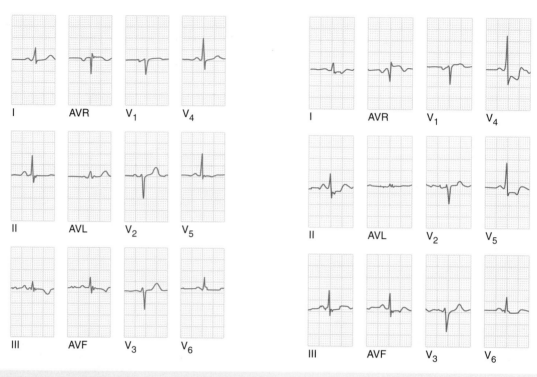

Fig. 5.55 A positive exercise test. The resting 12-lead ECG (left) shows some minor T wave changes in the inferolateral leads but is otherwise normal. After 3 minutes' exercise on a treadmill there is marked planar ST depression in leads II, V4 and V5 (right). Subsequent coronary angiography revealed critical 3-vessel coronary artery disease.

(e.g. smoking, hypertension, hyperlidaemia—see secondary prevention)

- the use of measures to control symptoms
- treatment to improve life expectancy.

Symptoms alone are a poor guide to the extent of coronary artery disease; exercise testing is therefore advisable in all patients who are potential candidates for revascularisation. A schema for the investigation and treatment of patients with angina is illustrated in the flow chart (Fig. 5.58).

The control of symptoms should start with an explanation of how they are caused. Most patients respond to a careful presentation of the problem emphasising the prospect of spontaneous improvement due to collateral development and can learn to help themselves by avoiding undue exertion and by using prophylactic sublingual nitrates.

Aspirin

Low dose (75–300 mg) aspirin reduces the risk of adverse events such as myocardial infarction and should be prescribed for all patients with coronary artery disease unless it causes troublesome dyspepsia or other side-effects.

Anti-anginal drug treatment

Three groups of drugs are used to help relieve or prevent the symptoms of angina: nitrates, beta-adrenoceptor antagonists (beta-blockers) and calcium antagonists.

- **Nitrates.** These drugs act directly on vascular smooth muscle to produce venous and arteriolar dilatation; their beneficial effects in angina are due to a reduction in myocardial oxygen demand (lower preload and afterload) and an increase in myocardial oxygen supply (coronary vasodilatation).

  Sublingual glyceryl trinitrate (GTN) administered

ADVICE TO PATIENTS WITH ANGINA

- Do not smoke
- Aim at ideal body weight
- Take regular exercise
  (exercise up to, but not beyond, the point of chest pain is beneficial and helps to promote collateral vessels)
- Avoid severe unaccustomed exertion, vigorous exercise after a heavy meal, or in very cold weather
- Take sublingual nitrate before undertaking exertion that may induce angina

Fig. 5.56   A thallium scan showing reversible anterior myocardial ischaemia. The images are cross-sectional tomograms of the left ventricle. The resting scans (right) show even uptake of thallium and look like doughnuts; during stress (in this case a dobutamine infusion) there is reduced uptake of thallium, particularly along the anterior wall (arrows), and the scans look like crescents (left). Subsequent angiography showed a severe stenosis in the left anterior descending coronary artery.

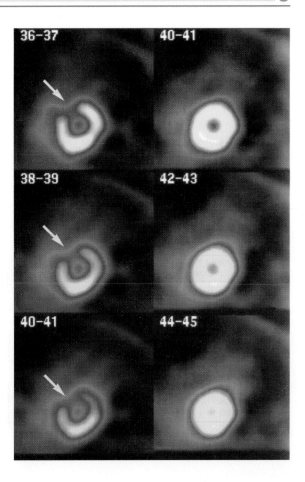

from a metered-dose aerosol (400 micrograms per spray) or as a tablet (500 micrograms) allowed to dissolve under the tongue or crunched and retained in the mouth, will usually relieve an attack of angina in 2–3 minutes. Unwanted side-effects include headache (which may be more distressing than the angina), symptomatic hypotension and, rarely, syncope. GTN tablets deteriorate when exposed to the atmosphere and should be replaced 8 weeks after the bottle has been opened; in contrast, sublingual nitrate sprays have a long shelf life and can be used for many years.

Patients often need to be reassured that GTN is not dangerous or habit forming and should be advised to use the drug prophylactically before engaging in exercise that is liable to provoke pain. The appropriate use of GTN (and other drugs) allows more exercise to be taken, which may help to promote the formation of collateral vessels.

As sublingual GTN has a short duration of action (see Table 5.6), there has been much interest in ways of giving more prolonged nitrate therapy. GTN can

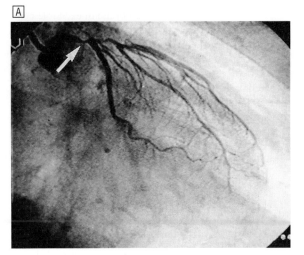

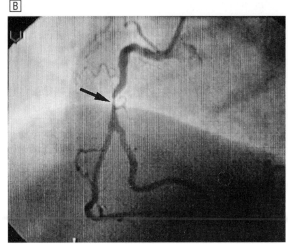

Fig. 5.57   Coronary angiograms from a patient with stable angina. A Left coronary angiogram showing a severe stenosis of the left main stem (arrow); there is also a severe stenosis in the proximal left anterior descending coronary artery. B Right coronary angiogram showing another severe stenosis (arrow).

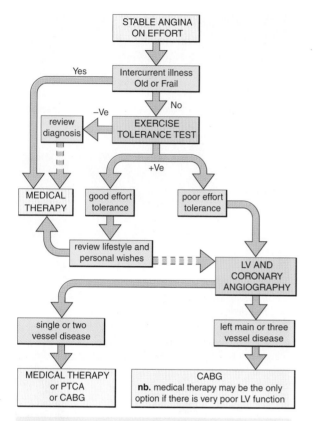

Fig. 5.58 A schema for the investigation and treatment of stable angina on effort.

Table 5.6 Duration of action of some nitrate preparations

Preparation	Peak action	Duration of action
Sublingual GTN	4–8 min	10–30 min
Buccal GTN	4–10 min	30–300 min
Transdermal GTN	1–3 h	Up to 24 h
Oral isosorbide dinitrate	45–120 min	2–6 h
Oral isosorbide mononitrate	45–120 min	6–10 h

N.B. slow release formulations of all these drugs are available.

giving set and the infusion rate must be adjusted carefully according to the clinical response.

- **Beta-adrenoceptor antagonists.** These drugs lower myocardial oxygen demand by reducing heart rate, blood pressure and myocardial contractility. Unfortunately they can exacerbate cardiac failure and peripheral vascular disease and may provoke bronchospasm in patients with obstructive airways disease. The properties and side-effects of the 'beta blockers' are discussed in detail on page 271.

    In theory non-selective beta-adrenoceptor antagonists may aggravate coronary vasospasm by blocking the coronary artery β_2-adrenoceptors and it is usually advisable to use a once daily cardioselective preparation (e.g. atenolol 50–100 mg daily; SR metoprolol 200 mg daily).

    A β-adrenoceptor antagonist drug should not be withdrawn abruptly because this may precipitate dangerous arrhythmias, worsening angina or myocardial infarction (**the β-blocker withdrawal syndrome**).

- **Calcium antagonists.** These drugs inhibit the slow inward current caused by the entry of extracellular calcium through the cell membrane of excitable cells, particularly cardiac and arteriolar smooth muscle, and lower myocardial oxygen demand by reducing blood pressure and myocardial contractility.

    Nifedipine, nicardipine and amlodipine often cause a reflex tachycardia; this may be counterproductive and it is often best to use these drugs in combination with a β-adrenoceptor antagonist. In contrast, verapamil and diltiazem are particularly suitable for patients who are not receiving a beta blocker because they inhibit conduction through the AV node and tend to cause a bradycardia. All the calcium antagonists reduce myocardial contractility and may aggravate or precipitate heart failure. Other unwanted effects include oedema, flushing, headache and dizziness.

    The dosage and some of the distinguishing features of these drugs are listed in Table 5.7.

be given percutaneously as a paste or plasters (5–10 mg once or twice a day), or as a slow-release buccal tablet (1–5 mg 6-hourly).

GTN is subject to extensive first pass metabolism in the liver and is therefore virtually ineffective when swallowed; however, other nitrates such as isosorbide dinitrate (10–20 mg, 3–6 times a day) and isosorbide mononitrate (20–40 mg, 2–3 times a day) can be given by mouth. Headache is common but tends to diminish if the patient perseveres with the treatment. Continuous nitrate therapy often causes pharmacological tolerance but this can be avoided by using a regimen that includes a nitrate-free period of 6–8 hours every day. A variety of once-daily proprietary preparations with a built-in nitrate-free period are available; it is usually best to schedule the medication so that drug levels are low during the night when the patient is inactive.

Intravenous nitrates (nitroglycerin 0.6 mg/hr or isosorbide dinitrate 1 mg/hr) are useful in the treatment of unstable angina and acute heart failure (p. 217). These drugs can be adsorbed and degraded in the

Although each of these groups of drugs can be shown to be superior to placebo in relieving the symptoms of angina, there is little convincing evidence that one group

Table 5.7 Calcium antagonists used for the treatment of angina

Drug	Dose	Feature
Nifedipine	5–20 mg 8-hourly*	May cause marked tachycardia
Nicardipine	20–40 mg 8-hourly	May cause less myocardial depression than the other drugs in this group
Amlodipine	2.5–10 mg daily	Ultra long acting
Verapamil	120–240 mg 8-hourly*	Commonly cause constipation; useful anti-arrhythmic properties (see p. 238)
Diltiazem	60–120 mg 8-hourly*	Similar antiarrhythmic properties to verapamil

* Once or twice daily slow release preparations are available

is more effective than another. Nevertheless, it is conventional to start therapy with low-dose aspirin, sublingual GTN, and a β-adrenoceptor antagonist and then add calcium channel antagonist or a long-acting nitrate later, if necessary. The goal of controlling angina with minimal side-effects and the simplest possible drug regimen is unlikely to be reached without a degree of trial and error.

Surgical treatment

'Surgical' options for the treatment of ischaemic heart disease include coronary angioplasty (sometimes called PTCA for percutaneous transluminal coronary angioplasty), reversed saphenous vein bypass grafting and internal mammary artery grafting (sometimes called CABG for coronary artery bypass grafting).

Coronary angioplasty (PTCA)

This is performed by passing a fine guidewire across a coronary stenosis under radiographic control and using it to position a balloon which is then inflated to dilate the stenosis (Fig. 5.59). PTCA has many applications and can be used to provide complete or partial ('culprit lesion' angioplasty) revascularisation in patients with stable angina, unstable angina or myocardial infarction.

Coronary angioplasty is an effective symptomatic treatment for chronic stable angina and is mainly used in single or two-vessel disease; there is no evidence that it improves survival. Stenoses in bypass grafts can be dilated as well as those in the native coronary arteries and the procedure is often used to provide palliative therapy for patients with recurrent angina after CABG.

The main complication of PTCA is occlusion of the vessel by thrombus or by a loose flap of intima (coronary artery dissection). This occurs in about 2–5% of procedures and may necessitate urgent coronary bypass grafting. The risk of complications and the likely success of the procedure are closely related to the morphology of the stenosis. Short, concentric, soft lesions on a straight segment of artery are ideal for this form of treatment. On the other hand, the outcome tends to be worse if the target lesion is complex, eccentric, calcified, lies on a bend or involves an important branch of the artery.

Recurrent angina is common (32% at 6 months in one study) and may require further angioplasty or bypass grafting. Re-stenosis is often due to smooth muscle proliferation and tends to occur within 3 months. Low-dose aspirin therapy is beneficial but does not prevent re-stenosis.

Coronary artery bypass grafting

This involves major surgery under cardiopulmonary bypass. The internal mammary arteries or reversed segments of the patient's own saphenous vein are used to bypass the major coronary artery stenoses (Fig. 5.60). In general, the operative mortality is less than 1%; however the risk is higher in elderly patients and those with poor left ventricular function.

Approximately 90% of patients are free of angina a year after surgery but less than 60% of patients are asymptomatic 5 or more years after CABG. Early postoperative angina is usually due to graft failure arising from technical problems during the operation or poor 'run off' due to disease in the distal native coronary vessels. Late recurrence of angina may be due to progressive disease in the native coronary arteries or graft degeneration. Less than 50% of vein grafts are patent 10 years after surgery although internal mammary artery grafts last much longer.

Low-dose aspirin (75–150 mg daily) has been shown to improve graft patency and should be prescribed indefinitely provided that it is well tolerated. Aggressive lipid-lowering therapy has also been shown to slow the progression of disease in the native coronary arteries and bypass grafts; total blood cholesterol should therefore be reduced to 5.2 mmol/l or less if possible (see pages 767–768). There is a substantial excess cardiovascular morbidity and mortality in patients who continue to smoke after bypass grafting. Persistent smokers are twice as likely to die in the ten years following surgery compared with those who quit at the time of their operation.

Coronary artery bypass grafting has been shown to improve survival in patients with left main coronary stenosis, and in symptomatic patients with 3-vessel coronary disease (i.e. disease involving left anterior descending,

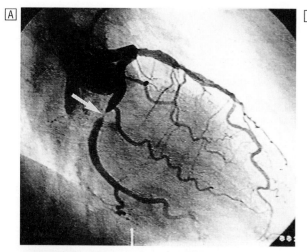

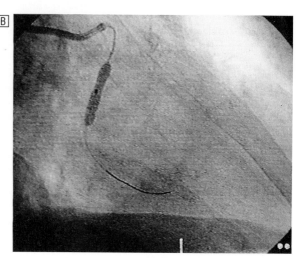

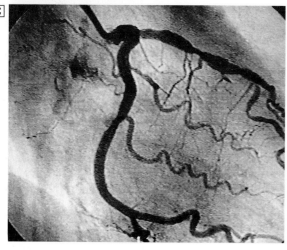

Fig. 5.59 A sequence of coronary angiograms illustrating a successful angioplasty. ▣A A severe stenosis of the circumflex coronary artery (arrow). ▣B A guide catheter is lying in the left coronary ostium, a fine wire has been passed through the stenosis, and a balloon has been positioned and inflated in the stenosis. ▣C Final appearance.

circumflex and right coronary arteries) or 2-vessel disease involving the proximal left anterior descending coronary artery. The improvement in survival is most marked in those who have undergone left internal mammary artery grafting and those with impaired left ventricular function prior to surgery.

Coronary angioplasty and coronary artery bypass grafting are compared in Table 5.8.

Prognosis

In general the prognosis of coronary artery disease is related to the number of diseased vessels (1-, 2- or 3-vessel coronary artery disease) and the degree of left ventricular dysfunction. A patient with single vessel disease and good LV function has an excellent outlook (5-year survival $>90\%$) whereas a patient with severe LV dysfunction and extensive 3-vessel disease has a poor prognosis (5-year survival $<30\%$).

More than half of a group of patients with angina will live for 5 years, and a third for 10 years from the time of diagnosis. Spontaneous symptomatic improvement due to the development of collateral vessels is common.

UNSTABLE ANGINA

Unstable angina is the term used to describe patients who present with rapidly worsening angina (crescendo angina), severe angina at rest or prolonged and severe ischaemic chest pain without ECG or enzyme evidence of significant myocardial infarction; it may present as a new phenomenon or against a background of chronic stable angina.

The culprit lesion is usually a complex ulcerated or fissured atheromatous plaque with adherent thrombus and local coronary artery spasm (Fig. 5.61); it is important to appreciate that coronary artery thrombosis is

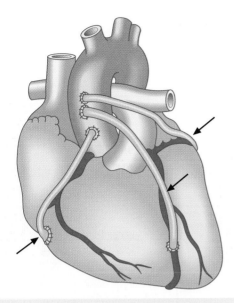

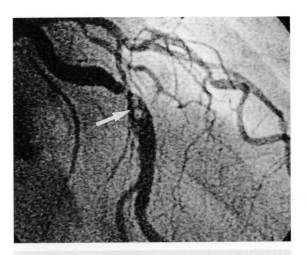

Fig. 5.61 Coronary angiogram from a patient with unstable angina demonstrating a complex stenosis of the circumflex coronary artery with a filling defect due to adherent thrombus (arrow).

Fig. 5.60 Diagram illustrating a triple coronary artery bypass graft operation.

a dynamic process whereby the lesion may expand by accretion, sometimes leading to complete occlusion of the vessel, or retract, sometimes only temporarily, due to the effects of endogenous thrombolysis. Episodes of myocardial ischaemia are due to an abrupt reduction in coronary blood flow caused by thrombosis or spasm (**supply-led ischaemia**). In contrast, stable angina is related to a fixed obstruction and is usually precipitated by an increase in myocardial oxygen demand (**demand-led ischaemia**).

The ECG usually shows acute ST segment elevation or depression during episodes of myocardial ischaemia; the ECG changes are sometimes prolonged.

Management

Patients should be admitted to hospital because there is a 10–15% risk of death or acute myocardial infarction during the unstable phase and clinical trials have shown that appropriate medical therapy can reduce the incidence of adverse events by at least 50%.

The initial treatment should include bed rest, aspirin (75–300 mg daily), and a β-adrenoceptor antagonist (e.g. atenolol 50–100 mg daily or metoprolol 50–100 mg 12-hourly). Nifedipine can be added to the β-adrenoceptor antagonist but may cause an unwanted tachycardia if it is used alone; verapamil or diltiazem are therefore preferable if a β-adrenoceptor antagonist is contraindicated.

Most patients respond rapidly to these measures and can be gradually mobilised. If there are no contra-

Table 5.8 Comparison between coronary angioplasty and coronary artery bypass grafting

	PTCA	CABG
Principal use	Single vessel disease; 2-vessel disease; unstable angina	Left main stem stenosis; 3-vessel disease
Mortality	<1%	<1%
Incidence of neurological complications	None	5% seldom permanent but stroke may occur
Hospital stay	24–36 hours	7–10 days
Return to work	2–5 days	2–3 months
Recurrence of angina	30% in 6 months. PTCA may be repeated	10% in 1 year, then 5% per year
Main complications	Myocardial infarction; emergency CABG; vascular damage related to the arterial puncture site	Diffuse left ventricular damage; peroperative MI; infection; wound pain

indications to surgery or angioplasty, exercise testing should be arranged 3–4 weeks later, when the plaque has stabilised, with a view to recommending coronary arteriography if the test is positive at a low work load.

If the pain persists or recurs, infusions of intravenous heparin (1000 Units/hour, adjusted according to the thrombin time) and intravenous nitrates (e.g. nitroglycerin 0.6–1.2 mg/hr or isosorbide dinitrate 1–2 mg/hr) may be helpful.

Coronary arteriography should be considered in patients who fail to settle on medical therapy, those with extensive ECG changes and those with severe pre-existing stable angina. This often shows single vessel disease that is amenable to angioplasty. Balloon dilatation of the culprit lesion may also be advisable in patients with multivessel disease. However, if the lesion is not suitable for angioplasty or there is a significant left main stem stenosis the patient should be referred for urgent coronary artery bypass grafting.

A plan for the management of unstable angina is illustrated in Figure 5.62.

MYOCARDIAL INFARCTION

Myocardial infarction is almost always due to the formation of occlusive thrombus at the site of rupture of an atheromatous plaque in a coronary artery (Fig. 5.63). The thrombus often undergoes spontaneous lysis over the course of the next few days although by this time the damage has been done; nevertheless, without treatment the infarct related artery remains permanently occluded in 30% of patients. Many early deaths are due to ventricular fibrillation but in patients who survive the first few hours the outcome is largely determined by the extent of myocardial damage. The process of infarction takes at least 8 hours and therefore most patients present when it is still possible to salvage myocardium and improve outcome (Fig. 5.64).

Clinical features

Pain is the cardinal symptom of myocardial infarction, but breathlessness, vomiting and collapse or syncope are common features. The pain occurs in the same sites as angina but is usually more severe and lasts longer; it is often described as a tightness, heaviness or constriction in the chest. At its worst the pain is one of the most severe which can be experienced and the patient's expression and pallor may vividly convey the seriousness of the situation.

Most patients are breathless and in some this is the only symptom. If syncope occurs it is usually due to an arrhythmia or profound hypotension. Vomiting and

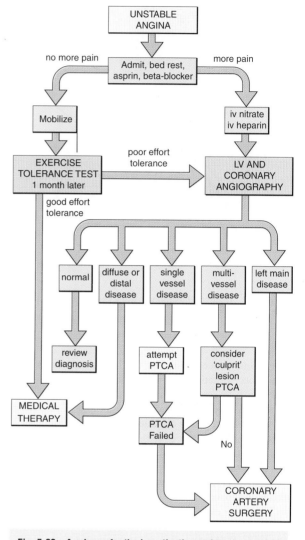

Fig. 5.62 A schema for the investigation and treatment of unstable angina on effort.

sinus bradycardia are often due to vagal stimulation and are particularly common in patients with inferior myocardial infarction. Nausea and vomiting may also be caused or aggravated by opiates given for pain relief.

Sometimes infarction occurs in the absence of physical signs.

Some myocardial infarcts pass unrecognised; these painless or 'silent' myocardial infarcts are particularly common in elderly and diabetic patients.

Sudden death, presumably from ventricular fibrillation or asystole, may occur immediately, and many deaths occur within the first hour. If the patient survives this most critical stage, the liability to dangerous arrhythmias remains, but diminishes as each hour goes by. The

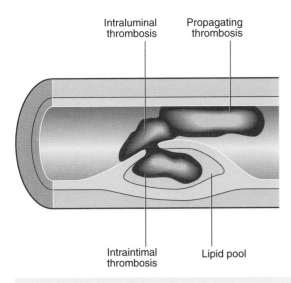

Intraluminal thrombosis

Propagating thrombosis

Intraintimal thrombosis

Lipid pool

Fig. 5.63 Coronary artery thrombosis. Myocardial infarction is caused by occlusion of a coronary artery due to thrombus propagating from a ruptured atheromatous plaque.

CLINICAL FEATURES OF MYOCARDIAL INFARCTION

Symptoms
- Prolonged cardiac pain:
    chest, throat, arms, epigastrium or back
- Anxiety:
    fear of impending death
- Nausea and vomiting
- Breathlessness
- Collapse/syncope

Physical signs
- Signs of sympathetic activation:
    pallor, sweating, tachycardia
- Signs of vagal activation:
    vomiting, bradycardia
- Signs of impaired myocardial function:
    hypotension, oliguria, cold peripheries
    narrow pulse pressure
    raised JVP
    3rd heart sound
    quiet 1st heart sound
    diffuse apical impulse
    lung crepitations
- Signs of tissue damage:
    fever, leucocytosis, high ESR
- Signs of complications:
    e.g. mitral regurgitation, pericarditis (see below)

development of cardiac failure reflects the extent of myocardial damage and is the major cause of death in those who survive the first few hours of infarction.

Differential diagnosis

The differential diagnosis is wide and includes most causes of chest pain or collapse (see pages 207–211).

Investigations

Electrocardiography

The ECG is usually a sensitive and specific way of confirming the diagnosis; however, it may be difficult to interpret if there is bundle branch block or evidence of previous myocardial infarction. Occasionally the initial ECG is normal and diagnostic changes appear a few hours later.

The earliest ECG change is usually ST elevation; later on there is diminution in the size of the R wave, and in transmural (full thickness) infarction a Q wave begins to develop. One explanation for the Q wave is that the myocardial infarct acts as an 'electrical window' trans-

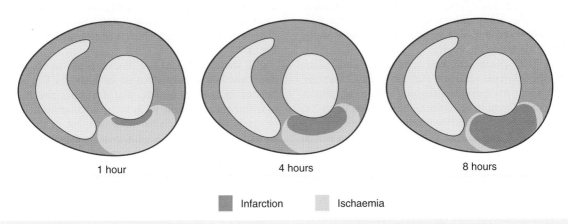

1 hour

4 hours

8 hours

Infarction   Ischaemia

Fig. 5.64 The time course of myocardial infarction. The relative proportion of ischaemic, infarcting and infarcted tissue slowly changes over a period of 8–12 hours. In the early stages of myocardial infarction a significant proportion of the myocardium in jeopardy is potentially salvageable.

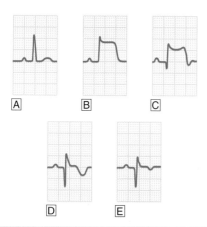

Fig. 5.65   The serial evolution of ECG changes in full thickness myocardial infarction. A Normal ECG complex. B Acute ST elevation ('the current of injury'). C Progressive loss of the R wave, developing Q wave, resolution of the ST elevation and terminal T wave inversion. D Deep Q wave and T wave inversion. E Old or established infarct pattern—the Q wave tends to persist but the T wave changes become less marked.

The rate of evolution is very variable. In general stage B appears within minutes, stage C is within hours, stage D within days and stage E after several weeks or months. This diagrammatic representation should be compared with the actual ECGs in Figures 5.67, 5.68 and 5.69.

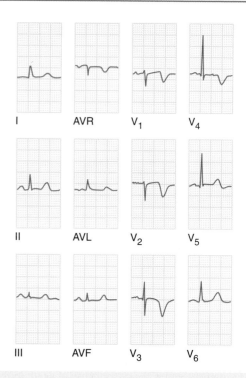

Fig. 5.66   Recent anterior subendocardial (partial thickness) infarction. There is deep symmetrical T wave inversion together with a reduction in the height of the R wave in leads V1, V2, V3 and V4.

mitting the changes of potential from within the ventricular cavity, and allowing the ECG to 'see' the reciprocal R wave from the other wall of the ventricle. Subsequently the T wave becomes inverted because of a change in ventricular repolarisation; this change persists after the ST segment has returned to normal. These features are shown diagrammatically in Figure 5.65 and their sequence is sufficiently reliable for the approximate age of the infarct to be deduced.

In contrast to transmural lesions, subendocardial infarction causes deep symmetrical T wave inversion to develop (Fig. 5.66) without Q waves or ST elevation; this is often accompanied by some loss of the R waves in the leads facing the infarct.

The ECG changes are best seen in the leads which 'face' the infarcted area (see Fig. 5.8 in ECG section). When there has been anteroseptal infarction, abnormalities are found in one or more leads from V1 to V4, while anterolateral infarction produces changes from V4 to V6, in aVL and in lead I. Inferior infarction is best shown in leads II, III and aVF, while at the same time leads I, aVL and the anterior chest leads may show 'reciprocal' changes of ST depression (Figs 5.67, 5.68 and 5.69). Infarction of the posterior wall of the left ventricle is not recorded in the standard leads by ST elevation or Q waves, but the reciprocal changes of ST depression and a tall R wave may be seen in leads V1–V4.

Plasma enzymes

Myocardial infarction causes a detectable rise in the plasma concentration of enzymes which are normally concentrated within cardiac cells. The enzymes most widely used in the detection of myocardial infarction are creatine kinase (CK), aspartate aminotransferase (AST) and lactate dehydrogenase (LDH). Serial (usually daily) estimations are particularly helpful because it is the change in enzyme levels which is of diagnostic value (see Fig. 5.70).

CK starts to rise at 4–6 hours, peaks at about 12 hours and falls to normal within 48–72 hours. CK is also present in skeletal muscle, and a modest rise in CK may sometimes be due to an intramuscular injection or vigorous physical exercise. Measurement of the myocardial isoenzyme of CK (CK-MB) is expensive but is more specific for myocardial damage.

AST starts to rise about 12 hours after infarction and reaches a peak on the first or second day, returning to normal within 3 or 4 days. LDH starts to rise after 12 hours, reaches a peak after 2 or 3 days and may remain elevated for a week or more (see Fig. 5.70); measurements of LDH are therefore appropriate when a patient presents several days after a possible infarct. Unfor-

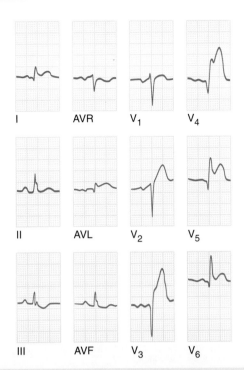

Fig. 5.67 Acute full thickness anterior myocardial infarction. This ECG was recorded from a 48-year-old man who had developed severe chest pain 6 hours earlier. There is ST elevation in leads I, aVL, V2, V3, V4, V5 and V6, and there are Q waves in leads V3, V4 and V5. Anterior infarcts with prominent changes in leads V2, V3 and V4 are sometimes called 'anteroseptal' infarcts as opposed to 'anterolateral' infarcts where the ECG changes are predominantly found in V4, V5 and V6.

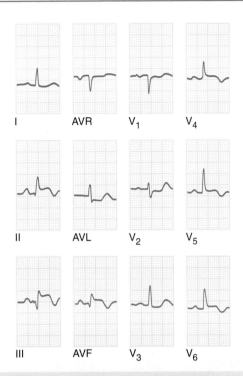

Fig. 5.68 Acute full thickness inferolateral myocardial infarction. This ECG was recorded from a 55-year-old woman who had developed severe chest pain 4 hours earlier. There is ST elevation in the inferior leads II, III and aVF and the lateral leads V4, V5 and V6. There is also 'reciprocal' ST depression in leads aVL and V2.

tunately, LDH is highly concentrated in red cells and abnormal results can be due to very mild haemolysis.

Other blood tests

A leucocytosis is usual, reaching a peak on the first day. The ESR becomes raised and may remain so for several days.

Chest radiography

This may demonstrate pulmonary oedema which is not evident on clinical examination (see Fig. 5.20, p. 215). The heart size is often normal but there may be cardiomegaly due to previous myocardial damage, coexisting cardiac disease or a pericardial effusion.

Cardiac ultrasound

Echocardiography can be performed at the bedside and is an invaluable technique for assessing left and right ventricular function and detecting important complications such as cardiac rupture, ventricular septal defect, mitral regurgitation, and pericardial effusion.

Radionuclide scanning

A radionuclide ventriculogram (p. 206) can be used to assess left ventricular function and may provide useful prognostic information.

Infarct 'avid' scanning is possible because some isotopes (e.g. pyrophosphate) are taken up by freshly infarcted myocardium. This may help to establish the diagnosis in patients who present after a cardiac arrest when it is sometimes difficult to interpret any ECG and enzyme changes.

Early management

The earlier a patient with suspected acute myocardial infarction is brought within reach of a defibrillator, the better. In the United Kingdom most front-line ambulances are equipped with a semi-automatic advisory defibrillator. A patient with severe chest pain also requires urgent medical assessment and analgesia so it is often appropriate to summon an ambulance and a general practitioner at the same time.

In general, all patients with suspected myocardial infarction should be admitted to hospital for further observation and monitoring. However, an exception may be made if the patient has a terminal illness, serious

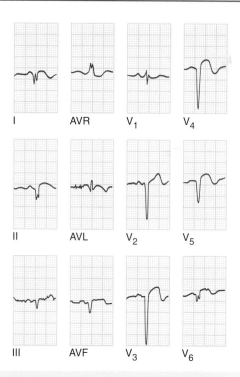

II   AVL   V$_2$ V$_5$

III   AVF   V$_3$ V$_6$

Fig. 5.69 Established anterior and inferior full thickness infarction. This ECG was recorded from a 70-year-old man who had presented with an acute anterior infarct 2 days earlier and had been treated for an inferior myocardial infarct 11 months before then. There are Q waves in the inferior leads (II, III and aVF) and Q waves with some residual ST elevation in the anterior leads (I, and V2–V6).

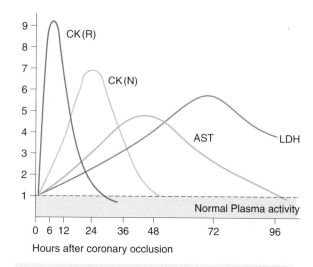

Hours after coronary occlusion

Fig. 5.70 Changes in plasma enzyme concentrations after myocardial infarction. Creatinine kinase (CK) is the first to rise, followed by aspartate aminotransferase (AST) and then lactate (hydroxybutyrate) dehydrogenase (LDH). In patients treated with a thrombolytic agent reperfusion is usually accompanied by a rapid rise in plasma creatinine kinase (curve CK(R)) due to a washout effect; if there is no reperfusion the rise is less rapid but the area under the curve is often greater (curve CK(N)).

concomitant disease, or the infarct occurred more than 24 hours earlier and there is adequate domestic support.

The essentials in the immediate management of acute myocardial infarction are summarised in the information box.

Many patients are treated initially in a dedicated coronary care unit simply because this offers a convenient way of concentrating the necessary expertise, monitoring and resuscitation facilities.

If there are no complications the patient can be mobilised from the second day and discharged from hospital on the sixth or seventh day.

Analgesia

Intravenous opiates (initially morphine sulphate 10 mg or diamorphine 5 mg) and antiemetics (initially cyclizine 50 mg or prochlorperazine 12.5 mg) should be administered through an intravenous cannula and titrated against the response by giving repeated small aliquots until the patient is comfortable.

Intramuscular injections should be avoided because

EARLY MANAGEMENT OF ACUTE MYOCARDIAL INFARCTION
• Bed rest
• Oral aspirin
• High flow oxygen
• i.v. access
• i.v. analgesia with opiates
• i.v. antiemetic
• Consider thrombolysis with i.v. streptokinase or alteplase
• Consider i.v. β-adrenoceptor antagonist
• Monitor ECG
• Detect and treat complications early

a painful haematoma may form if the patient receives anticoagulants or thrombolytic therapy.

Aspirin

Oral administration of 150–300 mg aspirin daily improves survival (30% reduction in short-term mortality) on its own, and enhances the effect of thrombolytic therapy. The first tablet should be given in a soluble or chewable form and the therapy should be continued indefinitely if there are no unwanted effects.

Thrombolytic drugs

Coronary thrombolysis helps restore coronary patency (Fig. 5.71), preserves left ventricular function, and

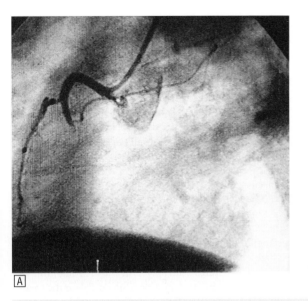 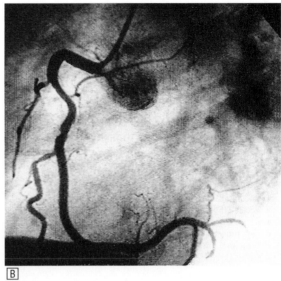

Fig. 5.71 Coronary angiograms from a patient with acute inferior myocardial infarction. Ⓐ complete occlusion of the proximal right coronary artery; Ⓑ appearance of the right coronary artery following successful thrombolytic therapy.

improves survival. Successful thrombolysis leads to reperfusion with relief of pain, resolution of acute ECG changes and sometimes transient arrhythmias. The sooner the patient is treated, the better the results; any delay will only increase the extent of myocardial damage—'minutes mean muscle'.

Clinical trials have shown that the appropriate use of these drugs can reduce the hospital mortality of myocardial infarction by between 25 and 50%. The benefit is greatest in those who receive treatment within the first few hours and the choice of agent is less important than the speed of treatment.

Streptokinase, 1.5 million Units in 100 ml of saline given as an intravenous infusion over 1 hour, is a widely used regimen. Streptokinase is relatively cheap (approximately £80 per dose in the UK) but is antigenic and occasionally causes serious allergic manifestations. The drug may also cause hypotension which can often be managed by stopping and restarting the infusion at a slower rate. Circulating neutralising antibodies are formed following treatment with streptokinase and may persist for 5 years or more. These antibodies can render subsequent infusions of streptokinase ineffective so it is advisable to use another agent if the patient requires further thrombolysis in the next few years.

Anistreplase (30 Units) can be given as a single intravenous injection over 5 minutes but is expensive and has no other advantages when compared to streptokinase.

Alteplase (human tissue plasminogen activator or tPA) is a genetically-engineered drug and is approxi-

mately 10 times more expensive than streptokinase; it is not antigenic and seldom causes hypotension. The standard regimen is a 3-hour intravenous infusion (a bolus of 10 mg followed by 50 mg in the first hour and then 40 mg over the next 2 hours); however, recent work suggests that an accelerated regimen sometimes known as fast tPA, given over 90 minutes (bolus dose of 15 mg, followed by 0.75 mg/kg of body weight, but not exceeding 50 mg, over 30 minutes and then 0.5 mg/kg body weight, but not exceeding 35 mg, over 60 minutes), may be preferable. Because it is so expensive many units only use tPA if streptokinase is contraindicated by virtue of allergy, previous exposure, or profound hypotension.

An overview of all the large randomised trials confirms that thrombolytic therapy significantly reduces short-term mortality in patients with suspected myocardial infarction if it is given *within 12 hours* of the onset of symptoms and the ECG shows *bundle branch block or characteristic ST segment elevation* of greater than 1 mm in the limb leads or 2 mm in the chest leads. In contrast, thrombolysis appears to be of little net benefit in other patient groups, specifically those who present more than 12 hours after the onset of symptoms and those with a normal ECG or ST depression.

In patients with ST elevation or bundle branch block the absolute benefit is approximately 30 lives saved per 1000 patients treated within 6 hours and 20 lives saved per 1000 patients treated between 7 and 12 hours after the onset of symptoms.

The major hazard of thrombolytic therapy is bleeding.

Cerebral haemorrhage causes 4 extra strokes per 1000 patients treated and the incidence of other major bleeds is between 0.5 and 1%. Accordingly, it may be wise to withhold the treatment if there is a significant risk of serious bleeding. Some potential contraindications to thrombolytic therapy are given in the information box below.

RELATIVE CONTRAINDICATIONS TO THROMBOLYTIC THERAPY

- Active internal bleeding
- Previous subarachnoid or intracerebral haemorrhage
- Uncontrolled hypertension
- Recent surgery (within 1 month)
- Recent trauma (including traumatic resuscitation)
- High probability of active peptic ulcer
- Pregnancy or current menstruation
- Severe diabetic proliferative retinopathy

The potential benefits and risks of thrombolytic therapy must be assessed in every case. For example, it would be reasonable to give thrombolytic therapy to a patient who presents early with evidence of extensive anterior infarction despite a history of peptic ulceration; on the other hand the risks of thrombolysis would probably exceed the benefits in a patient with a similar history of peptic ulceration who presents late with evidence of limited inferior myocardial infarction.

Angioplasty

Immediate or *primary* angioplasty of the infarct-related coronary artery is a relatively safe and effective alternative to thrombolytic therapy. This form of treatment is particularly suitable for patients in whom the hazards of thrombolysis are high, but it is only available in a few centres.

Similarly, *rescue* angioplasty is sometimes undertaken in patients who do not respond to thrombolytic therapy.

Anticoagulants

Subcutaneous heparin (12 500 units twice daily for 7 days or until discharge from hospital), given in addition to oral aspirin, may prevent reinfarction after successful thrombolysis and reduce the risk of thromboembolic complications. Clinical trials have shown that this form of therapy produces a small reduction in short-term mortality (approximately 5 lives saved per 1000 patients treated) but also increases the risk of cerebral haemorrhage (0.56% versus 0.4%) and other bleeding complications (1% versus 0.8%).

A period of treatment with warfarin should be considered if there is persistent atrial fibrillation, evidence of extensive anterior infarction, or if echocardiography shows mobile mural thrombus, because these patients are at increased risk of systemic thromboembolism.

β-adrenoceptor antagonists

Acute β-adrenoceptor antagonist use with intravenous atenolol (5–10 mg given over 5 minutes) or metoprolol (5–15 mg given over 5 minutes) relieves pain, reduces arrhythmias and improves short-term mortality, in patients who present within 12 hours of the onset of symptoms, but should be avoided if there is heart failure, heart block or severe bradycardia. Chronic β-adrenoceptor antagonist therapy improves long-term survival, and should be given to all patients who can tolerate it.

Nitrates and other agents

Sublingual glyceryl trinitrate (400–500 micrograms) is a valuable first-aid measure in threatened infarction and intravenous nitrates (nitroglycerin 0.6–1.2 mg/hour or isosorbide dinitrate 1–2 mg/hour) are useful for the treatment of left ventricular failure and recurrent or persistent ischaemic pain.

Large-scale trials have shown that there is little to be gained from the routine use of oral nitrate therapy, oral calcium antagonists or intravenous magnesium in patients with acute myocardial infarction.

Complications of infarction

Arrhythmias

Nearly all patients with acute myocardial infarction have some form of arrhythmia; in many cases this is mild and of no haemodynamic or prognostic significance. Various degrees of heart block (pp. 239–243) are also common. Some common arrhythmias are listed in the information box below; the diagnosis and management of these arrhythmias is discussed in detail on pages 225–245.

Pain relief, rest, reassurance and the correction of hypokalaemia can all play a major role in preventing arrhythmias.

Ventricular fibrillation occurs in about 5–10% of patients who reach hospital and is thought to be the major cause of death in those who die before receiving

---

COMMON ARRHYTHMIAS IN ACUTE MYOCARDIAL INFARCTION

- Ventricular fibrillation
- Ventricular tachycardia
- Accelerated idioventricular rhythm
- Ventricular ectopics
- Atrial fibrillation
- Atrial tachycardia
- Heart block

---

medical attention. Prompt defibrillation will usually restore sinus rhythm. Moreover, the prognosis of patients who are successfully resuscitated in this way is identical to the prognosis of patients with acute myocardial infarction that is not complicated by ventricular fibrillation. The need to recognise and treat ventricular fibrillation quickly is one of the main foundations on which the policy of acute coronary care is built.

Atrial fibrillation is common, frequently transient, and may not require treatment. However, if the arrhythmia causes a rapid ventricular rate with severe hypotension or circulatory collapse, cardioversion by means of an immediate synchronised DC shock should be considered. In other situations digoxin (see p. 239) is usually the treatment of choice. Atrial fibrillation (due to acute atrial stretch) is often a feature of impending or overt left ventricular failure and therapy may be ineffective if heart failure is not recognised and treated appropriately.

Sinus bradycardia does not usually require treatment, but if there is hypotension or haemodynamic deterioration, atropine (0.6 mg intravenously) may be given.

Heart block (see section on AV block complicating acute myocardial infarction in rhythms section) complicating *inferior* infarction is usually temporary and often resolves following thrombolytic therapy; it may also respond to atropine (0.6 mg intravenously repeated as necessary). However, if there is clinical deterioration due to second degree or complete heart block a temporary pacemaker should be considered. Heart block complicating *anterior* infarction is more serious, because asystole may suddenly supervene, and constitutes an indication for the insertion of a prophylactic temporary pacemaker (see page 244).

Ischaemia

Post-infarct angina occurs in up to 50% of patients. Most patients have a residual stenosis in the infarct-related vessel despite successful thrombolysis, and this may cause angina if there is still viable myocardium downstream; nevertheless there is no evidence that routine angioplasty improves outcome after thrombolysis. In some patients occlusion of a vessel may precipitate angina by disturbing a system of collateral flow that was compensating for disease in another vessel.

Patients who develop angina at rest or on minimal exertion following myocardial infarction should be managed in the same way as patients with unstable angina (see pp. 254–256). Intravenous nitrates (e.g. nitroglycerin 0.6–1.2 mg/hour or isosorbide dinitrate 1–2 mg/hour) and intravenous heparin (1000 units/hour, adjusted according to the thrombin time) may be helpful

and early coronary angiography with a view to angioplasty of the 'culprit' lesion should be considered.

Acute circulatory failure

Acute circulatory failure usually reflects extensive myocardial damage and indicates a bad prognosis. All the other complications of myocardial infarction are more likely to occur when acute heart failure is present.

The assessment and management of heart failure complicating acute myocardial infarction is discussed in detail on pages 213–214.

Pericarditis

This may occur at any stage of the illness but is particularly common on the second and third day. The patient may recognise that a different pain has developed, even though it is at the same site, and often finds that the pain is positional and tends to be worse, or sometimes only appears, on inspiration. A pericardial rub may be audible.

The post-myocardial infarction syndrome (**Dressler's syndrome**) is probably an autoimmune reaction to necrotic myocardium and is characterised by persistent fever, pericarditis and pleurisy. The symptoms tend to occur a few weeks or even months after the infarct and often subside after a few days; prolonged or severe symptoms may require treatment with high-dose aspirin, a non-steroidal anti-inflammatory drug or even corticosteroids.

Mechanical complications

Part of the necrotic muscle in a fresh infarct may tear or rupture with devastating consequences:

- Papillary muscle damage may cause acute pulmonary oedema and shock due to the sudden onset of severe mitral regurgitation with a loud pansystolic murmur and third heart sound. The diagnosis may be confirmed by Doppler echocardiography, and emergency mitral valve replacement may be necessary. Lesser degress of mitral regurgitation are common.
- Rupture of the interventricular septum may cause left-to-right shunting through a ventricular septal defect. This usually presents with sudden haemodynamic deterioration accompanied by a new loud pansystolic murmur and may be difficult to distinguish from acute mitral regurgitation; however, patients with an acquired ventricular septal defect tend to develop right heart failure rather than pulmonary oedema. Doppler echocardiography and right heart catheterisation will confirm the diagnosis and without prompt surgery the condition is usually fatal.
- Rupture of the ventricle may lead to cardiac tamponade and is usually fatal. (See p. 214.)

Embolism

Thrombus often forms on the endocardial surface of freshly infarcted myocardium; this may lead to systemic embolism and occasionally causes a stroke or ischaemic limb.

Venous thrombosis and pulmonary embolism may occur but have become less common due to the use of prophylactic anticoagulants and early mobilisation.

Ventricular aneurysm

A left ventricular aneurysm develops in approximately 10% of patients and is particularly common when there is persistent occlusion of the infarct-related vessel. Heart failure, ventricular arrhythmias, mural thrombus and systemic embolism are all recognised complications of aneurysm formation. Other clinical features include a paradoxical impulse on the chest wall, persistent ST elevation on the ECG, and an unusual bulge from the cardiac silhouette on the chest radiograph. Echocardiography is usually diagnostic. Surgical removal of a left ventricular aneurysm carries a high morbidity and mortality but is sometimes neccessary.

Late management

Patients who have survived a myocardial infarction are at risk of further ischaemic events; any management strategy should therefore aim to identify those patients at high risk and introduce effective secondary prevention measures.

Risk stratification and further investigation

The prognosis of patients who have survived an acute myocardial infarction is related to the degree of myocardial damage, the extent of any residual myocardial ischaemia and the presence of significant ventricular arrhythmias.

Left ventricular function. The degree of left ventricular dysfunction can be crudely assessed from the physical findings (tachycardia, third heart sound, crackles at the lung bases, elevated venous pressure, etc.), the ECG changes and the size of the heart on chest radiograph. However, formal measurements using echocardiography or radionuclide imaging are often valuable and may help to select patients for ACE inhibitor therapy (see below).

Ischaemia. Patients who are suitable candidates for revascularisation should undergo an exercise tolerance test approximately 4 weeks after the infarct; this will help to identify those individuals with significant residual myocardial ischaemia who require further investigation and may help to boost the confidence of the remainder.

If the exercise test is negative and the patient has a good effort tolerance the outlook is good with a 1–4% chance of an adverse event in the next 12 months. In contrast, patients with residual ischaemia in the form of chest pain or ECG changes at low exercise levels are at high risk with a 15–25% chance of suffering a further ischaemic event in the next 12 months.

Coronary arteriography, with a view to angioplasty or by pass grafting, should therefore be considered in any patient with a strongly positive exercise tolerance test or significant angina on effort.

Arrhythmias. The presence of ventricular arrhythmias during the convalescent phase of myocardial infarction may herald sudden death and is associated with a poor prognosis. Although empirical antiarrhythmic treatment appears to be of no value, and may even be hazardous, in this situation selected patients may benefit from sophisticated electrophysiological testing and specific antiarrhythmic therapy.

Recurrent ventricular arrhythmias are sometimes manifestations of myocardial ischaemia or impaired LV function and may respond to appropriate treatment directed at the underlying problem.

Routine drug therapy

Aspirin. Low-dose aspirin therapy reduces the risk of further infarction and other vascular events by approximately 25% and should be continued indefinitely if there are no unwanted effects.

β-adrenoceptor antagonists. Continuous treatment with an oral β-adrenoceptor antagonist has been shown to reduce long-term mortality by approximately 25% in the survivors of acute myocardial infarction. Unfortunately, patients with bradycardia, heart block, hypotension, overt cardiac failure, asthma, chronic obstructive airways disease and significant peripheral vascular disease do not usually tolerate beta-blockers.

Angiotensin-converting enzyme inhibitors. Acute full thickness myocardial infarction is often followed by thinning and stretching of the infarcted segment (**infarct expansion**); this leads to an increase in wall stress with progressive dilatation and hypertrophy of the remaining ventricle (**ventricular remodelling**— see Fig. 5.72). As the ventricle dilates it becomes less efficient and heart failure may supervene. Infarct expansion occurs over a few weeks but ventricular remodelling may take years. Accordingly, heart failure often develops many years after acute myocardial infarction. Several clinical trials have shown that long-term treatment with an ACE inhibitor (e.g. captopril 50 mg three times a day, enalapril 10 mg twice daily, or ramipril 2.5–5 mg twice daily) can counteract ventricular remodelling and prevent the onset of heart failure, and indicate that this form of therapy should be considered in any patient who has sustained a myocardial infarct complicated by transient heart failure or poor residual left ventricular function (e.g. LV ejection fraction <40%).

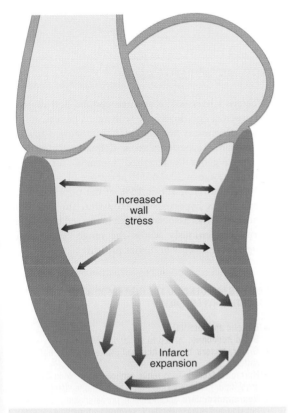

Fig. 5.72   Infarct expansion and ventricular remodelling.
Full thickness myocardial infarction causes thinning and stretching of the infarcted segment (infarct expansion) which leads to increased wall stress with progressive dilatation and hypertrophy of the remaining ventricle (ventricular remodelling).

Risk factor modification

Smoking. The 5-year mortality of patients who continue to smoke cigarettes is double that of those who quit smoking at the time of their infarct. Giving up smoking is the single most effective contribution a patient can make to his or her own future.

Lipids. There is often a temporary and potentially misleading fall in plasma cholesterol following myocardial infarction; however, measurements carried out within 24 hours or more than 3 months after the onset of symptoms are usually representative. Effective lipid-lowering therapy (see page 767) reduces the risk of further coronary events and ideally should aim to reduce the total cholesterol to 5.2 mmol/l or less and LDL cholesterol to less than 3.4 mmol/l or less.

Other risk factors. Maintaining an ideal body weight, taking regular exercise, and achieving good control of hypertension and diabetes may all improve the long-term outlook.

Mobilisation and rehabilitation

There is histological evidence that the necrotic muscle of an acute myocardial infarct takes 4–6 weeks to become replaced with fibrous tissue. Accordingly, it is conventional to restrict physical activities during this period. When there are no complications the patient can sit in a chair on the second day, walk to the toilet on the third day, return home in 5–7 days and gradually increase activity with the aim of returning to work in 6–8 weeks. The majority of patients may resume driving after 4–6 weeks; however, in the UK vocational (e.g. HGV and PSV) driving licence holders require special assessment.

Emotional problems such as denial, anxiety and depression are common and must be recognised and dealt with accordingly. Many patients are severely and even permanently incapacitated as a result of the psychological rather than the physical effects of myocardial infarction, and all benefit from thoughtful explanation, counselling and reassurance at every stage of the illness. The patient's spouse will also require emotional support, information and counselling.

Formal rehabilitation programmes based on graded exercise protocols with individual and group counselling are often very successful and in some cases have been shown to improve the long-term outcome.

Prognosis

In about a quarter of all cases of myocardial infarction death occurs within a few minutes without medical care. Half the deaths from myocardial infarction occur within 2 hours of the onset of symptoms and three-quarters within 24 hours. About 40% of all affected patients die within the first month.

Early death is usually due to an arrhythmia but later on the outcome is determined by the extent of myocardial damage. Unfavourable features include poor left ventricular function, heart block and persistent ventricular arrhythmias. The prognosis is worse for anterior than for inferior infarcts. Bundle branch block and high enzyme levels both indicate extensive myocardial damage. Old age, stress and social isolation are also associated with a higher mortality. In the absence of unfavourable features, the outlook is as good for those who survive ventricular fibrillation as for the others.

Of those who survive an acute attack, more than 80% live for a further year, about 75% for 5 years, 50% for 10 years and 25% for 20 years.

SUDDEN DEATH

This term can be applied when a person previously in apparent good health falls ill and dies within minutes or at most a few hours.

Approximately 30% of these patients have an identifiable non-cardiac cause of death such as cerebral haemorrhage or a ruptured aortic aneurysm. However, in most cases death is attributable to coronary artery disease and is usually due to an arrhythmia related to acute myocardial infarction, ischaemia, heart failure or scarring from a previous myocardial infarct. An arrhythmia is probably also the cause of sudden death in patients with other cardiac abnormalities such as acute myocarditis, severe aortic stenosis, critical pulmonary stenosis and hypertrophic cardiomyopathy. A small group of patients who die suddenly have no obvious pathological cause of death on postmortem examination; a cardiac arrhythmia seems the most likely cause in this group as well.

Observations on patients who have all died during ambulatory ECG monitoring suggest that ventricular fibrillation is the commonest arrhythmia causing sudden death. In many cases of ventricular fibrillation prompt resuscitation can restore effective cardiac action (see pp. 233–234).

The survivors of an 'out-of-hospital' cardiac arrest require careful evaluation. If there is no evidence of acute myocardial infarction there is a high chance of recurrent cardiac arrest and the patient may benefit from specific antiarrhythmic therapy. In patients with poor left ventricular function (ejection fraction < 20%) empirical therapy with amiodarone 200 mg daily may be the best option; others may benefit from drug treatment guided by electrophysiological studies, various forms of arrhythmia surgery or an automatic implantable defibrillator (see page 243).

Relatives of patients who have died suddenly often seek reassurance, and should be examined, if appropriate, for evidence of hypertrophic cardiomyopathy, Marfan syndrome and hyperlipidaemia. A family history of sudden death in childhood or young adult life is sometimes associated with prolongation of the QT interval on the ECG, and beta-blockade may improve prognosis in this group.

FURTHER READING

Davies M J (ed.) 1993 Atherosclerosis. British Heart Journal 69, S1–S73. *This supplement to the British Heart Journal contains 10 excellent review articles on the pathophysiology and prevention of coronary artery disease*
Fibrinolytic therapy trialists (FTT) collaborative group 1994 Indications for fibrinolytic therapy in suspected acute myocardial infarction: collaborative overview of early mortality and major morbidity results from all randomised trials of more than 1000 patients. Lancet 343: 311–322. *A useful summary of the benefits and hazards of thrombolytic therapy*
McMurray Y, Rankin A 1994 Treatment of myocardial infarction, unstable angina and angina pectoris. British Medical Journal 309: 1343–1350

VASCULAR DISEASE

SYSTEMIC HYPERTENSION

In Western societies the average systolic and diastolic blood pressures gradually rise with age. The distribution of blood pressure is not Gaussian, but skewed towards hypertension. Hypertension is defined arbitrarily at levels above generally accepted 'normals', for example 140/90 at the age of 20, 160/95 at the age of 50. According to these criteria, about 15% of the population can be regarded as hypertensive. However, the morbidity and mortality risks associated with increased blood pressure rise continuously across the range of pressures, although more steeply at higher pressures.

> **FACTORS INFLUENCING THE DEVELOPMENT OF ESSENTIAL HYPERTENSION**
>
> - **Genetic and familial**
> - **Socio-economic**: related to social deprivation
> - **Dietary factors**: obesity, high salt intake, high alcohol, caffeine
> - **Hormonal factors**: high renin, reduced nitric oxide (also atrial naturetic peptide, anti-diuretic hormone effects)
> - **Neurotransmitters**: acetylcholine, noradrenaline, substance P, neuropeptide Y, serotonin, dopamine, encephalin

The risks associated with a particular blood pressure are dependent upon the combination of risk factors in the specific individual. These include the risks associated with age (risk increases with age), gender (males > females), ethnic origin (blacks > whites), diet (high salt), smoking and concomitant disease (e.g. coronary artery disease).

Exercise, anxiety, discomfort and unfamiliar surroundings can all lead to a transient rise in blood pressure, and measurements should be repeated when the patient is resting and relaxed until consistent readings are obtained (ideally on 3 separate occasions). Patients who have an isolated recording of high blood pressure, which subsequently settles, may nevertheless be at increased risk and should be kept under review.

Aetiology

In more than 95% of cases a specific underlying cause of hypertension is not found. Such patients are said to have **essential hypertension**. In 70% of those with essential hypertension another member of the family is affected and inheritance is thought to be multifactorial. Essential hypertension is especially frequent in some ethnic groups, particularly American Blacks and Japanese, and is commoner in countries where there is a high salt intake.

The pathogenesis of essential hypertension is not clearly understood. However, it is known that the underlying defect is an increase in peripheral vascular resistance. Some authorities believe that this is due to an increase in sympathetic nervous activity while others believe that there is a fundamental defect in the vascular smooth muscle.

In about 5% of unselected cases, hypertension can be shown to be a consequence of a specific disease or abnormality. The causes are listed in the information box below.

CAUSES OF SECONDARY HYPERTENSION

- **Coarctation of the aorta**
- **Renal disease**
  Parenchymal renal disease, e.g. glomerulonephritis, chronic pyelonephritis, collagen vascular diseases
  Polycystic kidney disease
  Renal artery stenosis
- **Endocrine disorders**
  Phaeochromocytoma
  Cushing's syndrome
  Conn's syndrome (primary hyperaldosteronism)
  Hyperparathyroidism
  Acromegaly
  Primary hypothyroidism
  Congenital adrenal hyperplasia
  11 beta-hydroxylase, 17-hydroxylase deficiency
- **Drugs**
  e.g. Oral contraceptives containing oestrogens, anabolic steroids, corticosteroids, non-steroidal anti-inflammatory drugs, carbenoxolone, sympathomimetic agents
- **Pregnancy** $\pm$ pre-eclampsia

In phaeochromocytoma, hypertension results from an increased cardiac output and/or a raised peripheral resistance due to excessive catecholamines. Conn's syndrome is associated with sodium retention, and probably an alteration in the reactivity of vascular smooth muscle. Renal causes of hypertension are also often associated with sodium retention, and in many cases with high plasma concentrations of renin, which causes the production of the potent vasoconstrictor agent angiotensin II. The latter stimulates aldosterone secretion and thus also encourages sodium retention.

Pathophysiological changes

In an individual patient it may not be possible to distinguish factors responsible for the cause from those contributing to the perpetuation of hypertension. In larger arteries (>1 mm diameter) the internal elastic lamina is thickened, smooth muscle hypertrophied, and fibrous tissue deposited. The vessels dilate and become tortuous and their walls become less compliant. Atheroma is perpetuated. In smaller arteries (>1 mm) hyaline arteriosclerosis occurs in the wall, the lumen narrows and aneurysms may develop. These structural changes associated with long-standing hypertension affect peripheral resistance vessels and vessels in the kidneys. They lead to an increase in peripheral vascular resistance, a further rise in blood pressure, and acceleration of atheroma within vessel walls.

Reduced renal perfusion pressure, in the presence of renovascular disease, leads to the production of renin and angiotensin and further salt and water retention. Thus, a vicious circle may be established.

Malignant phase hypertension may be superimposed on hypertension of any aetiology. It is not a separate disease entity. An accelerated pattern develops with a rapid rise in pressure and severe damage to various organ systems. The characteristic pathological changes are necrosis in the walls of small arteries and arterioles ('fibrinoid necrosis') and intravascular thrombosis. Left ventricular failure may occur and also renal impairment with proteinuria and microscopic haematuria. Arterial pressure exceeds the limit of vascular autoregulation to the brain, and cerebral and retinal oedema supervene, leading to *hypertensive encephalopathy*. The clinical manifestations include headache, confusion, coma and fits. If untreated death occurs within months.

Clinical features of hypertension

Symptoms

Hypertension occasionally causes headache or polyuria but, provided there are no complications, most patients remain asymptomatic. Accordingly, the diagnosis is usually made at routine examination or when a complication arises. There may be a family history of hypertension and prior history of renal disease. Symptoms mainly relate to the complications of hypertension, including angina, left ventricular failure and cerebrovascular disease. A careful history should identify those patients with drug or alcohol induced hypertension and those at increased risk from smoking. Paroxysmal headache, palpitations and sweating should prompt a careful search for a phaeochromocytoma. Similarly, recurrent backache or urinary tract infection may be due to chronic pyelonephritis.

Physical signs

Most patients have no abnormal physical signs apart from the hypertension. Non-specific signs may include left ventricular hypertrophy (apical heave), accentuation of the aortic component of the second heart sound, and possibly a fourth heart sound. The optic fundi are often abnormal (see below).

The three main objectives of clinical examination in a hypertensive patient are to identify any underlying causes (most commonly found in young patients with no family history of hypertension), to recognise risk factors for the development of complications and to detect any complications already present.

Physical examination must include detection of the delay between radial and femoral pulses characteristic of coarctation of the aorta, and examination for enlarged kidneys in polycystic disease. The characteristic facies and habitus of Cushing's syndrome may be recognised, and a bruit is sometimes audible over the abdomen in renal artery stenosis.

It is important to identify signs of obesity and hyperlipidaemia which may interact with hypertension, particularly in the genesis of ischaemic heart disease.

Complications

The adverse effects of hypertension principally involve the central nervous system, the retina, the heart and the kidneys.

Central nervous system

Stroke may result from cerebral haemorrhage or from cerebral infarction and is a common complication of hypertension and a major cause of death in hypertensive patients. Carotid atheroma and transient cerebral ischaemic attacks are more common in hypertensive patients.

Hypertensive encephalopathy (see pathophysiology, above) is a rare condition characterised by a very high blood pressure and neurological symptoms including transient disturbances of speech or vision, paraesthesiae, disorientation, fits and loss of consciousness. Papilloedema is common. The neurological deficit is usually reversible if the hypertension is properly controlled. Subarachnoid haemorrhage is more common in hypertensive patients.

Retina

The optic fundi reveal a gradation of changes linked to the severity of hypertension and hence provide an indication of the arteriolar damage occurring elsewhere.

HYPERTENSIVE RETINOPATHY

- **Grade 1**: thickening, irregularity and tortuosity of arterioles. Increased reflection—'silver wiring'
- **Grade 2**: as above plus constriction of retinal veins at arterial crossings (arteriovenous nipping)
- **Grade 3**: as above plus flame-shaped haemorrhages and 'cotton wool' exudates
- **Grade 4**: as above plus papilloedema (bulging optic disc with blurred edges)

Malignant phase hypertension may be present prior to the full development of papilloedema, and demands urgent treatment. 'Cotton wool' exudates are associated with retinal ischaemia or infarction, and fade in a few weeks. 'Hard' exudates are small white dense deposits of lipid which may persist for years (see Fig. 5.73).

Heart

Hypertension places a pressure load on the heart and may lead to left ventricular hypertrophy and ultimately

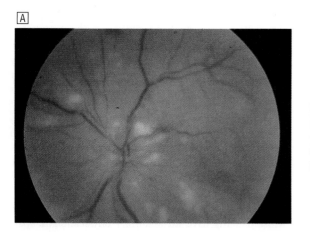

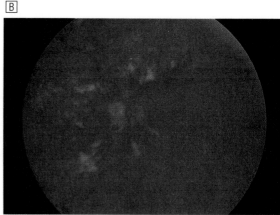

Fig. 5.73 [A] **Grade III/IV hypertensive retinopathy** showing swollen optic disc, retinal haemorrhages and multiple cotton wool spots (infarcts). [B] **Central retinal vein thrombosis** showing swollen optic disc and widespread fundal haemorrhage, commonly associated with systemic hypertension.

left ventricular failure (pp. 218–224). However, the excess cardiac mortality and morbidity associated with hypertension is largely due to a higher incidence of coronary artery disease (pp. 245–266). Hypertension is also implicated in the pathogenesis of aortic aneurysm and aortic dissection.

Kidneys

In addition to being a cause, renal disease may also be a result of hypertensive damage to the renal vessels. Long-standing hypertension may cause proteinuria and progressive renal failure.

Investigations

Some investigations need to be done on all patients, while others can be reserved for those with specific features of a particular condition or those who are refractory to the initial treatment.

INVESTIGATION OF HYPERTENSION: ALL PATIENTS

- Urine analysis: protein, glucose, haematuria
- Plasma urea/creatinine
- Chest radiograph (cardiomegaly, heart failure, rib notching)
- ECG (left ventricular hypertrophy, ischaemia)
- Plasma electrolytes (hypokalaemic alkalosis may indicate primary or secondary hyperaldosteronism **N.B.** diuretic therapy is commonest cause)
- Plasma cholesterol/triglycerides

INVESTIGATION OF HYPERTENSION: HIGH RISK PATIENTS

- **Intravenous urogram, ultrasound**
  —if renal disease suspected
- **Radionuclide renography or renal arteriography**
  —if there is evidence of renal artery stenosis
- **24-hour urine catecholamines (vanillylmandelic acid, VMA)**
  —if history suggests phaeochromocytoma
- **Plasma renin activity and aldosterone**
  —if Conn's syndrome suspected
- **Urinary cortisol, dexamethasone suppression test**
  —if signs of Cushing's syndrome
- **Angiography/MRI**
  —if coarctation suspected
- **Intravenous urogram, ultrasound**
  —if renal disease suspected

Special investigations are required when clinical evidence points to an underlying cause of the hypertension (for example < 45 years of age, malignant hypertension, or evidence of renal disease).

Renal artery stenosis often causes refractory hypertension and should be considered in patients with severe hypertension that is difficult to control or has developed rapidly. Renal arteriography provides the most detailed information about the renal vessels, and can permit percutaneous balloon dilatation of a renal artery stenosis.

Management

The object of treating systemic arterial hypertension is to reduce the risk of complications and to improve patient survival. The benefits of treatment have to be weighed against side-effects and inconvenience. In most instances, the discovery of hypertension commits the patient to a lifetime of supervision and treatment. It is important to treat the whole patient, and not just the blood pressure. Because of these considerations it is not particularly helpful to set up arbitrary levels of blood pressure at which treatment should be commenced (see introduction). There is agreement that hypertension should be treated with anti-hypertensive drugs if it is severe (e.g. over 160/100 at age 20, 170/110 in men aged 50) or if it is associated with retinal, cardiac or renal damage. There is now evidence of the benefits of such treatment in mild hypertensives, e.g. 140/90 at age 20, 160/95 at age 50. A large-scale trial conducted in Britain by the Medical Research Council tested the effects of treating mild hypertension with a beta-antagonist (propranolol), a thiazide diuretic or a placebo. Treatment reduced the incidence of non-fatal stroke, renal failure and other systemic complications. The trials which have shown the most consistent benefits of treatment have tended to be those in which the 'treated' group has been subject to close medical supervision, and attention has been paid to the correction of other risk factors.

In the elderly, hypertension can respond to treatment with gratifying clinical results; indeed, a large European trial showed that treatment produced a substantial fall in cardiovascular mortality.

General measures

Diet

Reducing alcohol consumption and correcting obesity are both effective anti-hypertensive measures. Very low sodium diets (10–20 mmol/d) lower blood pressure but are not well tolerated. Moderate sodium restriction (70–80 mmol/d) is helpful and patients should be advised to stop adding salt to food and to avoid foods with a very high sodium content.

Smoking

The effects of cigarette smoking and hypertension on cardiovascular morbidity are more than additive, and smoking should be strongly discouraged. *Stopping smoking constitutes the single most important and effective risk reduction.*

Exercise and relaxation

Regular exercise improves physical fitness and can lower blood pressure. Formal relaxation classes, meditation and biofeedback have all been shown to reduce blood pressure in small groups of patients; their efficacy is usually proportional to the enthusiasm of the teacher and the commitment of the participant; it is unusual, however, for such treatment to replace the need for anti-hypertensive drug therapy.

ANTI-HYPERTENSIVE DRUG THERAPY

Compliance is hampered by the fact that the patient is usually asymptomatic prior to treatment, but may be aware of side-effects following drug therapy. Many patients can be satisfactorily treated with a single anti-hypertensive drug, the choice of which will be determined by safety, convenience and freedom from side-effects. Another large group will require a combination of two or three anti-hypertensive agents to give good control with a low level of side-effects. A small minority will have severe hypertension refractory to conventional treatment and requiring intensive investigation and special treatment. The principal agents used in single drug treatment of hypertension are thiazide diuretics, beta-adrenoceptor antagonists and ACE inhibitors; calcium antagonists and some vasodilators are also effective.

A 'stepped care' approach to treatment was previously recommended by the WHO. Specific drug combinations were used in sequence, with additional drugs added if the pressure was not controlled. Current strategies favour tailoring drug therapy to the specific needs of the individual patient, especially in view of complicating medical conditions (asthma, vascular disease, diabetes), and withdrawing and replacing drugs if ineffective. Simplified dosing regimens improve compliance (ideally once daily).

Many physicians start treatment with a β-adrenoceptor antagonist or a thiazide diuretic, depending on the likely side-effects and the presence of any relevant additional pathology. For example, β-adrenoceptor antagonists commonly cause cold extremities, and thiazide diuretics may cause impotence. On the other hand a β-adrenoceptor antagonist is likely to benefit a patient with angina whereas a diuretic or ACE inhibitor may be more appropriate if there is evidence of heart failure. In some countries calcium antagonists are the most frequent first line therapy.

Thiazide diuretics

These diuretics and their adverse effects are discussed on page 602. The mechanism of their hypotensive action is incompletely understood, and it may take up to a month for the maximum effect to be observed. Thiazide diuretics may cause hyperuricaemia (precipitating gout), and may cause glucose intolerance, but seldom cause postural hypotension.

A daily dose of 5 mg bendrofluazide or 0.5 mg cyclopenthiazide is appropriate. More potent loop-acting diuretics such as frusemide (40 mg daily) or bumetanide (1 mg daily) have few advantages over thiazides in the treatment of hypertension unless there is substantial renal impairment or if they are used in conjunction with an ACE inhibitor, when their greater ability to cause sodium excretion may be useful. The loop diuretics have a more abrupt diuresis, may be less well tolerated, and are more costly. Potassium sparing diuretics (e.g. spironolactone 5–10 mg daily) are not very effective anti-hypertensive agents, except in the presence of hyperaldosteronism.

β-adrenoceptor antagonists

A large number of β-adrenoceptor antagonists ('β-blockers') are available and these differ in several important respects. Those with a short half-life are mostly available in slow release, once daily, formulations. Metoprolol (100–200 mg daily) and atenolol (50–100 mg daily) are cardioselective and therefore preferentially block the cardiac β_1-adrenoceptors as opposed to the β_2-adrenoceptors which mediate vasodilatation and broncho-dilatation. Pindolol (15–30 mg daily) and oxprenolol (160–320 mg daily) have partial agonist (intrinsic sympathomimetric) activity and therefore tend to cause less bradycardia. Propranolol is subject to extensive first pass metabolism which means that a large and variable proportion of the drug is destroyed in its first passage through the liver. The dose of propranolol must, therefore, be carefully titrated according to the patient's individual needs. Propranolol is lipid-soluble and crosses the blood-brain barrier; this may explain why it commonly causes CNS side-effects such as nightmares, drowsiness and depression. In contrast, atenolol and sotalol are water-soluble and largely excreted unchanged through the kidneys; CNS side-effects are therefore less common. 'Beta-blockers' may aggravate asthma, heart failure, and peripheral vascular disease and may cause fatigue and muscle discomfort. Metabolic side-effects of beta-blocking drugs include a tendency to increase plasma concentrations of cholesterol in low density lipoproteins. They are nevertheless widely used and are especially useful in the presence of angina.

Labetalol. This is a combined alpha and beta adrenoceptor antagonist which is sometimes more effective than pure beta-blockers and can be useful as an infusion in malignant phase hypertension.

Angiotensin converting enzyme (ACE) inhibitors
(p. 223)

These inhibit the conversion of angiotensin 1 to angiotensin 2 and thus have been a major advance in the treatment of moderate to severe hypertension. They have few side-effects and compliance tends to be good. They should be used with particular care in patients with impaired renal function and avoided with renal artery stenosis, as a sudden reduction in renal perfusion may precipitate renal failure. As in the treatment of cardiac failure it is best to start with a small dose (e.g. captopril 6.25 mg daily) and build up to an effective maintenance dose (e.g. captopril 25–75 mg twice daily, or enalapril 20 mg daily or lisinopril 10–20 mg daily). Their side effects include first dose hypotension and cough, and they may cause rashes, proteinuria and a metallic taste. *Electrolytes and creatinine should be checked before commencing therapy and 7–10 days after starting (creatinine and urea will rise in the presence of significant renal artery stenosis).*

Calcium antagonists

Diltiazem (60 mg 8-hourly or slow release), amlodipine (5–10 mg daily) or nifedipine (Adalat LA 30–90 mg once daily) are effective and usually well tolerated anti-hypertensive drugs. They are particularly useful when hypertension coexists with angina. Side-effects include flushing, palpitations, fluid retention and constipation. Diltiazem and verapamil may cause bradycardia.

Drug combinations

These may allow control of hypertension refractory to either drug alone, at doses insufficient to cause serious side-effects. In some respects the drugs have complementary actions—for example thiazides increase renin production while β-adrenoceptor antagonists depress it. On the other hand the complexity of combination therapy may discourage compliance and the risk of side-effects unrelated to the dose of drug is increased. A number of beta-blocker/thiazide combination tablets have been marketed, but the proportion of the two drugs is not necessarily optimal for every patient.

In severe hypertension the more potent vasodilator minoxidil (10–50 mg daily) may be useful. However, this produces marked fluid retention and increased facial hair and is therefore unsuitable for female patients.

The emergency treatment of hypertension

It is not appropriate to attempt to cause an instantaneous fall in blood pressure. Too rapid a fall may cause cerebral damage, including blindness, and may sometimes precipitate coronary or renal insufficiency. Even in the presence of cardiac failure or hypertensive encephalopathy a controlled reduction over a period of 30–60 minutes to a level of about 150/90 is adequate, and there is often less urgency.

The most effective agent for blood pressure reduction in an emergency is a controlled intravenous infusion of sodium nitroprusside (0.3–1.0 μg/kg body weight per minute), but this requires very careful supervision, preferably in an intensive care unit. Up to 6 μg/kg/min may be required (with intensive monitoring) in some instances. Alternatives are intravenous or intramuscular labetalol (2 mg/min to a maximum of 200 mg) or intramuscular hydralazine (5 or 10 mg aliquots repeated at half-hourly intervals and titrated against the blood pressure response). In some patients, however, it is possible to avoid parenteral therapy; for example, chewing a nifedipine 10 mg capsule is often sufficient to produce a graded reduction in blood pressure. Bed-rest, sedation and a diuretic are also helpful. Urinary output and plasma electrolytes should be monitored, and urgent enquiry made into the cause of the hypertension.

Hypertensive emergencies in young patients may result from acute glomerulonephritis or from an acute exacerbation of chronic renal failure. The latter is also an important cause of severe hypertension in older patients, but they are also likely to suffer from acute renal ischaemia caused by atheroma or embolism. The possibility of phaeochromocytoma should also be considered.

REFRACTORY HYPERTENSION

The common causes of treatment failure in hypertension are non-compliance with drug therapy, inadequate therapy, and failure to recognise an underlying cause such as renal artery stenosis or phaeochromocytoma; of these the first is by far the most prevalent. There is no easy solution to compliance problems, but a simple treatment regimen, attempts to improve rapport with the patient, and careful supervision may all help.

PERIPHERAL ARTERIAL DISEASE

Disease of the peripheral arteries is most commonly due to atheroma. Less common causes are thromboembolism, vasculitis, Raynaud's disease and cold injury (frostbite). A variant of atheromatous peripheral vascular disease occurs in diabetics: here the major arterial pulses may be preserved but soft tissue ischaemia, infection and ulceration are common, and diabetic peripheral neuropathy may affect sensation.

ATHEROMATOUS PERIPHERAL VASCULAR DISEASE

Clinical features

Atheromatous peripheral vascular disease is more common in men than women, is strongly associated with smoking, and affects the legs more than the arms. Patients are usually over 50 years old.

Symptoms

The commonest presenting symptom is intermittent claudication—a discomfort or ache in the calves or buttocks which comes on with walking and disappears with rest. Pulses in the leg and foot are absent or diminished. Patients may also complain of cold feet or legs and discolouration due to peripheral cyanosis.

Eventually the patient may develop rest pain in the affected limb. Characteristically this is worse at night, and the patient may get temporary relief by allowing the limb to hang over the side of the bed outside the bedclothes.

Signs

Characteristic features are coldness of the feet or lower limbs, diminished or absent peripheral pulses. There may be loss of hair over the affected limb, especially if the condition is long-standing. By the time the patient experiences rest pain in the limb it is common for the skin to be pale or discoloured, and for hair growth to be absent. Small patches of skin necrosis (leg ulcers) may appear, often related to pressure points or minor injury. Finally, frank gangrene may occur, usually starting with one or more toes. This is indicated by dark discolouration, spreading proximally, severe pain and often infection with a foul smelling discharge.

Investigations

Although radiographs may show calcification in arteries, they are not sensitive indicators of the degree of arterial narrowing nor of its localisation. Measurement of ratio of ankle to brachial cuff pressures has provided a useful marker of the extent of disease in epidemiological studies, but lacks sensitivity in an individual. Doppler ultrasound provides the initial investigation of choice. It enables peripheral pulse pressure to be measured and sites of stenosis and occlusion to be identified, and also helps to select patients for angiography and revascularisation. Ultrasound of the abdomen can detect vascular calcification and aneurysms in the abdominal aorta.

Angiography is necessary prior to balloon or surgical revascularisation to define the anatomy and allow an accurate assessment of the presence and extent of vascular stenoses (see Fig. 5.74). Percutaneous puncture of a non-affected artery under local anaesthesia permits the injection of radiographic contrast and conventional angiography or digital subtraction angiography performed. The latter subtracts background information to provide high definition angiograms of the lower limb vessels.

Management

Management advice is summarised in the information box below. It is important to assess the whole patient for

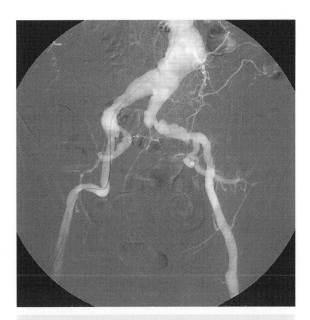

Fig. 5.74 Digital contrast angiogram of a patient with peripheral vascular disease showing marked tortuosity of the distal aorta, and iliac vessels with extensive atheroma leading to indentations and stenoses. There is an aneurysmal dilatation in the distal aorta prior to the bifurcation.

MANAGEMENT OF PERIPHERAL ARTERIAL DISEASE

General measures
- Stop smoking
- Lose weight if obese
- Stop vasoconstrictor drugs
- Optimise diabetic and hypertension control
- Encourage exercise (increases collateral flow)
- Avoid infection and trauma, arrange chiropody
- Vasodilators/anticoagulants are unhelpful

Indications for revascularisation
- Acute ischaemia of the limb. The hallmarks are: acute pain, pallor, pulseless, paralysis
  Embolectomy or surgical repair may be required and amputation may be necessary if intervention is delayed
- Chronic ischaemia with impaired skin and tissue viability, non-healing ulcers
- Disabling symptoms due to arterial stenoses or occlusions

---

evidence of coronary or cerebrovascular disease and for smoking-related lung disease.

Balloon angioplasty is particularly useful for iliac or femoral stenoses. Aorto-iliac surgical bypass grafts are effective, especially when disease is confined to vessels proximal to the inguinal ligament. Amputation may be necessary for a painful, infected and non-viable limb.

Medication has little role in atheromatous peripheral vascular disease. Vasodilators may only be useful where there is a substantial vasospastic component (nifedipine 5–10 mg 8-hourly). Severe pain, especially if there is a neuropathic component, may be helped by amitriptyline (25–50 mg at night).

The major cause of death in patients with atheromatous peripheral vascular disease is myocardial infarction. It is important to reduce risk factors for this.

SUDDEN OCCLUSION OF A MAJOR ARTERY

This is usually due to embolism from the heart as a result of mural thrombus after myocardial infarction, endocarditis, rheumatic heart disease, or, rarely, an atrial myxoma. Emboli that precipitate acute clinical symptoms lodge most frequently at the aortic, iliac or popliteal bifurcations. The limb becomes painful, cold, numb and pale, and pulses distal to the occlusion are absent. Surgical embolectomy should be considered without delay. A Fogarty balloon catheter is used to extract the embolus through a small arteriotomy, and the procedure is often performed under local anaesthesia. While preparations for surgery are being made, pain should be relieved and the limb kept at rest and at room temperature.

VASCULITIS

Vasculitis is a generic term for inflammatory diseases affecting blood vessels. Vasculitides affecting medium-sized or large vessels may cause symptoms of peripheral artery disease. The most important are polyarteritis nodosa (p. 921), giant cell arteritis (p. 924) and Takayasu's disease (pulseless disease or aortic arch syndrome, p. 925). The clinical presentation and management of this group of diseases is detailed in Chapter 15.

RAYNAUD'S PHENOMENON AND RAYNAUD'S DISEASE

Clinical features

Raynaud's phenomenon is caused by intense vasospasm of peripheral arteries. On exposure to cold the fingers (and less commonly the toes) become initially very pale from vasoconstriction. This is followed by cyanosis secondary to the poor blood flow. Eventually when the blood flow returns there is redness and discomfort. When the phenomenon occurs without other associated illness or precipitating cause it is called *Raynaud's disease*. This occurs more frequently in women than in men, and is common, affecting about 5% of the population. Other associations are listed in the information box below.

Management

Patients should stop smoking, and vasoconstrictor drugs or β-adrenoceptor antagonists should be withdrawn. Cold exposure should be avoided. Nifedipine (5–10 mg 8-hourly) is sometimes helpful. Severe cold injury causes occlusion of peripheral arterioles while leaving large vessels patent. Initially the limb or digits are white and anaesthetic; as warming occurs they become dusky and painful.

DISEASES OF THE AORTA

AORTIC ANEURYSM

An aortic aneurysm is an abnormal dilatation of the aortic wall. Dissecting aneurysm has a different pathology and is considered separately.

ANEURYSMS MAY BE DUE TO:

- Atheromatous disease—
  affects ascending or descending aorta
- Collagen vascular diseases—
  thoracic aorta: cystic medial necrosis, Marfan's syndrome, Ehlers–Danlos syndrome
- Syphilis—saccular aneurysms of ascending aorta with calcification

Aetiology

Atheromatous disease

Atheroma may weaken the aortic wall and lead to local aneurysm formation. The commonest site is the abdo-minal aorta between renal and iliac arteries, but the thoracic aorta may also be affected.

Marfan's syndrome

Aneurysms associated with this disorder may rupture directly, or cause dissection. Patients usually present in the third to fifth decade: they may have the characteristic facial and skeletal features of the fully fledged syndrome, but formes frustes occur. Marfan's syndrome is autosomal dominant and may also cause mitral regurgitation. Chest radiography, ultrasound or CT scanning may detect aortic dilatation at an early stage. Elective replacement of the ascending aorta may be considered, but carries a mortality of 5–10%. Use of β-adrenoceptor antagonists may also reduce the risk of dilatation and rupture. Pregnancy is particularly hazardous.

Syphilitic aortic aneurysm

This is now rare. It usually presents as a chance radiographic finding, as angina-like chest pain, or as heart failure due to aortic reflux. Besides a dilated ascending aorta, the radiograph may show fine 'egg-shell' calcification of the aorta. Serology is usually positive. Surgical treatment may be required for progressive enlargement, angina due to coronary ostial stenosis, or aortic reflux. Otherwise, treatment is that of the underlying syphilis (see page 184).

Clinical features

Clinically, 'expansile' pulsation of an aneurysm must be distinguished from 'transmitted' pulsation from a normal aorta.

CLINICAL FEATURES OF ABDOMINAL ANEURYSMS

- More common in men, especially over 60 years of age

Symptoms
- Commonly asymptomatic (especially small aneurysms <5 cm diameter)
- May present with backache, abdominal pain or limb claudication
- May present acutely with pain and hypotension from rupture

Signs
- Aneurysm may be palpable in abdominal aorta
- Evidence widespread vascular disease
- Stigmata of distal embolisation
- Haemodynamic collapse (hypotension, tachycardia, shock) with rupture of aneurysm

The diagnosis is made by ultrasound scanning or CT, and the abdominal or chest radiograph may reveal calcification. The natural history of an aneurysm is expansion, and it may eventually rupture.

Management

Elective surgical repair has a much lower mortality than emergency surgery for rupture. Suggested management for abdominal aneurysms is shown in the information box below. The mortality for surgical repair of thoracic aneurysms is higher than that of abdominal aneurysms. They are usually treated conservatively unless there are signs of progressive enlargement. In contrast, dissecting aneurysms of the ascending aorta usually require emergency surgical intervention (see below).

MANAGEMENT OF ABDOMINAL AORTIC ANEURYSMS

- **Symptoms of rupture:**
  Emergency surgery
- **Backache or abdominal pain**
  Ultrasound, CT or angiography, consider surgery
- **Asymptomatic:**
  Ultrasound—if <4 cm, serial ultrasound + follow up
  if >4 cm, consider surgery

DISSECTING ANEURYSM OF THE AORTA

A dissecting aneurysm is the result of a tear in the intima of the aorta followed by entry of blood into the plane of the media and separation of a 'flap' of intima from the rest of the aortic wall. This creates a false lumen and may go on to external rupture. The dissection may cause ischaemia of vital organs, especially the coronaries or the renal vessels, by occluding the origins of their supplying arteries.

Predisposing factors are hypertension, connective tissue disorders, pregnancy and congenital abnormalities of the aortic valve. Classification of dissecting aneurysms distinguishes *Type A aneurysms* which arise in the ascending aorta, with or without extension into the descending aorta, from *Type B aneurysms* which are confined to the descending aorta, distal to the origin of the left subclavian artery. Two-thirds are Type A aneurysms.

Clinical features

Symptoms

Clinical presentation is usually acute, with sudden onset of very severe pain in the chest and back, often starting between the shoulder blades and described as 'tearing'. The onset is often very abrupt.

Signs

On examination there may be hypertension and asymmetry of the brachial, carotid or femoral pulses. In Type A dissection there may be a diastolic murmur of aortic reflux. There is sometimes an inappropriate bradycardia from stimulation of aortic baroreceptors. The chest radiograph characteristically shows broadening of the upper mediastinum and distortion of the aortic 'knuckle', but these appearances are not invariable (they are absent in 40%). A left-sided pleural effusion is common. The most useful investigations are trans-oesophageal echocardiography or CT scanning. If neither is available or the results are inconclusive, then angiography is indicated.

Management

Initial management involves control of hypertension (maintain systolic pressure <100 mmHg) and definition of the site of origin and extent of the dissection. Type A dissecting aneurysms require emergency surgical repair under cardio-pulmonary bypass. Type B aneurysms can often be treated medically, with bed-rest and careful control of blood pressure. In Type B surgical intervention may be needed if there is evidence of leakage or extension, or for renal or bowel ischaemia from the intimal flap.

VENOUS THROMBOSIS

Thrombo-occlusive disease of peripheral veins may present as superficial thrombophlebitis or deep vein thrombosis.

SUPERFICIAL THROMBOPHLEBITIS

This is characterised by a tender painful superficial vein which may be reddened and palpable as a thickened cord. The condition usually occurs in patients with varicose veins and often affects the saphenous vein. Arm veins may be affected following infusion of irritant fluids. Pulmonary embolism is extremely rare. The problem usually resolves spontaneously but analgesics, limb elevation and a non-steroidal anti-inflammatory agent may be required.

DEEP VENOUS THROMBOSIS

This is most common in the lower limbs, particularly in the venous sinuses of the soleus muscle in the calf and in the femoral and iliac veins. It is much less frequent in the upper limb but the axillary vein may be involved as a complication of trauma, long venous infusion catheters, neoplasm or radiotherapy.

Pathology

At first the thrombus consists mainly of dense layers of platelets and fibrin; later it is a loose, friable, jelly-like mass of fibrin and red cells which may become detached to form an embolus. After a few days inflammatory changes occur in the wall of the vein. The thrombus may undergo lysis or organisation.

Aetiology

A number of factors may precipitate venous thrombosis and these are listed in the information box. Although deep vein thrombosis can occur in an otherwise normal individual, a careful search will usually uncover one or more aetiological factors. The condition is extremely common in elderly women with fractured neck of femur, and elderly hemiplegic patients; it is also a common complication of abdominal or gynaecological surgery and of myocardial infarction with prolonged bed rest.

A series of surgical risk factors have been defined (see information box).

FACTORS THAT MAY PREDISPOSE TO VENOUS THROMBOSIS

- **Venous stasis**
  Immobility (bed-rest, surgery, limb paralysis)
  Low cardiac output, varicose veins
- **Venous injury**
  Trauma
  Intravenous cannulation
- **Increased coagulability**
  Malignant disease, drugs (e.g. oestrogens, oral contraceptives), dehydration, polycythaemia, nephrotic syndrome, ulcerative colitis
- **Inherited coagulation defects**
  Antithrombin-III, protein C, protein S deficiency
- **Increasing age**

RISK FACTORS FOR DEEP VENOUS THROMBOSIS FOLLOWING SURGERY

- Abdominal or pelvic surgery
- Prolonged surgery and general anaesthesia
- Old age
- Obesity
- Malignancy
- Prior deep venous thrombosis
- Coagulation disorders (see p. 832)

Clinical features

Deep vein thrombosis may be clinically silent in up to 50% of cases. Some patients may present with pulmonary embolism (see below, p. 277) and, occasionally, hospitalised patients may present with a low-grade pyrexia. There may be pain, swelling, and cyanotic discolouration of the affected limb. If the lumen of the main vein is occluded there may be dilatation of the superficial

veins and the overlying skin may be warm (but not overtly inflamed, as in superficial thrombophlebitis). In the most severe cases the limb may become deeply cyanosed with gross oedema, and venous gangrene may supervene. However, thrombosis may spread proximally without clinical features, and involve ileo-femoral veins.

POST-PHLEBITIC SYNDROME

This is due to long-standing deep venous obstruction with destruction of the deep venous valves. This leads to high pressure in the remaining leg veins and can cause chronic pain, oedema, venous staining, eczema and ulceration.

Diagnosis

Unfortunately, the clinical features of deep vein thrombosis (DVT) are very variable and clinical diagnosis is notoriously unreliable. Clinical features of deep vein thrombosis are usually absent. Indeed, even in the presence of angiographically proven pulmonary embolus, half of the patients will have no clinical signs of DVT.

Ascending venography is the definitive investigation and will also help to define the extent and site of thrombus. Ileo-femoral thrombosis may be detected by ultrasound. Doppler can detect the presence of venous flow, and compression of the femoral vein can demonstrate the presence of thrombus. Definition of the extent of thrombosis influences the choice of treatment because thrombus that extends into the ileo-femoral vessels is more likely to lead to the post-phlebitic syndrome or pulmonary embolism.

Ultrasound examination may also help in the differential diagnosis in the lower leg; this includes simple muscle strain, haematoma and ruptured Baker's cyst (p. 892).

Management

Treatment is aimed at preventing the propagation of thrombus, pulmonary embolism, and damage to the valves of the vein leading to chronic venous insufficiency. Unless there is a major contraindication, such as active peptic ulceration or bleeding, treatment is initiated with heparin (using the same dose as in pulmonary embolism, see p. 279) and continued with warfarin. Thrombolysis with streptokinase, urokinase or t-PA (p. 279) has been shown to improve the outcome in selected cases and should be considered in patients with recent, extensive ileo-femoral thrombosis. See also indications for thrombolysis in pulmonary embolism. Surgical thrombectomy may occasionally be required.

Oral anticoagulants are commonly continued for three months, but this period has not been defined accurately. Indefinite therapy may be indicated in patients with persisting risk factors (see information box) or recurrent episodes of deep vein thrombosis. Most patients require a short period of bed-rest. Mobilisation and physiotherapy can begin as soon as the patient can walk without undue discomfort. Graduated elastic stockings accelerate venous flow and may reduce oedema and encourage recanalisation. However, care must be taken to avoid a constricting effect by the stocking rolling up. Support of this kind may also be necessary to control chronic venous insufficiency.

Prevention

Various measures have been shown to reduce the incidence of deep vein thrombosis and pulmonary embolism in patients at risk. These are most applicable to patients confined to bed or undergoing surgery, when the period of risk can be easily defined (see information box).

PREVENTION OF VENOUS THROMBOEMBOLISM

- **Avoid venous stasis**
  Calf muscle stimulation (during surgery)
  Early mobilisation and active leg exercises
  Graduated support stockings
- **Anticoagulants**
  Low dose heparin (or low molecular weight heparin)
  (e.g. 5000 units subcutaneously 8–12-hourly)
  Low dose warfarin/coumadin (INR 1.2–1.5:1)
  Full dose i.v. heparin or oral warfarin for patients at high risk.

PULMONARY THROMBOEMBOLISM

Aetiology and incidence

Pulmonary embolism most commonly results from detachment of vascular thrombus from the leg (70–80%) or pelvis (10–15%). Other rare causes of pulmonary embolism include amniotic fluid, placenta, air, fat, tumour (e.g. choriocarcinoma) and parasites such as schistosomula. Effectively, the prophylaxis of pulmonary embolism is that of the prophylaxis and treatment of deep venous thrombosis (above). Pulmonary thromboembolism is one of the most common acute severe pulmonary illnesses and accounts for at least 30 000 deaths per annum in the UK. Symptomatic pulmonary emboli occur in up to 1% of all postoperative patients. However, the autopsy incidence is 10–25% and in one-third of these, pulmonary embolism is a major cause of death. A significant proportion of these are not suspected in life. Thus continued awareness of the possibility of pulmonary embolism in high risk groups

and willingness to pursue the diagnosis on the grounds of clinical suspicion is likely to reduce morbidity and save lives.

Pathophysiology

The pathophysiological consequences, clinical presentations, physical signs and results of investigations can most easily be understood if pulmonary emboli are classified simply on a basis of size—massive; small or medium sized; and multiple microemboli.

Massive emboli become lodged in the proximal pulmonary arteries and chambers of the right heart, causing an acute and catastrophic reduction in cardiac output and right heart failure with major disruption in pulmonary ventilation-perfusion relationships due to massive areas of the lung being ventilated but not perfused.

Small and medium-sized emboli occlude segmental arteries, causing infarction of the segment, pleural pain, haemoptysis and reduction in surfactant. This is often associated with localised loss of lung volume and collapse. A fever, which is usually low grade, may be a feature in some patients with established infarction.

In the rare condition of multiple microemboli, showers of tiny emboli occlude the capillary beds of the lung. Due to collateral vascular supply there is no infarction but insidious loss of the microvascular bed supplying the gas exchange units of the lung (see Fig. 6.1, p. 314). Patients with this condition may present with atypical exertional dyspnoea but often the condition is not suspected until there are late complications including severe pulmonary hypertension and right ventricular failure.

Clinical features

Massive pulmonary thromboembolism

Patients classically present several days after a major operation or other predisposing event with central chest pain, acute dyspnoea and apprehension. Symptoms due to sudden loss of cerebral and coronary blood flow, secondary to obstruction of right ventricular outflow, are often prominent. These include faintness, syncope and circulatory arrest. Pleurisy and haemoptysis are uncommon although they may have occurred as a result of a previous 'sentinel' small embolus causing infarction (up to one-third of massive embolic events are preceded by a sentinel embolus). Unlike other causes of acute severe dyspnoea (p. 323), which are associated with orthopnoea, the patient with massive embolisation may be more comfortable lying flat. On examination, the patient, if conscious, will have a sinus tachycardia and other signs of low cardiac output including hypotension, impaired cerebration and peripheral vasoconstriction. Tachypnoea and central cyanosis will be obvious and the JVP will be elevated. A right ventricular gallop rhythm is an important physical sign in the first 24 hours and in established pulmonary embolus a widely split P_2 may be detected.

Despite the major disorder of gas exchange there may be few if any signs on percussion and auscultation of the chest. If a patient (particularly one with a predisposing condition) is tachypnoeic, cyanosed, without major chest signs but with signs of reduced cardiac output and raised JVP, the diagnosis is massive pulmonary embolism until proven otherwise.

Small/medium-sized embolus

The patient classically presents with pleuritic chest pain and dyspnoea which is proportional to the severity of pain and associated restriction of ventilation. In established infarction up to 50% of patients will exhibit haemoptysis. On examination cyanosis is not prominent unless there has been repeated or extensive embolisation, in which case the JVP may also be elevated. In established infarction, pyrexia and signs of a pleural effusion or elevation of the hemidiaphragm (which may mimic pleural effusion) may be present. A localised wheeze or a pleural rub may be heard, but the commonest signs in the first 36 hours are reduced air entry with a few coarse crepitations.

Multiple microemboli

This rare condition usually presents with a history of increasing exertional dyspnoea over several months and later weakness, angina and even syncope on exertion. Before severe pulmonary hypertension and right ventricular failure develop, physical signs may be absent (pulmonary hypertension does not develop until two-thirds of the pulmonary vascular bed has been destroyed) and such patients, with a potentially treatable disease, may be labelled as 'hysterical' until it is too late for a useful functional recovery.

Investigations

(i) Massive embolus

Bedside investigations can provide useful signs (Table 5.9, p. 281) supporting a clinical diagnosis. Echocardiography usually demonstrates a small and vigorously contracting left ventricle, and occasionally thrombus can be seen in the right ventricular outflow tract or main pulmonary artery. Chest radiograph features including oligaemia of affected areas and dilatation of the hilar pulmonary arterial trunk may be unimpressive, or subtle. Massive embolism can occur without infarct shadows or evidence of loss of lung volume if there have been no previous pulmonary infarcts due to sentinel emboli. A number of 'classical' ECG patterns have been described (see Table 5.9 and Fig. 5.75)

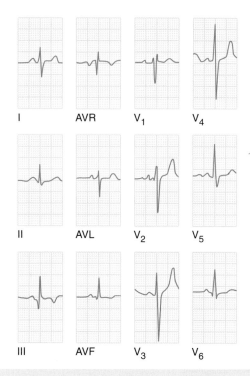

Fig. 5.75 ECG from patient with pulmonary embolism showing '$S_1Q_3T_3$' pattern.

($S_1Q_3T_3$) but these can change rapidly and often the only abnormality is sinus tachycardia. Arterial blood gases typically show severe hypoxaemia and often marked hypocapnia. This is an unusual combination, and while it may also occur in severe acute asthma and patients with left ventricular failure, these conditions are usually easy to distinguish from massive embolisation on clinical grounds.

In some cases pulmonary angiography is necessary to confirm the diagnosis. This technique not only provides 'gold standard' confirmation of the diagnosis but the catheter in situ can be used to measure haemodynamic effects and for the delivery of thrombolytic agents.

(ii) Small/medium-sized embolus

The chest radiograph may show a number of different features depending upon the age of the infarct(s) (see Fig. 5.76), but horizontal linear opacities (particularly if bilateral) strongly support a clinical diagnosis. During the evolution of infarction, the chest radiograph appearances can change rapidly over 24 hours. Arterial blood gases may show hypocapnia if hyperventilation is prominent but unless embolisation has been extensive hypoxaemia is not usually a feature. Similarly, the ECG is usually unhelpful, but if embolisation has been extensive there may be signs of right ventricular hypertrophy

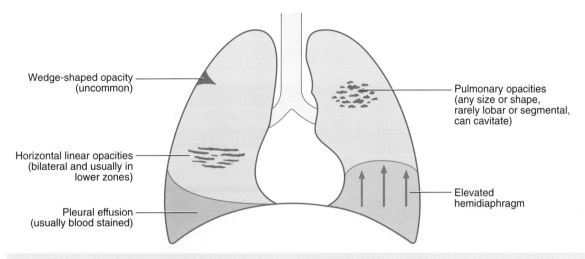

Wedge-shaped opacity
(uncommon)

Pulmonary opacities
(any size or shape,
rarely lobar or segmental,
can cavitate)

Horizontal linear opacities
(bilateral and usually in
lower zones)

Pleural effusion
(usually blood stained)

Elevated
hemidiaphragm

Fig. 5.76 Features of pulmonary thromboembolism/infarction on chest radiograph.

and strain (see p. 280). If a small pleural effusion is present this is usually (although not invariably) blood-stained and a diagnostic aspiration with a 21G needle can be useful since the only other common cause of a blood-stained pleural effusion is malignancy. In established, uncomplicated pulmonary infarction a peripheral blood leucocytosis (up to 20 000) may be detected. A ventilation-perfusion scan (p. 319) is usually required to support the diagnosis, although empirical anti-coagulation should be commenced while the investigation is awaited (see Fig. 5.77). In difficult cases pulmonary angiography (p. 319) may be necessary to establish a confident diagnosis.

(iii) Chronic microembolic disease

At an early stage before severe pulmonary hypertension or right ventricular failure sets in, most investigations will be unrevealing. The chest radiograph may show enlarged pulmonary arteries; at a later stage this sign together with oligaemia of the peripheral lung fields may become prominent. Exercise-induced hypoxaemia or desaturation upon formal exercise testing (p. 322) may be a very useful early sign, which may prompt cath-eterisation studies which could show raised pulmonary artery pressures. However, confirmation of the diagnosis in microvascular embolism may be very difficult since ventilation-perfusion scintigraphy, and even pulmonary angiography, may not demonstrate the microvascular lesions. Occasionally an open lung biopsy may be necessary to demonstrate the intravascular thrombi. It has been suggested recently that many if not all cases of so-called thromboembolic pulmonary hypertension may in fact represent primary pulmonary hypertension with super-added thrombus formation. At a late stage in the

disease the classical ECG and radiological features of pulmonary hypertension (p. 280) and right ventricular failure (p. 220) usually become obvious but by this stage the prognosis is poor.

Management

(i) Massive thromboembolism

In the shocked or collapsed patient, external cardiac massage/oxygen treatment, vasopressors and reversal of acidosis (p. 215) are often necessary. The central aims are to counter the haemodynamic consequences of the embolus and to prevent further embolisation. If initial resuscitation has not restored an adequate cardiac output, embolectomy may be necessary.

Thrombolytic therapy

The rationale for thrombolytic therapy in massive thromboembolism is based on the observation that patients who survive the acute event may die in the succeeding hours or days, presumably from the effects of continued haemodynamic disturbance or the effects of further emboli in a critically compromised circulation. The usual treatment is 250 000–500 000 Units of strep-tokinase in dextrose or saline given intravenously (or via a cannula inserted in the pulmonary artery) over 30 minutes. This is followed by a maintenance dose of 100 000–150 000 Units per hour for 72 hours. Clinical efficacy has been demonstrated with shorter infusions of tPA (alteplase) 100 mg over 2 hours. This will provide adequate treatment for the majority of patients, but the adverse effects obviously can include haemorrhage, and there are a number of relative contraindications to thrombolytic therapy (see p. 262).

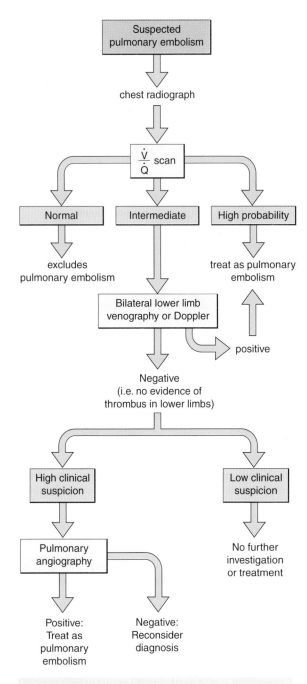

Fig. 5.77 Flow chart for the investigation of pulmonary thromboembolism.

Occasionally, patients need higher doses but this should be approached in close collaboration with the blood coagulation laboratory. Generally the maintenance dose of heparin is monitored by the thrombin time, which should ideally be maintained at around 3 x

normal (> 4 x carries the risk of haemorrhage and < 2 x may be insufficient to prevent re-thrombosis).

Prevention of further embolisation

Anticoagulation therapy (p. 840) has long been known to reduce the mortality rate from pulmonary thromboembolism, probably by preventing the extension of embolic occlusion from further localised pulmonary thrombosis and by arresting further deep venous thrombosis (see p. 275).

(ii) Small/medium-sized embolus

There is no specific treatment for the pulmonary effects of a small embolus leading to infarction, apart from pain relief. However, it must be remembered that such emboli may precede massive thromboembolism, and prompt anticoagulation (p. 840) is essential. Therefore early diagnosis by venography (p. 278) and decisions about other local measures (p. 277) and long-term anticoagulation will be necessary.

(iii) Chronic microembolisation

Patients with this uncommon, relentlessly progressive condition require prompt diagnosis, hopefully before severe pulmonary hypertension has set in, and long-term anticoagulation.

In patients for whom anticoagulation is contraindicated or who have persistent lower limb-derived thromboembolisation despite therapeutic anticoagulation, it may be necessary to consider interruption of the inferior vena cava by 'umbrellas' or other devices.

PRIMARY PULMONARY HYPERTENSION

This is a rare condition, occurring more frequently in females, particularly children and young adults. Some cases are probably caused by multiple small pulmonary emboli or a poorly understood thrombotic process occurring locally in the pulmonary arteries, but in many others the aetiology is obscure. The pathological features, which include medial hypertrophy and fibrinoid necrosis, occur in all branches of the pulmonary arterial tree and result in pulmonary vascular obstruction, severe pulmonary hypertension and right heart failure. Patients usually present with dyspnoea on exertion, but physical signs may be unimpressive until right heart failure sets in. The diagnosis may be suspected after exercise-induced desaturation, and is confirmed by unexplained severe pulmonary hypertension with right heart pressures which may exceed systemic levels. Most patients die within 2–3 years of the onset of symptoms and anticoagulation or treatment with vasodilators

Table 5.9 Categorisation of pulmonary thromboemboli

		Acute massive	Acute small/medium	Chronic microembolism
Pathophysiology		Major haemodynamic effects: $\downarrow$ Cardiac output; acute right heart failure; disordered ventilation/perfusion ratio	Occlusion of segmental pulmonary artery $\rightarrow$ infarction $\pm$ effusion	Chronic occlusion of pulmonary micro-vasculature; pulmonary hypertension, right heart failure
Symptoms		Sudden syncope, faintness, central chest pain, apprehension, severe dyspnoea	Pleurisy, restricted breathing, haemoptysis	Exertional dyspnoea. Late—exertional syncope, symptoms of RV failure
Signs	Cardiovascular	Major circulatory collapse; tachycardia; hypotension; $\uparrow$ JVP; gallop rhythm; P_2 widely split (late)		May be nil early. Late—RV heave, loud, split P_2. Terminal—signs of RV failure
	Respiratory	Severe cyanosis, otherwise no local signs	Pleural rub, raised hemidiaphragm, crepitations, effusion (usually blood-stained)	
	Other	$\downarrow$ urine output	Low grade fever	
Investigations	Chest radiograph	Often subtle; oligaemic lung fields, slight $\uparrow$ hilar shadows	Pleuro-pulmonary opacities; pleural effusion; linear shadows; raised hemidiaphragm	Enlarged pulmonary trunk; enlarged heart, prominent RV
	ECG	$S_1 Q_3 T_3$ (p.278) T wave $\downarrow V_1$-V_4 RBBB		Signs of RV hypertrophy and 'strain'
	Blood gases	$\downarrow PaO_2 \downarrow PaCO_2$	$(\downarrow PaCO_2)$	Exertional $\downarrow PaO_2$ or desaturation (on formal exercise testing)
	V/Q scan	Major areas of $\downarrow$ perfusion	Perfusion defect(s) not matched on the ventilation scan	May be no abnormality
	Pulmonary angiography	Definitive diagnosis	Definitive diagnosis	May be no abnormality. May need lung biopsy to confirm diagnosis

appears to have little efficacy. Heart-lung transplantation should be considered early.

FURTHER READING

Beard K, Bulpitt,C, Mascie-Taylor H, O'Malley K, Sever P et al 1992 Management of elderly patients with sustained hypertension. British Medical Journal 304: 412–416
Collins R, Peto R, MacMahon S, Herbert P, Fiebach M H et al 1990 Blood pressure, stroke and coronary heart disease. Lancet 335: 827–838
MRC Working Party 1992 Medical Research Council trial of treatment of hypertension in older adults: principal results. British Medical Journal 304: 405–412

PRINCIPAL CAUSES OF VALVE DISEASE

Valve regurgitation	Valve stenosis
• Congenital	• Congenital
• Acute rheumatic carditis	• Rheumatic carditis
• Chronic rheumatic carditis	• Senile degeneration
• Infective endocarditis	
• Syphilitic aortitis	
• Valve ring dilatation (e.g. dilated cardiomyopathy)	
• Traumatic valve rupture	
• Senile degeneration	
• Damage to chordae and papillary muscles (e.g. MI)	

DISEASES OF THE HEART VALVES

A diseased valve may be narrowed (stenosed) or it may fail to close adequately, and thus permit regurgitation of blood. The term 'incompetence' may be used synonymously with regurgitation or reflux, but the latter descriptions are preferable. The principal causes of valve disease are summarised in the information box (right).

The aetiology of individual valve lesions is considered separately below.

RHEUMATIC HEART DISEASE

ACUTE RHEUMATIC FEVER

Aetiology and prevalence

Acute rheumatic fever is triggered by infection with specific strains of streptococcus pyogenes which express antigens that cross-react with those of human connective tissue. A cell wall constituent (N-acetylglycosamine) of the group A streptococcus shares antigenic properties with heart valve glycoprotein.

The condition usually affects children or young adults, and there is a familial variation in susceptibility. Its prevalence in Western Europe and North America has progressively declined to very low levels, but it remains common in parts of Asia, Africa, South America and Eastern Europe. In developing countries rheumatic fever is still the most common cause of acquired heart disease in childhood and adolescence and the most common cause of death in the first five decades of life.

Clinical features

Rheumatic fever is a systemic illness typically presenting with fever, anorexia, lethargy and joint pains. Arthritis

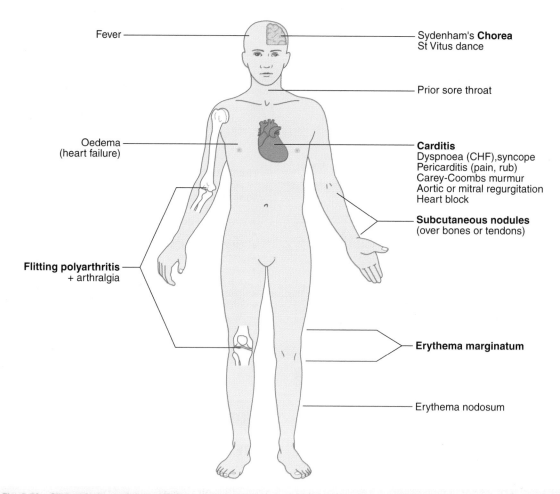

Fever — Sydenham's **Chorea** / St Vitus dance

Prior sore throat

Oedema (heart failure)

Carditis / Dyspnoea (CHF),syncope / Pericarditis (pain, rub) / Carey-Coombs murmur / Aortic or mitral regurgitation / Heart block

Subcutaneous nodules (over bones or tendons)

Flitting polyarthritis + arthralgia

Erythema marginatum

Erythema nodosum

Fig. 5.78 Clinical features of rheumatic fever. Bold labels indicate Duckett–Jones major criteria.

occurs in approximately 75% of patients and other features include skin rashes, carditis and neurological features (Fig. 5.78). According to the revised Duckett–Jones criteria, the diagnosis is based upon two or more major clinical manifestations; or one major and two or more minor manifestations. In both cases evidence of previous streptococcal infection is required. (*Evidence*: anti-streptococcal antibody; anti-streptolysin antibody; positive culture for group A streptococcus; recent scarlet fever).

Carditis

This is the most important manifestation of rheumatic fever. Carditis presents as breathlessness (due to heart failure or pericardial effusion), palpitations, or chest pain (usually due to peri- or pancarditis). Other features consist of tachycardia, cardiac enlargement and new or changed cardiac murmurs. A soft systolic murmur is common but non-specific. A soft mid-diastolic murmur (Carey–Coombs murmur) can be due to valvulitis with nodules forming on the mitral valve leaflets. There may be a pericardial friction rub—often intermittent. Cardiac failure may result either from impaired function of ventricular muscle or from mitral or aortic incompetence. Severe mitral or aortic incompetence occurs in a 'fulminant' form of rheumatic fever more common in developing countries. Electrocardiographic changes include ST or T wave changes; conduction defects sometimes occur which may cause syncope.

Sydenham's chorea (St Vitus dance)

Central nervous system involvement may manifest late after the initial infection (6 months or more), with those affected exhibiting spasmodic unintentional movements and possibly altered speech. Spontaneous recovery is usual, though it may be followed by chronic cardiac disease.

Arthritis

The arthritis of rheumatic fever is often symmetrical, affecting large joints with acute painful inflammation which characteristically 'flits' from joint to joint (i.e. a migratory polyarthralgia). The joints affected include those of the limbs, spine, and sometimes temporomandibular and costoclavicular joints. There is commonly, but not invariably, a history of sore throat 2–4 weeks before the onset of joint symptoms. In adults, joint symptoms tend to be more prominent than carditis; in children under six years old the converse may be true.

Skin lesions

The following may be present:

- **Erythema marginatum**, which occurs in 10–20% of children with rheumatic fever. It starts as red mac-

---

INVESTIGATIONS IN ACUTE RHEUMATIC FEVER

- **Evidence of a systemic illness** (nonspecific)
  Leucocytosis, raised ESR, raised C-reactive protein
- **Evidence of preceding streptococcal infection** (specific):
  Throat swab culture: group A beta haemolytic streptococci (also from family members and contacts)
  Antistreptolysin O antibodies (ASO titres): rising titres, or levels of >200 units (adults), >300 units (children)
- **Evidence of carditis**
  Chest radiograph: cardiomegaly; pulmonary congestion
  ECG: first and second degree heart block; features of pericarditis; T wave inversion; reduction in QRS voltages
  Echocardiography: cardiac dilatation and valve abnormalities

---

ules (blotches) which fade in the centre but remain red at the edges. The resulting red rings or 'margins' may coalesce or overlap.

- **Erythema nodosum**, dusky red raised papules or nodules, usually on the front of the shins; they are less common, and less specific.
- **Subcutaneous nodules** are uncommon, but associated with more severe carditis. They are small (<0.5 cm), firm, painless, and best felt over bone or tendons. Typically the nodules are much smaller than those of rheumatoid arthritis. Other systemic manifestations are rare, but include pleurisy, pleural effusion and pneumonia.

Investigations

These are listed in the information box below.

It is important to note that while the systemic markers are nonspecific, they may be useful in following progress of the disease. Furthermore, positive throat cultures are present only in a minority of patients at the time of clinical presentation and ASO titres are normal in about a fifth of adult cases of rheumatic fever and most cases of chorea.

Management

Treatment for acute rheumatic fever is directed towards limiting cardiac damage, relieving symptoms and eliminating the streptoccal infection.

Bed-rest and supportive therapy

During the acute phase of rheumatic fever or during active carditis the patient should be rested in bed, as otherwise there is a risk of recurrence of signs and symptoms. Later, the patient may feel well although temperature, leucocyte count and erythrocyte sedimentation rate (ESR) remain elevated. Bed-rest must be continued until these indices of continuing disease activity have settled. In patients who have had carditis, it is conventional to continue bed-rest for 2–6 weeks after the ESR and temperature have returned to normal.

Cardiac failure should be treated as necessary (see p. 222). Valve replacement may be required for severe mitral or aortic incompetence. Heart block is seldom progressive, and pacemaker therapy is rarely needed. Prolonged bed-rest, particularly in children or adolescents, produces problems of boredom and depression that need to be anticipated and managed.

Aspirin

In large regular doses aspirin is effective in providing symptomatic relief of arthritis. A reasonable starting dose is 60 mg/kg body-weight per day, divided into 6 doses. In adults up to 120 mg/kg/day may be needed, up to the limits of tolerance or a maximum of 8 g per day. Mild toxic effects include nausea, tinnitus and deafness, more serious ones are vomiting, tachypnoea and acidosis. Aspirin should be continued until the ESR has fallen, and then gradually tailed off.

Corticosteroids

These produce more rapid symptomatic relief than aspirin, and are indicated in cases with carditis or severe arthritis. There is no evidence that long-term steroids are beneficial. Prednisolone or prednisone 1.0–2.0 mg/kg per day in divided doses should be continued until ESR is normal, then gradually tailed off.

Antistreptococcal therapy

Eradication of streptococcal infections and prevention of recurrence are important. Benzathine penicillin 916 mg (1.2 million Units) should be given on diagnosis, once a week for 3 weeks, and then monthly for the first year. Subsequent prophylaxis may be with oral phenoxy-methyl–penicillin 500 mg continued for at least 5 years after the last attack and until the patient reaches at least 20 years of age (250 mg 12-hourly may be used, but the results are inferior to the higher oral dose or the intramuscular route). If compliance with an oral regimen is in doubt, then i.m. administration may be employed.

Recurrences are more common when cardiac disease is present and, if so, prophylaxis should continue until age 30. A sulphonamide, or erythromycin, may be used if the patient is allergic to penicillin.

Follow-up

Carditis most frequently occurs within 2 weeks of the onset of arthritis. Chronic rheumatic heart disease is much commoner in patients who have carditis during the initial attack or during a recurrence. It is important to prevent recurrence by continuing antistreptococcal prophylaxis, and to recognise and follow up chronic valve lesions, but at the same time it is important not to induce a cardiac neurosis. Echocardiography is valuable in assessing valve problems. If it is normal, yearly follow-ups can be extended to two-yearly, and discontinued ten years after the initial attack.

CHRONIC RHEUMATIC HEART DISEASE

Chronic valvular heart disease develops subsequently in at least half of those affected by rheumatic fever with carditis. The predominantly affected valve is the mitral (in > 90%) and then less commonly the aortic, tricuspid and pulmonary. The lesions develop after 10–20 years in 'Western' countries but much earlier in developing countries.

Pathology

The main pathological process in chronic rheumatic heart disease is a progressive fibrosis particularly affecting the heart valves. This is in contrast to the destructive lytic process in acute rheumatic fever. The condition also affects the pericardium and myocardium and may contribute to heart failure and conduction disorders. For the mitral valve the result is shortening of the chordae tendineae, fusion of the commisures and a reduction in size of the valve orifice. The haemodynamic result is mitral stenosis with or without regurgitation. Similar disorders of the aortic and tricuspid valves produce distortion and rigidity of the cusps, and in consequence, stenosis and incompetence. Once damage has developed on a valve, the altered haemodynamic stresses on the valve perpetuate and extend the damage even in the absence of a continuing rheumatic process.

MITRAL VALVE DISEASE

MITRAL STENOSIS

Aetiology and pathophysiology

Isolated mitral stenosis accounts for about 25% of all cases of rheumatic heart disease, and an additional 40% have mixed mitral stenosis and regurgitation. Two thirds of cases occur in women. Acquired mitral stenosis is almost entirely rheumatic in origin, but there is evidence that some cases may follow a viral carditis. Some cases of rheumatic fever may be unrecognised and it is only possible to elicit a history of rheumatic fever or chorea in about half of the patients.

The mitral valve orifice is normally about 5 cm^2 in diastole, and is reduced to 1 cm or less in severe mitral stenosis. Patients usually remain asymptomatic until the stenosis is moderate (approx 2 cm^2). With the reduction in size of the valve orifice, cardiac output can be maintained only by a rise in left atrial, pulmonary venous and

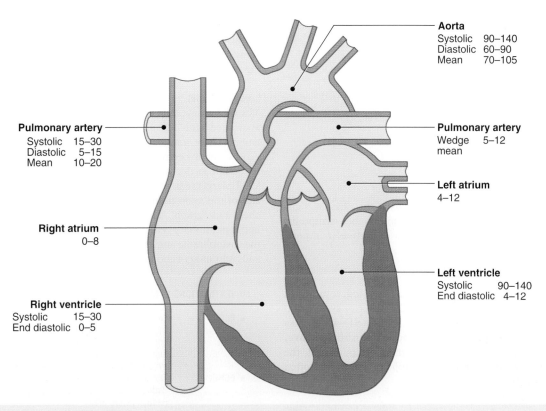

Aorta
Systolic   90–140
Diastolic 60–90
Mean   70–105

Pulmonary artery
Systolic   15–30
Diastolic 5–15
Mean   10–20

Pulmonary artery
Wedge   5–12
mean

Left atrium
4–12

Right atrium
0–8

Left ventricle
Systolic   90–140
End diastolic 4–12

Right ventricle
Systolic   15–30
End diastolic 0–5

Fig. 5.79   Line diagram of the heart with normal pressure values (mmHg).

pulmonary capillary pressures, with resulting loss of lung compliance and the development of exertional dyspnoea. With mild stenosis atrial pressure rises only on exercise, but as the stenosis becomes more severe ($1.0–1.5$ cm^2), raised left atrial pressure is required to maintain cardiac output even at rest, with further increases in pressure on exercise. The raised atrial pressure precipitates atrial fibrillation, which may be the first sign of clinical deterioration. Loss of co-ordinated atrial contraction, and shortened diastole in uncontrolled atrial fibrillation, both contribute to diminished ventricular filling. Conditions associated with an increase in cardiac output (e.g. pregnancy) are tolerated poorly.

A sudden increase in pulmonary venous pressure, caused perhaps by the onset of atrial fibrillation, may precipitate pulmonary oedema. The onset of atrial fibrillation may be accompanied by a 20% fall in cardiac output. With a more gradual rise in pressure, there tends to be an increase in pulmonary vascular resistance which protects against pulmonary oedema.

In about 80% of cases left atrial dilatation is prominent, and is usually accompanied by atrial fibrillation. A minority of patients remain in sinus rhythm; this is usually associated with a small fibrotic left atrium and severe

pulmonary hypertension. All cases may eventually develop pulmonary hypertension and right ventricular hypertrophy. The pulmonary hypertension results from a combination of passive back-pressure, arteriolar constriction, and obliterative changes in the pulmonary vasculature.

All patients with mitral stenosis are at risk from left atrial thrombosis and systemic thromboembolism, particularly those with atrial fibrillation. Prior to anticoagulant therapy, emboli caused a quarter of all deaths in this condition.

Clinical features
The main features of mitral stenosis are tabulated below.

Symptoms
The gradual reduction in the mitral valve orifice usually produces insidious onset of breathlessness, and pulmonary congestion may cause cough. The extra demands of pregnancy, or the impairment of function brought about by tachycardia or atrial fibrillation, may precipitate deterioration, and may bring on breathlessness even at rest. Acute pulmonary oedema or pulmonary hypertension can lead to haemoptysis. Systemic embolism is sometimes a presenting feature.

Asymptomatic mitral stenosis: the physical signs of mitral stenosis are often found before symptoms develop, and their recognition is of particular importance in pregnancy.

Signs

The stenotic valve prolongs atrial emptying, resulting in the leaflets remaining open at the onset of systole and closing with an unusually loud sound (S1) which may be palpable—the tapping apex beat. The turbulent flow, which is heralded by the opening snap, causes the characteristic low pitched diastolic murmur, and often a thrill (Fig. 5.80).

The murmur is accentuated by exercise and during atrial systole. In early or asymptomatic patients a presystolic murmur may be the only auscultatory abnormality. In patients with symptoms the murmur usually extends from the opening snap to the first heart sound. The opening snap gets closer to the second sound (S2) as the stenosis becomes more severe, but may be inaudible if the valve is heavily calcified. Accompanying mitral regurgitation causes a pansystolic murmur which radiates towards the axilla.

The development of pulmonary hypertension may be demonstrated by an abnormal pulsation felt to the left of the sternum, due either to right ventricular hypertrophy or to forward displacement of the heart by a dilated left atrium. Pulmonary hypertension may cause a loud pulmonary component of the second heart sound, and right atrial hypertrophy may produce a prominent *a*

wave in the jugular venous pulse (unless atrial fibrillation is present). Tricuspid regurgitation secondary to right ventricular dilatation causes a systolic murmur and systolic waves in the venous pulse.

Investigations

The ECG may show either the bifid p waves (p mitrale) associated with left atrial hypertrophy or atrial fibrillation. There may be evidence of right atrial and right ventricular hypertrophy; one of the earliest signs is a reduction in the size of the usual QS complex in lead VI. Enlargement of the left atrium and its appendage and of the main pulmonary artery may be seen on the chest radiograph. There may be enlargement of the upper pulmonary veins and horizontal linear shadows in the costophrenic angles as indications of a high left atrial and pulmonary venous pressure.

Echocardiography can provide the definitive evaluation of mitral stenosis; apart from confirming the diagnosis it allows an assessment of its severity and it also provides information on the rigidity and state of calcification of the valve cusps, the size of the left atrium, and the state of left ventricular function (Fig. 5.81).

Prior to the advent of echocardiography, cardiac catheterisation was used to confirm the severity of mitral stenosis by measurement of the gradient across the mitral valve from pressures recorded simultaneously in the left ventricle and left atrium (or pulmonary capillary wedge position). Cardiac catheterisation may still have a role in assessing coexisting mitral regurgitation and coronary disease.

Management

Patients with minor symptoms should be treated medically, but the definitive treatment of mitral stenosis is by mitral valvotomy, balloon valvuloplasty or mitral valve replacement. If the patient remains symptomatic despite medical treatment, if pulmonary congestion persists, or if pulmonary hypertension develops, valvuloplasty or surgery is indicated.

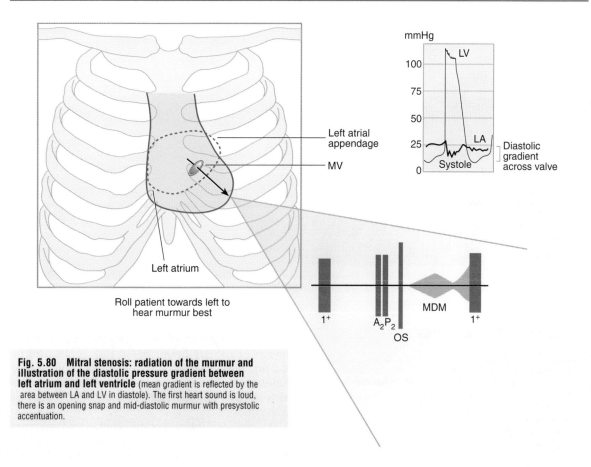

Roll patient towards left to
hear murmur best

Left atrial
appendage

MV

Left atrium

mmHg

LV

LA

Systole

Diastolic
gradient
across valve

1^+ A_2P_2 OS   MDM 1^+

**Fig. 5.80   Mitral stenosis: radiation of the murmur and
illustration of the diastolic pressure gradient between
left atrium and left ventricle** (mean gradient is reflected by the
area between LA and LV in diastole). The first heart sound is loud,
there is an opening snap and mid-diastolic murmur with presystolic
accentuation.

Medical management
This consists of anticoagulants (p. 840) to reduce the
risk of systemic embolism, digoxin (0.125–0.25 mg/d)
to control the ventricular rate in atrial fibrillation (or to
prevent a rapid ventricular rate if atrial fibrillation should
develop), diuretics to control pulmonary congestion (p.
222) and antibiotic prophylaxis against infective endocarditis (p. 299).

Mitral balloon valvuloplasty
This is the treatment of choice if the appropriate criteria
are fulfilled (see information box). Closed or open mitral
valvotomy may be used if the facilities or expertise for
valvuloplasty are not available.

Mitral valve replacement
If there is substantial mitral reflux, or if the valve is rigid
and calcified, then surgery rather than balloon valvuloplasty is indicated.

Monitoring and after care
Clinical symptoms are a guide to the severity of mitral re-
stenosis, but echocardiography provides a more accurate

CRITERIA FOR MITRAL VALVULOPLASTY

- Significant symptoms
- Isolated mitral stenosis
- No (or trivial) mitral regurgitation
- Mobile, non-calcified valve/sub-valve apparatus on echo
- Left atrium free of thrombus

assessment. The ECG gives evidence of increasing pulmonary hypertension and the heart size on chest radiography is a useful but not infallible guide to severity.
Patients who have had a mitral valvuloplasty or valvotomy should be followed up at 1–2 yearly intervals
because re-stenosis may eventually occur.

MITRAL REGURGITATION

Aetiology and pathophysiology
Chronic, gradual-onset mitral regurgitation produces
volume overload of the left atrium. Left atrial dilatation

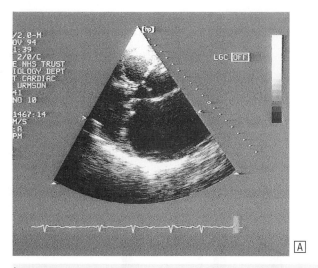

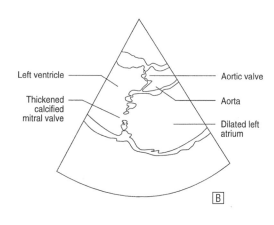

Left ventricle

Thickened
calcified
mitral valve

Aortic valve

Aorta

Dilated left
atrium

Fig. 5.81 A Echocardiogram of mitral stenosis. B Line diagram of main features.

CAUSES OF MITRAL REGURGITATION

- Mitral valve prolapse
- Dilatation of the mitral valve ring
  (e.g. rheumatic fever, myocarditis, cardiomyopathy)
- Damage to valve cusps and chordae
  rheumatic heart disease, endocarditis
- Damage to papillary muscle
- Myocardial infarction

---

occurs and there is little increase in pressure until heart failure ensues. In contrast, acute regurgitation results in a rapid rise in left atrial pressure because atrial compliance is normal. The raised atrial and pulmonary venous pressure leads to pulmonary oedema and can be measured invasively. As part of the left ventricular stroke volume regurgitates into the atrium the stroke volume has to increase to maintain cardiac output, and this results in ventricular enlargement.

Mitral prolapse

This is also known as 'floppy' mitral valve. It is one of the more common causes of mild mitral regurgitation, and is caused by congenital abnormality or degenerative myxomatous changes. Mitral prolapse is sometimes a feature of connective tissue disorders such as Marfan's syndrome.

In the mildest forms of mitral prolapse the valve remains competent but bulges back into the atrium during systole, causing a mid-systolic click, and no murmur. In the presence of a regurgitant valve the click is followed by a late systolic murmur. The murmur lengthens as regurgitation becomes more severe, and the com-

bination of a click and late systolic murmur provides the clinical hallmark of mitral prolapse. Occasionally, multiple clicks are heard, or the click is obscured by the first heart sound; the pansystolic murmur may be indistinguishable from other causes of mitral regurgitation. The physical signs may vary with posture or respiration.

Progressive elongation of the chordae tendineae may lead to increasing mitral regurgitation, while if chordal rupture occurs, regurgitation may suddenly become severe. These complications are rare before the fifth or sixth decade.

Mitral prolapse is associated with an increased incidence of arrhythmias—these are usually benign but a small minority of patients have frequent and bizarre arrhythmias. Some patients with atypical chest pain are found to have mitral prolapse but this association is not specific. Telling a patient there is an abnormal valve sometimes exacerbates or perpetuates a cardiac neurosis. Mitral prolapse is more common than would be expected in young people with embolic stroke or transient cerebral ischaemic attacks, but the overall risk of the complication is exceedingly small. Haemodynamically significant mitral prolapse can predispose to infective endocarditis, and hence requires antibiotic prophylaxis, but overall the long-term prognosis is good.

Other causes of mitral regurgitation

Regurgitation can result from dilatation of the mitral valve ring in association with diseases involving the myocardium, such as rheumatic fever, extensive infarction, diphtheria, myocarditis or cardiomyopathy. Papillary muscle dysfunction commonly follows myocardial infarction. Rupture of the papillary muscles or chordae may also occur with infarction, resulting in acute severe pulmonary oedema. The valve cusps may also be damaged gradually from chronic rheumatic heart disease, in which case there is often coexisting mitral stenosis and/or aortic valve disease. Mitral regurgitation can develop rapidly with infective endocarditis. The main features of mitral reflux are listed in the information box below.

SYMPTOMS OF MITRAL REGURGITATION

Acute mitral regurgitation
- Symptoms of acute pulmonary oedema and reduced cardiac output

Chronic progressive mitral regurgitation
- Exertional dyspnoea, nocturnal dyspnoea, palpitations (AF, atrial flutter, increased stroke volume)
- Symptoms of pulmonary oedema (esp. with pregnancy or AF)
- Symptoms of diminished cardiac output, e.g. fatigue, tiredness
- Ankle, leg oedema, abdominal swelling (right heart failure)

SIGNS OF MITRAL REGURGITATION

- Atrial fibrillation/flutter
- Cardiomegaly—displaced hyperdynamic apex beat
- Apical pansystolic murmur ± thrill
- Soft S1, apical S3
- Signs of raised pulmonary capillary pressure crepitations, pulmonary oedema, effusions
- Signs of pulmonary hypertension may be present

Clinical features

These are summarised in the information box.

The symptoms depend on how suddenly the regurgitation develops. When the valve damage is a slow process the symptoms are similar to those in mitral stenosis. After acute myocardial infarction, the mitral regurgitation may be severe, and should be differentiated from ventricular septal rupture.

The physical signs arise from the regurgitant jet which causes an apical systolic murmur. This often radiates into the axilla, and may be accompanied by a thrill. The apex beat is usually displaced to the left as a result of dilatation of the left ventricle. The abnormal valve closure is often associated with a quiet first heart sound, and the increased forward flow through the mitral valve may give rise to a loud third heart sound and even a short mid-diastolic murmur.

Investigations

The radiograph and ECG often give evidence of left atrial and/or left ventricular hypertrophy. Atrial fibrillation is common, as a consequence of atrial dilatation. Echocardiography provides information about the state of the mitral valve, but Doppler (or Colour Doppler) cardiography gives a better estimate of the extent of regurgitation (Fig. 5.16, p. 208). At cardiac catheterisation the severity of mitral regurgitation may be indicated by the size of the v waves in the left atrial or PAW trace, or by left ventricular angiography. However, this is not always reliable, as left atrial compliance may vary. In practice, the usual problem lies in deciding the extent to which cardiac failure is due to mitral regurgitation and the extent to which it reflects impaired left ventricular function.

Management

If mitral regurgitation is due to myocardial disease, treatment when available is directed to the latter. When the valve disease is predominant and symptoms severe, mitral valve replacement is indicated. Infective endocarditis should be treated if possible before surgery. Mitral regurgitation of moderate severity can be treated medically, as shown in the information box.

MEDICAL MANAGEMENT OF MITRAL REGURGITATION

- Diuretics
- Vasodilators, e.g. captopril (ACE inhibitors) (p. 223)
- Digoxin if atrial fibrillation is present
- Anticoagulants if atrial fibrillation is present
- Antibiotic prophylaxis

Patients who are being managed medically should be reviewed at regular intervals; worsening symptoms or progressive radiological cardiac enlargement are indications for surgical intervention. Similarly, diminished LV function or markers of raised LV end-diastolic pressure on echocardiography are indications for intervention.

INVESTIGATIONS IN MITRAL REGURGITATION

- **ECG**	Left atrial hypertrophy (if not in AF)
	Left ventricular hypertrophy
- **Chest radiograph**	Enlarged left atrium
	Enlarged left ventricle
	Signs of pulmonary venous hypertension
	Signs of pulmonary oedema (if acute)
- **ECHO**	Dilated LA, LV
	Dynamic LV (unless LVF predominates)
	Regurgitation detectable on Doppler or colour Doppler (Fig. 5.16, p. 208)
- **Cardiac catheterisation**	Dilated LA, LV, mitral regurgitation
	Pulmonary hypertension may be present (chronic MR)

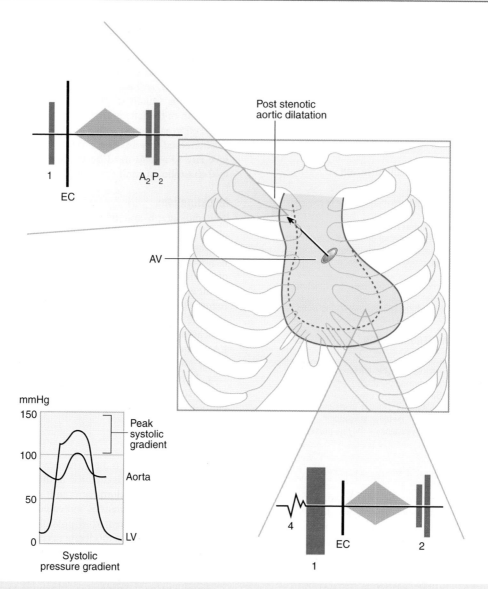

Fig. 5.82   Aortic stenosis: radiation of the murmur in aortic stenosis with left ventricular hypertrophy and enlargement of the ventricle. Pressure traces show the systolic gradient between left ventricle and aorta. The murmur may be heard in the aortic outflow and also at the apex; a 'diamond shape' murmur and an ejection click (EC) may be present with valvular aortic stenosis.

AORTIC VALVE DISEASE

AORTIC STENOSIS

Aetiology and pathophysiology

The likely aetiology of aortic stenosis varies with the age of the patient, and possible causes are summarised in the information box.

Except in the congenital forms, aortic stenosis develops slowly; the cardiac output is maintained at the cost of a steadily increasing gradient across the aortic valve. The left ventricle becomes increasingly hypertrophied, and coronary blood flow may become inadequate. The fixed outflow obstruction limits the increase in cardiac output required on exercise. Patients may develop angina, left ventricular failure and arrhythmias even in the absence of concomitant coronary disease. In elderly patients aortic stenosis and coronary atheroma frequently coexist.

CAUSES OF AORTIC STENOSIS

Infants, children, adolescents
- Congenital aortic stenosis
- Congenital subvalvular aortic stenosis
- Congenital supravalvular aortic stenosis

Young adults to middle-aged
- Calcification and fibrosis of congenitally bicuspid aortic valve
- Rheumatic aortic stenosis

Middle-aged to elderly
- Calcification of bicuspid valve
- Senile degenerative aortic stenosis
- Rheumatic aortic stenosis

SYMPTOMS OF AORTIC STENOSIS

- Exertional dyspnoea
- Angina
- Pulmonary oedema
- Exertional syncope
- Sudden death

SIGNS OF AORTIC STENOSIS

- Ejection systolic murmur
- Slow rising carotid pulse, reduced pulse pressure
- Left ventricular hypertrophy
- Thrusting left ventricle
- Signs of left ventricular failure (crepitations, pulmonary oedema)

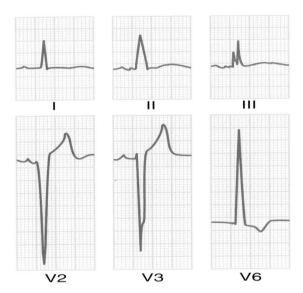

I   II   III

V2   V3   V6

Fig. 5.83   Left ventricular hypertrophy: QRS complexes in limb leads I, II and III are slightly widened and can have increased amplitude. In this illustration they are of normal amplitude but there is a very large S wave in V2 and a large R wave in V6 with T wave inversion in V6.

INVESTIGATIONS IN AORTIC STENOSIS

- **ECG**: Left ventricular hypertrophy (usually)
- **Chest radiograph**: May be normal. Sometimes enlarged left ventricle and dilated ascending aorta on PA view, calcified valve on lateral view
- **ECHO**: Calcified valve, hypertrophied LV, Doppler estimate of gradient
- **Cardiac catheterisation**: Systolic gradient between LV and aorta. Post-stenotic dilatation of aorta. Regurgitation of AV may be present

N.B. cardiac catheter may only be required to determine if coronary disease is present

Clinical features

Mild or moderate aortic stenosis is asymptomatic. The features are summarised in the information box below. The characteristic murmur is illustrated in Figure 5.82.

Investigations

The ECG may show left atrial and ventricular hypertrophy and ST changes, and in advanced cases features of hypertrophy are gross (Fig. 5.83). LBBB is common. Downsloping ST segments and T inversion ('strain pattern') may be seen in leads reflecting the left ventricle. However, especially in the elderly, the ECG may be normal despite severe stenosis. The postero-anterior chest radiograph is frequently normal, but may show left ventricular enlargement and post-stenotic dilatation of the ascending aorta (Fig. 5.84A). A lateral radiograph, or magnetic resonance image, may show valve calcification (Fig. 5.84B), but the diagnosis is more readily made on echocardiography.

Echocardiography will show an abnormal aortic valve, which may be heavily calcified and disorganised, and an hypertrophied left ventricle. Doppler cardiography permits calculation of the systolic gradient across the aortic valve from the velocity of the ejected jet of blood, and detects the presence or absence of aortic regurgitation. Cardiac catheterisation is indicated if the ultrasound studies are unsatisfactory or if it is necessary to assess the state of the coronary arteries.

Management

Patients with symptomatic aortic stenosis and a valve gradient indicative of moderate or severe stenosis (i.e. >60 mm mercury in the presence of a normal cardiac output at rest) should have aortic valve replacement. To wait too long exposes the patient to the risk of sudden

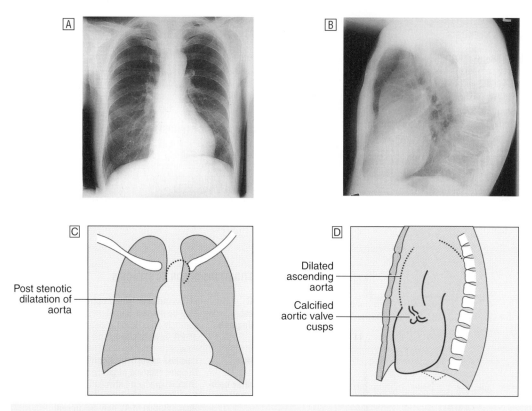

Fig. 5.84 Radiographs of aortic stenosis in [A] **the postero-anterior projection and** [B] **the lateral projection.** Cardiac enlargement may not be evident even in the presence of marked hypertrophy in the PA chest radiograph. There is post-stenotic dilatation in the ascending aorta and this is seen well in the lateral projection. [C], [D]: **line interpretations.**

death, or irreversible deterioration in ventricular function. However, prospective reviews of *asymptomatic* stenosis in the elderly have revealed a relatively benign prognosis without surgery, and in some patients conservative management may be appropriate. Patients should be kept under review, as the development of angina, symptoms of low cardiac output, or heart failure are indications for surgery. Old age, per se, is not a contraindication to valve replacement, and results remain very good in experienced centres even into the ninth decade.

Aortic balloon valvuloplasty may produce transient improvement in patients with severe heart failure or intercurrent illness, but does not substitute for valve replacement in this condition. It is useful in congenital aortic stenosis.

Patients with mild aortic stenosis should be followed up with regular cardiac ultrasound examination to detect progression of stenosis. Anticoagulants are only required in patients who have had a valve replacement with a mechanical prosthesis.

AORTIC REGURGITATION

Aetiology and pathophysiology

The condition results from congenitally abnormal aortic cusps (e.g. bicuspid valves), or from valve damage due to rheumatic heart disease or infective endocarditis, or other rarer causes (see information box).

When regurgitation is marked, the stroke output of

CAUSES OF AORTIC REGURGITATION

Congenital
- Bicuspid valve, or disproportionate cusps

Acquired
- Rheumatic disease
- Infective endocarditis
- Trauma
- Aortic dilatation: Marfan syndrome, atheroma, syphilis, ankylosing spondylitis

the left ventricle may be doubled or trebled. The major arteries are then conspicuously pulsatile—the left ventricle dilates and hypertrophies and initially compensates for the regurgitation. The left ventricular diastolic pressure rises, at first only with exercise, the pulmonary vascular pressures then also increase and breathlessness develops. In contrast to chronic gradual onset regurgitation, acute regurgitation may result from damage to the aortic leaflets (endocarditis, trauma), and auscultatory signs may be masked by the abrupt rise in LV end-diastolic pressure (shortening or even abolishing the typical murmur).

Clinical features

These are listed in the information box below. Until the onset of breathlessness the only symptom may be an awareness of the heartbeat, particularly when lying on the left side. This results from the increased stroke volume. Paroxysmal nocturnal dyspnoea may be the first symptom and peripheral oedema, or angina, may occur. The characteristic murmur is illustrated in Figure 5.85. Although it is usually best heard to the left of the sternum it is sometimes louder to the right. A thrill is uncommon. When the leak is small the murmur will be heard only if the steps shown in Figure 5.85 are followed: this is of crucial importance in the early detection of infective endocarditis affecting the aortic valve. A systolic murmur due to the increased stroke volume is common, and does not necessarily indicate stenosis. When the leak is large the diagnosis is usually easy, with gross pulsation in the large arteries, a collapsing pulse, a low diastolic and an increased pulse pressure. There is usually a thrusting apical impulse and often a presystolic impulse and a fourth heart sound. The regurgitant jet produces fluttering of the mitral leaflets and a soft mid-diastolic murmur called an Austin Flint murmur. In acute severe

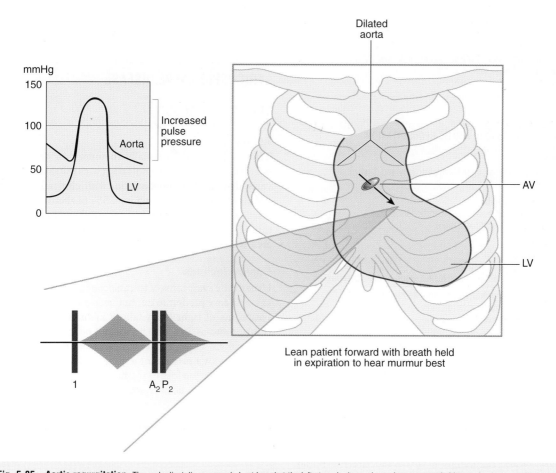

Fig. 5.85 Aortic regurgitation. The early diastolic murmur is best heard at the left sternal edge and may be accompanied by an ejection systolic murmur due to increased blood flow with the enlarged stroke volume. The murmur is best heard with the patient leaning forward and the breath held in expiration.

regurgitation the features of heart failure may predominate, the murmur may be short (or even absent), and

---

SYMPTOMS OF AORTIC REGURGITATION

Mild to moderate AR
- Often asymptomatic
- Awareness of heart-beat, 'palpitations'

Severe AR
- Symptoms of heart failure
- Angina

SIGNS OF AORTIC REGURGITATION

Pulses
- Large volume or 'collapsing' pulse
- Bounding peripheral pulses
- Capillary pulsation in nail-beds—Quincke's sign
- Femoral bruit ('pistol shot')—Durozier's sign
- Head nodding with pulse—de Musset's sign

Murmurs
- Early diastolic murmur
- Systolic murmur of increased stroke volume
- Austin Flint murmur (soft mid-diastolic)

Other signs
- Thrusting apex, 4th heart sound, enlarged LV
- Signs of heart failure

INVESTIGATIONS IN AORTIC REGURGITATION

ECG
- Initially normal, later LV hypertrophy and T wave inversion

Chest radiograph
- Cardiac dilatation, may be aortic dilatation
- Features of left heart failure

ECHO
- Dilated left ventricle
- Hyperdynamic ventricle
- Fluttering anterior mitral leaflet, Doppler detects reflux

Cardiac catheterisation (may not be required)
- Dilated LV, aortic regurgitation
- Dilated aortic root

---

there may be insufficient time for the ventricle to dilate. This possibility must be considered, especially in the context of endocarditis.

Investigations

The chest radiograph characteristically shows cardiac and aortic dilatation, together with signs of left heart failure. When regurgitation is marked the ECG may show left ventricular hypertrophy and ST changes. Echocardiography in aortic regurgitation shows a dilated ventricle with vigorous contraction (until heart failure

ensues). There may be fluttering of the anterior mitral leaflet in the regurgitant jet. Regurgitation is readily detected by Doppler or Colour Doppler cardiography. In severe aortic regurgitation the rise in diastolic pressure may cause mitral valve closure before the onset of ventricular systole. The echocardiogram may reveal vegetations in infective endocarditis, and gives information about left ventricular function. Cardiac catheterisation and aortography can be helpful in assessing severity, and dilatation of the aorta.

Management

Aortic valve replacement under cardiopulmonary bypass is indicated when aortic regurgitation is beginning to cause symptoms or when an enlarging heart or progressive ECG changes give evidence of increasing left ventricular overload. Treatment is required for underlying conditions (endocarditis, syphilis). Antibiotic prophylaxis against endocarditis is required for the damaged valve or the prosthetic replacement.

TRICUSPID VALVE DISEASE

TRICUSPID STENOSIS

Aetiology

Tricuspid stenosis is usually rheumatic in origin, and nearly always occurs in association with mitral and aortic valve disease. It is uncommon, with clinically evident tricuspid disease occurring in <5% of rheumatic heart disease. Isolated rheumatic tricuspid stenosis is very rare. Tricuspid stenosis and regurgitation are also associated with the carcinoid syndrome (p. 456).

Clinical features

Usually the symptoms of the associated mitral and aortic valve disease predominate, but tricuspid stenosis causes symptoms of right heart failure including hepatic discomfort and ascites, and peripheral oedema.

The main clinical feature is a raised jugular venous pressure with a prominent *a* wave, and a slow *y* descent on account of the loss of the normal rapid RV filling (p. 197). There may be presystolic hepatic pulsation, which represents a palpable *a* wave. There is a mid-diastolic murmur usually best heard at the lower left or right sternal edge; this is usually higher pitched than the murmur of mitral stenosis and increased by inspiration.

Management

In patients who require surgery to other valves, the tricuspid valve is either replaced or subjected to valvotomy at the time of surgery. Balloon valvuloplasty can be employed for the rare instances of isolated tricuspid stenosis.

TRICUSPID REGURGITATION

Aetiology and pathophysiology

Tricuspid regurgitation is common. The most frequent cause is described as 'functional', as the valve is not

structurally abnormal but is stretched as a result of right ventricular dilatation (e.g. following pulmonary hypertension or cor pulmonale).

Symptoms are usually nonspecific, and relate to reduced forward flow and venous congestion (tiredness, oedema, hepatic enlargement). The most prominent clinical feature is a large systolic wave in the jugular venous pulse (a *cv* wave replaces the normal *x* descent).

Management

Tricuspid regurgitation, which is due to right ventricular dilatation, gets better when the cause of right ventricular

overload is corrected, for example by mitral valve replacement or by diuretic and vasodilator treatment of left ventricular failure.

Patients with a normal pulmonary artery pressure tolerate isolated tricuspid reflux without ill effects, and valves damaged by endocarditis do not always need to be replaced. A few patients with organic tricuspid valve damage and elevated pulmonary artery pressure may need tricuspid valve repair (annuloplasty) or replacement.

PULMONARY VALVE DISEASE

PULMONARY STENOSIS

Aetiology

The condition is virtually always congenital. It may be isolated or associated with other abnormalities such as Fallot's tetralogy (p. 304).

Clinical features and management

The principal finding on examination is the ejection systolic murmur, loudest to the left of the upper sternum, and radiating towards the left shoulder. There may be a thrill, best felt when the patient leans forward and breathes out. The murmur is often preceded by an ejection sound. Delay in right ventricular ejection may cause wide splitting of the second heart sound (p. 198). Severe pulmonary stenosis is characterised clinically by: a loud harsh murmur; an inaudible pulmonary closure sound (P2); an increased right ventricular thrust, prominent *a* waves in the jugular pulse; ECG evidence of right ventricular hypertrophy; and post-stenotic dilatation in the pulmonary artery on the chest radiograph.

Mild to moderate isolated pulmonary stenosis is rela-

SYMPTOMS OF PULMONARY STENOSIS

- Symptoms of right heart failure
- Symptoms of the underlying cause of pulmonary stenosis—e.g. carcinoid syndrome (see p. 456)

SIGNS OF PULMONARY STENOSIS

- Giant *a* wave in the JVP
- RV hypertrophy and dilatation
- Systolic murmur (upper left sternum)—increases on inspiration with increased pulmonary flow
- Systolic thrill over pulmonary outflow
- P2 soft and delayed
- Valvular PS may have an ejection click

INVESTIGATIONS IN PULMONARY STENOSIS

Chest radiograph
- Prominent pulmonary artery (post-stenotic dilatation)

ECG
- Right atrial and RV hypertrophy

ECHO
- Abnormal PV
- Outflow gradient on Doppler

INFECTIVE ENDOCARDITIS ON NATIVE VALVES

Prevalence of organisms in Europe and North America

Bacteria
- Streptococci

viridans	30–40%
enterococci	10–15%
Other streptococci	20–25%

- Staphylococci

aureus	9–27%
Coagulase negative	1–3%

- Gram negative bacilli
- Haemophilus
- Anaerobes   Total 3–8%

Other organisms
Rickettsia, fungi   Less than 2%

---

tively common, does not usually progress, and does not require treatment. It is a low-risk lesion for infective endocarditis.

Severe pulmonary stenosis (resting gradient >50 mmHg with a normal cardiac output) is treated by percutaneous pulmonary balloon valvuloplasty or, if unavailable, by surgical balloon valvotomy. Long-term results are very good. Postoperative pulmonary regurgitation is common but benign.

PULMONARY REGURGITATION

Pulmonary regurgitation is rare as an isolated phenomenon. It is usually associated with pulmonary artery dilatation which is due to pulmonary hypertension, and may follow mitral stenosis. An early diastolic decrescendo murmur is heard at the left sternal edge and may be difficult to distinguish from aortic regurgitation (Graham Steell murmur). The pulmonary hypertension may also be secondary to other disease of the left side of the heart, to primary pulmonary vascular disease, or to Eisenmenger's syndrome. Trivial pulmonary regurgitation is a frequent echocardiographic Doppler finding in normal individuals and is not of clinical significance.

INFECTIVE ENDOCARDITIS

Aetiology

Infective endocarditis is due to microbial infection of a heart valve (native or prosthetic) or the lining of a cardiac chamber or blood vessel, or a congenital anomaly (e.g. septal defect). The causative organism is usually a bacterium, but may be a rickettsia (*Coxiella burnetii*—Q fever endocarditis), chlamydia, or fungus.

Streptococcus viridans (*S. mitis* and *S. sanguis*, alpha-haemolytic streptococci) are commensals in the upper respiratory tract and a common cause of periodontal infection. They may enter the blood-stream on chewing, teeth brushing or at the time of dental treatment. Other streptococci including *Streptococcus faecalis*, *S. milleri* and *S. bovis*, may enter the blood from the bowel or urinary tract. *S. milleri* and *S. bovis* are sometimes associated with large bowel neoplasms.

Staphylococcus aureus is a common cause of acute endocarditis, originating from skin infections, abscesses or vascular access sites (e.g. intravenous and central lines), and intravenous drug addiction. It is a highly virulent and invasive organism, usually producing florid vegetations, valve destruction greater than in subacute endocarditis, and abscess formation. Other causes of acute endocarditis include *Streptococcus pneumoniae* and *Neisseria gonorrhoeae*.

Postoperative endocarditis follows cardiac surgery and affects native or prosthetic heart valves or other prosthetic materials. The commonest organism is a coagulase negative staphylococcus (*Staphylococcus albus*). There is frequently a history of postoperative wound infection with the same organism.

In Q fever endocarditis (rickettsia) the patient often has a history of contact with farm animals. It commonly affects the aortic valve and may cause hepatic complications and purpura. Prolonged (lifelong) antibiotic therapy may be required.

Brucella is associated with a history of contact with goats or cattle and often affects the aortic valve.

Fungi (Candida, Aspergillus) may attack previously

normal or prosthetic valves. Abscesses and emboli are common, therapy is difficult (surgery often required) and the mortality is high. Concomitant bacterial infection may be present.

Prevalence

A community study of South East Scotland has revealed an incidence of 16 cases per million per annum. In a large British study, the underlying heart disease in 24% of patients was rheumatic heart disease, in 19% congenital heart disease, and in 25% some other cardiac abnormality (e.g. calcified AV, floppy MV). The remainder (32%) were not thought to have a pre-existing cardiac abnormality.

Pathophysiology

Endocarditis occurs at sites where the endothelium is damaged by a high pressure jet of blood (ventricular septal defect, persistent ductus arteriosus, or regurgitant mitral or aortic valves) or on damaged valves. In intravenous drug addicts right heart valves are affected (especially tricuspid). Endothelial damage leads to the deposition of platelets and fibrin, which are colonised by blood-borne organisms, creating vegetations. The avascular valve tissue and presence of fibrin aggregates help to protect the proliferating organisms from host defence mechanisms. Affected valves develop vegetations composed of organisms, fibrin and platelets, and the vegetations may become large enough to cause obstruction or may break away as emboli. Regurgitation may develop or increase owing to the perforation of a cusp or the disruption of chordae. Extracardiac manifestations result from emboli or from immune complexes, which may be responsible for vasculitis and skin lesions. Mycotic aneurysms may develop in arteries at the site of infected emboli. At postmortem it is common to find infarction of the spleen and kidneys, and sometimes an immune glomerulonephritis.

Clinical features

Possible clinical features in endocarditis, and their frequency, are given in Figure 5.86.

The clinical course of endocarditis

Prior to the advent of effective therapy, the illness often ran a stuttering course over several months accompanied by the striking clinical stigmata. This pattern is now rare. Clinically, endocarditis has been divided into an acute and a more insidious 'subacute' form. The designation of acute and subacute forms has been questioned as the clinical pattern is influenced not only by the organism, but also by the site of infection, prior antibiotic therapy and the presence of a valve or shunt prosthesis. Furthermore, the subacute form may abruptly develop acute

life-threatening complications including valve disruption or emboli.

Subacute endocarditis should be suspected when a patient known to have congenital or valvular heart disease develops a persistent fever or complains of unusual tiredness, night sweats, weight loss or develops new signs of valve dysfunction or heart failure. Less often, it presents as an embolic stroke or peripheral arterial embolism. Other features include purpura and petechial haemorrhages in the skin and mucous membranes, and splinter haemorrhages under the finger or toe nails. Osler's nodes are painful tender swellings at the finger tips, probably the result of vasculitis. They are rare. Digital clubbing is a late sign. The spleen is frequently palpable; in Coxiella infections both it and the liver may be considerably enlarged. Microscopic haematuria is common. The finding of any of these features in a patient with persistent fever or malaise is an indication for re-examination for hitherto unrecognised heart disease.

Acute endocarditis usually presents as a severe febrile illness with prominent and changing heart murmurs and petechiae. Clinical stigmata of chronic endocarditis are usually absent. Embolic events are common, and cardiac or renal failure may develop rapidly. Abscesses may be detected on echocardiography. Partially-treated acute endocarditis behaves like subacute endocarditis.

Postoperative endocarditis may resemble subacute or acute endocarditis depending on the virulence of the organism. The infection usually affects the valve ring. Any unexplained fever in a patient who has had heart valve surgery should be investigated for possible endocarditis.

Investigations

Blood culture is the crucial investigation. It should identify the infection and give guidance about management. Several specimens (>3) should be taken prior to commencing therapy, and these need not wait for episodes of pyrexia. Aseptic technique is essential and the risk of contaminants minimised by sampling from different venepuncture sites. An indwelling line should not be used for cultures. Aerobic and anaerobic cultures are required but new techniques can identify the organism immunologically, without culture. A knowledge of prior antibiotic treatment may allow an inactivating enzyme to be added and facilitate growth.

Elevation of the ESR, a normocytic, normochromic anaemia and leucocytosis are common but not invariable and thrombocytopenia may be present. Measurement of plasma C-reactive protein is more reliable than the ESR in assessing progress. Proteinuria may occur and microscopic haematuria is usually present.

Echocardiography is the key investigation for detect-

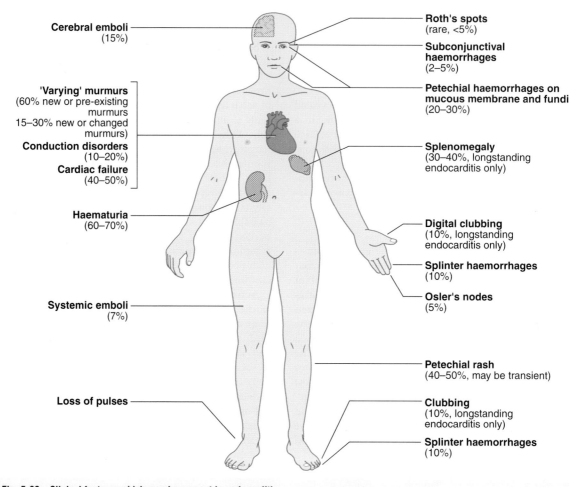

Cerebral emboli (15%)

Roth's spots (rare, <5%)

Subconjunctival haemorrhages (2–5%)

Petechial haemorrhages on mucous membrane and fundi (20–30%)

'Varying' murmurs (60% new or pre-existing murmurs 15–30% new or changed murmurs)
Conduction disorders (10–20%)
Cardiac failure (40–50%)

Splenomegaly (30–40%, longstanding endocarditis only)

Haematuria (60–70%)

Digital clubbing (10%, longstanding endocarditis only)

Splinter haemorrhages (10%)

Osler's nodes (5%)

Systemic emboli (7%)

Petechial rash (40–50%, may be transient)

Loss of pulses

Clubbing (10%, longstanding endocarditis only)

Splinter haemorrhages (10%)

Fig. 5.86 **Clinical features which may be present in endocarditis.**

ing and following the progress of vegetations, for investigating valve damage, and for detecting abscess formation. Vegetations (3–5 mm) can be detected by transthoracic echo, and even smaller (1–1.5 mm) by transoesophageal echo. Vegetations may be difficult to distinguish in the presence of an abnormal valve and the sensitivity of transthoracic echo is approximately 65%. Failure to detect vegetations does not exclude the diagnosis and should not delay treatment.

The ECG may show the development of conduction defects (abscess formation) and occasionally infarction due to emboli. Chest radiograph shows evidence of cardiac failure and cardiomegaly.

Management
Isolation of the organism allows minimum inhibitory concentrations (MIC) and minimum bacteriocidal concentrations (MBC) of the antimicrobial drug to be measured against the specific organism. Drug levels 4–8 times the MIC/MBC are effective in eradicating the organism. Any source of infection should be removed if possible; for example, a tooth with an apical abscess should be extracted.

Persisting infection is indicated by continuing fever, changing murmurs, and a persistently elevated ESR or CRP concentration. Antimicrobial therapy must be started before surgery.

Prevention
Patients with valvular or congenital heart disease may be susceptible to infective endocarditis. Patients should be aware of the risk of endocarditis, the need to avoid bacteraemia, and the importance of maintaining good dental health. Potential sources of infection should be treated promptly. Antibiotic prophylaxis requires that the drug and dose chosen should be sufficient to kill the

Table 5.10 Antimicrobial treatment in infective endocarditis

Organism	Antimicrobial	Dose	
Strep. viridans	Benzylpenicillin i.v.	2–4 g 6-hourly	2 wks
	plus gentamicin i.v.	1 mg/kg 8-hourly	2 wks
	then amoxycillin orally	6 g daily from	2–6 wks
Strep. faecalis	Benzylpenicillin i.v.	4–8 g 6-hourly	2 wks
	plus gentamicin i.v.	3 mg/kg 8-hourly	2–4 wks
	then amoxycillin orally	6–8 g daily from	2–6 wks
Staph. aureus	Flucloxacillin i.v.	2 g 6-hourly	2 wks
	then flucloxacillin 4 wks orally	2 g 6-hourly	4 wks
	or fusidic acid	580 mg 8-hourly	6 wks
	or clindamycin	Doses vary	6 wks
Staph. aureus (allergy or methicillin resistant)	Vancomycin i.v.	1 g 12-hourly	6 wks
	or rifampicillin orally	600 mg 12-hourly	6 wks
	plus erythromycin orally	500 mg 6-hourly	6 wks
Coxiella burnetii	Tetracycline i.v. orally	0.5–1 g 12-hourly	long term
	or rifampicillin orally	600 mg 12-hourly	—minimum 1 year
	plus doxycycline orally	100 mg 12-hourly	

N.B. Gentamicin—monitor renal function and adjust dose (consider netilmycin)
Vancomycin—adjust dose if renal function impaired

INDICATIONS FOR CARDIAC SURGERY IN INFECTIVE ENDOCARDITIS

- **Heart failure** due to valve damage
- **Failure of antibiotic therapy** (persistent or uncontrolled infection)
- **Large vegetations on left sided heart valves** with evidence of, or 'high risk' of, systemic emboli
- **Abscess formation**

N.B. Patients with prosthetic valve endocarditis or fungal endocarditis often require cardiac surgery

offending organism, but only be given shortly before bacteraemia in order to reduce resistance.

FURTHER READING

American Heart Association Special Writing Committee on Rheumatic Fever, Endocarditis and Kawasaki Disease of the Council of Cardiovascular Disease in the Young 1992 (update) Guidelines for the diagnosis of rheumatic fever: Jones criteria. Journal of the American Heart Association 268: 2069–2073
British Society for Antimicrobial Chemotherapy Endocarditis Working Party 1990 Antibiotic prophylaxis of infective endocarditis. Lancet 335: 88–89
Dajani A S, Bisno A L, Chung K J et al 1990 Prevention of bacterial endocarditis. Recommendations of the American Heart Association. Journal of the American Medical Association 264: 2919–2922

ANTIBIOTIC PROPHYLAXIS AGAINST ENDOCARDITIS

LOCAL ANAESTHETIC

- **Dental procedures or upper respiratory tract** — Amoxycillin 3 g orally 1 h before

  If allergic to penicillin: — Erythromycin 1.5 g orally 1 h before plus 0.5 g 6 h later **or** clindamycin 600 mg orally 1 h before

GENERAL ANAESTHETIC

- **Dental procedures or upper respiratory tract** — Amoxycillin 1 g i.m. in 2.5% lignocaine **plus** 0.5 g amoxycillin orally 6 h later

  If allergic to penicillin: — Vancomycin 1 g i.v. infusion over 1 h before, **plus** 120 mg gentamicin i.v.

- **Genitourinary procedures or high risk patients** — Amoxycillin 1 g i.m. in 2.5% lignocaine **plus** 120 mg gentamicin i.v., **plus** 0.5 g amoxycillin orally 6 h later

  If allergic to penicillin: — Vancomycin 1 g i.v. infusion over 1 h before, **plus** 120 mg gentamicin i.v.

N.B. Obstetric and gynaecological procedures or gastrointestinal surgery/instrumentation—treat only prosthetic valve patients (as for high risk patients, above)

CONGENITAL HEART DISEASE

Congenital heart disease may present at the time of birth when major anomalies result in failure to oxygenate venous blood in lungs (e.g. pulmonary atresia and right-to-left shunt), or separation of systemic and pulmonary circulations (e.g. complete transposition of the great vessels) and failure to provide oxygenated blood to the periphery. Presentation shortly after birth may follow closure of the ductus arteriosus, in situations where the ductus provides the major route for oxygenation (see below), or following onset of heart failure. Later in childhood or adult life congenital disease presents incidentally, or when pulmonary vascular disease supervenes, or following haemodynamic change (e.g. pregnancy). However, early recognition is important as 70% of deaths due to congenital heart disease occur in the first year of life.

PREVALENCE OF CONGENITAL CARDIAC MALFORMATIONS	
Overall prevalence	0.75% of live births
Lesion prevalence	**% of all CHD defects**
• Ventricular septal defect	25–30%
• Atrial septal defect (secundum)	10–15%
• Persistence of ductus arteriosus	10%
• Complete transposition	5%
• AV septal defect (ostium primum)	5%
• Hypoplastic left heart	5%

Aetiology

The incidence of haemodynamically significant congenital cardiac abnormalities is about 0.75% of live births. In most cases the cause of the abnormality is unknown, but some fetal defects are due to maternal infections in the early weeks of pregnancy. Rubella is associated with persistent ductus arteriosus and pulmonary valvular or artery stenosis. Maternal alcohol abuse is associated with septal defects, and intrauterine radiation or drug effects may cause various defects. Genetic or chromosomal abnormalities such as Down syndrome (p. 19) may cause septal defects, heart block or valve abnormalities. All degrees of severity occur. Some defects are not compatible with extrauterine life, or only for a short time. Early diagnosis is important because many types of congenital heart disease are amenable to surgical treatment, but this opportunity may be lost if secondary changes, for example pulmonary vascular damage, occur.

Clinical features

Symptoms may be absent, or the child may be noticed to be breathless, or may fail to attain normal growth and development. Clinical signs vary with the anatomical lesion. Cerebrovascular accidents and cerebral abscesses are complications of severe cyanotic congenital disease.
    Principal features are illustrated in Figure 5.87.

Central cyanosis and digital clubbing

Central cyanosis of cardiac origin occurs when desaturated blood enters the systemic circulation without passing through the lungs (i.e. there is a right-to-left shunt). In the neonate the commonest cause of this is transposition of the great arteries, in which the aorta arises from the right ventricle and the pulmonary artery from the left. In older children cyanosis is usually the consequence of a ventricular septal defect combined with severe pulmonary stenosis (Tetralogy of Fallot, p. 304) or with pulmonary vascular disease (Eisenmenger's syndrome, see below). Prolonged cyanosis is associated with finger and toe clubbing.

Pulmonary hypertension

Persistently raised pulmonary flow (e.g. with left-to-right shunt) leads to increased pulmonary resistance followed by pulmonary hypertension. When the shunt is reversed cyanosis is evident (Eisenmenger's syndrome).

Growth retardation

This is a feature of all severe congenital cardiac defects. There is also an increased frequency of intellectual impairment.

Syncope

In the presence of increased pulmonary vascular resistance or severe left or right outflow obstruction exercise may provoke syncope. Systemic vascular resistance falls on exercise but pulmonary vascular resistance may rise, worsening right-to-left shunting and cerebral oxygenation.

Eisenmenger's syndrome

This occurs when increased pulmonary flow due to an initial left-to-right shunt produces severe pulmonary hypertension and *reversal* of the shunt (i.e. right-to-left shunting). Progressive changes (including obliteration of distal vessels) take place in the pulmonary vasculature, and once established the increased pulmonary resistance is irreversible. Central cyanosis appears, and digital clubbing develops. The chest radiograph shows enlarged central pulmonary arteries and peripheral 'pruning' of the pulmonary vessels. The ECG shows right ventricular hypertrophy. Eisenmenger's syndrome is more common with large ventricular septal defects, or persistent ductus arteriosus, than with atrial septal defects. Patients with the syndrome are at particular risk from abrupt changes in afterload which exacerbate right-to-left shunting (vasodilatation, anaesthesia, pregnancy).

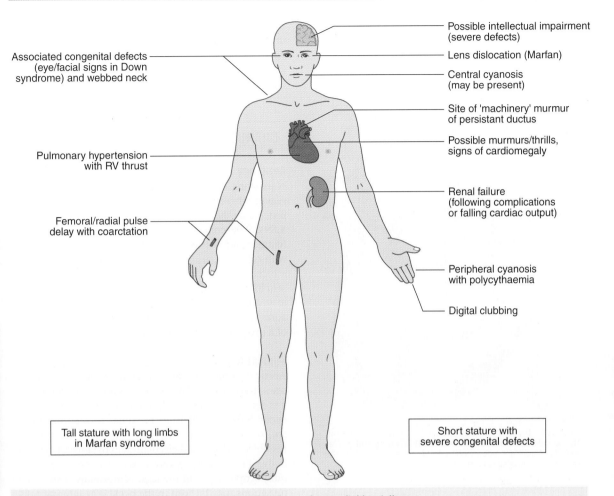

Possible intellectual impairment (severe defects)

Lens dislocation (Marfan)

Central cyanosis (may be present)

Site of 'machinery' murmur of persistant ductus

Possible murmurs/thrills, signs of cardiomegaly

Renal failure (following complications or falling cardiac output)

Peripheral cyanosis with polycythaemia

Digital clubbing

Associated congenital defects (eye/facial signs in Down syndrome) and webbed neck

Pulmonary hypertension with RV thrust

Femoral/radial pulse delay with coarctation

Tall stature with long limbs in Marfan syndrome

Short stature with severe congenital defects

Fig. 5.87   Clinical features which may be present in various forms of congenital heart disease.

PERSISTENT DUCTUS ARTERIOSUS

Aetiology

During fetal life, before the lungs begin to function, most of the blood from the pulmonary artery passes through the ductus arteriosus into the aorta just below the origin of the left subclavian artery. Normally the ductus closes soon after birth but sometimes it fails to do so. Since the pressure in the aorta is higher than that in the pulmonary artery there will be a continuous arteriovenous shunt, the volume of which depends on the size of the ductus. As much as 50% of the left ventricular output may be recirculated through the lungs, with a consequent increase in the work of the heart. When the ductus is structurally intact a prostaglandin synthetase inhibitor (indomethacin) may be used to induce closure. However, in the presence of a congenital defect with impaired lung perfusion (e.g. pulmonary stenosis and right-to-left shunt) oxygenation is improved by maintaining the ductus open with prostaglandin treatment. However, such treatments are ineffective in an abnormal ductus. Persistence of the ductus may be associated with other abnormalities, and is much commoner in females.

Clinical features

With small shunts there may be no symptoms for years, but when the ductus is large, growth and development may be retarded. Usually there is no disability in infancy, but cardiac failure may eventually ensue, dyspnoea being the first symptom. A continuous 'machinery' murmur is heard with late systolic accentuation, maximal in the second left intercostal space near the sternum (Fig. 5.88). It is frequently accompanied by a thrill. Enlargement of the pulmonary artery may be detected radiologically. The ECG is usually normal.

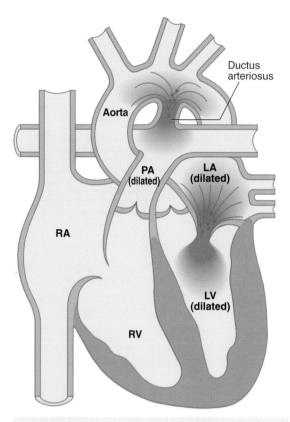

Fig. 5.88 Diagram of persistent ductus arteriosus showing the connection between the aorta and pulmonary artery. The intensity of shading is proportional to velocity of blood flow, and hence reflects the distribution of murmurs.

A large left-to-right shunt in infancy may cause a considerable rise in pulmonary artery pressure, and sometimes this leads to progressive pulmonary vascular damage. Pulses are increased in volume.

Persistent ductus with reversed shunting

With the resulting rise in pulmonary vascular resistance, pulmonary artery pressure rises further until it equals or exceeds aortic pressure. The shunt through the defect may then reverse, causing central cyanosis (Eisenmenger's syndrome, see p. 301). With a persistent ductus arteriosus this cyanosis may be more apparent in the feet and toes than in the upper part of the body. The murmur becomes quieter, may be confined to systole, or may disappear. The ECG shows evidence of right ventricular hypertrophy.

Management

The morbidity and mortality of surgical division is low, but most can now be closed by percutaneous occlusion with the Rashkind umbrella (which obstructs the ductus) or similar device. Closure should be undertaken in infancy if the shunt is significant and pulmonary resistance not elevated. In older children or adults with small shunts conservative management may be acceptable, but endocarditis prophylaxis is needed.

COARCTATION OF THE AORTA

Aetiology

Narrowing of the aorta most commonly occurs in the region where the ductus arteriosus joins the aorta, i.e. just below the origin of the left subclavian artery (Fig. 5.89). The condition is twice as common in males as females and occurs in 1:4000 children. It is associated with other abnormalities, of which the most frequent is a bicuspid aortic valve. 'Berry' aneurysms may be present in the cerebral circulation at the time of presentation in severe cases (p. 1071). Acquired coarctation of the aorta is rare; it may follow trauma, or be a complication of a progressive arteritis (Takayasu's disease, p. 925).

Clinical features

Aortic coarctation is an important cause of cardiac failure in the newborn, but symptoms are often absent when it is detected in older children or adults. Headaches may occur from hypertension proximal to the coarctation, and occasionally weakness or cramps in the legs may result from decreased circulation in the lower part of the body. The blood pressure is raised in the upper body but normal or low in the legs. Abnormally large arterial pulsations may be seen in the neck. The femoral pulses are weak, and delayed in comparison with the radial. A systolic murmur may sometimes be heard posteriorly, over the coarctation. There may also be an ejection systolic murmur in the aortic area due to the bicuspid valve. As a result of the aortic narrowing collaterals form, mainly involving the periscapular and intercostal arteries. These may be visible or even palpable in older children and adults, around the scapulae and below the ribs posteriorly.

Radiological examination in early childhood is often normal but at a later age may show changes in the contour of the aorta (indentation of the descending aorta, '3 sign'), and notching of the under surfaces of the ribs from collaterals (see Fig. 5.89). Magnetic resonance imaging will also demonstrate the lesion. The ECG may show left ventricular hypertrophy.

Management

In untreated severe cases, death may occur from left ventricular failure, dissection of the aorta or cerebral haemorrhage. Surgical correction is advisable in all but

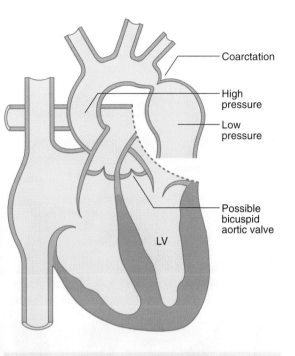

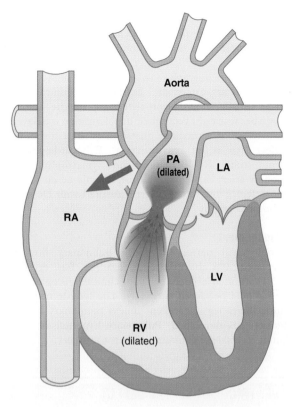

Fig. 5.89 Diagram of coarctation of the aorta.

the mildest cases. If this is done sufficiently early in childhood the risk of persistent hypertension may be avoided. Patients repaired in late childhood or adult life often remain hypertensive or become hypertensive again. Recurrence of stenosis may occur as the child grows and this may be managed by balloon dilatation. Coexistent aortic valve disease also requires long-term follow-up.

Fig. 5.90 Diagram of atrial septal defect illustrating the blood flow across the atrial septum (from left to right prior to the advent of pulmonary hypertension and Eisenmenger's syndrome). The murmur is produced by increased flow velocity across the pulmonary valve, as a result of left-to-right shunting and large stroke volume. The density of shading is proportional to velocity of blood flow.

ATRIAL SEPTAL DEFECT

Aetiology
Atrial septal defect is one of the commonest congenital heart defects, and occurs twice as frequently in females. Most are 'ostium secundum' defects, involving the fossa ovalis. Ostium primum defects result from a defect in the atrioventricular septum and are associated with a 'cleft mitral valve' (split anterior leaflet).

Since the normal right ventricle is much more compliant than the left, a large volume of blood shunts through the defect from the left to right atrium and then to the right ventricle and pulmonary arteries (Fig. 5.90). As a result there is gradual enlargement of the right side of the heart and of the pulmonary arteries. Pulmonary hypertension and shunt reversal sometimes complicate atrial septal defect, but are less common and tend to

occur later in life than with other types of left-to-right shunt.

Clinical features
Most children are free of symptoms for many years and the condition is often detected at routine clinical examination or following a chest radiograph. Dyspnoea, chest infections, cardiac failure and arrhythmias (e.g. atrial fibrillation) are other possible modes of presentation. The characteristic physical signs are the result of the volume overload of the right ventricle:

● Wide fixed splitting of the second heart sound:
—wide because of delay in right ventricular ejection, increased stroke volume and RBBB;
—fixed because the septal defect equalises left and right atrial pressures throughout the respiratory cycle
● A systolic flow murmur over the pulmonary valve.

In children with a large shunt there may be a diastolic flow murmur over the tricuspid valve. Unlike a mitral flow murmur, this diastolic murmur is usually high-pitched.

The chest radiograph shows enlargement of the heart, the pulmonary artery, and pulmonary plethora. The ECG usually shows incomplete right bundle branch block because right ventricular depolarisation is delayed as a result of ventricular dilatation (with a 'primum' defect there is left axis deviation). Echocardiography demonstrates RV dilatation and hypertrophy, pulmonary artery dilatation, and can directly demonstrate the defect. Flow velocities are measured with Doppler echocardiography.

Management

Atrial septal defects in which pulmonary flow is increased 50% above systemic flow (i.e. flow ratio of 1.5:1) are often large enough to be clinically recognisable and should be closed surgically. The long-term prognosis thereafter is excellent unless pulmonary hypertension has developed. Pulmonary hypertension and shunt reversal are contraindications to surgery.

VENTRICULAR SEPTAL DEFECT

Aetiology

Congenital ventricular septal defect occurs as a result of incomplete septation of the ventricles. Embryologically, the interventricular septum has a membranous and a muscular portion, and the latter is further divided into inflow, trabecular and outflow portions. Most congenital defects are 'perimembranous', i.e. at the junction of the membranous and muscular portions.

Ventricular septal defects are the most common congenital cardiac defect, occurring once in 500 live births. The defect may be isolated or part of complex congenital heart disease. Acquired ventricular septal defect may result from rupture of an infarcted interventricular septum as a complication of acute myocardial infarction, or rarely from trauma.

Clinical features

Flow from the high-pressure left ventricle to the low-pressure right ventricle during systole produces a pan-systolic murmur usually heard best at the left sternal edge but radiating all over the precordium (Fig. 5.91). A small defect often produces a loud murmur (maladie de Roger) in the absence of other haemodynamic disturbance. Conversely, a large defect may produce a softer murmur, particularly if pressure in the right ventricle is elevated. This may be the case immediately after

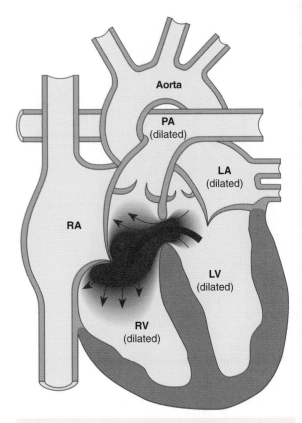

Fig. 5.91 Diagram of ventricular septal defect. The density of shading is proportional to velocity of blood flow. In this instance there is a relatively small septal defect with a high velocity of flow from the left ventricle to the right ventricle.

birth, while pulmonary vascular resistance remains high, or when the shunt is reversed—Eisenmenger's syndrome (described above).

Congenital ventricular septal defect may present as cardiac failure in infants, as a murmur with only minor haemodynamic disturbance in older children or adults, or rarely as Eisenmenger's syndrome. In a proportion of infants, the murmur gets quieter or disappears. This may be due to *spontaneous closure* of the defect or to the development of Eisenmenger's syndrome.

Cardiac failure is usually absent in the immediate postnatal period but becomes apparent in the first 4–6 weeks of life (large defect). In addition to the murmur, there is prominent parasternal pulsation, tachypnoea and indrawing of the lower ribs on inspiration. The chest radiograph shows pulmonary plethora and the ECG shows right and left ventricular enlargement.

Management

Small ventricular septal defects require no specific treatment apart from endocarditis prophylaxis. Cardiac failure caused by a ventricular septal defect in infancy is initially treated medically with digoxin (10–20 μg/kg per day) and frusemide (1–3 mg/kg per day). Persisting failure is an indication for surgical repair of the defect.

Echocardiography helps to predict the small septal defects that are likely to close spontaneously. Eisenmenger's syndrome is avoided by monitoring (repeated ECG and echocardiography) for signs of rising pulmonary resistance and carrying out surgical repair when appropriate. Fully developed Eisenmenger's syndrome is not benefited by surgical closure of the defect. Heart-lung transplantation may be the only method of surgical correction.

Prognosis

Except in the case of Eisenmenger's syndrome, long-term prognosis is very good in congenital ventricular septal defect. Most patients with Eisenmenger's syndrome die in the second or third decades of life, but a few survive to the fifth decade without transplantation.

TETRALOGY OF FALLOT

The four components (Fig. 5.92) of the tetralogy are given in the information box (overleaf).

The RV outflow obstruction is most often subvalvular (infundibular), but may be valvular, or supravalvular, or a combination of these. The VSD is usually large and similar in aperture to the aortic orifice. The combination results in elevated RV pressure and right-to-left shunting of cyanotic blood across the VSD. Tetralogy of Fallot is distinct anatomically and embryologically from the coincidence of pulmonary stenosis and ventricular septal defect in the same patient.

Aetiology

The embryological cause is abnormal development of the bulbar septum which separates the ascending aorta from the pulmonary artery, and which normally aligns and fuses with the outflow part of the interventricular septum. The defect occurs in about 1 in 2000 births and is the commonest cause of cyanosis in infancy (> 1 year).

Clinical features

The children are cyanosed but cyanosis may not be present in the newborn child. It is only when right ventricular pressure rises to equal or exceed left ventricular pressure that a large right-to-left shunt develops. The subvalvular component of the RV outflow obstruction is dynamic, and may increase suddenly under adrenergic stimulation. The affected child suddenly becomes increasingly cyanosed, often after feeding or a crying attack, and may become apnoeic and unconscious. These attacks are called 'Fallot's spells'. In older children Fallot's spells are uncommon, but cyanosis becomes increasingly apparent, with stunting of growth, digital clubbing and polycythaemia. Some children characteristically obtain relief by squatting after exertion. The natural history before the development of surgical correction was variable, but most patients died in infancy or childhood.

On examination the most characteristic feature is usually the combination of cyanosis with a loud ejection systolic murmur in the pulmonary area (as for pulmonary stenosis). Cyanosis may be absent in the newborn, or in patients where right ventricular outflow obstruction is mild ('acyanotic tetralogy of Fallot'). Growth may be impaired.

Investigations

ECG shows right ventricular hypertrophy, and the chest radiograph shows an abnormally small pulmonary artery and a 'boot-shaped' heart. Echocardiography is diagnostic and demonstrates that the aorta is not continuous with the anterior ventricular septum.

Management

The definitive management is total correction of the defect by surgical relief of the pulmonary stenosis and closure of the ventricular septal defect. Primary surgical correction may be undertaken prior to age 5, except if the pulmonary arteries are too hypoplastic, when a palliative shunt may be performed (for example an anastomosis between the pulmonary artery and subclavian artery). The shunt improves pulmonary blood flow and does not preclude definitive correction at a later stage.

The prognosis after total correction is good, especially if the operation is performed in childhood. Follow-up is needed to identify residual pulmonary stenosis, recurrence of the septal defect, or rhythm disorders.

OTHER CAUSES OF CYANOTIC CONGENITAL HEART DISEASE

Other causes of cyanotic congenital heart disease are summarised in Table 5.11. Echocardiography is usually the definitive diagnostic procedure, supplemented if necessary by cardiac catheterisation.

FURTHER READING

Sutton G C, Fox K M 1988 Clinical and investigative features of cardiac pathology of congenital heart disease. Current Medical Literature Ltd./Royal Society of Medicine, London

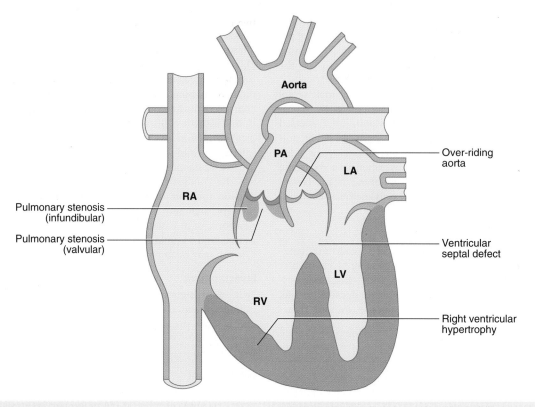

Fig. 5.92   Tetralogy of Fallot comprising pulmonary stenosis, a ventricular septal defect, overriding of the ventricular septal defect by the aorta, and right ventricular hypertrophy.

FALLOT'S TETRALOGY

- RV outflow obstruction (pulmonary stenosis)
- ventricular septal defect
- 'overriding' of the ventricular septal defect by the aorta
- right ventricular hypertrophy

DISEASES OF THE MYOCARDIUM

Although the myocardium is involved in most types of heart disease the terms myocarditis and cardiomyopathy are usually reserved for conditions that primarily affect the heart muscle. An international commission has recommended using specific terminology, e.g. 'sarcoid heart muscle disease', when the cause of heart muscle disease is known and using the term 'cardiomyopathy' only if a cause cannot be identified.

SPECIFIC DISEASES OF HEART MUSCLE

ACUTE MYOCARDITIS

This is an acute inflammatory and potentially reversible condition that may complicate a wide variety of infections; inflammation may be due to infection of the myocardium or circulating toxins. Viral infection is the commonest cause of myocarditis in the UK.

The clinical picture ranges from a symptomless disorder, sometimes recognised by the presence of an inappropriate tachycardia, to fulminant heart failure. ECG changes are common but non-specific. If necessary, the diagnosis can be confirmed by endomyocardial biopsy.

Although death may occur, due to a ventricular arrhythmia or rapidly progressive heart failure, the immediate prognosis is excellent. However, there is strong evidence that some forms of myocarditis may lead

Table 5.11   Other causes of cyanotic congenital heart diseases

Tricuspid atresia	Absent tricuspid orifice, hypoplastic RV. RA to LA shunt, VSD shunt, other anomalies. Surgical correction *may* be possible
Transposition of the great vessels	Aorta arises from the morphological RV, pulmonary artery from LV. Shunt via atria, ductus and possible VSD. Palliation by balloon atrial septostomy/enlargement. Surgical correction possible
Pulmonary atresia	PV atretic and pulmonary artery hypoplastic. RA to LA shunt, pulmonary flow via ductus. Palliation by balloon atrial septostomy. Surgical correction may be possible
Ebstein's anomaly	TV is dysplastic and displaced into RV, right ventricle 'atrialised'. Tricuspid regurgitation and RA to LA shunt. Spectrum of severity. Arrhythmias. Surgical repair possible, but significant risks
Hypoplastic left heart	Anomalies affecting left heart; atresia, stenosis of AV/MV. Hypoplastic aorta. Heart failure in first week. Palliation with atrial septostomy and maintaining ductus. Surgical repair very complex and high risk. Consider heart-lung transplant

SPECIFIC DISEASES OF HEART MUSCLE

- **Infections**
  Viral, e.g. coxsackie A and B, influenza, HIV
  Bacterial, e.g. diphtheria
  Protozoal, e.g. trypanosomiasis, p. 159

- **Endocrine and metabolic disorders**
  e.g. diabetes, hypo- and hyperthyroidism, acromegaly, carcinoid syndrome, inherited storage diseases

- **Connective tissue diseases**
  e.g. scleroderma, SLE, polyarteritis nodosa

- **Infiltrative disorders**
  e.g. haemochromatosis, haemosiderosis, sarcoidosis, amyloidosis

- **Endomyocardial fibrosis and eosinophilic heart disease**

- **Toxins**
  e.g. drugs, alcohol, irradiation

- **Neuromuscular disorders**
  e.g. dystrophia myotonica, Friedreich's ataxia

to chronic low grade myocarditis or dilated cardiomyopathy (see below); for example, in Chagas' disease (p. 159) the patient usually recovers from the acute infection but often develops a chronic and potentially fatal dilated cardiomyopathy 10 or 20 years later.

Specific antimicrobial therapy may be used if a causa-tive organism has been identified; however, this is rare and in most cases only supportive therapy is available. Treatment for cardiac failure or arrhythmias may be required and patients should be advised to avoid intense physical exertion because there is some evidence that this can induce potentially fatal ventricular arrhythmias. Clinical trials have failed to demonstrate any benefit from treatment with corticosteroids and immuno-suppressive agents.

SPECIFIC HEART MUSCLE DISEASE

Many forms of specific heart muscle disease produce a clinical picture that is indistinguishable from dilated cardiomyopathy (e.g. connective tissue disorders, sarcoidosis, haemochromatosis, alcoholic heart muscle disease). In contrast, amyloidosis and eosinophilic heart disease produce symptoms and signs similar to those found in restrictive cardiomyopathy (see below), whereas Friedreich's ataxia (p. 1112) can mimic hypertrophic cardiomyopathy (see below).

The treatment and prognosis is determined by the underlying disorder. Abstention from alcohol may lead to a dramatic improvement in patients with alcoholic heart disease.

CARDIOMYOPATHY

There are three types of cardiomyopathy (Fig. 5.93).

Dilated cardiomyopathy

In this condition there is impaired ventricular contraction (often affecting both ventricles) leading to progressive left-sided and, later, right-sided heart failure. Functional mitral and/or tricuspid regurgitation may occur; arrhythmias are also common. The ECG usually shows non-specific changes but echocardiography is useful in making the diagnosis. The differential diagnosis includes most forms of specific heart muscle disease (e.g. alcoholic heart disease) and ischaemic heart disease. Treatment is aimed at controlling the resulting heart failure. Although some patients remain well for many years the prognosis is generally poor and cardiac transplantation may be indicated.

Restrictive or obliterative cardiomyopathy

In this condition ventricular filling is impaired because the ventricles are 'stiff'. This leads to high atrial pressures with atrial hypertrophy, dilatation and later atrial fibrillation. The differential diagnosis includes endomyocardial fibrosis, eosinophilic heart muscle disease and amyloidosis. Diagnosis can be very difficult and may require complex Doppler echocardiography, CT or MRI scanning and endomyocardial biopsy. Treatment is usually symptomatic, but excision of fibrotic endocardium may benefit some patients.

Hypertrophic cardiomyopathy

This is a familial condition characterised by inappropriate and elaborate ventricular hypertrophy with malalignment of the myocardial fibres. The hypertrophy may be generalised or largely confined to the interventricular septum (asymmetric septal hypertrophy) or the apex (apical hypertrophic cardiomyopathy—a variant which is common in the Far East).

In approximately 50% of cases the disease is transmitted as an autosomal dominant trait. Recent genetic studies have suggested that in many patients the condition is due to an abnormality of the beta myosin heavy chain caused by a variety of single point mutations on chromosome 14.

Heart failure may develop because the stiff non-compliant ventricles impede diastolic filling. Hypertrophy of the septum may also cause dynamic left ventricular outflow tract obstruction (**HOCM—hypertrophic obstructive cardiomyopathy**) and mitral regurgitation due to abnormal systolic anterior motion of the anterior mitral valve leaflet.

The symptoms and signs are similar to those of aortic stenosis and are listed in the information box below.

The natural history of hypertrophic cardiomyopathy is variable but clinical deterioration is often slow. The risk of sudden death is greatest in patients who present early in life (<30 years) and those who have:

- non-sustained ventricular tachycardia detected by ambulatory ECG monitoring
- a history of syncope
- a family history of sudden death

Management

No treatment is definitely known to improve prognosis, but β-adrenoceptor antagonists help to relieve angina and sometimes prevent syncopal attacks. Arrhythmias are common and often respond to treatment with amiodarone. Dual chamber pacing and surgery (partial resection of the septum or mitral valve replacement) are useful in selected patients, particularly those with outflow tract obstruction. Digoxin and vasodilators may increase outflow tract obstruction and should be avoided.

CLINICAL FEATURES OF HYPERTROPHIC CARDIOMYOPATHY

Symptoms
- angina on effort
- dyspnoea on effort
- syncope on effort
- sudden death

Signs
- jerky pulse†
- palpable left ventricular hypertrophy
- double impulse at the apex
  (palpable fourth heart sound due to left atrial hypertrophy)
- mid-systolic murmur at the base†
- pansystolic murmur (due to mitral regurgitation) at the apex

† signs of left ventricular outflow tract obstruction which may be augmented by standing up (reduced venous return), inotropes and vasodilators (e.g. sublingual nitrate)

Investigations
- Chest radiograph—non-specific changes only
- ECG—left ventricular hypertrophy ± a wide variety of often bizarre abnormalities
- Echocardiography—usually diagnostic

CARDIAC TUMOURS

Primary cardiac tumours are rare (<0.2% of autopsies), but the heart and mediastinum may be the site of metastases.

Most primary tumours are benign (75%), and of these the majority are myxomas. The remainder are fibromas, lipomas, fibroelastomas and haemangiomas.

ATRIAL MYXOMA

Myxomas most commonly arise in the left atrium, as single or multiple polypoid tumours, attached by a pedicle to the interatrial septum. They are usually gelatinous but may be solid and even calcified, with superimposed thrombus.

The tumour may be detected incidentally (on echocardiography), or following investigation of pyrexia, syncope, arrhythmias or emboli. Occasionally the condition presents with malaise and features suggestive of a connective tissue disorder (p. 912) including a raised ESR.

On examination the first heart sound is usually loud and there may be a murmur of mitral regurgitation with a variable diastolic sound (tumour 'plop') due to prolapse of the mass through the mitral valve.

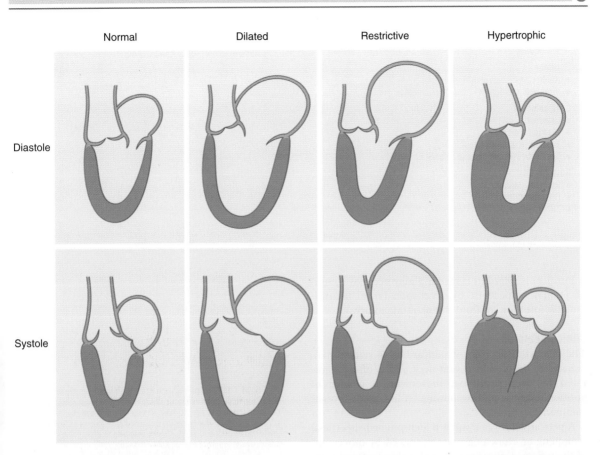

Fig. 5.93 **The three types of cardiomyopathy.**

The diagnosis is made on echocardiography and treatment is by surgical excision. If the pedicle is removed less than 5% of tumours recur.

FURTHER READING

Banatvala, J (ed) 1993 Viral infections of the heart. Edward Arnold, London
Stewart J T, McKenna W K 1992 Hypertrophic cardiomyopathy: diagnosis, prognosis and management. In: Rowlands D J (ed) Recent advances in cardiology. Churchill Livingstone, Edinburgh

DISEASES OF THE PERICARDIUM

The normal pericardial sac contains about 50 ml of fluid, similar to lymph, which lubricates the surface of the heart. The pericardium limits distension of the heart, contributes to the haemodynamic interdependence of the ventricles, and acts as a barrier to infection. Nevertheless, congenital absence of the pericardium does not appear to result in significant clinical or functional limitations.

ACUTE PERICARDITIS

Aetiology

Pericardial inflammation may be due to infection, immunological reaction, trauma or neoplasm and sometimes remains unexplained. Pericarditis and myocarditis often coexist, and all forms of pericarditis may produce a pericardial effusion (see below) which, depending on the aetiology, may be fibrinous, serous, haemorrhagic or purulent.

A fibrinous exudate may eventually lead to varying degrees of adhesion formation whereas serous pericarditis often produces a large effusion of turbid, straw-coloured fluid with a high protein content.

A haemorrhagic effusion is often due to malignant disease, particularly carcinoma of the breast, carcinoma of the bronchus and lymphoma.

AETIOLOGY OF ACUTE PERICARDITIS

Common
- Acute myocardial infarction
- Viral (e.g. coxsackie B, but often not identified)

Less common
- Uraemia
- Malignant disease
- Trauma (e.g. blunt chest injury)
- Connective tissue disease (e.g. SLE)

Rare (in UK)
- Bacterial infection
- Rheumatic fever
- Tuberculosis

Purulent pericarditis is rare and may occur as a complication of septicaemia, by direct spread from an intrathoracic infection, or from a penetrating injury.

Clinical features

The characteristic pain of pericarditis is retrosternal, radiates to the shoulders and neck and is often aggravated by deep breathing, movement, a change of position, exercise and swallowing. A low grade fever is common.

A pericardial friction rub is a high-pitched superficial scratching or crunching noise produced by movement of the inflamed pericardium, and is diagnostic of pericarditis; it is usually heard in systole but may also be audible in diastole and frequently has a 'to-and-fro' quality. A rub is often most easily detected by listening during both held inspiration and expiration to the praecordium with the stethoscope diaphragm.

Investigation

The ECG shows ST elevation with upward concavity (Fig. 5.94) over the affected area, which may be widespread. Later, there may be T wave inversion, particularly if there is a degree of myocarditis.

Management

The pain can usually be relieved by aspirin (600 mg 4-hourly), but a more potent anti-inflammatory agent such as indomethacin (25 mg 8-hourly) may be required. Corticosteroids may suppress symptoms but there is no evidence that they accelerate cure.

In viral pericarditis recovery usually occurs within a few days or weeks, but there may be recurrences (*chronic relapsing pericarditis*).

Purulent pericarditis requires treatment with antimicrobial therapy, paracentesis, and if necessary surgical drainage.

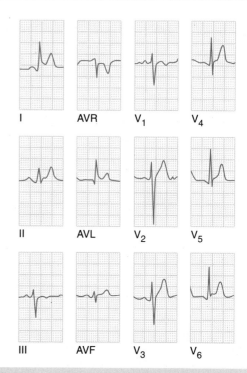

Fig. 5.94 ECG from a young man with acute pericarditis complicating acute myeloblastic leukaemia showing widespread ST elevation (leads I, II, aVL, V3–V6). The upward concave shape of the ST segments (see lead I) and the unusual distribution of ECG changes (involving anterior and inferior leads) may help to distinguish pericarditis from acute myocardial infarction.

PERICARDIAL EFFUSION

If a pericardial effusion develops there is sometimes a sensation of retrosternal oppression. An effusion is difficult to detect clinically; although the heart sounds may become quieter, pericardial friction is not always abolished.

The QRS voltages on the ECG are often reduced in the presence of a large effusion. Serial chest radiographs may show a rapid increase in the size of the cardiac shadow over days or even hours, and when there is a large effusion the heart often has a globular or pear-shaped appearance. Echocardiography is a useful and very sensitive means of detecting a pericardial effusion (Fig. 5.95A, B).

Cardiac tamponade

This term is used to describe acute heart failure due to compression of the heart by a large or rapidly developing effusion. Atypical presentations may occur when the effusion is loculated as a result of previous pericarditis or cardiac surgery. See also Shock, page 214.

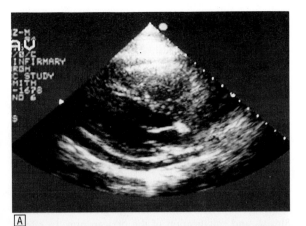

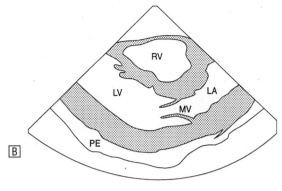

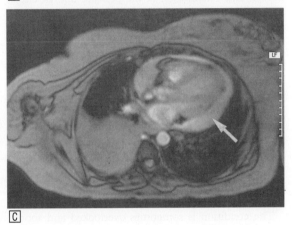

Fig. 5.95 **A** **Echocardiogram (long axis view) showing a large pericardial effusion.** **B** **line drawing:** PE = pericardial effusion, LV = left ventricle, RV = right ventricle, LA = left atrium, MV = mitral valve. **C** **MRI scan showing pericardial effusion.**

CLINICAL FEATURES OF CONSTRICTIVE PERICARDITIS

- Fatigue
- Rapid, low volume pulse
- Pulsus paradoxus (an excessive fall in blood pressure during inspiration)
- Elevated JVP with a rapid *y* descent
- Kussmaul's sign (a paradoxical rise in the JVP during inspiration)
- Loud early third heart sound or 'pericardial knock'
- Hepatomegaly
- Ascites
- Peripheral oedema

Pericardial aspiration

Paracentesis of a pericardial effusion may be indicated for diagnostic purposes or for the treatment of cardiac tamponade.

The fluid may be aspirated by introducing a needle just medial to the cardiac apex or by inserting a needle below the xiphoid process and directing it towards the left shoulder. The route of choice will depend on the experience of the operator, the configuration of the patient and the position of the effusion. Simultaneous echocardiography is very helpful.

Complications of paracentesis include arrhythmias, damage to a coronary artery, and bleeding with exacerbation of tamponade as a result of injury to the right ventricle.

A few millilitres of fluid may be sufficient for diagnostic purposes; however, if therapeutic drainage is required it is unwise to attempt aspiration of the whole effusion through a rigid needle and it may be safer to use a plastic cannula inserted over a needle or guidewire.

A viscous, loculated or recurrent effusion may require formal surgical drainage.

TUBERCULOUS PERICARDITIS

Tuberculous pericarditis may complicate pulmonary tuberculosis but may also be the first manifestation of the infection. In Africa a tuberculous pericardial effusion is a common feature of the acquired immunodeficiency syndrome (AIDS).

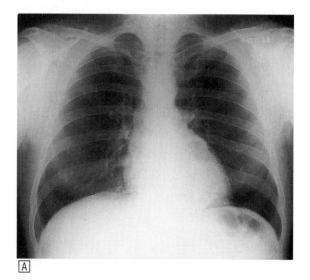

[A]

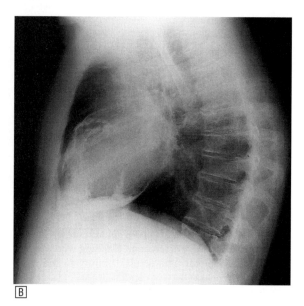

[B]

Fig. 5.96 [A] **PA and** [B] **lateral chest radiographs from a patient with severe heart failure due to chronic constrictive pericarditis.** The heart is not enlarged and there is heavy calcification of the pericardium that is most visible on the lateral film.

The condition typically presents with chronic malaise, weight loss and a low grade fever. An effusion usually develops and the pericardium may become thick and unyielding leading to pericardial constriction or tamponade. An associated pleural effusion is often present.

The diagnosis may be confirmed by aspiration of the fluid and direct examination or culture for tubercle bacilli. Treatment requires specific antituberculous chemotherapy (p. 361). Corticosteroids may help to prevent the development of constrictive pericarditis.

CHRONIC CONSTRICTIVE PERICARDITIS

Constrictive pericarditis is due to progressive thickening, fibrosis and calcification of the pericardium. In effect, the heart is encased in a solid shell and cannot fill properly; the calcification may extend into the myocardium so there may also be impaired myocardial contraction.

The condition often follows an attack of tuberculous pericarditis but can also complicate haemopericardium, viral pericarditis, rheumatoid arthritis and purulent pericarditis; it is often impossible to identify the original insult.

Clinical features

The symptoms and signs of systemic venous congestion are the hallmarks of constrictive pericarditis; atrial fibrillation is common and there is often dramatic ascites and hepatomegaly. Breathlessness is not a prominent symptom because the lungs are seldom congested.

The condition is sometimes overlooked and should be suspected in any patient with unexplained right heart failure and a small heart. A chest radiograph, which may show pericardial calcification (Fig. 5.96), and echocardiography often help to establish the diagnosis. CT scanning and magnetic resonance imaging are also useful techniques for imaging the pericardium.

Constrictive pericarditis is often difficult to distinguish from restrictive cardiomyopathy and the final diagnosis may depend on complex echo-Doppler studies and cardiac catheterisation.

Management

Surgical resection of the diseased pericardium can lead to a dramatic improvement but carries a high morbidity and produces disappointing results in up to 50% of patients.

Diseases of the respiratory system

The lungs, with their combined surface area of greater than 500 m², are directly open to the external environment. Thus, structural, functional or microbiological changes within the lungs can be closely related to epidemiological, environmental, occupational, personal and social factors. Primary respiratory diseases are responsible for a major burden of morbidity and untimely deaths, and the lungs are often affected in multisystem diseases.

Respiratory symptoms are the commonest cause of presentation to the family practitioner. Asthma occurs in more than 10% of British children; lung cancer caused 38 000 deaths in Great Britain in 1990; the lung is the major site of opportunistic infection in those immunocompromised by AIDS or by anti-allograft and anticancer chemotherapeutic regimens; and the spectre of tuberculosis, particularly the emergence of multiply drug-resistant strains, is back with us.

A number of important research advances have occurred in recent years. The discovery of the genetic mechanism of cystic fibrosis provides a novel opportunity to develop gene therapy strategies to replace the defective gene. The lung is especially favoured for gene therapy since its airway epithelial cells are accessible to nebulised particles and the extensive microvascular pulmonary capillary endothelium is available to intravenously-delivered agents. Finally, recent advances in our understanding of the cellular and molecular mechanisms underlying diseases such as asthma and the Adult Respiratory Distress Syndrome are likely to lead to rational, mechanism-based therapy within the foreseeable future.

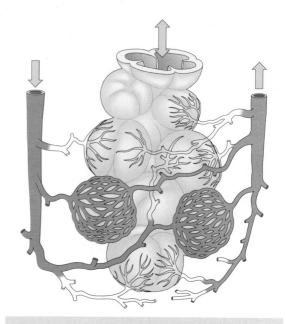

Fig. 6.1 **The acinus—the basic gas exchange unit of the lung.**

APPLIED ANATOMY AND PHYSIOLOGY

The upper respiratory tract includes the nose, nasopharynx and larynx. It is lined by vascular mucous membranes with ciliated epithelium on their surfaces. The lower respiratory tract includes the trachea and bronchi. These form an interconnecting tree of conducting airways eventually joining, via around 64 000 terminal bronchioles, with the alveoli to form the acini. The lower respiratory tract is lined with ciliated epithelium as far as the terminal bronchioles. The larynx and large bronchi are richly supplied with sensory nerve receptors involved in the cough reflex.

Some knowledge of the patterns of branching of the lobar and segmental bronchi is necessary for interpreting investigations, including CT scans, chest radiographs and bronchograms. The acinus is the gas exchange unit (see Fig. 6.1) of the lung and comprises branching respiratory bronchioles leading to clusters of alveoli. The alveoli are lined mostly with flattened epithelial cells

(type I pneumocytes), but there are some, more cuboidal, type II pneumocytes. The latter produce surfactant, a mixture of phospholipids which acts to reduce surface tension and counteract the tendency of alveoli to collapse. Type II pneumocytes also display a remarkable capacity to divide and reconstitute the type I pneumocytes after lung injury.

The interpretation of a variety of pulmonary function tests requires some understanding of the effects of physiological mechanisms, including ventilation and blood flow, gas exchange and control of breathing.

VENTILATION, BLOOD FLOW AND DIFFUSION

Major bronchial and pulmonary divisions are shown in Figure 6.2.

The muscular effort of inspiration overcomes elastic resistance of the lungs and chest wall and non-elastic resistance, chiefly in the airways. In normal subjects, the large central airways (see Fig. 6.2) contribute most of the resistance, and the peripheral airways contribute less despite their individually small calibre because of their large combined cross-sectional area. In disease, resistance of either kind may greatly increase and call into action accessory muscles of inspiration (sterno-mastoid and scaleni) or expiration (abdominals). Examples are listed in the information box.

Fatigue developing in muscles working against abnor-

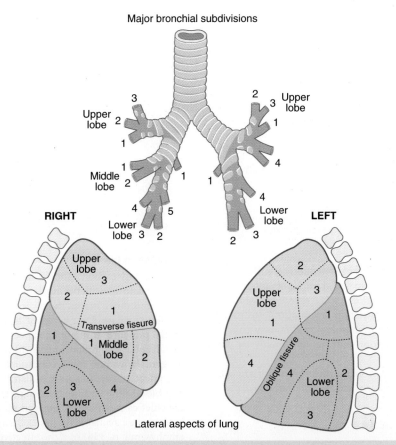

Major bronchial subdivisions

Lateral aspects of lung

Fig. 6.2 The major bronchial divisions and the fissures, lobes and segments of the lungs. The position of the oblique fissure is such that the left upper lobe is largely anterior to the lower lobe. On the right side the transverse fissure separates the upper from the anteriorly placed middle lobe which is matched by the lingular segment on the left side. The site of the lobe determines whether physical signs are mainly anterior or posterior. Each lobe is composed of two or more bronchopulmonary segments, i.e. the lung tissue supplied by the main branches of each lobar bronchus. BRONCHOPULMONARY SEGMENTS: **Right**—*Upper lobe* 1. Anterior 2. Posterior 3. Apical *Middle lobe* 1. Lateral 2. Medial. *Lower lobe* 1. Apical 2. Posterior basal 3. Lateral basal 4. Anterior basal 5. Medial basal **Left**—*Upper lobe* 1. Anterior 2. Apical 3. Posterior 4. Lingular. *Lower lobe* 1. Apical 2. Posterior basal 3. Lateral basal 4. Anterior basal.

EXAMPLES OF INCREASED RESPIRATORY RESISTANCE

Elastic resistance
- Pulmonary fibrosis
- Pulmonary oedema
- Kyphoscoliosis
- Ankylosing spondylitis

Non-elastic resistance
- Asthma
- Emphysema
- Chronic bronchitis
- Tumours of major bronchi

---

mal loads or at a mechanical disadvantage can contribute to respiratory failure (p. 326).

The right ventricle pumps blood against the relatively low pulmonary vascular resistance. Increased resistance, due for example to thromboembolism (p. 277) or to destructive changes caused by chronic bronchitis and emphysema (p. 334), imposes an additional load result-

ing in right ventricular hypertrophy, and eventually failure ensues.

Gas exchange

Gas exchange in the lungs is inefficient unless ventilation is distributed uniformly to different parts of the lungs and is matched by uniform distribution of blood flow.

It follows that if the range of ratios of ventilation to blood flow found throughout the lung is greater than normal, greater proportions of ventilation and blood flow will appear to be wasted. Abnormally large proportions of ventilation wasted on dead space mean more work to maintain the alveolar ventilation needed to match metabolic CO_2 production and hold arterial PCO_2 in normal limits (4.8–6.0 kPa; 36–45 mmHg), for these quantities are linked by the expression:

$$PaCO_2 \, \alpha \, \frac{CO_2 \, production}{alveolar \, (useful) \, ventilation}$$

This mechanism is, therefore, one of the causes of hypercapnia—($PaCO_2 > 6$ kPa (45 mmHg)): see the information box.

SOME CAUSES OF HYPERCAPNIA (RAISED $PaCO_2$)

Central
- Brain-stem lesion
- Central sleep apnoea

Neuromuscular
- Peripheral neuropathy
- Myasthenia gravis
- Myopathies

Chest wall
- Kyphoscoliosis
- Ankylosing spondylitis
- Trauma

Pulmonary
- Chronic bronchitis (and emphysema)

Blood flow wasted on perfusing poorly ventilated lung has the effect of a right-to-left shunt. This might occur by: bronchial obstruction (with secretions, mucosal oedema, broncho-constriction or tumours); destruction of elastic tissue (e.g. emphysema); pulmonary collapse; consolidation; fibrosis or oedema, and finally by chest wall deformities.

This mechanism is probably the most important cause of hypoxaemia in disease (see information box).

CAUSES OF HYPOXAEMIA

- Venous admixture effect (poorly ventilated lung)
- Alveolar underventilation (raised $PaCO_2$)   } Corrected by oxygen
- Impairment of diffusion (less important at rest)
- Right-to-left shunts (circulatory channels bypassing lungs)
- Reduced oxygen content (PaO_2 may be normal) (anaemia; inactivated haemoglobin)

Hypoxaemia due to all these causes, except that due to congenital heart disease or vascular anomalies (where shunted blood does not pass through the alveoli), is reversed by giving oxygen. Hypoxaemia also occurs if the oxygen capacity of the blood is reduced as, for example, in anaemia or carbon monoxide poisoning.

The normal arterial PaO_2 is over 12 kPa (90 mmHg) at the age of 20 and falls to around 11 kPa (82 mmHg) at 60. Above this age a further fall in PaO_2 of up to 1.3 kPa (10 mmHg) may occur on lying down because of closure of small airways in the dependent regions of the lungs.

Maldistribution of ventilation and blood flow has, therefore, important effects on gas exchange.

Table 6.1 Some influences on the respiratory centre

Stimulant	
Voluntary—	*Overbreathing*
Upper brain stem lesions—	*Central neurogenic hyperventilation*
Input from receptors—	*Pain; muscles and joints; pulmonary afferents*
Increased $PaCO_2$—	*Via central and peripheral chemoreceptors*
Increased arterial hydrogen ion concentration—	*Via peripheral chemoreceptors*
Decreased PaO_2— (< 8 kPa at rest)	*Via peripheral chemoreceptors*
Pyrexia	
Depressant	
Voluntary—	*Breath-holding*
Brain-stem lesions	
Sedative drugs (opiates; benzodiazepines)	
Hypothermia	

Diffusion in the lungs

Oxygen and carbon dioxide move along the terminal airways and alveoli by molecular diffusion in the gas phase and move across the alveolar wall by diffusion in the liquid phase from a site of higher to one of lower partial pressure. It might be expected that thickening of the alveolar wall might impair diffusion, particularly of oxygen. However, most conditions which might have this effect can also cause maldistribution of ventilation and blood flow and analysis suggests that this remains the chief cause of hypoxaemia in these conditions.

If the area available for gas exchange is reduced (as in emphysema, p. 334) or if the effective area is reduced by maldistribution of ventilation and perfusion, the overall ability of the lung to transfer gases will also diminish. Such a reduction may not be significant at rest, but may limit the amount of oxygen which can be taken up during exercise and so become a cause of hypoxaemia.

CONTROL OF BREATHING

Influences on the respiratory centre may be exerted either neurally, via CNS receptors, or chemically via peripheral chemoreceptors sensitive to the composition of blood and cerebrospinal fluid.

Their effects are summarised in Table 6.1. It follows that either hyper- or hypocapnia implies some alteration in respiratory control. In some patients with chronic bronchitis and chronic hypercapnia, relief of the concurrent hypoxaemia may, by removing one of the remaining stimuli to breathing, be followed by worsening of the hypercapnia.

LUNG DEFENCES

Each day our lungs are directly exposed to more than 7000 litres of air which contain varying amounts of inorganic and organic particles as well as potentially lethal bacteria and viruses. In general terms, physical mechanisms including cough are particularly important in defence of the upper airways, whereas the lower airways are protected by complex mucociliary mechanisms, the anti-microbial properties of surfactant and the lung lining fluids; and by the resident alveolar macrophages.

Physical defences

Most large particles are removed from inspired air by the nose, which is composed of a 'stack' of fine aerodynamic filters comprising fine hairs and columnar ciliated epithelium which cover the turbinate bones. The larynx acts as a sphincter during cough and expectoration and is an essential mechanism protecting the lower airways during swallowing and vomiting.

Mucociliary clearance

Particles with a diameter greater than 0.5 μm which survive passage through the nose will be trapped by the lining fluid of the trachea and bronchi to be cleared by the 'mucociliary escalator' (see Fig. 6.3). This highly effective small particle clearance mechanism works by a complex interaction between cilia, which are a series of small projections on the surface of respiratory epithelial cells, and mucus, which forms a 'raft' on top of the cilia. Particles are trapped by the mucus which is then swept by the cilia in a cephalic direction. Other important functions of mucus include: dilution of noxious substances; lubrication of the airways; and humidification of inspired air. Mucus, which is mostly secreted by goblet cells of the respiratory epithelium, is composed of 95% water, the mucus glycoproteins and a variety of other proteins (see information box) which, although present in low concentrations, are likely to play an important role in the defence of the bronchial tree. A number of factors may reduce mucociliary clearance by interfering with ciliary function or by causing actual ciliary damage. These include: pollutants, cigarette smoke, local and general anaesthetic agents, bacterial products and viral infection. There is also a rare autosomal recessive condition (1 in 30 000 live births) called primary ciliary dyskinesia which may be associated with male infertility and situs inversus (Kartagener's syndrome). Primary ciliary dyskinesia is characterised by repeated sinusitis and respiratory tract infections which progress to persistent lung suppuration and bronchiectasis, thus reinforcing the importance of ciliary clearance in antibacterial lung defences.

Surfactant and other defensive proteins

In addition to surface active properties which are so important in lung mechanics (see p. 314), surfactant contains a number of proteins, including surfactant

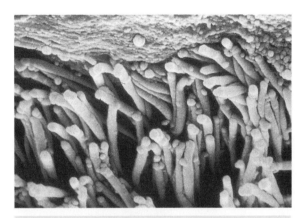

Fig. 6.3 The mucociliary escalator. Scanning electron micrograph of the respiratory epithelium showing large numbers of cilia overlaid by the mucus 'raft'.

PROTECTIVE AGENTS IN THE LUNG LINING FLUIDS

- Surfactant proteins—bacterial opsonisation
- Immunoglobulins (IgA, IgG, IgM)—bacterial opsonisation, generation of the immune response
- Complement—bacterial opsonisation, generation of the inflammatory response
- Bactericidal proteins—bacterial killing
- Proteinase inhibitors—protection of host tissues during the inflammatory response

protein A, which can opsonise bacteria and other particles, rendering them susceptible to phagocytosis by macrophages. Lung lining fluids also contain other defensive proteins (see information box above) including immunoglobulins, complement, defensins (powerful antibacterial peptides) and a variety of antiproteinases which play an important role in protecting healthy tissues from damage which would be incurred by the release of proteinases from inflammatory cells during the inflammatory response (see p. 40, Ch. 2).

Alveolar macrophages

These multipotent cells normally patrol the alveoli (see Fig. 6.4) where they demonstrate a formidable array of mechanisms with which they recognise and destroy bacteria and other foreign organic particles. The remarkably versatile resident macrophage can also 'call in reinforcements' by generating mediators which cause an inflammatory response and attract granulocytes and monocytes (see p. 41). It may also generate an immune response by presenting antigens and by releasing specific lymphokines (see p. 38, Ch. 2). Finally, the alveolar macrophage exerts important scavenging functions in the clearance of dead bacteria and other cells during the

Table 6.2 Summary of typical physical signs in the more common respiratory diseases

Pathological process	Movement of chest wall	Mediastinal displacement	Percussion note	Breath sounds	Vocal resonance	Added sounds
Consolidation as in lobar pneumonia	Reduced on side affected	None	Dull	High-pitched bronchial	Increased Whispering pectoriloquy	Fine crepitations early; coarse crepitations later
Collapse due to obstruction of major bronchus	Reduced on side affected	Towards lesion	Dull	Diminished or absent	Reduced or absent	None
Collapse due to peripheral bronchial obstruction	Reduced on side affected	Towards lesion	Dull	High-pitched bronchial	Increased Whispering pectoriloquy	None early; coarse crepitations later
Localised fibrosis and/or bronchiectasis	Slightly reduced on side affected	Towards lesion	Impaired	Low-pitched bronchial	Increased	Coarse crepitations
Cavitation (usually associated with consolidation or fibrosis)	Slightly reduced on side affected	None, or towards lesion	Impaired	'Amphoric' bronchial	Increased Whispering pectoriloquy	Coarse crepitations
Pleural effusion Empyema	Reduced or absent (depending on size) on side affected	Towards opposite side	Stony dull	Diminished or absent (occasionally bronchial)	Reduced or absent (occasionally increased)	Pleural rub in some cases (above effusion)
Pneumothorax	Reduced or absent (depending on size) on side affected	Towards opposite side	Normal or hyper-resonant	Diminished or absent (occasionally faint bronchial)	Reduced or absent	Tinkling crepitations when fluid present
Bronchitis: acute chronic	Normal or symmetrically diminished	None	Normal	Vesicular with prolonged expiration	Normal	Rhonchi, usually with some coarse crepitations
Bronchial asthma	Symmetrically diminished	None	Normal	Vesicular with prolonged expiration	Normal or reduced	Rhonchi, mainly expiratory and high-pitched
Bronchopneumonia	Symmetrically diminished	None	May be impaired	Usually harsh vesicular with prolonged expiration	Normal	Rhonchi and coarse crepitations
Diffuse pulmonary emphysema	Symmetrically diminished	None	Normal	Diminished vesicular with prolonged expiration	Normal or reduced	Expiratory rhonchi
Interstitial lung disease	Symmetrically diminished	None	Normal	Harsh vesicular with prolonged expiration	Usually increased	End-inspiratory crepitations uninfluenced by coughing

aftermath of infection and inflammation. Nevertheless, it is important to appreciate that the excessive or uncontrolled release of some of these powerful macrophage products may cause disordered inflammation or scarring responses which are likely to be important in the pathogenesis of a variety of inflammatory diseases including asthma, chronic bronchitis and emphysema and other inflammatory/scarring conditions of the lung, e.g. fibrosing alveolitis.

SPECIAL INVESTIGATIONS

It is essential to take a detailed history from the patient, and much can be learned from a careful physical exam-

ination (see Table 6.2). Routine haematological and biochemical investigations can provide indices of infection, immunosuppression and evidence of metastasis of lung tumours, but a number of special investigations are often helpful in the diagnosis and monitoring of lung disease.

IMAGING

The 'plain' chest radiograph

Many diseases, including bronchial carcinoma and pulmonary tuberculosis, cannot be detected at an early stage without a radiograph of the chest. A lateral film provides additional information about the nature and situation of a pulmonary, pleural or mediastinal abnor-

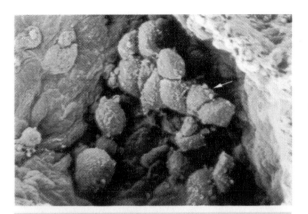

Fig. 6.4 Alveolar macrophages. Scanning electron micrograph showing alveolar macrophages (arrow) patrolling the alveolar spaces of the lung.

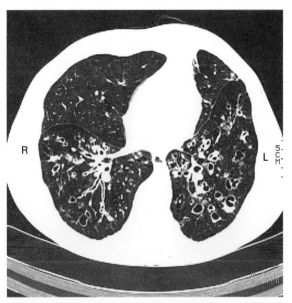

Fig. 6.5 Computed Tomography of the thorax showing extensive dilatation of the bronchi (bronchiectasis) in both lower lobes.

mality. Comparison with previous radiographs may help to distinguish between a 'new' or progressive change which is thus potentially serious, and 'old' or static abnormalities which may be of no importance. In some diseases, such as chronic bronchitis and asthma, there is often no radiographic abnormality. In these diseases functional assessment (p. 321) may be of much more value in detecting abnormality.

Computed tomography

This has virtually taken over from conventional tomography in centres where it is accessible. Conventional tomography was valuable in determining the position and size of the pulmonary nodule or mass and whether calcification or cavitation was present. It was also useful in localising lesions before percutaneous needle biopsy and in assessing the mediastinum and thoracic cage. But in all of these examples, except possibly for assessing the ribs, the CT scan is more sensitive and accurate. Computed tomography is now widely used in the pre-operative assessment of patients with lung cancer, particularly for assessing mediastinal spread, and the same examination will often indicate whether liver and adrenals are involved. Its value in imaging the mediastinum can be greatly enhanced by using an intravenous contrast which outlines the mediastinal vessels. The new high resolution CT scan is useful in diagnosing interstitial fibrosis, and in identifying bronchiectasis (Fig. 6.5).

Ventilation perfusion imaging

Its main value is in the detection of pulmonary thromboemboli. ^{133}Xe gas is inhaled (the ventilation scan) and ^{99m}Tc-labelled macroaggregates of albumin, or albumin microspheres, are injected intravenously, the particles becoming trapped in pulmonary microvessels

and providing the 'perfusion' scan. Pulmonary emboli can be detected as a 'filling defect' in the perfusion scan (Fig. 6.6), but patients with asthma, chronic bronchitis or other forms of obstructive airways disease may also have disordered pulmonary vascular distribution. However, in these patients the ventilation scan shows defects which match the areas of reduced perfusion on the perfusion scan, whereas the perfusion defects in pulmonary embolism are not matched to defects on the ventilation scan. Ventilation perfusion scanning may also be useful in pre-operative assessment of the functional effects of lung cancer and bullae.

Pulmonary angiography

This is the definitive method of diagnosing pulmonary emboli, particularly in the acutely ill and shocked patient or when ventilation perfusion scans are equivocal. Dye is passed down a catheter inserted via the femoral vein into the main pulmonary artery. This catheter can also be used to measure pulmonary artery pressure and instil thrombolytic agents such as streptokinase. Digital subtraction angiography (DSA) is a technique whereby images obtained before dye injection are digitised and subtracted from post-contrast images, thus removing bones and other background structures from the final digital images. This technique is more sensitive and requires much less contrast to obtain high quality images (Fig. 6.7).

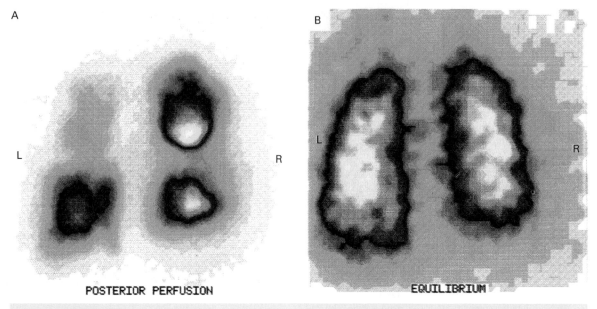

Fig. 6.6 **Lung ventilation and perfusion scintigraphy.** Multiple perfusion defects present in perfusion scan A with normal ventilation scan B. These appearances indicate a high probability of recent pulmonary embolism.

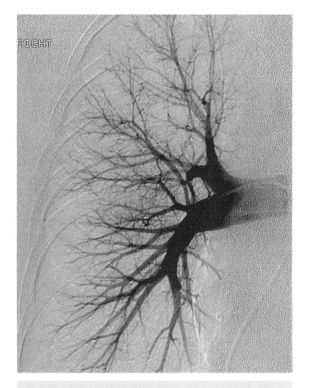

Fig. 6.7 **Normal digital subtraction pulmonary angiogram of the right lung.**

ENDOSCOPIC EXAMINATION

Laryngoscopy

The larynx may be inspected indirectly with a mirror or directly with a laryngoscope. Fibreoptic instruments allow a magnified view to be obtained.

Bronchoscopy

The trachea and larger bronchi are inspected by a bronchoscope of either flexible fibreoptic or rigid type. Structural changes, such as distortion or obstruction, can be seen. Abnormal tissue in the bronchial lumen or wall can be biopsied, and bronchial brushings, washings or aspirates can be taken for cytological or bacteriological examination. The range of direct vision is limited by the calibre of the sub-segmental bronchi, but peripheral lesions can sometimes be reached by flexible biopsy forceps directed under fluoroscopic control. Small biopsy specimens of lung tissue taken by forceps passed through the bronchial wall (transbronchial biopsy) may reveal sarcoid granulomata or malignant diseases, but are generally too small to be of diagnostic value in diffuse interstitial lung disease (p. 379 and p. 384).

Mediastinoscopy

In this surgical procedure the mediastinoscope is introduced through a small incision at the suprasternal notch to give a view of the upper mediastinum. Biopsy of some mediastinal nodes is possible, which may be of value in obtaining a diagnosis and in determining whether a bronchial carcinoma has spread to the mediastinum and is, therefore, inoperable.

Pleural aspiration and thoracoscopy

Pleural aspiration and biopsy using an Abram's needle will provide histological evidence of the cause of pleural effusion. Transthoracic needle biopsy (often with CT screening) may be useful in obtaining a cytological diagnosis from a peripheral lung lesion. In difficult cases, thoracoscopy may be necessary to obtain diseased tissue, and the recent introduction of video-assisted thoracoscopic lung biopsy is likely to obviate the need for surgical thoracotomy in cases of interstitial lung disease when an open lung biopsy is required (see p. 381).

SKIN TESTS

The tuberculin test (p. 360) and Kveim test (p. 382) may be of value in the diagnosis of tuberculosis and sarcoidosis respectively. Skin hypersensitivity tests are useful in the investigation of allergic disease (p. 336).

IMMUNOLOGICAL AND SEROLOGICAL TESTS

The presence of pneumococcal antigen (revealed by counter-immunoelectrophoresis) in sputum may be of diagnostic importance. Exfoliated cells colonised by Influenza A virus (p. 354) can be detected by fluorescent antibody techniques. In blood, high or rising antibody titres to specific organisms (such as *Legionella*, *Mycoplasma*, *Chlamydia* or viruses) may eventually clinch a diagnosis suspected on clinical grounds. Precipitating antibodies may be found as a reaction to fungi such as *Aspergillus* (p. 367) or to antigens involved in allergic alveolitis (p. 385).

MICROBIOLOGICAL INVESTIGATIONS

Sputum, pleural fluid, throat swabs, blood and bronchial washings and aspirates can be examined for bacteria, fungi and viruses. In some cases, as when *M. tuberculosis* is isolated, the information is diagnostically conclusive but in other circumstances the findings must be interpreted in conjunction with the results of clinical and radiological examination.

HISTOPATHOLOGICAL AND CYTOLOGICAL EXAMINATION

Histopathological examination of biopsy material (obtained endoscopically from pleura, lymph node or lung biopsy) often allows a 'tissue diagnosis' to be made. This is of particular importance in suspected malignancy or in elucidating the pathological changes in interstitial lung disease (p. 379). Important causative organisms, such as *M. tuberculosis*, *Pn. carinii* or fungi may be identified in bronchial washings, brushings or transbronchial biopsies.

Cytological examination of exfoliated cells in sputum, pleural fluid or bronchial brushings and washings or of fine-needle aspirates from lymph nodes or pulmonary lesions can provide rapid evidence of malignancy. Cellular patterns in bronchial lavage fluid may help to distinguish pulmonary changes due to sarcoidosis (p. 381) from those caused by fibrosing alveolitis (p. 383) or allergic alveolitis (p. 385)

LUNG FUNCTION TESTING

Most pulmonary function tests detect impairment and assess the effects of treatment or progress of the disease. (Some abbreviations used in pulmonary function testing are shown in Table 6.3).

Fewer tests, such as measurements of exercise tolerance, assess disability or handicap. Some tests require a high degree of skill and elaborate apparatus, but others are simple routine procedures which can be undertaken by any doctor without special training.

Measurements of ventilatory capacity

The forced expiratory volume in one second (FEV_1), forced vital capacity (FVC) and vital capacity (VC) are obtained from maximal forced and relaxed expirations into a recording spirometer and compared with predicted values based on age, sex and height and ethnic group. Typical patterns of abnormality known as

Table 6.3	Abbreviations used in pulmonary function testing
FEV_1	Forced expiratory volume in one second
FVC	Forced vital capacity
VC	Vital capacity (forced or relaxed)
PEF	Peak (maximum) expiratory flow
TLC	Total lung capacity
FRC	Functional residual capacity
RV	Residual volume
T_{co}	Gas transfer factor for carbon monoxide
D_{co}	Diffusing capacity for carbon monoxide
K_{co}	Transfer coefficient for carbon monoxide (T_{co}/litre lung volume)

Table 6.4 Patterns of abnormal ventilatory capacity

Test	Obstructive	Restrictive
FEV_1	$\downarrow\downarrow$	$\downarrow$
VC	$\downarrow$ or normal	$\downarrow\downarrow$
FEV_1/VC	$\downarrow$	Normal or $\uparrow$

obstructive and **restrictive** ventilatory defects are shown in Table 6.4.

If an obstructive ventilatory defect is found, the response to bronchodilators in standard doses (salbutamol 200 mcg from pressurised aerosol) or larger doses (salbutamol 2.5 mg by nebuliser) can be measured. Reversibility of airflow obstruction is found in asthma (p. 340) and in some patients with chronic bronchitis.

Peak expiratory flow (PEF) can be measured during forced expiration by a gauge or meter, which is simpler and cheaper than a spirometer. Reduced values indicate airflow obstruction, and serial measurements are of use in following circadian changes (p. 340) and responses to therapy or to occupational exposure to allergens or sensitising agents. PEF is of little value in restrictive ventilatory defects.

Measurements of lung volumes

Normal landmarks and patterns of abnormality of lung volumes in obstructive and restrictive ventilatory defects are shown in Figure 6.8. The values are obtained either by diluting helium (a non-toxic, non-absorbed gas) into the gas in the lungs, or in a whole body plethysmograph.

Measurements of gas transfer factor

The gas transfer factor (diffusing capacity) may be thought of as the conductance of the lungs for the gas being studied. It forms a useful overall estimate of the ability of the lungs to exchange gases, and is of particular value in interstitial lung disease (p. 379), sarcoidosis (p. 381) and emphysema (p. 334). It is normally estimated by measuring the uptake of carbon monoxide from a single breath of a 0.3% mixture in air.

Arterial blood gas analysis

Modern automatic analysers give a rapid direct read-out of PO_2, PCO_2 and hydrogen ion concentration in arterial blood, often supplemented by derived variables (such as oxygen saturation and bicarbonate concentration) which may be of value in assessment of hypoxaemia or acid-base balance (p. 603). Such measurements are of particular value in the management of respiratory failure (p.

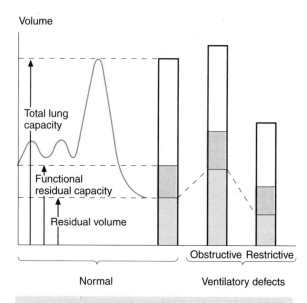

Fig 6.8 Normal lung volumes and the changes which occur in obstructive and restrictive ventilatory defects.

326) and asthma (p. 336) and adult respiratory distress syndrome (ARDS) (p. 388).

Ear or pulse oximeters allow continuous non-invasive measurement of arterial oxygen saturation, of value in assessing hypoxaemia and the effects of oxygen therapy.

Exercise tests

Exercise challenge is a self-evident test for detecting exercise-induced asthma (p. 340). Formal exercise tests, in which cardiac and respiratory responses to bicycle or treadmill exercise are measured in the laboratory, are of value in detecting exercise hypoxaemia and in assessing disability due to respiratory disease.

'Everyday' exercise tests, such as measurement of the distance the patient can walk in six minutes, require no complex apparatus and assist in the assessment of disability, handicap and the response to treatment.

FURTHER READING

Gibson G J 1995 Respiratory function tests. In: Brewis R A L et al, Respiratory Medicine. Baillière Tindall, London

Haslett C 1995 Non-immune defence mechanisms of the lung. In: Ledingham J et al (eds) The Oxford Textbook of Medicine. Oxford University Press, Oxford

Leach R M, Treacher D F 1992 Oxygen transport: the relationship between oxygen delivery and consumption. Thorax 47: 971–978

Wagner P D, Rodriguez-Roisin R 1991 Clinical advances in pulmonary gas exchange. American Review of Respiratory Disease 143: 883–889

MAJOR MANIFESTATIONS OF LUNG DISEASE

DYSPNOEA

Breathlessness or dyspnoea can be defined as an unpleasant subjective awareness of the sensation of breathing. It is a common symptom of cardiac disease and respiratory disease, but it may occasionally be prominent in diseases of other systems, e.g. exertional dyspnoea in severe anaemia or acute dyspnoea in diabetic ketoacidosis. The term 'dyspnoea', derived from the Greek roots *dys* 'difficult, painful' and *pnoia* (breathing), is often used ambiguously, since several types of disagreeable symptoms may be generated in the thorax. Those with asthma or chronic obstructive airways disease may describe a 'tight chest', a 'smothering' feeling may be described by patients with restrictive lung disease, patients with pulmonary oedema may feel they are 'drowning' and clearly any cause of pleural pain (p. 396) will cause limitation of breathing.

In broad physiological terms, patients usually perceive discomfort either from an increased ventilatory rate or drive, which can be provoked by a variety of factors, or from any disease which causes sufficient reduction of ventilatory capacity (see information box). Other factors, however, including the stimulation of J receptors leading to amplification of the ventilatory response in asthma or restrictive disorders, may also contribute.

PHYSIOLOGICAL BASIS OF DYSPNOEA

Increased ventilatory rate
- $\uparrow PaCO_2$—e.g. COPD
- $\downarrow PaO_2$—e.g. cyanotic congenital heart disease, asthma, COPD
- Acidaemia—e.g. diabetic ketoacidosis, lactic acidosis
- Exercise
- Fever

Reduced ventilatory capacity
- $\downarrow$Lung volume, e.g. restrictive lung diseases— pneumonia, pulmonary oedema, interstitial lung diseases
- $\uparrow$Resistance to airflow, e.g. asthma, COPD, upper airway or laryngeal obstruction
- Pleural pain

It will now be obvious that diseases presenting with dyspnoea may often have a multifactorial aetiology, e.g. acute respiratory infections may stimulate respiratory rate as a consequence of fever, hypoxaemia and, in severe cases, by acidaemia or hypercapnia. They may also reduce ventilatory capacity by increasing bronchial resistance and by restricting ventilation because of pleural pain.

While it is useful to understand the physiological basis of dyspnoea, patients often present either as an emergency with acute breathlessness (with prominent symptoms even at rest) or to the clinic with more chronic dyspnoea on exertion, and it is useful therefore to describe the causes of dyspnoea in this fashion (see Table 6.5 below).

AN APPROACH TO THE DIFFERENTIAL DIAGNOSIS IN PATIENTS WITH CHRONIC EXERTIONAL DYSPNOEA

Chronic obstructive pulmonary disease (COPD)

There is usually a history of exertional dyspnoea over many months or years, with a steady chronic decline in exercise capacity (e.g. exertional dyspnoea on hills, followed by stairs, followed by walking on the flat). Chronic persistent cough and daily production of sputum is the rule and there may be a history of recurrent acute exacerbations of bronchitis. Wheezing on exercise may be prominent. In late disease, particularly if cor pulmonale develops, orthopnoea, nocturnal breathlessness and ankle swelling may supervene.

On examination cyanosis may be apparent at rest or on trivial exertion, together with expiratory wheeze, pursing of the lips and intercostal indrawing. The antero-posterior diameter of the chest may be increased (barrel chest) and there may be a reduced crico-sternal distance with a 'tracheal tug' on inspiration. However, it is important to note that patients presenting with type II respiratory failure (see p. 326) may not be distressed. The chest radiograph may show signs of hyperinflation and/or bullae, arterial blood gases may reveal hypoxaemia, hypercapnia and a raised plasma bicarbonate, indicating compensated type II respiratory failure. There will often be a severe obstructive defect on spirometry, with a low FEV_1 which may or may not improve after inhaled bronchodilators.

Heart disease

It is often difficult to differentiate dyspnoea due to heart disease from that caused by lung disease. A history of cough, wheezing and nocturnal breathlessness may occur in cardiac failure as well as chronic obstructive pulmonary disease (COPD). A history of angina or hypertension may be useful in implicating a cardiac cause.

On examination, an increase in heart size as judged by a displaced apex beat, a raised JVP and cardiac murmurs may implicate cardiac disease (although these signs can occur also in severe cor pulmonale; see page 335). The chest radiograph and ECG may provide evidence of left ventricular or atrial enlargement. Arterial blood gases may be of value, since in the absence of intracardiac

Table 6.5 Some causes of dyspnoea

	Acute dyspnoea at rest	Chronic exertional dyspnoea
Cardiovascular system	Acute pulmonary oedema Pulmonary embolus Major neonatal congenital heart disease	Chronic cardiac failure Chronic pulmonary thromboembolism Congenital heart disease
Respiratory system	Acute severe asthma Acute exacerbation of COPD Pneumothorax Pneumonia Adult Respiratory Distress Syndrome Inhaled foreign body (especially in the child) Lobar collapse Laryngeal oedema (e.g. anaphylaxis)	COPD 'Chronic asthma' Bronchial carcinoma Interstitial lung diseases: sarcoidosis, fibrosing alveolitis, extrinsic allergic alveolitis, pneumoconiosis Lymphatic carcinomatosis (may cause intolerable dyspnoea) Large pleural effusion(s)

Others	Metabolic acidosis (e.g. diabetic ketoacidosis, lactic
	   acidosis, uraemia, overdose of salicylates or ethylene
	   glycol)
		Severe anaemia

shunts or severe, obvious pulmonary oedema, the PaO_2 in cardiac disease is not usually reduced significantly and the $PaCO_2$ is low or normal.

Interstitial or alveolar disease of the lung

A large number of conditions can cause interstitial lung disease (p. 380), which may be difficult to distinguish from other conditions including infiltrating malignancy and chronic opportunistic lung infections (see information box, p. 380). It is imperative to elicit a detailed history, including occupation and exposure to birds and other sources of organic agents which may provoke lung disease. The chest radiograph is nearly always abnormal, but early changes may be very subtle. Pulmonary function tests usually show a restrictive defect (reduced vital capacity) and reduced gas transfer (p. 322). Arterial blood gases may show hypoxaemia, or haemoglobin desaturation may be detected by oximetry, particularly during formal exercise testing, which may be valuable in early disease but $PaCO_2$ is seldom elevated even in advanced disease.

Diseases of the chest wall or respiratory muscles

These are usually obvious on history, examination and chest radiography. While other rarer causes of alveolar hypoventilation, e.g. brain stem defects, primary alveolar hypoventilation and alveolar hypoventilation in gross obesity may cause disordered breathing and cyanosis, these conditions are not usually associated with breathlessness.

Psychogenic breathlessness

The patient may present with other classical symptoms of an anxiety disorder, but it is essential to be confident of the diagnosis since anxiety is a highly prevalent symptom and various organic conditions (e.g. primary pulmonary hypertension and repeated pulmonary thromboembolism) may present with breathlessness alone and particularly in the early stages, few, if any, physical signs. Historical features, including absence of symptoms on exercise, relation to anxiety, the feeling of 'not being able to take a deep enough breath' and frequent 'sighing' breathing may all be suggestive of anxiety-induced symptoms. Specialist centres use a number of features to develop a 'points' score in favour of this type of psychogenic hyperventilation syndrome—see the information box below.

SOME FACTORS POINTING TO PSYCHOGENIC HYPERVENTILATION

- 'Inability to take a deep breath'
- Frequent sighing/erratic ventilation at rest
- Short breath-holding time in the absence of severe respiratory disease
- Difficulty in performing/inconsistent spirometry manoeuvres
- High score on Nijmegen questionnaire
- Induction of symptoms during submaximal hyperventilation
- Resting end-tidal $CO_2 < 4.5\%$

To exclude serious organic disease in difficult cases it may be necessary to proceed to formal exercise testing since psychogenic dyspnoea alone is not associated with desaturation or hypoxaemia even on exercise.

Occasionally this syndrome can develop into a full-blown acute 'hysterical' hyperventilation attack (see below) which may appear dramatic and even lead to rigidity and carpo-pedal spasm due to acute respiratory alkalosis, secondary to severe hyperventilation. This condition may need to be distinguished from other organic causes of acute severe breathlessness (see below).

AN APPROACH TO THE PATIENT WITH ACUTE SEVERE DYSPNOEA

Acute severe breathlessness is one of the commonest medical emergencies. The presentation is often dramatic and it is easy for the inexperienced clinician to be disconcerted. Although there are usually a number of possible causes, attention to the history and a rapid but careful examination will usually suggest a diagnosis which can often be confirmed by routine investigations, including chest radiograph, ECG, arterial blood gases and echocardiography. Some specific features aiding in the diagnosis of important causes of acute severe breathlessness are considered in detail in Table 6.6.

History
It is important to ascertain the rate of onset and severity of dyspnoea and whether associated cardiovascular (chest pain, orthopnoea, palpitations, sweating and nausea) or respiratory (cough, wheeze, haemoptysis, stridor) symptoms are present. A previous history of repeated episodes of left ventricular failure, asthma or exacerbations of chronic bronchitis is valuable. Recent intake of drugs or a history of renal disease, diabetes or anaemia should be established. In the severely ill patient it may be necessary to obtain a brief history from friends, relatives or ambulance personnel. In children, particularly pre-school toddlers, the possibility of inhalation of a foreign body should always be considered, and it is important to be aware that many objects, e.g. wax crayons, are radio-lucent and may not be detected on the chest radiograph.

Examination
The severity of the condition should immediately be established, in particular the patency of the airway, level of consciousness, ability to speak (in phrases or sentences), and cardiovascular status assessed by examining the pulse rate and rhythm, blood pressure and degree of peripheral perfusion. On further examination, signs of cyanosis, digital clubbing, anaemia, polycythaemia and any evidence of diabetes or renal failure should be noted. Urticaria or areas of angio-oedema, especially on the face, may support a diagnosis of anaphylaxis. A detailed examination of the respiratory system should include the respiratory rate, pattern of breathing, peak flow rate (if possible), the position of the trachea and whether there are areas of hyperresonance or dullness on percussion. Breath sounds should be compared on each side of the chest and at the bases, and the presence of ronchi or crepitations noted.

CHEST PAIN

See page 207, Chapter 5.

HAEMOPTYSIS

Haemoptysis is an alarming symptom and nearly always brings the patient to the doctor. A clear history should be taken in order to establish that it is true haemoptysis, and not haematemesis or epistaxis (this distinction is not always easy). A small isolated episode may remain without a diagnosis despite intensive investigation, but haemoptyses can also be the first sign of carcinoma, tuberculosis or other important lung disease (see box).

CAUSES OF HAEMOPTYSIS

Bronchial disease
- Carcinoma
- Bronchiectasis
- Acute bronchitis
  Bronchial adenoma
  Foreign body

Parenchymal disease
- Tuberculosis
- Suppurative pneumonia
  Lung abscess
  Parasites (e.g. hydatid disease, flukes)
  Trauma
  Actinomycosis
  Aspergilloma

Lung vascular disease
- Pulmonary embolus and infarction
  Polyarteritis nodosa
  Goodpasture's syndrome
  AV malformation
  Idiopathic pulmonary haemosiderosis

Cardiovascular disease
- Acute left ventricular failure
- Mitral stenosis
  Aortic aneurysm

Blood disorders
  Leukaemia
  Haemophilia
  Anticoagulants

- = more common causes

A history of repeated small haemoptyses over days or weeks is highly suggestive of lung carcinoma. Clearly, it is important to elicit a history of smoking, previous tuberculosis, etc. Chronic fever and weight loss may suggest tuberculosis. An acute episode of tracheitis or bronchitis may cause purulent sputum streaked with blood, and pneumonia may be associated with 'rusty' coloured sputum or frank haemoptysis. Bronchiectasis can cause catastrophic life-threatening pulmonary haemorrhage and there may be a history of previous tuberculosis or whooping cough in early life. Major risk factors for pulmonary embolus include malignancy, immobilisation and the post-partum period. A history of cardiovascular disease or mitral stenosis may suggest left ventricular failure, pulmonary embolism or infarction.

Physical examination may reveal clues as to the underlying diagnosis, e.g. finger clubbing in carcinoma or bronchiectasis; other signs of malignancy such as cachexia; fever or a pleural rub in lobar pneumonia or pulmonary infarction; the cardiac murmurs of mitral valve disease; a swollen leg in pulmonary embolism; and signs of systemic diseases including rash purpura, haematuria, splinter haemorrhages, lymphadenopathy or splenomegaly in systemic diseases which may be associated with haemoptysis.

Management

In catastrophic acute haemoptysis, the patient should be nursed on the side of the suspected lesion, resuscitated then bronchoscoped, ideally under general anaesthesia with a rigid bronchoscope which is necessary to optimise bronchial suction and can be used to ventilate the patient. Emergency angiography and embolisation to occlude the bleeding vessel or emergency lobectomy/pneumonectomy are potentially life-saving procedures in the acute setting.

In the vast majority of cases, however, the haemoptysis itself is not life-threatening and it is possible to follow a logical sequence of investigations which include:

- Chest radiograph which may give clear evidence of a localised lesion including malignant or benign tumour, pneumonia or tuberculosis.
- Full blood count and other haematological tests including clotting screen will be necessary.
- Bronchoscopy will often lead to a tissue diagnosis in bronchial tumours.
- Ventilation perfusion scan. This may be helpful in establishing a diagnosis in suspected pulmonary infarction. In some circumstances pulmonary angiography may be necessary (see p. 319).
- CT scan. This is particularly useful in investigating peripheral chest radiograph lesions which may not be accessible to bronchoscopy.

RESPIRATORY FAILURE AND SLEEP APNOEA

Respiratory failure results from a disorder in which lung function is inadequate for the metabolic requirements of the individual. Its classification into type I and type II relates to the absence or presence of hypercapnia (raised $PaCO_2$). A summary of respiratory failure and its characteristic blood gas abnormalities is shown in Table 6.7.

Management of acute type I respiratory failure

The patient should be treated with high concentration ($>35\%$) oxygen by oro-nasal mask. Young children may require to be treated in oxygen tents, since few of them tolerate masks. Very ill patients and those with ventilatory arrest may require immediate tracheal intubation or tracheostomy and mechanical ventilation (see p. 331). Effective management requires prompt treatment of the underlying disorder. An accurate history is important, yet may be difficult to obtain if the patient is distressed or confused because of hypoxia, when information from relatives or ambulance personnel may be invaluable. Patients should be closely monitored and arterial blood gases taken on presentation should be checked within 20 minutes to establish acceptable PaO_2 levels. If there is no improvement despite treating the underlying condition, an early decision about mechanical ventilation will be necessary in some conditions, particularly severe acute asthma. No matter how distressed or apparently hysterical the patient with acute type I respiratory failure may appear, with the exception of acute left ventricular failure and pleural pain due to pulmonary infarction or pneumonia, the administration of sedatives or other CNS depressants is absolutely contraindicated; in acute severe asthma such medication may have fatal results.

Management of type II respiratory failure

Acute

In acute type II respiratory failure, also known as asphyxia, CO_2 retention occurs and causes severe acute respiratory acidosis (see Table 6.7). Treatment is aimed at immediate or very rapid reversal of the precipitating event, for example dislodgement of a laryngeal foreign body or tracheostomy, fixation of ribs in a flail chest injury, reversal of narcotic poisons, treatment of acute severe asthma, etc. In some cases it will be necessary to support ventilation temporarily by intubation and mechanical ventilation if the condition cannot immediately be reversed.

SOME CAUSES OF 'ACUTE ON CHRONIC' TYPE II RESPIRATORY FAILURE

- Retention of secretions
- Bronchospasm
- Pulmonary embolus
- Cardiac failure
- Rib fractures/intercostal muscle tears
- Pneumothorax
- CNS depression (narcotic drugs)

Chronic

The most common cause of chronic type II respiratory failure is COPD. Here CO_2 retention may occur on a

Table 6.6 Differential diagnosis of acute severe dyspnoea

Condition	History	Signs	Chest radiography	Arterial blood gases	ECG	Other tests
Left ventricular failure	Chest pain, orthopnoea, palpitations, *a previous cardiac history	Central cyanosis, JVP ($\rightarrow$ or $\uparrow$), *sweating, cool extremities, *dullness and crepitations at bases	Cardiomegaly, *Upper zone vessel enlargement, *overt oedema/pleural effusions	$\downarrow PaO_2$ $\downarrow PaCO_2$	Sinus tachycardia, signs of myocardial infarction, arrhythmia	Echo-cardiography ($\downarrow$left ventricular function)
Massive pulmonary embolus	Recent surgery or other risk factors. Chest pain, previous pleurisy, *syncope, *dizziness	Severe central cyanosis, *elevated JVP, *absence of signs in the lung (unless previous pulmonary infarction), shock (tachycardia, reduced blood pressure)	May be subtle changes only, prominent hilar vessels, *oligaemic lung fields	$\Downarrow PaO_2$ $\downarrow PaCO_2$	Sinus tachycardia $S_1Q_3T_3$ pattern $\downarrow$ T (V1–V4) Right bundle branch block	*Echo-cardiography V/Q scan *Pulmonary angiography
Acute severe asthma	*History of previous episodes, asthma medications, wheeze	Tachycardia and pulsus paradoxus. Cyanosis (late) *JVP $\rightarrow$ *$\Downarrow$ peak flow rhonchi	*Hyperinflation only (unless complicated by pneumothorax)	$\downarrow PaO_2$ $\downarrow PaCO_2$ (until late)	Sinus tachycardia, (bradycardia with severe hypoxaemia—late)	
Acute exacerbation of COPD	*Previous episodes (admissions). If in Type II respiratory failure, may not be distressed	Cyanosis *Signs of COPD (barrel chest, intercostal indrawing, pursed lips, tracheal tug) *Signs of CO_2 retention (warm periphery, flapping tremor, bounding pulses)	*Hyperinflation, minor signs of emphysema, signs of events precipitating exacerbation (see p. 326)	$\downarrow$ or $\Downarrow PaO_2$. In type II failure $PaCO_2$ may be $\uparrow$, with $\uparrow$ [H$^+$] and $\uparrow$ bicarbonate	Nil, or signs of right ventricular failure (in cor pulmonale)	
Pneumonia	*Prodromal illness *Fever *Rigors *Pleurisy	Fever *Pleural rub *Consolidation Cyanosis (only if widespread)	*Pneumonic consolidation	$\downarrow PaCO_2$ $\downarrow PaO_2$	Tachycardia	
Metabolic acidosis	*Evidence of diabetes/renal disease *Overdose of aspirin or ethylene glycol	Fetor (ketones) *Hyperventilation without physical signs in heart or lungs *Dehydration Air hunger (Kussmaul's respiration)	Normal	*PaO_2 normal $\Downarrow PaCO_2$ $\Downarrow$pH ($\uparrow$ H$^+$)		
Psychogenic (a diagnosis of *exclusion*)	(Previous episodes)	***Not** cyanosed ***No** heart signs ***No** lung signs Carpo-pedal spasm	Normal	*PaO_2 normal $\Downarrow PaCO_2$ *pH (H$^+$) normal or $\uparrow$		End-tidal $PaCO_2$

* Denotes a valuable discriminatory feature

chronic basis, the potential for acidaemia being corrected by renal conservation of bicarbonate which results in the plasma pH remaining within the normal range. The status quo is often maintained until there is a further pulmonary insult (see information box) such as an exacerbation of bronchitis which precipitates an episode of 'acute on chronic' respiratory failure. The further acute increase in $PaCO_2$ results in acidaemia, and worsening hypercapnia may also lead to drowsiness and eventually coma. The central aim of treatment in type II respiratory failure is to keep the patient alive and achieve a safe PaO_2 without inducing extremes of $PaCO_2$ or pH, while identifying and treating the precipitating condition (see information box). It is important to note

Table 6.7 Respiratory failure

	Type I ($PaO_2 < 8.0$ kPa) ($PaCO_2 < 6.6$ kPa)		Type II ($PaO_2 < 8.0$ kPa) ($PaCO_2 > 6.6$ kPa)	
	Acute	Chronic	Acute	Chronic
Typical blood gases	$PaO_2\downarrow\downarrow$ $PaCO_2\leftrightarrow$ or $\downarrow$ pH$\leftrightarrow$ or $\downarrow\downarrow$ $HCO_3\leftrightarrow$	$PaO_2\downarrow$ $PaCO_2\leftrightarrow$ pH$\leftrightarrow$ $HCO_3\leftrightarrow$	$PaO_2\downarrow$ $PaCO_2\uparrow$ pH$\downarrow$ $HCO_3\leftrightarrow$	$PaO_2\downarrow$ $PaCO_2\uparrow$ pH$\downarrow$ or $\leftrightarrow$ $HCO_3\uparrow$
Causes	Asthma Pulmonary embolus Pulmonary oedema Adult respiratory distress syndrome Pneumothorax Pneumonia	Emphysema Lung fibrosis Lymphangitis carcinomatosa L→R shunts Anaemia	Severe acute asthma Acute epiglottis Inhaled foreign body Respiratory muscle paralysis Flail chest injury Sleep apnoea Brain stem lesion Narcotic drugs	Chronic bronchitis Primary alveolar hypoventilation Kyphoscoliosis Ankylosing spondylitis
Therapy	Treat underlying cause High concentration O_2 Mechanical ventilation if necessary	Treat underlying disorder Long-term O_2	Treat underlying disorder Controlled low concentration O_2 Mechanical ventilation or tracheostomy if necessary	Treat underlying disorder Controlled long-term O_2 delivery Mechanical ventilatory support if necessary

that in the patient who already has severe lung disease, only a small insult may be required to tip the balance towards catastrophic respiratory failure. Moreover, in contrast to acute severe asthma, in type II respiratory failure the patient, despite being critically ill with severe hypoxaemia, hypercapnia and acidaemia, may not be overtly distressed.

In the initial assessment it is important to assess the patient's conscious level and their ability to respond to commands, particularly the ability to cough effectively. This may give a preliminary indication of whether intubation and tracheal suction may be necessary to clear secretions or whether physiotherapy will be helpful. The decision regarding mechanical ventilation can be complex and difficult. It is better to make an early decision, based on whether there is a potentially remediable precipitating condition (see box) and whether the patient is likely to regain an acceptable quality of life, rather than wait until the patient suffers a respiratory arrest. At the initial assessment stage it is also important to remember that while physical signs of CO_2 retention (confusion, flapping tremor, bounding pulses, etc.) can be helpful if present, they are often unreliable and there is no substitute for arterial blood gases in the initial assessment and early progress of these patients.

Prompt intervention may occasionally be necessary for some precipitating conditions, e.g. intercostal tube drainage of pneumothoraces, injection with local anaesthetic for fractured ribs and torn muscles, which can result in dramatic improvement of respiratory function

(see information box above). Generally, however, the treatment is empirical and includes low concentration controlled oxygen therapy, physiotherapy, bronchodilators, broad-spectrum antibiotics, and diuretics if there is suspicion of cardiac failure. While the dangers of hypercapnia have not been exaggerated it is important to recognise that severe hypoxaemia **must** be reversed if the patient is not to suffer potentially fatal arrhythmias or severe cerebral complications. The aim of oxygen therapy is not necessarily to achieve a normal PaO_2; even a small increment of increase in the PaO_2 will often have a greatly beneficial effect on oxygen delivery to tissues since the arterial values of these patients are often on the very steep part of the oxygen saturation curve. If controlled oxygen treatment causes a serious increase in the $PaCO_2$, particularly if it is associated with a reduction in pH, the patient may require mechanical ventilation. Alternatively, treatment with respiratory stimulants can in some circumstances be used to stimulate ventilation over a 24–48 hour period while the precipitating condition is treated.

THE SLEEP APNOEA/HYPOPNOEA SYNDROME

In the past decade it has been realised that 2–4% of the middle-aged population suffer consequences of recurrent upper airway obstruction during sleep. They experience daytime sleepiness, especially in monotonous situations, and this results in a 3-fold risk of road traffic accidents and a 9-fold risk of single vehicle accidents.

ASSESSMENT AND MANAGEMENT OF 'ACUTE ON CHRONIC' TYPE II RESPIRATORY FAILURE

Initial assessment
NB: Patient may not appear distressed despite being critically ill.

- Conscious level (response to commands, ability to cough)
- CO_2 retention (warm periphery, bounding pulses, flapping tremor)
- Airways obstruction (wheeze, intercostal indrawing, pursed lips, tracheal 'tug')
- Right heart failure (oedema, raised JVP, hepatomegaly, ascites)
- Background functional status and quality of life
- Physical signs of precipitating event (see information box above)

Investigations
- Arterial blood gases (severity of hypoxaemia, hypercapnia and acidaemia)
- Chest radiograph

Management
- Maintenance of airway
- Treat specific precipitating event (see information box above)
- Frequent physiotherapy and pharyngeal suction
- Nebulised bronchodilators
- Controlled oxygen therapy:
  Start with 24% Ventimask.
  Aim for a PaO_2 of around 7 kPa (a $PaO_2 < 5$ is very dangerous)
- Antibiotics
- Diuretics

Progress
- If $PaCO_2$ continues to rise or patient cannot achieve a safe PaO_2 without severe hypercapnia and acidaemia, respiratory stimulants (see p. 333) or mechanical ventilation may be required

---

Difficulty with concentration, impaired work performance and impaired cognitive function, along with depression and irritability, are other features. The patient usually feels that he has been asleep all night but wakes feeling unrefreshed. Bed-partners will report loud snoring in all body postures and often will have noticed multiple breathing pauses.

The problem results from recurrent occlusion of the back of the throat during sleep, most often starting at the level of the soft palate. On inspiration the pressure in the throat is sub-atmospheric. During wakefulness upper airway dilating muscles—including palatoglossus and genioglossus—actively contract during each inspiration to preserve airway patency. During sleep muscle tone generally declines, including that in the upper airway dilating muscles, and their ability to maintain patency falls. In most people sufficient tone persists to result in uncompromised breathing during sleep. However, in those who for some reason have a narrow throat when awake, upper airway opening muscle action is more important and when it falls during sleep the airway narrows. If the narrowing is slight, turbulent flow and the vibration and noise of snoring occurs—around 40% of middle-aged men and 20% of middle-aged women snore. If the upper airway narrowing during sleep progresses to the point of occlusion or near occlusion, the sleeping subject increases respiratory effort to try to breathe until the increased effort transiently awakens them, so briefly that they have no recollection but long enough for the upper airway dilating muscles to open the airway again. Then a series of deep breaths are taken before the subject rapidly returns to sleep, snores and becomes apnoeic once more. This recurrent cycle of apnoea, awakening, apnoea, awakening ... may repeat itself many hundreds of times per night and the sleep fragmentation results in the daytime sleepiness and impaired daytime performance. The awakenings are associated with surges in blood pressure which result over years in an increased frequency of hypertension, ischaemic heart disease and stroke.

Predisposing factors to the sleep apnoea/hypopnoea syndrome include being male, which doubles the risk probably due to a testosterone effect on the upper airway, and obesity, found in about half the patients and having the effect of narrowing the throat by parapharyngeal fat deposits. Acromegaly and hypothyroidism also predispose by submucosal infiltration narrowing the upper airway. The condition is often familial, and in these families the maxilla and mandible are back-set thus narrowing the upper airway. Alcohol and sedatives predispose to snoring and apnoeas by relaxing the upper airway dilating muscles.

Investigation

Any person who falls asleep once per day when not in bed, who complains that his work is impaired by sleepiness or who is a habitual snorer with multiple witnessed apnoeas should be referred to a sleep or respiratory specialist, provided that the sleepiness does not result from inadequate time in bed or from shift work. Overnight studies of breathing, oxygenation and sleep quality are diagnostic (Fig. 6.9) but the level of complexity of investigation will vary depending on probability of diagnosis, differential diagnosis and resources. The currently accepted threshold for abnormality is 15 apnoeas + hypopnoeas per hour of sleep, where an apnoea is a 10 second or longer breathing pause and a hypopnoea a 10 second or longer 50% reduction in breathing.

Differential diagnosis

Narcolepsy is a much rarer cause of sleepiness, occurring in 0.05% of the population and associated sometimes

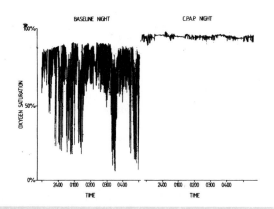

Fig. 6.9 Sleep apnoea/hypopnoea syndrome: overnight oxygen saturation trace in 46-year-old patient showing on left panel a night when he slept without CPAP and had 53 apnoeas plus hypopnoeas/hour, with 55 brief awakenings/hour and marked oxygen desaturation. Right panel shows the next night when he slept with a CPAP pressure of 10 cm H_2O which abolished his breathing irregularity and awakenings and improved his oxygenation.

with cataplexy (when muscle tone is lost in fully conscious people in response to emotional triggers and they may flop over), hypnogogic hallucinations (hallucinations at sleep onset), and sleep paralysis. Idiopathic hypersomnolence occurs in younger individuals and is characterised by long nocturnal sleeps.

Management

In a few patients advice to avoid evening alcohol and lose weight suffices, but most need to use continuous positive airway pressure (CPAP) delivered by nasal mask every night at home. CPAP blows the throat open by making the upper airway pressure above atmospheric. The pressure for CPAP is set in the laboratory to the lowest that will prevent apnoeas, hypopnoeas and awakenings. The effect is dramatic (Fig. 6.9) and CPAP results in marked improvements in symptoms, daytime performance, quality of life and survival. There is no evidence that upper airway surgery currently has any role in the management of the syndrome.

OXYGEN THERAPY

Principles

The delivery of oxygen to tissue mitochondria is controlled by factors exerting influences at various levels, including: inspired oxygen concentration (FIO_2); alveolar ventilation; ventilation/perfusion distribution within the lung; haemoglobin and concentrations of agents such as carbon monoxide which may bind to haemoglobin; influences on the oxygen haemoglobin

dissociation curve; cardiac output; and distribution of capillary blood flow within the tissues.

Many of the causes of hypoxaemia (see information box p. 316) are corrected by increasing the FIO_2, but right to left shunting, either through circulatory channels bypassing the lung or through parts of the lung in which the alveoli are inaccessible to inspired oxygen, is less susceptible to such therapeutic approaches. The increased amount of dissolved oxygen carried by the blood which has perfused alveoli with a high PaO_2 can saturate the haemoglobin in small quantities of shunted blood, but persistence of cyanosis when 100% oxygen is breathed indicates that the shunt is larger than 20% of the cardiac output.

The consequences of severe hypoxaemia include: systemic hypotension, pulmonary hypertension, polycythaemia, tachycardia, and undesirable cerebral consequences ranging from confusion to coma.

Objectives

1. To overcome the reduced partial pressure and quantity of oxygen in the blood in hypoxaemia.
2. To increase the quantity of oxygen carried in solution in the plasma, even when the haemoglobin is fully saturated.

Adverse effects

100% oxygen is both irritant and toxic if inhaled for more than a few hours. Premature infants develop retrolental fibroplasia and blindness if exposed to excessive concentrations. In adults, pulmonary oxygen toxicity (as manifested by pulmonary oedema) would not be expected to occur unless the patient had been treated with a concentration of greater than 40% oxygen for more than 24 hours.

Administration

Oxygen should always be prescribed in writing with clearly specified flow rates or concentrations.

- **High concentrations for short periods**, such as 60% via an MC mask, are particularly useful in acute type I respiratory failure such as commonly occurs in left ventricular failure or asthma.
- **Low concentrations,** either via a 24% or 28% Ventimask, provide the most accurate method of delivering controlled oxygen therapy, particularly in type II respiratory failure. However, when low concentration oxygen is required continuously for more than a few hours, 1–2 litres per minute via nasal double cannulae allows the patients to eat and to undergo physiotherapy, etc., while continuing to receive oxygen.

When MC masks are used, the oxygen should be

humidified by passing it over warm water (as in the East–Radcliffe humidifier). This is not necessary with Ventimasks or the nasal cannulae, as a high proportion of atmospheric air is mixed with oxygen.

- **Chronic oxygen delivery**: long-term oxygen from cylinders delivered to the home, or more conveniently from an oxygen concentrator, is often given via a low concentration mask or through nasal cannuli. Assessment for long-term oxygen therapy usually requires that the patients should have a PaO_2 of less than 7.3 kPa breathing air and an FEV_1 of less than 1 litre in the steady state (i.e. usually at least 1 month since the previous exacerbation).

Long-term chronic oxygen delivery has also been achieved by transtracheal microcatheters which have proven to be both oxygen-saving and of cosmetic benefit for the patient.

MECHANICAL VENTILATION

Patients with any type of respiratory failure may require treatment with mechanical ventilation. This is usually achieved through a cuffed endotracheal tube introduced via the mouth or nose under general anaesthesia (see information box). IPPV (Intermittent Positive Pressure

---

SOME TERMS AND ABBREVIATIONS IN RESPIRATORY SUPPORT

- **CPAP**   **Continuous Positive Airways Pressure**—can be achieved with an ET tube or with tightly-fitting face or nasal mask. May be useful in preventing pharyngeal collapse in obstructive sleep apnoea (see p. 328).
- **IMV**   **Intermittent Mandatory Ventilation**—delivery of an obligatory number of breaths, mechanically imposed on spontaneous breathing (a technique which is useful when 'weaning off' ventilator)
- **IPPV**   **Intermittent Positive Pressure Ventilation**—no spontaneous breathing
- **MMV**   **Mandatory Minute Volume**—mechanically imposed breaths to augment spontaneous breathing in order to achieve a pre-determined minute ventilation
- **PEEP**   **Positive End-Expiratory Pressure**—prevents complete lung deflation, resulting in increased FRC and increased oxygenation, especially in areas of oedema/atelactasis. However, may compromise left ventricular function and enhances the risk of barotrauma

---

COMPLICATIONS OF MECHANICAL VENTILATION

- Barotrauma (pneumothorax, pneumomediastinum) especially with high PEEP
- Increased susceptibility to infection
- Tracheal damage after prolonged ventilation
- Difficulty in 'weaning off' some chronic type II respiratory failure patients
- Bronchopulmonary dysplasia in infants

Ventilation) is still the commonest form of mechanical ventilation. In some cases of type I respiratory failure, PEEP (Positive End-Expiratory Pressure) may be useful to correct maldistribution of ventilation and blood flow. (See information box for use of terms.) Powerful ventilators delivering a fixed volume are used for patients with type II respiratory failure associated with airflow obstruction. The volume and oxygen concentration of the air supplied by the ventilator is adjusted to bring arterial PaO_2 and $PaCO_2$ towards normal values, and ventilatory assistance should be gradually reduced, if possible, as soon as the cause of respiratory failure has been successfully treated.

FURTHER READING

Douglas N J, Polo O 1994 Pathogenesis of obstructive sleep apnoea hypopnoea syndrome. Lancet 344: 653–655
Ingbar D H (ed) 1994 Respiratory emergencies. Clinics in Chest Medicine: 383–551
Polo O, Berthon-Jones M, Douglas N J et al 1994 Management of obstructive sleep apnoea/hypopnoea syndrome. Lancet 344: 656–660

OBSTRUCTIVE PULMONARY DISEASES

CHRONIC BRONCHITIS AND EMPHYSEMA

Chronic bronchitis and emphysema are pathologically distinct but they frequently co-exist as a syndrome commonly termed Chronic Obstructive Pulmonary Disease (COPD) and it may be difficult or impossible to determine the relative importance of each condition in the individual patient. Generalised airflow obstruction is the dominant feature of both diseases.

Chronic bronchitis and emphysema are often grouped together and can be regarded as forming a spectrum with 'pure' chronic bronchitis at one end and 'pure' emphysema at the other. For descriptive purposes, however, it is convenient to deal with them separately, with emphasis on their similarities and differences, and on the relationships which frequently exist between them.

CHRONIC BRONCHITIS

Definition
This is clinical and is based on the history. A patient can be assumed to have chronic bronchitis if sputum has been coughed up on most days of at least three consecutive months for more than two successive years, providing other causes of productive cough such as bronchiectasis and untreated chronic asthma have been excluded.

Aetiology
Chronic bronchitis develops in response to the long-continued action of various types of irritant on the bronchial mucosa. The most important of these is cigarette tobacco smoke, but others include dust, smoke and fumes occurring as specific occupational hazards or as part of a general atmospheric pollution in industrial cities and towns. Infection is sometimes a precipitating factor in the onset of chronic bronchitis but its main role is in aggravating the established condition. Exposure to dampness, sudden changes in temperature and to fog may cause exacerbations of chronic bronchitis.

Chronic bronchitis occurs most commonly in middle and late adult life and is much more common in smokers than in non-smokers, and in urban than in rural dwellers.

Strep. pneumoniae and/or *H. influenzae* can be isolated from sputum in most patients at some time, particularly during exacerbations associated with purulent sputum.

Pathology
In all cases there is hypertrophy of the mucus-secreting glands and an increase in the number of goblet cells in the bronchi and bronchioles with a consequent decrease in ciliated cells. There is, therefore, less efficient transport of the increased mucus in the airways. Mucosal oedema and permanent structural damage of the airway walls reduces the calibre of the air passages. A major proportion of airflow obstruction in chronic bronchitis is irreversible, unlike the airflow obstruction in chronic asthma. Air is 'trapped' in the alveoli because the degree of obstruction is greater during expiration. Over-distension of the alveoli results and disruption of their walls may occur (emphysema, p. 334).

Clinical features
The disease generally starts with repeated attacks of productive cough, usually after colds during the winter months, which show a steady increase in severity and duration with successive years until cough is present all the year round. Wheeze, breathlessness and tightness in the chest are also common complaints, especially in the morning, before the excessive bronchial secretions are cleared by coughing. Sputum may be scanty, mucoid and tenacious and occasionally streaked with blood. Frankly purulent sputum is indicative of bacterial infection which often occurs in these patients.

Breathlessness is caused by airflow obstruction and is aggravated by infection, excessive cigarette smoking and adverse atmospheric conditions. Clinically apparent airflow obstruction is not a feature of all patients but when it does occur it worsens the prognosis.

Variable numbers of inspiratory and expiratory rhonchi, mainly low and medium pitched, are audible in most patients. Crepitations which usually, but not always, disappear after coughing may be audible over the lower lobes. Physical signs attributable to emphysema may co-exist (p. 334).

Investigations

Chest radiograph
No characteristic abnormality. Often normal, but may show features suggesting co-existing emphysema (p. 335).

Pulmonary function tests
Ventilatory capacity. The forced expiratory volume in one second (FEV_1) is reduced in many cases and the ratio of FEV_1 to vital capacity (VC) is in consequence subnormal. Peak expiratory flow (PEF) may also be reduced and, in contrast to asthma, serial measurements show little or no diurnal variation (p. 339).

Lung volumes. An overall increase in lung volumes (p. 322) is seen, dependent upon the degree of associated hyperinflation (emphysema).

Gas transfer. This is normal or slightly impaired. Marked reduction suggests the presence of significant coexisting emphysema.

Arterial blood gas measurement. In severe cases there is a permanent increase in $PaCO_2$ and fall in PaO_2 reflecting generalised alveolar underventilation. This is often preceded by hypoxaemia.

Exercise tests. Simple assessments of exercise ability such as the six-minute walking test give valuable estimates of everyday disability.

COMPLICATIONS OF CHRONIC BRONCHITIS

- Type I and II respiratory failure
- Pulmonary hypertension
- Right ventricular failure
- Secondary polycythaemia

Prognosis

Chronic bronchitis is usually a progressive disease, punctuated by acute exacerbations and remissions and eventually causing respiratory and right heart failure. Some patients die within a few years of the onset of symptoms; others survive for many years with gradually diminishing respiratory reserve.

A productive cough continues in some patients, without severe airflow obstruction. Their prognosis is very much better than those who have airflow obstruction.

Management

Reduction of bronchial irritation

It is of extreme importance that bronchial irritation should be reduced to a minimum. The patient who smokes should be urged to stop completely and permanently. Dusty and smoke-laden atmospheres should be avoided, which may involve a change of occupation.

Treatment of respiratory infection

Respiratory infection must be treated promptly because it aggravates breathlessness and may precipitate Type II respiratory failure in patients with severe airflow obstruction. Purulent sputum is treated with oral oxytetracycline or ampicillin in a dose of 250 mg 6-hourly or co-trimoxazole 960 mg 12-hourly. A 5–10-day course of treatment is usually effective and the sputum becomes mucoid. Well-informed, reliable patients can be given a supply of one of these drugs and be permitted to start a course of treatment on their own initiative when the need arises.

Because the vast majority of bacterial infections in chronic bronchitis are caused by *Strep. pneumoniae* or *H. influenzae*, bacteriological examination of sputum is essential only when the response to empirical treatment is unsatisfactory and the sputum remains purulent. In that event a change of antibiotic, guided by the results of bacterial sensitivity tests, will be indicated. Continuous suppressive antibiotic treatment is not advised as it is apt to promote the emergence of drug-resistant organisms within the respiratory tract.

Bronchodilator therapy

Bronchodilators are much less effective in chronic bronchitis than in bronchial asthma but should be given to all patients with reversible airflow obstruction. Regular treatment with an inhaled β_2-adrenoceptor agonist (salbutamol 200 mcg or terbutaline 500 mcg, 4–6 hourly) may be sufficient in patients with mild to moderate disease. The anticholinergic bronchodilator drug ipratropium bromide in a dose of 40–80 mcg 6-hourly should be added in patients with more severe airflow obstruction. Theophylline therapy often has little measurable effect on the airways obstruction associated with chronic bronchitis but it will improve quality of life in some patients.

Symptomatic measures

These may be required to control unproductive cough during the night. An unproductive nocturnal cough is often less troublesome if the patient sleeps in a warm bedroom. A hot drink or the inhalation of steam helps to liquefy sputum and make it easier to cough up. The so-called expectorant cough mixtures and drugs which claim to reduce sputum viscosity are of little or no value. Cough suppressants are usually contraindicated.

CHRONIC BRONCHITIS: HOSPITAL TREATMENT OF SEVERE EXACERBATIONS

- **Antibiotic treatment**
  Oral amoxycillin (250–500 mg 8-hourly) or intravenous ampicillin (500 mg 6-hourly), or oral co-trimoxazole (960 mg 12-hourly) are effective in most patients. Antistaphylococcal treatment should be given, initially at least, during influenza epidemics (p. 354)
- **Bronchodilator therapy**
  Nebulised salbutamol (5 mg) or terbutaline (10 mg) in combination with ipratropium bromide (0.5 mg) 6-hourly
- **Diuretic therapy**
  Frusemide (40–120 mg daily) or bumetanide (1–5 mg daily) orally or intravenously according to the extent of oedema
- **Oxygen therapy**
  Controlled oxygen therapy (p. 330) monitored by arterial blood gas measurements
- **Respiratory stimulants**
  Doxapram hydrochloride by intravenous infusion (1.5–4 mg per minute) may be of value in patients with profound respiratory acidosis
- **Physiotherapy**
  Assisted expectoration is of value in patients who are drowsy because of CO_2 retention (carbon dioxide narcosis)
- **Mechanical ventilation**
  Rarely justified unless the patient was leading an active life prior to the acute exacerbation

---

Long-term domiciliary oxygen therapy

Long-term low concentration oxygen therapy (2 l/min by nasal cannulae) decreases pulmonary hypertension and prolongs life in hypoxaemic chronic bronchitic patients who have developed right heart failure. The most efficient method of providing oxygen in this way is by an oxygen concentrator. Low-concentration oxygen should be administered for 15 hours or more per 24 hours.

Prevention

Stopping smoking is the most important preventative measure. The control of atmospheric pollution in urban areas and the increased use of measures to prevent the inhalation of dust by industrial workers will also help to reduce the prevalence of chronic bronchitis.

EMPHYSEMA

The word 'emphysema' means 'inflation' in the sense of abnormal distension with air. Although usually confined to a pathological process in the lungs, 'emphysema' is also sometimes used to describe simple overinflation of normal lung, and the abnormal presence of air in body tissues other than the lungs.

Aetiology

Emphysema is closely related to cigarette smoking. It is thought that over many years, the persistent inflammation in the airways and alveolar septa caused by smoking causes irreparable damage to the supporting connective tissue of the alveolar septa, particularly at their attachments to the small airways. Oxidants and proteinases, released from activated inflammatory cells, have been implicated in this process. The rare genetic abnormality of alpha-1-antiproteinase deficiency, which leads to severe emphysema in young adults, led to the concept that emphysema may arise from loss of the normal balance between proteinases in the lung and the antiproteinases which protect tissues from their effects. Cigarette smoking may alter the balance not only by attracting inflammatory cells and stimulating the release of proteinases but also by inactivating antiproteinases and the enzymes responsible for repair of damaged interstitial proteins, e.g. elastin.

Pathology

In some cases generalised destruction of the alveolar walls ('panacinar' emphysema) is the dominant lesion (Fig. 6.10). Where emphysema occurs together with a major component of chronic bronchitis, it is 'centrilobular' or 'centriacimar', and principally affects those alveoli which are most closely related to the respiratory bronchioles. The overinflation of lung tissue which occurs distal to an almost complete bronchial obstruction (e.g. by foreign body or tumour) has been termed 'obstructive emphysema'.

CLINICAL SYNDROMES OF EMPHYSEMA AND CHRONIC BRONCHITIS

Although the two types of emphysema develop in different ways, factors such as bacterial infection, alveolar over-distension and distortion of the airways may eventually blur their features. Two distinctive clinical patterns, however, have been recognised. In one (the 'blue and bloated' type) predominant features are cough

and sputum, infective exacerbations, cyanosis with arterial hypoxaemia and hypercapnia, and right ventricular failure with peripheral oedema. In the other (the 'pink and puffing' type) disabling exertional dyspnoea may antedate by many years the onset of respiratory and cardiac failure and cough and cyanosis are not prominent. A mixed syndrome of chronic bronchitis and emphysema is, however, much more commonly seen than either of the two individual syndromes, and computed tomography studies (p. 335) do not support the original supposition that the pathological changes of bronchitis predominated in the 'blue and bloated' type and those of emphysema in the 'pink and puffing'.

Clinical features

Most patients with pulmonary emphysema complain of exertional breathlessness but because other causes of airflow obstruction, such as chronic bronchitis and bronchial asthma, often co-exist it is seldom possible to assess the contribution of emphysema per se to the production of this symptom. There is a progressive increase in respiratory disability but the tempo of deterioration varies widely from one patient to another.

Clinical abnormalities found in the advanced stages of any chronic condition causing airflow limitation (including chronic bronchitis, emphysema and chronic asthma) are given in the information box below.

CLINICAL ABNORMALITIES FOUND IN PATIENTS WITH ADVANCED AIRFLOW OBSTRUCTION

- A reduction in the length of the trachea palpable above the sternal notch
- Tracheal descent during inspiration (tracheal 'tug')
- Contraction of the sternomastoid and scalene muscles on inspiration
- Excavation of the suprasternal and supraclavicular fossae during inspiration
- Jugular venous filling during expiration
- Indrawing of the costal margins and intercostal spaces during inspiration
- An increase in the antero-posterior diameter of the chest relative to the lateral diameter

---

These signs of generalised abnormality contrast with the signs of lateralised disease (Table 6.2). Purse-lip breathing is characteristic of emphysema and is assumed to be adopted by patients to aid expiration by breathing out against a resistance in an attempt to prevent air trapping.

The physical signs in the chest are caused by pulmonary hyperinflation (Table 6.2). Chest expansion is symmetrically diminished, as are the breath sounds. There is decreased cardiac dullness.

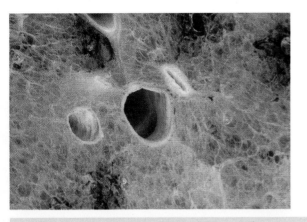
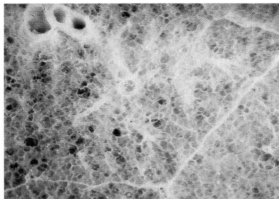

Fig. 6.10 The pathology of emphysema. Normal (left) and emphysematous (right) lung showing gross loss of the normal surface area available for gas exchange.

Investigations

Imaging
Chest radiograph abnormalities in emphysema are:

- bullae
- hypertranslucent lung fields with loss of peripheral vascular markings
- low flat diaphragm or 'terracing' of the hemi-diaphragms
- prominent pulmonary arterial shadows at both hila.

It is rarely possible to make a confident diagnosis of emphysema unless bullae are clearly seen.

High resolution computed tomography (CT) can detect emphysema with certainty but this investigation is rarely used for routine diagnostic purposes.

Pulmonary function tests
FEV_1 and VC show an obstructive defect with a reduced FEV_1/VC ratio. PEF is reduced and serial measurements show little or no diurnal variation.

Lung volumes show an increase in TLC and RV.

The transfer factor and transfer co-efficient for carbon monoxide are markedly reduced in emphysema in contrast with chronic asthma, and chronic bronchitis not complicated by emphysema.

Arterial blood gas measurements tend to be relatively normal until a late stage of the disease compared with chronic bronchitis.

Complications
Pulmonary bullae are thin-walled air spaces created by rupture of alveolar walls. They may be single or multiple, large or small and tend to be situated subpleurally. Rupture of bullae may cause pneumothorax (p. 400) and

occasionally bullae increase in size, compress functioning lung tissue and further embarrass pulmonary ventilation (Fig. 6.11).

Respiratory failure and cor pulmonale (right heart failure secondary to lung disease) are generally late complications in patients in whom emphysema predominates.

Loss of weight is common in patients with severe emphysema and often stimulates unnecessary investigation.

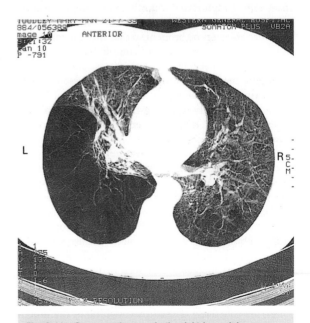

Fig. 6.11 Gross emphysema in the right lower lobe. High resolution CT scan showing emphysema most evident in the left lower lobe.

Management

There is no specific treatment for emphysema. Associated chronic bronchitis should be treated (p. 333) and late complications of respiratory failure (p. 326) and right heart failure require treatment as they develop (p. 333).

Physiotherapy may be helpful during exacerbations associated with bronchial infection to encourage expectoration. Regular exercise should be encouraged to increase mobility.

Ablation of giant bullae may bring about considerable improvement in symptoms and lung function. This type of surgical treatment should be considered when large bullae compress adjacent lung tissue. Single lung transplantation can allow patients disabled by breathlessness to regain virtually normal activities.

Prognosis

Progressive increase in exertional breathlessness is the rule unless the patient stops smoking at an early stage of the illness. Respiratory and right heart failure are usually late complications but when they develop, death usually ensues within a few years.

BRONCHIAL ASTHMA

The symptoms of bronchial asthma are caused by an inflammatory reaction within the bronchial wall involving many cells, mediators and cytokines. Eosinophils, mast cells, lymphocytes and other cells are involved in this inflammatory process which results in hyper-responsiveness of the bronchi so that they narrow easily in response to a wide range of stimuli. This may result in coughing, wheezing, chest tightness, and shortness of breath, these symptoms often being worse at night. Narrowing of the airway is usually reversible, but in some patients with chronic asthma the bronchial wall inflammation may lead to irreversible obstruction of airflow.

Characteristic pathological features include the presence in the airway of inflammatory cells, plasma exudation, oedema, hypertrophy of smooth muscle, mucus plugging, and shedding of the epithelium (Fig. 6.12). These changes may be present even in patients with mild asthma when they have few symptoms. The airflow obstruction, which characteristically fluctuates markedly, causes mismatch of alveolar ventilation and perfusion and increases the work of breathing. Being more marked during expiration it also causes air to be 'trapped' in the lungs. A narrowed bronchus can no longer be effectively cleared by coughing of the mucus formed by the disease process, and many of the bronchi become obstructed by mucus plugs. This is usually a conspicuous finding at autopsy. Respiratory arrest may occur within a few minutes after the onset of a severe episode, or death from asthma may occur from alveolar hypoventilation and severe arterial hypoxaemia in the patient exhausted by a prolonged attack.

Bronchial asthma is a common disease affecting 10–20% of the population. In the vast majority of cases the disease is mild and often unrecognised. There is evidence that the prevalence of asthma is increasing, the reason for this being unknown. In spite of better understanding of the pathophysiological processes involved in this disease, which has led to apparently improved treatment, mortality from asthma has not been influenced and in some countries has increased.

Aetiology

Early onset asthma (atopic)

It is common for asthma to have its onset in childhood, and generally it occurs in atopic individuals who readily form IgE antibodies to commonly encountered allergens. Asthma in these individuals is often referred to as 'atopic' asthma. They can be identified by skin hypersensitivity tests (p. 339) which produce positive reactions to a wide range of common allergens. Other allergic disorders such as allergic rhinitis and eczema are often present, and a family history of these disorders and of 'early onset' asthma is common. It is unusual for a single allergen to be the sole cause of asthma.

The allergens responsible for asthma in atopic individuals generally enter the bronchi with the inspired air and are derived from organic material such as pollen, mite-containing house dust, feathers, animal dander and fungal spores. Previous exposures to these agents will have stimulated the formation of IgE and an anaphylactic antigen-antibody reaction in the bronchi may follow further exposure to specific allergen. This causes the release, from cells, such as the mast cell, in the bronchial wall, of pharmacologically active substances which provoke bronchial constriction and an inflammatory reaction of allergic type in the bronchial wall. Much less frequently similar effects may be produced by ingested allergens derived from certain foods such as fish, eggs, milk, yeasts and wheat, which presumably reach the bronchi via the bloodstream.

The mast cell does not play such a major role as was once thought. The traditional view was that inhaled allergen interacted with surface mast cells through IgE-dependent mechanisms, causing these cells to release mediators, such as histamine, which then act on receptors on smooth muscle cells and lead to bronchoconstriction. This is probably a mechanism of the early asthmatic reaction, but several different cells are involved in the perpetuation of the chronic inflammatory reaction in the bronchial wall characteristic of asthma.

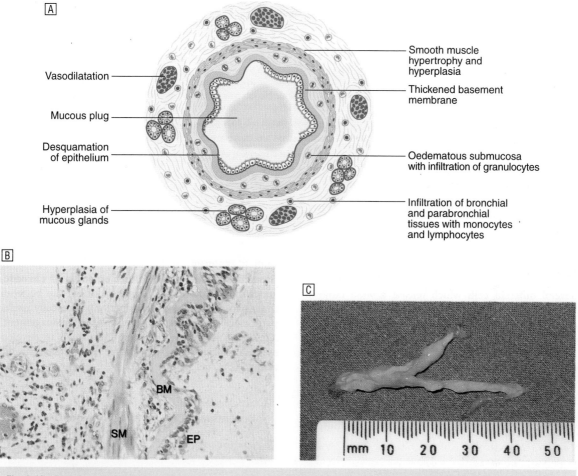

Fig. 6.12 Pathological changes in asthma. [A] Diagram to illustrate pathological changes seen in the bronchus of an asthmatic; [B] Histological section of bronchus in patient with asthma, demonstrating pathological changes as illustrated in [A]. (SM = smooth muscle, BM = basement membrane, EP = epithelium.) [C] Mucus plug expectorated by patient with acute severe asthma.

Eosinophils play an important role, the asthmatic inflammatory reaction being characterised by a cellular infiltration rich in activated eosinophils. These cells release several mediators including lipid mediators and oxygen radicals, and their granules also contain basic proteins including major basic protein, eosinophil cationic protein, eosinophil-derived neurotoxin and eosinophil peroxidase. T-lymphocytes are present in increased numbers in asthmatic airways and immunological markers suggest that they are activated. They play an important role in orchestrating and perpetuating the chronic asthmatic response. To do this they must be programmed to release appropriate cytokines, such as interleukin-5. Alveolar macrophages and other inflammatory cells may be more important than mast cells in chronic asthma. The number of macrophages is increased in

asthma and may be activated via a number of mechanisms including a low-affinity IgE receptor. They release a wide range of mediators including lipid mediators and oxygen radicals, but also many cytokines which may have important effects in determining the type of inflammatory response which ensues. Epithelial shedding is commonly observed in airway biopsies from asthmatic patients, and this has long been recognised as a feature of fatal asthma. Epithelial damage may contribute to airway hyperresponsiveness in a number of ways including the exposure of sub-epithelial nerve endings. Microvascular leakage is also an important feature of asthma and may be triggered by many inflammatory mediators. Some of its consequences are plasma exudation into the lumen of the airways contributing to mucus plugging, decreased mucociliary clearance,

Table 6.8   Allergens and other substances liable to provoke attacks of asthma

Causative agent	Preventive measures	Efficacy
Pollens	Try to avoid exposure to flowering vegetation Keep bedroom windows closed	Low
Mites in house dust	Vacuum clean mattress daily Shake out blankets daily Dust bedroom thoroughly	Doubtful
Animal dander	Avoid contact with dogs, cats, horses or other animals	High
Feathers in pillows or quilts	Substitute latex foam pillows and terylene quilts	High
Drugs (e.g. beta-adrenoceptor antagonists)	Avoid all preparations of relevant drugs	High
Foods	Identify and eliminate from diet	Low[1]
Industrial chemicals (e.g. isocyanates, epoxy resins)	Avoid exposure to chemical, or change occupation	High

[1] More effective in control of eczema.

release of kinins and complement fragments, and oedema of the airway wall giving rise to epithelial stripping. Several different cells which release a wide range of inflammatory mediators are involved in the production of the characteristic pathophysiological changes of asthma. The means of interaction are not understood, but cytokines are thought to play an important role together with mediators from eosinophils and other cells which lead to the changes which involve all components of the bronchial wall and its lumen. Asthma can, therefore, no longer be regarded as simple bronchoconstriction produced by contraction of bronchial muscle.

Late onset asthma (non-atopic)

Asthma can begin at any age in non-atopic individuals and because the majority of these patients are adults this type of asthma is often called late onset asthma. There is no clinical evidence that external allergens play a part in the production of the disease, to which the term 'intrinsic asthma' is sometimes applied (Fig. 6.13).

Triggers of the asthmatic response

Allergens can trigger episodes of asthma in atopic patients but asthma is often aggravated by non-specific factors such as cold air, tobacco smoke, dust and acrid fumes, respiratory viral infection and emotional stress. In children and young adults asthma almost invariably follows strenuous exertion (exercise-induced asthma) or exposure to cold air. Acute attacks of asthma may be caused by drugs such as beta-antagonists, aspirin and non-steroidal anti-inflammatory drugs. Asthma may develop because of exposure to dusts, organic materials, fumes and chemical substances in the working environment (occupational asthma).

Clinical features

Bronchial asthma may be either **episodic** or **chronic**, and although there is a good deal of overlap between these two syndromes the distinction is clinically useful particularly in terms of prognosis and management. There is a tendency for atopic individuals to develop episodic asthma, and non-atopic individuals chronic asthma (Fig. 6.13).

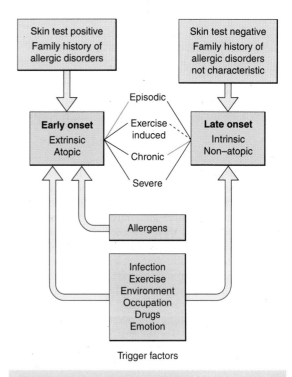

Fig. 6.13   Aetiology and types of asthma.

Episodic asthma

In this form of the disease the patient has no respiratory symptoms between episodes of asthma. Paroxysms of wheeze and dyspnoea may occur at any time and can be of sudden onset. Episodes of asthma can be triggered by allergens, exercise, viral infections such as the common cold, or may be apparently spontaneous. Attacks may be mild or severe and may last for hours, days or even weeks.

Severe acute asthma

This term has replaced 'status asthmaticus' as the description of life-threatening attacks of asthma. The patient usually adopts an upright position fixing the shoulder girdle to assist the accessory muscles of respiration. There is often an unproductive cough which aggravates respiratory distress. The respiratory symptoms are accompanied by tachycardia, pulsus paradoxus (p. 197), sweating and, in severe cases, central cyanosis.

Chronic asthma

Symptoms of chest tightness, wheeze and breathlessness on exertion, together with spontaneous cough and wheeze during the night, may be chronic unless controlled by appropriate therapy. Episodes of severe acute asthma can occur, and cough productive of mucoid sputum with recurrent episodes of frank respiratory infection is common in this type of asthma, which in adults may be difficult to distinguish from chronic bronchitis.

Clinical features

During an attack the chest is held near the position of full inspiration and the percussion note may be hyperresonant. Breath sounds when not obscured by numerous high-pitched polyphonic expiratory and inspiratory rhonchi are vesicular in character with prolonged expiration. In very severe asthma airflow may be insufficient to produce rhonchi; a 'silent chest' in such patients is an ominous sign. There are usually no abnormal physical signs between attacks except in patients with untreated chronic asthma who are seldom without expiratory rhonchi. Severe asthma persisting from childhood may cause a 'pigeon chest' deformity (p. 403).

Investigations

Radiological examination

In an acute attack of asthma the lungs appear hyperinflated. Between episodes the chest radiograph is usually normal. In long-standing cases the appearances may be indistinguishable from hyperinflation caused by emphysema and a lateral view may demonstrate a 'pigeon chest' deformity. Occasionally, when a large

bronchus is obstructed by tenacious mucus, there is an opacity caused by lobar or segmental collapse.

A chest radiograph should be performed, if possible, in all patients with severe acute asthma if there is poor response to treatment and assisted ventilation is being contemplated, to exclude pneumothorax, a rare but potentially fatal complication of the pulmonary hyperinflation produced by severe airflow obstruction in asthma. The chest radiograph may show mediastinal and subcutaneous emphysema in very severe disease.

Pulmonary function tests

Measurement of the forced expiratory volume in one second (FEV_1) and vital capacity (VC) or peak expiratory flow (PEF) provide a fairly reliable indication of the degree of airflow obstruction (p. 321), and can also be used to determine whether and to what extent it can be relieved by bronchodilator drugs (Fig. 6.14) or corticosteroids, or to confirm that the abnormality is provoked by exercise (Fig. 6.15) or hyperventilation or occupational exposure. Such tests have an important place in the diagnosis and treatment of asthma. Serial recordings of PEF are useful in distinguishing patients with chronic asthma from those with fixed or irreversible airflow obstruction associated with chronic bronchitis. In asthma there is usually a marked diurnal variation in PEF, the lowest values being recorded in the mornings ('morning dipping') (Fig. 6.16). Serial PEF recordings are also invaluable in the assessment of a patient's response to corticosteroid drugs and in the long-term monitoring of patients with poorly controlled disease. Also they are essential in monitoring response to treatment of severe acute asthma.

Measurement of bronchial reactivity can be of value in diagnosis and assessment of the effects of treatment. This can be achieved by administering increasing concentrations of substances such as histamine and methacholine by inhalation until there is a 20% fall in FEV_1 or PEF. This concentration is called the PC_{20}. Patients with asthma show evidence of bronchoconstriction at much lower concentrations than normal subjects.

Arterial blood gas analysis

Measurements of arterial blood gas pressures (PaO_2 and $PaCO_2$) are indispensable in the management of patients with severe acute asthma.

Skin hypersensitivity tests

A prick is made in the skin with a fine needle through a drop of an aqueous extract of the substance to be tested. A positive reaction is indicated by the development of a wheal and flare, which begin to appear within a few minutes. Tests are usually performed with a group of

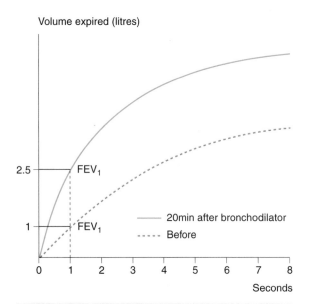

Fig. 6.14 Reversibility test. Forced expiratory manoeuvres before and 20 min after inhalation of a β_2-adrenoceptor agonist. Note the increase in FEV_1 from 1.0 to 2.5 litres.

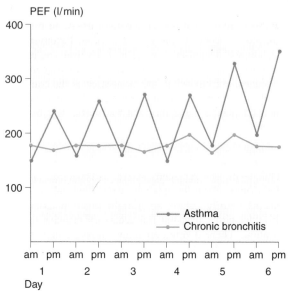

Fig. 6.16 'Morning dipping'. Serial recordings of peak expiratory flow (PEF) in patients with chronic bronchitis and asthma. Note sharp overnight fall (morning dip) and subsequent rise during the day in patient with asthma which does not occur in patient with chronic bronchitis.

common allergens known to cause bronchial asthma. It is seldom possible with these tests to identify one particular allergen as the cause of asthma in an individual

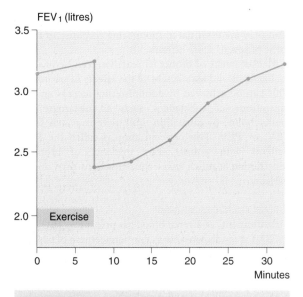

Fig. 6.15 Exercise-induced asthma. Serial recordings of forced expiratory volume in one second (FEV_1) in patient with bronchial asthma before and after 6 minutes of strenuous exercise. Note initial slight rise on completion of exercise, followed by sudden fall and gradual recovery.

patient and their chief value is to distinguish atopic from non-atopic subjects.

Management

The principles of management of asthma are based closely on the guidelines for the management of asthma produced by the British Thoracic Society and also the International Consensus Report on the diagnosis and management of asthma.

Avoidance

There are a few instances in which a single agent can be identified as the cause of attacks of asthma. These include allergens such as grass pollens, house dust mites, animal dander, drugs, industrial chemicals such as isocyanates and certain articles of diet. The measures which can be taken to prevent or reduce exposure to these agents, and the degree of success likely to be achieved, are summarised in Table 6.8. The vast majority of asthmatic patients are hypersensitive to a wide range of allergens and attempts to avoid them all are impracticable.

Avoidance of day-to-day triggers such as exercise and cold air generally imposes inappropriate restrictions on lifestyle, and it may be preferable to adjust treatment to cover exposure to these. Smoking should be discouraged.

Hyposensitisation

This involves the subcutaneous injection of initially very small, but gradually increasing doses of extracts of allergens believed to be responsible for the patient's asthma. Hyposensitisation may be of some value when only a single allergen is implicated but it is not without risk of producing an acute anaphylactic reaction. This form of therapy has largely been abandoned in Britain because of the attendant risks. Hyposensitisation with a mixture of allergens is irrational and cannot be recommended.

Management of chronic persistent asthma

Step 1 Occasional use of inhaled short acting β_2-adrenoceptor agonist bronchodilators. Short acting bronchodilators, such as salbutamol or terbutaline, by inhalation used as required for relief of minor symptoms. If more than occasional use (more often than once daily or three times each week) is necessary, treatment with inhaled drugs which have a beneficial effect on the underlying asthmatic inflammatory disease process should be prescribed (Step 2 treatment). β_2-adrenoceptor agonist therapy alone is only recommended if it is used occasionally and when this allows the patient to lead an active normal life free from nocturnal and exercise-induced asthmatic symptoms.

Step 2 Regular inhaled anti-inflammatory agents. Inhaled short acting β_2-adrenoceptor agonists as required **plus** an inhaled steroid (beclomethasone dipropionate, budesonide or fluticasone propionate) in dose up to 800 mcg daily. Alternatively sodium cromoglycate or nedocromil sodium can be used instead of an inhaled steroid, but these drugs are rarely effective and they are mainly used in the treatment of childhood asthma.

Step 3 High dose inhaled steroids. Inhaled short acting β_2-adrenoceptor agonists as required **plus** an inhaled steroid in the dose range 800–2000 mcg daily. When steroids in high dose are inhaled via a conventional pressurised metered dose inhaler (MDI) the routine use of a large volume spacer (holding chamber) is recommended. When dry powder inhalers are used, mouth rinsing with spitting out of the rinsing liquid after each treatment should be encouraged. Spacers and rinsing are recommended to decrease gastro-intestinal absorption of swallowed drug, and to lower the risk of developing the local side-effect of oropharyngeal candidiasis.

Step 4 High dose inhaled steroids and regular bronchodilators. Inhaled short acting β_2-adrenoceptor agonists as required with an inhaled steroid (800–2000 mcg daily) **plus** a sequential therapeutic trial of one or more of:

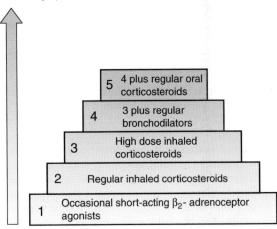

Severity of chronic asthma symptoms

5 — 4 plus regular oral corticosteroids
4 — 3 plus regular bronchodilators
3 — High dose inhaled corticosteroids
2 — Regular inhaled corticosteroids
1 — Occasional short-acting β_2- adrenoceptor agonists

Fig. 6.17   A stepwise approach to the therapy of chronic asthma.

- inhaled long acting β_2-adrenoceptor agonist (salmeterol or formoterol)
- sustained release theophylline
- inhaled ipratropium bromide or oxitropium bromide
- long acting oral β_2-adrenoceptor agonist (sustained release salbutamol or terbutaline preparations)
- high dose inhaled bronchodilators
- sodium cromoglycate or nedocromil sodium.

Step 5 Addition of regular oral steroid therapy. Inhaled short acting β_2-adrenoceptor agonists as required with an inhaled steroid in high dose (800–2000 mcg) and one or more of the long acting bronchodilators **plus**: regular prednisolone tablets in the lowest dose necessary to control symptoms in a single daily dose.

Using this type of 'step' approach to asthma management (see Fig. 6.17), initial treatment for each patient should be chosen individually depending upon severity of disease. In general it is better to start with a treatment regimen which is likely to achieve disease control and then 'step down' rather than to start with inadequate treatment and then have to 'step up'. Patient compliance is likely to be better when control of symptoms is achieved rapidly. Regular review is important and if there has been good symptomatic control for 3–6 months a step down of treatment should be made. This is of particular importance in those patients taking oral and high dose inhaled steroids (Steps 3–5).

Short course oral steroid treatments

Short courses of 'rescue' oral prednisolone are often required to regain control of symptoms. For adults

30–60 mg of prednisolone can be given initially and the same dose continued in single daily doses each morning until 2 days after control has been re-established. In children a dose of 1–2 mg/kg body weight can be used. Tapering of the dose to withdraw treatment is not necessary. Indications for 'rescue' courses of prednisolone include:

- symptoms and peak expiratory flow (PEF) progressively worsening day by day
- fall of PEF below 60% of the patient's best known recording
- onset or worsening of sleep disturbance by asthma
- persistence of morning symptoms until midday
- progressively diminishing response to an inhaled bronchodilator
- symptoms severe enough to require treatment with nebulised or injected bronchodilators.

Increase in dose of inhaled steroid

Doubling the dose of inhaled steroid is often advised to control minor exacerbations of asthma not severe enough to warrant treatment with oral prednisolone. This appears to be effective in many cases.

Management of acute severe asthma

The aims of management are to prevent death, to restore pulmonary function to the patient's best as quickly as possible, to maintain optimal pulmonary function and to prevent early relapse. The features of severe acute asthma are shown in the information box.

PEF should be recorded immediately in all patients

IMMEDIATE ASSESSMENT OF ACUTE SEVERE ASTHMA

Features of severity
- Pulse rate > 120 per min
- Pulsus paradoxus
- Unable to speak in sentences
- Peak flow < 50% of expected

(NB: *apparent* distress and respiratory rate may be misleading.)

Life-threatening features
- Can't speak
- Central cyanosis
- Exhaustion, confusion, reduced conscious level
- Bradycardia
- 'Silent chest'
- Unrecordable peak flow

Arterial blood gases in life-threatening asthma
- A normal (5–6 kPa) or high CO_2 tension
- Severe hypoxaemia (< 8 kPa) especially if being treated with oxygen
- A low pH or high [H⁺]

---

unless they are too ill to co-operate initially. PEF measurements are most easily interpreted when expressed as a percentage of the predicted normal value or of the previous best obtained value on optimal treatment. When neither of these is known, decisions have to be made on the absolute value recorded, remembering that normal values vary with age, sex and height. In previously fit asthmatics recordings of < 200 litres/min are indicative of severe disease, and values of < 100 litres/min must be taken as evidence of life-threatening asthma.

Immediate treatment
See Figure 6.18.

Oxygen
The highest concentration available should be used and set at a high flow rate. High concentration oxygen therapy does not cause or aggravate carbon dioxide retention in asthma, and the presence of carbon dioxide retention must not be interpreted as a contraindication for high concentration oxygen treatment. The concentration of oxygen used can be adjusted according to the arterial blood gas measurements. A PaO_2 of > 8.5–9 kPa should be maintained if possible.

High doses of inhaled β_2-adrenoceptor agonists
When possible beta-agonists should be nebulised in oxygen. Salbutamol 2.5–5 mg or terbutaline 5–10 mg should be given initially and repeated within 30 minutes if necessary. When treatment is given outside hospital and oxygen is not available an air compressor can be used to drive the nebuliser. An alternative method of giving high doses of beta-agonists in general practice is multiple actuations of a metered dose inhaler into a large volume spacer device.

Systemic steroids
Systemic steroids are necessary for the treatment of all cases of severe acute asthma. Intravenous hydrocortisone 200 mg and/or oral prednisolone 30–60 mg should be given initially.

If features of severity persist:

- Ipratropium bromide 0.5 mg should be added to the nebulised beta-agonist
- Aminophylline (250 mg i.v. over 20 minutes) can be given to patients who are not already taking oral theophyllines, and/or salbutamol or terbutaline (250 μg i.v. over 10 minutes).

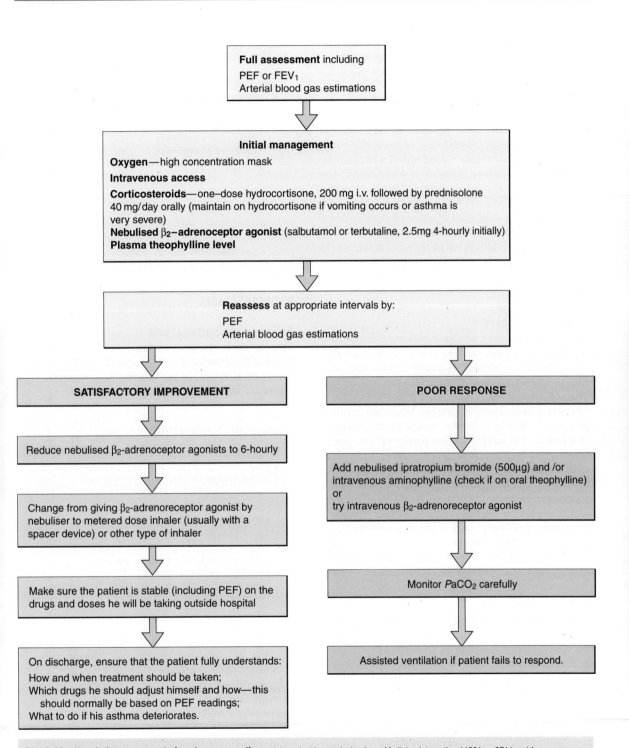

Fig. 6.18 Hospital management of acute severe asthma. Adapted with permission from *Medicine International* 1991, p. 3711 and from Prof. A. Tattersfield.

Subsequent management

All patients must be closely supervised and oxygen therapy continued. Systemic steroid treatment with oral prednisolone 30–60 mg daily is recommended for patients responding to treatment, but intravenous hydrocortisone 200 mg 6-hourly should be continued in the seriously ill. If there is little or no improvement nebulised β_2-adrenoceptor agonist therapy can be repeated after 15–20 minutes and as necessary thereafter. Ipratropium bromide 0.5 mg mixed with the beta-agonist in the nebuliser chamber is recommended 6-hourly until there is clinical response. For the few patients who do not respond well to this treatment a continuous intravenous infusion of aminophylline (0.5–0.9 mg/kg hourly) may be necessary. Continuous intravenous infusion of salbutamol or terbutaline can also be considered. When there has been a good response to the initial therapy, nebulised β_2-adrenoceptor agonist treatment can be given 4-hourly or as necessary.

Monitoring of treatment

PEF recordings every 15–30 minutes to assess early response and as necessary thereafter. In hospital PEF values should be charted 6-hourly before and after inhaled bronchodilator treatments throughout the period of hospital stay.

Repeat measurement of arterial blood gas tensions and pH or H^+ within 1–2 hours is necessary in all patients if the first arterial sample showed markers of life-threatening disease (see information box on page 342). Continuous monitoring of oxygen saturation by pulse oximetry is valuable in all patients to help assess response, especially in the very ill. Oximetry may also prevent the need to repeat an arterial puncture in many patients. When aminophylline is used in the treatment regimen, continuous therapy should be monitored by theophylline serum levels with the aim of achieving and maintaining a concentration of 55–110 μmol/l.

Assisted ventilation

Mechanical ventilation is necessary as a life-saving procedure in few patients. Indications for endotracheal intubation and intermittent positive ventilation are shown in the information box.

Prognosis

The prognosis of the individual attack is good. There is occasionally a fatal outcome especially if treatment is inadequate or delayed. Spontaneous remission is fairly common in episodic asthma particularly in children but rare in chronic asthma, which can lead to irreversible airflow obstruction. Seasonal fluctuations can occur in both types of asthma. Atopic subjects with episodic

---

> **INDICATIONS FOR ASSISTED VENTILATION IN ACUTE SEVERE ASTHMA**
>
> - Coma
> - Respiratory arrest
> - Exhaustion, confusion, drowsiness
> - Deterioration of arterial blood gas tensions despite optimal therapy:
>
> PaO_2 <8 kPa and falling
> $PaCO_2$ >6 kPa and rising
>   pH <7.3 and falling

asthma are usually worse in the summer when they are more heavily exposed to antigens while chronic asthmatics are usually worse in winter months because of the increased frequency of viral infections.

BRONCHIECTASIS

Aetiology and pathogenesis

Bronchiectasis, the term used to describe abnormal dilatation of the bronchi, may be produced in different ways. It may be acquired, or less commonly, congenital. The causes are listed in the information box below.

> **CAUSES OF BRONCHIECTASIS**
>
> **Congenital**
> - Ciliary dysfunction syndromes, cystic fibrosis, primary hypogammaglobulinaemia
>
> **Acquired—children**
> - Pneumonia (whooping cough and measles), primary tuberculosis, foreign body
>
> **Acquired—adults**
> - Suppurative pneumonia, pulmonary tuberculosis, pulmonary eosinophilia, bronchial tumours
> - Ciliary dysfunction syndromes
>   Primary ciliary dyskinesia (immotile cilia syndrome), Kartagener's syndrome, Young's syndrome

Bronchiectasis is usually secondary to severe bacterial infection in childhood, often as a complication of whooping cough or measles.

Bronchiectasis may be due to bronchial distension resulting from the accumulation of pus beyond a lesion obstructing a major bronchus, such as a tuberculous hilar lymph node, an inhaled foreign body or a bronchial carcinoma. Recurrent infection and chronic obstruction by viscid mucus are both factors in causing bronchiectasis in cystic fibrosis (p. 346). Rarely, it may be the result of congenital dysfunction of the cilia, which is a feature of, for example, Kartagener's syndrome (bronchiectasis, sinusitis and transposition of the viscera).

Pathology

The bronchiectatic cavities may be lined by granulation tissue, squamous epithelium or normal ciliated epithelium. There may also be inflammatory changes in the deeper layers of the bronchial wall and hypertrophy of the bronchial arteries. Chronic inflammatory and fibrotic changes are usually found in the surrounding lung tissue.

Clinical features

Bronchiectasis may involve any part of the lungs but the more efficient drainage by gravity of the upper lobes usually produces less serious symptoms and complications than when bronchiectasis involves the lower lobes.

The three groups of clinical features that occur in more severe cases are shown in the information box below.

SYMPTOMS OF BRONCHIECTASIS

Due to accumulation of pus in dilated bronchi
- Chronic productive cough usually worse in mornings and often brought on by changes of posture. Sputum often copious and persistently purulent in advanced disease

Due to inflammatory changes in lung and pleura surrounding dilated bronchi
- Fever, malaise and increased cough and sputum volume when spread of infection causes pneumonia, which is frequently associated with pleurisy. Recurrent pleurisy in the same site often occurs in bronchiectasis

Haemoptysis
- Can be slight or massive and is often recurrent. Usually associated with purulent sputum or an increase in sputum purulence. Can, however, be the only symptom in so-called 'dry bronchiectasis'

General health
- When disease is extensive and sputum persistently purulent a decline in general health occurs with weight loss, anorexia, lassitude, sleep sweating, and failure to thrive in children. In these patients digital clubbing is common

---

Physical signs in the chest may be unilateral or bilateral and are usually basal. If the bronchiectatic cavities are dry without lobar collapse there may be no abnormal physical signs. In the presence of large amounts of secretion numerous coarse crepitations will be heard over the affected areas. When collapse is present the character of the physical signs depends on whether or not the proximal bronchi supplying the collapsed lobe are patent (Table 6.2).

Investigations

Bacteriological and mycological examination of sputum

This is necessary in all patients but is especially important in bronchiectasis associated with cystic fibrosis and in any patient who has received repeated antibiotic courses.

Radiological examination

Bronchiectasis, unless very gross, is not usually apparent on the conventional chest radiograph. In advanced disease the cystic bronchiectatic spaces may be visible. Abnormalities produced by associated pulmonary infection and/or collapse are evident. A diagnosis of bronchiectasis can only be made with certainty by computed tomography or bronchography.

Assessment of ciliary function

A screening test can be performed in patients suspected of having a ciliary dysfunction syndrome by assessing the time taken for a small pellet of saccharin placed in the anterior chamber of the nose to reach the pharynx, when the patient can taste it. This time should not exceed 20 minutes and is greatly prolonged in patients with ciliary dysfunction. It is possible to assess ciliary function by measuring ciliary beat frequency using biopsies taken from the nose. Whenever possible the ciliary ultrastructure should also be determined by electron microscopy.

Management

Postural drainage

The aim of this measure is to keep the dilated bronchi emptied of secretions. Efficiently performed it is of great value both in reducing the amount of cough and sputum and in preventing recurrent episodes of bronchopulmonary infection. In its simplest form, postural drainage consists of adopting a position in which the lobe to be drained is uppermost, thereby allowing secretions in the dilated bronchi to gravitate towards the trachea from which they can readily be cleared by vigorous coughing. 'Percussion' of the chest wall with cupped hands aids dislodgement of sputum, and a number of mechanical devices are available which cause the chest wall to oscillate, thus achieving the same effect as postural percussion and chest wall compression. The optimum duration and frequency of postural drainage depends on the amount of sputum but 5–10 minutes once or twice daily is a minimum for most patients.

Antibiotic therapy

The policy governing the use of antibiotics in most patients with bronchiectasis is the same as that in chronic bronchitis (p. 333). Some, especially those with cystic fibrosis, present difficult therapeutic problems because of secondary infection with bacteria such as staphylococci and Gram-negative bacilli, in particular pseudomonas species. In these circumstances it may prove necessary to use oral ciprofloxacin (250–750 mg twice daily) or ceftazidime by intravenous injection or infusion (100–150 mg/kg daily in 3 divided doses). The bronchi of some patients with cystic fibrosis also become colonised by *Aspergillus fumigatus*.

Surgical treatment

It is essential to demonstrate exactly the extent of bronchiectasis by CT scanning (or bronchography if CT is not available). Pulmonary function must also be carefully assessed. The most suitable cases for pulmonary resection are young patients in whom bronchiectasis is unilateral and confined to a single lobe or segment. Unfortunately, many of the patients in whom medical treatment proves unsuccessful are also unsuitable for pulmonary resection either because of extensive bronchiectasis or co-existing chronic bronchitis. Resection of areas of bronchiectatic lung has no role in the management of the progressive forms of bronchiectasis, for example those associated with ciliary dysfunction and cystic fibrosis.

Prognosis

The disease is progressive when associated with ciliary dysfunction and cystic fibrosis and inevitably causes respiratory failure and right ventricular failure. In many patients the prognosis is relatively good if postural drainage is performed regularly and antibiotics are used judiciously.

Prevention

Because bronchiectasis commonly starts in childhood following measles, whooping cough or a primary tuberculous infection, it is essential that these conditions receive adequate prophylaxis and treatment. The early recognition and treatment of bronchial obstruction is particularly important.

CYSTIC FIBROSIS

Epidemiology and pathogenesis

Cystic Fibrosis (CF) is the most common severe autosomal recessive disease in Caucasians, occurring with a frequency of about 1 in 2500 live births. Carriers have no disease or other phenotypic marker, but the identification of the CF gene will now permit carrier detection and DNA analysis in utero. In 1985 it was recognised that the CF gene was located on the long arm of chromosome 7. In 1989 the gene was sequenced and its protein, which is now called the cystic fibrosis transmembrane conductance regulatory protein (CFTR), was identified. This genetic defect is associated with disordered ion transport in epithelial cells resulting in increased sodium chloride in sweat and increased electrical potential difference across the respiratory epithelium (see Fig. 6.19). This somehow predisposes to ciliary dysfunction and repeated infection and colonisation with bacteria in the lung leading to a vicious cycle of bacterial colonisation, lung inflammation and scarring, resulting in severe bronchiectasis (p. 344) which progressively destroys lung function.

There are also disorders in the gut epithelium and in the pancreas. 80% of patients with cystic fibrosis have both pulmonary disease and pancreatic disease, but 15% have lung sepsis with apparently normal pancreatic function.

Clinical features

Lung function is normal at birth, which leads to the hope that if the basic defect can be corrected many of the sequelae (see below) might be avoided. Males are nearly always infertile with aspermia secondary to disordered vas deferentia and seminal vesicles. Patients with CF develop symptoms of bronchiectasis early in life and usually have chronic pseudomonas infection by their teens. Repeated lung infection, inflammation and scarring eventually destroys the lungs. Pancreatic insufficiency caused by inflammatory damage to pancreatic acinar cells leads to malabsorption. In many cases this can be corrected with pancreatic enzyme supplements. In addition to repeated infections a number of important complications may occur in cystic fibrosis patients (see information box).

COMPLICATIONS OF CYSTIC FIBROSIS

Respiratory
- Spontaneous pneumothorax
- Haemoptysis
- Nasal polyps
- Respiratory failure
- Cor pulmonale

Gastrointestinal
- Malabsorption
- Adult meconium ileus equivalent
- Biliary cirrhosis
- Increased frequency of gallstones

Others
- Diabetes (11% of adults)
- Delayed puberty
- Male infertility
- Psycho-social problems
- Amyloidosis
- Arthropathy

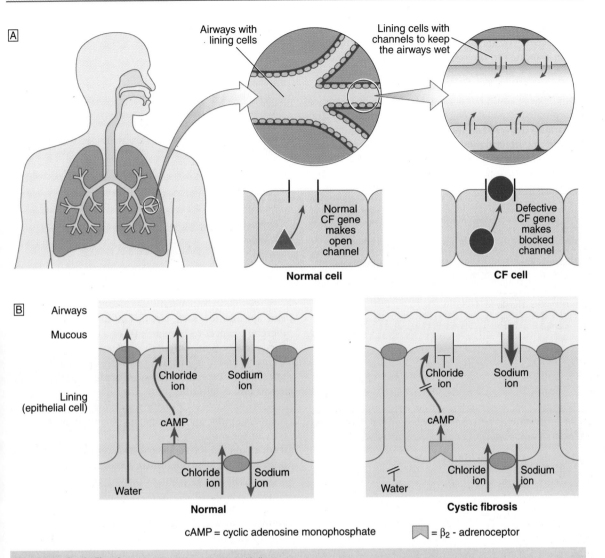

Fig. 6.19 **Cystic fibrosis:** basic defect in the pulmonary epithelium.

Management

The management of established cystic fibrosis is that of severe bronchiectasis (p. 345). All patients with cystic fibrosis who produce sputum should have physiotherapy twice each day and more frequently during exacerbations of respiratory infection. Postural drainage and manual percussion may be helpful. Lung infections are usually associated with *Pseudomonas aeruginosa*, *Haemophylus influenzae* and *Staphylococcus aureus*. Most adults become chronically colonised with *Pseudomonas aeruginosa*. Infections with *Haemophylus influenzae* can be treated with a number of antibiotics and *Staphylococcus aureus* should be treated with flucloxacillin or erythromycin. In some centres, patients are treated with intravenous antibiotics every three months, and patients can be taught how to give their own antibiotics at home through an indwelling central venous cannula implanted subcutaneously in the chest wall. Aerosolised and nebulised antibiotics have also been used. A number of patients with cystic fibrosis develop symptoms of bronchospasm which can be treated effectively with bronchodilators following appropriate reversibility tests. Prognosis has greatly improved in cystic fibrosis with recent developments in the control of bronchial sepsis and a better maintenance of nutrition, and many patients now survive into adult life. In cases of inexorable respiratory failure, organ transplantation may be necessary.

The potential for somatic gene therapy

The discovery of the CF gene and the fact that the lung defect is located in the respiratory epithelium (which is accessible by instillation of fluid or nebulisation) presents a special opportunity for correction of this disease. The CF gene could be 'packaged' within a liposome or incorporated by genetic engineering into a modified viral vector and delivered to the respiratory epithelium with the aim of correcting the genetic defect. The feasibility of this approach is currently under investigation.

FURTHER READING

Barnes P J, Pedersen S 1993 Efficacy and safety of inhaled corticosteroids in asthma. American Review of Respiratory Disease 148: S1–S26

Bochner B S et al 1994 Immunological basis of allergic asthma. Annual Review of Immunology: 707–735

Hodgkin J E (ed) 1990 Chronic obstructive pulmonary disease. Clinics in Chest Medicine 11(3): 363–573

Porteous D J, Dorin J R 1991 Cystic fibrosis 3: Cloning the cystic fibrosis gene—implications for diagnosis and treatment. Thorax 46: 46–55

British Thoracic Society et al 1993 Guidelines on the management of asthma. Thorax 48 (Suppl 2): S1–S24

INFECTIONS OF THE RESPIRATORY SYSTEM

Infections of the respiratory tract may be caused by viruses, bacteria or fungi. Viruses are frequently responsible for upper respiratory illnesses. Although viral infection is a relatively uncommon specific cause of pneumonia, it is often complicated by bacterial infection of the bronchi and lungs, as for example in influenza. The bacteria most frequently responsible for respiratory infection, including pneumonia, are *Streptococcus pneumoniae* often in association with *Haemophilus influenzae*, *Staphylococcus aureus*, various species of Gram-negative bacilli and *Legionella pneumophila*. Organisms such as mycoplasma, coxiella and chlamydia are other but less common causes of acute pneumonia. Pulmonary infection by *Mycobacterium tuberculosis*, atypical mycobacteria and fungi results in diseases of a more chronic type, which are described separately.

UPPER RESPIRATORY TRACT INFECTIONS

The vast majority of these illnesses, of which acute coryza (common cold) is by far the most common, are caused by viruses (Table 6.9). Immunity is short-lived,

Table 6.9 Respiratory infections caused by viruses

Clinical syndrome	Usual cause (other causes in parentheses)
Epidemic influenza	Influenza A and B
'Flu-like' illness	Adenoviruses, rhinoviruses. (Enteroviruses)
Sore throat	Adenoviruses. (Enteroviruses, parainfluenza viruses, influenza A and B in partially immune)
Common cold (coryza)	Rhinoviruses. (Coronaviruses, enteroviruses, adenoviruses, respiratory syncytial virus)
'Feverish' cold	Rhinoviruses, enteroviruses. (Influenza A and B, parainfluenza viruses, respiratory syncytial virus)
Croup	Parainfluenza 1, 2, 3. (Rhinoviruses, enteroviruses)
Bronchitis	Rhinoviruses, adenoviruses. (Influenza A and B)
Bronchiolitis	Respiratory syncytial virus. (Parainfluenza 3)
Pneumonia	Influenza A and B. (Respiratory syncytial virus and parainfluenza viruses in adults)

and specific for each virus. The average person can therefore expect to have at least two or three attacks of coryza every year. Other viral infections include acute laryngitis and acute laryngotracheobronchitis. Bacterial infection is the usual cause of acute tonsillitis, otitis media and epiglottitis.

Most patients with upper respiratory tract infections recover rapidly and specific investigation is indicated only in the more severe illness. Viruses can be isolated from exfoliated cells collected on throat swabs, and viral infections may be identified retrospectively by serological tests. In sputum exfoliated cells colonised by certain viruses can be identified by the fluorescent antibody technique, allowing the pathogen to be rapidly defined. Culture of throat swabs and pharyngeal exudate may be helpful if streptococcal sore throat is suspected, and examination of the blood will identify infectious mononucleosis. Radiographic examination may be required to confirm the presence of chronic sinus infection. The clinical features, complications and management of the common and most important upper respiratory tract infections are summarised in Table 6.10.

THE PNEUMONIAS

Pneumonia is the term used to describe inflammation of the lungs associated with acute lower respiratory tract infection and recently developed radiological signs. There are many different kinds of pneumonia, some common, others rare (see Table 6.11).

Aetiology

The pneumonias can be divided into primary and secondary, as shown in the information box below. This is a somewhat artificial distinction, but in general the primary pneumonias encompass those caused by community-acquired organisms such as *Streptococcus pneumoniae* and mycoplasma whereas the 'secondary pneumonias' (e.g. nosocomial pneumonia and aspiration pneumonia) occur when the lung or host have been compromised by prior disease.

Occasionally in some types of both primary and secondary pneumonia, prominent features are destruction of lung tissue by the inflammatory process, a high incidence of abscess formation and the subsequent development of pulmonary fibrosis and bronchiectasis. The term **suppurative pneumonia** has been applied to this group of conditions (p. 356).

Investigations

Sputum

An attempt should always be made to establish a positive microbiological diagnosis, though this is not always possible, particularly if antibiotics have been given before specimens are submitted for examination. Direct smear examination of sputum by Gram and Ziehl–Neelsen stains may give an immediate indication of possible pathogens and indicate what treatment should be prescribed. Culture (including anaerobic culture where indicated) and sensitivity testing should be carried out.

Where a microbiological diagnosis is essential, as in severely ill immunosuppressed patients, and a specimen of sputum cannot be obtained, an attempt should be made to aspirate secretions or washings from the trachea or bronchi either by bronchoscopy or by inserting a needle through the cricothyroid membrane. Some patients can be induced to produce sputum by the administration of nebulised hypertonic saline.

Blood culture

Blood culture should be performed in patients with severe pneumonia and may yield a positive result when sputum examination is negative, particularly in pneumococcal pneumonia.

Serological tests

Pneumococcal antigen may be detected in serum. Serological tests may be helpful in the diagnosis of mycoplasma, chlamydia, legionella and viral infections, specimens being examined at ten-day intervals. A four-fold rise of antibody titre suggests recent infection.

Nose and throat swabs

Swabs of the nose and throat, and post-nasal and bronchial aspirates, can be cultured for viruses or examined by immunofluorescence or electron microscopy.

Total and differential white blood count

The total white cell count is often below $5.0 \times 10^9/l$ in patients with viral infection. A high neutrophil polymorph leucocytosis favours bacterial infection but in overwhelming bacterial infections the total white cell count may be low.

Arterial blood gas measurements

The PaO_2 and $PaCO_2$ and the hydrogen ion concentration or pH of arterial blood should be measured in all patients who are seriously ill and in those with a previous history of chronic respiratory disease.

Radiological examination

This is necessary for confirmation of the diagnosis and for the early detection of complications such as pleural effusion and empyema. Follow-up radiological examination is important because if a pneumonia fails to resolve it may be secondary to bronchial obstruction, e.g. by a carcinoma.

THE PRIMARY PNEUMONIAS

The organisms which cause primary pneumonias are listed in the information box below.

PNEUMONIA INVESTIGATIONS

Achieving a microbiological diagnosis

An attempt to identify the organism causing pneumonia should be undertaken in all cases.

Sputum

Sputum should be examined in the laboratory as quickly as possible after expectoration. Pathogens may not be cultured from sputum if antibiotic therapy has been started. Direct examination of sputum smears by Gram and Ziehl–Neelsen (or auramine) stains may give an immediate indication of possible pathogens and thus aid the choice of initial antibiotic treatment. Anaerobic culture should also be performed where indicated. Examination by specific immunofluorescence techniques should be requested when organisms such as legionella and pneumocystis are suspected. About one-third of patients with pneumonia may not be able to produce sputum initially. In these, inhalation of nebulised hypertonic saline may induce sputum production. If this fails, bronchoscopy should be considered at an early stage to allow bronchial lavage and brushings of the lobes or segments most obviously involved on the chest radiograph. Needle aspiration through the cricothyroid membrane is an alternative method of obtaining tracheal secretions.

Blood

Blood culture should be performed in all seriously ill patients since this may yield a positive result when sputum examination is negative, especially in pneumococcal pneumonia. Examination for pneumococcal antigen may be positive even in patients who have received prior antibiotic treatment. Serological tests are also of value in the retrospective diagnosis of mycoplasma, chlamydia, legionella and viral infections. A fourfold rise in antibody titre between specimens examined at 7–10-day intervals suggests a recent infection, as does a single very high titre in serum taken late in the disease.

Urine

Identification of pneumococcal antigen in urine indicates pneumococcal infection.

Pleural fluid

Whenever pleural fluid is present in less than a trivial amount this should be sampled to exclude empyema formation, and to provide a specimen for microbiological examination.

Nose and throat swabs

Swabs of the nose and throat, and post-nasal and bronchial aspirates, can be cultured for viruses or examined by immunofluorescence or electron microscopy.

Assessment of severity of disease and detection of underlying disease and/or complications

Chest radiograph. Extent of consolidation, cavitation, effusion. Presence of evidence of bronchial obstruction, developing empyema or cardiomegaly.

Arterial blood gas analysis. Assessment of degree of hypoxaemia (and hypercapnia) to determine concentration of oxygen required for treatment.

Haematological indices. White cell count of $> 15\,000 \times 10^9/l$ makes a bacterial pathogen likely, but the WBC may be low in viral infection or overwhelming bacterial infection. Detection of underlying haematological disease, anaemia and haemolysis.

Biochemistry and urinalysis. Assessment of severity and identification of underlying or associated renal or hepatic disease and diabetes.

PNEUMOCOCCAL PNEUMONIA

Pneumococcal pneumonia is characterised by homogeneous consolidation of one or more lobes or segments.

Table 6.10   Common and most important upper respiratory tract infections: clinical features, complications, management

	Clinical features	Complications	Management
Acute coryza (common cold)	Rapid onset. Burning and tickling sensation in nose. Sneezing. Sore throat. Blocked nose with watery discharge. Discharge usually green/yellow after 24/48 h (secondary infection). Nasal allergy can give rise to similar clinical features	Sinusitis. Lower respiratory tract infection (bronchitis/pneumonia). Hearing impairment, otitis media (due to blockage of Eustachian tubes)	Most do not require treatment. Paracetamol 0.5–1 g 4–6-hourly for relief of systemic symptoms. Nasal decongestant in some cases. Antibiotics not necessary in uncomplicated coryza
Acute laryngitis	Often a complication of acute coryza. Dry sore throat. Hoarse voice or loss of voice. Attempts to speak cause pain. Initially, painful and unproductive cough. Stridor in children (croup) because of inflammatory oedema leading to partial obstruction of a small larynx	Complications rare. Chronic laryngitis. Downward spread of infection may cause tracheitis, bronchitis or pneumonia	Rest voice. Paracetamol 0.5–1 g 4–6-hourly for relief of discomfort and pyrexia. Steam inhalations may be of value. Antibiotics not necessary in simple acute laryngitis
Acute laryngotracheo-bronchitis (croup)	Initial symptoms like common cold. Sudden paroxysms of cough accompanied by stridor and breathlessness. Contraction of accessory muscles and indrawing of intercostal spaces. Cyanosis and asphyxia in small children, if appropriate treatment not given	Asphyxia. Death. Superinfection with bacteria, especially *Strep. pneumoniae* and *Staph. aureus*. Viscid secretions may occlude bronchi	Inhalations of steam and humidified air/high concentrations of oxygen. Endotracheal intubation or tracheostomy to relieve laryngeal obstruction and allow clearing of bronchial secretions. Intravenous antibiotic therapy for seriously ill (Co-amoxiclav or erythromycin). Maintain adequate hydration
Acute epiglottitis	Fever and sore throat, rapidly leading to stridor because of swelling of epiglottis and surrounding structures (infection with *H. influenzae*). Stridor and cough in absence of much hoarseness may distinguish acute epiglottitis from other causes of stridor	Death from asphyxia which may be precipitated by attempts to examine the throat — AVOID USING A TONGUE DEPRESSOR OR ANY INSTRUMENT unless facilities for endotracheal intubation or tracheostomy are immediately available	Intravenous antibiotic therapy essential. Co-amoxiclav or chloramphenicol. Other measures as for acute laryngo-tracheobronchitis
Acute bronchitis	Often follows acute coryza. Irritating unproductive cough accompanied by retrosternal discomfort of tracheitis. Chest tightness, wheeze and breathlessness when bronchi become involved. Sputum is initially scanty, mucoid, viscid and may be streaked with blood. After a day or so sputum becomes mucopurulent and more copious. Acute bronchial infection may be associated with a pyrexia of 38–39°C and a neutrophil leucocytosis. Spontaneous recovery occurs over a few days in the majority of patients	Bronchopneumonia. Exacerbation of chronic bronchitis which often results in Type II respiratory failure in patients with severe chronic obstructive airways disease. Acute exacerbation of bronchial asthma	Specific treatment rarely necessary in previously healthy individuals. Cough may be eased by pholcodeine 5–10 mg 6–8-hourly. In patients with chronic bronchitis (p. 331) and asthma (p. 336) aggressive treatment of exacerbations may be required. Amoxycillin 250 mg 8-hourly should be given to previously healthy patients who are thought to be developing bronchopneumonia (see also p. 355)
Influenza (A specific acute illness caused by a group of myxoviruses—two common type A and B)	Sudden onset of pyrexia associated with generalised aches and pains, anorexia, nausea and vomiting. Degree of ill health ranges from mild to rapidly fatal. Usually harsh unproductive cough. Most patients do not develop complications and acute symptoms subside within 3–5 days, but may be followed by 'post-influenzal asthenia' which can persist for several weeks. During epidemics the diagnosis is usually easy. Sporadic cases may have to be diagnosed by virus isolation, fluorescent antibody techniques or serological tests for specific antibodies	Tracheitis, bronchitis, bronchiolitis and bronchopneumonia. Secondary bacterial invasion by *Strep. pneumoniae*, *H. influenzae* and *Staph. aureus* may occur. Toxic cardiomyopathy may cause sudden death (rare). Encephalitis, demyelinating encephalopathy and peripheral neuropathy are also rare complications	Bed rest is advisable until fever has subsided. Paracetamol 0.5–1 g 4–6-hourly can be used to relieve headache and generalised pains. Pholcodeine 5–10 mg 6–8-hourly may be given to suppress cough. Specific treatment for pneumonia (p. 352) may be necessary

The disease occurs at all ages but most frequently in early and middle adult life. The highest incidence is in winter. It is usually a sporadic disease spread by droplet infection.

Clinical features

The onset is sudden, often with rigors, or with vomiting or a convulsion in children. The temperature rises in a few hours to 39–40°C. Loss of appetite, headache and

Table 6.11 Frequency of identifiable pathogens in pneumonia in the U.K.

Pathogen	%
Bacterial	80–90
Streptococcus pneumoniae	60–75
Mycoplasma pneumoniae	5–18
Haemophilus influenzae	4–5
Legionella sp.	2–5
Chlamydia psittaci	2–3
Staphylococcus aureus	1–5
Gram-negative bacilli	rare
Anaerobes	rare
Rickettsial	1
Coxiella burnetii	
Viral	10–20
Influenza	8
Other viruses	2–8

aching pains in the body and limbs accompany the pyrexia. Localised chest pain of pleural type often develops at an early stage in the illness. Occasionally it may be referred to the shoulder or to the abdominal wall. There is a short, painful cough, dry at first but later productive of tenacious sputum which is characteristically rust-coloured and occasionally frankly blood-stained. Breathing is rapid (30–40/min. in adults, 50–60 in children), and shallow when pleural pain is present. The pulse is rapid, the skin is hot and dry, the face is flushed, and central cyanosis may be observed in severe cases. Herpes labialis is often present. A marked neutrophil leucocytosis is characteristic. *Strep. pneumoniae* can usually be isolated from the sputum, and a positive blood culture may be obtained.

Physical signs in the chest
In the first 24–48 h of the illness there is diminution of respiratory movement, slight impairment of the percussion note and often a pleural rub on the affected side. At a variable time after the onset, generally within two days, signs of consolidation appear (p. 318), with breath sounds of high-pitched bronchial type. When resolution begins, numerous coarse crepitations are heard, indicating liquefaction of the alveolar exudate. If a pleural effusion develops physical signs of fluid in the pleural space are usually found, but bronchial breath sounds can persist and the presence of an effusion may be suspected only from stony dullness on percussion and recurrence or persistence of pyrexia.

Radiological examination
Radiographs show a homogeneous opacity localised to the affected lobe or segment appearing within 12–18

hours of the onset of the illness (Fig. 6.20, p. 353). Radiological examination is particularly helpful if a complication such as pleural effusion or empyema is suspected.

Management
Most patients respond promptly to antibiotic treatment and recovery is usual within a week. Delayed recovery

---

FEATURES ASSOCIATED WITH A HIGH MORTALITY IN PNEUMONIA

Clinical
- Age 60 years or older
- Respiratory rate >30/min.
- Diastolic blood pressure 60 mmHg or less
- Atrial fibrillation
- More than 1 lobe involved on chest radiograph
- Presence of underlying disease

Laboratory
- Hypoxaemia (PaO_2 <8 kPa)
- Leucopenia (WBC <4000 × 10^9/l)
- Leucocytosis (WBC >20 000 × 10^9/l)
- Raised serum urea (>7 mmol/l)
- Positive blood culture

---

suggests either that some complication such as empyema has developed or that the diagnosis is incorrect.

Antibiotic treatment
When a clinical diagnosis of pneumonia is made, provided the patient is not seriously ill, the initial treatment should consist of amoxycillin, 500 mg 8-hourly, erythromycin, 500 mg 6-hourly, or co-trimoxazole, 960 mg 12-hourly by mouth. Patients who are gravely ill and in whom a staphylococcal or a Gram-negative infection is considered should receive, together with ampicillin by intravenous injection, antibiotics to which the causative organism is unlikely to be resistant, for example, flucloxacillin, 250–500 mg 6-hourly intravenously and gentamicin 2–5 mg/kg daily in divided doses 8-hourly intravenously. If *Strep. pneumoniae* is isolated or no pathogenic organisms are reported on culture, and the patient appears to be making satisfactory clinical progress, flucloxacillin and gentamicin can be withdrawn and treatment with oral ampicillin, erythromycin or co-trimoxazole continued. In most cases of uncomplicated pneumococcal pneumonia a 7–10-day course of treatment is usually adequate.

Oxygen
Oxygen should be administered to all hypoxaemic patients. High concentrations should be used in all patients who do not have hypercapnia or advanced obstructive airways disease.

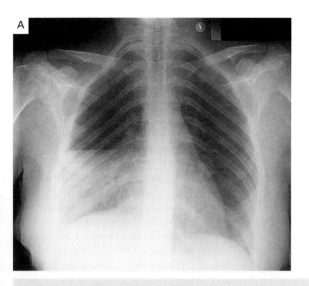
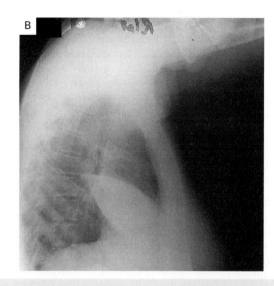

Fig. 6.20 Pneumonia of the right middle lobe. Ⓐ Postero-anterior (PA) view: consolidation in right middle lobe with characteristic opacification beneath the horizontal fissure and loss of normal contrast between the right heart border and lung. Ⓑ Lateral view: consolidation confined to the anteriorly-situated middle lobe.

Treatment of pleural pain

It is important to relieve pleural pain in order to allow the patient to breathe normally and cough efficiently. Mild analgesics such as paracetamol are rarely adequate and most patients require pethidine 50–100 mg or morphine 10–15 mg by intramuscular or intravenous injection. Opiates, however, must be used with extreme caution in patients with poor respiratory function.

Physiotherapy

Assisted coughing is important especially in patients who suppress cough because of pleural pain. The administration of analgesic drugs should be coordinated with physiotherapy to allow optimum patient cooperation.

STAPHYLOCOCCAL PNEUMONIA

Pneumonia due to *Staph. aureus* may occur either as a primary respiratory infection or as a blood-borne infection from a staphylococcal lesion elsewhere in the body, for example, osteomyelitis. The second condition is essentially one of pyaemic abscess formation in the lungs and is much less common than staphylococcal pneumonia.

Primary staphylococcal pneumonia, although it occurs much less frequently than pneumococcal pneumonia, is a relatively common illness, especially as a complication of influenza. Staphylococcal infection must also be assumed when pneumonia develops in debilitated patients in hospital and in patients with cystic fibrosis. It may present as a lobar or segmental pneumonia, which may be difficult to distinguish clinically from a severe pneumococcal infection, or as a suppurative pneumonia (p. 356) with multiple lung abscesses which may persist as thin-walled cysts after the acute infection has subsided.

Management

Intravenous flucloxacillin 0.25–1 g 6-hourly or erythromycin 2–4 g daily in divided doses. In severe infections sodium fusidate 500 mg intravenously over 6 hours, 3 times daily should be administered as well as flucloxacillin or erythromycin. Antibiotic therapy often has to be given for 14 days or longer. Oral therapy can be substituted for intravenous (flucloxacillin and erythromycin) when pyrexia has subsided and the patient is obviously recovering.

KLEBSIELLA PNEUMONIA

Pneumonia due to *Kl. pneumoniae* is an uncommon disease with a high mortality. There is usually massive consolidation and excavation of one or more lobes, the upper lobes being most often involved, with profound systemic disturbance and the expectoration of large amounts of purulent sputum, sometimes chocolate-coloured. The diagnosis is made by the radiological appearances of pulmonary suppuration often associated with increase in size of the affected lobe and the isolation of the causative organism from sputum.

Management

Gentamicin 2–5 mg/kg intravenously daily in divided doses 8-hourly with peak and trough blood level monitoring, ceftazidime 1 g intravenously 8-hourly or ciprofloxacin 200 mg 12-hourly by intravenous infusion over 30–60 min. Treatment may have to be continued for 2 to 3 weeks.

LEGIONELLA PNEUMONIA (LEGIONNAIRES' DISEASE)

Legionnaires' disease is caused by a bacillus (*L. pneumophila*) which appears to be transmitted in water droplets often originating in infected humidifier cooling towers and perhaps from stagnant water in cisterns and showerheads. Epidemics traced to institutions such as hospitals receive much publicity but sporadic cases infected from unknown sources are common. It can be a serious or even fatal illness, but most patients survive. Gastrointestinal symptoms, mental confusion, hyponatraemia and proteinuria often accompany the pneumonia and if present raise the suspicion of legionella infection.

Management

Erythromycin 0.5–1 g 6-hourly (intravenously in severely ill). Rifampicin 600 mg twice daily by mouth or intravenous injection should be given in combination with erythromycin to all severely ill patients in whom the diagnosis has been confirmed or thought to be likely, e.g. during epidemics. At least 14 days of antibiotic treatment is usually required in Legionnaires' disease.

ACTINOMYCOSIS

Formerly included amongst the fungal diseases, this is now regarded as a bacterial infection. It is caused by *A. israeli*, an anaerobic organism which exists as a commensal in the mouth. When local defences are impaired, actinomycosis can cause cervicofacial, abdominal or, occasionally, pulmonary infection such as a widespread suppurative pneumonia (p. 356). Empyema, often bilateral and associated with persistent chest wall sinuses, may develop. The pus may contain 'sulphur grains'. Sinus formation is also a feature of cervicofacial and abdominal infection.

Management

Benzylpenicillin 2–4 g intravenously 6-hourly. The duration of therapy depends upon response.

PNEUMONIA CAUSED BY VIRUSES AND OTHER ORGANISMS

A distinctive form of pneumonia may be produced by certain viruses, and also by unclassified organisms such as mycoplasma and chlamydia which have some features of viruses and bacteria. The clinical picture differs from that of the bacterial pneumonias in that fever and toxaemia usually precede respiratory symptoms by several days. Severe headache, malaise and anorexia are characteristic features in the early stages. The physical signs in the chest, if there are any, appear later and are seldom gross. The existence of a pulmonary lesion may not be recognised without a chest radiograph. The spleen may be palpable in the first week, the white blood count is generally normal and the pyrexia does not respond to penicillin. The diagnosis can often be confirmed by isolation of the causal organism or by serological tests.

The disease is often self-limiting. Pyrexia usually subsides by lysis after 5–10 days and complete recovery and radiographic resolution follow, the latter sometimes being slow. Very rarely death takes place from widespread extension of the pneumonia or from viral encephalitis.

Influenza, parainfluenza and measles

These illnesses are occasionally complicated by pneumonias (primary viral pneumonias) which are frequently complicated by bacterial infection. The combination of influenza and staphylococcal pneumonia is often fatal. There is no specific therapy available.

Varicella (chickenpox)

In adults pneumonia caused by varicella (chickenpox) virus is a serious complication of the disease and usually has characteristic radiographic features. The chest radiograph shows numerous miliary nodular shadows which may eventually calcify.

Varicella can be treated with oral acyclovir 200 mg 5 times daily for 5 days (half dose for children under age of 2) or intravenous vidarabine 10 mg/kg daily for at least 5 days. These antiviral agents are usually reserved for the treatment of chickenpox in immunocompromised patients.

Respiratory syncytial virus

This is the most important respiratory pathogen of early childhood, especially in the first two months of life. It causes bronchiolitis and occasionally pneumonia, and carries a risk of death. The infant is fevered, and cough, wheezy breathing and occasionally an erythematous rash are prominent features. There is no specific treatment available for infection by RSV.

Chlamydia psittaci

This organism is the cause of psittacosis (ornithosis), a systemic illness contracted from infected birds. The pneumonia associated with it may be extensive, and severe systemic upset and death are common. Headache is a prominent early symptom.

Management

Tetracycline 500 mg 6-hourly orally or 500 mg 12-hourly by intravenous infusion.

Mycoplasma pneumoniae

Outbreaks of pneumonia caused by this organism are common in barracks and institutions. Most cases occur in children and young adults. Maculo-papular rashes, haemolytic anaemia and meningo-encephalitis occur rarely.

Cold agglutinins (p. 798) can be demonstrated in a high proportion of cases. Antibodies can be detected and haemagglutination and complement-fixation tests are available for diagnosis.

Management

Tetracycline 500 mg 6-hourly or erythromycin 500 mg 6-hourly. In severe infections treatment should be given intravenously.

Coxiella burnetii

This organism causes **Q fever** which may be complicated by pneumonia and endocarditis.

Management

Tetracycline 500 mg 4-hourly orally.

Lack of response to treatment in pneumonia

- **Incorrect diagnosis/resistant organism**
  Consider: pulmonary infarction, pulmonary oedema, tuberculosis, pulmonary eosinophilia, allergic alveolitis, connective tissue disorder, Wegener's granulomatosis.

- **Complication of disease or therapy**
  Pleural effusion or empyema, retention of sputum causing lobar collapse, development of thromboembolic disease, pyrexia due to drug hypersensitivity.

THE SECONDARY PNEUMONIAS

This group, sometimes described as 'non-specific' bronchopneumonia, and aspiration pneumonia, comprises a large number of different conditions. Their common features are the existence of some abnormality of the respiratory system. This predisposes to the invasion of the lung by organisms of relatively low virulence derived from the upper respiratory tract or from the mouth, for example streptococci, certain types of pneumococci, *H. influenzae* and various species of anaerobic bacteria.

Infection may reach the lungs in various ways. Pus may be aspirated from an infected nasal sinus, or septic matter may be inhaled during tonsillectomy or dental extraction under general anaesthesia. Vomitus or the contents of a dilated oesophagus may enter the larynx during general anaesthesia, coma or even sleep and aspiration may also occur in patients with gastro-oesophageal reflux (p. 417). Pus from acute bronchitis, dilated bronchi or a lung abscess may also be carried into the alveoli by the air stream or by gravity.

Ineffective coughing caused by post-operative or post-traumatic thoracic or abdominal pain, by debility or immobility, or by laryngeal paralysis may also predispose to the development of a secondary (aspiration) pneumonia.

Partial bronchial obstruction, as for example by a tumour, is another potential cause of secondary pneumonia, because it allows infection derived from the upper air passages to become established in the inadequately drained portion of lung beyond the obstruction.

ACUTE BRONCHOPNEUMONIA

Bronchial infection can be 'aspirated' into the alveoli and result in widespread patches of consolidation. This tends to occur at the extremes of life, as a complication of measles and whooping cough in children or in the elderly and debilitated when it is often called 'hypostatic pneumonia'.

Pathology

Acute inflammation of the bronchi and terminal bronchioles is present, with associated collapse and consolidation of the distal alveoli. The lesions are patchy and distributed bilaterally, and tend to be more widespread in the lower lobes.

Clinical features

Symptoms of acute bronchitis are followed after two or three days by increased cough and sputum purulence associated with a rise in temperature. Breathlessness and central cyanosis may then appear, but pleural pain is uncommon. In the early stages the physical signs are those of acute bronchitis and then numerous crepitations become audible. There is a neutrophil leucocytosis and the chest radiograph shows mottled opacities in both lung fields, chiefly in the lower zones.

Course and complications

Onset is more insidious than pneumococcal pneumonia and the disease tends to run a more protracted course. Mortality is higher at the extremes of life and if the disease supervenes on chronic bronchitis and emphysema or any debilitating illness.

Management

Amoxycillin 250–500 mg 8-hourly by mouth or co-trimoxazole 960 mg 12-hourly are usually effective. Physiotherapy is of particular importance in the debilitated and the elderly, and oxygen (p. 330) may be required.

ASPIRATION AND SUPPURATIVE PNEUMONIA (INCLUDING PULMONARY ABSCESS)

Suppurative pneumonia is the term used to describe a form of pneumonic consolidation in which there is destruction of the lung parenchyma by the inflammatory process. Although microabscess formation is a characteristic histological feature of suppurative pneumonia, it is usual to restrict the term 'pulmonary abscess' to lesions in which there is a fairly large localised collection of pus, or a cavity lined by chronic inflammatory tissue, from which pus has escaped by rupture into a bronchus.

Suppurative pneumonia and pulmonary abscess may be produced by infection of previously healthy lung tissue with *Staph. aureus* or *Kl. pneumoniae*. These are, in effect, primary bacterial pneumonias associated with pulmonary suppuration. More frequently, suppurative pneumonia and pulmonary abscess are forms of secondary pneumonia. They may develop after the inhalation of septic material during operations on the nose, mouth or throat under general anaesthesia, or of vomitus during anaesthesia or coma. In such circumstances gross oral sepsis may be a predisposing factor. Aspiration into the lungs of acid gastric contents can give rise to a severe haemorrhagic pneumonia complicated by ARDS (p. 388) which is often fatal.

Bacterial infection of a pulmonary infarct or of a collapsed lobe may also produce a suppurative pneumonia or a lung abscess. The organisms isolated from the sputum may include *Strep. pneumoniae, Staph. aureus, Strep. pyogenes, H. influenzae*, and in some cases anaerobic bacteria. In many cases, however, no pathogens can be isolated, particularly when antibiotics have been given.

Clinical features

These are listed in the information box below.

CLINICAL FEATURES OF SUPPURATIVE PNEUMONIA

Onset
- Acute or insidious

Symptoms
- Cough productive of large amounts of sputum which is sometimes fetid and blood-stained. Pleural pain common. Sudden expectoration of copious amount of sputum occurs if abscess ruptures into a bronchus

Clinical signs
- High remittent pyrexia. Profound systemic upset. Digital clubbing may develop quickly (10–14 days). Chest examination usually reveals signs of consolidation; signs of cavitation rarely found. Pleural rub common. Rapid deterioration in general health with marked weight loss can occur if disease not adequately treated

---

Radiological examination

There is a homogeneous lobar or segmental opacity consistent with consolidation or collapse. A large, dense opacity, which may later cavitate and show a fluid level, is the characteristic finding when a frank lung abscess is present.

Management

In many patients oral treatment with ampicillin 500 mg 6-hourly or co-trimoxazole 960 mg 12-hourly is effective. If an anaerobic bacterial infection is suspected (e.g. from fetor of the sputum) oral metronidazole 400 mg 8-hourly should be added. Antibacterial therapy should be modified according to the results of microbiological examination of sputum. Prolonged treatment for 4–6 weeks may be required in some patients with lung abscess.

Physiotherapy is of great value especially when large abscess cavities have formed. It may not be possible to drain lower lobe cavities without postural coughing.

In most patients there is a good response to treatment and although residual fibrosis and bronchiectasis are common sequelae, these seldom give rise to serious morbidity. Empyema (p. 399) may complicate the acute phase of the disease.

Prevention

Every precaution should be taken during operations on the mouth, nose and throat to prevent the inhalation of blood, tonsillar fragments and other material. Oral sepsis should be eradicated, especially if a general anaesthetic is contemplated.

NOSOCOMIAL PNEUMONIA

Pneumonia developing in hospital in a patient who has been admitted for more than 48 h should be considered to be hospital-acquired. The spectrum of pathogenic organisms involved is different from community-acquired pneumonia in which *Strep. pneumoniae* is common, and other pathogenic bacteria, *Mycoplasma pneumoniae*, and *Legionella pneumophila* have to be considered. In nosocomial pneumonia there is a predominance of Gram-negative bacteria such as pseudomonas species, *Escherichia* species and *Klebsiella* species. Infections caused by *Staph. aureus* are also common in hospital and anaerobic organisms are much more likely than in pneumonia acquired at home.

FACTORS PREDISPOSING TO NOSOCOMIAL PNEUMONIA

Reduced host defences against bacteria

- Reduced immune defences (e.g. steroid treatment, diabetes)
- Reduced cough reflex (e.g. post-operative)
- Disordered mucociliary clearance (e.g. anaesthetic agents)

Aspiration of nasopharyngeal secretions

- Immobility
- Reduced conscious level
- Vomiting
- Dysphagia
- Nasogastric intubation

Gastro-oesophageal aspiration

- Achlorhydria due to acid-suppressing drugs

Bacteria introduced into lower respiratory tract

- Endotracheal intubation/tracheostomy
- Infected ventilators/nebulisers

Bacteraemia

- Abdominal sepsis
- Intravenous cannula infection
- Infected emboli

PNEUMONIA IN THE IMMUNOCOMPROMISED PATIENT

Pulmonary infection is common in patients receiving immunosuppressive drugs and in those with diseases causing defects of cellular or humoral immune mechanisms. For example, patients with the acquired immune deficiency syndrome (AIDS) (p. 89) are susceptible to many types of pneumonia, and pulmonary infection with *Pneumocystis carinii* is a common cause of death in patients with AIDS. The common pathogenic bacteria are responsible for the majority of lung infections in immunocompromised patients, but Gram-negative bacteria, especially *Pseudomonas aeruginosa*, are more of a problem than Gram-positive organisms, even *Staph. aureus*. However, in such patients unusual organisms or those normally considered to be of low virulence or non-pathogenic may become 'opportunistic' pathogens. *Pneumocystis carinii* and other fungi such as *Aspergillus fumigatus*, viral infections, cytomegalovirus and herpes viruses, and infections with *M. tuberculosis* and other types of mycobacteria are all common causes of infection in patients with AIDS and in those being treated with immunosuppressive drugs.

Clinical features

Diagnosis is often very difficult because all the normally pathogenic organisms and the 'opportunists' tend to cause a similar clinical and radiological picture. The onset of disease, however, tends to be less rapid in *Pneumocystis carinii* and mycobacterial infections than with pathogenic bacteria. In *Pneumocystis carinii* pneumonia symptoms of cough and breathlessness can be manifestations of the disease days before the onset of systemic symptoms or even a chest radiograph abnormality.

Diagnosis

Open-lung biopsy offers the greatest chance of establishing a diagnosis if examination of sputum has not been of any diagnostic help or patients do not have sputum. This, however, is a major high-risk invasive procedure and should be reserved for patients in whom less invasive procedures fail to establish a diagnosis and in whom there has been no response to wide spectrum antibiotic treatment. Some patients who cannot produce sputum can be induced to do so by the inhalation of nebulised hypertonic saline. Fibreoptic bronchoscopy should be performed early since a diagnosis can often be established by examination of lavage fluid, bronchial brushings or transbronchial biopsies. Sputum, bronchial aspirates and bronchoalveolar lavage fluid should be examined for *Pneumocystis carinii*, bacteria, mycobacteria, fungi and viruses.

Management

Whenever possible treatment should be based on an established aetiological diagnosis. In practice, however, the cause of the pneumonia is frequently not known when treatment has to be started. A combination of antibiotics to provide a wide spectrum of antibacterial activity is often given (e.g. a third generation cephalosporin, or a quinolone, plus an anti-staphylococcal antibiotic, or an anti-pseudomonal penicillin plus an aminoglycoside) and bronchoscopy is performed if there is no response to such treatment.

Treatment of Pneumocystis carinii *pneumonia*

Co-trimoxazole 120 mg/kg daily in divided doses intravenously or by mouth. In patients who do not respond to high-dose co-trimoxazole the use of intravenous pentamidine should be considered.

TUBERCULOSIS

This disease, which a few years ago was considered to be almost under control in Western Europe and North America, has once again become a serious worldwide problem because of AIDS and the predicted spread of this specific communicable disease to the normal population. However, in Western countries there is still a tendency for tuberculosis to be overlooked, the diagnosis being made late or only at autopsy.

Aetiology

Three types of mycobacteria are responsible for disease in man as shown in the information box.

TYPES OF MYCOBACTERIA CAUSING DISEASE IN MAN

- **Mycobacterium tuberculosis**
  Cause of most infections
- **Mycobacterium bovis**
  Endemic in cattle. Spread to man by milk. Now rarely responsible for human disease in UK
- **Atypical or opportunistic mycobacteria**
  Rare. Cause pulmonary and generalised infections in immunocompromised; cervical lymph node infection in children. Are primarily resistant in vitro to many drugs used for treatment of *M. tuberculosis*

Entry of the tubercle bacillus into the body or the alimentary or respiratory tract is not necessarily followed by a clinical illness, the development of which is dependent upon several other factors. Those of most practical importance are:

Age and sex

In Europe and North America tuberculosis was becoming a disease of the middle-aged and elderly population, but because of AIDS the age spectrum is changing.

Natural resistance

Susceptibility to tuberculosis is not inherited in the strict sense of the word, but the observation that certain races and even certain regional groups are more prone to develop the disease suggests that natural resistance varies between races and from region to region. The natural resistance of a community tends to rise as the period of exposure increases. Immigrants to Britain from Asia are more prone to have the disease than the indigenous population and also tend to have more florid types of tuberculosis. Resistance is, of course, low in immunocompromised patients.

Standard of living

The prevalence of tuberculosis diminishes as social and economic conditions improve. Poor housing with associated overcrowding increases the risk of massive infection or reinfection.

Conditions affecting individual patients

Diabetes mellitus, gastric surgery, silicosis and alcoholism all predispose to the development of tuberculosis, as does AIDS and treatment with corticosteroids or immunosuppressive drugs.

THOSE AT GREATEST RISK OF ACQUIRING TUBERCULOSIS

- Children, adolescents and young adults
- Contacts of patients with smear-positive pulmonary disease
- Immunocompromised individuals (e.g. AIDS patients and those on immunosuppressive therapy)
- Those in close contact with many potential patients (e.g. health workers)
- Underprivileged people living in overcrowded conditions

Pathology

The initial **'primary' tuberculosis infection** usually occurs in the lung but occasionally in the tonsil or alimentary tract, especially the ileocaecal region. The primary infection differs from subsequent infections in that the primary focus in lung, tonsil or bowel is almost invariably accompanied by caseous lesions in the regional lymph nodes, such as the mediastinal, cervical or mesenteric groups respectively.

In most people the primary infection and the associated lymph node lesions heal and calcify. In a few, healing, particularly in lymph nodes, is incomplete and viable tubercle bacilli may enter the bloodstream. In consequence tuberculous lesions may develop elsewhere. **'Haematogenous' lesions** of this kind are more common in the lungs, bones, joints and kidneys and lesions may develop months or even years after the primary infection.

Sometimes the primary infection does not heal. A pulmonary lesion, particularly when it occurs during adolescence or early adult life, may lead to progressive pulmonary tuberculosis. A tuberculous mediastinal lymph node, in children especially, may compress a lobar or segmental bronchus (rarely a main bronchus) and produce pulmonary collapse. Occasionally the node may ulcerate through the bronchial wall and discharge caseous material into the lumen with the production of acute tuberculous lesions in the related lobe or segment. Infection may also be carried by lymphatics from tuberculous mediastinal lymph nodes to the pleura or pericardium with the production of tuberculous pleurisy or pericarditis. Comparable complications may occur when the primary lesion is in the tonsil or gut, for example 'cold abscess' of the neck or tuberculous peritonitis.

Rarely a caseous tuberculous focus ruptures into a vein and produces acute dissemination throughout the body, a condition known as **acute miliary tuberculosis**. Meningitis often complicates this condition.

Progressive pulmonary tuberculosis may develop directly from a primary lesion or it may occur later following reactivation of an incompletely healed primary focus. Alternatively it may be the result of re-infection.

Post-primary pulmonary tuberculosis is the term used to describe lung disease, the characteristic pathological feature of which is the tuberculous cavity, formed when the caseated and liquefied centre of a tuberculous pulmonary lesion is discharged into a bronchus. Extension of infection to the pleura causes tuberculous pleurisy, which is sometimes accompanied by effusion and is occasionally followed by the development of a tuberculous empyema. Blood-borne dissemination to other organs is uncommon in post-primary pulmonary tuberculosis.

Clinical features

The two groups of clinical features in tuberculosis are shown in the information box below.

CLINICAL FEATURES OF TUBERCULOSIS

Systemic effects
- Anorexia, weight loss, lassitude, sleep sweats, evening pyrexia

Local effects
- Cough, sputum and haemoptysis

Case-finding
Mass radiography is an expensive method of case-finding and should in developed countries be used in a selective manner concentrating on certain specific groups. The highest yield by far is from patients referred by general practitioners because of symptoms. Open access to chest radiography for general practitioners and minimum waiting time for patients are essential for success.

Sputum-smear examination (Ziehl–Neelsen stain or auramine-phenol fluorescent test) is an important method of case-finding in developing countries.

Contact examination achieves a high yield in case-finding. Efforts should be concentrated on the immediate examination of household contacts of sputum-smear positive patients, especially contacts under 25 years of age.

Chemotherapy
Proper use of modern highly-effective chemotherapy, by rendering patients non-infectious rapidly, makes a very important contribution to the control of the disease.

Isolation of patients
Isolation is rarely considered necessary nowadays even in smear-positive patients, except where young children are at risk, provided the source case is being properly treated by chemotherapy.

BCG vaccination
This is carried out by the administration of freeze-dried vaccine, reconstituted at the time of use, injected by the intradermal route (0.1 ml) at the junction of the upper and middle thirds of the upper arm. Complications such as local abscess formation and enlargement of regional lymph nodes are very rare. Bacille Calmette–Guérin (BCG) vaccine should not be given in the presence of immunodeficiency. The duration of protection is up to seven years. Vaccination reduces the incidence of pulmonary tuberculosis in young adults by 80% and minimises the risk of serious disseminated disease—miliary tuberculosis and tuberculous meningitis.

Policy in relation to BCG vaccination in a community depends upon the size of the problem locally. If the infection rate is very low (1% or less) mass vaccination is inappropriate on the grounds of cost and the fact that BCG interferes with the diagnostic value of the tuberculin test in such a situation. Where there are many positive tuberculin reactors, as occurs in communities with low living standards, vaccination of the newborn is usually indicated. Where infection rates remain at low levels, vaccination at puberty, as is still performed in the UK, is practical.

Chemoprophylaxis
The concept of administering chemotherapy to individuals in order to try to prevent the development of tuberculosis is adopted in different communities with varying degrees of enthusiasm (p. 362).

Elimination of bovine infection

Although such infection is now extremely rare in Western countries, constant vigilance will be required to ensure that it remains so.

Tuberculin test

With the Mantoux technique a solution of Old Tuberculin or purified protein derivative (PPD) tuberculin is injected intradermally on the flexor aspect of the forearm. The test is regarded as positive if, 2–4 days after the injection, there is a reaction consisting of a raised area of inflammatory oedema not less than 5 mm in diameter, with surrounding erythema.

The test should first be performed with one tuberculin unit (TU) in 0.1 ml of normal saline. If there is no reaction it should be repeated with 10 TU in the same volume of saline. In order to obtain accurate results it is essential to use freshly prepared dilutions of tuberculin. Differential tuberculin testing with antigens prepared with other mycobacteria, e.g. PPD-A (*Myco. avium*) or PPD-Y (*Myco. kansasii*) is often a satisfactory method of distinguishing atypical mycobacterial infection from tuberculosis.

The younger the patient, the greater is the diagnostic significance of a positive tuberculin test. A repeatedly negative test over a period of 6 weeks from the onset of symptoms practically rules out tuberculosis except in the elderly, or after acute exanthemata, or in the later stages of miliary tuberculosis and tuberculous meningitis in patients taking immunosuppressive drugs. The tuberculin test is usually negative in patients with sarcoidosis.

Tuberculin testing is an essential part of the examination of family contacts. If positive it is of value as a diagnostic measure and if negative it indicates which of the contacts should be vaccinated with BCG. When large numbers of individuals are being tested, particularly children, a multiple puncture technique, which is quick and almost painless, is preferable to the Mantoux test (Heaf or tine test).

The test should be read after three days, and four grades of positivity are recognised (Table 6.12).

Reactions in grades III and IV indicate infection with mammalian tubercle bacilli and a grade I reaction may indicate infection with atypical mycobacteria. The significance of a grade II reaction is uncertain. Individuals previously vaccinated with BCG usually have a positive reaction of Grade II or III.

Management: general principles

Antituberculosis chemotherapy

Specific chemotherapy is by far the most important measure in the treatment of all forms of tuberculosis and should be given to every patient with active disease.

Rest

Rest is unimportant except in a few specific circumstances and the majority of patients are now ambulant throughout treatment, many of them remaining at work. Immobilisation is necessary in certain forms of skeletal tuberculosis.

Isolation

Isolation of patients who are excreting tubercle bacilli and who are therefore potentially infectious has previously been an important principle. The observation made in Madras that the frequency of disease amongst contacts was no greater when the patient was being treated at home than in a sanatorium has led to the adoption of a policy whereby the majority of patients are treated wholly as out-patients. However, many authorities still prefer to isolate patients from contact with young children. An initial period of treatment in hospital, as distinct from isolation, may be recommended for patients who cannot be relied upon to take their drugs regularly and for those who present difficult therapeutic problems.

Surgical treatment

Pulmonary resection, nephrectomy or removal of superficial lymph nodes is rarely required, but drainage of an abscess from tuberculous lymph nodes or of an empyema may be necessary. Surgical treatment of tuberculosis of the spine may be essential to prevent paraplegia.

Chemotherapy

Effective treatment of tuberculosis is based on detailed knowledge of the drugs available so that the most appropriate regimen for the individual patient can be devised.

In Britain four drugs—rifampicin, isoniazid, pyrazinamide and ethambutol—are used as first line treatment in most cases. Streptomycin is now rarely used except in patients with multiple drug resistance or

Table 6.12	Positive Heaf test grades
Grade	
I	One or two faint papules
II	Four discrete papules
III	The area encircled by the papules is completely indurated
IV	Any reaction which is greater than III, including central necrosis

Table 6.13   Daily doses and side-effects of commonly used antituberculosis drugs

Drug	Clinical setting	Dose	Side-effects
Rifampicin[1]	Children Adults weighing less than 50 kg and in the elderly Adults weighing more than 50 kg	10–20 mg/kg 450 mg 600 mg	Drug interactions, hypersensitivity hepatitis, vasculitis, fever, skin flushing, nausea and abdominal pain, breathlessness and wheeze (intermittent regimens only). Rifampicin should not be given again to any patient in whom it has caused vasculitis
Isoniazid	Children Adults Intermittent regimen Miliary TB/meningitis	10 mg/kg 200–300 mg 15 mg/kg[2] 10–12 mg/kg[2]	Hypersensitivity, polyneuropathy, lack of mental concentration
Ethambutol	Children and adults: initial 8 weeks Subsequently In renal failure	25 mg/kg 15 mg/kg According to serum levels	Optic neuritis, hypersensitivity
Pyrazinamide	Children and adults	20–35 mg/kg (max 2.5 g)	Hepatitis, gout, hypersensitivity
Streptomycin sulphate	Children Adults under 40 years and weighing more than 45 kg Adults 40–60 years or weighing less than 45 kg Adults over 60 years or in patients with renal failure Intermittent regimens	30 mg/kg 1 g 0.75 g According to serum levels 0.75–1 g	Vestibular disturbance, hypersensitivity Deafness (rare)

[1] Taken at least 30 minutes before breakfast.
[2] Plus pyridoxine 10 mg to prevent peripheral neuropathy.

hypersensitivity. Thiacetazone, which is cheap, is widely used in developing countries. Pyrazinamide is particularly useful in the treatment of tuberculous meningitis because it diffuses well into the cerebrospinal fluid. The role of drugs such as ciprofloxacin, which have in vitro activity against the tubercle bacillus but which have not been formally assessed in clinical trials, is uncertain. Apart from a few minor variations in dose the duration of treatment and the policy governing the use of antituberculosis drugs is the same for all forms of the disease.

These drugs should be used in once daily doses as shown in Table 6.13.

Adverse effects

In choosing a suitable drug regimen for individual patients it is important to bear in mind those side-effects which are particularly liable to cause serious chronic disability, such as vestibular disturbance due to streptomycin which accordingly must be prescribed with caution. Even in the relatively low dose recommended for ethambutol, a few patients develop optic neuritis and some are left with a permanent visual defect. This potential hazard must be taken into consideration whenever ethambutol is prescribed, particularly in children.

Streptomycin and occasionally isoniazid, ethambutol and rifampicin may produce a hypersensitivity reaction, comprising pyrexia and an erythematous skin eruption which usually but not invariably develops 2–4 weeks after treatment is started. Rifampicin, which colours the urine orange-pink, is a potent liver enzyme inducer and should be used with appropriate caution when prescribed with other drugs such as oestrogens (e.g. oral contraceptives), warfarin, corticosteroids, oral hypoglycaemic drugs, phenytoin and digoxin. It should, if possible, be avoided in patients with liver disease. The principal adverse effects of the most commonly prescribed drugs are shown in Table 6.13.

Drug regimens

The 'short course' regimens shown in the information box are virtually 100% effective in the treatment of tuberculosis.

Any patient who cannot be trusted to take antituberculosis drugs regularly should be kept in hospital for the initial (2 months) phase of treatment or be given supervised out-patient therapy. Thereafter for 10 months, the following should be given at home twice weekly (at 3- and 4-day intervals): streptomycin sulphate 1 g intramuscularly, and isoniazid 15 mg/kg orally in a single dose, plus pyridoxine 10 mg. Pyridoxine is given to prevent peripheral neuropathy. This type of chemotherapy should be wholly supervised, the tablets being administered at the same time as the injection.

SIX- AND NINE-MONTH DRUG REGIMENS

Duration 6 months
Initial phase 2 months
- Ethambutol or streptomycin plus isoniazid plus rifampicin plus pyrazinamide
Continuation phase 4 months
- Isoniazid plus rifampicin

Duration 9 months
Initial phase 2 months
- Ethambutol, pyrazinamide or streptomycin plus isoniazid plus rifampicin
Continuation phase 7 months
- Isoniazid plus rifampicin

Inexpensive treatment regimens

In developing countries it is sometimes impossible for economic reasons to adhere to ideal chemotherapeutic regimens.

12-MONTH REGIMENS, INEXPENSIVE AND REASONABLY EFFECTIVE

Twice weekly
- Streptomycin 1 g i.m.
- Isoniazid 15 mg/kg plus pyridoxine 10 mg orally

The effectiveness of this regimen is nearly 100% in the absence of primary drug resistance if daily treatment with standard doses of streptomycin and isoniazid can be afforded for the first 2–3 months

Daily
- Isoniazid 300 mg
- Thiacetazone 150 mg } single doses by mouth

Very cheap regimen which is 80–95% effective

Response to treatment

It is most unusual, even in advanced cases, for sputum cultures to remain positive for longer than 6 months if bacilli at the start of treatment are fully sensitive to the drugs used. Reliance must be placed on smear examination where facilities for sensitivity testing do not exist.

Drug-resistant tubercle bacilli

The treatment of patients infected with drug-resistant tubercle bacilli presents a problem requiring specialised knowledge. Additional drugs available for the treatment of such cases are: sodium aminosalicylate (commonly referred to as PAS—*p*-aminosalicylic acid), 5 g 12-hourly by mouth, ethionamide or prothionamide (0.75–1 g daily by mouth), capreomycin (0.7–1 g intramuscularly daily) and cycloserine (0.75–1 g daily by mouth) and ciprofloxacin.

Corticosteroid drugs

These agents suppress the cell-mediated reaction induced by the tubercle bacillus and may promote a rapid dissemination of infection by interfering with tissue defence mechanisms. If, however, a corticosteroid drug is given in conjunction with effective antituberculous chemotherapy, it may exert a favourable influence on the course of the disease by reducing the severity both of the local inflammatory reaction and of the associated systemic disturbance. In acute pulmonary tuberculosis such treatment will rapidly relieve pyrexia and will often produce a dramatic improvement in the radiological appearances. The effect is temporary and ceases when the corticosteroid drug is withdrawn, but it may save the lives of patients with fulminating infection by enabling them to survive until antituberculous chemotherapy has had time to exert its influence. Prednisolone is given in a dose of 20 mg daily for 6–12 weeks.

Corticosteroid drugs in combination with chemotherapy may prevent or minimise the formation of fibrous tissue and be of value in tuberculosis affecting the pleura, pericardium, intrathoracic or superficial lymph nodes, the eye and meninges. Whenever there is evidence of ureteric obstruction, corticosteroids should be administered in addition to chemotherapy because such treatment significantly reduces the need for surgery.

Chemoprophylaxis

Some indications for chemoprophylaxis using isoniazid are listed in the information box below.

CHEMOPROPHYLAXIS OF TUBERCULOSIS

Isoniazid (5 mg/kg by mouth) daily for 1 year should be considered in:

- Non-BCG vaccinated tuberculin-positive children under age 3 years—vulnerable in respect of miliary TB and TB meningitis
- Unvaccinated contacts who have recently become tuberculin positive
- Immunosuppressed patients
- Adolescents with high degree of tuberculin sensitivity

Isoniazid (5 mg/kg by mouth) daily for 6 weeks should be considered in:

- Infants of highly infectious patients—isoniazid-resistant BCG vaccine can be used with isoniazid chemoprophylaxis

---

PRIMARY PULMONARY TUBERCULOSIS

The pathological features of this type of tuberculosis are outlined on page 358. The primary infection usually

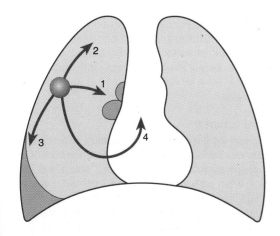

Fig. 6.21 Primary pulmonary tuberculosis. 1: Spread from primary focus to hilar and mediastinal lymph glands to form the 'primary complex' which in most cases heals spontaneously. 2: Direct extension of the primary focus—'progressive pulmonary tuberculosis'. 3: Spread to the pleura—tuberculous pleurisy and pleural effusion. 4: Blood-borne spread: *few bacilli*—pulmonary, skeletal, renal, genito-urinary infection often months or years later; *massive spread*—miliary tuberculosis and meningitis.

occurs in childhood. A history of contact with a case of active pulmonary tuberculosis is obtained in many instances.

Clinical features

In the vast majority of patients the primary infection produces no symptoms or signs and passes unnoticed unless routine radiological examination of the chest happens to be performed at the appropriate time or serial tuberculin tests show conversion from negative to positive.

In a few patients the primary infection produces a febrile illness which is generally mild and lasts for no more than 7–14 days. It is unusual for gross focal symptoms or signs to develop but a slight dry cough is occasionally present. The leucocyte count is normal but the ESR is raised.

The primary infection may be accompanied by erythema nodosum which is characterised by bluish red, raised, tender, cutaneous lesions on the shins, and less commonly on the thighs, and is associated in some patients with pyrexia and polyarthralgia. Erythema nodosum may be the first clinical indication of a tuberculous infection. The tuberculin reaction is always strongly positive in these patients and evidence of primary tuberculosis can usually be detected on the chest radiograph. Erythema nodosum is, however, seen in conditions other than primary tuberculosis, for example sarcoidosis, streptococcal infections and drug reactions.

Occasionally the primary pulmonary infection pursues a progressive course (p. 359). Symptoms and signs due to its complications (Fig. 6.21) may appear either during the course of the initial illness or after a latent interval of weeks or months. Such complications include pleurisy or pleural effusion (p. 396), lobar or segmental collapse, acute miliary tuberculosis, tuberculous meningitis (p. 1095) and post-primary pulmonary tuberculosis (p. 364).

Prognosis

Because primary pulmonary tuberculosis and its complications respond satisfactorily to antituberculous chemotherapy (p. 361), which should be given in every case, the prognosis is excellent.

MILIARY TUBERCULOSIS

The pathogenesis of this condition has already been described (p. 358). Hitherto it has occurred chiefly in children and young adults but with the changing age-structure of tuberculosis in many countries miliary tuberculosis is affecting persons in older age groups in whom it tends to take the form of an insidious illness—the 'cryptic' type—which is often difficult to diagnose. Before the introduction of chemotherapy the disease was invariably fatal but most treated patients now recover completely.

Clinical features

The disease may start suddenly or may be preceded by a few weeks of vague ill-health. In children and young adults systemic disturbance rapidly becomes profound. In particular there is a high pyrexia with drenching sweats during sleep, marked tachycardia, loss of weight and usually progressive anaemia. Cough and breathlessness are only occasionally present. There may be no abnormal physical signs in the lungs, although widespread crepitations may be heard late in the disease. The liver is often enlarged and the spleen may be palpable. Choroidal tubercles may be visible on ophthalmoscopy but are rarely present in the elderly. Leucocytosis is usually absent or slight. If chemotherapy is not given, death takes place within days or weeks.

'Cryptic' miliary tuberculosis

Diagnosis of this form of disseminated disease is shown in the information box.

Investigations

The diagnosis of acute miliary tuberculosis can be made with confidence only when radiological examination of the chest shows the characteristic 'miliary' mottling symmetrically distributed throughout both lung fields or when choroidal tubercles are seen. The diagnosis can often be suspected at an earlier stage by the symptoms, progressive clinical deterioration, persistent pyrexia and splenomegaly.

Bacteriological confirmation should be sought by culture of sputum, urine or bone marrow. A liver biopsy may be diagnostic in difficult cases. Although the tuberculin reaction is usually positive in young patients a negative result does not exclude acute miliary tuberculosis as tuberculin sensitivity is occasionally depressed in the later stages of the illness.

A therapeutic trial of chemotherapy with ethambutol or pyrazinamide and isoniazid in conventional doses (p. 361) is indicated in patients suspected to have the cryptic form of miliary tuberculosis. Clinical improvement is usually evident within 10 days if the diagnosis is correct.

Prognosis

Antituberculosis chemotherapy (p. 361) has reduced the mortality of miliary tuberculosis from 100% to virtually zero providing the diagnosis is made at an early stage.

POST-PRIMARY PULMONARY TUBERCULOSIS

Most of the morbidity and mortality from tuberculosis is caused by this form of the disease. In Western Europe and North America the majority of cases occur in middle-aged and elderly subjects, but AIDS has caused an increase among young adults. In developing countries it is most prevalent in adolescence and early adult life.

The lesions are most frequently situated in the upper lobes. The disease is often bilateral and occasionally a whole lobe may be consolidated in acute pneumonic tuberculosis.

Clinical features

The onset of post-primary pulmonary tuberculosis is usually insidious, with the gradual development of general symptoms or cough and sputum. Sometimes a dramatic event such as haemoptysis, pleural pain or a spontaneous pneumothorax marks the onset but the diagnosis is now frequently made by radiography before any symptoms have appeared.

At first no abnormal physical signs may be present but despite this an extensive lesion may be visible radiologically. The earliest physical signs consist of a few crepitations usually situated over one or other lung apex posteriorly. Ultimately, physical signs of consolidation, cavitation and fibrosis may develop, and occasionally those of pleurisy with or without effusion, or spontaneous pneumothorax (Table 6.2, p. 318).

Radiological examination

This is of paramount importance for diagnosis in the early stages before physical signs appear and for assessment of the extent and progress of the disease.

The earliest radiological change is an ill-defined opacity or opacities usually situated in one of the upper lobes (Fig. 6.22). In more advanced cases opacities are larger and more widespread and may be bilateral. Occasionally there is a dense homogeneous shadow involving the whole lobe ('pneumonic tuberculosis'). An area or areas of translucency within the opacities indicates cavitation; very large cavities may be visible in some cases. The presence of cavitation in an untreated patient usually indicates that the disease is active. When fibrosis is marked the trachea and heart shadow are displaced towards the side of the lesion.

The radiological appearances of pleural effusion and pneumothorax, which may accompany those of pulmonary tuberculosis, are described on pages 397 and 401.

Diagnosis

The grounds on which pulmonary tuberculosis should be suspected are listed in the information box below.

The presence of any of these symptoms demands immediate radiological examination of the lungs and, if an abnormality is found, the examination of at least three specimens of sputum for tubercle bacilli. The diagnosis can readily be made by microscopic examination of sputum smears stained by the Ziehl–Neelsen method when

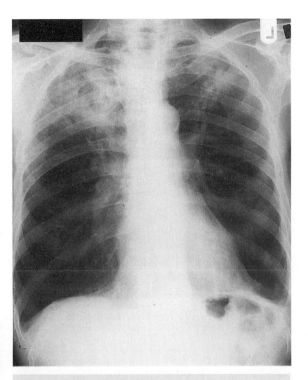

Fig. 6.22   Bilateral pulmonary tuberculosis. Upper lobe shadowing more obvious on the right.

SYMPTOMS AND SIGNS WHICH SHOULD ALWAYS RAISE THE SUSPICION OF TB

- Persistent cough
- Haemoptysis
- Pleural pain not associated with an acute illness
- Spontaneous pneumothorax
- Lethargy
- Weight loss

---

bacilli are numerous, whereas the auramine-phenol fluorescent test is of value in the detection of small numbers of tubercle bacilli. Culture of sputum, or of bronchoalveolar lavage fluid, fasting gastric washings or laryngeal swabs if no sputum can be obtained, is necessary when smears are negative and is essential for the detection of drug resistance (p. 362). Cultural methods are thus of great practical value and should be used in the examination of every specimen if facilities permit. Drug-sensitivity tests can now be conducted rapidly by use of the Bactec radiometric method.

In the vast majority of patients the diagnosis of pulmonary tuberculosis can be made with confidence by radiological examination of the chest and examination of the sputum. In some patients it is necessary to perform further radiological examination after a course of treat-ment with an antibiotic, such as ampicillin, in order to exclude an acute inflammatory cause for an abnormal radiograph shadow.

Complications

The complications are shown in the information box below.

COMPLICATIONS OF TUBERCULOSIS

- **Pleurisy**
  With or without pleural effusion
- **Pneumothorax**
  May follow rupture of cavity into pleural space
- **Empyema or pyopneumothorax**
  Serious complications of rupture of a tuberculous lesion into the pleural space
- **Tuberculous laryngitis**
  Usually only occurs in advanced pulmonary disease
- **Tuberculous enteritis**
  Follows swallowing heavily infected sputum in some patients with extensive pulmonary disease
- **Ischiorectal abscess**
  Consider TB in all cases. Tubercle bacilli can pass through rectal mucosa
- **Blood-borne dissemination**
  Uncommon complication of post-primary pulmonary disease except in the immunosuppressed
- **Respiratory failure and right ventricular failure**
  Late complications when disease has caused extensive pulmonary destruction and fibrosis
- **Fungal colonisation of cavities**
  Cavities which persist after antituberculosis treatment may become colonised with *Aspergillus fumigatus* and a ball of fungus (aspergilloma) may develop

---

Prognosis

There has been a remarkable decline in the mortality from pulmonary tuberculosis with the advent of effective chemotherapy. Provided the tubercle bacilli are not initially drug-resistant and chemotherapy is used correctly, a fatal outcome is uncommon even if the disease has reached an advanced stage when it is first recognised. Late complications of respiratory failure and secondary infection with pyogenic bacteria or fungi can be prevented if pulmonary tuberculosis is diagnosed at a reasonably early stage and is efficiently treated.

EXTRA-PULMONARY TUBERCULOSIS

Tuberculosis can affect any organ and tissue of the body (see Fig. 6.23).

Gastrointestinal tuberculosis

Tuberculous ulceration of the tongue can occur but is rare. Diarrhoea, malabsorption, intestinal obstruction

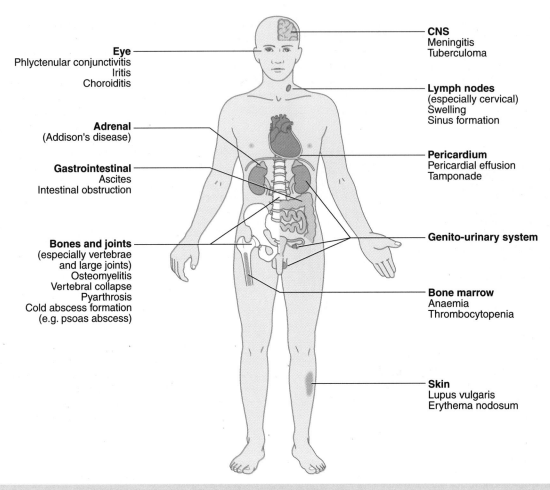

Eye
Phlyctenular conjunctivitis
Iritis
Choroiditis

Adrenal
(Addison's disease)

Gastrointestinal
Ascites
Intestinal obstruction

Bones and joints
(especially vertebrae
and large joints)
Osteomyelitis
Vertebral collapse
Pyarthrosis
Cold abscess formation
(e.g. psoas abscess)

CNS
Meningitis
Tuberculoma

Lymph nodes
(especially cervical)
Swelling
Sinus formation

Pericardium
Pericardial effusion
Tamponade

Genito-urinary system

Bone marrow
Anaemia
Thrombocytopenia

Skin
Lupus vulgaris
Erythema nodosum

Fig. 6.23 **Some of the extra-pulmonary tissues which can be affected by tuberculosis.**

and ascites can result from tuberculosis of the intestines and peritoneum. Peritoneal involvement is a common autopsy finding in patients who have died from undiagnosed disseminated disease.

Pericardium

Infection of the pericardial sac is uncommon but can give rise to pericardial effusion and tamponade (p. 214). Constrictive pericarditis can be a late result of infection and is the consequence of fibrosis and calcification.

Genito-urinary tuberculosis

Renal tuberculosis is a fairly common form of non-pulmonary tuberculosis but rarely gives rise to symptoms until the renal lesions are extensive. Haematuria and increased frequency of micturition can be caused by renal tuberculosis. Patients with 'sterile pyuria' should always be suspected of having tuberculosis and at least

three early morning urine specimens should be examined.

Infection of the fallopian tubes was a common cause of infertility; it can also give rise to salpingitis and tubal abscess. Epididymal tuberculosis presents as a painless craggy swelling which subsequently can form a sinus.

Central nervous system tuberculosis

Tuberculous meningitis is an extremely serious form of infection which can be associated with miliary tuberculosis but can also present in the absence of generalised disease. Headache, neck stiffness, vomiting and disordered consciousness are features of the disease, which can be fatal or result in permanent neurological deficit if not diagnosed and treated at an early stage. Cerebral tuberculomata are uncommon and may or may not present with focal neurological signs.

Lymph node tuberculosis

This is a very common manifestation of tuberculous disease, especially in Asians. Lymph node enlargement in any site can occur but cervical node involvement is most common. The enlargement of lymph nodes is usually painless. When caseation and liquefaction of the nodes occur the swellings become fluctuant and sinus formation is common.

Bone and joint tuberculosis

Skeletal infection is relatively common and can lead to vertebral collapse, pyarthrosis, osteomyelitis and 'cold' abscess formation.

Tuberculous infection in other sites

Destruction by infection of the adrenal glands can give rise to Addison's disease (p. 715). Tuberculous infection of the skin is referred to as lupus vulgaris and erythema nodosum can be a manifestation of primary tuberculosis. Phlyctenular kerato-conjunctivitis, iritis and choroiditis can occur in patients who have a tuberculous infection.

Management

Treatment of non-pulmonary tuberculosis

The principles of chemotherapy and duration of treatment are the same as for the treatment of pulmonary tuberculosis. Corticosteroid therapy is usually used in combination with specific antituberculosis treatment in most forms of non-pulmonary tuberculosis.

NON-*M. TUBERCULOSIS* COMPLEX MYCOBACTERIA (ATYPICAL MYCOBACTERIA)

Mycobacteria of the non-*M. Tuberculosis* complex are ubiquitous in the environment and have in the past been called atypical or opportunistic mycobacteria. Clinically important disease caused by these organisms is uncommon compared with tuberculosis, but there has been a recent increase in pulmonary and non-pulmonary infections, which is in part explained by the susceptibility of immunocompromised individuals to infection with these organisms. Disseminated mycobacteriosis is a problem in AIDS. In general these mycobacteria show in vitro resistance to many of the antituberculosis drugs, and treatment is often difficult.

The organisms which most often cause disease in man are: *M. malmoense, M. kansasii, M. xenopi* and members of the *M. avium/intracellulare* group of mycobacteria.

RESPIRATORY DISEASES CAUSED BY FUNGI

Most fungi encountered by man are harmless saprophytes but some species may, in certain circumstances, infect human tissue or promote damaging allergic reactions.

The term *mycosis* is applied to disease caused by fungal infection. Predisposing factors include metabolic disorders such as diabetes mellitus, toxic states, for example chronic alcoholism, diseases in which immunological responses are disturbed such as AIDS, treatment with corticosteroids and immunosuppressive drugs, and radiotherapy. Local factors such as tissue damage by suppuration or necrosis and the elimination of the competitive influence of a normal bacterial flora by antibiotics may also facilitate fungal infection.

Diagnosis

The diagnosis of fungal disease of the respiratory system is usually made by mycological examination of sputum—microscopic examination of stained films for fungal hyphae being extremely important—supported by serological tests and in some cases by skin sensitivity tests.

ASPERGILLOSIS

Most cases of bronchopulmonary aspergillosis are caused by *Aspergillus fumigatus*, but other members of the genus (*A. clavatus, A. flavus, A. niger* and *A. terreus*) occasionally cause disease. The conditions associated with aspergillus species are listed in the information box below.

CLASSIFICATION OF BRONCHOPULMONARY ASPERGILLOSIS

- Allergic asthma (p. 336)
- Allergic bronchopulmonary aspergillosis (asthmatic pulmonary eosinophilia)
- Extrinsic allergic alveolitis
- Intracavitary aspergilloma
- Invasive pulmonary aspergillosis

ALLERGIC BRONCHOPULMONARY ASPERGILLOSIS (ABPA)

Caused by hypersensitivity reactions to *A. fumigatus* involving the bronchial wall and peripheral parts of the lung. In the vast majority of patients it is associated with bronchial asthma, but it can occur in non-asthmatic patients and is a recognised complication of cystic fibrosis. It is one of the causes of pulmonary eosinophilia (p. 390), since it is characterised by fleeting radiographic abnormalities associated with peripheral blood eosinophilia.

Clinical features

Fever, breathlessness, cough productive of bronchial casts and worsening of asthmatic symptoms can all be manifestations of ABPA, but frequently the diagnosis is suggested by abnormalities on routine chest radiographs of patients whose asthmatic symptoms are not worse than usual. When repeated episodes of ABPA have caused bronchiectasis, the symptoms and complications of that disease often overshadow those of asthma.

Investigations

The disease is characterised by recurrent transient radiograph abnormalities of two main types: diffuse pulmonary infiltrates and lobar or segmental pulmonary collapse. Permanent radiographic changes of bronchiectasis ('tram-line', ring and 'gloved-finger' shadows) are seen predominantly in the upper lobes in patients with advanced disease.

The diagnostic criteria are shown in the information box.

DIAGNOSTIC CRITERIA FOR ABPA

- Asthma (in the majority of cases)
- Peripheral blood eosinophilia $> 0.5 \times 10^9/l$
- Presence or history of chest radiograph abnormalities
- Positive skin test to an extract of *A. fumigatus*
- Serum precipitating antibodies to *A. fumigatus*
- Elevated total serum IgE
- Fungal hyphae of *A. fumigatus* on microscopic examination of sputum.

Management

In the absence of effective safe antifungal agents which can be given long-term, the main aims of therapy are:

- Suppression of the immunopathological responses to *A. fumigatus* with low dose oral corticosteroid therapy (prednisolone 7.5–10 mg daily)
- Optimal control of associated asthma
- Prompt effective management of exacerbations associated with new chest radiograph changes—prednisolone 40–60 mg daily and physiotherapy. If lobar collapse persists for more than 7–10 days bronchoscopy to remove impacted mucus should be performed to prevent the development of bronchiectasis.

Extrinsic allergic alveolitis

Hypersensitivity to *A. clavatus* is one of the many causes of extrinsic allergic alveolitis (p. 385).

INTRACAVITARY ASPERGILLOMA

Inhaled air-borne spores of *A. fumigatus* may lodge and germinate in damaged pulmonary tissue, and an 'asper-

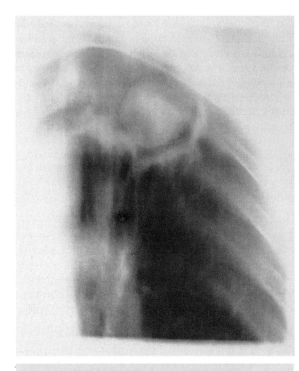

Fig 6.24 Aspergillomata in left upper lobe cavity, as demonstrated using conventional tomography. Rounded fungal ball separated from the wall of the cavity by a 'halo' of air.

gilloma' (a ball of aspergillus fungus) can form in any area of damaged lung in which there is a persistent abnormal space. The most common cause of such pulmonary damage is tuberculosis, (see Fig. 6.24), but an aspergilloma can develop in an abscess cavity, a bronchiectatic space or even a cavitated tumour. Most, but not all, are caused by *A. fumigatus*.

Clinical features

An aspergilloma often produces no specific symptoms but may be responsible for recurrent haemoptysis which is often severe. The presence of a fungus ball in the lung can also give rise to non-specific systemic features such as lethargy and weight loss.

Radiological examination

The development of a fungal ball within a cavity produces a tumour-like opacity on radiograph. An aspergilloma can usually be distinguished from a peripheral bronchial carcinoma by the presence of a crescent of air between the fungal ball and the upper wall of the cavity. Aspergillomata may be multiple.

Diagnosis

The diagnosis is usually suspected because of the chest radiograph findings. Serum precipitins to *A. fumigatus* can be demonstrated in virtually all patients. Sputum contains hyphal fragments on microscopy which are often only scanty, and is usually positive on culture. Less than 50% of patients exhibit skin hypersensitivity to extracts of *A. fumigatus*.

Management

Specific antifungal therapy is of no value. Surgical removal of the aspergilloma is indicated in patients who have massive haemoptysis and in whom thoracotomy is not contraindicated because of poor respiratory reserve. Bronchial artery embolisation is an alternative approach to the management of recurrent haemoptysis in those patients.

INVASIVE PULMONARY ASPERGILLOSIS

Invasion of previously healthy lung tissue by *A. fumigatus* is uncommon but can produce a serious and often fatal condition which usually occurs in patients who are immunocompromised either by drugs or disease. The source of the infection can be an aspergilloma but this is by no means always so.

Clinical features

Spread of the disease throughout the lungs is usually rapid with the production of consolidation, necrosis and cavitation. There is grave systemic disturbance. The formation of multiple abscesses is associated with the production of copious amounts of purulent sputum which is often blood-stained.

A much more indolent form of invasive pulmonary aspergillosis is now recognised.

Diagnosis

Invasive pulmonary aspergillosis should be suspected in any patient thought to have severe suppurative pneumonia (p. 356) which has not responded to antibiotic therapy. The diagnosis can be established by the demonstration of abundant fungal elements in stained smears of sputum. Serum precipitins can be demonstrated in some, but not all, patients.

Management

If the diagnosis is established at an early stage anti-fungal therapy can be successful. Amphotericin 0.25–1 mg/kg daily by slow intravenous infusion over 6 hours should be given in combination with flucytosine 150–200 mg/kg daily by mouth or by intravenous infusion, in 4 divided doses. The combination of flucytosine and amphotericin prevents resistance to flucytosine developing and allows a smaller daily dose of amphotericin to be used than would be possible if this drug was used on its own. Liposomal amphotericin is recommended when toxicity precludes the use of conventional amphotericin. Itraconazole has been used successfully in the treatment of invasive aspergillosis.

HISTOPLASMOSIS

Histoplasmosis is caused by *Histoplasma capsulatum* or a variant, *Histoplasma duboisii,* found in soil. Infection with these fungi is by inhalation of infected dust. Occasionally infection passes through the buccal or intestinal mucosa or through the skin. The disease attacks dogs, rats and mice, and the fungus multiplies in soil enriched by the droppings of chickens, pigeons and bats. Infection has proved a hazard for explorers of caves.

Histoplasma capsulatum is found in all parts of the United States of America, especially in the East Central states and less commonly in Latin America from Mexico to Argentina, in Europe, North, South and East Africa, Nigeria, Malaysia, Indonesia and Australia.

Pathology

The parasite in its yeast phase multiplies mainly in monocytes and macrophages and produces areas of necrosis in which the parasites may abound. From these foci the bloodstream may be invaded, causing metastatic lesions in the liver, spleen and lymph nodes. Pulmonary histoplasmosis may produce pathological changes similar to those of tuberculosis.

Clinical features

The majority, perhaps 90%, of pulmonary infections are benign, producing no symptoms, but more severe infections may closely simulate pulmonary tuberculosis, including the production of a primary complex with enlarged regional lymph nodes, multiple small discrete lesions and occasionally cavitation. Healed lesions may calcify.

The severity of the symptoms of histoplasmosis varies from, in the majority of cases, a slight fever of short duration like influenza, to a severe and prolonged pyrexial illness which ultimately proves fatal.

Diagnosis

In those geographical areas where the disease occurs, histoplasmosis should be suspected in every obscure infection in which there are pulmonary signs or where there are enlarged lymph nodes with or without hepatosplenomegaly. Tissue is obtained by biopsy for impression smear, histology, culture and animal inoculation. Radiological examination in long-standing cases may show calcified lesions in the lungs, spleen or other organs. In the more acute phases of the disease single or multiple soft pulmonary shadows with enlarged mediastinal nodes may be seen.

Delayed hypersensitivity to the intradermal injection of histoplasmin develops in patients with either active or healed infections but is usually negative in the rapidly progressive form of the disease. Complement-fixing antibodies are detected within 3 weeks of the onset of an acute primary infection and increase in titre as the disease progresses. Precipitating antibodies may also be detected.

Histoplasma duboisii. The fungus of African histoplasmosis is considerably larger than the classical *H. capsulatum*. It is found throughout East, Central and West Africa. This disease differs in several ways from *H. capsulatum* infection. The bones, skin, lymph nodes and liver develop granulomatous lesions or cold abscesses resembling tuberculosis but the lungs are seldom involved. The disease is treated in the same way as *H. capsulatum* infections.

Management
Specific treatment with amphotericin is only indicated in severe infection. The dosage of 0.5 mg/kg is given intravenously over a 6-hour period gradually increasing to a maximum of 1.0 mg/kg combined with an oral antifungal imidazole. Amphotericin treatment can be given on alternate days and may have to be continued for a prolonged period, which will almost inevitably result in renal toxicity. Recovery from generalised histoplasmosis is rare.

Coccidioidomycosis
See p. 147, Chapter 4.

Blastomycosis
See p. 147.

Cryptococcosis
See p. 147.

FURTHER READING

British Thoracic Society 1993 Guidelines for the management of community-acquired pneumonia in adults admitted to hospital. British Journal of Hospital Medicine 49: 346–350
Court C A, Garrard C S 1992 Nosocomial pneumonia in the Intensive Care Unit—mechanisms and significance. Thorax 47: 465–473
Neville K, Bromberg A, Bromberg R et al 1994 The third epidemic—multidrug-resistant tuberculosis. Chest 105: 45–48

TUMOURS OF THE BRONCHUS AND LUNG

Bronchial carcinoma is by far the most common lung tumour, accounting for more than 90% of all lung tumours. Benign tumours are rare. A primary carcinoma of any organ, but particularly of the breast, kidney, uterus, ovary, testes and thyroid may give rise to pulmonary metastatic deposits, as may an osteogenic or other sarcoma.

Bronchial tumours represent the commonest cause of obstruction to a major bronchus (see information box).

CAUSES OF LARGE BRONCHUS OBSTRUCTION

COMMON
- Bronchial carcinoma or adenoma
- Enlarged tracheobronchial lymph nodes (malignant or tuberculous)
- Inhaled foreign bodies (especially right lung and in children)
- Bronchial casts or plugs consisting of inspissated mucus or blood clot (especially asthma, haemoptysis, debility)
- Collections of mucus or mucopus retained in the bronchi as a result of ineffective expectoration

RARE
- Aortic aneurysm
- Giant left atrium
- Pericardial effusion
- Congenital bronchial atresia
- Fibrous bronchial stricture (e.g. post-TB)

The clinical and radiological manifestations of bronchial obstruction (Figs 6.25 and 6.26, pp. 372 and 373) depend on the site of the obstruction, whether the obstruction is complete or partial, the presence or absence of secondary infection and the effect on pulmonary function. Signs of displacement of the mediastinum or elevation of the diaphragm only occur if a major portion of the lung becomes collapsed. Bacterial infection is almost inevitable whenever a major bronchus is significantly obstructed. This explains why pneumonia may often be the first clinical manifestation of a bronchial carcinoma, even when the degree of obstruction is insufficient to cause collapse. The cause of bronchial obstruction can be determined at bronchoscopy, which also enables biopsy of abnormal tissue and removal of foreign bodies, casts, plugs or tenacious secretions.

PRIMARY TUMOURS OF THE LUNG

Aetiology
Cigarette smoking is by far the most important single factor in the causation of lung cancer. It is probably directly responsible for at least 90% of lung carcinomas, the risk being directly proportional to the amount smoked and to the tar content of cigarettes. For example, the death rate from the disease in heavy cigarette smo-

kers is 40 times that in non-smokers. There is now a great deal of interest in the effect of 'passive' smoking, and 5% of all lung cancer deaths have been attributed to this cause, although hard evidence for the magnitude of the effect is still awaited. The incidence of lung cancer is slightly higher in urban than in rural dwellers, presumably as a result of atmospheric pollution. Another reason for the higher incidence of lung cancer in urban areas is the increased risk of the disease in certain occupations. Asbestos exposure is by far the most important, but a number of other industrial products and processes have been associated with lung cancer

BRONCHIAL CARCINOMA

Bronchial carcinoma has emerged as a major cause of death this century (see Fig. 6.27). It accounts for more than 50% of all male deaths from malignant disease and in 1991 was responsible for 8% of all male deaths. (see box).

LUNG CANCER IN GREAT BRITAIN 1991

- 38,000 deaths
- 8% of all male deaths and 4% of all female deaths
- More than threefold increase in deaths since 1950
- Most rapidly increasing cause of cancer death in women
- Commonest cause of cancer death in men
- Commonest cause of cancer death in women in Scotland
- After breast cancer, the second commonest cause of cancer death in women in England and Wales

---

Pathology

Bronchial carcinomas arise from the bronchial epithelium or mucous glands. The common cell types are listed in Table 6.14.

When the tumour obstructs a large bronchus it causes pulmonary collapse and infection and symptoms arise early. A tumour of a peripheral bronchus may, however, attain a very large size without producing symptoms. Such a tumour, which is usually of the squamous type, may undergo central necrosis and cavitation, when it may have similar radiographic features to a lung abscess (Fig. 6.28, p. 376).

Bronchial carcinoma may involve the pleura either directly or by lymphatic spread. It may also extend into the chest wall and cause severe pain by invading the intercostal nerves or the brachial plexus. The tumour or its lymph node metastases may spread into the mediastinum where the phrenic and left recurrent laryngeal nerves may be affected. Lymphatic spread may occur to supraclavicular ('scalene') as well as to the mediastinal lymph nodes. Blood-borne metastases occur most com-

monly in liver, bone, brain, adrenals and skin. Even a small primary tumour may cause widespread metastatic deposits. A carcinoma of the small cell type has often spread beyond the lung by the time of diagnosis.

Clinical features

Lung cancer may present clinically in many ways, most often due to local involvement of the bronchus, but symptoms may also arise from spread to the chest wall or mediastinum, from distant blood-borne spread or less commonly as a result of a variety of non-metastatic paraneoplastic syndromes (see information box p. 374).

Cough is the most common early symptom; sputum is purulent if there is secondary infection. Bronchial obstruction often causes distal infection because there is interference with bronchial drainage. This may lead to pneumonia, and a recurrent pneumonia at the same site or one which is slow to respond to treatment, particularly in a cigarette smoker, should immediately suggest the possibility of bronchial carcinoma. A lung abscess may sometimes develop, leading to cough productive of large volumes of purulent sputum. A change in the character of the 'regular' cough of a smoker, particularly if it is associated with other new respiratory symptoms, should also alert the general practitioner to the possibility of bronchial carcinoma.

Haemoptysis is a common symptom in tumours arising in large bronchi, but it is less frequent in peripheral tumours. Occasionally, central tumours may invade large vessels, causing massive haemoptysis which may be fatal. Repeated episodes of scanty haemoptysis or blood-streaking of sputum in a smoker are highly suggestive of bronchial carcinoma.

Breathlessness may occur early where the tumour occludes a large bronchus, resulting in collapse of a lobe or lung. Rapid development of a large pleural effusion may also cause dyspnoea of sudden onset and **stridor** may occur where spread of the tumour to the subcarinal and paratracheal glands causes compression of the main bronchi or lower end of the trachea.

Additional symptoms may suggest spread to the pleura and chest wall. **Pleural pain** is quite common and is usually due to malignant invasion of the pleura, although it may also follow distal infection/pneumonia. Involvement of the intercostal nerves or brachial plexus may cause pain in the chest or upper limb along the appropriate nerve root distribution. Bronchial carcinoma in the apex of the lung may cause Horner's syndrome. The combination of pain in the shoulder and arm, together with unilateral Horner's syndrome, is often referred to as 'Pancoast's syndrome'.

Evidence of direct mediastinal spread or involvement of mediastinal lymph glands almost invariably means that the tumour is inoperable.

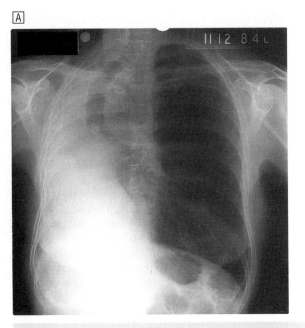

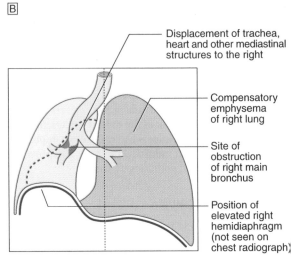

Displacement of trachea, heart and other mediastinal structures to the right

Compensatory emphysema of right lung

Site of obstruction of right main bronchus

Position of elevated right hemidiaphragm (not seen on chest radiograph)

Fig. 6.25 Collapse of the right lung—effects on neighbouring structures. A Chest radiograph; B artist's impression.

Table 6.14 Common cell types of bronchial carcinoma

	Percentage
Squamous	50%
Small cell	25%
Adenocarcinoma	15%
Large cell	10%

The patient may also present with symptoms due to blood-borne metastases, such as focal neurological defects, epileptic seizures, personality change, jaundice, bone pain or skin nodules. Lassitude, anorexia and weight loss are usually late symptoms, indicating the presence of extensive metastatic spread.

Finally, the patient may present with symptoms referable to the presence of a number of non-metastatic extrapulmonary manifestations (see information box p. 374).

Physical signs

In the chest

Examination is usually normal unless significant bronchial obstruction has been produced, or spread to the pleura or mediastinum has taken place. A tumour obstructing a large bronchus produces the physical signs of collapse or occasionally obstructive emphysema. Pulmonary infection beyond an obstructing tumour gives rise to pneumonia that usually responds slowly to treatment; an underlying bronchial carcinoma is suspected

from the relative absence of physical signs usually associated with pneumonia. Involvement of the pleura produces the physical signs of pleurisy or of pleural effusion (p. 396). Occasionally a massive tumour may cause the signs of a large pleural effusion.

Clubbing of the fingers

Digital clubbing is often seen and some patients present with the features of hypertrophic pulmonary osteoarthropathy (HPOA). In this syndrome there is pain, which may be severe, usually in the wrists and ankles but also in the knees and shins. The distal parts of the long bones of the wrists and ankles may be exquisitely tender to touch and pitting oedema is often present over the anterior aspect of the shin. Finger clubbing is present in most patients with HPOA and is usually gross. Radiographs of the painful bone show subperiosteal new bone formation. HPOA is most frequently associated with bronchial carcinoma but can occur with other tumours and has been described in association with cystic fibrosis.

Digital clubbing and HPOA can also be regarded as paraneoplastic or non-metastatic syndromes. Two endocrine syndromes, inappropriate ADH secretion and ectopic ACTH secretion (p. 708) are associated with small cell carcinoma. Hypercalcaemia is usually caused by a squamous carcinoma. Associated neurological syndromes (p. 374) may occur with any type of bronchial carcinoma but perhaps most often with small cell tumours.

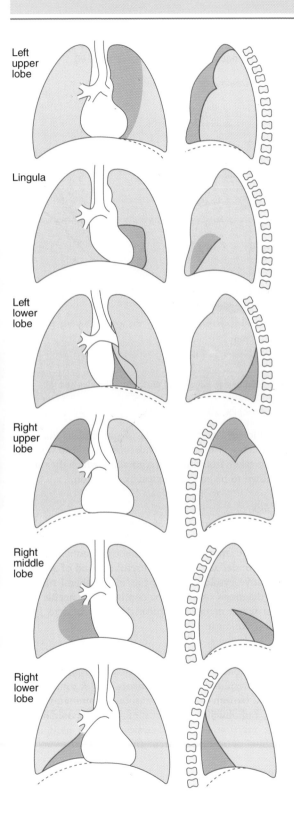

Left
upper
lobe

Lingula

Left
lower
lobe

Right
upper
lobe

Right
middle
lobe

Right
lower
lobe

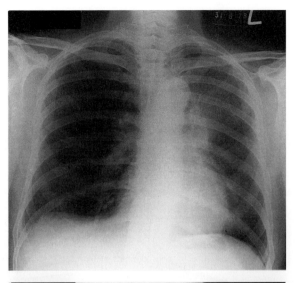

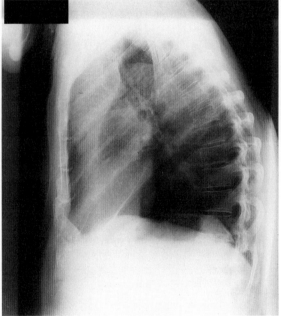

Fig. 6.26   Radiological features of lobar collapse caused by bronchial obstruction. The dotted line in the drawings represents the normal position of the diaphragm. Radiographs show example of left upper lobe collapse which is often the most difficult to identify: this is due to the hazy, ill-defined shadowing on the PA view. The collapsed lobe is more easily seen on the lateral view.

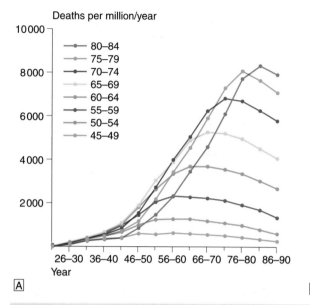

Male mortality from lung cancer by age and year of death, England and Wales 1921–90

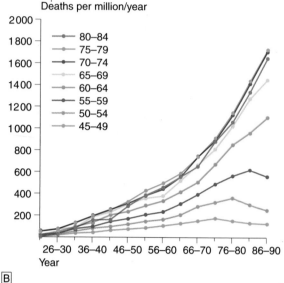

Female mortality from lung cancer by age and year of death, England and Wales 1921–90

A

B

Fig. 6.27 Mortality trends from lung cancer in England and Wales, 1921–1990 by age and year of death, for A males and B females.

NON-METASTATIC EXTRA-PULMONARY MANIFESTATIONS OF BRONCHIAL CARCINOMA

Endocrine
- Inappropriate secretion of antidiuretic hormone (ADH)
- Ectopic ACTH secretion
- Hypercalcaemia
- Carcinoid syndrome
- Gynaecomastia

Neurological
- Polyneuropathy
- Myelopathy
- Cerebellar degeneration

Other
- Digital clubbing
- Hypertrophic pulmonary osteoarthropathy
- Nephrotic syndrome
- Myasthenia
- Polymyositis and dermatomyostis

Investigations

Radiology
The conditions which radiological examination can reveal are shown in the information box. Bronchial carcinoma often presents as a 'solitary nodule' on the chest radiograph and may need to be distinguished from other conditions.

Bronchoscopy
Inspection of the intrabronchial portion of the tumour and removal of tissue for pathological examination is possible in about two-thirds of patients. If abnormal tissue is not visible at bronchoscopy, bronchial washings can be taken from the lung segment in which the tumour is shown to be on radiological examination.

Cytology
Cytological examination of sputum, bronchial brushings or bronchial washings for malignant cells is a valuable diagnostic measure. Percutaneous needle aspiration biopsy under screening is a useful method of obtaining a positive cytological diagnosis in peripheral tumours. The diagnosis can often be confirmed by needle aspiration when metastatic spread has occurred to lymph nodes, skin or liver.

Other investigations
Scalene node biopsy, mediastinoscopy or pleural biopsy may be required in some patients. CT scanning of the thorax, barium swallow, ultrasound examination of the liver, radionuclide bone scanning and examination of bone marrow trephine biopsies may be used in the 'staging' of bronchial carcinoma (p. 851).

Specific management
Curative treatment is almost exclusively achieved by surgical resection. Unfortunately the majority of patients present with evidence of tumour spread at the time of

RADIOLOGICAL PRESENTATIONS OF BRONCHIAL CARCINOMA

Unilateral hilar enlargement
- Central tumour. Hilar glandular involvement. Peripheral tumour in apical segment of a lower lobe can look like an enlarged hilar shadow on the straight radiograph

Peripheral pulmonary opacity
- Usually irregular but well circumscribed. May have irregular cavitation within it. Can be very large (Fig. 6.28)

Lung, lobe or segmental collapse
- Usually caused by tumour within the bronchus causing occlusion. Whole lung collapse can be produced by compression of main bronchus by enlarged lymph glands

Pleural effusion
- Usually indicates tumour invasion of pleural space; very rarely a manifestation of infection in collapsed lung tissue distal to a bronchial carcinoma

Broadening of mediastinum, enlarged cardiac shadow, elevation of a hemidiaphragm
- Manifestations of mediastinal invasion. If a raised hemidiaphragm is caused by phrenic nerve palsy, screening will show it to move paradoxically upwards when patient sniffs

Rib destruction
- Direct invasion of the chest wall or blood-borne metastatic spread can cause osteolytic lesions of the ribs

SOME CAUSES OF A SOLITARY PULMONARY NODULE ON THE CHEST RADIOGRAPH

Common
- Primary bronchial carcinoma
- Localised pneumonia
- Tuberculosis
- Pulmonary infarction

Uncommon
- Solitary metastasis (breast, sarcoma, kidney, testis)
- Bronchial adenoma
- Arterio-venous malformations
- Hamartoma
- Rheumatoid nodule
- Localised Wegener's granuloma
- 'Pseudo-tumour'—fluid in a lung fissure
- Foreign body

to the lung, the results of surgical resection are poor in undifferentiated and poorly differentiated tumours. By contrast the 5-year survival rate after resection of squamous carcinoma can be as high as 50%.

Staging of the tumour (p. 851) is essential prior to surgical resection and it is also important to assess pulmonary function because many patients have poor function from associated chronic bronchitis. These patients have a high risk of post-operative complications and surgical resection is usually not considered (if their pulmonary function is very poor).

Radiotherapy

Radiotherapy is much less effective than surgery in the curative treatment of bronchial carcinoma. It is of greatest value in the palliation of distressing complications such as superior vena caval obstruction, recurrent haemoptysis, and pain caused by chest wall invasion or by skeletal metastatic deposits. Obstruction of the trachea and main bronchi can also be relieved temporarily by radiotherapy. Undifferentiated tumours (e.g. small cell) or poorly differentiated tumours are usually more susceptible to radiotherapy than well differentiated tumours, especially adenocarcinoma. Radiotherapy is used in conjunction with chemotherapy in the treatment of small cell carcinoma.

Chemotherapy

The treatment of small cell carcinoma with combinations of cytotoxic drugs, sometimes in combination with radiotherapy, can increase the median survival of patients with this highly malignant type of bronchial carcinoma from 3 months to well over a year. Different combinations of chemotherapeutic agents, adjuvant therapy and radiotherapy have been and are being assessed in order to improve the prognosis of patients with small cell lung cancer. In a good prognosis group (age <70, normal serum sodium and albumin concentration, weight loss $<10\%$ and disease limited to one hemithorax) the combination of doxorubicin, cyclophosphamide and etoposide (doxorubicin 60 mg/m^2 i.v. bolus, day 1; cyclophosphamide 750 mg/m^2 i.v. infusion, day 1; etoposide 120 mg/m^2 i.v. infusion, days 1, 2 and 3) has minimal toxicity except for alopecia and is effective in 75% or more of patients. The above regimen is given every 3 weeks for 6 cycles. For patients in a poor prognosis group, oral etoposide (50 mg 12-hourly for 10 days every 3 weeks for 6 cycles) offers good palliation.

The use of combinations of chemotherapeutic drugs requires considerable medical skill and expertise and it is recommended that such treatment should only be given under the supervision of clinicians experienced

diagnosis and can only be offered palliative therapy. Radiotherapy, and in some cases chemotherapy, can relieve distressing symptoms.

Surgical treatment

Regrettably, few patients are suitable for surgery. Even if after investigation the tumour appears to be localised

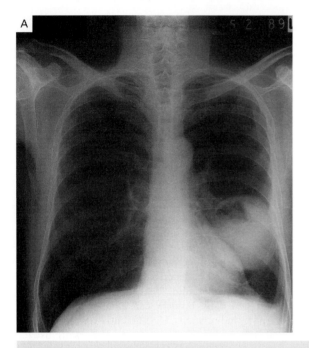

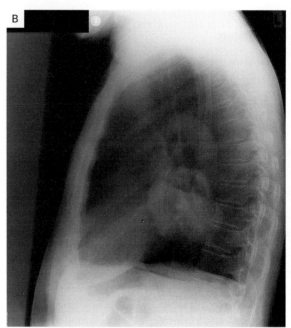

Fig. 6.28   Large cavitated bronchial carcinoma. [A] Posterior-anterior (PA) view [B] Lateral view of A showing tumour in the left lower lobe.

in such treatment. In general, chemotherapy is far less effective in non-small cell bronchial cancers.

Laser therapy

Laser treatment via a fibreoptic bronchoscope is essentially palliative, the aim being to destroy tumour tissue occluding major airways to allow re-aeration of collapsed lung. The best results are achieved in tumours of the main bronchi.

General management

As in other forms of advanced carcinoma, pain relief and attention to diet are important. Hypercalcaemia is an uncommon but important complication of lung cancer, particularly squamous cell carcinoma. Symptoms include polyuria, nocturia, fatigue, confusion and occasionally coma. Treatment in the acute situation involves intravenous rehydration, maintenance of a good urine output and administration of disphosphonates. Thereafter, steroids may be effective and mithramycin or disodium pamidronate may be necessary to maintain a normal blood calcium.

Prognosis

The overall prognosis in bronchial carcinoma is very poor. Less than 10% of patients survive 5 years after diagnosis. The best prognosis is with well-differentiated

squamous tumours which have not metastasised and are amenable to surgical treatment.

BRONCHIAL ADENOMA

This is an uncommon tumour occurring in a younger age group than carcinoma and affecting equally females and males. Although classified as a benign tumour it possesses some of the properties of a malignant growth and may eventually metastasise. There are two histological types of bronchial adenoma, the relatively more common bronchial carcinoid and the rare cylindroma (adenoid cystic carcinoma) which often arises at the tracheal bifurcation.

Clinical features

A bronchial adenoma may produce symptoms over several years. Recurrent haemoptysis due to the vascularity of tumour is common, as is recurrent bronchopulmonary infection distal to bronchial obstruction caused by the adenoma. Very rarely, and usually when metastatic spread has occurred, the bronchial adenoma may give rise to the carcinoid syndrome. The physical signs are usually those of pulmonary collapse. The tumour may be suspected if the patient is young and symptoms have been present over a prolonged period;

but confirmation of the diagnosis can only be made by bronchoscopy, biopsy and histology.

Management

Treatment is by resection of the lobe or segment containing the tumour along with the bronchus from which it arises. Occasionally when surgical resection is not possible local removal of tumour tissue from the bronchial lumen or laser therapy may be an alternative.

SECONDARY TUMOURS OF THE LUNG

Blood-borne metastatic deposits in the lungs may be derived from many primary tumours (p. 370). The secondary deposits are usually multiple and bilateral. Often there are no respiratory symptoms and the diagnosis is made by radiological examination. Breathlessness may be the only symptom if a considerable amount of lung tissue has been replaced by metastatic tumour. Occasionally, haemoptysis occurs in patients with metastatic pulmonary malignant disease.

PULMONARY LYMPHATIC CARCINOMATOSIS

Lymphatic infiltration may develop in patients with carcinoma of the breast, stomach, bowel, pancreas or bronchus. This grave condition causes severe and rapidly progressive breathlessness. The diagnosis is often suggested by the chest radiograph, which shows diffuse pulmonary shadowing radiating from the hilar regions often associated with septal lines in the costophrenic angles.

TUMOURS OF THE MEDIASTINUM

The mediastinum can be divided into four major compartments with reference to the lateral chest radiograph (Fig. 6.29):

1. **Superior mediastinum**—above a line drawn between the 5th dorsal vertebral body and the upper end of the body of the sternum
2. **Anterior mediastinum**—in front of the heart
3. **Posterior mediastinum**—behind the heart
4. **Middle mediastinum**—between the anterior and posterior compartments.

A variety of conditions can present radiologically as a mediastinal mass (see box).

COMMON MEDIASTINAL MASSES

Superior mediastinum
- Retrosternal goitre
- Vascular lesion:
  Persistent left superior vena cava
  Prominent left subclavian artery
- Thymic tumour
- Dermoid cyst
- Lymphoma
- Aortic aneurysm

Anterior mediastinum
- Retrosternal goitre
- Dermoid cyst
- Thymic tumour
- Lymphoma
- Aortic aneurysm

- Pericardial cyst
- Hernia through the diaphragmatic foramen of Morgagni

Posterior mediastinum
- Neurogenic tumour
- Paravertebral abscess
- Oesophageal lesion
- Aortic aneurysm
- Foregut duplication

Middle mediastinum
- Bronchial carcinoma
- Lymphoma
- Sarcoidosis
- Bronchogenic cyst
- Hiatus hernia

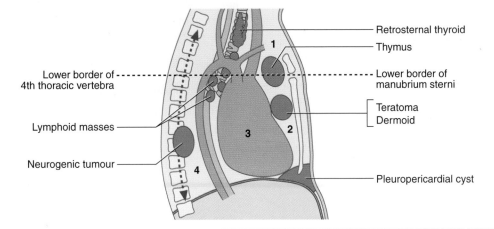

Fig. 6.29 The divisions of the mediastinum described in the diagnosis of mediastinal masses. (1) Superior mediastinum; (2) Anterior mediastinum; (3) Middle mediastinum; (4) Posterior mediastinum. Sites of the more common mediastinal tumours are also illustrated.

BENIGN TUMOURS AND CYSTS

These include intrathoracic goitre (see Fig. 6.30), vascular lesions, benign thymic tumours, dermoid cysts, pericardial cysts, diaphragmatic hernias, neurogenic tumours and developmental cysts. They may compress but do not invade vital structures. The diagnosis is usually made by chance when radiological examination of the chest is undertaken for some other reason. The tumour may cause dyspnoea by compression of lung tissue or occasionally by narrowing of the trachea. A benign tumour in the upper part of the thorax occasionally compresses the superior vena cava. A dermoid cyst very occasionally ruptures into a bronchus.

MALIGNANT TUMOURS

Included in this category are mediastinal lymph node metastases, lymphomas, leukaemia, malignant thymic tumours and mediastinal sarcoma. Aortic and innominate aneurysms have destructive features resembling those of malignant mediastinal tumours. All these conditions, except lymph node malignancies, are uncommon. The distinguishing feature of this group of tumours is their power to invade as well as to compress mediastinal structures, bronchi and lungs. As a result even a small malignant tumour can produce symptoms although as a rule the tumour has attained a considerable size before this happens. The structures which may be invaded or compressed and the symptoms and signs produced in each case are outlined in the information box below.

Investigation

Radiological examination

A benign mediastinal tumour generally appears as a sharply circumscribed opacity situated mainly in the mediastinum but often encroaching on one or both lung fields (Fig. 6.30). A malignant mediastinal tumour seldom has a clearly defined margin and often presents as a general broadening of the mediastinal shadow. Fluoroscopic examination of the hemidiaphragms and oesophagus (barium swallow) should be undertaken in all suspected cases of mediastinal tumour.

CT scanning

CT scanning of the thorax is a useful investigation for mediastinal tumours and has virtually replaced conventional tomography in the investigation of these lesions.

SYMPTOMS AND SIGNS PRODUCED BY MALIGNANT INVASION OF THE STRUCTURES OF THE MEDIASTINUM

Trachea and main bronchi
- Stridor, breathlessness, paroxysmal cough, pulmonary collapse

Oesophagus
- Dysphagia, oesophageal displacement or obstruction on barium swallow examination

Phrenic nerve
- Diaphragmatic paralysis

Left recurrent laryngeal nerve
- Paralysis of left vocal cord giving rise to hoarseness and 'bovine' cough

Sympathetic trunk
- Horner's syndrome

Superior vena cava
- SVC obstruction results in non-pulsatile distension of neck veins, oedema and cyanosis of head, neck, hands and arms. Dilated anastomotic veins on chest wall

Pericardium
- Pericarditis and/or pericardial effusion

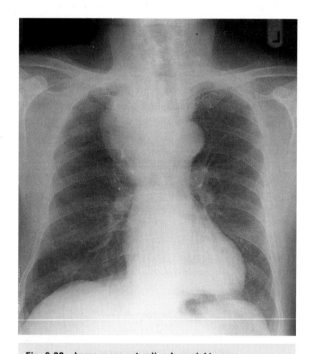

Fig. 6.30   Large mass extending from right upper mediastinum—intrathoracic goitre.

Bronchoscopy

Bronchoscopy should be carried out in most patients because bronchial carcinoma is a common cause of mediastinal tumour by secondary lymphatic spread.

Mediastinoscopy

If enlarged lymph nodes are suspected in the anterior mediastinum, tissue from these nodes can be removed for histological examination by this technique.

Surgical exploration

An exact diagnosis cannot be made in some patients without surgical exploration of the chest and removal for histological examination of part or all of the tumour.

Management

Benign mediastinal tumours should be removed surgically once they are discovered because most produce symptoms sooner or later. Some of them, particularly cysts, may become infected while others, especially neural tumours, may become malignant. The operative mortality is low providing there is not a relative contraindication to surgical treatment such as co-existing cardiovascular disease, chronic obstructive airways disease or extreme age.

The treatment of lymphoma and leukaemia is described on pages 819 and 806 respectively. A malignant thymoma usually responds dramatically to radiotherapy and lymph node metastases from bronchial carcinoma respond well though temporarily to radiotherapy or to chemotherapy in the case of small cell carcinoma. Complications such as superior vena caval obstruction and tracheal obstruction can also be treated with radiotherapy or a combination of radiotherapy and chemotherapy.

FURTHER READING

Talbot D C, Smith I E 1992 New drugs in lung cancer. Thorax 47: 188–194
Woll P J 1991 Growth factors and lung cancer. Thorax 46: 924–929

INTERSTITIAL AND INFILTRATIVE PULMONARY DISEASES

Interstitial lung diseases are a heterologous group of conditions caused by diffuse thickening of the alveolar walls with inflammatory cells and exudate (e.g. the adult respiratory distress syndrome—ARDS), granulomas (e.g. sarcoidosis), haemorrhage (e.g. Goodpasture's syndrome, p. 643) and/or fibrosis (e.g. fibrosing alveolitis). Some are the result of exposure to known agents, for example asbestos, whereas in others, such as sarcoidosis, the cause is unknown. Lung disease may occur in isolation, or as part of a systemic connective tissue disorder, for example in rheumatoid arthritis and systemic lupus erythematosus. Interstitial lung diseases may present acutely, as in acute drug reactions, ARDS or the early stages of extrinsic allergic alveolitis, but more often the natural history is one of slowly progressive loss of alveolar-capillary gas exchange units over months or even years. This relentless progression of increased lung stiffness, disordered matching of ventilation and perfusion and gas transfer defects results in worsening exertional dyspnoea which in many cases eventually progresses to respiratory failure, pulmonary hypertension, cor pulmonale and death.

Aetiology

There is a very wide range of causes of interstitial lung disease (see information box). Some, like sarcoidosis, are quite common whereas others such as berylliosis are rare but nevertheless important in those industries where beryllium exposure may occur. Despite the different causes and pathological processes involved, many interstitial lung diseases give rise to similar symptoms, physical signs, radiological changes and disturbances of pulmonary function and are therefore worthy of collective consideration. Nevertheless, the various underlying aetiologies present very different implications for prognosis and therapy. Moreover, interstitial lung diseases may be confused with other conditions (see information box) with similar clinical and radiological features. Therefore, a general approach to interstitial lung disease will be considered before a more detailed description of some specific disorders.

Diagnosis of interstitial lung disease: a general approach

The first task is to differentiate the disorder from other conditions which can mimic interstitial lung diseases (ILDs) (see information box below), and then to determine which of the many causes of ILD is implicated (second information box). Establishing a diagnosis is important for a number of reasons. Firstly, there are prognostic implications; for example, sarcoidosis is usually self-limiting, whereas lymphatic carcinomatosis is invariably fatal. Secondly, establishing a specific diagnosis will avoid inappropriate treatment, for example the powerful immunosuppressive regimes used for some ILDs (such as cryptogenic fibrosing alveolitis) would be undesirable if the underlying condition is an unsuspected infection. Thirdly, some ILDs can be expected

SOME CAUSES OF INTERSTITIAL LUNG DISEASE

- **Sarcoidosis**
- **Cryptogenic fibrosing alveolitis**
- **Exposure to organic dusts** e.g. farmer's lung, bird fancier's lung
- **Exposure to inorganic dusts** e.g. asbestosis, silicosis
- **As part of systemic inflammatory disease** e.g. adult respiratory distress syndrome, fibrosing alveolitis in connective tissue disorders
- **Pulmonary eosinophilia**
- **Exposure to irradiation and drugs**
- **Rare disorders** e.g. alveolar proteinosis, histiocytosis

to respond better than others to treatment, e.g. a good response to corticosteroids could be predicted in sarcoidosis (p. 381) whereas the prognosis would need to be more guarded in cryptogenic fibrosing alveolitis (p. 383). Finally, an open lung biopsy taken when the patient is already established on empirical immunosuppressive therapy is not only associated with a higher morbidity and mortality but the tissue obtained is more difficult to interpret histologically.

CONDITIONS WHICH MIMIC INTERSTITIAL LUNG DISEASES

Infection	Malignancy
• Viral pneumonia	• Leukaemia and lymphoma
• Pneumocystis carinii	• Lymphatic carcinomatosis
• Mycoplasma pneumonia	• Multiple metastases
• Tuberculosis	• Alveolar cell carcinoma
• Parasites, e.g. filariasis	**Pulmonary oedema (cardiac failure)**
• Fungal infiltration	

Pulmonary haemorrhage

Aspiration

Establishing a diagnosis often presents a considerable clinical challenge, necessitating meticulous attention to the history and physical signs together with the judicious and selective use of investigations.

History

The duration of disease may sometimes be difficult to ascertain. In the early stages particularly, shortness of breath or cough may only be noticed on significant exertion, therefore the condition may not present clinically until there is quite extensive lung pathology. It is clearly important to elicit a detailed history of exposure to organic dusts, inorganic dusts and drugs, including the degree and duration of exposure. Extrinsic allergic alveolitis may be suspected in pigeon fanciers, but also in those who keep budgerigars and cockatiels as pets. A

history of rashes or joint pains may suggest an underlying connective tissue disorder. It may be possible in the history to implicate disorders which may mimic ILD; for example there may be a history suggestive of repeated cardiac failure, or aspiration. Chronic opportunistic infections and infiltrating malignancy, particularly lymphoma, may be extremely difficult to distinguish from other causes of ILD. With the increased incidence of AIDS it is important to take a full sexual history and a history of possible intravenous drug misuse.

Physical signs

In many cases, especially in early disease, there may be few, if any, physical signs. In advanced disease the patient may be tachypnoeic and cyanosed on minor exertion. Digital clubbing may be prominent, particularly in cryptogenic fibrosing alveolitis or asbestosis. There may be restriction of lung expansion, particularly at the bases, with dullness to percussion and showers of inspiratory crepitations on auscultation. Extrapulmonary signs, including lymphadenopathy or uveitis, should suggest sarcoidosis (see information box on p. 382) and arthropathies or rashes may suggest fibrosing alveolitis occurring as part of a connective tissue disorder such as lupus erythematosus or rheumatoid arthritis. In advanced disease there may be dyspnoea and cyanosis at rest, and signs of pulmonary hypertension or right heart failure due to cor pulmonale may be apparent.

Laboratory investigation

No single blood test is diagnostic for a particular interstitial lung disease. Some laboratory tests may be useful in indicating systemic disease or providing crude indices of disease activity. Routine biochemical liver function tests and tests of renal function may be disordered in systemic connective tissue diseases or sarcoidosis. The ESR and C-reactive protein may be non-specifically elevated. Serological tests including antinuclear antibodies, rheumatoid factor, etc., may be elevated in connective tissue diseases associated with fibrosing alveolitis. Serum levels of angiotensin-converting enzyme (ACE) may be elevated in sarcoidosis; however, this test is not specific for this disorder. Special tests including HIV serology or antibodies to antiglomerular basement membrane (anti GBM) may be carried out in suspected AIDS, or Goodpasture's syndrome (see p. 643).

Radiology

The chest radiograph may show a fine reticular shadowing, a reticulo-nodular or even a nodular pattern of infiltration at the bases and peripherally (Fig. 6.31A). In

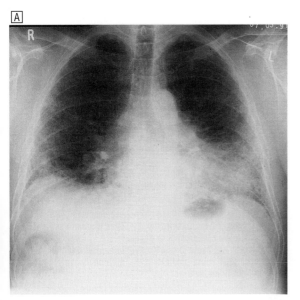

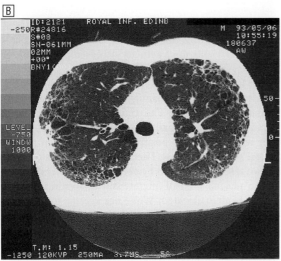

Fig. 6.31 Cryptogenic fibrosing alveolitis. [A] Chest radiograph showing bilateral, predominantly lower zone and peripheral coarse reticular-nodular shadowing and small lungs. [B] The CT scan shows honeycombing and scarring which is most marked peripherally.

advanced disease there may be cystic areas and honeycombing.

High resolution CT scanning may be useful in detecting early interstitial lung disease and assessing the extent and type of involvement (Fig. 6.31B) and is also helpful in identifying hilar and paratracheal lymphadenopathy, particularly in sarcoidosis. Gallium[67] scanning has been used to monitor the progress and response to treatment of sarcoidosis, but positive Gallium scanning occurs in

other interstitial lung diseases and is not therefore of any diagnostic value.

Bronchoscopy and bronchoalveolar lavage

Cytology

Bronchoalveolar lavage is not often of diagnostic value, but there are some important exceptions. Increased numbers of lymphocytes in bronchoalveolar lavage fluid occur in sarcoidosis and extrinsic allergic alveolitis, whereas a neutrophilia is suggestive of cryptogenic fibrosing alveolitis or pneumoconiosis. Occasionally bronchoalveolar lavage may provide specific diagnostic information, as exemplified by the recovery of specific organisms in pneumocystis or fungal infections or by the finding of copious lipoproteinaceous material in alveolar proteinosis or the large numbers of iron-laden macrophages in pulmonary haemosiderosis.

Histology

Examination of biopsy material is an important diagnostic procedure in most cases. A transbronchial biopsy obtained via the fibreoptic bronchoscope will often establish the diagnosis in sarcoidosis, lymphatic carcinomatosis and certain infections. However, it provides only a small sample of tissue and in less specific disorders such as cryptogenic fibrosing alveolitis a larger biopsy sample is usually necessary to yield a confident diagnosis. This used to necessitate a thoracotomy and open lung biopsy. However, the advent of video-assisted thoracoscopic lung biopsy has considerably refined this procedure, with a marked reduction in associated discomfort, morbidity and mortality.

SARCOIDOSIS

Sarcoidosis is a multi-system granulomatous disease. It is associated with imbalance between subsets of T lymphocytes and other disturbances of cell-mediated immunity, but the relationship between these phenomena and sarcoidosis has not yet been explained. The lesions are histologically similar to tuberculous follicles, apart from the absence of caseation and tubercle bacilli, but there is no convincing evidence that the disease is caused by any of the mycobacteria. Chronic beryllium poisoning produces a disease which mimics sarcoidosis both pathologically and clinically but exposure to beryllium is now extremely uncommon. Histological changes resembling those of sarcoidosis are occasionally seen in individual organs, such as lymph nodes, in conditions such as carcinoma and fungal infections, but these localised 'sarcoid reactions' are not associated with systemic sarcoidosis.

Pathology

The mediastinal and superficial lymph nodes, lungs, liver, spleen, skin, eyes, parotid glands and phalangeal bones are most frequently involved, but all tissues may be involved (see Figs 6.32, 6.33). The characteristic histological feature consists of non-caseating epithelioid follicles which usually resolve spontaneously, but fibrosis occurs in up to 20% of cases of pulmonary sarcoidosis and it is presently impossible to identify this group of patients prospectively. Sarcoidosis is seldom fatal unless it affects vital organs such as the heart or the central nervous system. Calcium metabolism may be disturbed causing hypercalcaemia and, rarely, nephrocalcinosis and renal failure.

Clinical features

Since sarcoid lesions can develop in almost any tissue, there may be a number of unusual presentations, such as cardiac arrhythmias or cranial nerve palsies (see the information box). However, in most tissues the granulomas are usually 'silent' and the disease is most commonly detected by an abnormal chest radiograph revealing bilateral hilar lymphadenopathy in an asymptomatic patient. However, with more extensive lung involvement there may be exertional dyspnoea or cough. Patients may also present with an 'acute' form of sarcoidosis, with erythema nodosum, arthropathy, uveitis and bilateral hilar lymphadenopathy. At the other extreme, patients with chronic extensive sarcoidosis may complain of lassitude, fatigue, breathlessness and cough.

PRESENTATION OF SARCOIDOSIS

- Asymptomatic—abnormal routine chest radiograph (c. 30%)
- Respiratory and constitutional symptoms (20–30%)
- Erythema nodosum and arthralgia (20–30%)
- Ocular symptoms (5–10%)
- Skin sarcoids (5%)
- Superficial lymphadenopathy (5%)
- Other (1%), e.g. hypercalcaemia, diabetes insipidus

Investigations

Skin sensitivity to tuberculin is depressed or absent in most patients, and the Mantoux reaction is, therefore, a useful 'screening' test; a strongly positive reaction to one TU virtually excludes sarcoidosis. Although the diagnosis can often be made with a fair measure of confidence from the clinical and radiological features (see information box) and the tuberculin test it should, if possible, be confirmed histologically by biopsy of a superficial lymph node or of a skin lesion when these are present. Transbronchial lung biopsy frequently (in 70–

CHEST RADIOGRAPH CHANGES IN SARCOIDOSIS

Stage I
- Radiograph shows bilateral hilar enlargement, usually symmetrical; paratracheal nodes often enlarged
- Spontaneous resolution usually within one year in majority of cases. Often asymptomatic, but may be associated with erythema nodosum and arthralgia

Stage II
- Radiograph shows a combination of hilar glandular enlargement and pulmonary opacities which are often diffuse, but not always
- Patients usually asymptomatic. Spontaneous improvement occurs in majority

Stage III
- Radiograph shows diffuse pulmonary shadows without evidence of hilar adenopathy. Evidence of pulmonary fibrosis may be present or develop
- Disease less likely to resolve spontaneously. Pulmonary fibrosis can cause breathlessness, pulmonary hypertension and cor pulmonale

---

85% of cases, even in those with apparently normal radiology) confirms the diagnosis. Bronchoalveolar lavage usually yields fluid with an increased proportion of lymphocytes.

The Kveim test is also a helpful diagnostic procedure, provided that a potent antigen can be obtained from human sarcoid tissue. The antigen (0.1 ml) is injected intradermally and a small nodule develops about 4 weeks later when the test is positive, biopsy of which reveals typical sarcoid follicles. The development of a positive Kveim test is suppressed by corticosteroid therapy.

The plasma level of angiotensin-converting enzyme (ACE) is often elevated. While not specific for sarcoidosis, this test may be valuable in the assessment of disease activity and response to treatment. The chest radiographical features have been used to stage sarcoidosis (see box).

When parenchymal lung disease is significant there may be disordered pulmonary function tests with a reduction in gas transfer and typical restrictive abnormalities occurring in more advanced disease, particularly if fibrosis has occurred.

In Stage 3 sarcoidosis assessment of disease progression is by repeated measurement of lung volumes, carbon monoxide transfer factor and serial chest radiographs.

Hypercalcaemia may occur but seldom causes symptoms. Corticosteroid treatment may be necessary to avert renal complications of hypercalcaemia.

Management

Stage 1 and Stage 2 disease usually resolve spontaneously and treatment is seldom required but

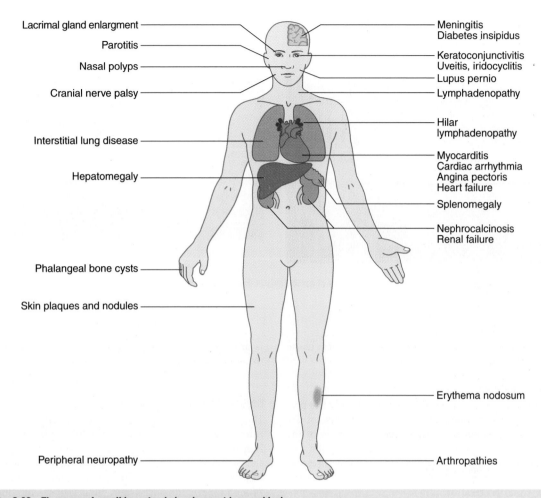

Lacrimal gland enlargment

Parotitis

Nasal polyps

Cranial nerve palsy

Interstitial lung disease

Hepatomegaly

Phalangeal bone cysts

Skin plaques and nodules

Peripheral neuropathy

Meningitis
Diabetes insipidus

Keratoconjunctivitis
Uveitis, iridocyclitis

Lupus pernio

Lymphadenopathy

Hilar
lymphadenopathy

Myocarditis
Cardiac arrhythmia
Angina pectoris
Heart failure

Splenomegaly

Nephrocalcinosis
Renal failure

Erythema nodosum

Arthropathies

Fig. 6.32   The range of possible systemic involvement in sarcoidosis.

occasionally patients with persistent erythema nodosum, pyrexia and arthralgia, or iridocyclitis require oral corticosteroid therapy for a short period.

Symptomatic Stage 3 pulmonary sarcoidosis and sarcoidosis involving the eyes or other vital organs usually needs to be treated with corticosteroids which may have to be continued for several years. Sarcoidosis usually responds rapidly to prednisolone 20–40 mg daily for 4 weeks; thereafter the disease is usually suppressed by a maintenance dose of 7.5–10 mg daily, or 20 mg daily on alternate days.

CRYPTOGENIC FIBROSING ALVEOLITIS

Fibrosing alveolitis exemplifies many of the typical features of interstitial lung disease. It may be a manifestation of one of the connective tissue disorders such as rheumatoid disease (see Table 6.17) or it may occur as an isolated pulmonary abnormality (cryptogenic fibrosing alveolitis).

Cryptogenic fibrosing alveolitis is probably not a single disease entity but a group of diseases with similar pathological changes. Cryptogenic fibrosing alveolitis is characterised histologically by cellular infiltration, thickening of alveolar walls together with large mononuclear cells in alveolar spaces. There is a variable degree of fibrosis and in most cases progressive fibrosis occurs. Whatever the cause of fibrosing alveolitis, lung macrophages appear to become 'activated' and produce chemotactic and activating factors for neutrophils which injure tissues by the release of proteinases and oxidants (see p. 38). Lung macrophages are probably also involved in fibrosis by their release of fibronectin and a range of pro-fibrotic cytokines and growth factors which

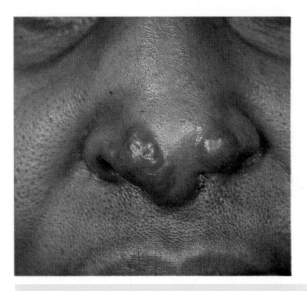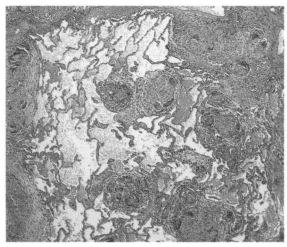

Fig. 6.33 Cutaneous sarcoid lesions (left). Histology of sarcoidosis in the lung (right).

stimulate fibroblasts to proliferate and secrete scar tissue matrix proteins.

Clinical features

Progressive exertional breathlessness is usually the presenting symptom, often accompanied by persistent dry cough. In most patients there is gross clubbing of the fingers and toes. Chest expansion may be poor and numerous bilateral end-inspiratory crepitations (crackles) are audible on auscultation, particularly over the lower zones posteriorly.

Radiological examination

The chest radiograph shows diffuse pulmonary opacities which are usually most obvious in the lower zones. The hemidiaphragms are high and the lungs appear small. In advanced disease the chest radiographs may show 'honey-comb lung' in which diffuse pulmonary shadowing is interspersed with small cystic translucencies. 'Honeycomb lung' is also a characteristic feature of rare diseases such as histiocytosis X and tuberous sclerosis (Fig. 6.31). High resolution CT scanning can reveal a dramatic picture in late disease (see p. 381). It may be particularly useful in early disease when chest radiograph changes may be slight or absent.

Pulmonary function tests

These show a restrictive ventilatory defect with proportionate reduction in FEV_1 and VC (p. 321). The carbon monoxide transfer factor is low and there is an overall reduction in lung volume. In early disease there is arterial hypoxaemia on exercise; later, arterial hypoxaemia and hypocapnia are present at rest.

Bronchoalveolar lavage and lung biopsy

Bronchoalveolar lavage fluid usually contains increased numbers of neutrophils and eosinophils. Transbronchial biopsy is often of no help because the small size of the biopsy specimens does not allow the pathologist to differentiate between fibrosing alveolitis and other forms of pulmonary fibrosis. Open lung biopsy, or video-assisted thoracoscopic lung biopsy, may be necessary to establish a diagnosis, particularly in patients with atypical clinical or radiological features.

Diagnosis

The diagnosis can often be made with confidence from the history, clinical findings, chest radiograph, pulmonary function test abnormalities and in some cases the bronchoalveolar lavage fluid cell counts. Serological tests for antinuclear and rheumatoid factor may be positive even in patients without evidence of a connective tissue disorder.

Management

Treatment with corticosteroids is beneficial in about 30% of patients but is of little value or no value in the remainder, few of whom survive for more than 5 years. A trial of prednisolone is indicated in most patients with progressive disease and should be given in a daily dose of 40–60 mg for 6–8 weeks. Assessment of response to this treatment is by repeat measurement of lung volumes, transfer factor and chest radiograph. Prednisolone should be withdrawn rapidly over a few weeks if there is no response. Should objective evidence of improvement be demonstrated the dose can be reduced gradually to a maintenance dose of 10 or 12.5 mg daily. In patients in whom it is not possible to reduce the dose of prednisolone below 15 or 20 mg daily without evidence of relapse, azathioprine in a dose of 1.5–2 mg/kg daily should be added in an attempt to reduce the dose of prednisolone to levels which are less likely to give side-effects. An alternative regimen is oral cyclophosphamide (2–3 mg/kg) daily with 20 mg prednisolone orally on alternate days.

Prognosis

The median survival time of untreated cases is about 4 years. The rate of progression of pulmonary changes varies considerably from death within a few months to survival with minimal symptoms for many years. Occasionally the disease process may 'burn out', but in the majority of patients the disease is progressive, even in those who have responded to treatment. Single lung transplantation may improve the outlook for some patients.

LUNG DISEASES DUE TO EXPOSURE TO ORGANIC DUSTS

A wide range of organic agents may cause respiratory disorders (see Table 6.15). Disease results from a local immune response to animal proteins (e.g. bird fancier's lung) or fungal antigens in mouldy vegetable matter. The most common presentation has been termed extrinsic allergic alveolitis.

EXTRINSIC ALLERGIC ALVEOLITIS

In this condition the inhalation of certain types of organic dust produces a diffuse immune complex reaction in the walls of the alveoli and bronchioles.

The pathogenic mechanisms concerned in the production of extrinsic allergic alveolitis are not fully understood. It is thought that the disease develops in sensitised individuals mainly through a Type III Arthus reaction, although Type IV mechanisms are probably also important. When the antigen is inhaled the immune complexes formed in antibody excess are precipitated very rapidly. Deposition of these immune complexes results in complement activation, causing a localised inflammatory reaction in the alveolar walls. Immunofluorescence has shown IgG, IgA and complement to be fixed in the

Table 6.15 Some examples of lung diseases caused by organic dusts

Disorder	Source	Antigen/agent
Farmer's lung*	Mouldy hay, straw, grain	*Micropolyspora faenae* *Aspergillus fumigatus*
Bird fancier's lung*	Avian excreta, proteins and feathers	Avian serum proteins
Malt worker's lung*	Mouldy maltings	*Aspergillus clavatus*
Byssinosis	Textile industries	Cotton, flex, hemp dust
Air conditioner/ humidifier lung	Contamination of air conditioning	Thermophilic actinomycetes
Cheese worker's lung*	Mouldy cheese	*Aspergillus clavatus* *Penicillium casei*
Maple bark stripper's lung*	Bark from stored maple	*Cryptostroma corticale*

* Denotes lung disease presenting as extrinsic allergic alveolitis

pulmonary tissues when biopsy specimens are examined in the acute stages. The presence of granulomata in the alveolar walls provides some evidence for a Type IV response to antigen being involved. Bronchoalveolar lavage fluid from patients with extrinsic allergic alveolitis usually shows an increase in the number of lymphocytes.

Some of the agents which produce extrinsic allergic alveolitis, their source, and the names given to the resulting diseases are shown in Table 6.15. If patients with this disorder continue to be exposed to the relevant antigen for long periods they may eventually develop permanent pulmonary damage and progressive lung scarring, leading to severe respiratory disability, pulmonary hypertension and cor pulmonale.

Clinical features

Extrinsic allergic alveolitis should be suspected when a person, regularly exposed to a heavy concentration of organic dust, complains, within a few hours of re-exposure to the same dust, of flu-like symptoms including headache, muscle pains, malaise, pyrexia, dry cough and breathlessness without wheeze. A chronic form is also recognised and is distinguished by the development of irreversible fibrosis. This may follow recurrent acute episodes or it may occur following continuous exposure to low concentrations of antigens, as in some cases of budgerigar fancier's lung. In this variant, breathlessness on exertion and sometimes weight loss are prominent, but fever and systemic symptoms are often absent.

Investigation

In the acute stage of the disease there may be end-inspiratory crepitations (crackles) audible over both lungs. The chest radiograph shows diffuse micronodular shadowing, often more pronounced in the upper zones. Pulmonary function studies reveal a restrictive ventilatory defect with preservation of the FEV_1/VC ratio. The PaO_2 is reduced and the $PaCO_2$ is often below normal because of over-ventilation. Diffusion capacity is impaired.

The diagnosis of extrinsic allergic alveolitis is usually based on the characteristic clinical and radiological features together with the identification of a potential source of antigen at the patient's home or place of work. Reduction in the transfer factor (TLCO) is the most sensitive functional abnormality and its magnitude often correlates closely with the degree of radiological abnormality. The diagnosis may be supported by a positive precipitin test or by more sensitive serological tests based on the ELISA technique. However, it is also important to recognise that the great majority of farmers with positive precipitins do not have farmer's lung, and up to 15% of pigeon breeders may have positive serum precipitins and yet remain healthy. Where the diagnosis is suspected but the cause is not readily apparent it may be helpful to visit the patient's home or workplace. Occasionally, such as where a new agent is suspected, it may be necessary to prove the diagnosis by a provocation test: if positive, the inhalation of the relevant antigen is followed after 3–6 hours by pyrexia and a reduction in VC and gas transfer factor. Rarely lung biopsy may be necessary to establish a diagnosis.

Management

Mild forms of extrinsic allergic alveolitis rapidly subside when exposure to the antigen ceases. In acute cases prednisolone should be given for 3 to 4 weeks starting with an oral dose of 40–60 mg per day. Severely hypoxaemic patients may require high concentration oxygen therapy initially. Most patients recover completely, but the development of interstitial fibrosis causes permanent disability when there has been prolonged exposure to antigen.

BYSSINOSIS

Not all inhaled organic dusts cause interstitial infiltration. In byssinosis the initial lesion is acute bronchiolitis associated with symptoms and signs of generalised airflow obstruction, more in keeping with asthma. Initially, symptoms tend to recur after the weekend break ('Monday fever') but eventually become continuous. There is usually no radiological abnormality. Recovery follows removal from the dust hazard in most cotton workers. Smokers have a greater incidence of byssinosis than non-smokers.

HUMIDIFIER FEVER

This is a disease with a similar pattern of symptoms to byssinosis. Fever and breathlessness may be a problem at the beginning of the week but often subside at the weekend. It is thought to be caused by water-borne micro-organisms from contaminated humidifiers in air conditioning systems.

LUNG DISEASES DUE TO EXPOSURE TO INORGANIC DUSTS

In certain occupations, the inhalation of dusts, fumes or other noxious substances may give rise to specific pathological changes in the lungs. Generally, prolonged exposure to inorganic dusts (see Table 6.16) leads to diffuse pulmonary fibrosis (the pneumoconioses), although berylliosis causes an interstitial granulomatous

Table 6.16   Some lung diseases caused by exposure to inorganic dusts

Cause	Occupation	Description	Characteristic features
Coal dust	Coal mining	Coal-worker's pneumoconiosis	Focal and interstitial fibrosis, centrilobular emphysema, progressive massive fibrosis
Silica	Mining, quarrying, stone dressing, metal grinding, pottery, boiler scaling	Silicosis	
Asbestos	Demolition, shipbreaking, manufacture of fireproof insulating materials and brake-pads, pipe and boiler lagging	Asbestos-related disease	Interstitial fibrosis, pleural disease
Iron oxide	Arc welding	Siderosis	Mineral deposition only
Tin oxide	Tin mining	Stannosis	
Beryllium	Aircraft, atomic energy and electronics industries	Berylliosis	Granulomata, interstitial fibrosis

disease similar to sarcoidosis. The dusts themselves cause little direct damage to the lung parenchyma and the pathological result depends largely on the inflammatory and fibrotic responses to the particular dust. The fibrogenic properties of mineral dusts vary, silica being markedly fibrogenic whereas iron and tin are almost inert. The most important types of pneumoconioses are coal worker's pneumoconiosis, silicosis and asbestosis.

Industrial inorganic gases and fumes can cause other respiratory diseases including acute pulmonary oedema and asthma (see information box). Industrial lung dis-

---

SOME LUNG DISEASES DUE TO INORGANIC GASES AND FUMES

Cause	Occupation	Disease
• **Irritant gases** (chlorine, ammonia, phosgene, nitrogen dioxide)	Various (industrial accidents)	Acute lung injury ARDS
• **Cadmium**	Welding and electroplating	Chronic bronchitis and emphysema
• **Isocyanates** (e.g. epoxy resins)	Plastic, paints; manufacture of epoxy resins and adhesives	Bronchial asthma, eosinophilic pneumonia

---

eases may also arise from exposure to organic dusts, e.g. farmer's lung and other extrinsic allergic alveolitides.

Clearly, it is essential to elicit a detailed occupational history, both present and past, since a diagnosis of occupational lung disease can easily be overlooked and the patient may be eligible for compensation. It must also be emphasised that in many types of pneumoconiosis a long period of dust exposure is required before radiological changes appear, and these may precede clinical symptoms.

Notes on diagnosis and claims for benefits in pneumoconiosis, occupational asthma and other related occupational diseases in Britain are contained in government pamphlets. New industrial processes are constantly being introduced and it is necessary to remain alert to the possibility that they may be associated with occupational lung disease.

COAL-WORKER'S PNEUMOCONIOSIS

This disease follows prolonged inhalation of coal dust. The condition is subdivided into simple pneumoconiosis and progressive massive fibrosis for clinical purposes and for certification. It must be emphasised that for certification purposes in Britain the diagnosis rests at present on radiological and not clinical features.

Simple coal-worker's pneumoconiosis
This is categorised radiologically into three grades, depending on the size and extent of the nodulation present. It does not progress if the miner leaves the industry.

Progressive massive fibrosis
In this form of the disease, large dense masses, single or multiple, occur mainly in the upper lobes. These may be irregular in shape and may cavitate. Tuberculosis may be a complication. The disease can be disabling, may shorten life expectancy and may progress even after the miner leaves the industry.

Cough and sputum from associated chronic bronchitis are frequently present. The sputum may be black (melanoptysis). Progressive breathlessness on exertion occurs in the later stages and respiratory and right ventricular failure supervene as terminal events. There may be no abnormal physical signs in the chest but where present they are those of chronic obstructive airways disease.

Antinuclear factor is present in the serum of about 15% of patients with coal-worker's pneumoconiosis. Rheumatoid factor is present in some patients in whom rheumatoid arthritis coexists, with rounded fibrotic nodules 0.5–5 cm in diameter. These are mainly in the periphery of the lung fields and the association is known as **Caplan's syndrome**. This syndrome may also occur in other types of pneumoconiosis.

SILICOSIS

This disease is becoming rare as the standards of industrial hygiene improve. It is caused by the inhalation of fine free crystalline silicone dioxide (silica) dust or quartz particles.

Silica is a most fibrogenic dust and causes the development of hard nodules which coalesce as the disease progresses. Tuberculosis may modify the silicotic process with ensuing caseation and calcification. The radiological features are similar to those seen in coal-worker's pneumoconiosis though the changes tend to be more marked in the upper zones. The hilar shadows may be enlarged, and 'egg-shell' calcification in the hilar lymph nodes is a distinctive feature but does not occur in all patients. The disease progresses even when exposure to dust ceases. The patient should, therefore, be removed from the offending environment as soon as possible. Clinical features are similar to those of coal-worker's pneumoconiosis.

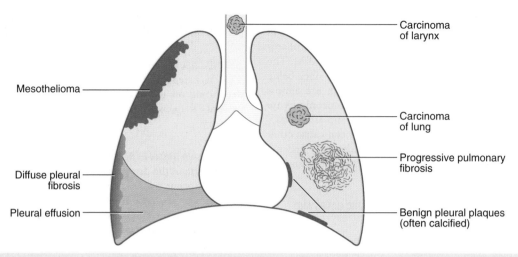

Fig. 6.34   Asbestos: the range of possible effects on the respiratory tract.

ASBESTOSIS

The main types of the fibrous mineral, asbestos, are chrysotile (white asbestos), which accounts for 90% of the world's production, crocidolite (blue asbestos) and amosite (brown asbestos). Exposure occurs in the mining and milling of the mineral and in a variety of occupations (see p. 386).

Asbestos may cause laryngeal carcinoma and a variety of lung pathologies (see p. 398).

Of these only asbestosis and mesothelioma automatically qualify for industrial injury benefit in Britain. Asbestosis was defined by the Advisory Committee on Asbestos (1979) as 'Fibrosis of the lungs caused by asbestos dusts which may or may not be associated with fibrosis of the parietal or pulmonary layer of the pleura'.

Pulmonary fibrosis caused by the inhalation of asbestos fibres is characterised by increasing exertion breathlessness. Digital clubbing is usually present and end-inspiratory crepitations (crackles) are audible over the lower zones of both lungs.

The radiological changes are usually confined to the lower two-thirds of the lung fields and comprise mottled shadows with some streaky opacities and sometimes 'honeycombing' (see Fig. 6.34). The cardiac silhouette often appears 'shaggy'.

The most important physiological abnormalities are a reduced carbon monoxide transfer factor, decreased lung volumes and a restrictive ventilatory defect.

Respiratory and right ventricular failure eventually supervene. The incidence of bronchial carcinoma is much increased, and is at least tenfold in persons suffering from asbestosis who also smoke.

The diagnosis is usually easy to establish from the history of exposure to asbestos, the clinical features of end-inspiratory crepitations and digital clubbing, the pulmonary function test abnormalities and the chest radiograph which also often shows pleural plaques (see p. 398). Open lung biopsy may be required to confirm the diagnosis but is not without risk and should not be undertaken solely for the purposes of allowing patients to claim benefit.

Management
No specific treatment is available. Corticosteroids are of no value in the management of asbestosis.

Prevention
Improvements of standards of industrial hygiene are now enforced by law in many countries; such measures as wearing respirators, damping dust and efficient ventilation systems are already proving effective in a number of industries.

LUNG DISEASES DUE TO SYSTEMIC INFLAMMATORY DISEASE

THE ADULT RESPIRATORY DISTRESS SYNDROME

The adult respiratory distress syndrome (ARDS) is a catastrophic form of acute inflammatory lung injury. It characteristically develops in a small proportion of patients several hours to a day or more following a variety of predisposing disorders, most commonly Gram-negative septicaemia, multiple trauma or pneumonia (see information box). Although it was fully described only

SOME CONDITIONS PREDISPOSING TO ARDS

Common
- Gram-negative septicaemia
- Multiple trauma
- Pneumonia (bacterial, viral, pneumocystis, mycoplasma)
- Pancreatitis
- Severe burns
- Gastric aspiration
- Perforated viscus

Uncommon
- Multiple blood transfusions
- Cardiopulmonary bypass
- Inhaled toxic gases
- Fat embolisation
- Raised intracranial pressure
- Drugs, e.g. thiazides, methadone, barbiturates

25 years ago, pulmonary oedema had been recognised as a complication of multiple trauma in both World Wars when it was called 'shock lung'. It is now clear that ARDS forms the major component of a systemic disorder which often includes renal failure, liver failure, and in its later stages even loss of gut and skin integrity—multiple organ failure (MOF).

Pathology
In the early stages there is pulmonary microvascular endothelial and alveolar type I epithelial damage. This results in exudation of protein-rich fluid into the interstitium of the alveolar septae and into the alveoli themselves (non-cardiogenic pulmonary oedema). There is the rapid development of interstitial and alveolar fibrosis. The damaged lung is prone to ventilator-induced barotrauma (pneumothoraces) and secondary infection, particularly with Gram-negative organisms.

Clinical features
The syndrome usually presents as rapidly progressive dyspnoea and hypoxaemia. On examination there are often crepitations in both lungs, and the chest radiograph shows widespread bilateral fluffy shadowing and the 'ground glass' appearance of alveolar oedema (see Fig. 6.35). In some cases the cardiophrenic angles may remain clear at an early stage. Swan–Ganz catheterisation, to confirm a low pulmonary wedge pressure, may be helpful in establishing a diagnosis of ARDS and ensuring that left ventricular failure or hypervolaemia is not contributing to the pulmonary oedema.

Management
When ARDS is fully established, mechanical ventilation is mandatory to correct hypoxaemia, and often a combination of high inflation pressures, high concentration oxygen and PEEP (see p. 331) are required to maintain adequate tissue oxygenation. There is no specific treat-

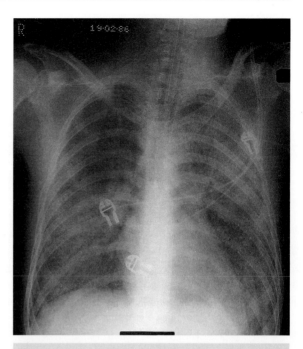

Fig. 6.35 Adult respiratory distress syndrome: diffuse bilateral pulmonary opacification in a young patient requiring assisted ventilation.

ment, and it is generally considered that the potentially beneficial anti-inflammatory effects of high dose corticosteroid treatment are outweighed by detrimental effects, particularly the increased susceptibility to secondary infection.

Prognosis
The mortality rate in established ARDS is around 70%, often from multiple organ failure, but secondary lung infections and the development of progressive lung scarring may contribute to mortality. Perhaps surprisingly, given the severity of lung injury and later scarring in ARDS, many of those who survive appear to make a significant functional recovery over the ensuing months.

RESPIRATORY INVOLVEMENT IN CONNECTIVE TISSUE DISORDERS

Fibrosing alveolitis is a recognised complication of most connective tissue diseases. The clinical features are usually indistinguishable from cryptogenic fibrosing alveolitis (see p. 383) and the response to immunosuppressive drugs is similarly unpredictable. Connective tissue disorders may also cause disease of the pleura, diaphragm and chest wall muscles (see Table 6.17). Pulmonary hypertension and cor pulmonale may result from

Table 6.17   Respiratory complications of connective tissue disorders

	Airways	Parenchyma	Pleura	Diaphragm and chest wall
Rheumatoid arthritis	Bronchitis, obliterative bronchiolitis, bronchiectasis, crico-arytenoid arthritis, stridor	Fibrosing alveolitis, nodules, upper lobe fibrosis, infections	Pleurisy, effusion, pneumothorax	Poor healing of intercostal drain sites
Systemic lupus erythematosus	—	Fibrosing alveolitis, 'vasculitic' infarcts	Pleurisy, effusion	'Shrinking lungs'
Systemic sclerosis	Bronchiectasis	Pulmonary fibrosis, aspiration pneumonia	—	'Hidebound chest'
Dermatomyositis/polymyositis	Bronchial carcinoma	Fibrosing alveolitis	—	Intercostal and diaphragmatic myopathy
Rheumatic fever	—	Pneumonia	Pleurisy, effusion	Diaphragmatic paralysis

advanced fibrosing alveolitis associated with connective tissue disorders.

Indirect associations between connective tissue disorders and respiratory complications include: those due to disease in other organs, e.g. thrombocytopenia causing haemoptysis; pulmonary toxic effects of drugs used to treat the connective tissue disorder; and secondary infection due to the disease itself, neutropenia or immunosuppressive drug regimens.

Rheumatoid disease

Fibrosing alveolitis is the most common pulmonary manifestation (rheumatoid lung). The clinical features, investigations, treatment and prognosis are similar to those of cryptogenic fibrosing alveolitis, although a rare variant of localised upper lobe fibrosis and cavitation has been described.

Pleural effusion is common, especially in men with seropositive disease. Effusions are usually small and unilateral but can be large and bilateral. Most resolve spontaneously. Biochemical testing shows an exudate (p. 397) with markedly reduced glucose levels and raised lactate dehydrogenase (LDH). Serology of the fluid may reveal a high titre of rheumatoid factor. Effusions that fail to resolve spontaneously may respond to a course of high dose (40 mg per day) oral prednisolone.

Pulmonary nodules are often seen on the chest radiograph. They display the same histopathological features as subcutaneous nodules and are usually of little significance. However, they can cause pneumothorax, or cavitate and cause haemoptysis, thus mimicking bronchial carcinoma or pulmonary tuberculosis. Caplan's syndrome (p. 387) occurs when pneumoconiosis is complicated by the development of rheumatoid nodules which are visible on the chest radiograph.

Finally, rheumatoid disease is associated with disorders of the airways. Bronchitis and bronchiectasis are both more common in rheumatoid patients. Rarely, the potentially fatal condition, obliterative bronchiolitis, may develop.

Systemic lupus erythematosus

Fibrosing alveolitis is a relatively uncommon manifestation of systemic lupus erythematosus. Pleuropulmonary involvement is more common in lupus than any other connective tissue disorder. Up to two-thirds of patients have repeated episodes of pleurisy, with or without effusions. The characteristic effusion is an exudate with a normal glucose level and tests for ANF and LE cells are often positive.

Some patients with systemic lupus erythematosus present with exertional dyspnoea and orthopnoea without overt signs of fibrosing alveolitis. The chest radiograph reveals elevated diaphragms, and pulmonary function testing shows reduced lung volumes. This condition has been described as 'shrinking lungs' and is thought to be caused by diaphragmatic myopathy.

Systemic sclerosis

Most patients with systemic sclerosis eventually develop diffuse pulmonary fibrosis; at necropsy more than 90% have evidence of lung fibrosis. In some patients it is indolent, but when progressive, like cryptogenic fibrosing alveolitis, the median survival time is around 4 years. Pulmonary fibrosis is rare in the CREST variant (p. 917) of progressive systemic sclerosis.

Other pulmonary complications include recurrent aspiration pneumonias secondary to oesophageal disease. Rarely, sclerosis of the skin of the chest wall may be so extensive and cicatrising as to seriously restrict chest wall movement—the so-called 'hidebound chest'

PULMONARY EOSINOPHILIA AND VASCULITIDES

This term is applied to a group of disorders of different aetiology in which lesions in the lungs produce a chest radiograph abnormality associated with an increase in the number of the eosinophil leucocytes in the peripheral blood. There is no satisfactory classification of this disparate group of disorders, but they can be divided into two main categories: see box.

PULMONARY EOSINOPHILIA

Extrinsic (cause known)
- Helminths
  (e.g. Ascaris, Toxocara, Filaria)
- Drugs
  (Nitrofurantoin, para-aminosalicylic acid,
  sulphasalazine, imipramine, chlorpropamide,
  phenylbutazone)
- Fungi
  (e.g. *Aspergillus fumigatus*)

Intrinsic (cause unknown)
- Cryptogenic eosinophilic pneumonia
- Churg–Strauss syndrome
- Hypereosinophilic syndrome
- Polyarteritis nodosa (rare)

Some causes of extrinsic pulmonary eosinophilia are given in the information box. The most common disorder of this type in western countries is allergic bronchopulmonary aspergillosis (p. 367) and in tropical countries the presence of microfilariae in the pulmonary capillaries (p. 175) has to be considered.

CRYPTOGENIC EOSINOPHILIC PNEUMONIA

Cryptogenic eosinophilic pneumonia is more common in middle-aged females, and usually presents with malaise, fever, breathlessness and unproductive cough. The chest radiograph can show a variety of abnormal shadows, but they tend to be peripheral, often involve the upper zones and may be difficult to distinguish from the radiological features of pulmonary tuberculosis. Unless corticosteroids have been given, the peripheral blood eosinophil count is almost always very high, the ESR and total serum IgE are elevated. Bronchoalveolar lavage reveals a very high proportion of eosinophils in the lavage fluid. Response to prednisolone (20–40 mg daily) is usually dramatic. Prednisolone treatment can usually be withdrawn after a few weeks without relapse, but long-term low dose therapy is occasionally necessary to control the disease.

LUNG DISEASES DUE TO IRRADIATION AND DRUGS

Radiotherapy

The lungs are exposed during radiotherapy treatment of lung tumours and also tumours of the breast, spine and oesophagus. The pulmonary effects of radiation are exacerbated by treatment with cytotoxic drugs, oxygen delivery and previous radiotherapy. Radiotherapy may cause acute damage to the lung, and also a chronic insidious scarring disease.

After pulmonary irradiation, acute radiation pneumonitis may present with cough and dyspnoea within 6–12 weeks. This acute form of lung damage may resolve spontaneously or respond to corticosteroid treatment. Chronic interstitial fibrosis presents later, usually with symptoms of exertional dyspnoea and cough. Established post-irradiation fibrosis does not usually respond to corticosteroid treatment.

Drugs

Drugs may cause a number of parenchymal reactions including ARDS (see Table 6.18), eosinophilic reactions, and diffuse interstitial inflammation/scarring. Drugs can also cause other lung disorders including asthma (see p. 338), haemorrhage (e.g. anticoagulants, penicillamine) and occasionally pleural effusions and pleural thickening (e.g. hydralazine, isoniazid, methysergide). An ARDS-like syndrome of acute non-cardiogenic pulmonary oedema may present with dramatic onset of breathlessness, severe hypoxaemia and signs of alveolar oedema on the chest radiograph. This syndrome has been reported most frequently in cases of opiate overdose in drug addicts, but also after salicylate overdose, and there are occasional reports of its occurrence after therapeutic doses of drugs including hydrochlorothiazides and some cytotoxic drugs.

Pulmonary fibrosis may occur in response to a variety of drugs, such as bleomycin and methotrexate, amiodarone and nitrofurantoin. Eosinophilic pulmonary reactions can also be caused by drugs. The pathogenesis may be an immune reaction similar to that in extrinsic allergic alveolitis, which specifically attracts large numbers of eosinophils into the lungs. This type of reaction is well described as a rare reaction to a variety of antineoplastic agents (e.g. bleomycin), antibiotics (e.g. sulphonamides), sulphasalazine and the anticonvulsants phenytoin and carbamazepine. Patients usually present with breathlessness, cough and fever. The chest radiograph characteristically shows patchy shadowing. Most cases resolve completely on withdrawal of the drug, but if the reaction is severe, rapid resolution can be obtained with corticosteroids.

RARE INTERSTITIAL LUNG DISEASES

IDIOPATHIC PULMONARY HAEMOSIDEROSIS

This is a rare disease of unknown cause in which spontaneous intrapulmonary haemorrhage causes recurrent

Table 6.18   Drug-induced respiratory disease

Non-cardiogenic pulmonary oedema (ARDS)	Hydrochlorothiazide Thrombolytics (streptokinase) i.v. β-adrenoceptor agonists (e.g. treatment of premature labour) Aspirin (in overdose) Opiates (in overdose)
Non-eosinophilic alveolitis	Amiodarone, tocainide, flecainide, gold, nitrofurantoin, cytotoxic agents—especially bleomycin, busulphan, mitomycin C, methotrexate
Pulmonary eosinophilia	Antibiotics (nitrofurantoin, penicillin, tetracyclines, sulphonamides, nalidixic acid) Antirheumatic agents (gold, aspirin, penicillamine, naproxen) Cytotoxic drugs (bleomycin, methotrexate, procarbazine) Psychiatric drugs (chlorpromazine, dothiepin, imipramine) Anticonvulsants (carbamazepine, phenytoin) Others (sulphasalazine, nadolol)
Pleural disease	Bromocriptine, amiodarone, methotrexate, methysergide, nitrofurantoin Via induction of SLE—phenytoin, hydralazine, isoniazid, procainamide
Asthma	Via pharmacological mechanism (—β adrenoceptor antagonists, cholinergic agonists, e.g. pilocarpine, cholinesterase inhibitors, aspirin and NSAIDs) Idiosyncratic reaction (tamoxifen, dipyridamole)

episodes of haemoptysis and iron-deficiency anaemia. If the patient survives the acute haemorrhagic episodes, interstitial fibrosis may eventually cause respiratory failure and cor pulmonale. Pulmonary haemorrhage may also be associated with acute glomerulonephritis (Goodpasture's syndrome—p. 643). This disease should be suspected if haemoptysis is associated with disordered renal function, systemic hypertension and haematuria.

ALVEOLAR PROTEINOSIS

In this condition, which is more common in males, the basic defect appears to result from the excessive production of abnormal surfactant material which is not cleared by alveolar macrophages and pulmonary lymphatics. It is usually idiopathic but has been described after exposure to organic dusts and immunosuppressive drugs. Patients usually present with cough and exertional dyspnoea, but weight loss and fever are also common. Diffuse interstitial radiographic shadowing occurs early and may precede the onset of symptoms. Alveolar proteinosis can be diagnosed by bronchoalveolar lavage or lung biopsy. Bronchoalveolar lavage

fluid is opalescent and contains large amounts of PAS-positive material. Mortality in adults is now low, if treatment with whole lung lavage is employed to remove the abnormal material.

HISTIOCYTOSIS X

This rare condition is more common in young adult males. It may affect the lungs alone but is usually a generalised disorder including bone dysfunction and diabetes insipidus. It is characterised by the pulmonary accumulation of Langerhans histiocytes which are presumed to release mediators that provoke a diffuse scarring reaction and multiple cyst formation. Affected individuals usually present with cough and exertional breathlessness, and repeated pneumothoraces can be a major problem. Lung biopsy is often necessary to differentiate the condition from other interstitial lung diseases. About half of the patients respond to aggressive treatment with anti-inflammatory drugs.

LYMPHANGIOLEIOMYOMATOSIS

This condition occurs only in women, most of whom are of child-bearing age. The pulmonary disorder is due to massive proliferation of the smooth muscle of lymphatics and lung parenchyma, possibly under the influence of hormonal effects. Recurrent pneumothorax and haemoptysis are the main clinical problems initially, but as the disease progresses all the complications of a severe restrictive lung disease supervene. Pleurodesis may be necessary, and hormonal manipulation with drugs (tamoxifen) and oophorectomy is used as treatment, but their value is uncertain. As with other progressive lung disease in young adults, lung transplantation may be the only available treatment option.

PULMONARY NEUROFIBROMATOSIS

Bilateral lung fibrosis is a rare complication of neurofibromatosis (Von Recklinghausen's disease—see p. 1112). The pulmonary lesions are usually slowly progressive and there is no effective treatment.

PULMONARY TUBEROUS SCLEROSIS

About 1% of patients with this genetic disorder develop reticulonodular shadowing and cystic changes on the chest radiograph. There is no effective treatment and most patients die within 5 years of the development of pulmonary complications.

FURTHER READING

Donnelly S C, Haslett C 1992 Cellular mechanisms of acute lung injury: implications for future therapy in the adult respiratory distress syndrome. Thorax 47: 260–263

Dubois R M 1993 Idiopathic pulmonary fibrosis. Annual Review of Medicine: 441–451

Rom W N, Travis W D, Brody A R 1991 Cellular and molecular mechanism of asbestos-mediated disease. American Review of Respiratory Disease 143: 408–422

Rose C, King T E 1992 Controversies in hypersensitivity pneumonitis. American Review of Respiratory Disease 145:1–2

Seaton A 1994 Management of the patient with occupational lung disease. Thorax 49: 627–629

DISEASES OF THE NASOPHARYNX, LARYNX AND TRACHEA

DISEASES OF THE NASOPHARYNX

Acute infections have already been described (p. 351). Other disorders of the larynx include chronic laryngitis, laryngeal tuberculosis (p. 365), laryngeal paralysis and laryngeal obstruction. Tumours of the larynx are relatively common. For detailed information on these conditions the reader should refer to a textbook of disease of the ear, nose and throat.

ALLERGIC RHINITIS

This is a disorder in which there are episodes of nasal congestion, watery nasal discharge and sneezing. It may be **seasonal** or **perennial**.

Aetiology

Allergic rhinitis is due to an immediate hypersensitivity reaction in the nasal mucosa (p. 42). The antigens concerned in the seasonal form of the disorder are pollens from grasses, flowers, weeds or trees. Grass pollen is responsible for **hay fever (pollenosis)**, the most common type of seasonal allergic rhinitis in Northern Europe; this disorder is at its peak between May and July.

Perennial allergic rhinitis may be a specific reaction to antigens derived from house dust, fungal spores or animal dander but similar symptoms can be caused by physical or chemical irritants, for example pungent odours or fumes including strong perfumes, cold air and dry atmospheres. The term **vasomotor rhinitis** is often used for this type of nasal problem because in this context the term 'allergic' is a misnomer.

Clinical features

In the seasonal type there are frequent sudden attacks of sneezing with profuse watery nasal discharge and nasal obstruction. These attacks last for a few hours and are often accompanied by smarting and watering of the eyes and conjunctival injection. In the perennial variety the symptoms are similar but more continuous and generally less severe. Skin hypersensitivity tests with the relevant antigen are usually positive in seasonal allergic rhinitis and are thus of diagnostic value; but these tests are less useful in perennial rhinitis.

Management

The following symptomatic measures, singly or in combination, are usually effective in both seasonal and perennial allergic rhinitis:

- an antihistamine drug such as terfenadine 60 mg twice daily by mouth
- sodium cromoglycate nasal spray, one metered dose of a 2% solution into each nostril 4–6 times daily
- beclomethasone dipropionate or budesonide nasal spray, one or two metered doses of 50 μg into each nostril twice daily.

Patients failing to respond to these measures may obtain symptomatic relief from intramuscular injection of a long-acting corticosteroid preparation but this form of treatment should be reserved for occasional use in patients whose symptoms are very severe and interfere seriously with school, business or social activities. Vasomotor rhinitis is often difficult to treat, but may respond to ipratropium bromide administered from metered dose inhaler 0.02 mg into each nostril 3 or 4 times daily.

Prevention

In the seasonal type an attempt should be made to reduce exposure to pollen, for example by avoiding country districts and keeping indoors as much as possible with windows closed during the pollen season, especially when pollen counts are reported to be high. Some patients with hay fever may obtain benefit from pre-seasonal hyposensitisation (p. 341) with grass pollen extract, but this therapy is now rarely used in Britain because of the risk of anaphylactic reaction. The prevention of perennial rhinitis consists of avoiding, as far as possible, exposure to any identifiable aetiological factors but this is often difficult or impossible.

LARYNGEAL DISORDERS

CHRONIC LARYNGITIS

The common causes of this condition are listed in the information box below.

SOME CAUSES OF CHRONIC LARYNGITIS

- Repeated attacks of acute laryngitis
- Excessive use of the voice, especially in dusty atmospheres
- Heavy tobacco smoking
- Mouth-breathing from nasal obstruction
- Chronic infection of nasal sinuses

Clinical features

The chief symptom is hoarseness and the voice may be lost completely (aphonia). There is irritation of the throat and a spasmodic cough. The disease pursues a chronic course frequently uninfluenced by treatment, and in long-standing cases the voice is often permanently impaired.

Differential diagnosis

The causes of chronic hoarseness are listed in the information box below.

CAUSES OF CHRONIC HOARSENESS

Consider if hoarseness persists for more than a few days:
- Tumour of larynx
- Tuberculosis
- Laryngeal paralysis
- Inhaled corticosteroid treatment

These conditions must be considered in the differential diagnosis if hoarseness does not improve within a few weeks. In some patients a chest radiograph may bring to light an unsuspected bronchial carcinoma or pulmonary tuberculosis. If no such abnormality is found laryngoscopy should be performed, usually by a specialist in otolaryngology.

Management

The voice must be rested completely. This is particularly important in public speakers. Smoking should be prohibited. Some benefit may be obtained from frequent inhalations of medicated steam.

LARYNGEAL PARALYSIS

Aetiology

Paralysis is due to interference with the motor nerve supply of the larynx. It is nearly always unilateral and, by reason of the intrathoracic course of the left recurrent laryngeal nerve, usually left-sided. One or both recurrent laryngeal nerves may be damaged at thyroidectomy or by carcinoma of the thyroid. Rarely, the vagal trunk itself is involved by tumour, aneurysm or trauma.

Clinical features

Hoarseness

This always accompanies laryngeal paralysis whatever its cause. Paralysis of organic origin is seldom reversible, but when only one vocal cord is affected hoarseness may improve or even disappear after a few weeks following a compensatory adjustment whereby the unparalysed cord crosses the midline and approximates with the paralysed cord on phonation.

'Bovine cough'

A characteristic feature of organic laryngeal paralysis is a cow-like cough which results from the loss of the explosive phase of normal coughing consequent upon the failure of the cords to close the glottis. Difficulty in bringing up sputum, which some patients experience, is also explained on the same basis. A normal cough in patients with partial loss of voice or aphonia virtually excludes laryngeal paralysis.

Stridor

Stridor is occasionally present but is seldom severe except when laryngeal paralysis is bilateral.

Diagnosis

Laryngoscopy

This is necessary to establish the diagnosis of laryngeal paralysis with certainty. The paralysed cord lies in the so-called 'cadaveric' position, midway between abduction and adduction.

Management

The cause of laryngeal paralysis should be treated if that is possible. In unilateral paralysis the voice may be improved by the injection of teflon into the affected vocal cord. In bilateral organic paralysis, tracheal intubation, tracheostomy or a plastic operation on the larynx may be necessary.

HYSTERICAL HOARSENESS AND APHONIA

Hoarseness or complete loss of voice may occur as a manifestation of hysteria. There are often clues in the history to suggest a diagnosis of hysteria but laryngoscopy may be necessary to exclude a pathological cause of the voice abnormality. In hysteria only the voluntary movement of adduction of the vocal cords is seen to be impaired.

LARYNGEAL OBSTRUCTION

Laryngeal obstruction is more liable to occur in children than in adults because of the smaller size of the glottis. Some important causes are given in the information box below.

CAUSES OF LARYNGEAL OBSTRUCTION

- Inflammatory or allergic oedema, or exudate
- Spasm of laryngeal muscles
- Inhaled foreign body
- Inhaled blood clot or vomitus in an unconscious patient
- Tumours of the larynx
- Bilateral vocal cord paralysis
- Fixation of both cords in rheumatoid disease

Clinical features

Sudden complete laryngeal obstruction by a foreign body produces the clinical picture of acute asphyxia—violent but ineffective inspiratory efforts with indrawing of the intercostal spaces and the unsupported lower ribs, accompanied by cyanosis. Unrelieved, the condition progresses rapidly to coma and death within a few minutes. When, as in most cases, the obstruction is incomplete at first, the main clinical features are progressive breathlessness accompanied by stridor and cyanosis. There is indrawing of the intercostal spaces and lower ribs on both sides with each inspiratory effort. In such cases the great danger is that complete laryngeal obstruction may occur at any time and result in sudden death.

Management

Transient attacks of laryngeal obstruction due to exudate and spasm, which may occur with acute laryngitis in children (p. 351) and with whooping cough, are potentially dangerous but can usually be relieved by the inhalation of steam.

Laryngeal obstruction from all other causes carries a high mortality and demands prompt treatment. The following measures may have to be employed.

The relief of obstruction by mechanical measures

When a foreign body is known to be the cause of the obstruction in children it can often be dislodged by turning the patient head downwards and squeezing the chest vigorously. In adults this is often impossible, but a sudden forceful compression of the upper abdomen (Heimlich manoeuvre) may be effective. In other circumstances the cause of the obstruction should be investigated by direct laryngoscopy which may also permit the removal of an unsuspected foreign body, or the inser-

tion of a tube past the obstruction into the trachea. Tracheostomy must be performed without delay if these procedures fail to relieve laryngeal obstruction, but except in dire emergencies this operation should be performed in an operating theatre by a surgeon.

Treatment of the cause

In cases of diphtheria, antitoxin should be administered and for other infections the appropriate antibiotic should be given. In angioedema complete laryngeal occlusion can usually be prevented by treatment with adrenaline 0.5–1 mg (0.5–1 ml of 1:1000) intramuscularly, chlorpheniramine maleate 10–20 mg by slow intravenous injection and intravenous hydrocortisone sodium succinate 200 mg.

TRACHEAL DISORDERS

ACUTE TRACHEITIS

This is a common complication of viral and bacterial infection of the upper respiratory tract, and is usually associated with acute bronchitis (p. 351).

TRACHEAL OBSTRUCTION

External compression by enlarged mediastinal lymph nodes containing metastatic deposits, usually from a bronchial carcinoma, is a more frequent cause of tracheal obstruction than the uncommon primary benign or malignant tumours. Rarely, the trachea may be compressed by an aneurysm of the aortic arch, or in children by tuberculous mediastinal lymph nodes. Tracheal stenosis is an occasional complication of tracheostomy, prolonged intubation or trauma.

Clinical features

Stridor can be detected in every patient with severe tracheal narrowing. Endoscopic examination of the trachea should be undertaken without delay to determine the site, degree and nature of the obstruction.

Management

Localised tumours of the trachea can be resected, but reconstruction after resection may present complex technical problems. Laser therapy and radiotherapy are alternatives to surgery. The choice of treatment depends upon the nature of the tumour and the general health of the patient. Radiotherapy or chemotherapy may temporarily relieve compression by malignant lymph nodes and tracheal stents kept clear of secretions by suction through a tracheostomy may be of temporary value.

Tracheal strictures can sometimes be dilated but may have to be resected.

TRACHEO-OESOPHAGEAL FISTULA

This may be present in new-born infants as a congenital abnormality. In adults it is usually due to malignant lesions in the mediastinum, such as carcinoma or lymphoma, eroding both the trachea and oesophagus to produce a communication between them. Swallowed liquids enter the trachea and bronchi through the fistula and provoke coughing.

Management

Surgical closure of a congenital fistula if undertaken promptly is usually successful. There is usually no curative treatment for malignant fistulae and death from overwhelming pulmonary infection rapidly supervenes.

DISEASES OF THE PLEURA, DIAPHRAGM AND CHEST WALL

DISEASES OF THE PLEURA

PLEURISY

Pleurisy is not a diagnosis but simply the term used to describe the result of any disease process involving the pleura and giving rise to pleuritic pain or evidence of pleural friction. Pleurisy is a common feature of pulmonary infarction and may be an early manifestation of pleural invasion in pulmonary tuberculosis or by a pulmonary tumour.

Clinical features

Pleural pain is the characteristic symptom. On examination rib movement is restricted and a pleural rub is present in many cases, particularly when the patient takes a deep breath. It is not heard when the breath is held except near the pericardium, where a so-called pleuropericardial rub may be present. The other clinical features depend upon the nature of the disease causing the pleurisy. There may be complete clinical recovery or an effusion may develop, depending upon the underlying cause.

Every patient must have a chest radiograph but a normal radiograph does not exclude a pulmonary cause for the pleurisy. A preceding history of cough, purulent sputum and pyrexia is presumptive evidence of a pulmonary infection which may not have been severe enough to produce a radiographic abnormality or which may have resolved before the chest radiograph was taken.

Management

The primary cause of pleurisy must be treated. The symptomatic treatment of pleural pain is described on page 353.

PLEURAL EFFUSION

This term is used when serous fluid accumulates in the pleural space. The condition of purulent effusion or empyema is described on page 399. The passive transudation of fluid into the pleural cavity (hydrothorax) occurs in cardiac failure, and conditions causing hypoproteinaemia such as nephrotic syndrome, liver disease and severe malnutrition. Some causes of pleural effusion are shown in the information box.

CAUSES OF PLEURAL EFFUSION

Common	**Uncommon**
• Pneumonia	• Hypoproteinaemia (nephrotic syndrome, liver disease, malnutrition)
• Tuberculosis	
• Pulmonary infarction	• Connective tissue diseases
• Malignant disease	• Acute rheumatic fever
• Sub-diaphragmatic disorders (sub-phrenic abscess, pancreatitis, etc.)	• Post myocardial infarction syndrome
• Cardiac failure	• Meigs' syndrome (ovarian tumour plus effusion)
	• Myxoedema
	• Uraemia
	• Asbestos-related benign pleural effusion
	• Yellow nail syndrome

Pleural effusion may be unilateral or bilateral. Bilateral effusions often occur in cardiac failure, but are also seen in the much less common disorders such as the connective tissue diseases and hypoproteinaemia. The cause of the majority of pleural effusions can be identified if a careful history is taken and a comprehensive clinical examination performed.

Where the cause is obscure a lead may be given by enquiry regarding travel abroad, occupation, for example exposure to asbestos, contact with tuberculosis, or causes of thromboembolism such as oral contraception, recent immobilisation or operation. Detailed investigations as described below may, however, be necessary.

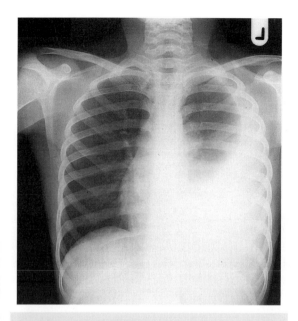

Fig. 6.36　Large pleural effusion. Chest radiograph showing the characteristic opacification.

Clinical features

The symptoms and signs of pleurisy often precede the development of effusion but the onset in some patients may be insidious. Breathlessness is the only symptom related to the effusion and the severity depends on the size and rate of accumulation of the fluid. The physical signs in the chest are those of fluid in the pleural space (p. 318).

Investigations

Radiological examination

The chest radiograph shows a dense uniform opacity in the lower and lateral parts of the hemithorax shading off above and medially into translucent lung. Occasionally the fluid is localised below the lower lobe, the appearances simulating an elevated hemidiaphragm. A localised opacity is seen when the effusion is loculated, for example in an interlobar fissure.

Ultrasonography

This investigation is valuable to differentiate between a loculated pleural effusion and pleural tumour and also helps to localise an effusion prior to aspiration and pleural biopsy.

Pleural aspiration and pleural biopsy

Absolute proof that an effusion is present can be obtained only by the aspiration of fluid. Pleural biopsy is always indicated whenever a diagnostic aspiration of pleural fluid is performed because the chances of obtain-ing a diagnosis from pleural biopsy material are much greater than by examination of the pleural liquid alone. A pleural biopsy needle should be inserted through an intercostal space at the area of maximum dullness on percussion and at the site of maximum radiological opacity as shown by postero-anterior and lateral films, or at a site determined by ultrasound. At least 50 ml of fluid should be withdrawn, aliquots being placed in separate containers for microbiological examination including culture for tuberculosis, cytological examination and biochemical examination. Whenever there is a strong suspicion of tuberculosis a large volume of pleural liquid should be submitted to the laboratory for examination. Pleural biopsies should be taken after pleural liquid has been aspirated for diagnostic purposes.

The appearance of the fluid is straw-coloured, blood-stained, purulent or chylous. The protein content gives an indication as to whether the effusion is an exudate (>30 g/l) or a transudate (<30 g/l). The predominant cell type (neutrophil, eosinophil, lymphocyte, red blood cell) provides useful information, and fluid should always be examined for malignant cells.

There is a high amylase level in effusions secondary to acute pancreatitis and a high concentration of cholesterol in most chronic rheumatoid effusions.

Other investigations

Estimation of the total and differential peripheral blood leucocyte count, a tuberculin test, and examination of the sputum for tubercle bacilli and malignant cells should be routine in most situations. A chest radiograph may disclose an underlying pulmonary lesion and indicate its nature. If the lung is obscured by a massive effusion the radiograph should be repeated after a large volume of fluid has been aspirated. Other investigations which may be of help include bronchoscopy, biopsy or aspiration of the scalene lymph node, thoracoscopy and serological tests for antinuclear and rheumatoid factors.

The main diagnostic features and more important causes of pleural effusion are shown in Table 6.19.

Management

Aspiration of pleural fluid may be necessary to relieve breathlessness. It is inadvisable to remove more than 1 litre on the first occasion because pulmonary oedema occasionally follows the aspiration of larger amounts. A pneumothorax may be produced even by a careful operator, and a chest radiograph must always be taken after the procedure.

Treatment of the underlying cause, for example heart failure, pneumonia, pulmonary embolism and sub-phrenic abscess, will often be followed by resolution of the effusion. However, certain conditions require special measures as detailed below.

Table 6.19   Pleural effusion: main causes and features

	Appearance of fluid	Type of fluid	Predominant cells in fluid	Other diagnostic features
Tuberculous	Serous, usually amber-coloured	Exudate	Lymphocytes (occas. polymorphs)	Positive tuberculin test Isolation of *Myco. tuberculosis* Positive pleural biopsy (80%)
Malignant disease	Serous, often blood-stained	Exudate	Serosal cells and lymphocytes Often clumps of malignant cells	Positive pleural biopsy (40%) Evidence of malignant disease elsewhere
Cardiac failure*	Serous, straw-coloured	Transudate	Few serosal cells	Other evidence of left heart failure Response to diuretics
Pulmonary infarction*	Serous or blood-stained	Exudate	Red blood cells Eosinophils	Contralateral evidence of infarction Source of embolism Factors predisposing to venous thrombosis
Rheumatoid disease*	Serous Turbid if chronic	Exudate	Lymphocytes (occas. polymorphs)	Rheumatoid arthritis Rheumatoid factor in serum Cholesterol in chronic effusion. Low glucose
Systemic lupus erythematosus*	Serous	Exudate	Lymphocytes and serosal cells	Other manifestations of SLE ANF or anti-DNA in serum
Acute pancreatitis	Serous or blood-stained	Exudate	No cells predominate	High amylase (greater than in serum)
Obstruction of thoracic duct	Milky	Chyle	None	Chylomicrons

* Effusion often bilateral.

Post-pneumonic pleural effusion

Pleural effusions complicating pneumonia may require aspiration to ensure that an empyema has not developed, and to prevent pleural thickening.

Tuberculous pleural effusion

Patients with tuberculous effusions should always receive antituberculosis chemotherapy (p. 361). Aspiration is required initially if the effusion is large and causing breathlessness. The addition of prednisolone 20 mg daily by mouth for 4–6 weeks will promote rapid absorption of the fluid and obviate the need for further aspiration, and may prevent fibrosis.

Malignant effusions

Effusions caused by malignant infiltration of the pleural surfaces re-accumulate rapidly. To avoid the distress of repeated aspirations, an attempt should be made to obliterate the pleural space (pleurodesis) by the injection of substances into the pleural fluid which produce an inflammatory reaction and extensive pleural adhesions. The agents most frequently used are inactivated *Corynebacterium parvum*, tetracycline and mustine hydrochloride.

ASBESTOS-RELATED PLEURAL DISEASE

Benign pleural plaques

These areas of pleural thickening do not produce clinical symptoms and are usually identified on routine chest radiograph. They are often calcified and in the early stage are best seen on oblique films. They are most commonly observed on the diaphragm and anterolateral pleural surfaces.

Benign pleural effusion

This is considered to be a specific asbestos-related entity and may be associated with pleural pain, fever and leucocytosis. The pleural liquid may be blood-stained, and differentiation of this benign condition from a malignant effusion caused by mesothelioma can be difficult. The disease is self-limiting but may cause considerable pleural fibrosis which sometimes leads to breathlessness.

Mesothelioma of the pleura

This malignant tumour of the pleura is usually caused by exposure to asbestos which may be trivial. Blue asbestos is thought to be the most potent cause of mesothelioma. Clinical presentation is frequently with chest pain. A pleural effusion, often blood-stained, may develop and cause breathlessness. A diagnosis can be confirmed histologically by pleural biopsy in some patients, but tumour masses may later develop in the chest wall at the site of the biopsy. Thoracotomy is seldom justified as a diagnostic procedure in patients with suspected mesothelioma. There is no curative treatment and chest wall pain is often difficult to control.

Diffuse pleural fibrosis

Diffuse pleural fibrosis is a much more important pleural manifestation of asbestos fibre inhalation than pleural plaque formation, since it can restrict chest expansion and cause breathlessness. The restrictive defect caused by diffuse pleural fibrosis tends to progress.

EMPYEMA

The term empyema is used to describe the presence of pus in the pleural space. The pus may be as thin as serous fluid or so thick that it is difficult or impossible to aspirate even through a wide-bore needle. Microscopically neutrophil leucocytes are present in large numbers. The causative organism may or may not be isolated from the pus. An empyema may involve the whole pleural space or only part of it ('loculated' or 'encysted' empyema) and is almost invariably unilateral.

Aetiology

Empyema is always secondary to infection in a neighbouring structure, usually the lung. The principal infections liable to produce empyema are the bacterial pneumonias and tuberculosis. Other causes are infection of a haemothorax and rupture of a subphrenic abscess through the diaphragm. Empyema has become a relatively rare disease because pulmonary infection can now be so readily controlled by antibacterial therapy.

Pathology

Both layers of pleura are covered with a thick, shaggy inflammatory exudate. The pus in the pleural space is often under considerable pressure and if the condition is not adequately treated there may be rupture into a bronchus from which pus is expectorated, or through an intercostal space with the formation of a subcutaneous abscess or sinus. A bronchopleural fistula is produced and a pyopneumothorax is formed when an empyema ruptures into a bronchus.

The only way in which an empyema can heal is by apposition of the visceral and parietal pleural layers with obliteration of the empyema space by organisation of the intervening exudate. This cannot occur unless re-expansion of the compressed lung is secured at an early stage by removal of all the pus from the pleural space. Re-expansion of the lung cannot take place if:

- there is delay in treatment or inadequate drainage and the visceral pleura becomes grossly thickened and rigid
- the pleural layers are kept apart by air entering the pleura through a bronchopleural fistula
- if disease in the lung, such as bronchiectasis, bronchial carcinoma or pulmonary tuberculosis, renders it incapable of re-expansion.

In all these circumstances an empyema tends to become chronic and healing may not take place without recourse to major thoracic surgery.

Clinical features

An empyema should be suspected in patients with pulmonary infection if there is a recurrence of pyrexia despite the continued administration of a suitable antibiotic. In other cases the illness produced by the primary infective lesion may be so slight that it passes unrecognised and the first definite clinical features are due to the empyema itself.

Once an empyema has developed two separate groups of clinical features are found. These are shown in the information box.

Investigation

Radiological examination

The appearances are indistinguishable from those of pleural effusion. When air is present in addition to pus (pyopneumothorax) a horizontal 'fluid level' marks the interface of liquid and air if the film is taken in the erect position.

CLINICAL FEATURES OF EMPYEMA

Systemic features
- Pyrexia; usually high and remittent
- Rigors, sweating, malaise and weight loss
- Polymorphonuclear leucocytosis; usually high

Local features
- Pleural pain; breathlessness; cough and sputum usually because of underlying lung disease; copious purulent sputum if empyema ruptures into a bronchus (bronchopleural fistula)
- Clinical signs of fluid in the pleural space

Aspiration of pus

This confirms the presence of an empyema. A wide-bore needle is inserted through an intercostal space over the area of maximum dullness on percussion. The position of the empyema should have previously been confirmed whenever possible by postero-anterior and lateral radiographs or by ultrasonography.

Bacteriological examination of pus

This may help to determine the cause of the empyema. The pus is frequently sterile when antibiotics have been given. The distinction between tuberculous and non-tuberculous disease can usually be made from the radiological changes in the lungs or by the isolation of tubercle bacilli from pus.

Management

Treatment of non-tuberculous empyema

1. **Acute**: When the patient is acutely ill and the pus is thin in consistency:

   (a) An intercostal tube should be inserted into the most dependent part of the empyema space and connected to a water seal drain system.
   (b) An antibiotic should be given to which the organism causing the empyema is sensitive.

An empyema can often be aborted if these measures are started early enough and the organisms are drug-sensitive. If, however, the intercostal tube is not providing adequate drainage, which can happen when the pus thickens, a short segment of rib is resected, the empyema cavity cleared of pus, and a wide-bore tube inserted to allow prolonged drainage.

2. **Chronic**: If the diagnosis is made before any drainage procedure is carried out it may be feasible to resect the empyema sac in toto, provided the patient is fairly fit and the underlying lung is healthy. 'Decortication' may be required if open drainage has been performed, and re-expansion of the lung is prevented by gross thickening of the visceral pleura. This procedure allows the lung to re-expand to fill the pleural space.

Treatment of tuberculous empyema

Antituberculosis chemotherapy must be started immediately and the pus in the pleural space should be aspirated through a wide-bore needle until it ceases to re-accumulate. In many patients no other treatment is necessary but surgery is occasionally required to ablate a residual empyema space.

SPONTANEOUS PNEUMOTHORAX

Aetiology

The two chief causes of spontaneous pneumothorax are:

1. rupture of a subpleural emphysematous bulla or pleural bleb, or of the pulmonary end of a pleural adhesion
2. rupture of a subpleural tuberculous focus into the pleural space.

   The first cause is very much more common in Britain. Other conditions which rarely give rise to pneumothorax include staphylococcal lung abscess, pulmonary infarction and bronchial carcinoma.

Pathology

There are three types of spontaneous pneumothorax (Fig. 6.37):

1. **Closed**: The communication between pleura and lung seals off as the lung deflates and does not reopen. The air is gradually absorbed and the lung re-expands (Fig. 6.37A).
2. **Open**: The communication is generally with a bronchus (bronchopleural fistula) and does not seal off when the lung collapses. The air pressure in the pleural space approximates to atmospheric pressure both on inspiration and expiration and the lung cannot re-expand. Moreover, the large bronchial communication facilitates the transmission of infection from the air passages into the pleural space and empyema is a common complication. The term 'open' is also applied to a pneumothorax resulting from a penetrating wound of the chest wall (Fig. 6.37B).
3. **Tension (valvular)**: The communication between pleura and lung persists but is small and acts as a one-way valve which allows air to enter the pleural space during inspiration and coughing but prevents it from escaping. Very large amounts of air may be trapped in the pleural space and the intrapleural pressure may rise to well above atmospheric levels. This causes not only compression of the underlying deflated lung but also mediastinal displacement towards the opposite side with consequent compression of the opposite lung (Fig. 6.37C).

Clinical features

The onset is usually sudden, with pain or a feeling of tightness on the affected side of the chest that may be aggravated by deep breathing. The patient becomes increasingly breathless and in severe cases cyanosed. Physical signs in the chest are of air in the pleural space (p. 318) but when the pneumothorax is small and localised there may be no abnormal signs and it may be revealed only by a radiograph.

Closed spontaneous pneumothorax

Breathlessness, which is seldom severe unless there is underlying bronchopulmonary disease, gradually abates over the course of a few days. Progressive spontaneous absorption of air takes place and re-expansion of the lung is usually complete within a few weeks depending upon the initial size of the pneumothorax. Pleural infection is uncommon in this type of pneumothorax.

Open spontaneous pneumothorax

This usually follows rupture of an emphysematous bulla, or a small pleural bleb, or a tuberculous cavity, or a lung

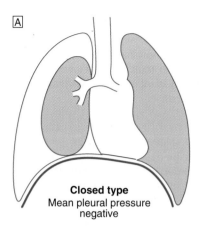

Closed type
Mean pleural pressure
negative

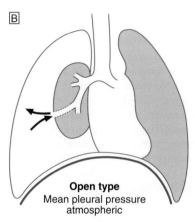

Open type
Mean pleural pressure
atmospheric

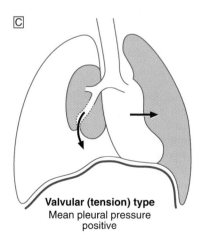

Valvular (tension) type
Mean pleural pressure
positive

Fig. 6.37 Types of spontaneous pneumothorax. A closed
type; B open type; C valvular (tension) type.

abscess into the pleural space. The onset is similar to
that of the closed type but breathlessness does not
improve and, when the cause is tuberculosis or lung
abscess, pyrexia and systemic disturbance soon ensue.
There are the physical and radiological signs of air and
fluid in the pleural space. Acid-fast bacilli can be isolated
from the pleural fluid in tuberculosis.

Tension pneumothorax

A tension or valvular pneumothorax produces the most
dramatic clinical picture. Breathlessness is rapidly progressive and is accompanied by central cyanosis. Death
may occur from asphyxia within a few minutes, but
usually the course of events is less rapid and medical
attention can be obtained in time to avert a fatal
outcome.

Recurrent spontaneous pneumothorax

Recurrence of pneumothorax is not uncommon,
especially in patients with emphysematous bullae. Subsequent incidents are usually on the same side.

Radiological examination

The chest radiograph shows a sharply defined edge of
the deflated lung which may be more easily seen, when
the pneumothorax is small, on a film taken in expiration.
There is complete translucency between this and the
chest wall, with no lung markings. The degree of pulmonary deflation varies. Care must be taken to differentiate between large emphysematous bullae and
pneumothorax, especially when radiographs are over-
penetrated. Radiographs also show the degree of mediastinal displacement and give information regarding the
presence or absence of pleural fluid and underlying pulmonary disease.

Management

Closed spontaneous pneumothorax

The patient is asymptomatic or only has slight breathlessness when the pneumothorax is small, and no treatment is required but radiographic observation should be
continued until re-expansion of the lung is complete. If
the pneumothorax is large and there is breathlessness it
is essential to employ more active measures. Rapid and
complete re-expansion of the lung is obtained by inserting a catheter into the pleural cavity through an intercostal space and connecting it to a water-seal drainage
system or a non-return (Heimlich) valve. In this type of
pneumothorax evacuation of air can be attempted using
a syringe and needle, a three-way tap and an underwater-
seal system.

Specific chemotherapy should be started immediately
if a tuberculous aetiology is suspected. The fluid may

be drained through the catheter, if a pleural effusion develops, by suitable posturing or aspirated with a needle and syringe.

Open spontaneous pneumothorax

There is a large bronchopleural fistula and pleural infection can rapidly supervene. Such patients are less amenable to medical treatment and the expertise of a thoracic surgeon is often required.

Tension pneumothorax

This constitutes an acute medical emergency. An intercostal catheter is immediately connected to a waterseal drainage system. Symptomatic relief is prompt and dramatic. A wide-bore plastic cannula should be used instead of an intercostal catheter if suitable equipment or medical expertise for this procedure is not immediately available. This should be attached to a length of tubing, the end of which should be placed underwater in a bottle or basin.

Recurrent spontaneous pneumothorax

Recurrent pneumothorax, particularly if bilateral, should be treated by obliteration of at least one pleural space. This can be achieved by introduction of an irritant substance such as kaolin, or by pleural abrasion or parietal pleurectomy at thoracotomy.

DISEASES OF THE DIAPHRAGM

Abnormalities of the diaphragm are common and may be congenital or acquired. Both hemidiaphragms are displaced downwards and functionally impaired by diseases which cause pulmonary hyperinflation, notably emphysema (p. 334). Diaphragmatic function can also be impaired in neuromuscular disorders, connective tissue diseases and skeletal deformities such as thoracic scoliosis. Paralysis of the diaphragm is usually unilateral and caused by lesions of one phrenic nerve. Bilateral hemidiaphragm weakness or paralysis can occur in polyneuropathies, the most common being the Guillain-Barré syndrome (infective polyneuropathy).

CONGENITAL DISORDERS

Diaphragmatic hernias

Congenital defects of the diaphragm can allow herniation of abdominal viscera. Posteriorly-situated hernias through the foramen of Bochdalek are more common than anterior hernias through the foramen of Morgagni.

Eventration of the diaphragm

Abnormal elevation of one hemidiaphragm, more often the left, results from total or partial absence of muscular development of the septum transversum. Most eventrations are asymptomatic and are detected by chance on radiograph in adult life, but severe respiratory distress can be caused in infancy if the diaphragmatic muscular defect is extensive.

Other oesophageal abnormalities

Defects of the oesophageal hiatus, congenital absence and duplication of the diaphragm. The diaphragm may be involved in most primary muscle disorders.

ACQUIRED DISORDERS

Diaphragmatic paralysis

Phrenic nerve damage leading to paralysis of a hemidiaphragm is most often produced by bronchial carcinoma (p. 375) but can also be the result of a number of neurological disorders, injury or disease of cervical vertebrae and tumours of the cervical cord. Trauma to the neck, including birth injuries, surgery and stretching of the phrenic nerve by mediastinal masses and aortic aneurysms may also lead to diaphragmatic paralysis. Sometimes no cause can be found.

Paralysis of one hemidiaphragm results in loss of approximately 20% of ventilatory capacity, but this is not usually noticed by otherwise healthy individuals.

Diagnosis is suggested by elevation of the hemidiaphragm on chest radiograph and is confirmed by screening or ultrasonography which show paradoxical movement of the paralysed hemidiaphragm on sniffing.

Other acquired diaphragmatic disorders

Hiatus hernia is common (p. 416) and diaphragmatic rupture usually caused by a crush injury may not be detected until years after the injury. Peripheral neuropathies of any type can involve the diaphragm, as can disorders affecting the anterior horn cells, e.g. poliomyelitis. Connective tissue disorders such as systemic lupus erythematosus, and hypothyroidism and hyperthyroidism, may cause diaphragmatic weakness. Respiratory disorders which cause pulmonary hyperinflation e.g. emphysema, and those which result in small stiff lungs, e.g. diffuse pulmonary fibrosis, decrease diaphragmatic efficiency and predispose to fatigue. Severe skeletal deformity such as kyphosis cause gross distortion of diaphragmatic muscle configuration and gross mechanical disadvantage.

CAUSES OF ELEVATION OF A HEMIDIAPHRAGM

- Phrenic nerve paralysis
- Eventration of the diaphragm
- Decrease in volume of one lung, e.g. lobectomy, unilateral pulmonary fibrosis
- Severe pleuritic pain
- Pulmonary infarction
- Subphrenic abscess
- Large volume of gas in the stomach or colon
- Large tumours or cysts of the liver

DEFORMITIES OF THE CHEST WALL

THORACIC KYPHOSCOLIOSIS

Abnormalities of alignment of the dorsal spine and its consequent effects on thoracic shape may be caused by:

- congenital abnormality
- vertebral disease including tuberculosis, osteoporosis and ankylosing spondylitis
- trauma
- neuromuscular disease such as poliomyelitis.

Simple kyphosis causes less pulmonary embarrassment than kyphoscoliosis.

Kyphoscoliosis, if severe, restricts and distorts expansion of the chest wall, causing maldistribution of the ventilation and blood flow in the lungs. Patients with severe deformity may develop Type II respiratory failure, pulmonary hypertension and right ventricular failure; survival beyond middle age is uncommon. The tempo of deterioration is often accelerated by bacterial infection in the bronchi and lungs.

PECTUS CARINATUM

Pectus carinatum (pigeon chest) is almost always caused by severe asthma during childhood. Very occasionally this deformity can be produced by rickets or occurs without any obvious explanation.

PECTUS EXCAVATUM

In pectus excavatum (funnel chest) the body of the sternum, usually only the lower end, is curved backwards. The heart is displaced to the left and may be compressed between the sternum and the vertebral column but only rarely is there associated disturbance of cardiac function. The deformity may restrict chest expansion and reduce vital capacity. The impairment of cardiac or pulmonary function is seldom sufficient to warrant surgical correction but an operation may be indicated for cosmetic reasons.

D. J. C. Shearman

Diseases of the alimentary tract and pancreas

THE ALIMENTARY TRACT

The alimentary tract is a coordinated structure with the function of ingesting and absorbing nutrients and excreting unabsorbed and waste products. It should not be regarded as a series of separate organs since the role of each component is closely related to that of other parts of the tract.

CONTROLLING AND COORDINATING MECHANISMS

The enteric nervous system

The wall of the gut contains millions of enteric neurons which are organised into two major plexuses, the myenteric (Auerbach's) plexus and the submucous (Meissner's) plexus. The former is situated between the circular and longitudinal muscle and is continuous from the upper oesophagus to the anus, while the latter is present continuously only in the small and large intestines. Many pharmacologically active substances are released by these enteric neurons to transmit messages within the plexuses or to epithelial, secretory or muscle cells; the most universal of these are acetylcholine, substance P and vasoactive intestinal peptide, although many others including some opioids have been demonstrated. The autonomic nervous system has input into the enteric plexuses via the vagus nerves and their mediator acetylcholine which in general is stimulatory, and via the sympathetic nerves with their mediator norepinephrine which are inhibitory.

Gastrointestinal peptides

These act in concert with the enteric nervous system to control the functions of the gastrointestinal tract.

Many hormones have been described. For example, gastrin, secretin, cholecystokinin and motilin are found in the upper gastrointestinal tract. They stimulate secretion and motility and are released as soon as food is ingested. By contrast peptides located in the ileum and colon such as neurotensin, peptide YY and enteroglucagon are in general inhibitory to secretion and motility and are released when some nutrients reach the distal intestine. Insulin and glucagon which regulate glucose homeostasis are localised to the pancreas.

Paracrine peptides (which act on cells adjacent to the cell producing the peptide), for example somatostatin, are widespread throughout the gastrointestinal tract.

Neurocrine peptides are released from nerve endings and play an important role in the transmission of messages within the myenteric plexuses (see above).

MOTILITY

Oesophagus

The upper oesophageal sphincter is formed by the striated cricopharyngeus muscle which exerts constant tone to keep the sphincter closed except during swallowing. Once the upper oesophageal sphincter relaxes, peristalsis sweeps along the length of the body of the oesophagus. The lowest few centimetres of the oesophagus form the lower oesophageal sphincter. This has a high resting tension which prevents reflux of gastric contents into the oesophagus (p. 416). Normally the sphincter relaxes when the peristalsis is initiated. Residual material is cleared from the lower half of the oesophagus by secondary peristaltic contractions. The sphincter is controlled by nervous and hormonal mechanisms.

Stomach

The normal tonic contraction of the fundus is inhibited by the arrival of food, probably by means of a centrally mediated vagal reflex. The gastric slow wave controls the frequency and direction of antral peristalsis, which is responsible for the thorough mixing of the gastric contents and their progressive emptying into the duodenum. Chemoreceptors for fat and acid and osmoreceptors in the duodenal mucosa control gastric emptying by means of local reflexes and the release of secretin, cholecystokinin and other enteric hormones.

Small intestine

Here the coordination is due to the slow wave initiated by the interstitial cells of Cajal situated between nerve fibres and muscle cells. They are the pacemaker which dictates the times at which any given segment of the gut can contract. The frequency of the slow wave in the duodenum is greater than in the ileum, thus enabling the proximal bowel to override more distal areas. By this means contractions are coordinated both to mix and propel the small bowel content so that all nutrients can be exposed to the absorptive cells. It is thought that the myenteric plexus and the enteric hormones determine the local response to the slow wave so that contractions may or may not occur depending on the state of affairs in the lumen at any one time.

Colon

Two main types of contraction occur in association with two different functions. First, there is segmentation which consists of contraction rings forming and disappearing over long periods; these produce a slow mixing of faeces but no propulsion, thus facilitating the absorption of water and electrolytes. Second, propulsion occurs through 'mass movement', a peristaltic wave which occurs several times a day. This action carries out the second function of the colon, namely the elimination of faeces. All activity in the colon is increased after eating, and defecation is more likely to occur post-prandially. The enteric hormones may be responsible for this activity.

Defecation

The arrival of faecal material in the rectum is followed by relaxation of the rectum. Soon, there is a sensation of fullness and a desire to defecate is recognised. At defecation there is a release of cortical inhibition and a voluntary increase in intra-abdominal pressure; the angle between the rectum and anal canal is straightened and the internal anal sphincter and pelvic floor relax; there is reflex contraction of the pelvic colon and rectum and relaxation of the external anal sphincter.

SECRETION

Gastric secretion

The vagus stimulates acid and pepsin secretion by a direct effect on the parietal and peptic cells and also initiates the release of gastrin from the antrum. More sustained output of this hormone is produced by a rise in pH and by ingested protein. The parietal cell has receptors for gastrin, acetylcholine (vagal stimulation) and for histamine (the H_2-receptor). Each receptor has a secondary messenger system within the parietal cell, but the proton pump H^+K^+adenosine triphosphatase is the final common pathway for acid secretion. Mechanisms are also required to turn off gastric secretion once digestion within the stomach is complete. These are largely the same as those which slow gastric emptying, that is the release of secretin and other enteric hormones and also the presence of a low pH in the gastric antrum which inhibits the further release of gastrin. Intrinsic factor is also secreted by the parietal cell in response to the same stimuli as acid.

Pancreatic secretion

The pancreas produces exocrine secretions which are important for digestion and also endocrine secretions which regulate carbohydrate metabolism. The exocrine tissue, composed of acinar cells grouped in lobules and drained by a duct system, forms almost the entire mass of the gland. The exocrine secretion is discharged into the intestine through the pancreatic duct, which usually enters the duodenum together with the common bile duct at the papilla of Vater (see also p. 475).

Pancreatic juice is an alkaline secretion which is iso-tonic with plasma, the main cations being sodium and potassium while the main anion is bicarbonate which is produced by the cells lining the duct system. The juice also contains enzymes which digest carbohydrate, fat and protein, the main ones being amylase, lipase and trypsin. These enzymes are synthesised by the acinar cells; they all require an alkaline medium for optimal efficiency, so that theoretically digestion may be impaired if the bicarbonate content of the pancreatic juice is reduced. Exocrine pancreatic secretion is stimulated partly through the autonomic nervous system and partly through hormonal mechanisms, particularly secretin and cholecystokinin in response to food. Over 24 hours, 1–3 litres of pancreatic juice are secreted.

The endocrine tissue is composed of specialised cells collected together in the small islets of Langerhans scattered throughout the gland, and accounts for only 1% of the mass of the pancreas. The A cells produce glucagon, the B cells insulin and the D cells gastrin, somatostatin and pancreatic polypeptide.

ABSORPTION

The area for absorption in the small intestine is increased several hundredfold by the presence of villi and microvilli. Under normal circumstances nutrients are transported from the absorptive cell by the lymphatic system (e.g. fat and fat-soluble vitamins) or by the portal venous system (e.g. amino acids and hexoses).

Fat

The digestion and absorption of fat takes place predominantly in the duodenum and upper jejunum. Dietary fat occurs largely in the form of insoluble long-chain triglycerides which are emulsified mechanically in the stomach and by detergents, mainly bile acids, in the small intestine. Bile acids are re-absorbed by the terminal ileum, returned to the liver and re-excreted in the bile—an enterohepatic circulation. Pancreatic lipase hydrolyses the triglycerides to monoglyceride and fatty acids. Pancreatic bicarbonate is required to maintain the optimum pH for this hydrolysis and for the next step in fat absorption, the solubilisation of the monoglycerides and fatty acids by bile acids. This consists of their incorporation into micelles which orientate the fatty acid and monoglyceride in such a way that they can be presented to the intestinal mucosal cell for absorption. After absorption by the enterocyte the monoglycerides are re-esterified with fatty acids to form triglycerides which are coated with phospholipid and protein to form chylomicrons or converted into very low-density lipoproteins. Both chylomicrons and lipoproteins leave the cell via the lymphatic system and are transported into the blood.

Carbohydrate

Dietary carbohydrate is in the form of starch (60%), lactose (10%) and sucrose (30%). These are digested by saccharidases to glucose, galactose and fructose. Glucose and galactose are absorbed into the cell by active transport mechanisms, the process requiring sodium ions and energy. The fructose molecule is too large to move across the cell membrane by simple diffusion and it is thought that its absorption might be facilitated by a carrier.

Protein

Initial hydrolysis of dietary protein molecules is performed by gastric pepsin and pancreatic enzymes. Further hydrolysis of peptides occurs at the brush border and a mixture of peptides and amino acids is absorbed into the cell. A large amount of protein enters the lumen of the gastrointestinal tract each day derived from sources other than dietary, such as various secretions, desquamated cells and the exudation of plasma proteins. These are absorbed by the same mechanisms as dietary protein.

Vitamins

The fat soluble vitamins A, D and K are incorporated into micelles and are then absorbed by passive diffusion, mainly in the proximal jejunum.

Folic acid is absorbed by an active process throughout the length of the small intestine.

Vitamin B_{12} is bound to gastric intrinsic factor. It proceeds along the intestine to the terminal ileum where B_{12} binds to a specific receptor and is absorbed.

Water and electrolytes

Each day 9 litres of water and 800 mmol sodium enter the gastrointestinal tract (Table 7.1) and are subsequently re-absorbed from the jejunum, ileum and

colon, so that finally only 150 ml water is excreted in the stool. In the small intestine and colon there are active transport mechanisms for the absorption of sodium and chloride, and water accompanies this movement. In the colon, these processes ensure that fluid ileal contents are converted into semi-solid faeces.

The cells of the small intestinal crypts also secrete electrolytes and it is this process which is stimulated in cholera (p. 129).

DEFENCE MECHANISMS

The epithelium

The epithelium of the entire gastrointestinal tract provides a barrier which prevents entry to the body by enzymes, hydrogen ions, food antigens and microorganisms. The barrier consists of the plasma membranes of the epithelial cells and the tight junctions between them; their integrity is maintained by a variety of mechanisms. For example, in the case of the stomach (p. 425) the secretion of bicarbonate ions into a surface mucus layer provides an alkaline barrier to the entry of hydrogen ions. Because the integrity of the surface epithelial cell is so important it follows that renewal of ageing or injured cells is an important defensive mechanism. The epithelial cells of the gastrointestinal tract are constantly renewed so that, for example, the epithelial surface of the small intestine is replaced every 48 hours.

The entire epithelium of the gastrointestinal tract is coated with mucus produced by specialised cells within or beneath the epithelium. The gel structure of mucus reduces attrition to the surface epithelium and its carbohydrate structures have a role in the prevention of colonisation by bacteria.

Immunological system

This has an important role in controlling the intestinal bacterial flora and in eliminating any micro-organisms which enter the mucosa. Recognition of antigens is undertaken by the specialised M cells of Peyer's patches. In turn these cells prime lymphoblasts which migrate to, and circulate in, the systemic circulation, to home to the lamina propria of the intestine. B cells then synthesise secretory IgA which is resistant to digestion by intestinal enzymes and has a role in protecting mucosal surfaces from bacterial invasion. The primed T cells return to reside between the epithelial cells as 'intraepithelial' lymphocytes where they have specific cell-mediated immune functions.

Table 7.1 Input of water and electrolytes into the gut in 24 hours				
	Volume (ml)	Sodium (mmol)	Potassium (mmol)	Chloride (mmol)
Diet	2000	150	50	200
Saliva	1000	50	20	40
Gastric secretion	2000	100	15	280
Bile	1000	200	5	40
Pancreatic secretion	2000	150	5	40
Intestinal secretion	1000	150	5	100

INVESTIGATION OF THE ALIMENTARY TRACT

RADIOLOGICAL EXAMINATION

Plain radiographs

These show the normal soft tissue shadows due to the liver, spleen and kidneys and also abnormal shadows. Gas in the intestine acts as a contrast medium so that the distribution of the bowel within the abdomen can be assessed. In obstruction there may be an excessive amount of gas and fluid in the bowel above the obstruction and films with the patient erect will demonstrate fluid levels. Finally, areas of opacification due to stones or to calcification in the liver, pancreas, cysts or blood vessels may provide important diagnostic information.

A chest radiograph will show the diaphragm. Free gas under the diaphragm indicates a perforation but may also be seen for the first few days following a laparotomy. Gas with a fluid level may be associated with a subphrenic abscess. Pulmonary lesions, from which pain may be referred to the abdomen, can also be identified.

Barium studies

These will demonstrate a break in the continuity of the outline of the gut, abnormalities in the appearance of the mucosa and disorders of motility.

The barium swallow and meal examination

Because pharyngeal swallowing is rapid, video recording or rapid sequence films are often necessary. The oesophagus is studied while barium is being swallowed so that it is seen distended with barium. Mucosal films are taken immediately after the barium has passed through the area. The procedure may demonstrate a disorder of motility, a filling defect caused by a tumour or varices, a stricture, a diverticulum or a hiatus hernia (Fig. 7.1).

The mucosa of the stomach is usually examined by a double-contrast study in which a small amount of barium is used together with the introduction of gas to distend the stomach. An ulcer is usually seen face on as a small collection of barium with radiating folds of mucosa (Figs 7.2 and 7.3). It may also appear as a projection beyond the normal outline while tumours cause filling defects. Small cancers can be detected by irregularity in the mucosal pattern. Observation of the motility of the stomach may indicate an inert area caused by infiltrating carcinoma. The duodenal cap is examined by studying its contours when it is completely filled with barium, and its mucosal pattern when it is distended with gas and the mucosa coated with barium.

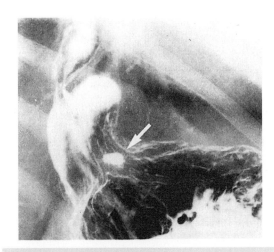

Fig. 7.1 **Hiatus hernia** with an ulcer (arrow) in the herniated portion of the stomach.

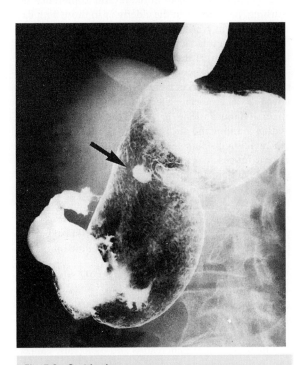

Fig. 7.2 **Gastric ulcer.**

Small bowel meal or follow-through examination

When disease of the small intestine is suspected, barium is observed during its passage through the small intestine and radiographs are taken at intervals. The outline of the barium may indicate structural abnormalities such as diverticula or strictures. When there is malabsorption, excess secretions may cause the barium to clump and flocculate.

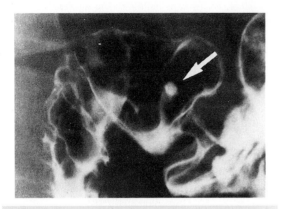

Fig. 7.3 Duodenal ulcer.

Barium enema

This procedure is uncomfortable and sometimes exhausting, particularly in the elderly or in those with cardiac disease in whom arrhythmia may be induced. A barium enema must always have been preceded by digital examination of the rectum and preferably also by sigmoidoscopy a few days earlier. The colon must be meticulously cleared of faeces by means of laxatives followed by a cleansing enema just before the barium enema. Barium alone or, for double-contrast examination, barium and air, is run into the bowel through a self-retaining catheter. Radiographs are taken with the colonic mucosa coated with barium and the lumen distended with air. In this way the colonic mucosa can be studied in detail and polyps or small tumours identified (Fig. 7.19, p. 470). In inflammatory bowel disease mucosal abnormalities are readily recognised (Fig. 7.14, p. 460). In some patients there will be a reflux of barium into the terminal ileum which can be outlined.

Computed tomography (CT) and magnetic resonance imaging (MRI)

CT is an important technique for defining certain intra-abdominal diseases, particularly those involving inaccessible organs or regions. Thus it is used in the diagnosis and management of pancreatitis and pancreatic cancer, and in diagnosing diseases of the retroperitoneal space and lymph nodes. It is also of importance in assessing the spread of tumour, e.g. gastric cancer, so that decisions can be made on whether surgery should be palliative or curative. MRI has not yet proven to be superior to CT for any intra-abdominal diagnostic problem.

Arteriography

In this procedure the coeliac axis, superior and inferior mesenteric arteries are selectively catheterised and con-

trast medium is infused. The procedure is used to detect active bleeding when contrast medium may pool in the lumen, or when bleeding has ceased, vascular abnormalities, e.g. angiodysplasia, may be detected by their characteristic vascular pattern.

Interventional radiology

This term embraces the combined use of imaging techniques to guide catheters or biopsy needles to abdominal masses or fluid collections. Thus small numbers of cells are obtained for cytopathology and cysts and abscesses may be drained without having to proceed to laparotomy.

ULTRASONOGRAPHY

This non-invasive technique, which can be used safely in pregnancy, is of great value in assessing the abdomen. It can be used in the diagnosis of liver, pancreatic and gallbladder disease and to identify ascites.

RADIONUCLIDE IMAGING

This is used in the following circumstances:

- For **imaging** the liver, spleen and biliary tract (p. 494).
- To **assess gastric emptying**. In this assessment a radiolabelled meal is eaten, the liquid being labelled with ^{111m}In DTPA and the solid with ^{99m}Tc-sulphur colloid labelled chicken liver. A scintillation camera records the emptying. The test is used particularly to diagnose gastroparesis (p. 437).
- To **assess inflammatory bowel disease**. A sample of the patient's blood is incubated with ^{99m}Tc which is taken up by the neutrophils and macrophages. On reinjection the labelled cells move to the inflamed bowel where they can be detected by scanning. The labelled cells are also lost into the intestinal lumen through the inflamed mucosa and so the radioactivity in a 48 hour collection of stools gives a measure of the total activity of the disease.
- To **detect Meckel's diverticulum**. ^{99m}Tc pertechnicate is given and is concentrated in gastric mucosa which is usually present in the diverticulum. It is detected by scanning.
- In the **detection of gastrointestinal bleeding**. The patient's red cells are labelled with ^{99m}Tc and are reinjected. Their accumulation at the site of bleeding is detected by scanning over the subsequent 24 hours.

ENDOSCOPY

The oesophagus, stomach, duodenum and colon are easily examined with fibreoptic instruments. Endoscopic instruments can also be used for therapeutic procedures which would otherwise require laparotomy, such as removal of a polyp.

Rigid instruments are used to examine the rectum and lower pelvic colon (sigmoidoscope) and occasionally the oesophagus (oesophagoscope).

Upper alimentary tract

It is usual to carry out the procedure with the patient under sedation, often as an outpatient. After a 12-hour fast the pharynx is anaesthetised with a spray or gargle. The endoscope is passed with the assistance of the patient in swallowing, and the procedure, whilst uncomfortable, should be no more so than any other intubation. Possible complications are perforation of the oesophagus or stomach whilst passing the instrument or during biopsy, the inhalation of secretions, cardiac arrhythmias or arrest, and the transmission of infections. All these are rare when appropriate precautions are used but resuscitation and after-care facilities must be available in endoscopy units.

Where possible, the oesophagus, stomach and duodenum are all inspected at the same examination because the presence of one lesion does not exclude another and double lesions are not uncommon, e.g. oesophagitis and duodenal ulcer. This is particularly important when endoscopy is carried out in patients with haematemesis or melaena because there may be more than one source of bleeding. In therapeutic endoscopy, the bleeding lesion is directly coagulated (p. 440).

Oesophagoscopy

This should be performed when there is dysphagia or when barium examination suggests a tumour or stricture. Other indications include suspected oesophagitis, varices or a motility disorder. Therapeutic procedures that can be carried out include dilatation of a stricture and injection of sclerosing material into oesophageal varices to control bleeding.

Gastroscopy

This is always indicated when a gastric ulcer has been demonstrated on barium studies so that biopsies can be taken to exclude malignancy; subsequent healing of the ulcer should also be confirmed. Gastroscopy is also necessary following a haematemesis, when there is upper abdominal pain or dyspepsia, and in the investigation of patients with symptoms after gastric surgery because the appearances are difficult to define radiologically.

Endoscopic retrograde cholangiopancreatography (ERCP)

At duodenoscopy the papilla of Vater is cannulated with a fine-bore catheter passed through the shaft of the instrument and radio-opaque dye is injected into the biliary and pancreatic ducts. The procedure is of great value in patients suspected of having pancreatic disease because distortion or obstruction of the ductal system may indicate a diagnosis of chronic pancreatitis or pancreatic carcinoma. It is of value in the diagnosis of pancreas divisum (p. 475). Obstruction or distortion of the common bile duct by a stone or a tumour can also be demonstrated and sphincterotomy can be performed to allow removal of stones.

Lower alimentary tract

Proctoscopy and sigmoidoscopy

These simple procedures should always be carried out in patients with symptoms referable to the lower bowel or anus. Both terms are inaccurate because proctoscopy visualises the anal canal and only 2–3 cm of the rectum, and sigmoidoscopy examines the rectum and the lower few centimetres of the pelvic colon. It is usual to perform the procedures without preparation but if the rectum contains faeces endoscopy must be repeated after the bowel has been emptied. Digital examination of the rectum should always precede endoscopy and the instruments should be warmed and well lubricated. Proctoscopy is used for the demonstration and injection of haemorrhoids. Sigmoidoscopy is necessary for the diagnosis of polyps, cancer of the rectum, ulcerative proctitis or colitis and Crohn's disease of the large bowel. Biopsy of the mucosa or a lesion may also be taken.

Colonoscopy

The fibreoptic colonoscope permits inspection of the entire colon but the procedure is time-consuming and occasionally difficult. More often a short colonoscope (flexible sigmoidoscope) is used to examine the sigmoid and left colon where most lesions occur. The bowel must be carefully prepared. During colonoscopy it is possible to take a biopsy of suspicious lesions and polyps can be removed using a diathermy snare.

Radiology or endoscopy?

The investigation of the oesophagus, stomach, duodenum and colon can be undertaken with either technique; how is the choice made?

Endoscopy has become the procedure of choice in examining the upper gastrointestinal tract because biopsies of lesions can be obtained. In addition it is much more accurate in the investigation of haematemesis and melaena. However, radiology has a role in the investigation of motility disorders of the oesophagus, particularly pharyngeal disorders. It is also of value when endoscopy has encountered technical difficulties due to strictures and hernias.

For the investigation of the colon, colonoscopy is time-consuming and fails to examine the entire colon in a proportion of cases. Thus radiology retains a significant role for this reason alone. Conversely, the colonoscope is better than radiology for examination of the recto-sigmoid region.

OTHER INVESTIGATIONS

Biopsy

The biopsy of lesions is an essential part of each endoscopic procedure. Biopsy of the small intestine is indicated if malabsorption is suspected and is carried out by means of the Crosby capsule. Because this is time-consuming, biopsy of the distal duodenum at endoscopy is often carried out in preference.

Secretory studies

The pentagastrin test

The acid output is measured in response to pentagastrin, a synthetic pentapeptide which exerts the biological effects of gastrin. Preparation consists of an overnight fast. H_2-receptor antagonist drugs must be stopped for at least 48 hours before the test and omeprazole seven days before. The fasting contents of the stomach are aspirated and their volume measured; then the secretions are collected continuously for one hour. This is termed the 'basal acid ouptut'. Pentagastrin is then injected subcutaneously and the gastric secretions are collected for a further hour. The acid output in this hour is termed the 'maximum acid output'.

USE OF THE PENTAGASTRIN TEST

- a large volume of fasting juice indicates obstruction of the gastric outlet
- a very high basal acid output suggests that the patient has the Zollinger–Ellison syndrome (p. 431)
- in patients with peptic ulcer it provides a preoperative base line
- achlorhydria can be demonstrated

The insulin test

This is used after gastric surgery to indicate the completeness of vagotomy.

Tests of exocrine pancreatic function

These are used to demonstrate exocrine insufficiency when diarrhoea or steatorrhoea is present in chronic pancreatitis or cystic fibrosis.

Exocrine function may be measured directly by passing a tube into the second part of the duodenum and collecting the secretory output of the gland in response to exogenous stimulation (secretin-cholecystokinin test) or endogenous stimulation by a meal (Lundh test). In the **secretin-cholecystokinin test** the hormones are injected intravenously and pancreatic secretions are collected for 1 hour. Measurements are made of the volume of secretion and the concentration of bicarbonate and amylase or lipase. A special double-lumen tube allows gastric and pancreatic secretions to be collected separately to prevent neutralisation of pancreatic bicarbonate by gastric hydrochloric acid. The **Lundh** test is simpler. A tube is passed into the duodenum and a liquid meal of fixed composition is given orally. The duodenal aspirate is collected by syphonage and the concentration of trypsin and amylase is recorded. Both tests detect the presence of established pancreatic insufficiency but usually provide no information as to the cause.

There is a variety of simple non-invasive tests of pancreatic function such as the **bentiromide** and **pancreolauryl tests** which depend upon the cleavage of an orally given marker by pancreatic enzyme and its excretion in the urine. Alternatively, serum trypsin-like immunoreactivity or serum isoamylase determinations may be made. When normal values for these tests are obtained, pancreatic insufficiency is excluded.

Tests for malabsorption

These are summarised in Table 7.2. Some are discussed in more detail below.

Bacteriological studies

The malabsorption syndrome (p. 451) may be due occasionally to bacterial colonisation of the small intestine. When this is suspected, intestinal secretion can be obtained for bacteriological studies by passing a fine sterile tube into the upper small intestine. A mercury bag attached to the tip of the tube ensures that the tube moves rapidly to the correct site. The patient should not be receiving antibiotics.

Breath tests

These are safe, simple, non-invasive methods of assessing absorption. Each test depends upon the metabolism by intestinal bacteria of a nutrient which may be labelled radioactively, followed by exhalation of radioactive metabolite carbon dioxide or hydrogen which is measured in the breath.

When lactose is ingested and remains unabsorbed, it is metabolised to hydrogen and there is a rise in hydrogen excretion in the breath.

When ^{14}C-xylose is given orally, $^{14}CO_2$ is excreted in excess if the small intestine is colonised with bacteria.

When cholyl-^{14}C glycine is given orally it is also metabolised to $^{14}CO_2$ by bacteria in the small intestine.

Table 7.2 Tests for malabsorption

	Test	Normal values
Fat	**Measurement of fat in a 5-day collection of stool** **SeHCAT test** This synthetic bile acid is given orally and its retention measured at 7 days by whole body counting	Excretion of less than 7g (22 mmol) per day Retention of more than 90% Severe ileal dysfunction = retention of less than 20%
Carbohydrate	**Xylose absorption test** 5 g xylose is given orally, and the urine is collected for 5 hours **Hydrogen breath test** 50 g lactose is given orally and breath hydrogen is measured every hour for 4 hours (see below)	Excretion of at least 2 g Less than 10ppm above baseline in any sample
Protein	**Faecal clearance of endogenous α_1-antitrypsin** This normal serum protein is excreted unchanged in the stool when there is any protein loss into the stool and is therefore measured in a 3-day collection of stool	No α_1-antitrypsin in the stool
Vitamins	**Vitamin B$_{12}$ absorption** 0.5 μg of radiolabelled vitamin B$_{12}$ is given orally followed 2 hours later by 1000 μg of non-radioactive vitamin B$_{12}$ given by intramuscular injection. Urine is collected for 24 hours	More than 16% of radioactivity appears in the urine
Breath tests	^{14}C-Xylose Cholyl-^{14}C-glycine Lactose H$_2$ (50 g orally)	$<0.0013\%$ of administered dose at 30 min $<1\%$ of administered dose within 4 hours <20 ppm rise in breath H$_2$ within 3 hours
Small intestinal culture **Small intestinal biopsy**		$<10^5$ organisms/ml (See Table 7.13)

Motility studies

Barium examination provides a poor demonstration of the motility of the oesophagus, stomach and small intestine. The isotope ^{99m}TC sulphur colloid incorporated into a solid or liquid bolus can be used to measure transit down the oesophagus. Radioactive markers incorporated into solid food and liquids are also used to measure emptying of the stomach (p. 410). Small intestinal motility can be estimated by administering a non-absorbable carbohydrate, and hydrogen gas excreted in the breath is measured. Motility can be studied more accurately by measuring the pressure changes in the lumen of the organ but this manometry is of diagnostic value only for oesophageal disorders.

Examination of the stool

In malabsorption the stool may be pale and frothy; in the irritable bowel syndrome it may be like pellets or ribbon with or without mucus. In mild ulcerative disease of the colon there may be flecks of blood in the mucus. Inspection of the stool is sufficient to diagnose fresh bleeding from the lower alimentary tract while the loss of over 60 ml of blood from a site proximal to the ascending colon will produce a black tarry stool. Microscopic examination is of value particularly in distinguishing amoebic dysentery and other parasitic diseases.

Faecal occult blood tests

Tests for occult blood using the guaiac test or immunological techniques detect small amounts in the stool and are performed for several successive days because bleeding from the gastrointestinal tract is often intermittent. Specimens obtained on the fingerstall at rectal examination can be readily examined.

Guaiac is a colourless compound which becomes coloured in the presence of peroxidase-like substances such as haemoglobin. It forms the basis of many commercial tests. It is positive to bleeding at any level in the gastrointestinal tract and so is the initial test of choice when occult bleeding is suspected. An immunological test detects only bleeding from the colon.

DISEASES OF THE MOUTH

DISORDERS OF THE TEETH

Mastication of food to a soft pulp is a prerequisite for good digestion. Inadequate mastication may cause dyspepsia. The teeth should be inspected to determine if they are healthy, present in adequate numbers and in correct apposition in the upper and lower jaws to allow efficient mastication. If dentures are worn it should be ascertained if they are comfortable and efficient.

Septicaemia may have its source in gingivitis or an apical abscess and is particularly liable to occur after dental manipulation. It may cause bacterial endocarditis in patients with valvular disease of the heart. All patients should be advised to consult a dentist regularly to conserve their teeth and to prevent or treat foci of infection in the mouth.

STOMATITIS

The mouth harbours a population of commensal microorganisms which normally is controlled by a reasonable standard of oral hygiene; if this is neglected the bacterial population may proliferate and cause stomatitis. Stomatitis may also occur when resistance to the commensal population is lowered by disease, especially in the immune-compromised host. Stomatitis may also be due to nutritional deficiencies or other factors.

ULCERATIVE STOMATITIS (VINCENT'S INFECTION)

This occurs mainly in adults with malnutrition and poor dental hygiene. Ulcers with ragged necrotic margins occur especially on the gums, but may involve the palate, the lips or the inner aspects of the cheeks; the ulcers are covered by a grey slough surrounded by an erythematous margin. A stained smear shows many spirochaetes and fusiform bacilli; these organisms are present in small numbers in the normal commensal population of the mouth and the condition may be regarded as an endogenous infection due to impairment of host resistance. The condition is infectious, so that the patient's food vessels and cutlery should be sterilised.

It is treated with metronidazole (200 mg 8-hourly for 4 days), or penicillin.

VIRAL INFECTIONS

Herpes simplex type I may cause the recurrent problem of herpes labialis in normal individuals. It can cause a much more severe stomatitis in AIDS (p. 99).

CANDIDOSIS

The fungus *Candida albicans* (p. 142) is a normal commensal in the mouth but it may proliferate to cause **thrush** in babies, in the aged and particularly in debilitated patients. Thrush is also common in those receiving prolonged treatment with oral antibiotics and in patients who are immunosuppressed by corticosteroids or AIDS.

White patches appear on the tongue and buccal mucosa and may enlarge and coalesce to form an easily detached membrane; there is little surrounding inflammation. In severe infection the pharynx and oesophagus may be affected, causing dysphagia (p. 415).

Treatment is discussed on p. 144.

STOMATITIS DUE TO DEFICIENCY OF NUTRITIONAL FACTORS

This may arise directly from an insufficient intake or indirectly as a result of impaired absorption of vitamins, especially niacin, riboflavin, folic acid and vitamin B_{12}. When the deficiency is acute and severe the tongue is red, raw and painful because of atrophy of the papillae. The tongue appears moist and unduly clean when the deficiency is chronic and less severe. Angular stomatitis often accompanies glossitis especially in the case of gross iron deficiency. In severe vitamin C deficiency the gums become swollen and spongy and bleed readily.

APHTHOUS ULCERATION

This is a common recurrent condition of unknown aetiology characterised by painful superficial ulcers in the mouth. The lesion begins as an indurated erythematous area followed in a day or so by ulceration. The ulcers are often multiple and remain painful for about a week before healing commences. They may recur every few weeks. Emotional stress may precipitate an attack, and in some women ulcers tend to recur in cyclical fashion during the premenstrual phase. While most patients are otherwise healthy, severe chronic aphthous ulceration may be found in association with Crohn's disease, ulcerative colitis, coeliac disease and Behçet's syndrome.

Hydrocortisone hemisuccinate lozenges (2.5 mg 8-hourly) may be effective in the early phase of lesions. Pain can be reduced with topical anaesthetics and secondary infection controlled with tetracycline mouth washes. A suspension of sucralfate (p. 429) may be tried to help healing.

OTHER FORMS OF STOMATITIS

An allergic reaction to chemicals in toothpaste, dentures, foodstuffs and many drugs, especially antibiotics, can cause stomatitis. A characteristic blue-black punctate line may be seen where the gum margins adjoin the teeth in lead poisoning. Skin diseases such as lichen planus, pemphigus and erythema multiforme involve the mouth sometimes before being seen on the skin. Stomatitis may be a manifestation of blood dyscrasias.

DISEASES OF THE TONGUE

In health the tongue is moist with only a slight white fur on the dorsum. The papillae are readily seen. Mouth breathing causes a dry tongue, but otherwise dryness of the tongue is an indication of dehydration. The tongue may be coated with whitish-yellow fur in those who smoke excessively but, in general, the presence of fur on the tongue has little clinical significance.

Glossitis

Glossitis may be a prominent feature of stomatitis resulting from nutritional deficiency.

Geographical tongue

This is the name given to a chronic migrating superficial glossitis; it looks odd but has no clinical significance.

Leukoplakia

Leukoplakia is a chronic condition characterised by white, firm, smooth patches beginning at the side of the tongue and later spreading over the dorsum. In the early stages the tongue is not painful but later the patches are split by fissures with resultant tenderness. The significance of leukoplakia is that it may precede the development of carcinoma. A biopsy of such lesions should always be undertaken. Hairy leukoplakia occurs in AIDS (p. 99).

Squamous carcinoma

In the mouth and tongue this is often related to excessive consumption of tobacco and alcohol and poor oral hygiene. It must be considered in all cases of chronic ulcer of the tongue and biopsy should be performed.

Kaposi's sarcoma

This is common in AIDS: see page 97.

Syphilis

Syphilis may present as a painful solitary ulcer usually on the tongue or palate.

Skin diseases

Tongue and oral ulceration occur in epidermolysis bullosa, pemphigus, pemphigoid and erythema multiforme. Lichen planus may also involve the mouth with white streaks and tiny papules.

FUNCTIONAL DISORDERS

Glossodynia refers to a painful tongue and glossopyrosis is a sensation of burning in the tongue. Burning may also occur in the gums and throat. If the tongue looks normal on inspection the cause is usually an underlying depression.

A complaint of a bad taste in the mouth is occasionally due to drugs or sinusitis but is usually a reflection of anxiety or depression. Halitosis, the complaint of bad breath, may be due to poor oral hygiene or to systemic disorders such as liver failure, uraemia or diabetes. The presence of halitosis should be confirmed by the physician. If it cannot be confirmed, the cause is likely to be psychological.

DISEASES OF THE SALIVARY GLANDS

XEROSTOMIA (DRYNESS OF THE MOUTH)

This may be due to dehydration or may be caused by anticholinergic or antidepressant drugs; but commonly it is due to anxiety. Xerostomia is one of the features of Sjögren's syndrome (p. 919). Excessive salivary secretion (ptyalism) may be a response to irritation or inflammation in the mouth, for example oral sepsis.

PAROTITIS

Parotitis may be due to the virus of mumps or a bacterial infection of the gland. The latter tends to develop during severe febrile illnesses or after major abdominal operations if adequate attention is not given to oral hygiene and to the prevention of dehydration and infection. The treatment consists of the parenteral administration of penicillin and surgical drainage if abscess formation has occurred.

Sarcoidosis is another cause of enlargement of the parotid glands.

SALIVARY CALCULI

These occur occasionally in the submandibular gland or its duct. They cause pain and swelling brought on by eating. Infection of the gland is a complication. Stones in the duct can be felt in the floor of the mouth and are removed by incision over the duct. Stones in the gland may require excision of the gland.

A 'MIXED' SALIVARY TUMOUR

This presents as a slow, painless enlargement of one salivary gland. The tumour is essentially of epithelial origin but may contain stromal elements and shows a variable degree of malignant change. It is treated either by excision or excision and radiotherapy.

DISEASES OF THE OESOPHAGUS

SYMPTOMS OF OESOPHAGEAL DISEASE

Dysphagia

Dysphagia is defined as difficulty in swallowing. Its causes are listed in Table 7.3 and are conveniently classi-

Table 7.3 Aetiology of dysphagia

Oral (painful mastication)	Oesophageal
Stomatitis	* Reflux oesophagitis or stricture
Aphthous ulceration	* Carcinoma (including carcinoma of cardia)
Candidosis	* Motility disorders (achalasia, diffuse spasm)
Herpes simplex	Dermatomyositis and scleroderma
Tonsillitis	Chagas' disease
Oral malignancy	Webs and rings, Sideropenic dysphagia, Lower oesophageal ring
	Candidiasis, herpes simplex
Pharyngeal	Mediastinal mass, Goitre, Bronchogenic carcinoma, Aortic aneurysm, Dilated left atrium
* Following cerebrovascular accident	Foreign bodies
Bulbar and pseudobulbar palsy	
Motor neurone disease	
Myasthenia gravis	
* Pharyngeal malignancy	
Pharyngeal diverticulum	
Globus hystericus	
* denotes most important cause	

fied into oral, pharyngeal and oesophageal. The oral causes are usually painful conditions of the oropharynx. With pharyngeal causes, dysphagia occurs immediately swallowing is attempted, and tracheal aspiration may cause coughing and laryngismus. In oesophageal dysphagia, there is a sensation of food sticking. When food does stick, relief is obtained by regurgitation or by sipping liquids until obstruction is relieved by the impacted bolus moving onwards. Sometimes the sensation of dysphagia is induced by food passing an abnormal area in the oesophagus without actual obstruction occurring. Dysphagia for solid food usually indicates organic obstruction. Dysphagia for both solids and liquids, which may be intermittent, suggests a motility disorder.

Painful dysphagia (odynophagia)

The usual cause is the bolus of food passing through an inflamed segment of the oesophagus. The cause of the inflammation may be severe reflux oesophagitis or an infection due to Candida or to herpes simplex. Some tablets may disintegrate in the lower oesophagus to cause local inflammation, ulceration and painful dysphagia.

Heartburn

This is a sensation of burning or a burning pain located high in the epigastrium or behind the lower end of the sternum often radiating upwards behind the sternum. Patients may indicate their discomfort with upward movements of the fingers over the chest. Heartburn is a common occasional symptom in the community but is prominent in reflux oesophagitis when the mucosa is inflamed (p. 418).

Oesophageal pain

Oesophageal pain is felt in dermatomes C8 to T10 which overlap with pain arising in the heart, stomach and biliary tree. It is well recognised that in some patients oeso-

phageal pain is impossible to distinguish from that of myocardial ischaemia. Thus oesophageal pain can be a central chest pain radiating to the neck, jaws and arms. Reflux oesophagitis or a motility disorder may cause such pain but sometimes no cause is found despite thorough investigation.

Regurgitation

This is the effortless return of gastric or oesophageal content into the mouth. Gastric content has a bitter taste, whereas oesophageal content regurgitated because of oesophageal obstruction is not bitter.

GASTRO-OESOPHAGEAL REFLUX AND HIATUS HERNIA

REFLUX OESOPHAGITIS

Oesophageal defence mechanisms

The lower oesophageal sphincter, which is a localised area of specialised smooth muscle sited at the distal end of the oesophagus, is the main barrier to reflux. This sphincter is normally contracted, thus creating a zone of high pressure so preventing the passage of gastric content into the oesophagus. In normal subjects the oesophageal sphincter relaxes during swallowing, but at other times there are spontaneous transient relaxations. Thus gastro-oesophageal reflux occurs to some degree in all individuals. In those with reflux oesophagitis, reflux is increased because the normal or resting pressure of the sphincter is reduced and the number of transient relaxations is increased.

Because the sphincter is normally situated below the diaphragm (Fig. 7.4A), its high pressure is reinforced by intra-abdominal pressure; moreover, the oblique entry

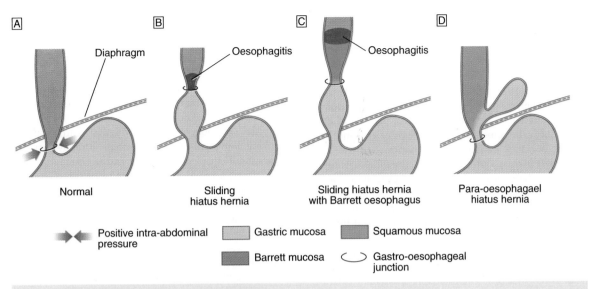

Fig. 7.4 **Hiatus hernia**, different types and Barrett's oesophagus.

of the oesophagus into the stomach ensures that the intra-abdominal oesophagus is closed when the stomach is distended. These mechanisms are lost when the lower oesophageal sphincter moves proximally to be situated above the diaphragm (Fig. 7.4B).

Once reflux has occurred, rapid clearance of acid from the oesophagus into the stomach limits its contact with the oesophageal mucosa. Effective clearance depends upon secondary peristalsis and the presence of saliva and is enhanced by the erect position. It is impaired in the supine position. Finally, the renewal and repair mechanisms of the oesophageal mucosa are important in preventing oesophageal damage.

Aetiology

The disorder may be defined as damage to the oesophageal mucosa due to the reflux of gastric contents. The injury is caused nearly always by hydrogen ions but pepsin and conjugated bile salts (refluxed from the duodenum) may play a role. Occasionally, when the patient is incapable of secreting acid, for example after gastric surgery, pancreatic enzymes and deconjugated bile salts may be the injurious agents.

Increased reflux of gastric contents into the oesophagus from reduced pressure in the lower oesophageal sphincter and an increased number of transient relaxations of the sphincter are the main factors in the development of reflux oesophagitis. Nevertheless there are many additional factors which may promote reflux (Table 7.4); some may have aetiological significance, whilst it is important to recognise the significance of others in management.

Role of hiatus hernia

A sliding hiatus hernia (Fig. 7.4B) is extremely common in the community and most of these individuals are asymptomatic and do not have reflux oesophagitis. However, most patients with oesophagitis do have a hiatus hernia which contributes to the impaired function of the lower oesophageal sphincter.

Incidence

Reflux oesophagitis is relatively common in Western countries, being present in 10% or more of patients undergoing endoscopy for upper gastrointestinal symptoms, an incidence similar to that of peptic ulcer.

Clinical features

There is a poor correlation between the severity of oesophageal symptoms and the degree of oesophagitis. Severe symptoms may be present and investigations may confirm reflux, yet oesophagitis is minimal or absent; in other patients, for example diabetics and the elderly, oesophageal symptoms may be absent despite severe oesophagitis and the patient may present with iron deficiency anaemia due to slow blood loss from the damaged mucosa.

Heartburn is the characteristic symptom. It occurs after meals and characteristically is brought on by bending and by lifting or straining due to an increase in the intra-abdominal pressure. Heartburn may also occur on lying down in bed at night, preventing sleep or awakening the patient several hours after the onset of sleep. It is sometimes precipitated immediately by acid food or drink—tomatoes, orange juice, cola—and by alcohol, especially fortified wines and spirits. Usually it is rapidly relieved by antacids. On occasions swallowing may be painful (odynophagia).

Oesophagitis may cause chest pain indistinguishable in character from cardiac pain but the time of the onset of pain may provide an important clue to its origin, for example when reflux occurs after meals and on bending.

Regurgitation of gastric content into the mouth may occur during bending, after large meals or at night. The patient becomes aware of regurgitation because of a bitter taste in the mouth or stains on the pillow. At night there may be aspiration into the trachea with laryngismus, coughing and aspiration pneumonia. Regurgitation may contribute to bronchitis and asthma. Sore throat, globus sensation ('lump in throat') and hoarseness are other consequences.

In long-standing oesophagitis the inflamed squamous mucosa may change to columnar or Barrett's mucosa (Fig. 7.4C) which is potentially pre-malignant because it is associated with an increased incidence of adenocarcinoma of the oesophagus. Oesophageal ulcers may occur, usually in the columnar mucosa close to the junction between squamous and columnar mucosa.

Transient dysphagia for solids in reflux oesophagitis may be the consequence of disordered motility. If the symptom persists a stricture may have developed, usually at the junction of columnar and squamous mucosa, or a tumour may have occurred within the columnar mucosa.

Investigations

The problem is investigated by endoscopy and biopsy of the oesophageal mucosa. The visual appearance of the mucosa in oesophagitis shows, with increasing severity, erythema, friability, exudate, erosions and bleeding. Ulcer, stricture and Barrett's mucosa are also detected.

When the visual changes are minimal or absent, biopsy may show evidence of inflammation; biopsy is also used to look for malignant change in Barrett's mucosa and in strictures. Barium studies are of particular value to assess an oesophageal stricture and ulcer but are of less value than endoscopy in assessing the characteristic mucosal changes of oesophagitis.

In a minority of patients in whom the diagnosis is uncertain, more complicated investigations may be required. In continuous pH monitoring a pH probe is fixed in the lumen 5 cm above the lower oesophageal sphincter. Monitoring for 24 hours allows symptoms to be correlated with posture, meals and reflux. The Bernstein test, in which acid or normal saline is perfused into the oesophagus, is sometimes useful in determining whether chest pain is oesophageal in origin. Pain occurs in response to acid but not saline.

Management

General measures

A number of factors are known to promote gastro-oesophageal reflux (Table 7.4), many of which can be modified or altered by practical measures which the patient can undertake. Their importance should be explained and emphasised. The most important are obesity and cigarette smoking. Weight reduction and stopping smoking alone will relieve symptoms in many patients. Meals should be of small volume and alcohol, fatty foods and caffeine avoided. No snacks must be taken after the evening meal, to reduce nocturnal reflux. Heavy lifting, stooping and bending at the waist should be avoided, especially after meals. The head of the bed should be elevated by 15 cm.

Drug therapy

Individual episodes of heartburn are promptly relieved by antacids, liquid preparations being best. Various alginate preparations are available which form a gel on the surface of the gastric contents preventing reflux in the upright position. Preparations are given when heartburn occurs or on retiring at night.

Histamine H_2-receptor antagonists relieve symptoms by reducing the volume and concentration of acid

Table 7.4 Factors which promote gastro-oesophageal reflux	
Mechanism	**Factor**
Impaired efficiency of the lower oesophageal sphincter (LOS)	Hiatus hernia Surgery to lower oesophagus, e.g. cardiomyotomy Diabetes mellitus Prolonged nasogastric intubation
Impaired efficiency of the LOS and secondary peristalsis	Scleroderma
Reduction in LOS pressure	Fatty foods Caffeine
Reduction in LOS pressure and impairment of oesophageal mucosal function	Cigarette smoking Alcohol
Increased intra-abdominal pressure and reduction in LOS due to circulating hormones	Pregnancy
Increased intra-abdominal pressure	Obesity Ascites Surgical corsets Bending and lifting

Increased gastric contents available for reflux	Impaired gastric emptying:
	  pyloric obstruction
	  gastroparesis
	  drugs, e.g. anticholinergics
	  fatty foods

	Increased volume of gastric contents
	  large meals
	  Zollinger–Ellison syndrome

secretion and they may also have a healing effect in the milder cases. Often they must be given in doses greater than those used for peptic ulcer (p. 429), e.g. ranitidine 300 mg 12-hourly or 8-hourly.

Omeprazole (p. 429) 20 mg in the morning is the drug of choice for reflux oesophagitis, particularly in severe cases. Usually healing is achieved, but relapse occurs when the drug is stopped. Thus the drug may need to be taken long-term in the same dosage.

Several other drugs probably have a marginal benefit in reflux oesophagitis. Sucralfate may be given in suspension, 1g four times a day. Metoclopramide and cisapride 10 mg 8-hourly may increase pressure in the lower oesophageal sphincter and increase gastric emptying, the latter drug acting without central nervous system side-effects.

Stricture

These are dilated during endoscopy, a procedure requiring repetition from time to time. Once dilatation has been achieved, acid suppression with H_2-receptor antagonists or omeprazole is essential to slow the rate of recurrence.

Surgery

This is indicated if severe symptoms persist despite adequate medical therapy. The aim of surgery is to return the lower oesophageal sphincter to the abdomen and to construct an additional valve mechanism. Symptoms are relieved in 85% of patients but recur in the long term in 10%. There is a 1% mortality rate with surgery, and 5% develop dysphagia or an inability to belch or vomit. Surgery is also required for severe strictures which cannot be dilated or which require frequent dilatation. The stricture is resected and an anti-reflux procedure performed.

Barrett's oesophagus

This premalignant condition (Fig. 7.4C) requires endoscopic surveillance for the assessment of dysplasia or carcinoma. The frequency of endoscopy has not yet been established.

PARAOESOPHAGEAL HERNIA

This is uncommon. The gastro-oesophageal junction and therefore the lower oesophageal sphincter remains in the normal position, but a knuckle of the greater curvature of the stomach passes through the oesophageal hiatus into the posterior mediastinum (Fig. 7.4D); it may be followed by the entire stomach and other abdominal organs.

Clinical features

Symptoms due to reflux do not occur because the position of the lower oesophageal sphincter is normal. There are complaints of epigastric fullness and pain whilst eating and for a period afterwards. Dysphagia may occur. Gastric ulcer or erosions in the hernia are common and lead to iron deficiency anaemia. When the hernia becomes large, dyspnoea may occur.

Paraoesophageal hernia is assessed by barium swallow and barium meal examination.

Volvulus of the herniated stomach is a serious complication. In twisting, the blood supply to the stomach is occluded and strangulation results. There is severe epigastric pain and distension.

Management

Small hernias require no treatment unless there is persistent blood loss. Ulcers within the hernia are treated as for peptic ulcer. Surgery is considered for large hernias within the thorax in order to resolve symptoms and prevent volvulus. This is a difficult decision because many patients are old and debilitated. In these patients a rigid regimen of small meals is recommended.

MOTILITY DISORDERS

PHARYNGEAL DYSPHAGIA

Some of the more common causes are shown in Table 7.3 and they may be usefully classified into diseases of the central nervous system, peripheral nerves, motor end plate or skeletal muscle. It should be remembered that pharyngeal dysphagia may be caused by thyroid enlargement or by tumours of the pharynx or cervical oesophagus (p. 421). The symptoms of pharyngeal dysphagia are discussed on page 416.

Central nervous system disorders

Stroke is a common cause of pharyngeal dysphagia. It is most frequently observed following infarction or bleeding of the vertebrobasilar or posteroinferior cerebellar arteries, but also occurs with a hemispheric stroke where cerebral oedema may be the causative factor. There is failure of pharyngeal peristalsis, dysfunction of the upper oesophageal sphincter and poor control of the tongue. The problem may resolve in 2–3 weeks, during which time nasogastric feeding may be given. Cricopharyngeal myotomy may be considered if the problem persists and if it can be demonstrated that this muscle is failing to relax. Percutaneous endoscopic gastrostomy may be necessary in the long term if the problem does not resolve.

Peripheral nerve and motor end plate disorders

These are motor neurone disease, Parkinson's disease, multiple sclerosis, and the motor end plate disorder myasthenia gravis. There is dysfunction of both the pharynx and the upper oesophageal sphincter.

Muscle disorders

These are polymyositis, dermatomyositis and the muscular dystrophies. There is reduced pharyngeal contraction and reduced upper oesophageal sphincter pressure so that aspiration is common.

ACHALASIA OF THE CARDIA
(achalasia; cardiospasm)

This is characterised by failure of peristalsis throughout the oesophagus and a failure of the lower oesophageal sphincter to relax on swallowing. The disease has an incidence of about 1 in 100 000.

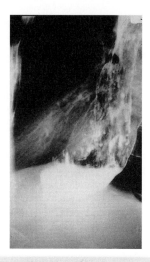

Fig. 7.5   Achalasia of cardia: dilated oesophagus with pointed termination.

Pathology

The oesophagus is dilated above a narrowed cardia but the muscle wall appears normal, except in long-standing disease when it becomes thin. On microscopic examination there is a marked loss of ganglion cells in Auerbach's plexus. There may also be changes in the vagus nerves and in the dorsal motor nucleus of the vagus. In Chagas' disease (American trypanosomiasis, p. 159) there are similar pathological changes in the oesophagus and its ganglion cells.

Clinical features

Dysphagia may at first be gradual and intermittent but later is persistent. It is caused initially by solids and later by both solids and liquids. It may be localised behind the lower end of the sternum. Retrosternal pain occurs in 50% of patients in the initial phases of the disease and is often precipitated by eating.

In the early stages, the patient continues to eat a normal diet but food accumulates in the capacious noncontractile oesophagus. The patient may notice a sense of fullness, and gurgling sounds can occur. Later the retained food cannot be expelled into the stomach and weight loss ensues. Regurgitation and inhalation of food and secretions may occur at night and cause recurrent pulmonary infection.

Investigations

A chest radiograph may be sufficient to show a dilated oesophageal outline, perhaps with a fluid level behind the heart shadow. There is absence of the usual gas shadow in the fundus of the stomach.

A barium swallow shows a dilated atonic oesophagus which fails to clear barium into the stomach. The oesophagus comes to a smooth pointed termination like a bird's beak (Fig. 7.5). While these appearances are typical they are not diagnostic because they can be mimicked by a carcinoma at the lower end of the oesophagus or in the cardiac portion of the stomach.

Oesophagoscopy is always required. Cleansing of the oesophagus is necessary, which may involve repeated lavage and aspiration at oesophagoscopy. The mucosa is usually normal but stagnation of food may lead to some inflammation and ulceration and there may be secondary infection with Candida. The oesophagus is dilated. With gentle pressure the endoscope can be passed into the stomach. Failure of passage should suggest the presence of carcinoma, and biopsies must be taken.

Motility studies will show reduced motility in the body of the oesophagus together with a raised pressure in the lower oesophageal sphincter, which fails to relax, and are used to establish the diagnosis and determine its severity.

Management

This may be by dilatation or cardiomyotomy. In the first a hydrostatic or pneumatic bag is positioned at the level of the diaphragm and then distended forcibly to weaken the lower oesophageal sphincter. One or more dilatations may be required to bring about adequate swallowing.

Failure of hydrostatic dilatation or inability to introduce the dilator are indications for operation which takes the form of cardiomyotomy (Heller's operation). Here the muscle at the lower end of the oesophagus, and for some distance above and below, is slit to expose but not to penetrate the mucosa. The procedure is relatively effective and safe even in the elderly. Both dilatation and cardiomyotomy may be complicated by reflux oesophagitis or occasionally by oesophageal perforation.

In patients who are unfit for dilatation or surgery, isosorbide dinitrate 5–10 mg sublingually just before meals or nifedipine 20 mg sublingually 1 hour before meals may assist swallowing.

Treated or untreated, patients with achalasia have an increased liability to squamous carcinoma of the oesophagus which makes periodic endoscopic review every 1 or 2 years desirable.

DIFFUSE SPASM OF THE OESOPHAGUS

In this condition there is muscular hypertrophy of the lower two-thirds of the oesophagus; Auerbach's plexus is normal, but there are degenerative changes in the vagus nerves.

Clinical features

The main symptom is pain precipitated by eating, by hot and cold liquids or by emotional stress. The pain is retrosternal but may radiate to the back, neck or arms thus mimicking angina pectoris. The pain is usually accompanied by dysphagia. The diagnosis is established by barium swallow which shows a hold-up of barium in the oesophagus due to multiple uncoordinated contractions. The appearance resembles a corkscrew. Manometry shows strong uncoordinated contractions.

Management

Gastro-oesophageal reflux is a precipitant of symptoms in some patients. This possibility is explored by endoscopic biopsy of the lower oesophagus to seek the histological changes of reflux oesophagitis (p. 418) and if necessary by 24-hour oesophageal pH monitoring to demonstrate a relationship of reflux to symptoms. A trial of antireflux therapy (p. 418) may be prescribed.

In general, treatment involves education in eating in a relaxed atmosphere with adequate mastication. Any emotional stress should receive attention. Glyceryl trinitrate sublingually, hydralazine (25 mg orally 12-hourly), nifedipine (5–20 mg orally 8-hourly) and anti-depressants may all relieve pain in some patients. Since most patients are over the age of 60, the physician has to persist with medical management. In the occasional young patient with intractable symptoms, pneumatic dilatation or an extended cardiomyotomy may be required.

Other spastic disorders of motility

Manometric studies in patients presenting with chest pain and dysphagia have revealed a number of motility disorders. **Nutcracker oesophagus** is defined by very high pressures in the distal oesophagus and **hypertensive lower oesophageal sphincter** by a high resting pressure in the sphincter.

These conditions present in the same way as diffuse spasm and share the same treatment regimens.

SCLERODERMA

Oesophageal involvement is common in this disease (see p. 915, Chapter 15). The smooth muscle of the lower two-thirds of the oesophagus atrophies and is replaced by fibrous tissue. There is a failure of oesophageal peristalsis and the lower oesophageal sphincter is incompetent. The patient complains of severe heartburn from gastro-oesophageal reflux. Dysphagia is common and may be due to stricture. Barium swallow shows a dilated aperistaltic oesophagus which empties normally in the erect position. Treatment is with omeprazole (p. 429) to abolish acid secretion.

Similar but less severe problems may occur in polymyositis (p. 918) and mixed connective tissue disease.

TUMOURS OF THE OESOPHAGUS

SQUAMOUS CELL AND ADENOCARCINOMA

There are wide geographic variations in the incidence of squamous cell carcinoma. It is very common around the Caspian Sea and some parts of southern Africa and China. Some aetiological factors are shown in Table 7.5. About 10% of these carcinomas are situated in the upper third of the oesophagus mainly in the post-cricoid region; the remainder are distributed fairly evenly in the middle and lower thirds. 10% to 20% of all oesophageal cancers are adenocarcinomas and these are sited in the lower oesophagus and at the gastro-oesophageal junction. The majority probably arise in Barrett's epithelium,

Table 7.5 Oesophageal cancer—predisposing factors
Squamous cell carcinoma
Tobacco (smoked or chewed)
Alcohol
Betel nut chewing
Tylosis—a hereditary disorder of squamous epithelium
Achalasia
Sideropenic dysphagia (Paterson–Kelly syndrome)
Head and neck squamous carcinoma
Adenocarcinoma
Barrett's epithelium
Smoking

the remainder being gastric cancers which have invaded the lower oesophagus.

Both histological forms extend circumferentially and longitudinally in the wall of the oesophagus to produce stenosing lesions or nodular or ulcerated masses.

Clinical features

Progressive dysphagia is typical. This starts with the 'sticking' of solid food, at first intermittently and then regularly, and proceeds to difficulty with semisolids and eventually liquids. There is discomfort, not amounting to pain, at the site of the obstruction which is usually well localised by the patient. Painful swallowing may occur. There may be aspiration or bleeding. The development of symptoms occupies some months so that by the time the patient first attends, weight loss is already a feature and there may be metastases in lymph nodes, liver and the mediastinum.

Investigations

Obstruction and an irregular narrowing of the oesophagus, seen at barium swallow, are highly suggestive of the diagnosis (Fig. 7.6). It may not be possible to distinguish between carcinoma of the oesophagus and achalasia of the cardia. Oesophagitis and a benign stricture may also simulate carcinoma.

Thus oesophagoscopy and biopsy are mandatory. Repeated biopsy may be required to obtain positive confirmation of the diagnosis, particularly when stricture formation prevents further insertion of the oesophagoscope or the biopsy forceps. In these circumstances the passage of a brush through the narrowed area dislodges cells which can be examined for malignancy.

Staging of the tumour by CT may be used to assess patients for surgery.

Management

The choice lies between palliation and radical measures, but five year survival is only 3%. In squamous carcinoma, particularly of the upper and middle thirds, high voltage radiotherapy is the treatment of choice in those centres possessing the necessary facilities. Otherwise, and with tumours of the lower third, oesophago-gastrectomy offers the best hope. There is the possibility that a combined approach of surgery with pre-operative radiotherapy may lead to enhanced survival.

Extensive tumours which are unsuitable for radical surgery or for intensive radiotherapy are treated palliatively, occasionally by bypass surgery, but more often by endoscopic insertion of a permanent tube (stent) into the oesophagus. This allows liquids to be taken and is effective in providing relief from the most distressing problem, the inability to swallow saliva. In some centres endoscopic laser therapy is available for tumour

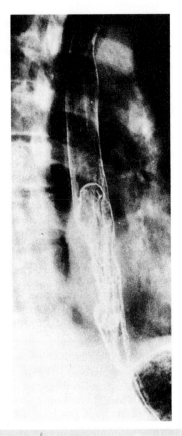

Fig. 7.6 Carcinoma of the oesophagus.

ablation. Treatment can be repeated as necessary and gratifying palliation with restoration of swallowing can be achieved. Hazards include perforation and bleeding.

LEIOMYOMA OF THE OESOPHAGUS

This is the commonest benign tumour of the oesophagus. It is usually single and sited in the lower oesophagus. It may be an incidental finding or it may present with dysphagia. On barium swallow or oesophagoscopy it is seen as a smooth rounded mass with intact overlying mucosa. Large tumours may be leiomyosarcomas. The treatment of symptomatic tumours is surgical.

MISCELLANEOUS DISORDERS

PHARYNGEAL POUCH

This develops at the site of the inferior constrictor of the pharynx probably as a result of incoordination of the cricopharyngeus muscle which leads to increased pressure acting on the weakest site in the posterior wall of the pharynx. The pouch causes dysphagia due to forward displacement of the oesophagus. There is swelling and gurgling in the neck on swallowing. The patient may present with recurrent attacks of stridor, and inhalation of contents of the sac may lead to pneumonia. The diagnosis is confirmed by barium swallow. Oesophagoscopy is hazardous. The pouch is removed surgically.

TRACTION DIVERTICULUM

This is most commonly situated in the anterior wall of the oesophagus just below the level of the tracheal bifurcation. It is due to chronic inflammation, usually tuberculous, in adjacent lymph nodes. By the time the diverticulum is discovered, often accidentally during a barium swallow, the disease in the lymph nodes has healed. It is seldom that the diverticulum itself causes symptoms and surgical treatment is rarely necessary.

MUCOSAL RING

The mucosal ring (or Schatzki ring) is an incomplete septum of mucosa at the junction of the squamous and columnar epithelium in the lower oesophagus. It presents with episodic dysphagia, usually when eating meat. The ring is diagnosed on barium swallow when the oesophagus is distended with barium. If necessary the ring may be treated with bougienage or pneumatic dilatation.

SIDEROPENIC DYSPHAGIA

This dysphagia (the Paterson–Kelly syndrome) is a very rare condition associated with iron deficiency anaemia, glossitis and koilonychia. A thin web of degenerated epithelial cells forms in the post-cricoid area and causes intermittent dysphagia to solids. The web is difficult to detect on barium examination or at endoscopy, but the dilatation caused by the passage of the endoscope is usually sufficient to relieve symptoms. The condition occurs usually in post-menopausal women. The lesion may be premalignant and endoscopic surveillance is required. Treatment is with iron replacement.

INFECTION OF THE OESOPHAGUS

Infection with Candida or herpes simplex occurs in malignancy, immunosuppression, and AIDS (p. 89). They cause acute, painful dysphagia and heartburn. The diagnosis is made by oesophagoscopy and biopsy. The treatment is discussed on page 96.

GLOBUS HYSTERICUS

The globus sensation is a 'lump in the throat', a sensation of dysphagia when food or fluid has not been ingested. The sensation probably arises in the cricopharyngeus muscle. In some patients the sensation may be precipitated by reflux into the lower oesophagus or a web. In the majority, however, this is probably a 'functional' disease.

CHEMICAL BURNS AND STRICTURE

Burns are usually caused by the ingestion of strong alkalis present in many cleaning fluids. By contrast the ingestion of strong acids usually spares the oesophagus and damages the distal stomach. With alkali ingestion, damage to the mucosa of the mouth, pharynx and oesophagus is immediate and there are no 'first aid' measures. There is severe pain in the mouth, pharynx and chest, and dysphagia and retching. The oesophagus may perforate, leading to shock and infection in the mediastinum. The problem is assessed by careful endoscopy. Commonly strictures result and in the long term there is an increased incidence of cancer in these patients.

PERFORATION OF THE OESOPHAGUS

This may occur at endoscopy, or spontaneously. Slow perforation can be caused by a foreign body.

Spontaneous perforation (Boerhaave's syndrome) results from a sudden increase in intra-oesophageal pressure caused by vomiting, straining or convulsions. There is severe chest and/or abdominal pain and shock. There may be subcutaneous emphysema, pleural effusion or pneumothorax. Perforation is confirmed by the ingestion of water soluble contrast medium and the treatment is surgical.

The perforation caused by endoscopy is usually much smaller, the symptoms are less dramatic and most can be treated conservatively with broad spectrum antibiotics and intravenous fluids.

FOREIGN BODIES IN THE OESOPHAGUS

Usually this is a coin in children or a fish or chicken bone in the adult. The object impacts in the cervical oesophagus, at the aortic arch or in the distal oesophagus. Usually there is a sharp pain at the level of the object, and dysphagia is common. A chest radiograph will localise a radio-opaque object. Most are located at endoscopy and can be removed directly. Food impaction almost always occurs in the lower oesophagus and indicates underlying disease.

FURTHER READING

Baehr P H, McDonald G B 1994 Esophageal infections: risk factors, presentation, diagnosis, and treatment. Gastroenterology 106: 509–532
Sagar P M, Gauperaa T, Sue-Ling H, McMahon M J, Johnston D 1994 An audit of the treatment of cancer of the oesophagus. Gut 35: 941–945

DISEASES OF THE STOMACH AND DUODENUM

SYMPTOMS OF GASTRIC DISEASE

Dyspepsia

This term is commonly used as a collective description for a variety of alimentary symptoms. The term 'ulcer dyspepsia', for example, is often used as an inclusive term for the symptoms of peptic ulcer. The symptoms are listed in the information box.

SYMPTOMS INCLUDED IN THE TERM DYSPEPSIA

- Upper abdominal pain which may or may not be related to food
- Gastro-oesophageal regurgitation and heartburn
- Anorexia, nausea and vomiting
- Early repletion or satiety after meals
- A sense of abdominal distension or 'bloating'
- Flatulence (burping, belching) and aerophagy

Although dyspepsia is most commonly associated with organic disease of the upper alimentary tract, for example reflux oesophagitis, peptic ulcer or gastric carcinoma, symptoms such as anorexia, nausea and vomiting with or without upper abdominal pain may be due to many other causes. These are included in the information box.

'Flatulent dyspepsia' is often used as a collective term for symptoms such as early satiety, flatulence, bloating and belching with or without abdominal pain.

Flatulence

This term is used to describe symptoms due to air in the gastrointestinal tract. This is often due to excessive swallowing of air (aerophagy). Under normal circumstances a small amount of air is swallowed with food, drink and saliva. Some of this gas may be expelled as a belch while the remainder passes into the intestine where it will be partially absorbed but the nitrogen will be expelled per rectum. Most of the colonic gas is the consequence of bacterial action in food residues in the lower small intestine and colon. A plain radiograph of the abdomen shows that gas is normally present in the

---

OTHER CAUSES OF DYSPEPSIA

- **Other organic disease of the digestive system**
  Pancreatic disease
  Crohn's disease
  Colon cancer and diverticular disease
- **Systemic disease**
  Cardiac, renal or hepatic failure
  Extra-abdominal malignancy such as lung carcinoma
- **Medication**
  Non-steroidal anti-inflammatory drugs (NSAIDs)
  Digoxin
  Analgesics
  Antibiotics
- **Alcohol abuse**
- **Pregnancy**
- **Psychiatric and functional disorders**
  Depressive illness
  Anxiety neurosis
  Non-ulcer dyspepsia
  Irritable bowel syndrome

---

stomach and colon but very little is seen in the small intestine.

Vomiting

This may occur in any acute disorder of the alimentary tract including intestinal obstruction. Numerous other conditions may also be responsible, for example, meningitis, uraemia, migraine, drugs such as digoxin or morphine and particularly in children, infection. The type, timing and related features of the vomiting are important diagnostically. Sudden vomiting without preceding nausea may be due to direct stimulation of the vomiting centre in the medulla and thus be an indication of intracranial disease. Vomiting in the morning may be due to pregnancy, alcoholism or anxiety. Vomiting of large quantities of food and secretions late in the day or night indicates gastric outlet obstruction. Vomiting which relieves pain is often due to a peptic ulcer. The complaint of persistent vomiting without loss of weight is nearly always indicative of psychological disturbance.

Waterbrash

This is the sudden filling of the mouth with saliva which is produced as a reflex response to a variety of symptoms from the upper gastrointestinal tract, e.g. peptic ulcer pain.

Loss of appetite (anorexia)

This may have a local cause such as carcinoma of the stomach but may also be a feature of any debilitating disease or of a psychological disturbance.

GASTRITIS

Gastritis refers to acute or chronic inflammation of the stomach which is often diffuse. It is sometimes recognised visually at endoscopy but is usually diagnosed histologically by gastric biopsy. The understanding of gastritis has been greatly enhanced by the recognition of *Helicobacter pylori* as the most important cause of chronic gastritis, and aspirin and other non-steroidal inflammatory drugs as a cause of acute (haemorrhagic) gastritis below.

Helicobacter pylori

This spiral Gram-negative bacterium colonises the epithelial mucous layer of the gastric antrum and body. It is seen close to the epithelial cell membranes and between epithelial cells but it does not invade. The organism produces urease which converts urea to ammonia thus creating its own localised alkaline milieu. Its presence induces an acute or chronic inflammatory response within the mucosa involving polymorphs and mononuclear cells. The surface epithelial cells show degeneration, detachment and necrosis. *H. pylori* is recognised as a cause of gastritis because gastric inoculation of volunteers causes acute inflammation of the mucosa and because established gastritis treated with therapy to eradicate helicobacter induces histological improvement.

H. pylori is common in all communities and is probably spread person to person. The presence of helicobacter correlates with histological gastritis, both increasing with age. In developed countries the prevalence of both is low in young adults but rises to over 50% in 50-year-olds. In developing countries infection is more frequent in younger age groups. Variations occur in relation to geographical site and ethnic background. Methods of diagnosis are given in the information box.

DIAGNOSIS OF H. PYLORI

- **histology**—the biopsy obtained at endoscopy is stained with haematoxylin and eosin or Giemsa stains
- **the urease activity** of the organism is utilised for diagnosis by placing the biopsy specimen in urea and assessing ammonia release (as in the commercial CLO test) or a radioactive urea breath test is used
- **an ELISA test** for the detection of serum IgG antibodies to helicobacter proteins is used

---

The gastric and mucosal barrier and non-steroidal anti-inflammatory drugs (NSAIDs)

Several mechanisms protect the gastric mucosa from hydrogen ions secreted into the lumen of the stomach.

The surface epithelial cells secrete bicarbonate which creates an alkaline milieu within the mucous layer at the surface of the mucosa; this bicarbonate secretion is under the influence of mucosal prostaglandins. The tight junctions between the epithelial cells and their surface lipoprotein layer provide a mechanical barrier and the normal turnover of epithelial cells and gastric mucus is also protective. The microvasculature of the mucosa is also important in maintaining these protective mechanisms. Collectively, all these mechanisms can be described as the 'gastric mucosal barrier'.

Several drugs will disrupt the barrier. When aspirin is in solution at a pH below 3.5 it is undissociated and fat-soluble, so that it is absorbed through the lipoprotein membrane of the surface epithelial cells; during absorption it damages the membrane and the tight junctions. It also inhibits prostaglandin synthesis thus reducing bicarbonate secretion by the surface epithelial cells. NSAIDs cause injury by decreasing the prostaglandin content of the mucosa.

The gastric damage after a few days' intake of aspirin or NSAIDs can be observed at endoscopy; there is erythema, mucosal haemorrhage and erosions, and these findings may also occur in the duodenum. Slow bleeding from the mucosa results in a positive faecal occult blood test.

ACUTE GASTRITIS

A variety of agents cause acute gastritis (Table 7.6), the unifying aetiological factor being disruption of the gastric mucosal barrier. Histological inflammation is secondary to this event. By contrast, infections of the mucosa cause injury by inducing an inflammatory response with polymorphs and other immunological cells which are attracted to the mucosa. This occurs in the initial infection with *H. pylori*. Phlegmonous gastritis, an infection with streptococci or other bacteria, progresses to suppuration and presents as an acute abdomen (p. 442). Several viral and fungal infections may produce acute gastritis especially in AIDS (p. 100).

ACUTE HAEMORRHAGIC GASTRITIS

This may result from any of the first six causes listed in Table 7.6. The appearances seen after the ingestion of

---

Table 7.6   Causes of acute gastritis

NSAIDs	Severe physiological stress
Alcohol	Uraemia
Drugs—iron, antimitotic agents	*H. pylori* (initial infection)
Bile	Other infections

NSAIDs (see p. 425) progress to erosions which vary in number and size and may become confluent and bleed; some may progress to acute ulcers. Whilst the most common cause is the ingestion of NSAIDs often in combination with alcohol, acute haemorrhagic gastritis and acute ulcers also occur after major surgery or injury to the central nervous system (Cushing's ulcers) or extensive burns (Curling's ulcers).

Clinical features

There are usually no symptoms referable to the stomach and the patient presents with gastrointestinal haemorrhage (p. 438). In a minority of patients there may be epigastric discomfort, anorexia and nausea.

CHRONIC GASTRITIS

The causes of chronic gastritis are shown in Table 7.7. The classification into Types A and B is histological with three stages which are progressive over many years. In **chronic superficial gastritis**, the mucosa is normal in thickness and there is patchy infiltration of lymphocytes and plasma cells. In **atrophic gastritis** there is a reduction in parietal and chief cells in the glands of the body and of mucous cells in the pyloric glands. There is epithelial metaplasia and an infiltrate of lymphocytes and plasma cells. The gastritis is termed active when there is also an infiltrate of polymorphs. In **gastric atrophy** glands are lost, the thickness of the mucosa is reduced, metaplasia to an intestinal form of epithelium is common but infiltration with lymphocytes and plasma cells is slight.

Type A gastritis

The gastritis involves the body of the stomach and spares the antrum and it is due to autoimmune activity against the parietal cell. Parietal cell antibodies in the serum are a marker of type A gastritis. In some patients the degree of gastric atrophy is so severe that the absence of parietal cells leads to failure to secrete intrinsic factor, and pernicious anaemia results. Type A gastritis is asymptomatic. It is important because it may lead to gastric cancer.

Type B gastritis (antral)

This common form of gastritis involves the antrum of the stomach but does spread to the body especially along the lesser curve. It is usually caused by *H. pylori*. Type B gastritis also occurs after gastric surgery when it may be caused by a loss of the trophic hormone gastrin and the reflux of bile, pancreatic and intestinal secretions into the stomach. It is not caused by *H. pylori* infection.

It is debatable whether Type B gastritis itself causes symptoms referable to the stomach. The condition is important as a precursor of gastric and duodenal ulceration (p. 427) and possibly gastric carcinoma (p. 435).

MÉNÉTRIER'S DISEASE (hypertrophic gastritis)

The gastric pits and glands are elongated and tortuous and the parietal and chief cells are replaced by mucus-secreting cells. As a result, the mucosal folds of the body and fundus of the stomach are greatly enlarged. Whilst some patients may have symptoms referable to the stomach the usual presentation is in middle age or later with protein-losing enteropathy (p. 453) due to protein leakage from the gastric mucosa. Treatment with antisecretory drugs (p. 429) may reduce the loss of protein but in non-responsive patients, gastric resection may be necessary.

PEPTIC ULCER

The term 'peptic ulcer' refers to an ulcer in the lower oesophagus, stomach, duodenum, in the jejunum after surgical anastomosis to the stomach, or rarely in the ileum adjacent to a Meckel's diverticulum. Ulcers in the stomach or duodenum may be acute or chronic; both penetrate the muscularis mucosae but the acute ulcer shows no evidence of fibrosis. Erosions do not penetrate the muscularis mucosae.

GASTRIC AND DUODENAL ULCER

Although the prevalence of peptic ulcer is decreasing in many Western communities it still affects, at some time, approximately 10% of all adult males. The male to female ratio for duodenal ulcer varies from 5:1 to 2:1 in different communities whilst that for gastric ulcer is 2:1 or less. Variations in the incidence of gastric and duodenal ulcer occur between different countries and between different parts of the same country. There have been remarkable changes in the prevalence of ulcer disease in Western communities over the last century. Gastric ulcer was the common form of ulcer disease in 1900. Then duodenal ulcer increased steadily from 1900 to the

Type	Cause
Table 7.7	Causes of chronic gastritis
Type A gastritis	Autoimmune
Type B gastritis	
Intact stomach	*H. pylori*
Postgastrectomy	?
Eosinophilic gastritis	?Allergy
Hypertrophic gastritis (Ménétrier's disease)	?Allergy

1950s when its prevalence peaked and is now declining. Mortality rates for both forms of ulcer are falling. By contrast, peptic ulcer is becoming more common in many developing countries.

Aetiology of chronic ulceration

Heredity

Patients with peptic ulcer often have a family history of the disease; this is particularly so with duodenal ulcers which develop below the age of 20 years. Gastric and duodenal ulcers are inherited as separate disorders. The relatives of gastric ulcer patients have three times the expected number of gastric ulcers, and duodenal ulcer relatives have three times the expected number of duodenal ulcers. The inheritance of blood group O, non-secretor status and elevated levels of serum pepsinogen I all confer an increased risk of duodenal ulcer.

Helicobacter pylori

This is the most important aetiological factor in peptic ulcer disease, accounting for 90% of duodenal ulcers and 70% of gastric ulcers. By causing Type B gastritis (p. 426) it reduces the resistance of the gastric mucosa to attack by acid and pepsin and a gastric ulcer may result. The sequence of events in the formation of duodenal ulcer is more difficult to explain; a key factor is probably the formation of gastric metaplasia in the first part of the duodenum in response to excess acid. This gastric epithelium allows colonisation of the duodenum by *H. pylori* already infecting the stomach. Duodenitis results. There is an inflammatory response in the mucosa with a predominance of polymorphs and it is in this area that an ulcer forms. Endoscopic observation in patients with duodenal ulcer disease shows ulcer, ulcer with duodenitis, or duodenitis alone at various times in the life-history of the disease. The presence of *H. pylori* in the gastric antrum stimulates the secretion of gastrin which in turn stimulates acid secretion and this may be an additional factor in the causation of duodenal ulcer.

NSAIDs

These damage the gastric mucosal barrier (p.425) and are an important aetiological factor in up to 30% of gastric ulcers. These drugs also reduce the integrity of the duodenal mucosa and are responsible for a very small proportion of duodenal ulcers.

Smoking

Smoking confers an increased risk of gastric ulcer and to a lesser extent duodenal ulcer. Once the ulcer has formed it is more likely to cause complications and less likely to heal on standard treatment regimens if the smoking continues.

Table 7.8 Role of other factors in chronic peptic ulcer

Factor	Degree of importance
Chronic stress	probably unimportant
Alcohol	unimportant
Diet	unimportant
Corticosteroids	probably unimportant except in very high doses
Duodenogastric reflux of bile	may play a role in gastric ulcer
Disorders of gastric emptying	
slow emptying	may play a role in gastric ulcer
fast emptying	may play a role in duodenal ulcer

Acid-pepsin versus mucosal resistance

An ulcer forms when there is an imbalance between aggressive factors, i.e. the digestive power of acid and pepsin, and defensive factors, i.e. the ability of the gastric and duodenal mucosa to resist this digestive power. This mucosal resistance constitutes the intact gastric mucosal barrier (p. 425). Ulcers occur only in the presence of acid and pepsin; they are never found in achlorhydric patients such as those with pernicious anaemia. On the other hand, severe intractable peptic ulceration nearly always occurs in patients with the Zollinger–Ellison syndrome which is characterised by very high acid secretion. However, in the majority of ulcer patients acid secretion is within the normal range or is only moderately raised. In these individuals, damage to the gastric mucosal barrier is necessary to facilitate the damaging effect of acid and pepsin. This initial damage results from *H. pylori* infection, NSAIDs and smoking.

The role of other factors in the aetiology of ulcer disease is detailed in Table 7.8.

Pathology

Chronic gastric ulcer is usually single; 90% are situated on the lesser curve within the antrum or at the junction between body and antral mucosa. Chronic duodenal ulcer is usually in the first part of the duodenum just distal to the junction of pyloric and duodenal mucosa; 50% are on the anterior wall. Gastric and duodenal ulcers coexist in 10% of all patients with peptic ulcers. More than one peptic ulcer is found in 10–15% of patients. The histology of chronic ulcer shows four layers: surface debris, an infiltrate of neutrophils, granulation tissue and collagen. A chronic ulcer extends to below the muscularis mucosa.

Clinical features

Peptic ulcer disease is a chronic condition with a natural history of spontaneous relapse and remission lasting for decades if not for life. Although they are different diseases, duodenal and gastric ulcers share common symptoms which will be considered together.

The commonest presentation is that of recurrent

abdominal pain which has three notable characteristics—localisation to the epigastrium, relationship to food and episodic occurrence. The pain is probably due to acid coming into contact with the ulcer but some patients continue to have pain when the ulcer is healed. Thus it is possible that acid contact with a mucosa damaged by gastritis or duodenitis may also cause pain.

Epigastric pain
Pain is referred to the epigastrium and is often so sharply localised that the patient can indicate its site with two or three fingers—the 'pointing sign'.

Hunger pain
Pain occurs intermittently during the day, often when the stomach is empty, so that the patient identifies it as 'hunger pain' and obtains relief by eating.

Night pain
Pain wakes the patient from sleep and may be relieved by food, a drink of milk or antacids; this symptom when present is virtually pathognomonic for ulcer.

Pain relief
Pain is relieved by food, milk or antacids and by belching and vomiting. The effect of vomiting is so striking that some patients learn to induce vomiting for pain relief.

Episodic pain ('periodicity')
Characteristically pain occurs in 'on again/off again' episodes, lasting one to three weeks at a time, three or four times in a year. Between episodes the patient feels perfectly well. To begin with, episodes may be quite brief and infrequent lasting only for a few days at a time, once or twice per year; as the natural history evolves, however, episodes of pain become more frequent and last longer. In temperate climates seasonal variations may be noted with an increased frequency of symptoms during winter and spring.

Other symptoms that occur, especially during episodes of pain, include waterbrash, heartburn, loss of appetite and vomiting. Occasional vomiting occurs in about 40% of ulcer subjects; persistent vomiting, occurring daily, suggests the possibility of gastric outlet obstruction.

In a third of patients the history is less characteristic. This is especially true in elderly subjects under treatment with non-steroidal anti-inflammatory drugs (NSAIDs). In these patients pain may be absent or so slight that it is experienced only as a vague sense of epigastric unease. Occasionally the only symptoms are anorexia and nausea, or a sense of undue repletion after meals. In some patients the ulcer is completely 'silent', presenting for the first time with anaemia from chronic undetected blood loss, or as an abrupt haematemesis or as acute perforation; in others there is recurrent acute bleeding without ulcer pain between the attacks.

Differential diagnosis
It is difficult to distinguish between gastric and duodenal ulcer on symptoms alone, nor is it important because any of the symptoms described above should alert the physician to the possibility of chronic ulcer and the need for appropriate investigation. Unfortunately, apart from haemorrhage all these symptoms may be present in non-ulcer dyspepsia and the importance of investigation is emphasised in making this distinction.

Investigations
The diagnosis can be made by double-contrast barium meal examination or by endoscopy. Endoscopy is the preferred investigation because it is more accurate and has the enormous advantage that suspicious lesions can be biopsied. Very occasionally a gastric ulcer may be malignant, therefore endoscopy and biopsy are mandatory when a gastric ulcer is detected on barium examination. Moreover in gastric ulcer disease endoscopy must be repeated after suitable treatment to confirm that the ulcer has healed and to obtain further biopsies if it has not.

Endoscopy is usually undertaken for the diagnosis of duodenal ulcer but unless symptoms persist or change it is not necessary to repeat the endoscopy to confirm healing after treatment. When the ulcer is diagnosed at endoscopy, biopsies are taken for the histological demonstration of *H. pylori* or the biopsy is subjected to the CLO-test (p. 425).

Management
The aims of treatment are to relieve symptoms and induce ulcer healing in the short term, and to prevent relapse in the long term. When *H. pylori* is found, an attempt should be made to eradicate it for this will prevent relapse and eliminate the need for long-term therapy.

General measures
Cigarette smoking is of aetiological importance in ulcer disease and prevents healing. It should be strongly discouraged. Aspirin and the non-steroidal anti-inflammatory drugs (NSAIDs) should be avoided because of the injurious effects on the gastroduodenal mucosa. Alcohol in moderation is not harmful and no special dietary advice is required.

Helicobacter pylori
This can be eradicated in 80% of cases by the concomitant therapy with colloidal bismuth subcitrate, one

Table 7.9   Drugs used in the healing of peptic ulcer

	Short-term treatment	Maintenance treatment	Side-effects
Drugs which reduce acid secretion			
Cimetidine	800 mg at night or 400 mg 12-hourly	400 mg at night	Delays elimination of warfarin, phenytoin and theophylline and should not be used concurrently with these drugs. Rarely causes confusion in the elderly, and gynaecomastia in males—both effects reversible on stopping the drug
Ranitidine	300 mg at night, or 150 mg 12-hourly	150 mg at night	Reversible confusion
Nizatidine	300 mg at night, or 150 mg 12-hourly	150 mg at night	Sweating, urticaria, somnolence (all rare, none serious)
Famotidine	40 mg at night or 20 mg 12-hourly	20 mg at night	Headache, dizziness, dry mouth (all rare, none serious)
Misoprostol	200 μg 6-hourly	Not recommended	Abortefacient activity. Avoid use in women of child bearing age. Diarrhoea
Omeprazole	20 mg once daily	Not recommended	Hypergastrinaemia
Drugs which enhance mucosal defence			
Bismuth chelate (tri-potassium dicitrato-bismuthate)	240 mg 12-hourly	Not recommended	Blackens tongue, teeth and faeces. Risk of Bismuth toxicity with prolonged use
Sucralfate	2 g 12-hourly	Not recommended	Reduces absorption of warfarin, phenytoin, tetracycline, digoxin

tablet four times a day, amoxycillin 500 mg 6-hourly and metronidazole 400 mg 8-hourly for two weeks. Unfortunately this regimen causes side-effects, nausea, diarrhoea, and dizziness, and compliance becomes a problem. Another programme, amoxycillin 500 mg 6-hourly and omeprazole 20 mg 12-hourly for four weeks, is under evaluation. Therapy for the eradication of *H. pylori* is undergoing rapid evolution, as are recommendations on the most appropriate time to give it, for example when the ulcer is diagnosed, or healed or recurs. Without the eradication of *H. pylori*, 80% of ulcers will recur within 12 months.

Short-term management

The initial aim of therapy is to relieve symptoms and to heal the ulcer as quickly as possible. The drugs used in the treatment of peptic ulcer, the recommended doses and their side-effects, are given in Table 7.9.

Histamine H₂-receptor antagonist drugs. These are competitive inhibitors of histamine at the H₂-receptor on the parietal cell. The H₂-receptor antagonist drugs available include cimetidine, ranitidine, famotidine and nizatidine; several others are under development. Although they differ in chemical structure, pharmacological properties and cost, for practical purposes the H₂-receptor antagonist drugs are all equally effective in reducing acid secretion and healing the ulcer when prescribed in recommended doses.

They may be prescribed in twice daily doses or as a single larger dose at night (see Table 7.9). Symptoms remit promptly, usually within days of starting treatment. Ulcer healing takes longer, but about 80% of duodenal ulcers will have healed after 4 weeks. Treatment should be prolonged for 6–8 weeks or longer in patients who persist in smoking and in patients who have to continue NSAIDs because of arthritic conditions. Gastric ulcers heal more slowly than duodenal ulcers so that treatment should be prolonged for 6 weeks and it is important to confirm ulcer healing by further endoscopy.

Worldwide experience suggests that the H₂-receptor antagonist drugs listed in Table 7.9 are safe.

Omeprazole. This is a substituted benzimidazole compound that specifically and irreversibly inhibits the proton pump hydrogen-potassium ATP-ase in the parietal cell. It is the most powerful inhibitor of gastric secretion yet discovered. Maximal inhibition of acid secretions occurs 3 to 6 hours after an oral dose and with repeated dosing, this inhibition increases over the first few days of treatment to reach virtual achlorhydria. The drug has the distinct advantage over others in the more rapid healing of both gastric and duodenal ulcer.

Colloidal bismuth compounds. Tri-potassium dicitratobismuthate is an ammoniacal suspension of a complex colloidal bismuth salt. Its ulcer healing effect is probably separate from its activity against *H. pylori*. It has no effect on gastric acid secretion. It acts by protecting the ulcer from acid and pepsin and by enhancing mucosal defence mechanisms.

Sucralfate. This is a basic aluminium salt of sucrose octasulphate. It has little effect on acid secretion but acts by protecting the ulcer and stimulating epithelial renewal and defence mechanisms.

Synthetic prostaglandin analogues (e.g. Misoprostol). Prostaglandins exert complex effects on the gastroduodenal mucosa. In low doses they protect against injury induced by noxious agents such as aspirin, an effect which is designated as 'cytoprotection'; at higher doses as in misoprostol, acid secretion is inhibited and bicarbonate and mucus secretion are stimulated.

Antacids. These are now prescribed mainly for symptomatic relief and are widely used for self-medication. Given in sufficiently large doses for 4–6 weeks antacids will induce ulcer healing; however, many patients find the side-effects and the inconvenience of frequent dosing unacceptable. Many preparations are available, varying in neutralising capacity, side-effects, palatability and cost. Sodium bicarbonate is the quickest acting and is widely used for self-medication. However, it is readily absorbed with the risk of alkalosis so that its use should be discouraged and it should not be prescribed.

The majority of antacids are based on combinations of calcium, aluminium and magnesium salts, all of which cause side-effects. Calcium compounds cause constipation, magnesium compounds cause diarrhoea and prolonged overdosage of either may rarely lead to hypercalcaemia or hypermagnesaemia. Aluminium compounds block absorption of digoxin, tetracycline and dietary phosphate. Most antacids have a high sodium content which may exacerbate congestive heart failure or ascites.

Antacids are available in tablet and liquid forms; although tablet forms are more convenient to take they are probably less effective than liquid preparations.

Choice of drug

The H$_2$-receptor antagonists, omeprazole, sucralfate and tri-potassium dicitratobismuthate are all equally effective and safe treatments for ulcer healing. The choice depends upon physician preference and cost. Omeprazole causes hypergastrinaemia due to its profound inhibition of acid secretion, the degree being proportional to the degree of acid inhibition; hypergastrinaemia occurs to some extent with H$_2$-receptor antagonists. It is not of consequence with the short term, for example the four week treatment of gastric or duodenal ulcer.

Maintenance treatment

Continuous maintenance treatments with small doses of H$_2$-receptor antagonists will prevent ulcer relapse; as many as 80% of patients remain ulcer free for as long as treatment is maintained. The indications for maintenance treatment are shown in the information box.

Long-term maintenance treatment with H$_2$-receptor antagonists is safe and effective. The effects and safety of long-term maintenance treatment with other ulcer healing agents is unknown.

Surgical treatment

It is very uncommon for elective surgery to be carried out for uncomplicated peptic ulcer. Surgery is indicated

---

INDICATIONS FOR MAINTENANCE TREATMENT IN PEPTIC ULCER

- In ulcer patients who do not have *H. pylori* and in those in whom *H. pylori* cannot be eradicated, e.g. patients who are not compliant of or cannot tolerate the triple therapy
- With frequent symptomatic relapse. By contrast, with only one or two episodes a year it is more convenient and cost-effective to give a 4–6 week course of therapy for each relapse
- When there is a history of life-threatening complications such as repeated bleeding or perforation
- When the risk of future complications or ulcer operation must be avoided if at all possible—for example in elderly subjects or patients with another serious condition such as respiratory, cardiac, renal or hepatic impairment. In such patients maintenance treatment should be considered for life

---

when ulcer healing is resistant to all forms of therapy including eradication of *H. pylori,* or when there are frequent relapses despite adequate maintenance therapy. The indications for surgery are strengthened if the ulcer has developed in adolescence or young adult life, if there is a strong family history, or if there has been a previous complication such as haemorrhage or perforation. Finally some patients fail to comply with medical therapy or express reservations about prolonged therapy, both points being in favour of elective surgical treatment. Other indications are when there is an ulcer which has produced gastric outlet obstruction, or an hour-glass stomach because of fibrosis, or in a recurrent ulcer following previous gastric surgery.

There is no single, ideal operation suitable for all ulcers and all patients. The operation of choice for a gastric ulcer is partial gastrectomy preferably with a Billroth I anastomosis, in which the ulcer itself and the ulcer-bearing area of the stomach are resected (Fig. 7.7). For duodenal ulcer the acid secretory capacity of the stomach may be reduced by vagotomy which eliminates nervous stimulation (Fig. 7.7). At truncal vagotomy the main nerves are divided and thereafter gastric emptying may be retarded so that a drainage operation such as pyloroplasty or gastroenterostomy has to be added. A drainage procedure is also required in selective vagotomy in which vagal innervation to the small intestine, pancreas and biliary tree is preserved.

The aim of highly selective vagotomy is to denervate only the acid-producing area of the stomach while leaving intact the vagal supply of the antrum and pylorus. Gastric emptying is not impaired and a drainage procedure is not required unless there is stenosis from ulcer scarring. The avoidance of a drainage procedure markedly reduces the incidence of post-cibal syndromes and

gastric secretion results in large volumes of gastric aspirate under 'basal' conditions. Pentagastrin does not increase the secretory rate much above 'basal' values because the stomach is already continuously secreting at or near maximal rates.

Clinical features

The ulcers are often multiple and severe and may occur in unusual sites such as the jejunum or oesophagus. There is a poor response to ulcer therapy. The history is usually short, and bleeding and perforations are common. The syndrome may present in the form of severe recurrent ulceration following a standard operation for peptic ulcer, the underlying cause not having been recognised.

The diagnosis should be suspected in all patients with unusual or severe peptic ulceration, especially if the barium meal examination shows abnormally coarse gastric mucosal folds. In about one third of patients there is a family history of multiple endocrine neoplasia Type 1 (MEN I) involving parathyroid, pituitary and pancreas.

Investigations

Hypersecretion of acid under basal conditions is confirmed by gastric aspiration and serum gastrin levels are elevated. An attempt is made to localise the tumour by CT, angiography or by measuring the gastrin concentration in blood samples from tributaries of the portal vein.

Management

A tumour which is small and can be localised can be resected surgically, with cure. In the majority of patients continuous therapy with omeprazole is effective but larger doses than those used to treat duodenal ulcer are required.

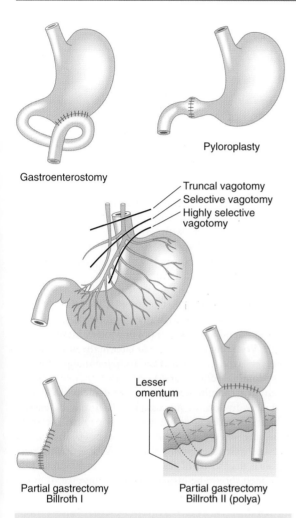

Gastroenterostomy

Pyloroplasty

Truncal vagotomy
Selective vagotomy
Highly selective vagotomy

Lesser omentum

Partial gastrectomy Billroth I

Partial gastrectomy Billroth II (polya)

Fig. 7.7   Operations for peptic ulcer.

in particular dumping (p. 433), but the risk of ulcer recurrence is greater. Vagotomy is preferred to partial gastrectomy because of the lesser mortality and lower incidence of long-term complications.

ZOLLINGER-ELLISON SYNDROME (GASTRINOMA)

This is a rare disorder in which severe peptic ulceration occurs due to a benign adenoma, or a malignant tumour or hyperplasia of the D cells of the islets of the pancreas. This 'gastrinoma' secretes large amounts of gastrin which stimulates the parietal cells of the stomach to secrete acid to their maximal capacity. The acid output may be so great that it reaches the upper small intestine, reducing the luminal pH to 2 or less. At this pH pancreatic lipase is inactivated and bile acids may be precipitated causing diarrhoea and steatorrhoea. Excessive

PERFORATION OF A PEPTIC ULCER

When free perforation occurs the contents of the stomach escape into the peritoneal cavity. The symptoms are those of peritonitis (p. 443) and they are in proportion to the extent of peritoneal soiling. If perforation occurs without loss of contents, as in the accidental perforation of the empty stomach at gastroscopy, few symptoms are produced and the accident may even pass unnoticed. Occasionally the symptoms of perforation appear and rapidly subside; presumably the perforation has closed spontaneously, or more probably the ulcer has perforated locally into an area confined by adhesions. Perforation occurs more commonly in duodenal than in gastric ulcers, and usually in ulcers on the anterior wall. About one quarter of all perforations occur in acute ulcers. There is evidence that NSAIDs are responsible for an increase in the number of perforations in the elderly.

Clinical features

Although perforation may be the first sign of ulcer, usually there is a history of recurrent-epigastric pain. The most striking symptom is sudden, severe pain; its distribution follows the spread of the gastric contents over the peritoneum. Thus initially the pain may be referred to the upper abdomen, but it quickly becomes generalised; shoulder tip pain may occur as a result of irritation of the diaphragm. The pain is accompanied by shallow respiration due to limitation of diaphragmatic movements, and by shock. The abdomen is held immobile and there is generalised 'board-like' rigidity. Intestinal sounds are absent and liver dullness to percussion may decrease due to the presence of gas under the diaphragm. Vomiting is common. After some hours the symptoms improve though the abdominal rigidity remains. However, the patient's condition deteriorates again as general peritonitis follows the initial peritoneal irritation.

A radiograph of the upper abdomen in the erect position may help to establish the diagnosis because free gas within the peritoneal cavity, if in sufficient amount, will show as a translucent crescent between the liver and diaphragm. However, radiological procedures should not be allowed to delay resuscitation and surgery based on the clinical findings.

Management and prognosis

After initial treatment of the patient for shock, the acute perforation is treated surgically either by simple closure, or by closure combined with vagotomy and drainage. More than half the patients who have a simple closure will eventually require a further elective operation for recurrence of ulcer symptoms, and for this reason the second option is usually taken.

Perforation carries a mortality of about 10%. The outlook is poorest in elderly patients in whom a large perforation results in extensive peritonitis or when operation is delayed.

GASTRIC OUTLET OBSTRUCTION

The causes are shown in Table 7.10. An ulcer in the region of the pylorus which causes a fibrous stricture or oedema, or a combination of both, presents as gastric outlet obstruction. The syndrome of gastric outlet obstruction is often loosely described as **'pyloric stenosis'**, even when the cause is chronic duodenal ulcer and therefore the pylorus is dilated.

Table 7.10 Gastric outlet obstruction

Cause	Treatment
Fibrous stricture from a duodenal ulcer, i.e. 'pyloric stenosis'	surgery
Oedema from pyloric channel or duodenal ulcer	standard medical therapy for ulcer
Carcinoma of the antrum	surgery
Adult hypertrophic pyloric stenosis	surgery
Gastroparesis	drugs to increase gastric motility

Clinical features

When duodenal or pyloric channel ulceration is the cause there may be a long preceding history of ulcer symptoms, whereas with cancer of the antrum, dyspepsia or loss of appetite is usually recent. In gastroparesis (p. 437) there is a history of epigastric fullness, nausea and intermittent vomiting.

Nausea and vomiting are the cardinal features of gastric outlet obstruction. Commonly, surprisingly large amounts of gastric content may be vomited and articles of food eaten 24 hours or more previously may be recognised. Vomiting tends to occur later in the day when the stomach is most distended and the patient may complain of abdominal fullness and heartburn.

Physical examination often shows evidence of wasting and dehydration. A succussion splash may be elicited 4 hours or more after the last meal or drink. Normally splashing occurs for less than an hour after meals because gastric emptying is rapid. Visible gastric peristalsis is diagnostic of gastric outlet obstruction and the abdomen should be inspected for its presence.

Investigations

The loss of gastric contents leads to dehydration with low serum sodium, chloride and potassium and raised bicarbonate and urea concentrations. The urine becomes alkaline. Aspiration of the stomach contents will confirm the diagnosis if the volume is in excess of 200 ml after fasting overnight or if the aspirate contains food residue.

Endoscopy is performed after the stomach has been lavaged to remove all food debris. The aim of endoscopy is to confirm or refute organic obstruction. Often obstruction due to fibrosis or carcinoma cannot be differentiated but this does not matter because surgical treatment is indicated for both. In the case of non-organic obstruction, i.e. gastroparesis, the pylorus appears normal and the endoscope can be passed into the duodenum.

Barium studies are rarely necessary for it is difficult to distinguish obstruction due to ulcer or cancer. Furthermore, when the obstruction is organic barium remains in the stomach and is difficult to remove.

Management

Nasogastric suction and the intravenous treatment of dehydration and metabolic alkalosis are commenced immediately. If there is uraemia or electrolyte disturbance, 4 litres of isotonic saline will be required in the first 24 hours and subsequently the potassium deficit will require 80 mmol per day.

Lavage of the stomach followed by endoscopy (see above) is performed as soon as dehydration is corrected. If necessary surgery is undertaken after 5–7 days of gastric aspiration to enable the dilated stomach to return to a more normal size. In patients with oedema as a cause of obstruction the volume of aspirate may decrease daily and it may be possible to commence oral fluids and food; a decision on surgery is then deferred until it is determined whether gastric emptying returns to normal. Obstruction secondary to ulcer is treated by vagotomy and gastroenterostomy. For cancer see page 436.

COMPLICATIONS FOLLOWING GASTRIC SURGERY

Although most operations performed for the relief of peptic ulcer are successful, 10% of patients will develop complications months or years afterwards. Some of these such as anaemia, nutritional impairment and bone disease develop insidiously, so that patients should be reviewed post-operatively at least once a year. Apart from recurrent ulcer those complications which develop soon after surgery are more common after gastric resection and are rare after highly selective vagotomy.

Recurrent ulcer ('stomal' ulcer)

When this occurs after surgery for duodenal ulcer, it is usually due to insufficient reduction of the secretory capacity of the stomach because of incomplete vagotomy or inadequate gastrectomy. A **jejunal ulcer** develops just distal to the jejunogastric anastomosis because the jejunal mucosa is more susceptible to acid-pepsin digestion than gastric or duodenal mucosa. About 15% of patients develop recurrent ulcer after highly selective vagotomy but the operation has the virtue of being free from the side-effects associated with resection, truncal vagotomy or drainage procedures.

Ulcer pain recurs, after months or years of freedom following the operation, or the patient may present with melaena or severe anaemia without any dyspeptic symptoms. Occasionally perforation occurs. Rarely a jejunal ulcer penetrates the colon causing a **gastro-jejunal-colic fistula.** Bacterial contamination of the small bowel follows causing diarrhoea, malabsorption and weight loss. The fistula can be demonstrated by barium enema.

Recurrent ulcer uncomplicated by perforation or fistula is best diagnosed by endoscopy, which will also reveal the occasional ulcer due to an unabsorbed suture which can be removed endoscopically. Usually recurrent ulcer can be treated by H_2-receptor antagonists or omeprazole but if this fails a more radical surgical procedure may be necessary.

Vomiting

Vomiting after gastric surgery is usually due to the presence of bile in the stomach ('bilious vomiting'). Epigastric cramping pain and nausea within an hour of eating are relieved by vomiting bitter yellow or green fluid. There may be loss of appetite and weight. The condition usually improves with time. It is treated with small dry meals and gastrokinetic drugs are given prior to meals, metoclopramide (10 mg 8-hourly), domperidone (10–20 mg 8-hourly), cisapride (10 mg 6-hourly or 8-hourly). Severe cases may require additional surgery. Occasionally vomiting is caused by obstruction to the afferent loop after a Billroth II operation (see Fig. 7.7) and the treatment is surgical.

In some patients the frequent presence of bile in the stomach after gastric surgery results in a superficial inflammation of the gastric mucosa which shows a chronic inflammatory exudate, with superficial haemorrhage and ulceration. The condition is often referred to as 'biliary gastritis'. It may be symptomless and observed only on routine post-operative endoscopy. However there may be epigastric discomfort, nausea, heartburn or vomiting of bile. It is treated in the same way as bilious vomiting.

The small stomach syndrome

This is a common but usually mild condition. Discomfort and distension with meals leads to diminished intake and weight loss or failure to regain weight. High energy small meals are indicated.

Dumping syndrome

In this condition there is a feeling of intense drowsiness with weakness and nausea after a meal and particularly after hot sweet foods. There may also be flushing, sweating and palpitations. The symptoms are due to the rapid passage of highly osmotic gastric contents into the intestine which promotes the rapid influx of fluid to dilute the osmotic load. The syndrome usually improves with time. The ingestion of small dry meals with the avoidance of fluids at meal times is often of value. Occasionally further surgery may be necessary.

Hypoglycaemia

Rarely, one or two hours after a meal, the patient experiences attacks of weakness, tremor and faintness. The hypoglycaemia responsible for these symptoms can be avoided by carbohydrate restriction. When symptoms do occur, the patient should use a readily available source of carbohydrate such as sweets.

Diarrhoea

This may occur after any operation on the stomach but especially after truncal vagotomy when most patients report some looseness of the stools. Moderate or severe diarrhoea occurs in about 5% and is characteristically episodic, several watery stools being passed daily for several days. A striking feature is the sense of urgency associated with the diarrhoea; defecation may be precipitate, and the patient becomes worried because of the fear of soiling. Loperamide (2 mg 8-hourly or more frequently) or codeine (30–60 mg 8-hourly) should be tried. Mild steatorrhoea (~ 10 g fat daily) is common after most ulcer operations and does not require treatment. If steatorrhoea is marked the patient may have a stagnant loop syndrome (p. 451).

Anaemia

Anaemia is a common sequel to operations on the stomach, particularly partial gastrectomy, because there is inadequate absorption of iron, or recurrent minor blood loss from gastritis or oesophagitis. Its incidence increases as the stores of iron become exhausted. The occurrence of anaemia reflects the adequacy of post-operative supervision because it is preventable by and responds to the administration of iron. Megaloblastic anaemia may also occur (p. 786) from vitamin B_{12} or folate deficiency. It is treated with appropriate vitamin replacement.

Nutritional impairment and osteomalacia

In a small proportion of patients some nutritional impairment follows gastric surgery and this increases with the extent of any resection. Severe weight loss is the most common manifestation. There may also be malabsorption or poor intake of vitamin D causing osteomalacia or a negative calcium balance leading to osteoporosis. These may develop for the first time 10 to 20 years after partial gastrectomy or occasionally after vagotomy and drainage. Their presentation and treatment is described on page 930.

FUNCTIONAL DISORDERS

NON-ULCER DYSPEPSIA

(Synonyms: Functional dyspepsia; Nervous dyspepsia; Non-organic dyspepsia)

In this common condition the patient complains of dyspepsia and other ulcer-like symptoms but investigation fails to detect an ulcer.

Aetiology

The condition of non-ulcer dyspepsia probably covers a spectrum of mucosal, motility and psychiatric disorders. The symptoms caused by motor dysfunction are analogous to the motility disturbances that occur in the irritable bowel syndrome (p. 470); indeed the symptoms of both disorders may be present suggesting a generalised motility disorder. Patients with mucosal disorder often have gastritis secondary to *H. pylori* but there is debate as to whether this chronic infection is symptomatic (p. 426).

Clinical features

Patients are usually young (< 40 years) and women are affected twice as commonly as men. Abdominal pain is associated with a variable combination of other 'dyspeptic' symptoms, the commonest being nausea and bloating after meals. Morning symptoms are characteristic and pain or nausea may occur on waking. Direct enquiry may elicit symptoms suggestive of colonic dysmotility such as pellet-like stools or a sense of incomplete rectal evacuation on defecation.

Generally the problem is to exclude peptic ulcer disease; in older subjects intra-abdominal malignancy is the prime concern. Features that suggest functional dyspepsia rather than organic disease are listed in the information box.

DISTINGUISHING FEATURES OF FUNCTIONAL DYSPEPSIA

- Pain/discomfort is not episodic but tends to occur daily for long periods at a time
- Pain may persist throughout the entire day from morning to night unaffected by food, antacids or bowel movement; food may provoke pain
- Pain is diffuse, described by sweeping movements of the hands over the abdomen, and may be referred to more than one site
- Vomiting brings no relief from pain and the patient cannot eat for hours afterwards; by contrast vomiting almost always relieves pain in ulcer subjects and they can eat almost immediately thereafter

---

There are no diagnostic signs apart perhaps from inappropriate tenderness on abdominal palpation. Symptoms appear disproportionate to clinical well-being and there is no weight loss. Patients may appear anxious and distraught. It is often possible to detect associated psychological factors. Many patients are self-admitted 'worriers', concerned about finance, employment, or family affairs. Older subjects may be fearful of developing cancer. There is often a history of previous psychotropic medication or a personal or family history of 'nerves'.

A drug history should be taken and the possibility of a depressive illness should be considered. Pregnancy should be ruled out in young women before radiological studies are undertaken. Alcohol abuse should be suspected when nausea and retching are prominent especially in the mornings. The presence of spider naevi or a palpable liver are suggestive and abnormal liver function tests or a raised mean corpuscular volume (MCV) support the diagnosis.

Investigations

The history will often suggest the diagnosis but especially in older subjects a barium meal or endoscopy should be performed to resolve doubt.

Management

The most important element is explanation and reassurance. Possible psychological factors should be explored and the concept of psychological influences on gut function should be explained so that it is respectable and acceptable to the patient. Cigarette smoking and alcohol abuse should be discouraged and sensible dietary advice may be necessary.

Drug treatment is not especially successful but merits trial. Antacids are sometimes helpful. Prokinetic drugs such as metoclopramide (10 mg 8-hourly) or domperidone (10–20 mg 8-hourly) or cisapride (10 mg 6-hourly or 8-hourly) may be given before meals if nausea, vomiting or bloating are prominent. Metoclopramide may induce extrapyramidal side-effects including tardive dyskinesia in young subjects. H_2-receptor antagonist drugs may be tried if night pain or heartburn are troublesome. *H. pylori* gastritis should be treated (p. 428).

Symptoms which can be associated with an identifiable cause of stress (impending marriage or divorce, financial or employment difficulties, for example) resolve with appropriate counselling. In many patients, however, symptoms may persist or recur over a lifetime so that formal psychotherapy should be considered if major psychological difficulties are identified.

PSYCHOGENIC VOMITING

Psychogenic vomiting may occur in anxiety neurosis. Usually it commences on wakening, or immediately after breakfast; only rarely does it occur later in the day. The disorder is probably a reaction to wakening and facing up to the worries of everyday life; in the young it can be due to school phobia. There may be retching alone or the vomiting of gastric secretions or food. Although psychogenic vomiting may occur regularly over long periods, there is little or no weight loss and this is of value in distinguishing it from vomiting due to organic disease of the alimentary tract. Early morning vomiting also occurs in pregnancy, alcohol abuse and depression.

In all patients it is essential to assess and, if possible, alleviate the underlying psychological disturbance. Tranquillisers and antiemetic drugs (e.g. metoclopramide 10 mg 8-hourly, domperidone 10 mg 8-hourly, prochlorperazine 5–10 mg 8-hourly) have only a secondary place in management.

TUMOURS OF THE STOMACH

CARCINOMA OF THE STOMACH

The incidence of this tumour varies considerably in different parts of the world—it is frequent in Japan, China and southern Europe but relatively uncommon in the USA. The incidence is falling in many countries. Japanese immigrants to America have a lower incidence than in Japan, indicating the possible importance of environmental factors such as trace elements in water or differences in methods of food preparation. It has been suggested that nitrites, often used as preservatives in food and present in drinking water, can be converted to the carcinogens nitrosamines in the milieu of the stomach. Patients with pernicious anaemia have an increased risk of developing gastric cancer and this may extend to gastric atrophy from other causes. The geographical incidence of *H. pylori*, leading to Type B gastritis (p. 426) parallels that of gastric cancer. There is an increased incidence of cancer of the stomach after partial gastrectomy or gastroenterostomy.

Pathology

Almost 50% of all gastric cancers occur at the pylorus or in the antrum; the lesion does not spread to the duodenum. Such growths may produce symptoms of obstruction to the gastric outlet. Cancer of the body of the stomach occurs in 20–30% of cases and often produces a fungating ulcerating mass. In 5–20% of patients, the tumour is at the cardia and produces dysphagia. Least common is a diffuse infiltrating scirrhous lesion spreading submucosally throughout the body of the stomach, which is defined as linitis plastica.

Gastric dysplasia is the term applied to precancerous lesions of the stomach; it is recognised by cytological changes in the epithelial cells. **Early gastric cancer** is defined as cancer confined to the mucosa, or mucosa and submucosa, regardless of the presence of lymph node metastasis. The lesion may be represented only by a depressed area with obliteration or distortion of the mucosal folds, irregular ulceration on an elevated base, or by a small polypoid lesion. Such changes can be seen and a biopsy taken during gastroscopy at a stage when the cancer is potentially curable.

The tumour is an adenocarcinoma of intestinal or diffuse type. The intestinal type has well-defined cells and a clear margin and it is this type which has shown a fall in incidence in several countries. The diffuse type consists of clusters of cells which spread widely within the mucosa. The tumour spreads by extension through the stomach wall, by lymphatic permeation and by embolism via the portal vein to the liver and thence to the systemic bloodstream. Gastric carcinoma may present as a malignant ulcer but this is rarely the result of malignant transformation of a benign ulcer. A chronic peptic ulcer rarely becomes malignant and malignant ulcers, however long they have been present, have always been malignant.

Clinical features

Loss of appetite, slight nausea and dyspepsia after meals occurring for the first time in middle age should always arouse suspicion. Sometimes there is epigastric pain suggestive of ulcer disease. If the diagnosis is to be made early such patients require careful investigation. Unfortunately, the majority of patients have advanced gastric carcinoma before they develop symptoms sufficient to seek advice. With advancement of the tumour, dyspepsia becomes troublesome with increasing anorexia and nausea, discomfort or pain, vomiting and weight loss. There may be cachexia and pallor, a mass may be palpable or peristalsis visible. The abdomen may be distended by ascites from peritoneal metastases. Sometimes it is acanthosis nigricans (p. 973) or the presence of metastases in the liver, pelvis or scalene lymph nodes which first brings the patient to the physician.

Carcinoma of the stomach should always be considered as a cause of unexplained iron deficiency anaemia in the middle-aged person. Tumours at the cardia may cause dysphagia, and tumours at the gastric outlet may cause vomiting. In the infiltrating type of tumour, diarrhoea may occur because of rapid emptying from the stomach.

Investigations

Early curable cancer is usually missed by a barium meal examination unless a double-contrast study is carried out to show distortion of the mucosal pattern. The only method of establishing a positive diagnosis is by gastroscopy and biopsy of suspicious areas. These procedures are also necessary to distinguish malignant from benign gastric ulceration. The commonest appearance

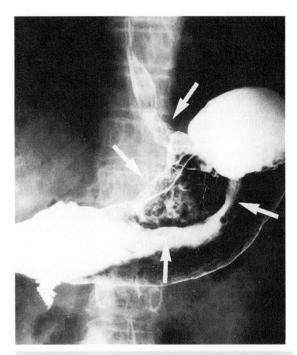

Fig. 7.8   Carcinoma of the stomach. Arrows indicate extent of tumour.

at barium meal is a filling defect in the antrum or body of the stomach (Fig. 7.8). In the rare diffuse infiltrating carcinoma, the stomach appears as a rigid tube through which the barium pours rapidly into the intestine. If dysphagia is the presenting symptom, a lesion in the cardia will probably be found, but symptomless lesions in this area can be easily missed. Exfoliative cytology may be used for diagnosis.

Management

The curative treatment is gastrectomy. It is usually only at laparotomy that the possibility of resection can be decided when about one-third of patients are found to have tumours capable of removal. In the remainder it is possible to perform only a palliative procedure which is worthwhile if pyloric obstruction is present even if there are secondary deposits. Such an operation relieves distressing vomiting and gives the patient some comfort.

A total gastrectomy may be required for tumours involving the upper part of the stomach. Careful preoperative treatment is essential, including the restoration of fluid and electrolyte balance and the correction of anaemia. Every effort should be made to improve nutrition, if necessary by parenteral or enteral feeding. A small proportion of patients with cancer of the stomach obtain worthwhile remission with a combination of cytotoxic drugs.

Prognosis

The prognosis in carcinoma of the stomach is poor and has hardly improved in the last 40 years. After an apparently successful resection the 5-year survival rate is about 20%. The overall 5-year survival rate is 5%. However, the 5-year survival rate is 85% for early gastric cancer. Thus, pending an entirely new approach to the problem, the only means currently available to improve outcome is the detection of gastric cancer when it is at a curable stage. This requires a vigorous approach to the problem of dyspepsia in the middle-aged including careful radiological and endoscopic examination and the careful follow-up of doubtful abnormalities.

OTHER TUMOURS OF THE STOMACH

Adenomatous polyps, leiomyomas and other benign neoplasms of the stomach are often found coincidentally at upper gastrointestinal endoscopy or barium studies. Occasionally they are the cause of dyspepsia, and leiomyoma may present with acute or occult bleeding. Some of these lesions may be removed at endoscopy, others may require resection. Primary lymphoma of the stomach usually has the radiological or endoscopic appearance of gastric cancer. The patient may present with abdominal pain, weight loss, nausea, vomiting and haematemesis and melaena. The treatment is gastric resection followed by radiotherapy.

MISCELLANEOUS DISORDERS OF THE STOMACH AND DUODENUM

GASTROPARESIS

This occurs in 50% of patients with long-standing diabetes mellitus, pseudo-obstruction (p. 454), anorexia nervosa, in diseases of the smooth muscle—progressive systemic sclerosis, dystrophia myotonica—and in dermatomyositis/polymyositis. It can also occur after gastric surgery. In a proportion of patients no underlying cause is apparent.

Clinical features

The symptoms range from epigastric fullness, early satiety, nausea and anorexia to uncontrollable nausea and vomiting. In some patients vomiting is infrequent because the patient learns to adapt to a liquid diet. As in organic obstruction (p. 432) there may be large volumes of vomitus, and food ingested more than 12 hours previously may be recognised.

Investigations

Endoscopy is performed to exclude organic obstruction. A radioisotopic gastric emptying study is also performed to confirm the diagnosis.

Management

The treatment is with prokinetic drugs, metoclopramide, domperidone and cisapride (p. 433), given 30 minutes before food.

BEZOARS

These are usually composed of plant material and occur in gastroparesis or after gastric surgery. They present with pain, nausea and vomiting and there may be a palpable epigastric mass. The bezoar is sometimes diagnosed on the plain radiograph of the abdomen but the diagnosis is usually made at endoscopy or by a barium meal. Treatment is by disruption at endoscopy or by enzyme ingestion.

DUODENAL DIVERTICULUM

This is an outpouching of the duodenal mucosa acquired at a point of weakness on the medial duodenal wall. It is generally single. Usually the diverticulum is asymptomatic but it may perforate retroperitoneally, it may obstruct the bile or pancreatic ducts or it may bleed. The treatment of all these complications is surgical.

EOSINOPHILIC GASTRITIS AND ENTERITIS

This condition usually involves the gastric antrum and pylorus but it may affect the small intestine and occasionally the colon. The term 'gastritis' is a misnomer because the characteristic eosinophilic infiltration is of the submucosa and muscle layers rather than the mucosa. There is also eosinophilia in the peripheral blood.

Clinical features

Patients with gastric involvement have nausea and vomiting, and a barium meal or endoscopy shows diffuse ulceration or narrowing of the gastric antrum. When the intestinal mucosa is involved there may be nausea, vomiting, pain, diarrhoea and weight loss. The diagnosis is made by jejunal biopsy. A barium follow-through examination may show solitary or diffuse involvement of intestine which may simulate Crohn's disease.

Management

Treatment is with prednisolone 20 mg/day until the symptoms resolve. Usually this is a matter of weeks.

FURTHER READING

Graham D Y, Go M F 1993 *Helicobacter pylori:* current status. Gastroenterology 105: 279

McColl K E L, Fullarton G M 1993 Duodenal ulcer pain—the role of acid and inflammation. Gut 34: 1300

Taha A S, Russell R I 1993 *Helicobacter pylori* and non-steroidal anti-inflammatory drugs: uncomfortable partners in peptic ulcer disease. Gut 34: 580

Talley N J 1992 Chronic peptic ulceration and nonsteroidal anti-inflammatory drugs: more to be said about NSAIDs? Gastroenterology 102: 1074

GASTROINTESTINAL HAEMORRHAGE

ACUTE UPPER GASTROINTESTINAL HAEMORRHAGE

This is an important condition because the incidence is approximately 150/100 000 per year and because there is a mortality of 10% in those admitted to hospital and 30% in the elderly.

Aetiology

The common causes of upper gastrointestinal bleeding in Western communities are shown in Table 7.11. The relative importance of each diagnosis varies from country to country. The regular consumption of aspirin or NSAIDs increases the incidence and consequently the mortality from upper gastrointestinal bleeding particularly in elderly females. About 3 per 1000 of such patients consuming these drugs are admitted for haemorrhage from haemorrhagic gastritis (p. 425) or a chronic ulcer.

There are also a number of uncommon causes of upper and lower gastrointestinal bleeding which are

Table 7.11 Common causes of upper gastrointestinal bleeding

Cause	%
Chronic duodenal ulcer	25
Chronic gastric ulcer	20
Gastric erosions	20
Varices	10
Mallory–Weiss tear	7
Oesophagitis	5
Duodenal erosions	5
Cancer of the stomach	3
Miscellaneous	5

nevertheless important because their correct management needs prompt recognition (Table 7.12).

Clinical features

Gastroduodenal haemorrhage is recognised by **haematemesis** (vomiting of blood) and/or **melaena** (passage of black stools). Haematemesis and melaena may occur together with a sudden large bleed whereas melaena alone indicates that bleeding is slower and less in amount. If blood remains in the stomach it becomes partially digested and appears brown and granular in the vomit or gastric aspirate, like coffee grounds. Blood passing through the intestinal canal is also altered in appearance, so that the faeces become black and sticky (a melaena, or 'tarry' stool), but occasionally in severe bleeding transit may be so rapid that the blood in the rectum is bright red. A melaena stool may be produced by bleeding as distal as the ascending colon.

In severe bleeding from whatever cause, the patient complains of weakness, faintness, nausea, and sweating, and may be agitated, restless and disorientated from cerebral anoxia. These signs may be absent in the young patient in whom compensatory mechanisms are more effective.

Serial recordings of the pulse rate and blood pressure give some indication of the severity of bleeding but for a more accurate assessment in patients who continue to bleed, measurement of central venous pressure is necessary. A postural hypotension of greater than 10 mmHg is an indication of the loss of more than 20% of the blood volume. The measurement of urinary output by catheterisation is helpful in patients with severe bleeding.

The initial haemoglobin level and haematocrit will not alter until haemodilution has occurred, which may not take place for some hours nor be complete for some days. A reduced haematocrit on admission to hospital suggests chronic bleeding prior to the acute episode. A raised urea with a normal serum creatinine indicates blood loss of at least one litre. There is no simple laboratory procedure which will give a reliable estimate of the amount of blood loss until haemodilution is complete. The passage of a nasogastric tube is of value in assessing the persistent rate of bleeding. It may also have a diagnostic value by indicating the source of bleeding to be in the upper gastrointestinal tract.

Investigations

Upper gastrointestinal endoscopy is undertaken to determine the site of bleeding and if possible the lesion causing it. If bleeding has stopped the endoscopist may see signs of recent bleeding such as adherent clot in an ulcer crater. A radionuclide scan with radiolabelled red cells may provide an important clue as to the possible

Table 7.12   Less common causes of gastrointestinal bleeding

Cause	Diagnostic points
Haemobilia	Bleeding from biliary tree; usually accompanied by jaundice and biliary colic
Aortic aneurysm	Usually bleeds into duodenum via aortic-duodenal fistula
Pancreatitis and pancreatic cancer	Diagnosed on the presence of other features of pancreatic disease
Duodenal and jejunal diverticula	Diagnosed by barium follow-through examination
Meckel's diverticulum	Painless lower gastrointestinal haemorrhage
Hereditary disorders of small blood vessels	Diagnosed on history and examination
Coagulation disorders	Diagnosed on family history, consumption of anticoagulants, or a low platelet count

location of bleeding in patients in whom repeated endoscopy has failed to find the site. Angiography is also used under these circumstances.

Management

A history of acute gastrointestinal blood loss within the previous 48 hours is an indication for immediate admission to hospital when the current practice is for most patients to be assessed by a physician and surgeon in a unit dedicated to this problem. The emergency nature of the condition is emphasised by the plan of management (Fig. 7.9). The emphasis is on resuscitation and monitoring. There are no pharmacological means of stopping bleeding except in patients with varices.

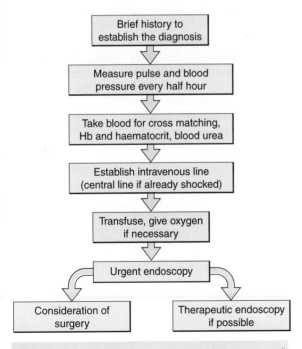

Fig. 7.9   Plan of management—acute gastrointestinal bleeding.

Transfusion

This commences immediately with normal saline. Colloidal solutions may then be used if blood is not immediately available. Blood is given as whole blood but if significant saline or expander has already been infused, packed red cells are preferable especially in the elderly. The decision to transfuse is based on clinical judgement but some of the salient criteria are shown in the information box.

> **GUIDELINES FOR TRANSFUSION IN UPPER GASTROINTESTINAL HAEMORRHAGE**
>
> Transfusion is required
> - if there is evidence of continued acute bleeding as shown by
>   a. nasogastric aspiration
>   b. increasing pulse rate or falling blood pressure
> - if the patient is clinically shocked
> - if the pulse rate is consistently >100/minute
> - if the systolic pressure is <100 mmHg
> - if the haemoglobin is <10 dl

Transfusion must keep pace with the estimated loss, which may be difficult in the elderly patient when under-transfusion is liable to lead to cardiac or renal failure, cerebral anoxia, angina or even myocardial infarction. Over-transfusion may lead to left ventricular failure. Therefore transfusion is usually monitored by central venous pressure measurements in the elderly and shocked patients.

Sedation

Great care is taken with the use of sedatives, for they may precipitate hepatic coma if the patient has portal hypertension and cirrhosis. If there are any indications that liver disease may be present (history of alcohol, jaundice, presence of hepato- or splenomegaly, stigmata of liver disease) no sedation should be considered prior to endoscopy. Morphine should never be given because

Table 7.13 Poor prognostic factors in gastrointestinal bleeding

Severe initial bleed based on transfusion requirements and presence of shock
Continued bleeding
Recurrence of bleeding once bleeding has stopped
Onset of bleeding during hospitalisation
Age over 60 years
Presence of other disease (cardiac, respiratory, renal)
Variceal bleeding

CAUSES OF ACUTE BLEEDING FROM THE LOWER GASTROINTESTINAL TRACT

Common
- Diverticular disease
- Angiodysplasia

Less common
- Ischaemic colitis
- Inflammatory bowel disease
- Carcinoma

Rare
- Solitary ulcer
- Meckel's diverticulum
- Polyps

it may cause vomiting. Diazepam (2 mg 8-hourly) may be given to control restlessness and anxiety.

Therapeutic endoscopy

Endoscopic methods for the control of upper gastro-intestinal bleeding have been developed because of the risks associated with emergency surgery. Techniques by which coagulating electrodes, heater probes and laser energy can be applied to a bleeding lesion under direct vision at endoscopy are all successful on some occasions. All require the lesion to be accessible to endoscopic instrumentation to enable the vessel responsible for bleeding to be identified. Hazards include perforation and re-bleeding.

Surgery

Judgement regarding whether and when surgery is necessary is based upon several factors which are known to imply a poor prognosis (Table 7.13). The presence of one or more of these factors is usually an indication for surgery. There is some controversy in that the elderly and those with concomitant diseases withstand bleeding poorly and it is argued that surgical intervention should be undertaken early. However, operative mortality is much higher in these patients.

Every attempt is always made to stop variceal bleeding without recourse to surgery. Excision of the bleeding gastric ulcer, or exposure and suture of the duodenal ulcer coupled in either case with vagotomy, is usually safer than partial gastrectomy which should be reserved for the complicated patient and requires an expert surgeon.

Management of other gastrointestinal lesions

Haemorrhagic gastritis (p. 425)

Many of the patients at risk will be in intensive care units where it is usual practice to use prophylactic treatment with oral sucralfate or intravenous H_2-receptor antagonists (p. 429) to prevent haemorrhagic gastritis and the acute Curling's or Cushing's ulcers. Therapeutic endoscopy and the use of intravenous or intra-arterial vaso-

pressin should be attempted prior to surgery. Every attempt is made to avoid surgery but gastric resection and vagotomy may be required.

Mallory-Weiss tear

The mucosa at the gastro-oesophageal junction is torn as a result of retching, vomiting or occasionally coughing. Often there is a history of recent intake of alcohol followed by the vomiting of food and then bright red blood. Bleeding nearly always stops spontaneously with conservative management. In a few patients therapeutic endoscopy or intra-arterial vasopressin may be required.

Vascular lesions (ectasias)

Localised vascular lesions in the stomach are responsible for a small percentage of bleeding lesions particularly in the elderly. Therapeutic endoscopy is the treatment of choice but if the lesion is extensive, resection of the affected area may be indicated.

Varices

See page 503.

ACUTE LOWER GASTROINTESTINAL HAEMORRHAGE

This is much less frequent than acute bleeding from the upper gastrointestinal tract, shock is less common and the bleeding usually ceases spontaneously.

Aetiology

The usual causes of such bleeding are shown in the information box. In about 10% of cases the cause of bleeding is not found.

Angiodysplasia

These ectasias probably result from venous obstruction. The mechanism is thought to be a degenerative process, the lesions being commoner in patients over the age of 65. It is thought that with ageing there is obstruction of the blood flow through the mucosal veins which can be occluded because of the lower pressure which exists within them while the higher arterial pressure maintains arterial inflow. Ultimately the repeated episodes of transient elevated pressure result in a dilatation and tortuosity of the submucosal veins and subsequently of the venules and capillaries of the mucosal units draining into the veins.

Lesions affect the right colon in 80% of patients and take the form of vascular abnormalities. The ectasias are of both the submucosal veins and the mucosal arteriolar-capillary-venular unit. Ectasias may also occur in the small bowel.

Diverticular disease

Bleeding results from rupture of an artery in the diverticulum (see p. 465), usually from the right side of the colon.

Clinical features

Blood is defecated and is red or plum coloured, and is usually mixed with clots, faeces or mucus. The bleeding is often recurrent. It is important not to confuse this bleeding with that of haemorrhoids (p. 474). Acute lower gastrointestinal bleeding from the small intestine, the caecum and right colon may occasionally appear as melaena. Abdominal pain is unusual.

The majority of patients are elderly. Those with angiodysplasia may have aortic valve disease. Those with diverticular disease are commonly hypertensive and it is unusual for them to have had other symptoms of diverticular disease.

The approach to the assessment of shock is the same as in acute upper gastrointestinal bleeding (p. 439).

Investigations

Colonoscopy is the investigation of choice, when vascular ectasias can be seen as dilated vessels but may be missed when the patient is shocked. It may also demonstrate a bleeding diverticulum. In patients in whom colonoscopy has failed to locate the bleeding lesion, and in those with very rapid bleeding, angiography is performed. Upper gastrointestinal endoscopy is performed if it is thought that the bleeding could be from oesophagus, stomach or duodenum.

Management

The emphasis is on non-surgical management. Transfusion is organised, sedation and bed rest are instituted

and investigation organised once the patient has been stabilised. If bleeding stops at this stage investigations may be deferred. Endoscopic coagulation of angiodysplastic lesions may be possible if bleeding continues and colonoscopy is performed. If the bleeding site is located by angiography it may be possible to treat angiodysplasia or bleeding from a diverticulum with intra-arterial vasopressin or embolisation. Continued bleeding unresponsive to the above measures requires surgical resection.

Bleeding from haemorrhoids

This is common but rarely severe and arises from internal haemorrhoids. There is painless passage of bright red blood characteristically at the beginning and end of defecation and it often squirts. The blood is on the stool but is not mixed with it. Similar bleeding may occur with an anal fissure but this is accompanied by acute localised pain whilst the motion is passed. The problem is investigated by proctoscopy. Sigmoidoscopy is also performed to ensure the bleeding is not due to a polyp or carcinoma.

OCCULT GASTROINTESTINAL HAEMORRHAGE

'Occult' means that blood or its breakdown products are present in the stool but cannot be seen. Bleeding into the upper gastrointestinal tract of up to 200 ml per day may be occult. The importance of occult bleeding is that it may signify a serious gastrointestinal lesion and that it may be a cause of severe anaemia.

Aetiology

All causes of acute upper and lower gastrointestinal haemorrhage (Tables 7.11 and 7.12, pp. 438–439 and information box, p. 440) may also cause occult bleeding. Hookworm is the most important cause worldwide but the following causes merit particular attention in Western communities.

Tumours

Tumours, benign or malignant, of any site in the gastrointestinal tract may cause occult bleeding. Colorectal cancer is the commonest.

Peptic ulcer and oesophagitis

Occult bleeding is extremely common and may occur when ulcer symptoms are absent.

Non-steroidal anti-inflammatory drugs

Occult bleeding occurs in all users. While the site is usually the stomach or duodenum it may also occur from the small intestine or colon.

Vascular lesions

Angiodysplasias of the colon or ectasias elsewhere in the gastrointestinal tract are an important cause of occult bleeding which is difficult to locate.

Clinical features

The problem comes to light because of iron deficiency (p. 783). There may be manifestations of other underlying disease but these are not usually present, hence the patient presents ultimately with anaemia.

Investigations

The presence of occult bleeding can be confirmed by an occult blood test (p. 413) but usually the presence of iron deficiency anaemia is sufficient to warrant a full gastrointestinal investigation for the site of the blood loss. The investigation commences with colonoscopy or barium enema followed by upper gastrointestinal endoscopy. If these are negative a decision may be made to treat the iron deficiency to determine if the problem recurs because further tests have a much lower chance of success. Such procedures include barium follow-through, angiography and CT of the abdomen.

FURTHER READING

Lieberman D 1994 Colon cancer screening: beyond efficacy. Gastroenterology 106: 803–812

Pasricha P J, Fleischer D E, Kalloo A N 1994 Endoscopic perforations of the upper digestive tract: a review of their pathogenesis, prevention, and management. Gastroenterology 106: 787–802

Quine M A, Bell G D, McCloy R F, Devlin H B, Hopkins A et al 1994 Appropriate use of upper gastrointestinal endoscopy—a prospective audit. Gut 35: 1209–1214

Sayer J M, Long R G 1993 A perspective on iron deficiency anaemia. Gut 34: 1297

ACUTE ABDOMEN

The term acute abdomen is used to define a group of abdominal conditions in which prompt surgical treatment must be considered to treat perforation, peritonitis and vascular and other intra-abdominal catastrophes. Some important causes are listed in the information box.

Clinical features

The history depends on the cause. Abdominal pain is the most prominent symptom. Visceral abdominal pain

CAUSES OF ACUTE ABDOMEN

Bowel
- Acute appendicitis
- Perforated peptic ulcer or abdominal viscus
- Diverticular disease
- Intestinal obstruction and strangulation
- Meckel's diverticulum
- Terminal ileitis due to *Yersinia* infection

Vascular
- Acute vascular insufficiency
- Ruptured aortic aneurysm

Gynaecological
- Ruptured ectopic pregnancy
- Ruptured ovarian cyst
- Acute salpingitis

Others
- Cholecystitis
- Acute pancreatitis
- Acute mesenteric adenitis

is experienced in that region of the abdominal wall innervated by spinal nerves with the same segmental origin as the sympathetic nerves of the obstructed or inflamed viscus (Fig. 7.10). Parietal abdominal pain results from irritation of the parietal peritoneum innervated by spinal nerves supplying the overlying abdominal wall. Thus, parietal pain is localised to the area of abdomen affected.

Abdominal tenderness, muscle guarding and rigidity are signs of peritonitis. Inflammation of the dia-

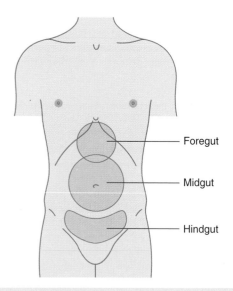

Fig. 7.10 Site of appreciation of abdominal pain according to the area of gut involved.

phragmatic peritoneum is suggested by shoulder-tip pain and hyperaesthesia. Inflammation of the pelvic peritoneum may produce tenderness which is detected on rectal examination. Other clinical features are described with the appropriate diseases.

Medical conditions which may simulate the acute abdomen include pleurisy, pneumonia and myocardial infarction, all of which may cause upper abdominal pain. These conditions are listed in the information box.

MEDICAL CONDITIONS WHICH MAY MIMIC ACUTE ABDOMEN

- Myocardial infarction
- Pneumonia
- Pleurisy
- Acute pyelonephritis
- Irritable bowel syndrome
- Tonsillitis, otitis media in children

Uncommon

- Diabetic ketoacidosis
- Acute porphyria
- Henoch–Schönlein purpura
- Haemophilia
- Sickle-cell disease
- Arteritis (polyarteritis nodosa or SLE)
- Herpes zoster
- Gastroenteritis

PERITONITIS

Peritonitis is the reaction of the peritoneum to an irritant. Usually this is infection although sometimes the irritation is chemical, at least initially, when bile or duodenal contents leak into the peritoneal cavity. Appendicitis is one of the commonest causes of peritonitis, *E. coli* being the organism usually responsible. Infection or chemical irritation causes the peritoneum to become congested and oedematous. There is an exudation of fluid containing large quantities of leucocytes, protein and antibodies. Dilution and destruction of the irritant is accompanied by its localisation and by the formation of adhesions. Failure of these defence mechanisms is characterised by spread of the infection, septicaemia, and toxaemia.

Clinical features

In perforations (for example peptic ulcer, p. 431), the onset is sudden with severe abdominal pain, vomiting, tenderness, rigidity and shock. Reflex guarding and muscle rigidity occur in relation to the area of peritoneum which is inflamed. Pelvic peritonitis is associated with tenderness on rectal examination. These initial severe features gradually decrease; the patient appears to

improve and the diagnosis can be missed. Subsequently paralytic ileus develops and fluid collects in the peritoneal cavity. There is increasing distension, the rigidity lessens, the tenderness remains and toxaemia develops.

When peritonitis is secondary to inflammation of a viscus, such as appendicitis, the initial signs are those of the underlying disease, later to be replaced by the features of peritonitis. Vomiting is common at the onset of peritonitis, but later diminishes in frequency and severity only to return with the onset of toxaemia and paralytic ileus.

Management

Shock is common in diffuse peritonitis and resuscitation must be undertaken before surgery. Blood cultures are obtained and parenteral treatment with a broad spectrum antibiotic and metronidazole is commenced. The surgical treatment of established peritonitis is by removal of the contaminating source such as in appendicitis, or perforated bowel or gallbladder, together with peritoneal toilet and lavage.

General peritonitis may resolve completely, but often inflammation localises to form an abscess at the primary site, or in the subphrenic region or in the pelvis. Persistence of fever, or continued elevation of pulse rate, white blood count and ESR, should lead to efforts to locate such residual loci of infection, for example by ultrasonography.

Pelvic abscess

This usually follows the localisation of a general peritonitis and forms in the lower part of the peritoneal cavity in front of the rectum. The abscess may irritate the bladder causing urinary frequency or involve the bowel causing diarrhoea with the passage of mucus and a feeling of incomplete emptying. It is evident on rectal or vaginal examination as a tender mass, which may discharge rectally or vaginally. Treatment with metronidazole (400 mg 8-hourly) is usually effective.

Subphrenic abscess

The localisation of pus between diaphragm and liver on the right side or between the diaphragm and the liver, spleen and stomach on the left is a complication of peritonitis most commonly following perforation of the stomach, duodenum or gallbladder, or after an operation on these organs. There are signs of persistent infection. There may be dullness at the base of the lung and tenderness over the lower ribs posteriorly. Diagnosis is aided by ultrasonography or a radiograph of the diaphragmatic region which may show elevation of the diaphragm with a fluid level below or an effusion above. Treatment is by drainage either at laparotomy or by insertion of a drain under ultrasound control.

ACUTE APPENDICITIS

Acute appendicitis occurs in all age groups. It is usually obstructive, the lumen of the appendix being narrowed by swelling of lymphoid tissue in its wall or by stricture from previous inflammation. Obstruction is made complete by impaction of a faecolith causing gangrene, perforation and a local abscess or generalised peritonitis. Another outcome is the formation of an oedematous inflammatory appendix mass.

Clinical features

The classical history is the sudden onset of vague central abdominal pain followed within a few hours by a shift of the pain to the right iliac fossa where it becomes localised to McBurney's point (one third of the distance along a line from the anterior superior iliac spine to the umbilicus). There is nausea and malaise. There may be vomiting but this is seldom severe and is often absent. The pulse rate is increased. In the early stages there is little elevation of temperature and the occurrence of rigors and a high fever make the diagnosis of appendicitis unlikely. There is tenderness and guarding in the right iliac fossa progressing to rigidity as peritonitis develops. Rectal examination may disclose tenderness in the right side of the pelvis.

The 'classical' history and findings occur in less than 50% of patients. Because of variations in its anatomical position the inflamed appendix may simulate other diseases of the abdomen. The patient may present with diarrhoea or with urinary or gynaecological symptoms and other causes of acute abdomen may be mimicked. The differential diagnosis is shown in the information box.

Investigations

The diagnosis is made on clinical findings. There may be a polymorphonuclear leucocytosis.

DIFFERENTIAL DIAGNOSIS OF ACUTE APPENDICITIS

- Acute mesenteric adenitis
- Terminal ileitis
    Yersinia infection
    Crohn's disease
- Meckel's diverticulum
- Irritable bowel syndrome
- Salpingitis or ovarian disease
- Perinephric abscess or acute cholecystitis when the appendix is retrocaecal

---

Management

The diseased appendix should be removed as early in the acute stage as possible. Even in the absence of obvious peritonitis the acutely ill patient should receive intra-operative antibiotic cover with rectal metronidazole and where there is obvious peritonitis, the systemic administration of ampicillin and metronidazole. A conservative policy is acceptable only when a clearly defined appendix mass is present without generalised abdominal signs. Once the mass has subsided, probably within 2 or 3 weeks, the appendix should be removed.

ACUTE MESENTERIC ADENITIS

There is enlargement of the mesenteric nodes secondary to viral infection. The patient, usually between 5 and 15 years, presents with features of acute appendicitis and while acute mesenteric adenitis may be suspected a laparotomy is undertaken because of the danger that there is an acutely inflamed appendix.

MECKEL'S DIVERTICULUM

This remnant of the vitelline duct which occurs in about 2% of the population is found on the anti-mesenteric border of the ileum about 50 cm from the ileocaecal valve. It may contain gastric mucosa which may secrete acid to cause mucosal ulceration and bleeding. The diverticulum may cause obstruction or inflammation and present as an acute appendicitis.

LESS COMMON FORMS OF PERITONITIS

Granulomatous peritonitis

This is caused by talc and occasionally starch used as surgical glove powder. Symptoms and signs of peritonitis begin within weeks of operation. Unfortunately a laparotomy may be required to exclude other causes of peritonitis.

Primary, spontaneous peritonitis

There is no recognisable source for peritonitis and it is assumed that bacteria enter the peritoneal cavity via the genital tract or during bacteraemia. The organisms involved are pneumococci, haemolytic streptococci or gonococci.

Tuberculous peritonitis

Although rare in Britain it is still relatively common elsewhere, notably in tropical countries. Peritonitis is secondary to a tuberculous focus in the abdomen, usually a mesenteric lymph node. The disease is characterised by wasting, malaise and gradually increasing abdominal distension and tenderness. Masses caused by matted omentum and loops of bowel may be palpable. The abdomen contains a straw-coloured fluid from which tubercle bacilli may be cultured. The fluid shows a protein concentration greater than 2.5 g/100 ml and large numbers of lymphocytes. Diagnosis may also be made by biopsy of granulomas seen at laparotomy or laparoscopy. In the adult, the condition may be confused with advanced malignant disease and an unnecessarily hopeless prognosis given. The response to anti-tuberculous chemotherapy (p. 361) is good and often dramatic.

Malignant ascites

Carcinoma of the stomach and other intra-abdominal tumours, including carcinoma of the colon and ovary, may be associated with the exudation of fluid into the peritoneal cavity. This follows the deposition of malignant cells on the peritoneal surface and is a sign of extensive spread of the disease. The process can be regarded as a low grade peritonitis. The fluid is rich in protein and its sediment contains malignant cells which may be identifiable on microscopy. Treatment is palliative. Relief of abdominal distension can be obtained by paracentesis, whilst instillation of an antimitotic agent such as methotrexate may slow the rate of re-accumulation.

INTESTINAL OBSTRUCTION

Intestinal obstruction may be complete or incomplete, acute or chronic, intermittent or continuous. The most important issue to decide is whether the obstruction is **simple** or associated with **strangulation**. The latter occurs when there is interference with the intestinal blood supply as when the bowel is trapped or twisted. Urgent relief is required if gangrene, perforation and peritonitis are to be avoided. A simple classification is provided in the information box. Mechanical causes will in general require surgical relief while paralytic ileus may respond to conservative measures.

Clinical features

The pain of mechanical obstruction is colicky and the distribution reflects the region of gut obstructed. Episodes of pain are accompanied by borborygmi. The advent of constant severe pain with abdominal tenderness is indicative of strangulation. Paralytic obstruction is characterised by a dull constant pain in an abdomen which is ominously silent. Vomiting is copious in high obstruction and may be late or absent in obstructions of the lower small bowel or colon. Distension may be absent or confined to some loops of the bowel which can be seen as ridges across the abdomen forming the so-called ladder pattern. Diffuse distension is late and may indicate chronic large bowel obstruction or paralytic

---

CAUSES OF INTESTINAL OBSTRUCTION

Mechanical obstruction
Luminal obstruction (obturation)
- Faecal impaction
- Gallstone ileus
- Worms, e.g. ascariasis

Intrinsic lesions of the bowel wall
- Tumours of the large intestine*
- Strictures, e.g. Crohn's disease
- Diverticular disease
- Intussusception

Extrinsic compression
- Adhesions*
- Hernias*
- Volvulus

Strangulation obstruction
Paralytic ileus
- Peritonitis
- Postoperative
- Vascular

* Common in Western communities

---

ileus. In complete obstruction neither faeces nor flatus is passed. In high obstruction, the bowel may move unaided or with enemas because of residual contents below the obstruction, while in large bowel obstruction spurious diarrhoea may be due to the discharge of faecal-stained mucus.

Physical examination

A careful examination is vital. The seven points to be assessed are listed in the information box.

CHECKLIST ON EXAMINATION FOR SUSPECTED OBSTRUCTION

- Is there evidence of inguinal or femoral hernias?
- Are there scars from previous operations?
- Is the abdomen distended, especially caecal distension?
- Is the abdomen tender?
- Is there a mass present?
- Are bowel sounds increased and tinkling (mechanical obstruction) or absent (paralytic ileus)?
- Is the rectum empty on rectal examination or is there faecal impaction?

Investigations

Plain radiographs taken in the erect and supine positions will reveal the diagnosis in most patients by displaying gaseous distension and fluid levels. However, gas may not be seen with high intestinal obstruction and in such patients a barium contrast study of the upper gastrointestinal tract is performed. A barium enema is indicated when large bowel obstruction is suspected. Barium examination is contraindicated if the clinical evidence suggests perforation, and Gastrografin should be used instead.

Management

The mainstays of treatment are decompression by gastrointestinal drainage via a nasogastric tube and the intravenous replacement of fluids and electrolytes. Once resuscitation is completed urgent surgery is performed for hernia, mechanical obstruction of the large bowel and strangulation. An initial non-surgical approach is adopted for paralytic ileus, obstruction due to adhesions and postoperative obstruction. Sigmoid volvulus, which is usually recognised on the plain radiograph, can often be treated at sigmoidoscopy by the insertion of a soft rubber tube into the twisted loop.

ISCHAEMIA OF THE ALIMENTARY TRACT

Aetiology

The intestines are supplied by the coeliac, superior mesenteric and inferior mesenteric arteries. The superior mesenteric, which supplies the mid-gut, has poor collateral support from the other two arteries. It follows that intestinal ischaemia is usually due to sudden or slow occlusion of the superior mesenteric artery. However, ischaemia may also arise from obstruction to the venous outflow from the intestine, or from a reduction in blood flow due to shock or cardiac failure without evidence of obstruction to the arterial or venous supply. The usual causes of blockage of the superior mesenteric artery are atheroma, thrombosis due to blood diseases, and embolism. Most cases of intestinal ischaemia occur in the elderly and in those with cardiac failure or arrhythmias.

ACUTE INTESTINAL FAILURE

This term describes the consequences of acute occlusion of the superior mesenteric artery. However, a third of patients do not have evidence of vascular occlusion and the cause of intestinal failure is poor blood supply from hypotension or cardiac failure. A variable length of the small intestine undergoes necrosis of the superficial epithelium and over several hours this progresses to gangrene. There may be a prodromal period of episodic or chronic abdominal pain often related to meals. This progresses to more severe abdominal pain, vomiting, watery and later bloody diarrhoea. Signs of peritonitis and hypovolaemic shock develop.

The diagnosis is essentially clinical but is assisted by the finding of a leucocytosis of up to 20 000–30 000/mm^3. The findings on a plain abdominal radiograph are usually nonspecific. Arteriography may be used to confirm the diagnosis provided it does not delay the urgent vascular surgery necessary to prevent gangrene. Unfortunately extensive resection of the small intestine is necessary in many patients and the overall mortality is 50%.

ISCHAEMIC COLITIS

Occlusion of the inferior mesenteric artery leads to ischaemia of the left colon particularly when blood flow in the superior mesenteric artery is also reduced.

The patient presents with colicky lower abdominal pain, nausea, vomiting and diarrhoea with the passage of blood and mucus. On examination there is tenderness and guarding on the left side of the abdomen and particularly in the left iliac fossa. Bowel sounds are usually present. In some patients the episode is transient; in others there may be persistent bleeding and pain suggesting progression to stricture formation. About 10% of patients progress to shock with generalised abdominal pain indicative of peritonitis secondary to gangrene.

Investigations

Several investigations are helpful. Leucocytosis is common. Sigmoidoscopy usually shows a normal rectal mucosa but blood may be seen descending from above. A plain radiograph of the abdomen shows 'thumb printing' at the splenic flexure and descending colon which are indentations of the bowel wall from submucosal haemorrhage and oedema. A double-contrast barium enema usually demonstrates the characteristic distribution of maximal involvement at the splenic flexure and sigmoid colon. The mucosal features are 'thumb printing' and ulceration. A stricture develops in up to 50% of patients and is demonstrated by a barium enema repeated after 2–3 weeks.

Management

Most patients recover with conservative management. Surgery is necessary when there are signs of peritonitis or when symptomatic stricture develops.

CHRONIC INTESTINAL ISCHAEMIA

This occurs when there is a gradual reduction of blood flow in the superior mesenteric artery with resulting impairment of the normal postprandial increase in blood flow to the small bowel. There is abdominal pain ('abdominal angina') some 30 minutes after each meal and the patient is afraid to eat and loses weight. The condition is rare.

FURTHER READING

Robert J H, Mentha G, Rohner A 1993 Ischaemic colitis: two
distinct patterns of severity. Gut 34: 4

DISEASES OF THE SMALL INTESTINE

SYMPTOMS OF SMALL INTESTINAL DISEASE

Pain
Pain originating in the small intestine is mid-abdominal
(Fig. 7.10, p. 442), usually colicky, even if obstruction
is not present, and is often accompanied by borborygmi.

Loss of weight
This may be due to reduced intake of food because of
anorexia, malabsorption of nutrients or loss of protein
from diseased bowel. However, it should be remembered that carcinoma at other alimentary sites is the
most important cause of loss of weight.

Symptoms of anaemia
These are common in small intestinal disease.

Diarrhoea
This is common because of malabsorption of nutrients
or in the case of resection or disease of the terminal
ileum because of the stimulation of colonic secretion.
Often the diarrhoea is painless and blood is not seen.

MALABSORPTION

A number of disorders result in malabsorption of one or
more of the essential nutrients, electrolytes, minerals or
vitamins. Some or all of the following features may
ensue; diarrhoea, abdominal pain and distension, loss of
weight, anaemia, or other evidence of specific deficiency.
However, some patients complain only of vague ill-
health, and the diagnosis may not be made for many
years.

Aetiology
Malabsorptive disorders can be classified according to
whether the primary disturbance is within the intestinal
lumen due to insufficiency of digestive enzymes or bile

acids, or within the intestinal mucosa. The classification
is listed in the information box.

CLASSIFICATION OF MALABSORPTIVE DISORDERS

Disorders of intraluminal digestion
- **Pancreatic insufficiency**
  chronic pancreatitis
  cystic fibrosis
  carcinoma of the pancreas
- **Deficiency of bile acids**
  interruption of the enterohepatic circulation of bile acids
  due to resection or disease of the terminal ileum
  colonisation of the small intestine with bacteria which
  deconjugate bile acids, which reduces their efficiency
  (stagnant loop syndrome)
- **Uncoordinated gastric emptying** which delivers gastric
  chyme too quickly to the intestine
  gastroenterostomy
  partial gastrectomy

Disorders of transport in the intestinal mucosa
- **Generalised mucosal abnormalities.** The mucosa is
  abnormal histologically
  coeliac disease
  tropical sprue
  lymphoma
  radiation enteritis
  Whipple's disease
- **Malabsorption of specific substances.** The mucosa is
  normal histologically
  lactase deficiency

Investigation
The commonly used absorption tests are detailed in
Table 7.2, page 413, and on page 412. In addition low
serum levels of folate, iron, calcium and vitamin B_{12} are
often used to infer malabsorption of these substances.
The barium follow-through examination is helpful in
two ways. It may show nonspecific features such as
dilated loops with flocculation and segmentation of barium and it may show specific structural abnormalities
which can cause malabsorption, e.g. Crohn's disease (p.
456), diverticula (p. 451) or strictures.

Biopsy of the jejunum with a Crosby capsule or of the
duodenum via an endoscope is important in making
the diagnosis of coeliac disease, and valuable diagnostic
information may be found in other disorders (Tables
7.14 and 7.15). Pancreatic function tests may be necessary if the intestinal biopsy is normal.

COELIAC DISEASE

Aetiology
Coeliac disease is characterised by an abnormal mucosa
in the small intestine induced by a component of the

Table 7.14   Findings on biopsy of the small intestine

Disease	Usual findings
Coeliac disease	Subtotal or partial villous atrophy
Dermatitis herpetiformis	Subtotal or partial villous atrophy
Tropical sprue	Partial villous atrophy
Whipple's disease	PAS positive macrophages
Intestinal lymphomas	Infiltrate of abnormal lymphoid cells
Parasitic infections	Giardia, strongyloides or coccidia may be seen
Lymphangiectasia	Dilated lymphatics

Table 7.15   Conditions in which subtotal villous atrophy has been described in a jejunal biopsy

Coeliac disease	Chronic inflammatory bowel disease
Dermatitis herpetiformis	Allergy to cow's milk or soy protein
Tropical sprue	Infections with bacteria, viruses or
Hypogammaglobulinaemia	giardia in children
Eosinophilic gastroenteritis	Whipple's disease
Kwashiorkor	Zollinger–Ellison syndrome
Cytotoxic drugs	Radiotherapy

gluten protein of wheat, barley, rye and probably oats. Local immunological responses to the gluten component are responsible for the damage to the mucosa. Antibodies to gliadin are found in the peripheral blood and splenic atrophy is common. The disease shows a high association with the histocompatibility antigens B8 DR3, DR7 and DQ2 and a family history of the disorder may be obtained in up to a quarter of patients.

Incidence

The incidence of the disease in Great Britain is 1 in 2000 to 1 in 8000, but may be higher because many cases remain undiagnosed.

Pathology

The mucosa of the normal small intestine has finger-like or leaf-like villi (Fig. 7.11A). In coeliac disease the mucosa at the duodeno-jejunal flexure is always abnormal and the abnormality extends distally for a variable distance. The appearance is either that of:

1. convolutions, like the surface of the cerebrum, which, when sectioned, appear as short wide villi ('partial villous atrophy', Fig. 7.12B)
2. a totally flat mucosa which is termed 'subtotal villous atrophy' (Fig. 7.11B and Fig. 7.12C).

In addition, the height of the epithelial cells is reduced and there is an increase in the number of plasma cells in the lamina propria and intraepithelial lymphocytes. The appearance may be patchy. All these histological features

return to normal during treatment with a gluten-free diet.

Clinical features

The disease usually presents in children under 2 years old and within 6 months of starting cereals. The child ceases to thrive and becomes fractious and irritable. The stools become voluminous and pale and the abdomen distended. As the disorder progresses growth is retarded and anaemia develops.

Less commonly the disorder may manifest for the first time in adult life and occasionally even in the elderly, when the presenting symptoms range from those of a mild anaemia and listlessness of long duration to a florid malabsorptive state developing rapidly over a period of weeks. The commonest features are diarrhoea, weight loss and anaemia, usually due to combined deficiency of folate and iron. There may be peripheral neuropathy, evidence of vitamin deficiency or hypoproteinaemia, oedema from hypoalbuminaemia, and bone pain and tetany due to hypocalcaemia secondary to vitamin D deficiency. Other clinical features are digital clubbing, glossitis, angular stomatitis, aphthous ulceration, skin pigmentation, amenorrhoea and infertility. There may be neuropsychiatric manifestations. On examination features of malnutrition and anaemia are common and the abdomen may be slightly distended and tympanitic.

Dermatitis herpetiformis

This is a variant of coeliac disease and has the same histocompatibility associations. It consists of itchy red papules on the extensor surfaces of the body together with a jejunal mucosa which shows the same histological features as coeliac disease but the changes are less severe.

Lymphoma and carcinoma

Lymphoma of the small intestine is a recognised complication of coeliac disease. In contrast to primary lymphoma of the intestine it primarily involves the jejunum. The complication presents with a return of weight loss, diarrhoea and abdominal pain after previous good control of the coeliac disease; obstruction or perforation may occur. There is also an increased incidence of gastrointestinal carcinoma in coeliac disease.

Ulcerative jejuno-ileitis

Coeliac patients with this complication respond poorly to a gluten-free diet and develop multiple ulcers in the jejunum which may bleed or perforate. Resection of the affected bowel may be necessary and mortality is high.

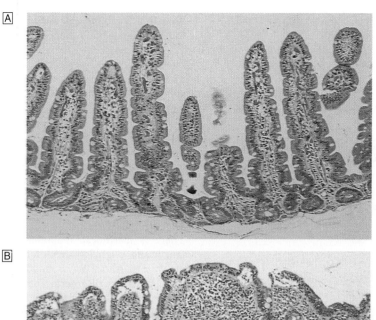

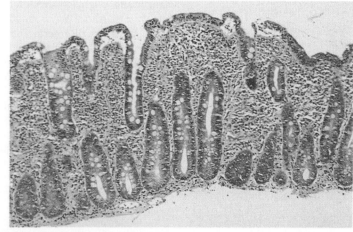

Fig. 7.11 Jejunal mucosa. Ⓐ **Normal.** Ⓑ Jejunum in coeliac disease showing subtotal villous atrophy and marked inflammatory infiltrate.

Investigations

An abnormal jejunal biopsy and a good clinical response to a strict gluten-free diet are sufficient for the diagnosis to be made. In children more strict diagnostic criteria are applied because there are other common causes of subtotal villous atrophy such as milk-protein intolerance, giardiasis and following gut viral infections. An initial biopsy is followed by a gluten-free diet and once the biopsy returns to normal as indicated by a second biopsy, a gluten challenge (an oral load of gluten) is given followed by a further biopsy.

In untreated coeliac disease, tests of carbohydrate, fat and vitamin absorption are frequently abnormal but return to normal after treatment with a gluten-free diet. These tests are not essential for diagnosis but indicate deficiencies which often require treatment during the initial weeks of the diet. Anaemia is common with evidence of iron deficiency and a high MCV due to folate deficiency.

Management

A gluten-free diet must be taken indefinitely. This requires the exclusion of wheat, rye, oats and barley, and imposes severe restrictions which must be fully explained to the patient. Booklets produced by Coeliac Societies in many countries containing diet sheets and recipes for the use of gluten-free flour are of great value in this respect. Initially frequent dietary counselling is required to make sure the diet is being observed. Mineral and vitamin supplements are also given when indicated but are seldom necessary if a strict gluten-free diet is adhered to. There is a case for offering investigation to

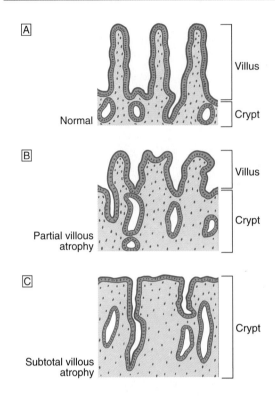

Fig. 7.12 Pathology of the mucosa at the duodenojejunal flexure. [A] Normal. [B] partial villous atrophy. [C] subtotal villous atrophy.

first degree relatives and non-invasive screening tests for more distant relatives, e.g. antigliadin antibody and intestinal permeability tests.

While the skin lesions of dermatitis herpetiformis improve with dapsone (50–100 mg/day), a strict gluten-free diet improves the skin and intestinal lesions and reduces the need for dapsone.

TROPICAL SPRUE

Tropical sprue is defined as malabsorption due to small intestinal disease in a patient in or from the tropics, in the absence of other intestinal disease or parasites. Its manifestations resemble those of coeliac disease.

Aetiology

The prevalence of sprue in certain well-defined tropical countries and localities, and its epidemiological pattern, including occasional epidemics, suggest that an infective agent or agents may be involved. It is thought that these are toxigenic *E. coli*. The disease occurs mainly in the West Indies and in Asia, including Sri Lanka, southern India, Malaysia and Indonesia.

Pathology

The changes closely resemble those of coeliac disease although partial villous atrophy rather than subtotal villous atrophy is the usual lesion. Mild changes in the jejunal mucosa, without gross malabsorption, are common in asymptomatic indigenous peoples throughout the tropics (tropical enteropathy), and for this reason the diagnosis of tropical sprue is made on a combination of clinical and laboratory findings as well as the jejunal histology.

Clinical features

There is diarrhoea, abdominal distension, anorexia, fatigue and weight loss. In visitors to the tropics the onset of severe diarrhoea may be sudden and accompanied by fever. When the disorder becomes chronic, the features of megaloblastic anaemia from folic acid malabsorption and subsequent deficiency are common. Remissions and relapses may occur. There may be oedema, glossitis and stomatitis. On investigation it is usual to find several of the abnormalities listed in the information box.

LABORATORY FINDINGS IN TROPICAL SPRUE

- Steatorrhoea
- Xylose malabsorption
- Vitamin B_{12} malabsorption
- Megaloblastic anaemia
- Hypoalbuminaemia
- Partial villous atrophy on jejunal biopsy

The differential diagnosis in the indigenous population in the tropics is from other infective, usually parasitic, causes of diarrhoea. The important differential diagnosis in visitors to the tropics is from giardiasis (p. 155). A barium follow-through examination, which may show a non-specific malabsorptive pattern, is only necessary to exclude other causes of malabsorption, e.g. Crohn's disease.

Management

Dehydration and electrolyte deficiencies must be corrected in severe diarrhoea. Tetracycline or oxytetracycline, 1 g daily in divided doses for 28 days, is the treatment of choice in all patients. In addition folic acid, 5 mg daily (10 mg intramuscularly in severe cases), and vitamin B_{12}, 1000 μg intramuscularly, is given because this seems to improve absorption as well as relieving symptoms due to folate deficiency. The jejunal mucosa soon returns to normal.

STAGNANT LOOP SYNDROME

This term is used to describe the intestinal abnormality associated with bacterial overgrowth in the small intestine and causing steatorrhoea and vitamin B_{12} malabsorption, both of which are improved by oral broad spectrum antibiotics. The syndrome is also called the contaminated bowel syndrome, blind loop syndrome and small intestine stasis syndrome.

Aetiology

The normal duodenum and jejunum contain less than 10^4/ml organisms which are usually derived from the saliva. The count of coliform organisms never exceeds 10^3/ml. In the stagnant loop syndrome there may be 10^8–10^{10} organisms/ml and these are organisms which are normally found only in the colon. The stagnant loop syndrome is predisposed to by conditions which impair the normal physiological mechanisms controlling bacterial proliferation in the intestine, for example gastric acidity which acts as a barrier to orally ingested bacteria, intestinal motility which clears bacteria, and antibodies to bacteria in the intestinal juice which control bacteria. Bacterial proliferation is also predisposed to by structural abnormalities which deliver colonic bacteria to the small intestine (fistulas) or which provide a secluded haven away from the main peristaltic stream (Table 7.16).

Clinical features

The patient presents with diarrhoea and/or steatorrhoea with anaemia due to vitamin B_{12} deficiency. These arise because of deconjugation of bile acids and utilisation of vitamin B_{12} by bacteria. There is also malabsorption of protein and carbohydrate. There may also be symptoms from the underlying intestinal lesion(s).

Investigations

The diagnosis is usually made clinically by reversal of the malabsorption of fat and vitamin B_{12} by broad spectrum antibiotics and by the demonstration of a causative lesion, for example by barium meal for jejunal diverticula or strictures and by barium enema for enterocolic fistula. If confirmation of the diagnosis is thought to be necessary, more sophisticated tests are required (Table 7.2, p. 413).

Management

Tetracycline 1–2 g orally daily is given and usually the steatorrhoea and vitamin B_{12} malabsorption are corrected within 3–4 days, while diarrhoea can be alleviated if the antibiotic is administered for 7–10 days every 4–6 weeks. Surgical resection is advocated when the abnormality is localised, for example stricture or fistula.

SOME SPECIFIC CAUSES OF STAGNANT LOOP SYNDROME

Jejunal diverticula

These are often seen on barium follow-through examinations in patients over the age of 50 years. The diverticula are usually asymptomatic but in addition to stagnant loop syndrome they may occasionally cause acute or chronic gastrointestinal bleeding or colicky abdominal pain. Obstruction and perforation may also occur. Surgery is avoided unless there is acute bleeding, obstruction or perforation.

Diabetic diarrhoea

This may result from diabetic autonomic neuropathy (p. 756) which reduces small intestinal motility resulting in the stagnant loop syndrome. Diarrhoea may also be due to pancreatic insufficiency or to coeliac disease, the latter being more common in diabetes. The patient complains of intermittent, watery diarrhoea which is often severe and may occur at night. Treatment is with tetracycline for stagnant loop syndrome and diphenoxylate, 5 mg 3 times daily orally or loperamide, 6–8 mg daily orally for diarrhoea. Clonidine, an α_2-adrenergic agonist, may also be of value (50–100 μg 8-hourly).

Table 7.16 Causes of stagnant loop syndrome

Cause	Mechanism
Gastric surgery	Reduction in acid
	Duodenal blind loop after Polya operation
Jejunal diverticula	Diverticula act as blind loop
Enterocolic fistulas, e.g. in Crohn's disease	Delivery of colonic bacteria to small intestine via the fistula
Strictures, e.g. in Crohn's disease	Delay of the faecal stream
Extensive bowel resection	Proximity of remaining small intestine to the colon
Diabetic autonomic neuropathy	Abnormal small intestinal motility
Scleroderma	Abnormal small intestinal motility
Hypogammaglobulinaemia	Lack of antibody in the intestine

Progressive systemic sclerosis (scleroderma)

In this condition the circular and longitudinal layers of the intestinal muscle are fibrosed and motility is abnormal. Malabsorption due to the stagnant loop syndrome is common. The patient may also present with intestinal pseudo-obstruction in which the clinical and radiographic features of obstruction are present but there is no mechanical cause.

Acquired hypogammaglobulinaemia

This rare disorder is characterised by a markedly reduced or absent IgA and IgM antibodies in the serum and jejunal secretion. Chronic diarrhoea, malabsorption and respiratory infections are common. The diarrhoea is due to the stagnant loop syndrome and recurrent gastrointestinal infections particularly with giardiasis.

The diagnosis is made on measurement of serum immunoglobulins and on intestinal biopsy which shows that plasma cells are reduced or absent and there may be nodules of lymphoid tissue (nodular lymphoid hyperplasia). Some patients have the histological features of coeliac disease.

Treatment involves control of giardiasis (p. 155) and if necessary regular parenteral replacement of immunoglobulins.

INTESTINAL RESECTION

Resection of the small intestine, sometimes extensive, may be necessary in Crohn's disease and in vascular insufficiency with gangrene. The significant consequences of ileal resection are shown in Table 7.17. By contrast, resection of the jejunum with preservation of the ileum may not produce such severe consequences because the enterohepatic circulation of bile acids and the ileocaecal valve are preserved. After such resections, the mucosa undergoes hyperplasia. After massive resections there may be gastric hypersecretion of acid.

Clinical features

There is severe diarrhoea with fluid and electrolyte loss in the post-operative period following extensive resec-

tions. Even when the resection involves only the terminal ileum, diarrhoea can be severe.

Investigations

The degree of ileal insufficiency can be tested by the measurement of vitamin B_{12} absorption and SeHCAT retention (Table 7.2).

Management

Parenteral fluids and feeding may be necessary initially in the post-operative period together with the anti-diarrhoeal agents loperamide (6–8 mg daily orally) and diphenoxylate (5 mg 8-hourly orally). Subsequent oral feeding should be accompanied by attempts to reduce gastrointestinal secretions so as to reduce the volume of diarrhoea. H_2-receptor antagonists will reduce the volume of gastric secretion and an elemental diet provides some of the nutritional requirements with minimal stimulation of digestive secretions. Enteral feeding may be required after massive resections. Cholestyramine given in a dose of 4 g orally at mealtimes binds bile acids in the intestine and prevents their cathartic effect in the colon. Supplements of calcium and all the vitamins are necessary.

LACTOSE INTOLERANCE

Aetiology

This is due to a deficiency of the enzyme lactase which is normally present in the brush border of the small intestinal mucosa. Lactose cannot be hydrolysed and it passes into the colon where it is fermented by bacteria producing volatile short-chain fatty acids, H_2 and CO_2, which cause discomfort and diarrhoea. In primary lactose deficiency the intestinal biopsy is normal; the enzyme deficiency is racial, being common in Blacks, Asians and South Americans. Primary deficiency is an uncommon cause of diarrhoea in Western communities because the lactase deficient individual learns to avoid milk. On the other hand secondary lactase deficiency is frequent in conditions associated with an abnormal

Table 7.17	Consequences of ileal resection
Result	**Cause(s)**
Diarrhoea	Bile acids cannot be absorbed and enter the colon where they inhibit water and electrolyte absorption Stagnant loop—see Table 7.16 Steatorrhoea and fatty acids in the colon
Steatorrhoea	When the ileal resection is greater than 100 cm the loss of bile acids in the stool leads to their insufficiency in the jejunum
Gallstones	Supersaturated bile because of diminished bile acid pool
Oxalate nephrolithiasis	Increased absorption of oxalate because calcium, which normally binds to oxalic acids, binds instead to the excess fatty acids in the intestine

intestinal biopsy, for example coeliac disease, tropical sprue and Crohn's disease of the small intestine; it also occurs transiently after gastrointestinal infections, particularly giardiasis and viral gastroenteritis.

Clinical features

The patient complains of colic, abdominal distension, increased flatus and sometimes diarrhoea after ingesting milk or milk products. Irritable bowel syndrome may be suspected. The diagnosis is suggested by an improvement in symptoms on lactose withdrawal. Useful investigations include the hydrogen breath test and the measurement of lactase activity in a jejunal biopsy specimen.

Management

A lactose-free or a lactose-restricted diet is recommended depending on the severity of the symptoms.

Diarrhoea due to other sugars

Diarrhoea can be caused by sorbitol, an unabsorbable carbohydrate, which is used as a sweetener in chewing gum and other sweets. Fructose, present in fruits and fruit juices, may also cause diarrhoea if consumed in greater quantities than can be absorbed.

PROTEIN-LOSING ENTEROPATHY

This term is used when there is excessive loss of protein into the lumen of the gastrointestinal tract, the loss being sufficient to cause hypoproteinaemia. Protein-losing enteropathy occurs in many gastrointestinal disorders but is most common in those with ulceration of the intestine, for example inflammatory bowel disease (Table 7.18). In some other disorders, e.g. Ménétrier's disease and intestinal lymphangiectasia, the consequences of protein loss are the presenting features.

Table 7.18 Diseases producing protein-losing enteropathy

Diseases of the stomach	e.g. Ménétrier's disease
Disorders of intestinal lymphatics	Intestinal lymphangiectasia, primary or secondary
Inflammatory disease of the gut	Inflammatory bowel disease
	Parasitic infections
	Stagnant loop syndrome
Tumours	Gastric, small intestinal, colonic, familial polyposis
Miscellaneous	Coeliac disease
	Tropical sprue
	Radiation enteritis
	Collagen-vascular disease
	Whipple's disease
	Allergic gastroenteropathy
	Constrictive pericarditis

Clinical features

The patient has peripheral oedema and hypoproteinaemia in the presence of normal liver function, (i.e. no evidence of failure of hepatic synthesis of plasma proteins), no evidence of proteinuria, and no cardiac failure.

Investigations

The diagnosis is confirmed by measurement of the faecal clearance of endogenous α_1-antitrypsin (Table 7.2).

Management

Treatment is that of the underlying condition.

INTESTINAL LYMPHANGIECTASIA

A congenital malunion of the lymphatics causes impaired drainage of the intestinal lymphatics, and the lymph which contains protein and fat is discharged into the lumen of the intestine. The condition presents with oedema of the lower limbs and investigation demonstrates hypoalbuminaemia, lymphocytopenia and steatorrhoea. The diagnosis is confirmed by intestinal biopsy which shows greatly dilated lymphatics and by lymphangiography in which a radio-opaque dye is introduced into the lymphatic system via lymphatics in the feet.

RADIATION DAMAGE TO THE INTESTINE

Radiation enteritis, colitis and proctitis are common after radiotherapy to the abdomen for malignancy.

Pathology

The rectum, sigmoid colon and terminal ileum are most frequently involved. Acute radiation damage causes an acute inflammation with crypt abscess formation. Over subsequent months and years the bowel may become fibrotic and stenotic. The underlying lesion appears to be damage to the endothelial cells of the submucosal arterioles. An endarteritis develops which causes ischaemia, atrophy of the mucosa, and ulceration which can lead to fistulas and abscesses.

Clinical features

In the acute phase which occurs within days of the commencement of radiotherapy there is abdominal pain and diarrhoea. When the rectum or colon is the main site of injury, blood and mucus occur in the stool. Small intestinal injury (enteritis) is associated with nausea, colic and watery diarrhoea. The chronic phase commences 6–12 months after radiotherapy and the patient may have one or more of the problems listed in the information box.

CHRONIC COMPLICATIONS OF RADIATION DAMAGE TO THE INTESTINE

- Proctitis
- Proctocolitis
- Small intestinal strictures
- Fistulas
    Rectovaginal
    Colovesical
    Enterocolonic
- Obstruction due to strictures
- Malabsorption due to:
    damage to terminal ileum
    stagnant loop syndrome

On examination there is often evidence of weight loss and malnutrition and it can be difficult to decide whether this is due to recurrence of a tumour or radiation damage. There are no specific findings on examination of the abdomen.

Investigations

In the acute phase, the rectal changes at sigmoidoscopy resemble those of ulcerative proctitis (p. 460). The extent of the lesion is determined by sigmoidoscopy, colonoscopy and barium enema. Characteristically there are ulcers with surrounding telangiectasia. The mucosa may be granular. Barium follow-through examination is used to seek structural changes such as strictures and fistulas in the small intestine. A 5-day stool is collected to detect steatorrhoea and the absorption of vitamin B_{12} and SeHCAT is tested to determine whether terminal ileal function is abnormal (Table 7.2).

Management

There is no specific treatment. Diarrhoea in the acute phase is treated with codeine phosphate, diphenoxylate or loperamide in standard dosage (see information box on drug therapy for Crohn's disease, p. 462). The drug therapy recommended for ulcerative colitis may bring improvement for chronic disease of the colon and rectum. Antibiotics may be required for stagnant loop syndrome and nutritional supplements are usually necessary when malabsorption is present. Surgery is avoided because the injured intestine is difficult to resect and anastomose, but may be necessary when obstruction supervenes.

MOTILITY DISORDERS

Small intestinal motility may become disordered in conditions which affect the smooth muscle or nerves of the intestine.

PRIMARY INTESTINAL PSEUDO-OBSTRUCTION

The cause is unknown but histological abnormalities are seen in the myenteric plexus and smooth muscle. Some cases are familial.

Clinical features

There are recurrent attacks of nausea, vomiting, abdominal colic and distension, often worse after food, constipation and diarrhoea. There is weight loss due to malabsorption and fear of eating.

Investigations

Plain radiographs of the abdomen show air-fluid levels and distended loops of bowel. The absence of mechanical obstruction is demonstrated by barium studies or more commonly by laparotomy undertaken initially because of the fear of mechanical obstruction. At laparotomy a full-thickness biopsy of the intestinal wall is taken to search for secondary causes of intestinal pseudo-obstruction.

Management

Further laparotomies are avoided. Drugs such as cisapride (10 mg orally 6-hourly or 8-hourly) are used to enhance small intestinal motility. Stagnant loop syndrome is treated.

SECONDARY INTESTINAL PSEUDO-OBSTRUCTION

The usual causes are the disorders of intestinal smooth muscle, scleroderma, dermatomyositis and amyloidosis, endocrine disorders such as hypothyroidism, or pharmacological causes, tricyclic antidepressants, opiates.

The clinical features and treatment are similar to the primary form.

FOOD INTOLERANCE

Whilst this may have an allergic basis (p. 44), most cases are unrelated to immunological mechanisms. There is an adverse reaction to an ingested food involving abdominal pain, vomiting and diarrhoea. The mechanism is usually psychological but may be pharmacological or due to food constituents (monosodium glutamate or sulphites) or to enzyme deficiency (e.g. lactase, p. 452).

MISCELLANEOUS DISORDERS

ULCERATION OF THE SMALL INTESTINE

This occurs in the conditions listed in the information box.

In primary ulcer, enteric-coated potassium tablets or NSAIDs are implicated. The area of ulceration may be caused by dissolution of the tablet. Fibrosis and stricture may result in partial small intestinal obstruction. Perforation or haemorrhage may also occur.

CAUSES OF ULCERATION OF THE SMALL INTESTINE

- Inflammatory bowel disease
  Crohn's disease
- Ulcerative jejunoileitis in coeliac disease
- Infections
  typhoid
- Lymphoma and carcinoma
- Vascular diseases
- Non-specific ulceration (primary ulcer)

INFECTIONS OF THE SMALL INTESTINE

GIARDIASIS (p. 155)

TRAVELLERS' DIARRHOEA (p. 71)

WHIPPLE'S DISEASE

This rare multisystem disease is important because it is curable and is now thought to be caused by the Gram-positive organism *Trophyrema whippelli*. Characteristically there is infiltration of the intestinal mucosa and other organs with macrophages which stain positively with periodic acid-Schiff (PAS). Electron microscopy shows numerous intracellular Gram-positive bacilliform bodies.

Clinical features

The patient presents with malabsorption and steatorrhoea consequent upon the infiltration of macrophages which interfere with lymph flow and restrict the absorption of nutrients. There is polyarthritis, fever, weight loss, abdominal pain and respiratory symptoms. Joint symptoms, most commonly affecting the knee or ankle, may precede other clinical manifestations by months or years and sacroiliitis and ankylosing spondylitis may occur. In addition to the arthropathy, examination may reveal lymphadenopathy, skin pigmentation and abdominal distension and tenderness. The diagnosis is made by jejunal biopsy.

Management

Treatment consists of prolonged oral therapy with antibiotic, tetracycline (1 g per day for 1 year) usually being the drug of choice. Arthralgias and arthritis settle within a month of starting treatment. Relapses occur and the patient must be followed-up permanently.

TUMOURS OF THE SMALL INTESTINE

LYMPHOMA

Lymphomatous tumours which involve the small intestine are shown in Table 7.19.

The condition tends to occur in children or young adults. There is abdominal pain, fever and weight loss and some patients have diarrhoea and steatorrhoea. On examination there may be an abdominal mass due to enlarged glands, and oedema from protein-losing enteropathy. The diagnosis is suspected on barium follow-through examination but the radiographic findings may be confused with Crohn's disease. Staging is performed as with other lymphomas which provides important information on optimal treatment and prognosis. Treatment involves a combination of surgery, abdominal radiotherapy and chemotherapy.

CARCINOMA

Adenocarcinoma arises predominantly in the duodenum or jejunum. It may be associated with coeliac disease, Crohn's disease or some of the multiple polyposis syndromes (familial polyposis, Gardner's syndrome). There is abdominal pain, weight loss, bleeding leading to iron deficiency anaemia, obstruction or intussusception. The diagnosis is made on barium follow-through examination. The treatment is surgical.

Leiomyosarcomas occur at any level in the small intestine; their presentation and treatment are similar to adenocarcinoma.

BENIGN TUMOURS

These are usually adenomas, leiomyomas or lipomas. Many are asymptomatic but they may present with abdominal pain, obstruction or bleeding and are diagnosed by barium follow-through examination.

Table 7.19 Lymphomatous tumours of the small intestine

Tumour	Features
Primary	Commonly in the ileum
Secondary	The intestine is involved as part of a generalised lymphomatous process which began elsewhere in the body
In coeliac disease	Commonly in the jejunum and multicentric
Immunoproliferative (α-heavy chain disease)	Multicentric

CARCINOID TUMOURS

This tumour occurs at many sites in the gastrointestinal tract but is most common in the appendix, the ileum and the rectum. Carcinoids are almost always benign in the appendix but may lead to appendicitis.

Carcinoids in the small intestine are multiple in 20% of cases and show low-grade malignancy with metastases to the abdominal lymph nodes and the liver.

Clinical features

The term 'carcinoid syndrome' refers to the systemic symptoms produced when the secretory products of the neoplastic enterochromaffin cells which comprise the tumour are released into the systemic circulation. These do not usually reach the systemic circulation unless they are produced by liver metastases. Serotonin (5HT) is released, and its metabolite 5-HIAA appears in the urine. Many kinins and hormones are also released and these cause diarrhoea and peripheral symptoms. The clinical features are shown in the information box.

The diagnosis is made by measuring urinary 5-HIAA in a 24-hour collection of urine.

CLINICAL FEATURES OF THE CARCINOID SYNDROME

- Symptoms due to:
  Local invasion of the bowel
  Hepatic metastases
- Flushing   Often precipitated by food,
- Diarrhoea   alcohol or exercise
- Right heart valve lesions
- Facial telangiectasia
- Hepatomegaly due to metastases

Management

The treatment of a carcinoid tumour is surgical resection. The treatment of patients with carcinoid syndrome is palliative because hepatic metastases have usually occurred. Surgical removal of the primary tumour is attempted, and the hepatic metastases are excised if possible for the reduction of tumour mass reduces symptoms. A variety of pharmacological agents are available which block some of the effects of serotonin, kinins and other secretory products. The most promising are the long-acting somatostatin analogues which inhibit the release of these mediators. Octatrein can be given by subcutaneous injection in a dose of 200 μg three times a day.

FURTHER READING

Bjarnason I, Hayllar J, MacPherson A J, Russell A S 1993 Side effects of nonsteroidal anti-inflammatory drugs on the small and large intestine in humans. Gastroenterology 104: 1832

Gordon J I 1993 Understanding gastrointestinal epithelial cell biology: lessons from mice with help from worms and flies. Gastroenterology 104: 315

Sollid L M, Thorsby E 1993 HLA susceptibility genes in celiac disease: genetic mapping and role in pathogenesis. Gastroenterology 105: 910

INFLAMMATORY BOWEL DISEASE

CROHN'S DISEASE AND ULCERATIVE COLITIS

Crohn's disease and ulcerative colitis are nonspecific inflammatory conditions of the alimentary tract. The former can affect any part of the alimentary tract whereas ulcerative colitis is confined to the large intestine. However, the diseases will be considered together because of similarities in their presentation, pathology, investigations, complications and treatment. In 10–20% of patients the two cannot be distinguished.

Epidemiology

The incidence for ulcerative colitis in Western populations is 5–10 per 100 000 persons at risk and for Crohn's disease 2–6 per 100 000 and is probably increasing. There are racial differences. Both disorders are less common in black races and more common in American Jews. The sex distribution is approximately equal. Both diseases occur in any age group with a peak between ages 15 and 20.

Aetiology

Genetics

There is strong evidence to support a genetic influence in both diseases because 10–15% of patients have a first degree relative with inflammatory bowel disease. A patient with Crohn's disease may have relatives with Crohn's or ulcerative colitis and vice versa. There is a high concordance rate for monozygotic twins to be affected, particularly for Crohn's disease. There are no HLA associations for inflammatory bowel disease. However, there is an increased association of both Crohn's and ulcerative colitis with ankylosing spondylitis and most of these patients have the HLA–B27 histocompatibility antigen (p. 905).

Infective agents

A variety of infective agents, bacterial and viral, have been proposed, particularly for Crohn's disease, but there is a lack of supportive evidence. A similar chronic inflammatory disorder of the ileum, Johne's disease in sheep and cattle, is caused by infection with *M. paratuberculosis*.

Immunological findings

There are a large number of abnormalities of the cellular and humoral immune systems but these are probably secondary phenomena. Nevertheless they may be responsible for some of the systemic features of the disease, for example circulating immune complexes causing uveitis and arthritis. The histological features suggest that the cells in the lamina propria are reacting to an antigen, but no antigen has been identified. Thus 'autoimmunity' (p. 44) remains an aetiological possibility.

Smoking

Smoking is more common in Crohn's disease and less common in ulcerative colitis than in the general population. The significance of this finding is not understood.

Pathology

Crohn's disease

The sites most commonly involved, in order of frequency, are terminal ileum and right side of colon, colon alone, terminal ileum alone, ileum and jejunum. The macroscopic features of Crohn's disease at different sites in the gastrointestinal tract are shown in Table 7.20.

Characteristically the entire wall of the bowel is oedematous and thickened. There are deep ulcers which often appear as linear fissures, thus the mucosa between them is described as 'cobblestone'. The deep ulcers may penetrate through the bowel wall to initiate abscesses or fistulas. Fistulas may develop between adjacent loops of bowel or between affected segments of bowel and the bladder, uterus or vagina and may appear in the perineum.

Characteristically the changes are patchy. Even when

Table 7.20 Macroscopic features of Crohn's disease at different sites

Site	Appearance
Common	
Small intestine	Narrowing, ulceration and cobblestone appearance of terminal ileum
Large intestine	Diffuse involvement resembling ulcerative colitis
	Short segments of disease
	Strictures
	Proctitis alone
Anus	Chronic fissures
	Fistula
	Ulceration
Less Common	
Duodenum	Ulceration, thickened folds, narrowing, stricture
Stomach	Thickening of antrum which may resemble carcinoma
Mouth	Aphthous-like ulcers
Uncommon or rare	
Oesophagus	Ulcers
	Thickened folds of epithelium
Skin	Ulceration in perineum, genitalia or abdominal wall

a relatively short segment of bowel is affected, the inflammatory process is interrupted by islands of normal mucosa and the change from the affected part is abrupt. A small lesion separated in this way from a major area of involvement is referred to as a 'skip' lesion. The mesenteric lymph nodes are enlarged and the mesentery thickened.

The microscopic features of Crohn's disease are of great importance because they allow confirmation of the diagnosis to be made on rectal and colonoscopic biopsies (Table 7.21). Non-caseating granulomas are characteristic of Crohn's disease. These are focal aggregates of epithelioid histiocytes which may be surrounded by lymphocytes and contain giant cells. Lymphoid aggregates or microgranulomas are also seen and when these are near to the surface of the mucosa they often ulcerate to form tiny aphthous-like ulcers.

Ulcerative colitis

The disease almost always involves the rectum (proctitis) and may also involve a variable part of the colon

Table 7.21 Microscopic features of the large intestine in ulcerative colitis and Crohn's disease

Ulcerative colitis	Crohn's disease
Inflammation is mucosal and submucosal	Inflammation is transmural
Granulomas absent	Granulomas present in bowel and lymph nodes
Crypt abscesses common	Crypt abscesses infrequent
Loss of goblet cells	Normal population of goblet cells
Width of the mucosa is normal or reduced	Width of mucosa is normal or increased

or the entire colon; but the colonic disease is always continuous with that in the rectum, in contrast to Crohn's disease which is often discontinuous.

In the early stages the mucosa is haemorrhagic and granular; thereafter ulceration develops. The ulcers may be superficial or penetrate to spread longitudinally beneath the mucosa. In severe disease the mucosa may slough in parts to expose granulation tissue while the remaining mucosa becomes oedematous, hyperplastic and raised, giving the appearance of pseudopolyposis. In **acute fulminant disease** the bowel, especially the transverse colon, may be greatly dilated (**toxic dilatation**) and the bowel wall becomes thin and may rupture. In long-standing disease the colon is shortened and generally narrowed with a lack of haustrations. Strictures are uncommon compared to Crohn's disease and anal lesions such as fissure and fistula are also less severe and less common.

The important microscopic features are listed in Table 7.21 where they are compared to those of Crohn's disease of the colon. The lamina propria is uniformly infiltrated with lymphocytes and plasma cells whilst polymorphs accumulate around ulcerated areas. Crypt abscesses consist of a collection of polymorphs in a crypt.

In 10–20% of patients it is not possible to distinguish ulcerative colitis from Crohn's disease of the colon on the histological criteria. The term **colitis intermediate** has been used for such patients.

In a small proportion of patients with chronic ulcerative colitis and Crohn's disease of the colon, multicentric precancerous lesions can be found on histological examination. Some of these are invisible to the naked eye. Thus surveillance for cancer depends upon multiple biopsies taken at colonoscopy.

Clinical features

Crohn's disease

Crohn's disease is a chronic disorder with unpredictable exacerbations and remissions. The presentation and symptoms depend in part on the site and extent of the bowel affected. Crohn's disease of the small intestine or ileum and right colon (ileocolitis) has a spectrum of features which may be considered together.

Pain is the commonest symptom due either to peritoneal involvement, or bowel obstruction, or both. It occurs most frequently in the right lower quadrant and may be associated with local tenderness or guarding. A mass is palpable on abdominal or rectal examination being formed of inflamed loops of bowel bound together, possibly including an abscess. It may be of any size. Colicky pain which is usually situated in the mid or lower abdomen suggests obstruction, and may be associated with nausea and vomiting and excessive borborygmi. Indeed, recurrent episodes of colic due to attacks of subacute obstruction are a prominent feature in the life history of a patient with Crohn's disease.

Exacerbations of pain may be accompanied by diarrhoea and fever. The diarrhoea is seldom as severe as in ulcerative colitis. The stools may be formed or loose, and rarely contain frank blood, mucus or pus unless the colon is involved.

Steatorrhoea and malabsorption of nutrients and drugs are common. Their cause is multifactorial (see the information box). Most patients suffer from malnutrition and weight loss, contributing factors being reduced food intake because of anorexia, malabsorption and increased catabolism. Malabsorption of iron, folic acid and vitamin B_{12} commonly leads to anaemia. In children growth retardation may be the principal presentation. In patients with chronic diarrhoea, sodium, potassium and water depletion are common and deficiency of magnesium and zinc may occur.

CAUSES OF MALABSORPTION IN CROHN'S DISEASE

Fat
- Reduction in absorptive surface due to
    extensive disease
    resection of bowel
- Bacterial colonisation of the small intestine due to
    strictures
    fistulas from the colon
- Interruption of the enterohepatic circulation of bile acids due to
    disease of the terminal ileum
    resection of the terminal ileum

Vitamin D
- Due mainly to the interruption of the enterohepatic circulation of bile acids

Protein
- Protein-losing enteropathy is common due to loss of protein through the ulcerated mucosa

Carbohydrate
- Lactase deficiency is common due to damage to the mucosa

Vitamin B_{12}
- Due to disease or resection of the terminal ileum

A diagnostic feature, when present, is the occurrence of anal lesions such as oedematous skin tags or perianal abscesses and fistulas; they are more common when the colon is affected.

Crohn's disease confined to the small intestine or duodenum presents with mid-abdominal or epigastric pain, sometimes simulating peptic ulceration. Crohn's disease of the large intestine presents with the same features as ulcerative colitis (see below).

Intra-abdominal complications. Abscess is common following slow penetration of the intestine by an ulcer. It may discharge into the intestinal lumen or elsewhere into the intestine, bladder or vagina to create a fistula. Ileovesical fistula may lead to recurrent urinary infections, symptoms of cystitis, and pneumaturia may be noticed in males. Free perforation of the intestine may occur. There is an increased incidence of carcinoma of the intestine in those segments affected by Crohn's disease.

Ulcerative colitis

The first attack is often the most severe and thereafter the disease is characterised by exacerbations and remissions although a minority of patients develop chronic symptoms. The clinical features and the management are largely determined by the extent of colonic involvement, the severity of the inflammation and the duration of the disease.

The principal symptom is diarrhoea with loose bloody stools containing mucus and pus. Defecation is often accompanied by lower abdominal discomfort although severe pain is uncommon. Tenesmus may occur because of proctitis. Tenderness may be present on palpation of the colon, especially in the left iliac fossa. Peritoneal irritation when present signifies that the serosa is involved in the inflammatory process.

In severe ulcerative colitis or Crohn's colitis, there is exhausting diarrhoea with up to 20 liquid stools per 24 hours, dehydration, fever and tachycardia. **Toxic dilatation** represents the most serious complication with tachycardia, a high swinging temperature and abdominal distension and tenderness. The patient is at grave risk of dying from colonic perforation.

In chronic ulcerative colitis the bowel is permanently damaged by fibrosis and behaves as a rigid tube incapable of absorbing fluid properly or of acting as a faecal reservoir. There is no toxaemia, but the patient lives in chronic ill-health and with persistent diarrhoea.

The symptoms may be trivial when the disease is confined to the rectum, and consist of loose motions and perhaps blood-streaking of the stool. A severe proctitis will cause tenesmus, frequent small loose stools, and bleeding and mucus per rectum, but systemic disturbance is absent. Paradoxically, in distal colitis, spasm may result in constipation with retention of faeces in the proximal colon and small hard stools.

Relapse is often associated with emotional stress, intercurrent infection or the use of antibiotics. There is no special risk to the patient during pregnancy in either ulcerative colitis or Crohn's colitis.

Cancer of the colon in chronic ulcerative colitis occurs with an increased frequency in patients with extensive or total colitis of more than 10 years' duration and an early age of onset. The cancer risk is also increased in Crohn's disease. The onset of colonic cancer is difficult to detect clinically when the patient has chronic bowel symptoms.

Stricture of the colon, anal fissure, abscess and fistula occur in ulcerative colitis but are much less common than in Crohn's colitis.

Systemic complications of inflammatory bowel disease

These are shown in the information box and most are common to both ulcerative colitis and Crohn's disease.

EXTRAINTESTINAL MANIFESTATIONS OF CROHN'S AND ULCERATIVE COLITIS

- **Hepatic**
  Fatty change
  Pericholangitis
  Granulomas
  Cirrhosis
  Amyloidosis
  Abscess
  Carcinoma of the biliary tree
  Sclerosing cholangitis
- **Skin**
  Erythema nodosum
  Pyoderma gangrenosum

- **Ocular lesions**
  Uveitis
  Episcleritis
  Conjunctivitis
- **Aphthous stomatitis**
- **Arthritis**
  Ankylosing spondylitis
  Seronegative arthritis
- **Clubbing of the fingers**
- **Thrombosis and embolism**

EXTRAINTESTINAL MANIFESTATIONS OF CROHN'S DISEASE

- **Renal disease**
  Urolithiasis
  Pyelonephritis
  Cystitis
  Hydronephrosis
  Amyloidosis
- **Gallstones**

General investigations

Blood tests

These may show a moderate anaemia (normochromic, normocytic or hypochromic), a raised erythrocyte sedimentation rate (ESR), a leucocytosis, abnormal liver function and hypoproteinaemia.

Stool cultures and blood cultures

The stool should be cultured for pathogenic bacteria and a search of the mucus made for amoebae to exclude an infective cause for colitis both on initial presentation and on relapses. Blood cultures are required if septicaemia is suspected.

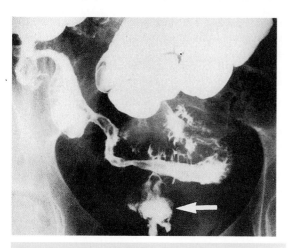

Fig. 7.13 Crohn's disease of the ileum showing marked narrowing and a fistula between the ileum and the bladder (arrow).

Investigation of Crohn's disease

The extent of the disease is assessed by barium meal and follow-through, and barium enema examination which may show alteration of the mucosal pattern, deep ulceration or the pathognomonic 'string sign' due to marked narrowing of a segment of affected bowel (Fig. 7.13). In long-standing cases there may be stricture formation. The lesions tend to be discontinuous along the length of the bowel.

Endoscopy of the stomach and duodenum is performed if the barium studies indicate any abnormality in these organs. Sigmoidoscopy and colonoscopy are usually required and may detect rectal and colonic abnormalities when the barium enema is normal. In Crohn's colitis the rectal mucosa shows focal inflammation and ulceration with the intervening mucosa appearing normal or oedematous; but in some patients the appearance is indistinguishable from that of ulcerative proctitis. Biopsies of the rectum and/or colon are always taken and often confirm the diagnosis by showing granulomas even when the mucosa is macroscopically normal. Similarly, biopsies or excision of perianal skin tags may show granulomas.

Another helpful investigation is the use of white cells labelled with ^{111}In or ^{99m}Tc to locate areas of active disease by scanning.

Investigation of ulcerative colitis

Sigmoidoscopy

This is essential in most patients. The mucosa appears engorged and hyperaemic and the normal vascular pattern is obliterated. In severe disease spontaneous bleeding will be seen; in less severe involvement the mucosa appears intact and bleeds only when it is gently rubbed; in mild cases the only abnormality is the absence of the normal vascular pattern.

Plain radiograph of the abdomen

This is essential in the diagnosis of suspected toxic dilatation and is also of value at the initial presentation as the colon will usually contain sufficient air to outline an abnormal mucosal pattern.

Barium enema and colonoscopy

The double-contrast barium enema will demonstrate the extent and severity of the disease. The earliest radiological change is a granular appearance of the colonic mucosa. In more severe disease ulceration and pseudopolyps will be seen (Fig. 7.14). In long-standing disease there may be shortening of the colon with narrowing of the lumen. Some of these features may be seen in Crohn's colitis but in Crohn's colitis the disease is often discontinuous, the ulcers are deeper and the ileum is narrow and irregular.

Colonoscopy is frequently used to assess the extent and severity of colitis because barium enema may underestimate the extent of the disease. In addition colonoscopic biopsies are important in distinguishing ulcerative colitis and Crohn's disease from each other and from other diseases which may cause colitis. Barium

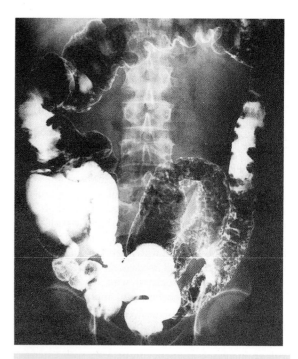

Fig. 7.14 Severe ulcerative colitis with deep ulcers and pseudopolyps affecting mainly the sigmoid colon.

enema or colonoscopy should not be performed in the acute disease and where toxic dilatation is suspected, because of the risk of perforation.

Activity of the disease

The degree of inflammatory activity can be assessed routinely without repeated radiological or endoscopic studies. Estimates of ESR and C reactive protein are of value. The stools may be collected after labelling of white cells (p. 410) to determine if there is an increased excretion of radioactivity.

Toxic dilatation

This may occur during an acute attack of ulcerative or Crohn's colitis. The abdomen may become increasingly tender and distended and the number of stools may decrease. The plain radiograph shows a dilated gas-filled colon with a diameter greater than 5 cm.

Differential diagnosis

Crohn's disease

The other common diseases in the ileocaecal region are appendicitis, appendix abscess and mesenteric adenitis. It may be impossible to decide between these possibilities in an acutely ill patient and a laparotomy may be necessary. Less commonly infections such as *Yersinia*, tuberculosis and actinomycosis, and lymphoma of the ileum or colon may mimic Crohn's disease. Ileocaecal tuberculosis may be indicated by evidence of tuberculosis elsewhere, for example on the chest radiograph. A 'negative' tuberculin test is common in patients with Crohn's disease whereas it is often strongly positive in tuberculosis. Carcinoma in the caecal region may sometimes be confused with Crohn's disease. Table 7.22 lists other colonic diseases to be considered.

Table 7.22   Conditions which must be differentiated from ulcerative and Crohn's colitis

Infective	Non-infective
Salmonellosis	Ischaemic colitis
Shigellosis	Radiation proctitis and colitis
Campylobacter gastroenteritis	Diffuse lymphoma
Haemorrhagic colitis due to *E. coli*	Vasculitides
Gonorrhoeal proctitis	Cathartic colon
Chlamydial proctitis	
Proctitis due to herpes simplex	
Pseudomembranous colitis	
Amoebiasis	
Yersinia infections	
Other parasitic infections	

Ulcerative colitis

A large number of diseases may cause inflammation of the colon and rectum (Table 7.22). Many of these are infective and their occurrence in homosexuals and in patients with acquired immunodeficiency syndrome (AIDS) makes it essential that these possibilities are kept in mind. The infective conditions are diagnosed visually (e.g. membranes seen coating the mucosa in pseudomembranous colitis, or amoebae seen microscopically in fresh stools), on biopsy (e.g. herpes simplex) or culture of stool. The non-infective conditions are suspected from the history (abuse of laxatives or previous irradiation) or radiological features.

Management of Crohn's disease

Diet and nutrition

It is essential to restore and maintain the patient's nutritional status. This is particularly difficult but of considerable importance in children. Great care and encouragement are needed to ensure that the patient takes a high-protein, high-energy diet, if necessary by providing supplemental dietary preparations. Enteral feeding by nasoenteric tube can be tolerated for prolonged periods even in the young. In addition to improving nutrition the inflammatory process may possibly benefit and the symptoms of partial obstruction may be relieved. Enteral feeding is particularly useful in the pre-operative preparation of patients, especially in those with external fistulas. Total parenteral nutrition may occasionally be required in very severely ill patients. In addition, plasma or blood transfusion may be used to correct anaemia or severe hypoproteinaemia.

A low-fat diet or milk-free diet may improve symptoms which are due to steatorrhoea or lactase deficiency and a low-residue diet is often of value for colic and subacute obstruction. When bacterial colonisation is suspected as the cause of steatorrhoea, intermittent courses of oral antibiotics are indicated using either metronidazole and/or broad spectrum antibiotics. Supplements of iron, folic acid, calcium, zinc, vitamins D and B_{12} and electrolytes, especially potassium, will be required when deficiencies occur. Many countries have Crohn's disease voluntary organisations where the exchange of information and mutual support are important.

Drugs

Diarrhoea may be helped by appropriate dietary management and by treatment with corticosteroids. Diarrhoea can be treated with oral doses of diphenoxylate or loperamide (see information box). Corticosteroids are beneficial when there is extensive active disease which does not improve with the general medical measures outlined above. However, they do not alter the long-term course of the disease. Prednisolone is given in a dose of 40–60 mg daily in divided doses for 2 to 4 weeks depending on response, and then gradually reduced and withdrawn over 4 to 6 weeks. Every effort should be made to stop steroids but this may be difficult in the occasional patient because of an early relapse when the dose is reduced. The drug therapy is shown in the information box.

DRUG THERAPY FOR CROHN'S DISEASE

- **Diphenoxylate**
  5 mg orally 8-hourly
- or **Loperamide**
  2 mg orally 6-hourly or 8-hourly   } for diarrhoea
- or **Codeine phosphate**
  30 mg orally 6-hourly or 8-hourly
- or **Prednisolone**
  40–60 mg orally daily
- **Sulphasalazine**
  1 g 8-hourly for colonic disease only—long-term maintenance
- **Azathioprine**
  2 mg/kg BW orally for those who fail to respond to steroids
- **Metronidazole**
  400 mg 12-hourly for perineal Crohn's disease

Surgical treatment

Although episodes of subacute obstruction can usually be managed by nasogastric suction and intravenous feeding, surgery may be necessary if obstruction occurs frequently. The majority of patients will require surgery at some time and often multiple operations are necessary. As the disease is multicentric extensive resections cannot eradicate it and the principle of surgery is to use only minimal resections for strictures and fistulas. Surgery may also be necessary for abscess, perforation and for extensive and severe involvement of the colon (see below).

Management of ulcerative colitis and Crohn's colitis

General measures

Admission to hospital is required for patients with severe bowel symptoms, especially when there are general disturbances such as weight loss, anaemia, fever or tachycardia. Such patients may require intensive supportive treatment either until the disease remits or as a preparation for surgery. Parenteral nutrition through a central venous line allows correction of nutritional deficiencies in the severely wasted patient and will do much to hasten recovery after operation. The measures should include the correction of dehydration and elec-

trolyte deficiencies, especially hypokalaemia; blood and plasma infusions to correct anaemia and hypoproteinaemia; and a high-protein, low-residue diet.

Blood cultures are obtained initially and repeated throughout the course of the illness if fever persists. Gram-negative bacteria are the commonest organisms cultured. Parenteral administration of broad spectrum antibiotics is necessary if septicaemia is suspected. However, antibiotics have no place in the primary management of ulcerative colitis; indeed a broad spectrum antibiotic may precipitate a relapse. Candidosis of the mouth and upper pharynx is common, especially in ill patients on corticosteroids, and must be treated (p. 144). There is no satisfactory drug for controlling diarrhoea. Codeine phosphate (30 mg 6-hourly or 8-hourly) or loperamide (2 mg 6-hourly) may be helpful in the chronic illness, but these drugs must be avoided in severely ill patients because they may precipitate toxic dilatation of the colon.

Corticosteroids

There is no specific treatment for ulcerative colitis but corticosteroids are very effective in inducing remission.

Local treatment. The preparations commonly used are prednisolone-21-phosphate or betamethasone. When sigmoidoscopic examination confirms that only the rectum is involved topical treatment with corticosteroid suppositories is all that is required; the patient is instructed to insert one, 2 times daily, retaining the material for as long as possible.

Topical treatment with corticosteroid enemas used once or twice daily may also be administered for distal colitis when symptoms are mild—not more than 4 stools per day with intermittent bleeding and little or no systemic upset. When symptoms are more severe, patients with distal colitis may require systemic corticosteroids. Systemic or local treatment may be continued for 3 to 6 weeks, the duration being judged from the sigmoidoscopic appearances and the clinical response.

Mesalazine can also be used for topical treatment and in a dose of 3–6 suppositories daily is as effective as corticosteroids.

Systemic treatment. Prednisolone is given in doses of between 40 and 60 mg daily by mouth for 3 to 6 weeks depending on the response. In severe disease corticosteroids may have to be administered intravenously as hydrocortisone (100–200 mg 6-hourly). The usual contraindications to the use of these drugs must be observed and potassium supplements should be given. Used in this way, corticosteroids will induce remission in the majority of patients, the dose being reduced at weekly intervals over four weeks as improvement takes place. Corticosteroids give rise to a sense of well-being and improve appetite, enabling the problem of persuading the patient to eat sufficient food to be solved.

Sulphasalazine. This is less effective than corticosteroids in the acute phase of the disease but may be used in mild or moderate attacks in oral doses of 2–4 g daily. Its principal value is that it reduces the liability to relapse. Once remission has been induced by corticosteroids all patients with colitis should be maintained on a small dose of sulphasalazine (0.5 g 6-hourly) for 2 years or longer. Sulphasalazine is a combination of 5-aminosalicylic acid which is the active agent linked to sulphapyridine acting as a 'carrier'. The compound is broken down by bacterial action in the colon, liberating 5-aminosalicylic acid which acts locally. Side-effects attributed to the sulphapyridine moiety include nausea, headache, rashes, reversible sterility in the male, and very rarely haemolytic anaemia and agranulocytosis.

Oral 5-ASA is not effective because it is absorbed from the small intestine and therefore does not reach the colon. Several preparations have been developed which deliver 5-ASA to the colon without using sulphapyridine as carrier. Mesalazine (250–500 mg 8-hourly) uses 5-ASA with an enteric coating and azodisalicylate (500 mg 12-hourly) joins 2 molecules of 5-ASA by an azo bond which is split by bacteria in the colon. 5-ASA may also be administered as an enema.

Azathioprine. In a dose of 2.5 mg/kg daily, azathioprine may be helpful in patients with chronic disease for whom surgery is inappropriate. It has a major role in allowing the dose of corticosteroids to be reduced in those patients with troublesome side-effects. Serious side-effects may occur including suppression of the bone marrow with pancytopenia and patients must be carefully supervised. The drug is used more frequently for Crohn's disease than ulcerative colitis.

Surgical management

If the appropriate medical measures are carried out assiduously the majority of patients with proctitis or moderately severe colitis will pass into remission. In severe forms of ulcerative colitis, or where there is toxic dilatation of the colon or perforation, and in the occasional patient with severe haemorrhage, emergency surgical treatment is required. A proctocolectomy is performed but in some urgent circumstances surgery will be restricted to a colectomy with ileostomy, the rectum and distal colon being removed at a later stage when the crisis is over.

Acute ulcerative colitis which fails to respond to medical treatment, or which relapses frequently in spite of adequate treatment, is also an indication for proctocolectomy. This operation is also indicated in chronic illness, or when the disease 'burns out' leaving a permanently damaged bowel, perhaps with stricture forma-

tion. Long-standing disease carries a risk of carcinoma; accordingly total bowel involvement, with activity extending over more than 10 years, should lead to serious consideration of proctocolectomy—especially when precancerous lesions are detected on biopsy during surveillance by a colonoscopy. The colonoscopy should be performed every one or two years.

At all stages of the disease, the timing of and preparation for surgery are important and require collaboration between the medical and surgical staff. In emergency situations intensive pre-operative replacement of blood, fluid and electrolytes is needed and an operation is performed as soon as the patient is fit to withstand surgery. In less urgent situations, the timing of surgery depends on the degree of improvement in the patient's general condition.

Whenever possible, in addition to a full explanation of ileostomy and its management with a demonstration of the actual appliance to be used, the patient should have the opportunity before operation of meeting someone with an established ileostomy. Modern surgical techniques and the range of ileostomy appliances available make for easy management of the stoma and allow the patient to live an almost normal life with little restriction of physical activity.

When the rectum is not grossly involved it may be preserved and ileorectal anastomosis performed. In selected patients ileo-anal anastomosis with formation of an ileal pouch can be used. Such methods are gaining in acceptance because of the avoidance of a stoma but are only used to treat ulcerative colitis and not Crohn's colitis. They are not without complications and the pouch itself may become inflamed.

A summary of therapeutic measures required for colitis of varying severity is listed in the information box.

SUMMARY OF MANAGEMENT OF ULCERATIVE AND CROHN'S COLITIS

Severe disease
- Hospitalisation
- Parenteral fluid, nutrition and blood
- Systemic corticosteroids
- Surgery for non-response and toxic dilatation

Mild disease or proctitis
- Corticosteroid enemas
- Oral sulphasalazine

Chronic disease
- Oral corticosteroids
- Azathioprine
- Surgery for chronic ill health

Disease in remission
- Oral 5-Aminosalicylic acid preparation
- Surveillance for cancer of colon after 10 years

Ileostomy management

Patients should be encouraged to join an ileostomy association or be enrolled in a stoma therapy clinic in order to be kept in touch with advances in techniques of ileostomy care. The ileostomy bag is emptied 2–3 times per 24 hours and with proper care should not be odorous. Ileostomy may lead to problems with self-image and marital difficulties which may require counselling.

Ileostomy patients are very prone to dehydration in hot climates and to gastrointestinal infections. A greatly increased oral fluid and salt intake is required under these circumstances. Hospital admission is often advisable during gastrointestinal infections.

Prognosis

In Crohn's disease, relapses are common and most patients will require surgery at some time. Despite this 75% of patients will remain at work and are socially integrated.

In population studies on ulcerative colitis one quarter to a half of patients have proctitis and one quarter have or develop extensive colitis. Life expectancy is normal in patients with proctitis; a third have only one attack, the remainder follow a chronic relapsing course. With more extensive disease, there is an increased mortality in the first year, but thereafter mortality is probably no greater than in the general population. Similar population studies have not been performed for Crohn's colitis but surgery is more commonly necessary and the mortality rate is twice that expected in the general population.

FURTHER READING

Lashner B A, Kirsner J B 1992 The epidemiology of inflammatory bowel disease: are we learning anything new? Gastroenterology 103: 696

Sofaer J 1993 Crohn's disease: the genetic contribution. Gut 34: 869

DISEASES OF THE LARGE INTESTINE

SYMPTOMS OF LARGE INTESTINAL DISEASE

Constipation

In Britain fewer than 20% of people have less than one bowel motion per day and only 4% have a bowel movement less frequently than three times a week. The latter should be regarded as constipated. In addition, if the stool is hard and difficult to pass the patient should be regarded as constipated whatever the frequency of bowel movement.

Diarrhoea

In contrast, less than 1% of the population have more than three bowel movements daily and this should be

regarded as abnormal, particularly if the stool is not formed. When the stool is liquid or semi-formed it is considered to be diarrhoea whatever the frequency of bowel movement. The diet in Western countries is low in roughage; where a high residue diet is usual, more than three bowel movements daily may be normal. An explanation must be sought for any change in bowel habit.

Urgency and incontinence

Urgency may reflect the presence of liquid stool but it may also occur with colonic and rectal inflammation. In these circumstances urgency may sometimes be followed by incontinence. Incontinence of normal stool may occur in anorectal disorders.

Bleeding

The appearance of recognisable blood in the stool is usually indicative of colonic or rectal disease. In rectal or anal disease the blood is bright red. In colonic disease it may be red, purple or plum coloured.

Mucus

Mucus in the stool may indicate colonic or rectal dysfunction or disease.

Pain

Colonic pain is hypogastric (Fig. 7.10, p. 442) and midline. It may localise laterally when there is colonic inflammation affecting the peritoneum.

Tenesmus

This is a pain or disagreeable sensation, sometimes likened to burning, which is felt in the rectum. The patient can localise the pain which is usually related to bowel movements. It can also be described as a sensation of incomplete evacuation.

DIVERTICULAR DISEASE

Though diverticula occur throughout the gastrointestinal tract, they are most common in the large bowel of middle-aged or elderly subjects. The presence of diverticula is known as **diverticulosis**; when they are inflamed the condition is known as **diverticulitis**. Such inflammation occurs almost exclusively in colonic diverticula. Because it is often difficult to separate the two conditions on clinical or radiological evidence, they are grouped together under the term 'diverticular disease'.

Aetiology

In diverticulosis the muscular coat of the bowel is often greatly thickened, suggesting that the diverticula have formed as a result of increased intracolonic pressure. Manometric measurements support this view. Pressure in the bowel is high and there is an area of spasm or failure to relax at the recto-sigmoid junction.

Dietary factors may be at least partly responsible. Diverticulosis is rare in areas of the world such as Africa and Asia where the usual diet is one of high residue; by contrast the incidence is increasing in Western countries where natural fibre is removed from the diet in the processes of food refining. Moreover there is evidence that intracolonic pressures vary with the bulk of faecal residue, a high faecal residue being associated with a low intraluminal pressure and vice versa.

Incidence

The incidence in Western communities is between 5 and 10% and in those over the age of 60 it is 30%, though only a small proportion of patients have symptoms.

Pathology

The pelvic colon is most commonly involved. Its muscle wall is thickened but the diverticula themselves are pouchings of the mucosa and have no muscle coat (Fig. 7.15). It is not clear how they become inflamed. Radiological examination frequently shows the presence of a faecolith in a diverticulum and it may be that faeces collect because of the inability of the diverticulum to contract. Faecal retention may then cause a local inflammatory reaction which may resolve spontaneously or progress to cause perforation, local abscess formation, fistula and peritonitis. The bowel wall becomes thickened with narrowing of the lumen when there are repeated attacks of diverticulitis, leading eventually to obstruction.

Clinical features

Pain or discomfort felt in the hypogastrium or in the left iliac fossa is common and there may be associated local tenderness. Acute diverticulitis can give rise to severe pain, guarding and rigidity on the left side, the signs of peritonitis and obstruction being combined. Change of bowel habit, either increasing constipation or constipation alternating with diarrhoea, is frequent. Complications are shown in Figure 7.16. On examination, the thickened tender colon may be palpable in the left iliac fossa and a mass may be present in those patients who have developed diverticulitis, with or without abscess formation.

Investigations

Sigmoidoscopy

This is necessary to exclude cancer of the rectum or lower sigmoid colon. Usually there are no positive fea-

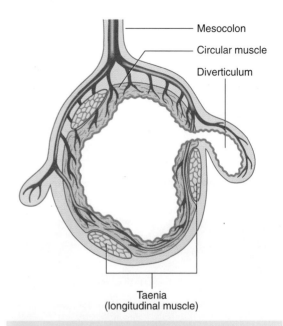

Mesocolon

Circular muscle

Diverticulum

Taenia (longitudinal muscle)

Fig. 7.15 The human colon in diverticulosis. The colonic wall is weak between the taeniae. The blood vessels that supply the colon pierce the circular muscle and weaken it further by forming tunnels. Diverticula usually emerge through these points of least resistance.

tures apart from possible discomfort and tenderness at the rectosigmoid junction.

Barium enema examination

This shows characteristic sacs along the contour of the gut in diverticulosis (Fig 7.17). After evacuation barium frequently remains in the diverticula which are clearly outlined. The barium enema must be postponed for 2–3 weeks in acute diverticulitis until the inflammation has settled when narrowing, rigidity and loss of normal haustration of a segment of colon can be identified. Evidence of fistula or abscess formation may be seen. Whether or not there are diverticula present, the main diagnostic difficulty is to distinguish the appearances from those of carcinoma. Radiological differentiation may be impossible and cancer and diverticular disease may coexist.

Flexible sigmoidoscopy

Flexible sigmoidoscopy is used to inspect the affected segment of bowel for visual evidence of cancer, and biopsies are taken. Colonoscopy is indicated when there is frank bleeding for it will determine whether the bleeding arises from a diverticulum or from a more proximal lesion such as angiodysplasia (p. 441).

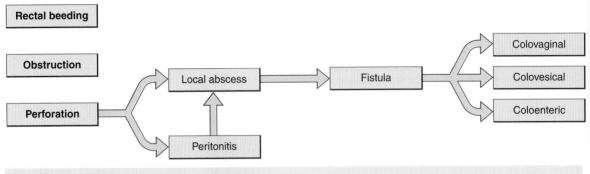

Fig. 7.16 Complications of diverticulitis.

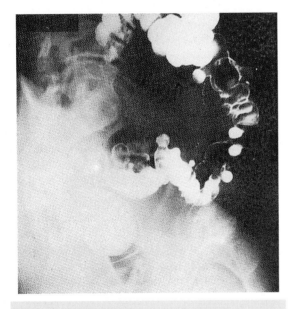

Fig. 7.17 Diverticular disease of the sigmoid colon.

Computed tomography

Computed tomography is used in the assessment of complicated diverticular disease when there are abscesses and fistulas.

Management

Asymptomatic diverticulosis is common, is often found accidentally and requires no treatment. A high-fibre diet is usually sufficient to relieve constipation. If not, a bulk laxative such as methylcellulose, 1–4 teaspoons daily in a liberal quantity of water, should be used in addition. Purgatives are avoided.

An attack of acute diverticulitis may require bed-rest, metronidazole (400 mg 8-hourly orally for 7 days), and ampicillin (500 mg 6-hourly for 7 days), intravenous and oral fluids, or even cessation of feeding and nasogastric suction. Most attacks resolve but a few require emergency surgery which usually is a temporary defunctioning proximal colostomy followed later by local resection. Many centres prefer resection and primary anastomosis. An emergency partial colectomy may be required for acute bleeding (p. 441).

Elective surgery is indicated after recovery from an acute attack in those patients who have developed obstructive features, in those who have complications such as fistula, and those in whom the possibility of carcinoma cannot be excluded. The treatment of choice is resection of the involved segment of pelvic colon with primary anastomosis.

ANTIBIOTIC-ASSOCIATED DIARRHOEA

Diarrhoea is quite common in patients receiving antibiotics and it usually stops when the antibiotic is ceased. In about 40% of patients with diarrhoea *C. difficile* can be cultured from the stool and it is assumed that the condition is caused by a disturbance of the intestinal flora. In a small proportion of patients, the condition progresses to an antibiotic-associated colitis. In some of the latter patients, the inflammation of the colon is so severe that a pseudomembrane forms over the mucosa, hence the name pseudomembranous colitis.

PSEUDOMEMBRANOUS COLITIS

Clostridium difficile is the major cause of antibiotic associated colitis and pseudomembranous colitis. This organism produces at least two exotoxins, A and B, which cause intestinal damage. The infection occurs most often in hospital where the organism resides in rooms and toilets and is transmitted by hand to the patient. It proliferates in the colon when the intestinal flora is disturbed by the administration of antibiotics, particularly broad spectrum antibiotics such as clindamycin.

Pathology

Antibiotic-associated colitis and pseudomembranous colitis can be regarded as a continuum. Initially the mucosa shows focal areas of inflammation and ulceration. The ulcers become covered by a membrane of fibrin, debris and polymorphs, which may spread to cover the entire mucosa.

Clinical features

Symptoms usually begin during the first week of antibiotic therapy but sometimes they arise later or even when antibiotic therapy is finished. The onset is often insidious with lower abdominal pain and increased frequency of bowel movements. The diarrhoea may become profuse and watery and the condition of the patient may resemble one with acute ulcerative colitis (p. 461). Indeed, the condition may progress to toxic dilatation.

Investigations

The diagnosis is made on the rectal appearance at sigmoidoscopy with erythema, white plaques or a confluent pseudomembrane. Biopsy may confirm the diagnosis if the focal inflammation and membrane is seen but in some cases it is indistinguishable from ulcerative colitis. However, a normal rectal mucosa does not exclude the disorder, for in some patients the condition is limited to the right colon. Confirmation is by a cytotoxicity assay for toxin A and B performed on a filtrate of diarrhoeal stool. The organism may also be cultured from the stool. When there is disparity between these results, they are interpreted in the context of the clinical findings.

Management

The offending antibiotic should be stopped. The patient should be isolated, and supportive therapy as for ulcerative colitis (p. 462) is given. The treatment of choice for mild to moderate disease is metronidazole 200–400 mg 8-hourly or bacitracin 20 000 U 6-hourly for 7–10 days. Severe disease is treated with oral vancomycin 125 mg 6-hourly for 10–14 days. Relapse is common and a further course of vancomycin is given.

PNEUMATOSIS CYSTOIDES INTESTINALIS

In this disease multiple gas-filled cysts line the colonic wall. The gas may track via the alveoli, mediastinum and retroperitoneal tissues when there is chronic lung or heart disease with severe bouts of coughing. Other patients are found to have pyloric obstruction or disease of the small intestine.

There is constipation, diarrhoea, rectal bleeding and mucus. The cysts are recognised on sigmoidoscopy, plain radiograph of the abdomen or barium enema.

Underlying gastrointestinal conditions are treated and the cysts resolve with high-flow oxygen therapy.

ENDOMETRIOSIS

Endometrial tissue can become embedded in the bowel, most frequently the sigmoid colon and rectum. A cystic mass develops which expands toward the lumen of the bowel, but the mucosa remains intact. If endometrial tissue surrounds the bowel, obstruction may ensue. There is cyclical rectal pain, discomfort, constipation or diarrhoea. Bimanual examination may reveal a tender nodule. Endoscopic and barium studies reveal intact mucosa over the mass. Large lesions are treated surgically. Other lesions can be treated by hormone therapy.

TUMOURS OF THE COLON

NEOPLASTIC (BENIGN) POLYPS

Aetiology and incidence

In population studies the incidence of neoplastic polyps closely parallels that of colonic cancer. Polyps precede cancer by five years, the average ages being 58 and 63 respectively, and it is believed that polyps are premalignant. In Western countries, neoplastic polyps occur in up to 10% of the population over the age of 40. The aetiological factors are the same as for cancer of the colon (see p. 469).

Pathology

Polyps are classified histologically into tubular adenoma, tubular-villous adenoma and villous adenoma, the risk of malignancy being greater in the latter two and greatest in the villous form (Table 7.23). The risk of malignancy is also related to size and all polyps of diameter greater than 2 cm have an average 50% risk. Multiple polyps are common.

Clinical features

Polyps are mostly asymptomatic and may be found incidentally on barium enema or colonoscopy. Occasionally

Table 7.23 Classification of benign colonic polyps

Type	Solitary	Multiple
Neoplastic	Adenoma	Familial polyposis
Hamartomatous	Juvenile	Juvenile polyposis
	Peutz–Jeghers	Peutz–Jeghers syndrome
Inflammatory	Benign lymphoid polyp	Benign lymphoid polyposis
		Inflammatory polyposis in colitis
Metaplastic		Multiple metaplastic polyps

they may cause bleeding, discharge of mucus or intussusception. A small proportion of polyps are responsible for occult bleeding.

Investigations and management

The mainstays of investigation and treatment are flexible sigmoidoscopy, double-contrast barium enema and colonoscopy; polypectomy is often carried out during the endoscopic procedure.

Polyps in the rectum can be removed at sigmoidoscopy. Flexible sigmoidoscopy is important because polyps at the rectosigmoid region can be detected more successfully than by the double-contrast enema. The double-contrast enema and colonoscopy are probably equally accurate in detecting polyps in the rest of the colon. Colonoscopy has an advantage in allowing immediate polypectomy; however the double-contrast enema can examine the right colon which is sometimes not seen at colonoscopy.

At colonoscopy the polyp which is usually pedunculated is removed with a snare and recovered for histological examination to assess the completeness of removal and the presence of premalignancy or invasive malignancy. Surgical polypectomy is necessary if there has been incomplete removal of a malignant polyp, or when the polyp is sessile, particularly if it is a villous adenoma.

Repeat colonoscopy is recommended at 6–12 months after removal of a benign polyp or polyps and thereafter every two years.

OTHER FORMS OF BENIGN TUMOURS

These exist in single or multiple forms (Tables 7.23 and 7.24). The multiple forms, apart from metaplastic polyps, tend to be associated with gastrointestinal malignancy. Juvenile polyps nearly always present with bleeding. In the Peutz–Jeghers syndrome, polyps are present throughout the gastrointestinal tract and there is melanin pigmentation at the mucocutaneous junctions. Metaplastic (hyperplastic) polyps are present in 75% of patients over the age of 40. They are pale, flat-topped sessile plaques of less than 5 mm.

Other polypoid lesions which may occur in the colon are lipomas, carcinoids (p. 456) and leiomyomas.

FAMILIAL ADENOMATOUS POLYPOSIS (FAP)

This condition has an incidence of 1 in 24 000 and it is transmitted by autosomal dominant inheritance. The responsible gene is localised to the long arm of chromosome 5. Gardner's syndrome, which has osteomas of the jaw and sebaceous cysts as well as colonic polyps, shares the same genetic abnormality and is considered to be part of the disease spectrum.

Pathology

There are 100 or more adenomas in the colon, usually 1000 and sometimes 5000. The rectum is always involved. Histologically the adenomas are usually tubular but occasionally are villous. The polyps appear at adolescence and become malignant in about 15 years; the patient often dies from carcinomatosis before the age of 40. Gastric, duodenal and periampullary polyps are also common.

Clinical features

Symptoms usually begin in the mid-30s. There may be abdominal pain, diarrhoea and blood and mucus in the stool.

Investigations

Carcinoma is usually present by the time symptoms arise. Because the rectum is always involved the diag-

Table 7.24 Gastrointestinal polyposis syndromes

	Familial polyposis (includes Gardner's syndrome)	Peutz–Jeghers syndrome	Turcot's syndrome	Cronkhite–Canada syndrome	Cowden's disease
Oesophageal polyps	–	–	–	+	+
Gastric polyps	+	++	–	+++	+++
Small intestinal polyps	+	+++	–	++	++
Colonic polyps	+++	++	+++	+++	+
Other features	Osteomas, soft tissue tumours, congenital retinal pigment hyperplasia	Pigmentation of lips, fingers	Malignant central nervous tumours	Hair loss, hyperpigmentation, nail dystrophy	Multiple congenital abnormalities, orocutaneous hamartomas, thyroid tumours, breast hypertrophy

nosis is established by sigmoidoscopy and biopsy. The barium enema shows multiple small filling defects unevenly distributed throughout the colon. Upper gastro-intestinal endoscopy is carried out for gastric, duodenal and periampullary polyps.

All relatives must be traced and kept under review by annual sigmoidoscopy after the age of 10.

Management

Total colectomy and ileorectal anastomosis is rec-ommended by some centres, with follow-up to detect rectal cancer. It is therefore safer to remove the rectum with the procedure of proctocolectomy and ileostomy.

CARCINOMA OF THE COLON AND RECTUM

Aetiology and incidence

Carcinoma of the large intestine is the most common malignant tumour of the alimentary tract in most West-ern communities and has an incidence approaching 60 per 100 000. It is rare in Africa and Asia. The vari-ation in incidence of the disease between different coun-tries has led to speculation that dietary factors and differences in bacterial flora of the bowel may be of aetiological significance. However, genetic factors are increasingly recognised. Cancer of the colon occurs three to five times more often amongst first degree rela-tives than in the general population and 'cancer family syndromes' have been described. Diseases known to be clearly associated with colonic carcinoma are long-standing ulcerative colitis and familial polyposis, but in the majority of patients the cancer arises from a malig-nant transformation of a benign adenomatous polyp.

Pathology

In communities with a high incidence of large bowel cancer, the distribution of tumours is shown in Figure 7.18. Concomitant (synchronous) multiple tumours are present in 2% of patients and the risk of a second cancer is higher in those who also have adenomatous polyps.

Macroscopically the tumour may be proliferative and fungating, ulcerative and infiltrating, polypoidal or encircling as a 'string' stricture. Perforation may occur at the site of the tumour leading to peritonitis, localised abscess or a fistula.

Spread occurs directly into and through the bowel wall, by lymphatics and by the bloodstream through both portal and systemic circulations. Colonic car-cinoma is capable of direct implantation on exposed surfaces, such as a suture line or area of trauma in the bowel. Metastases most commonly involve the liver.

Tumours are classified by the Dukes' system which has important prognostic implications (Table 7.25).

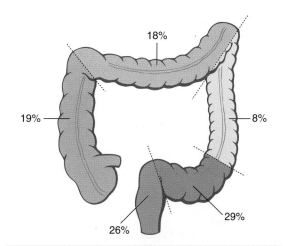

Fig. 7.18 Distribution of cancer of the large intestine.

Table 7.25 Dukes' classification of large bowel cancer

Stage	Definition	% of cases	Prognosis (5-year survival)
A	Spread not beyond muscularis No lymph node metastases	4	80%
B	Spread is beyond muscularis into pericolic tissues but no lymph node metastases	28	58%
C	Spread to lymph nodes	27	36%
D	Metastases present	41	6%

Clinical features

Symptoms vary depending on the site of the carcinoma. In tumours of the left colon, frank blood in the stool is common and obstruction is early. Tumours of the right colon present with anaemia due to occult bleeding, cachexia and alteration of bowel habit but obstruction is late because of the relatively fluid nature of the bowel contents. As a consequence left-sided tumours tend to be diagnosed earlier. Some patients may present with perforation, and caecal carcinoma may mimic acute appendicitis. Pain occurs in two-thirds of patients. It may vary from abdominal discomfort to colicky lower abdominal pain related to bowel movements.

Change in bowel habit, anaemia, weight loss and sometimes excessive borborygmi, abdominal distension and colicky pains indicating subacute obstruction, all point to a large bowel tumour. Some, however, are rela-tively symptomless until the patient presents as an emer-gency with obstruction.

Carcinoma of the rectum will almost always cause early bleeding with mucous discharge; later there is ten-esmus and a feeling of incomplete emptying of the bowel. Obstruction is a feature of tumours of the pelvi-rectal junction but not the rectum proper which is capacious and distensible.

The findings on physical examination range from no obvious abnormality to the signs of advanced malignancy with cachexia and signs of extra-colonic spread. A mass may be palpable. Rectal tumours may be palpated on digital examination. Fresh blood in the stool should always suggest the possibility of a tumour of the rectum or pelvic colon. Occult blood is found in the stool if an ulcerating lesion is present in the proximal colon.

Investigations

In most communities the initial investigations are a rigid sigmoidoscopy which will detect approximately one third of tumours, followed by a double-contrast barium enema examination. A barium enema will demonstrate advanced cancer as a filling defect or stricture (Fig. 7.19). However, the barium enema is not as accurate as colonoscopy in detecting small tumours and polyps and thus in many centres, flexible sigmoidoscopy and colonoscopy have become the investigations of choice. There is a tendency for carcinomas of the caecum to be missed because the filling with barium may be incomplete and the colonoscopy may not reach the area in a small proportion of cases. When caecal cancer is suspected, a barium follow-through examination may help to define the tumour.

Computed tomography is a valuable technique to search for hepatic metastases prior to surgery so that appropriate treatment can be planned.

Management

The treatment of choice is resection of the tumour as a one-stage procedure. If there is no colonic obstruction, or if it can be overcome by enemas, time should be spent in preparing the bowel by washouts and antibiotics. Anaemia should be corrected by pre-operative transfusion.

Carcinoma of the rectum may require total removal of the rectum with permanent colostomy and for this the patient requires pre-operative explanation of colostomy and its management. However, advances in suture techniques allow preservation of continuity in many more patients by means of a colorectal or colo-anal anastomosis. In addition, some centres are instituting local treatment of rectal cancers with irradiation, electrocoagulation or laser therapy in order to avoid colostomy.

Hepatic secondary tumour can sometimes be treated by resection in the hope of cure and the symptoms from multiple metastases can be palliated with hepatic artery ligation, embolisation and infusion chemotherapy.

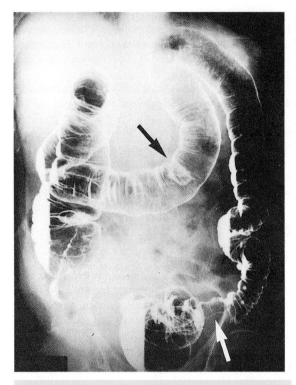

Fig. 7.19 Carcinoma of the sigmoid colon and a polyp in the transverse colon.

Screening for colon cancer

Screening programmes utilising faecal occult blood tests and regular endoscopy have been instituted in an attempt to diagnose the tumour at an early stage. They are not yet recommended.

Family cancer syndromes account for about 5% of all colon cancers and must be distinguished from familial adenomatous polyposis. They have an autosomal dominant inheritance and the onset of tumours between the ages of 20 and 40. All members of these families should have colonoscopic screening every 2 years from the age of 25. Colonoscopic screening is also recommended when the individual has more than one affected first-degree relative or if a first-degree relative has colon cancer under the age of 40. The interval between screening examinations has not yet been decided.

FUNCTIONAL DISORDERS

IRRITABLE BOWEL SYNDROME

Aetiology

One of the commonest disorders of the alimentary tract is that of long-standing bowel dysfunction associated with abdominal pain for which no organic cause can be found. Bowel habit is disturbed by diarrhoea or constipation occurring alone, or alternating. Some forms of this irritable bowel syndrome have in the past been called *spastic colon* and *idiopathic or nervous diarrhoea*.

Whilst it is generally accepted that disturbed motility in the colon forms the basis of the symptoms, consistent changes which would be helpful diagnostically have not been found. Patients with irritable bowel syndrome have a lowered threshold to pain induced by inflation of a balloon in the rectum and the referral of pain is more widespread to different parts of the abdomen than in normal individuals. Disturbances of motility have also been demonstrated in the small intestine, stomach, lower oesophagus and bladder and these help to explain the widespread nature of the symptoms.

The aetiology of the irritable bowel syndrome is uncertain. However in some patients psychological disturbances, especially anxiety and hypochondriasis, are evident. Patients may be tense, conscientious individuals who worry excessively about family or financial affairs. Social learning in relation to illness behaviour may explain why these patients consult their doctors. Some patients relate the onset of their symptoms to an attack of infective diarrhoea; in others certain foods may precipitate symptoms.

Clinical features

The syndrome is most frequent in women between the ages of 20 and 40 years. The commonest symptom is pain referred to the left or right iliac fossa or the hypogastrium, sometimes varying in site. Dyspepsia is also part of the syndrome in many patients. Pain often occurs in attacks usually relieved by defecation and sometimes provoked by food, and may be severe. Bowel habit is variable. Almost all patients at some time notice pellet-like or ribbon-like stools with or without mucus. Diarrhoea may be painless and characteristically occurs in the morning, and almost never at night. An urge to defecate after meals may be the consequence of an exaggerated gastrocolic reflex. Other symptoms include abdominal distension, a sensation of incomplete emptying of the rectum, excessive flatus and audible borborygmi. There may be urinary frequency and dysuria.

On examination there is tenderness over one or more areas of the colon and often the pelvic colon is easily palpated and tender.

Investigations

Although the diagnosis is usually suggested by the history alone, organic bowel disease has to be excluded, especially in patients developing symptoms for the first time over the age of 40 years. Sigmoidoscopy may be required to exclude an organic lesion in the rectum or rectosigmoid junction. The mucosa appears normal in the irritable bowel syndrome but the bowel may show marked motor activity, contracting and relaxing quite unlike the normal inert bowel. In appropriate circumstances a barium enema may be indicated to exclude organic disease. There are no diagnostic radiological features in the irritable bowel syndrome. The possibility of lactose intolerance, hyperthyroidism or alcohol excess should not be overlooked in patients whose principal complaint is painless diarrhoea.

Management

The patient must be reassured that no organic disease is present as anxiety may precipitate or aggravate the condition and there is sometimes an underlying fear of cancer. An explanation for the symptoms must be offered and this is best based upon a simple description of intestinal motility and its disorder, spasm, which can cause pain. In patients with persistent or troublesome symptoms, measures designed to modify the intestinal dysmotility are required. The patient with constipation and pain should be encouraged to increase the roughage content of the diet and one of the bulk laxatives such as methyl-cellulose should be prescribed in a dose sufficient to ensure normal bowel movement. It is important that the patient should stop chemical laxatives.

An anticholinergic drug such as dicyclomine (10 mg 3 times daily) or an anti-spasmodic such as mebeverine hydrochloride (135 mg 3 times daily) may be tried for pain and diarrhoea. For patients with painless diarrhoea, improvement is commonly obtained with some dietary restriction, particularly in the avoidance of milk, fresh fruits and salads. Codeine phosphate (30 mg 3–4 times daily) and loperamide (6–8 mg daily) are useful drugs which act quickly and can be carried by the patient to use either in emergency or before any event which is known to precipitate diarrhoea. Many patients, particularly those in whom abdominal pain is marked, benefit from small doses of antidepressants, tryptanol 10–20 mg at night or prothiadin 25–50 mg at night.

PROCTALGIA FUGAX

This is an episodic, often excruciating pain which arises in the rectum and can be localised to just above the anus; it lasts for a few seconds or minutes. It is unrelated to bowel movements or organic disease. The condition is fairly common and may occur in association with irritable bowel syndrome.

The probable cause is spasm of the pubococcygeus muscle or other muscles. There are no abnormal findings on examination. The patient is reassured. Heat or pressure applied to the perineum may abort an attack.

CONSTIPATION

This may be defined as less than 3 motions per week or as difficult or painful defecation. The causes are classified in the information box. Constipation is a common complaint and initially it is important to determine if there is true constipation. The normal bowel habit of many individuals is less than one stool per day; this does not constitute constipation. The clinical approach to true constipation is based on the possible causes (see upper information box). Important information to be obtained from the patient is shown in the lower information box.

CAUSES OF CONSTIPATION

- Inadequate diet and lifestyle ('simple constipation'), e.g. lack of fibre and exercise
- Irritable bowel syndrome
- Drugs
  Analgesics
  Anti-inflammatory agents
  Aluminium-containing antacids
  Antidepressants
  Diuretics
  Iron and many more
- Psychiatric and neurological disorders
  Ignoring call to stool
  Physical disability
- Organic diseases of the anus, rectum and colon
- Disorders of intestinal motility which may be secondary to metabolic problems
  Hypothyroidism
  Pseudo-obstruction

IMPORTANT INFORMATION IN A CONSTIPATED PATIENT

- Is the constipation of recent origin? If so full G.I. investigation is needed in those over 30 years old
- Is the diet well-balanced and containing fibre?
- What drugs is the patient receiving—particularly opiates, antacids, psychotropic agents?
- Are laxatives being used?
- Are there any psychiatric, neurological or systemic diseases?

SIMPLE CONSTIPATION

This is constipation due to an inadequate diet and lifestyle; there is no underlying organic disease and the condition responds to improvement in diet or the use of bulking agents (see Table 7.26). Investigation is not usually required but a rectal examination must be performed.

Management

The diet is reviewed and additional roughage is advised, e.g. fruit and vegetables. Unprocessed bran is recommended in increasing amounts, 1–3 tablespoons per day mixed with cereals. Some patients will complain of flatulence due to increased fermentation in the colon; in these patients, a hydrophilic bulking agent is recommended. Some constipated patients, particularly the elderly, have an inadequate fluid intake and this must be corrected.

SEVERE IDIOPATHIC CONSTIPATION

An occasional patient, usually a young woman, will fail to respond to a high-residue diet; indeed this may exacerbate symptoms. There is a reduction in propagative motor activity in the colon together with inappropriate contraction of the pelvic floor muscles on straining. The condition usually begins in childhood or adolescence and is resistant to all treatments. The diagnosis is made on the history and confirmed by motility studies. Treatment is difficult; saline laxatives may help but subtotal colectomy may become necessary in some patients.

MEGACOLON

Megacolon is a condition characterised by dilatation of the colon and obstinate constipation. The patients may be separated into two groups, congenital (Hirschsprung's disease) and acquired megacolon.

HIRSCHSPRUNG'S DISEASE

This is a familial disorder with an incidence of 1/5000. The cause is a congenital absence of the myenteric nerve plexus in the wall of the pelvic colon and upper rectum. Occasionally the defect extends proximally. The internal sphincter fails to relax. There is a family history in one third of cases.

Symptoms of colonic obstruction (constipation, abdominal distension and vomiting) usually date from birth, but in a few cases the condition may present in childhood or in the young adult. On examination there may be persistent abdominal swelling. The rectum is empty on digital examination.

Radiological examination with small amounts of barium shows a small rectum, a narrow segment above and then wide dilatation of the colon full of retained faeces.

Table 7.26 Laxatives

Laxative	Use
Chemical anthracine and phenylmethane derivatives, e.g. bisacodyl dioctyl sodium sulphosuccinate	Elderly or bed-bound individuals Pre-operative preparation
Saline laxatives	Radiological preparation
Hydrophilic agents ('bulk laxatives'), e.g. methylcellulose	Routinely used in chronic constipation especially in individuals who cannot tolerate dietary roughage

The diagnosis can be confirmed by a suction rectal biopsy which is taken near to the anus. The biopsy is of sufficient thickness to include muscle of the bowel wall in which the ganglion cells are situated. Acetylcholinesterase staining is used to identify ganglion cells. Rectal manometry may be helpful in some patients; the lower part of the rectum fails to relax when a balloon is distended in the upper rectum.

Treatment is by excision of the abnormal segment of colon and rectum.

ACQUIRED MEGACOLON

This may present in childhood when its usual cause is the withholding of stool during the toilet training period, that is *after* the first year of life. It is distinguished from Hirschsprung's disease by the presence of the urge to defecate and the presence of stool in the rectum. It responds to osmotic laxatives.

Acquired megacolon has several causes in the adult (Table 7.27). Abnormalities of sphincter muscle, pelvic floor and innervation are recognised in some patients. Radiologically acquired megacolon usually shows no narrowed segment and the dilatation extends down to the anus. The rectum is full of faeces. Most patients can be managed conservatively by treatment of the cause where identifiable, by high-residue diets, laxatives and perhaps saline enemas. The response will depend on the underlying pathogenesis. In a few patients colonic resection has been used as a last resort in the relief of obstinate constipation.

Table 7.27 Acquired megacolon in the adult

Disorder	Cause
Psychogenic megacolon	Disregard for urge to defecate; antidepressant drugs
Prolonged laxative abuse	Degeneration of myenteric plexus
Neurological disorders	Interruption of sensory and/or motor nerve supply
Smooth muscle disorders, e.g. scleroderma	Degeneration of colonic smooth muscle
Metabolic disorders, e.g. hypothyroidism	Delay in colonic transit

FAECAL IMPACTION

This occurs in acquired megacolon but also in patients who become bedridden. There may be a sensation of abdominal or rectal fullness and abdominal pain. Symptoms of large bowel obstruction (p. 445) may supervene. There may be spurious diarrhoea. Examination may reveal a firm abdominal mass. Rectal examination reveals the diagnosis. Olive oil retention enemas are used to soften the mass. Manual removal of the faecal masses may be necessary.

LAXATIVE ABUSE SYNDROMES

The prolonged consumption of chemical laxatives (see Table 7.25) may lead to degeneration of the myenteric plexus of the colon. The patient complains of increasing constipation despite large doses of laxatives. A barium enema demonstrates a featureless mucosa, loss of haustration and pseudostrictures, the 'cathartic colon'. When the patient has used prolonged anthraquinone purgatives, sigmoidoscopy may show a brown or black mucosa termed **melanosis coli**. Treatment of constipation is very difficult. The aim is to gradually replace chemical laxatives with saline and then bulk laxatives. This may take many months and some patients do not respond.

Surreptitious laxative abuse may occur particularly in women who complain of diarrhoea, abdominal discomfort and tiredness. They strongly deny taking laxatives and may continue even during investigation in hospital. Hypokalaema is common and there may be malabsorption due to the effect of laxatives on the small intestine.

ANORECTAL DISEASES

ANAL CONTINENCE AND INCONTINENCE

Continence depends upon an intact internal sphincter, external sphincter and puborectalis muscles and their efferent innervation. It also depends on training and on rectal sensation whereby the need to defecate is appreciated. The anal canal is sensitive to pain and touch, as is well demonstrated by the severe pain caused by fissures and inflamed haemorrhoids. The rectum is insensitive to painful stimuli so that the injection of a sclerosing agent for the treatment of haemorrhoids is painless. Rectal 'sensation' implies an ability to appreciate distension and contraction.

The more usual causes of incontinence are shown in the information box. Diarrhoea predisposes to incontinence, and can occur in the irritable bowel syndrome.

CAUSES OF INCONTINENCE

- Damage to the innervation of pelvic floor muscles during childbirth
- Anorectal disease
  Haemorrhoids
  Rectal prolapse
  Inflammatory bowel disease
- Neurological and psychiatric disease
  Spina bifida
  Spinal trauma
  Senile dementia
- Faecal impaction
- Congenital abnormalities of the anorectal region

Clinical features

Partial incontinence is minor soiling only and occurs commonly in the elderly, in those with some degree of faecal impaction and when there are prolapsing haemorrhoids. In major incontinence there is significant loss of control even when the stool is formed.

Management

This is usually very difficult. With diarrhoea or loose stools, a reduction in stool volume by the use of loperamide (6–8 mg daily) or lomotil (5 mg 3 times daily) may help all patients. If the patient is constipated, this must be treated. Thereafter, the use of electrophysiological tests to detect activity in the muscles of continence often identifies the main problem. Programmes of regular defecation help in the debilitated. Biofeedback techniques help in some patients. Repair operations can sometimes be instituted when the primary abnormality is identified as muscle damage.

HAEMORRHOIDS ('piles')

Internal haemorrhoids arise in the upper anal canal and lower rectum from the internal venous haemorrhoidal plexus. They enlarge to involve the skin-lined lower anal canal and the external haemorrhoidal venous plexus to become visible externally.

Bright red bleeding (p. 441) is common, as is prolapse of the piles on defecation, which may lead to permanent prolapse. Piles may cause pain and discomfort, mucous discharge and partial incontinence. The patient is investigated by proctoscopy and then by sigmoidoscopy to ensure that no other lesion is responsible for the bleeding. Symptomatic piles are treated on an outpatient basis by injection of sclerosant, or by rubber band ligation. Haemorrhoidectomy is reserved for more severe cases.

RECTAL PROLAPSE

This usually occurs in adult women. It occurs during defecation and is predisposed to by constipation and straining. There is bleeding and mucous discharge from the engorged mucosa. The treatment is surgical. Minor degrees of prolapse of the rectal mucosa may cause the solitary ulcer syndrome.

SOLITARY ULCER SYNDROME

In this disorder the mucosa of the anterior wall of the rectum undergoes partial prolapse and ulcerates. The ulcer is irregular and is surrounded by a halo of hyperaemia. The patient complains of the passage of mucus and small amounts of blood. There may be pain in the perineum and tenesmus. Ulceration is diagnosed at sigmoidoscopy, and biopsy of the ulcer shows characteristic histological features. Treatment is by the avoidance of constipation and straining. Marked prolapse is treated surgically.

PRURITUS ANI

This is a common condition and the aetiological factors are listed in the information box. The common factor in most cases is the contamination of the perianal skin with faecal constituents.

CAUSES OF PRURITUS ANI

Skin Diseases
- Contact eczema—due to local creams
- Lichen planus
- Psoriasis

Infections
- Candidosis, especially in those on corticosteroids and broad-spectrum antibiotics
- Threadworms

Gastroinestinal diseases which cause anorectal discharge
- Piles
- Fistula
- Fissure
- Irritable bowel syndrome
- Diarrhoea from any cause

Clinical features

The itch varies from a nuisance to overwhelming misery. The skin is damaged by scratching which causes further itching and pain.

Investigations

The entire perianal skin surface must be inspected. Proctoscopy and sigmoidoscopy determine if there is underlying disease. The urine is examined for glucose. Candidosis and fungal infection can be confirmed on skin scrapings.

Management

When no underlying cause is found, all local applications including medicated soaps are stopped. Personal hygiene is essential with careful washing after defecation. Bulk laxatives may stop perianal soiling with mucous discharge. Post-menopausal women may benefit from oestrogen therapy especially if there is associated genital pruritus.

FISSURE-IN-ANO

This is a tear in the sensitive skin-lined lower anal canal. It presents with severe pain commencing on defecation and continuing for some time afterwards. There may be bleeding, discharge of mucus and pruritus. The diagnosis is made on the history and the presence of a 'sentinel pile' which is an oedematous skin tag on the adjacent anal verge. The majority of fissures are cured by anal dilatation under general anaesthesia or by division of the internal sphincter.

FURTHER READING

Friedman G (ed) 1991 The irritable bowel syndrome: realities and trends. Gastroenterology Clinics of North America 20 (2): June. W. B. Saunders, Philadelphia
Hamilton S R 1993 The molecular genetics of colorectal neoplasia. Gastroenterology 105: 3
Lynch H T, Smyrk T C, Watson P, Lanspa S J, Lynch J F, et al 1993 Genetics, natural history, tumor spectrum, and pathology of hereditary nonpolyposis colorectal cancer: an updated review. Gastroenterology 104: 1535
Lynn R B, Friedman L S 1993 Irritable bowel syndrome. New England Journal of Medicine 329: 1940
Scott N, Quirke P 1993 Molecular biology of colorectal neoplasia. Gut 34: 289
Zighelboim J, Talley N J 1993 What are functional bowel disorders? Gastroenterology 104: 1196

DISEASES OF THE PANCREAS

SYMPTOMS OF PANCREATIC DISEASE

Pain

Abdominal pain is a feature of acute and chronic pancreatitis. Pain is referred to the epigastrium, to the mid-abdomen and to the back, often in the region of the lower thorax. It is usually constant, severe and can be relieved by flexion of the trunk.

Jaundice

Obstructive (cholestatic) jaundice (p. 500) is a feature of disease of the head of the pancreas and papilla of Vater.

Other symptoms

These arise from the development of diabetes mellitus (p. 724) and from pancreatic exocrine insufficiency which causes steatorrhoea and diarrhoea.

CONGENITAL AND GENETIC ABNORMALITIES

PANCREAS DIVISUM (DOMINANT DORSAL DUCT SYNDROME)

This occurs in up to 10% of the population and results from a failure of the dorsal and ventral pancreas to unite; consequently most of the pancreas is drained through the accessory papilla which is proximal to the papilla of Vater. Such patients are more prone to pancreatitis for the condition appears to be associated with stenosis of the opening of one or other papilla.

The diagnosis is made on endoscopic retrograde cholangiopancreatography (ERCP). Since most patients present with pancreatitis, the treatment is that of the pancreatitis.

ANNULAR PANCREAS

The ventral pancreas surrounds the second part of the duodenum and it is frequently associated with other congenital defects such as malrotation of the intestine, atresias and cardiac defects. The pancreas can constrict the duodenum causing obstruction soon after birth or in adult life and it may predispose to duodenal ulcer and acute pancreatitis. The diagnosis is made by barium studies and the treatment is surgical bypass of the constriction.

ECTOPIC PANCREATIC TISSUE

This may occur in the gastric antrum or duodenum and takes the form of a smooth nodule. It is usually asymptomatic and requires no treatment. If found coincidentally at surgery, the nodule is excised for it is subject to the same conditions, including carcinoma, as the pancreas itself.

CYSTIC FIBROSIS

This disease is considered on page 346. Here, the gastrointestinal manifestations are described.

Pathology

The pathological findings and their clinical features result from the obstruction by abnormal, viscid secretions of ducts in the salivary glands, digestive and biliary tracts and pancreas, causing atrophy and fibrosis.

Clinical features

Exocrine insufficiency leading to steatorrhoea and diarrhoea is almost universal in childhood. If the patient survives to adulthood, malabsorption tends to be less troublesome. Intestinal obstruction, often called 'meconium ileus equivalent', can occur in children and adults, caused by inspissated food and secretions. Rectal prolapse is common in children due to the large bulky stools and frequent coughing.

Recurrent episodes of acute pancreatitis may occur and the incidence of diabetes mellitus increases with age. Eventually chronic pancreatitis may supervene. Disease of the liver or biliary tract may also occur (p. 520).

Investigations

The diagnosis of cystic fibrosis is detailed on page 346. The gastrointestinal complications are investigated according to the suspected problem.

Management

Optimal treatment in the adolescent and adult depends on a team approach to complicated respiratory, nutritional and hepatobiliary problems. Many centres have established special clinics for such patients with appropriate specialist care (p. 346).

Patients with cystic fibrosis need 120–150% of the recommended daily energy allowance because of malabsorption and the catabolism induced by acute and chronic respiratory infections. Nutritional counselling and supervision are therefore very important and depend on high-energy supplements and snacks. Fat restriction is not advised because it limits calorie and essential fatty acid intake. Supplements of fat-soluble vitamins are required.

All patients with pancreatic insufficiency require oral pancreatic enzyme supplements; 'Creon' or 'Neutrizym' 1–2 capsules with meals. The dose, which may need to be increased to 30 capsules daily, is titrated to reduce steatorrhoea to a point at which stool frequency and offensiveness are reduced. Gastric acid neutralisation with antacid or H_2-receptor antagonists (p. 429) are often indicated to ensure a neutral pH in the duodenum which is necessary for the proper functioning of the pancreatic enzyme supplements.

While partial or complete intestinal obstruction may require surgery, the administration of N-acetylcysteine orally and rectally may relieve some obstructions.

PANCREATITIS

ACUTE PANCREATITIS

This is an acute inflammatory condition typically presenting with abdominal pain, and usually associated with raised pancreatic enzymes in blood or urine. In Western communities the incidence is 5–10 per 100 000.

Aetiology

In Britain about 50% of cases are associated with biliary disease and about 20% with alcoholism while in about 20% no cause can be identified. Alcoholism accounts for a much higher proportion in some countries, especially the USA and South Africa. The risk factors are listed in the information box.

RISK FACTORS FOR ACUTE PANCREATITIS

- Alcohol
- Gallstones
- Local obstructive factors
  Pancreas divisum
  Duodenal diverticulum
  Stenosis of the papilla of Vater
  Carcinoma in the head of the pancreas
- Drugs
  Azathioprine and many others
- Infections
  Mumps and other viruses
- Hyperlipoproteinaemia
- Major surgery or procedures
  ERCP
- Diffuse vascular diseases
- Hypercalcaemia
- Fulminant hepatic failure
- Abdominal trauma

The pancreas secretes the digestive enzymes as pro-enzymes which are activated in the intestinal lumen. Acute pancreatitis may result when activation occurs in the pancreatic duct system or even in the pancreatic acinar cells. The pathogeneses of gallstone or alcoholic pancreatitis are not understood. Under normal circumstances digestive and lysosomal enzymes are separated within the acinar cell. It is possible that contact between them activates the digestive enzyme to cause acute pancreatitis and this may explain the mechanism of action of some of the risk factors such as drugs and infections.

Pathology

The pancreas shows oedema, necrosis of the acinar and duct cells and an infiltration with inflammatory cells. With progression, the entire pancreas may become an inflammatory mass with haemorrhage into and around it. The release of enzymes leads to fat necrosis both in the pancreas and in the peritoneal cavity. Pancreatic secretions may subsequently collect to form one or more pseudocysts which have no epithelial lining and are lined with granulation and fibrous tissue. A pseudocyst communicates with a pancreatic duct—it may increase in size because of continued pancreatic secretion. A pancreatic abscess may form when the pseudocyst or the inflammatory mass becomes infected.

Clinical features

The onset is usually sudden with severe pain in the epigastrium or right hypochondrium. It often occurs within 12–24 hours following a large meal and alcohol. The pain is usually persistent and radiates most frequently through to the back, to either shoulder or to one of the iliac fossae before spreading to involve the whole abdomen. Nausea and vomiting are common. In severe cases profound shock supervenes and there is tachycardia, hypotension, cardiac arrhythmias and renal failure. An increased respiratory rate and hypoxia are common. Many other serious complications may arise either in the first few days or weeks of the disease (see Table 7.28).

Table 7.28 Complications of acute pancreatitis and their causes

Complication	Cause
Systemic	
Shock and renal failure	Loss of fluid into the pancreas and surrounding tissues
Respiratory failure	Shock lung syndrome (adult respiratory distress syndrome)
Diabetes mellitus	Destruction of pancreatic tissue
Hypocalcaemia	Sequestration of calcium in areas of fat necrosis
Subcutaneous fat necrosis	Release of pancreatic lipase
Pancreatic	
Abscess	Infection of necrotic pancreatic tissue
Pseudocyst	Collection of pancreatic debris and secretions
Gastrointestinal	
Haemorrhage	Gastric and duodenal erosions
Intestinal ileus	Local inflammation due to spread of pancreatic enzymes
Obstruction of the duodenum	Mechanical compression from the pancreatic mass
Obstructive jaundice	Compression of the common bile duct

Despite the severity of the pain there may be little or no guarding of the abdominal muscles at first. Later the upper abdomen becomes tender and rigid as peritoneal irritation increases and the initial shock passes off. Acute pancreatitis may simulate acute cholecystitis (with which it may coexist) and myocardial infarction. The disease may be recognised for the first time at laparotomy, the patient having been diagnosed with perforated peptic ulcer or acute appendicitis.

Pancreatic abscess

This presents 2–5 weeks after the onset of acute pancreatitis. The patient deteriorates with further abdominal pain, fever and weight loss. On examination there is abdominal tenderness but a palpable mass is uncommon.

Pancreatic pseudocyst

This develops 1–2 weeks after the onset of acute pancreatitis. There is abdominal pain, nausea and vomiting and weight loss. On examination there is often a smooth, round, tender mass in the upper abdomen. Frequently there is obstruction to the duodenum and common bile duct.

Pancreatic ascites

This follows pancreatic duct disruption or leaking of a pancreatic pseudocyst in patients with acute or chronic pancreatitis. The secretions may track into the mediastinum to cause a pleural effusion. The ascites presents with abdominal pain and an increase in girth.

Investigations

Amylase activity

Serum amylase activity (normal 50–300 u/l) is elevated on the first day of the disease and thereafter falls rapidly because of renal clearance. Urinary amylase activity measured on a 24-hour collection of urine may be helpful when the serum level is not diagnostic. A persistently raised serum amylase suggests the development of pseudocyst or pancreatic abscess or a non-pancreatic cause (Table 7.29). Very high levels of amylase activity also occur in ascitic fluid in pancreatic ascites and in pleural effusion secondary to pancreatic ascites.

Plain radiographs

Whilst changes may be seen on a plain radiograph of the abdomen, these are often non-specific. The plain radiograph is used to diagnose ileus or obstruction secondary to acute pancreatitis. A plain radiograph of the chest often shows a left pleural effusion, collapse or consolidation of the lung.

Table 7.29 Non-pancreatic causes of a raised serum amylase activity

Other causes of acute abdomen	
Intestinal obstruction with gangrene Cholecystitis Ruptured ovarian cyst Perforated duodenal ulcer	Like acute pancreatitis the rise in serum amylase is short-lived, but rarely above 1200 u/l
Abnormal amylase	
Macroamylasaemia Raised salivary amylase in alcoholics	The elevation in serum amylase is persistent

Imaging

Ultrasound scanning and computed tomography are used to confirm the diagnosis and are vital in monitoring the progress of the pancreatitis and in detecting the development of pseudocyst, abscess and haemorrhage. The procedures are complementary. Computed tomography best indicates the degree of damage to the pancreas itself, is helpful in defining haemorrhage into and around the pancreas, and identifies gas which is an important sign of pancreatic abscess formation. Ultrasonography is suited to the identification and serial assessment of pseudocysts, the assessment of biliary obstruction and the identification of gallstones.

Laparotomy

This may be performed when a condition requiring surgery such as a perforated duodenal ulcer cannot be excluded. The diagnosis is then made on the appearance of the pancreas and the absence of any other acute intra-abdominal disease.

Management

The reduced mortality from acute pancreatitis in recent years is due to an understanding of the mechanisms for the complications and the application of effective supportive therapy. The immediate requirements are the energetic treatment of shock and respiratory failure and the relief of pain. A central venous line is used to monitor the need for fluid replacement, and to avoid overloading the circulation. Serial arterial oxygen pressures are recorded because endotracheal intubation and positive pressure ventilation will be required if respiratory failure becomes a major factor. The bladder is catheterised to measure urinary output. Intravenous saline, plasma, plasma expanders or whole blood may be required in large volumes as determined by the clinical response, urinary output and central venous pressure. Oral feeding is withheld until pain, tenderness, fever and leucocytosis have resolved; parenteral alimentation is necessary in all but the milder cases. Gastric intubation and aspiration are used for symptomatic benefit.

Pain is best relieved by intravenous or intramuscular administrations of pethidine (100 mg); morphine should be avoided because of its undesirable effect of causing spasm of the sphincter of Oddi. Ileus is almost inevitable in the acute phase and nasogastric suction is continued until distension is relieved and active peristalsis has returned. When obstruction continues a Gastrografin meal will indicate if the duodenum is obstructed. Haemorrhage from the upper gastrointestinal tract is investigated and treated; bleeding into a cyst or the peritoneal cavity can be confirmed by computed tomography. Selective arteriography and therapeutic embolisation may be necessary to control haemorrhage.

Surgery

This is necessary for a pancreatic abscess and when there is cholecystitis the gallbladder should be drained or removed. Endoscopic sphincterotomy may be of value in acute pancreatitis caused by gallstones in the common bile duct. If the diagnosis of acute pancreatitis is made when laparotomy is undertaken for diagnostic uncertainty, no direct surgical intervention should be attempted unless there are gallstones. Surgical resection of the pancreas may be attempted when there is severe necrosis of the entire pancreas but the mortality rate is high.

Once the attack of acute pancreatitis has subsided it is essential to identify cholelithiasis and obstructive causes of pancreatitis (see information box, p. 476) in order to prevent further attacks.

Pseudocysts

These are treated expectantly for 4–6 weeks because many will resolve spontaneously. Surgery is necessary when the cyst enlarges rapidly or persistently obstructs the duodenum or common bile duct. The cyst is drained into the stomach or intestine. Surgical resection of the damaged pancreas is usually necessary for pancreatic ascites.

Prognosis

This depends upon the severity of the attack. Overall, the mortality is 10–20%. Patients with haemorrhagic pancreatitis have a mortality of over 50% whereas when there is only oedema of the pancreas, the mortality is less than 5%. Of the deaths, 75% occur in the first week. A variety of indices or scoring systems are used in an attempt to grade the severity of an attack.

CHRONIC PANCREATITIS

Chronic pancreatitis is defined as a continuing inflammatory disease of the pancreas characterised by irreversible morphological change and typically causing pain and/or permanent impairment of function.

Aetiology

The majority of cases of chronic pancreatitis in the Western world occur as a result of a persistent high alcohol consumption. It is possible that a small number result from cholelithiasis. It is very rare for acute attacks of pancreatitis to proceed to chronic pancreatitis. Chronic pancreatitis may occasionally be caused by stenosis or disease of the sphincter of Oddi and rarely the condition may be familial. In some parts of the tropics chronic pancreatitis is common and malnutrition may be an aetiological factor. Chronic pancreatitis is common in cystic fibrosis (p. 476).

Pathology

Plugs of protein and calcium carbonate crystals form in the ducts forming the nidus for stones which lead to duct obstruction and dilatation. On microscopy the pancreas shows fibrosis around the ducts and acina which are gradually replaced. By contrast, there is usually preservation of the islets of Langerhans. The end result is an atrophic pancreas with dilated cystic ducts, retention cysts and calcification.

Clinical features

The disease is most common in males between the ages of 35 and 45 years. Nearly all patients present with abdominal pain. Recurrent attacks occur at intervals of several weeks or months often within a few hours to two days of taking alcohol. In contrast to acute pancreatitis the pain may begin gradually and persist for days or weeks. Pain is located in the epigastrium, right or left subcostal areas or around the umbilicus; characteristically it may radiate to the back between T10 and T12 and relief may be obtained by crouching forward or leaning forward over a chair. Weight loss is common

due to malnutrition secondary to pancreatic pain, steatorrhoea and diabetes mellitus. Diarrhoea is common.

Diabetes mellitus develops in about a fifth of patients and steatorrhoea in a third and may occasionally be the presenting feature. Both these complications are more likely when the pancreas is calcified. Jaundice may arise from obstruction to the common bile duct by fibrosis within the pancreas and such obstruction is a possible cause of abdominal pain. Pseudocysts may develop and cirrhosis is common.

On examination there may be diffuse tenderness in the upper abdomen and features of malnutrition and weight loss.

Investigations

A variety of investigations may be used in chronic pancreatitis (Table 7.30 and Fig. 7.20). They may be conveniently classified into radiographic and imaging techniques which demonstrate the structural changes in the gland, and function and metabolic studies which indicate whether the function of the gland is inadequate for normal physiological processes.

Management

Pancreatic extracts (p. 476) are indicated when there is loss of weight, diarrhoea or abdominal discomfort; an average of 10 000–12 000 lipase units per meal is given (usually 5–6 tablets or capsules). The effectiveness of this therapy is assessed by improvement in symptoms and a reduction in faecal fat excretion. In patients who respond poorly, antacids and H_2-receptor antagonists prevent the inactivation of the pancreatic extract by gastric acid. The diet should be normal and nutritious. Fat may be restricted to 25% of total calories except in the case of cystic fibrosis (p. 476). Supplements of fat-soluble vitamins are often required. Oral hypoglycaemic

Table 7.30 Investigations for chronic pancreatitis	
Investigation or test	**Use or indication**
Radiographic	
Plain radiograph of the abdomen	Calcification of pancreas
Ultrasonography and computed tomography	To demonstrate atrophy and calcification, temporary enlargement in acute attacks and stricture of the common bile duct
ERCP	For planning surgery
Function tests	
N-benzoyl-tyrosyl-p-amino benzoic acid test	A normal test excludes pancreatic insufficiency
Secretin/CCK/stimulation test	To confirm pancreatic insufficiency
Glucose tolerance test	To demonstrate diabetes mellitus
5-day stool collection for fat excretion	To demonstrate steatorrhoea as the cause of diarrhoea and as a basis for monitoring treatment
Liver function tests	Raised serum alkaline phosphatase may indicate biliary obstruction

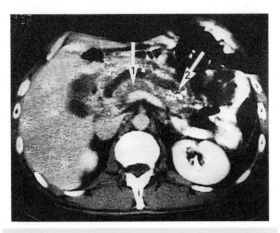

Fig. 7.20 Chronic pancreatitis. Abdominal CT scan showing a large dilated pancreatic duct (arrow 1). and pancreatic calcification (arrow 2).

agents are usually of no value in patients with diabetes mellitus and patients are managed with diet and insulin.

The treatment of pain is difficult. Abstinence from alcohol is absolutely essential for it reduces the frequency and sometimes the severity of pain. Some authorities believe that therapy with pancreatic extracts reduces the frequency and severity of pain and that these should be tried even if they are not required for reasons of malabsorption. The use of analgesics (aspirin, paracetamol) is often indicated especially before meals in order to counteract the postprandial increase in pain. Failing these, opiate analgesics may have to be used and occasionally percutaneous coeliac plexus block may be necessary. Addiction to the analgesic drugs can be a problem.

Surgery should be contemplated for the relief of intractable pain. Drainage of the pancreatic duct into the small bowel or removal of part or most of the pancreas are the most usual procedures. Surgery is also necessary for pseudocysts and for biliary obstruction. The ultimate result is so dependent on the alcoholic's ability to stop consuming alcohol that an operation is not worthwhile in the patient who cannot abstain.

Prognosis

Over a 10-year period, approximately one third of patients will obtain relief from pain without surgical treatment, pain will stabilise in one third and will worsen in one third. There is an increased mortality with only 50% survival at 7–10 years. Patients with chronic pancreatitis have an increased frequency of cancer of the pancreas.

TUMOURS OF THE PANCREAS

CARCINOMA

Incidence

The incidence of carcinoma of the pancreas is increasing in many Western countries and in males in the USA has reached 15 per 100 000. It is more common in males than in females and it occurs most frequently in the seventh decade.

Aetiology

Aetiological factors are smoking, high dietary fat and occupational exposure in chemical and metal industries.

Pathology

Ductal adenocarcinoma is by far the commonest tumour and is located in the head of the pancreas in about 60% of patients, the body or tail in 20% and in a combination of sites in the remainder. Tumours of the papilla of Vater obstruct the common bile duct; they are usually amenable to surgery and have a far better prognosis. Islet cell carcinoma (p.481), cystadenocarcinoma and papillary cystic neoplasms are rare forms of pancreatic cancer but are important because they have a better prognosis than adenocarcinoma.

Clinical features

All cancers of the pancreas are advanced by the time they cause symptoms apart from carcinoma of the ampulla which may bleed into the duodenum, or cause jaundice at a relatively early stage. Epigastric pain is common, but occasionally it may be absent throughout the course of the disease. The pain is variable in type but is characteristically dull and boring and radiates through to the back. It is often intensified by eating and by lying supine, especially at night. Pain may be relieved by crouching forward. Other symptoms include anorexia, nausea, discomfort and sometimes vomiting. Weight loss is common. The symptoms of diabetes mellitus may occasionally be the presenting feature.

Other clinical features depend largely on the site of the growth. In the majority of cases with involvement of the head of the pancreas, jaundice is the presenting feature and may be painless and progressive. Gastrointestinal haemorrhage and diarrhoea due to steatorrhoea may occur. A large firm liver eventually develops. An abdominal mass is present in one-quarter of patients and occasionally a distended gallbladder is palpable or ascites can be detected. Jaundice may not appear when the lesion affects mainly the body and tail of the pancreas.

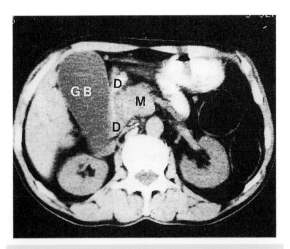

Fig. 7.21 Carcinoma of the head of the pancreas. Abdominal CT scan showing a large mass in the head of the pancreas (M) which is causing a dilated gallbladder (GB) and a displaced duodenal loop (D).

Investigations

The clinical diagnosis is supported by a raised serum alkaline phosphatase, a diabetic glucose tolerance test and a barium meal or endoscopy which may show distortion or displacement of the stomach or duodenum with possible invasion by tumour. Ultrasonography is a good initial screening test for pancreatic disease but computed tomography (Fig. 7.21) is the preferred method for confirming the diagnosis and deciding upon operability. It is impossible to distinguish cancer from chronic pancreatitis in a minority of patients. Fine-needle aspiration biopsy performed percutaneously under guidance with ultrasound, computed tomography or ERCP are helpful in such patients. Duodenoscopy is important in detecting cancer of the ampulla. It is important to emphasise that all these investigations will detect only advanced cancer because there is presently no means of making an earlier diagnosis.

Management

A Whipple operation which is a curative resection is rarely possible because most patients have extensive disease, are elderly and too ill. The procedure consists of removal of the duodenum and head of the pancreas and is only attempted when tumour is confined to the head of the pancreas. Thus in the majority of patients only palliative measures are considered. The aim of surgical palliation is to relieve or prevent obstructive jaundice by anastomosing the gallbladder to the jejunum (cholecystojejunostomy). Gastroenterostomy is usually performed to prevent duodenal obstruction. Alternatively, relief of obstructive jaundice may be achieved by the insertion of a stent along the obstructed bile duct via an endoscope in the duodenum and this is becoming the favoured palliative approach.

Relief of pain is very important. Initially oral methadone 5–10 mg may be used but the use of systems for the continuous delivery of morphine, or blockade of the coeliac ganglion, may be necessary.

Prognosis

Mean survival is 14 months after resection and 5 months after palliative surgery. Of all patients with this cancer, less than 10% survive for one year and five-year survival is rare.

PERIAMPULLARY TUMOURS

These arise from the papilla of Vater, from the terminal parts of the pancreatic or common bile ducts or from the duodenal mucosa adjacent to the papilla. Usually the tumour is an adenocarcinoma.

Most patients present with obstructive jaundice and half also have pain. Less common presentations are with iron deficiency anaemia due to bleeding from the tumour, or acute pancreatitis. The diagnosis is usually made at duodenoscopy. Computed tomography is used to assess the resectability of the tumour. The treatment is Whipple resection or transduodenal excision. The importance of the tumour lies in its relatively good prognosis in comparison with carcinoma of the pancreas. On average 40% of patients survive for five years.

ISLET CELL TUMOURS

These tumours which arise from the islet cells of the pancreas may be benign or malignant. The majority produce an excess of insulin, or gastrin (Zollinger–Ellison syndrome, (p. 431) and rarely glucagon. The remainder are termed 'non-functioning' because they do not release any physiologically active hormone and these usually present with pain and jaundice. They are diagnosed by the same methods as pancreatic cancer. In contrast to pancreatic cancer there is a 40% survival at five years.

FURTHER READING

Ihse I 1990 Pancreatic pain. Br. J. Surg. 77: 121–122

N. D. C. Finlayson, I. A. D. Bouchier

8

Diseases of the liver and biliary system

ANATOMY, PHYSIOLOGY AND INVESTIGATION

The liver is a principal organ for maintaining the body's internal environment, and it is in a key position to fulfil this as it receives virtually all the portal blood flowing from the intestines where most foreign material enters the body. The liver has a major influence on the flow of nutrients to the rest of the body as it controls the release of absorbed material into the systemic circulation and has a central role in carbohydrate, protein and fat metabolism. In addition, it stores substances such as minerals and vitamins which can be released as and when required. The liver metabolises endogenous substances such as bilirubin and exogenous substances such as drugs which are then excreted via the kidney or the biliary system. It is also the biggest reticuloendothelial organ in the body and as such has important immune functions in maintaining body integrity.

ANATOMY

LIVER

The liver is the heaviest internal organ in the body (1200–1500 g), and traditionally it has been divided into right and left lobes by the falciform ligament, the fissure of the ligamentum teres and the fissure of the ligamentum venosum, but advances in hepatic surgery have determined a more useful division into right and left **hemilivers** separated by the course of the middle hepatic vein lying roughly on a line between the inferior vena cava and the gallbladder bed and passing through the porta hepatis (Fig. 8.1). The right and left hemilivers are further subdivided into a total of eight segments in accordance with further subdivisions of the hepatic vasculature. Each segment is in turn made up of histological units known as **lobules**, and each lobule comprises a central vein, radiating sinusoids separated from one another by liver cell (hepatocyte) plates, and peripheral portal tracts. This histological unit has no functional significance. The portal tracts comprise the main connective tissue stroma of the liver. They originate in the porta hepatis, divide progressively as they branch out into the liver parenchyma, and contain branches of the hepatic artery and portal vein, the bile ducts (below) and the main hepatic lymphatics draining to the nodes in the porta hepatis. The branches of the hepatic vein contain little connective tissue, and they unite progressively to form three main veins which enter the inferior vena cava. Lymphatics are associated with the hepatic veins.

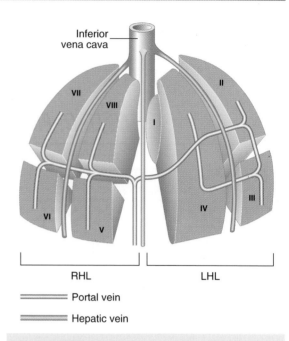

Fig. 8.1 Schematic representation of liver. RHL = right hemiliver; LHL = left hemiliver.

The functional unit of the liver is the **hepatic acinus** which comprises a group of hepatocytes receiving blood from single terminal branches of the hepatic artery and portal vein in a terminal portal tract. The anatomy of the hepatic acinus is almost the reverse of the hepatic lobule above, as the blood passing through the sinusoids of the acinus drains to branches of the hepatic veins located on its periphery. All hepatocytes appear capable of performing the many metabolic functions of liver cells, but under physiological conditions the metabolic activities of individual hepatocytes vary in relation to their location in the acinus. This may be determined by the microenvironment created for the hepatocyte by the composition of the blood in the adjacent sinusoids.

BILIARY SYSTEM

The biliary tract begins in the biliary canaliculi, which are integral parts of the hepatocytes, and the intrahepatic bile ducts derived from them join progressively to form the right and left hepatic ducts. These ducts join as they emerge from the liver to form the common hepatic duct which then forms the common bile duct by joining the cystic duct. The common bile duct is approximately 5 cm long and has a thin-walled wide-lumened proximal part and a thick-walled narrow-lumened distal part surrounded by the choledochal sphincter. The distal common bile duct usually joins the pancreatic duct before it enters the duodenum. The gallbladder is a pear-shaped sac lying under the right hemiliver with its fundus anteriorly behind the tip of the ninth costal cartilage. Its body and neck pass posteromedially towards the porta hepatis and the cystic duct then joins it to the common hepatic duct. The cystic duct mucosa has prominent crescentic folds (valves of Heister) giving it a beaded appearance on cholangiograms.

PHYSIOLOGY

The liver performs a wide variety of functions, the more important of which are listed in the information box. These functions are subserved by a unique blood supply including arterial and venous blood which flows to a system of highly permeable capillaries (sinusoids). The liver also has important immunological functions. The biliary tract conveys bile to the duodenum.

Carbohydrate metabolism
The main function of the liver in carbohydrate metabolism is the maintenance of the blood glucose concentration. Hepatocytes are rich in membrane receptors for insulin, and as a result the liver takes up a half or more of glucose absorbed during feeding, thereby preventing marked hyperglycaemia. The glucose taken up is stored as glycogen or metabolised to glycerol and fatty acids. Fructose and galactose can also be used for glycogen synthesis. Glucose derived from the breakdown of glycogen or from gluconeogenesis is released into the blood during fasting. Glycogen stores (70–80 g) suffice for some 24 hours of fasting, but thereafter gluconeogenesis, particularly from amino acids, becomes the main source of glucose.

Protein metabolism
Dietary proteins enter the portal vein as amino acids and most of the straight chain amino acids are taken up by the liver. The liver utilises amino acids for endogenous hepatic protein and plasma protein synthesis, and amino acid breakdown leads to the production of urea. A substantial proportion of the amino acids is released into the blood for the use of other tissues. During fasting, amino acids, including those reaching the liver from extrahepatic tissues, are used more for gluconeogenesis while endogenous protein synthesis, urea production and amino-acid release to the blood are suppressed. All the plasma albumin and most of its globulins, other than the gammaglobulins, are produced in the liver (see information box).

IMPORTANT LIVER FUNCTIONS

- **Nutrient metabolism**
  Carbohydrate
  Protein
  Fat
- **Protein synthesis**
  Albumin
  Coagulation factors and inhibitors (except von Willebrand factor)
  Complement factors
  Transferrin
  Haptoglobin
  Caeruloplasmin
  Protease inhibitors (α_1-antitrypsin)
  α-Fetoprotein
- **Metabolism and excretion**
  Exogenous material (drugs, alcohol, copper)
  Endogenous material (bilirubin, hormones)
- **Storage**
  Vitamins (vit. A, vit. B_{12}, folate)
  Minerals (iron)

Bilirubin
Unconjugated bilirubin is produced from the catabolism of haem after removal of its iron component. Some 425–510 μmol (250–300 mg) is produced daily, and most is derived from haemoglobin breakdown by Kupffer cells in the liver and other macrophages in the spleen and bone marrow. The rest is formed from catabolism of other haem-containing proteins, particularly myoglobin, cytochrome enzymes and free haem in the liver, and ineffective erythropoiesis in the marrow. Bilirubin normally present in the blood is almost all unconjugated and, as it is not water-soluble, it is bound to albumin and does not pass into the urine. It is taken up by hepatocytes, conjugated with glucuronic acid by the enzymes of the smooth endoplasmic reticulum (p. 517) to form bilirubin mono- and diglucuronide which renders it water-soluble, and excreted into the bile (Fig. 8.2). The uptake and excretion of bilirubin by hepatocytes into the bile is probably carrier-mediated.

Conjugated bilirubin is not absorbed in the small intestine. Bacteria in the terminal ileum and colon reduce it to a group of colourless chromogens (stercobilinogen) most of which are excreted in the stool (100–200 mg/d). Some are absorbed from the gut and pass to the liver where most are re-excreted in the bile; a small amount (4 mg/d) passes through the liver and is excreted in the urine where it is known as urobilinogen. Urobilinogen and its oxidation product urobilin in the urine are identical, respectively, with stercobilinogen and its oxidation product, stercobilin, in the faeces.

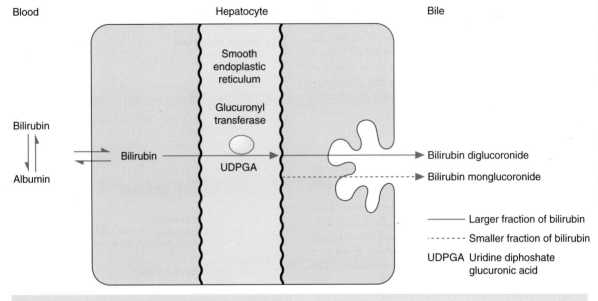

Fig. 8.2   The transport of bilirubin from the blood to the bile.

Bile acids.

Cholic and chenodeoxycholic acids, the **primary bile acids**, are produced in the liver from cholesterol and are conjugated with glycine or taurine. They are secreted into the bile, where they generate bile flow (p. 488), and they are carried in the bile to the duodenum. Most conjugated bile acids are conserved in the jejunal and ileal lumen and are actively reabsorbed in the terminal ileum, but glycine-conjugated chenodeoxycholate is also absorbed from the jejunum. The absorbed bile acids pass to the liver and are almost completely re-excreted in the bile. Small amounts reach the colon where bacterial deconjugation and dehydroxylation result in the pro- duction of **secondary bile acids**, deoxycholic acid from cholic acid, and lithocholic acid from chenodeoxycholic acid. Most of the secondary bile acids are excreted in the faeces, but small amounts are absorbed, reach the liver where they are conjugated with glycine or taurine, and are excreted in the bile (Fig. 8.3). This **entero- hepatic circulation** allows large amounts of bile acid to be delivered to the intestine daily from a relatively small total bile acid pool owing to almost complete reab- sorption and to frequent recycling of bile acids passing through the bowel. At any time about 85% of the bile acid pool is either in the gallbladder (fasting) or in the intestinal lumen (feeding). Synthesis of new bile acid compensates only for that lost in the faeces. The hepatic capacity for bile acid synthesis is limited, and large losses from the bowel cannot be replaced. Little bile acid reaches the systemic circulation normally, but the amount increases in liver disease.

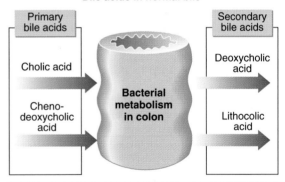

Fig. 8.3   Bile acids in normal bile.

Bile acids, as they enter bile, combine with cholesterol and phospholipids to form mixed micelles (Fig. 8.4). In the small intestine, provided the bile acid concentration remains sufficient to maintain the micellar state, this greatly increases the efficiency of fat absorption. Insuf- ficiency of bile acids results in poor absorption of dietary fat and fat-soluble vitamins, notably vitamins A, D and K. Such deficiency may result from impaired synthesis in chronic liver disease, biliary obstruction, small intestinal overgrowth of bacteria capable of deconjugating and dehydroxylating bile acids, and loss of bile acids into the colon in disease of the terminal ileum or after its

A

Longitudinal section

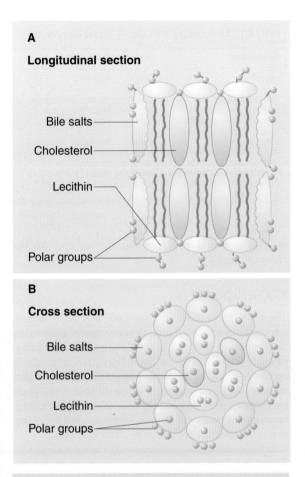

Bile salts

Cholesterol

Lecithin

Polar groups

B

Cross section

Bile salts

Cholesterol

Lecithin

Polar groups

Fig. 8.4 The structure of mixed micelles in bile.

resection. In this last instance, the bile acids interfere with colonic water and electrolyte metabolism causing choleretic diarrhoea, while their absence from the small intestine can result in steatorrhoea (p. 451).

Vitamins and minerals

Vitamins A, D and B_{12} are stored in large amounts; vitamin K and folate are stored in smaller amounts which soon disappear if dietary intake is deficient. The liver can convert tryptophan to nicotinic acid (p. 553) and can activate vitamins by phosphorylation of thiamin (p. 565), by 25-hydroxylation of vitamin D (p. 572) and by the production of tetrahydrofolate. Vitamin K is required by hepatocytes for converting the fully synthesised procoagulants of factors II (prothrombin), VII, IX and X into active coagulation factors. The liver stores iron as ferritin and haemosiderin and excretes excess copper into the bile (p. 529).

Hormones

The liver is an important site of hormone action and of hormone degradation. Some hormones such as insulin, glucagon, growth hormone, glucocorticoids, oestrogens and parathormone are catabolised mainly in the liver.

Drug and alcohol metabolism

The hepatic metabolism of drugs (p. 517) and alcohol (p. 526) is considered elsewhere.

Blood supply and lymphatic drainage

The hepatic artery and the portal vein supply about 1.5 litres of blood/minute to the liver, and both vessels are distributed throughout the liver in the portal tracts. The hepatic artery supplies about 25% of the total liver blood flow and about 50% of the total oxygen supply. The portal venous pressure is normally 3–5 mmHg, although portal blood flow varies considerably from a maximum postprandially to a minimum during fasting. Auto-regulation of blood flow by the hepatic artery ensures that the total liver blood flow remains constant. The hepatic arterial and portal venous blood flows into the hepatic sinusoids, which are devoid of basement membranes and lined by fenestrated endothelial cells making them highly permeable capillaries. All the plasma constituents pass through the sinusoidal walls into the space of Disse, which is the interstitial space of the liver. The sinusoids contain the phagocytic Kupffer cells, and the space of Disse contains unique stellate (Ito) cells responsible for vitamin A storage and for collagen synthesis. Lymph flow is considerable, as about half the lymph flowing through the thoracic duct comes from the liver.

Mononuclear phagocyte (reticuloendothelial) function

The functions of the liver include the activities of about 15% of its cells which are not hepatocytes. Foremost among these are the Kupffer cells, derived from blood monocytes, which have important immunological functions. They constitute the largest single mass of mononuclear phagocytes in the body and account for about 80% of the phagocytic capacity of this system. They phagocytose damaged and ageing red blood cells, bacteria, viruses, antigen-antibody complexes and endotoxin and produce numerous substances involved in inflammatory and immune reactions (p. 38). They also take up antigenic material, but unlike macrophages elsewhere in the body they do not produce processed antigen and thus prevent antigen from eliciting immunological responses. These cells therefore seem capable of preventing undesirable immunological responses, particularly for antigens which gain repeated access to the body from the gut. Failure of this function may contribute to hyperglobulinaemia in chronic liver disease (p. 490).

Age and the liver

The liver begins to function early in fetal life, but many functions require several weeks or months of postnatal development before their full functional capacities are reached. Examples of limited functional capacity at birth include reduced ability to transport bilirubin across the liver cell and to conjugate bilirubin, limited capacity to synthesise and secrete bile acids into bile, which may in turn limit bile flow (below), and limited ability to synthesise coagulation factors.

Changes in the liver occur only slowly in adult life, but significant changes have occurred in those over 70 years. The liver gradually gets smaller due mainly to a reduction in the number of hepatocytes, and liver blood flow falls to about half its normal level in the elderly due in part to a fall in cardiac output. The potential for toxic reactions to drugs metabolised by the liver may therefore be increased. The values for liver function tests remain within normal adult ranges. The liver in the elderly is probably no more susceptible to disease than in younger people, but its reserve is less and this may be an important cause of the increased mortality of acute liver diseases in older people.

Bile

The liver secretes 1–2 litres of bile daily, and the hepatocytes provide the driving force for bile flow by creating osmotic gradients of bile acids which form micelles in bile (bile acid dependent bile flow) and of sodium (bile acid independent bile flow). Common bile duct pressure is maintained by rhythmic contraction and relaxation of the choledochal sphincter and this pressure exceeds gallbladder pressure in the fasting state so that bile normally flows into the gallbladder where it is concentrated some ten-fold by resorption of water and electrolytes. Cholecystokinin released from the duodenal mucosa during feeding causes gallbladder contraction and reduces choledochal sphincter pressure and consequently bile flows into the duodenum. Vagal activity maintains gallbladder tone, but sympathetic activity has little or no effect on the gallbladder.

THE INVESTIGATION OF HEPATOBILIARY DISEASE

Investigations in liver disease are used to detect hepatic abnormality, to measure its severity, to define its structural effect on the liver, to look for specific causes of liver disease, and to investigate such consequences of liver

Table 8.1 Liver function tests used to assess liver disease

Measurement	Fluid	Assessment
Bilirubin	Plasma Urine	Transport
Aminotransferases	Plasma	Hepatocellular damage
Alkaline phosphatase	Plasma	Biliary obstruction
Gamma-glutamyl transferase	Plasma	Enzyme induction
Proteins (total and albumin)	Plasma	Synthesis
Coagulation tests	Plasma	Synthesis

Note: Bilirubin detected in the urine identifies conjugated hyperbilirubinaemia and indicates hepatobiliary disease. Alanine aminotransferase is more specific for liver damage than aspartate aminotransferase.

disease as portal hypertension, ascites and hepatic encephalopathy.

BIOCHEMICAL TESTS

The terms 'liver function tests' and 'liver tests' refer to a group of biochemical investigations useful in revealing or confirming that the liver is diseased, in indicating whether hepatic cells or the biliary tree is primarily involved, in giving an indication of the extent of liver damage, and in assessing progress (Table 8.1). There are no patterns of abnormality indicative of specific diagnoses and normality of all the commonly used liver function tests does not prove that the liver is normal.

Bilirubin

Hyperbilirubinaemia may be due to increased concentrations of unconjugated or conjugated bilirubin. Estimates of unconjugated and conjugated bilirubin in the blood are seldom necessary and routine clinical chemical methods are inaccurate when the total plasma bilirubin is less than 70 μmol/l (4 mg/dl).

Unconjugated hyperbilirubinaemia without any abnormality of other liver function tests may result from increased bilirubin production, as in haemolysis or ineffective erythropoiesis (p. 777), or from inability to transport bilirubin across the liver, as in Gilbert's syndrome (p. 498). Except in the newborn, the hyperbilirubinaemia rarely exceeds 100 μmol/l (6 mg/dl), and there is no bilirubin in the urine as the normal plasma albumin can bind about 400 μmol/l of unconjugated bilirubin. Conjugated bilirubin is also found in the blood in unconjugated hyperbilirubinaemia, but it does not exceed 20% of the total plasma bilirubin and is insufficient to cause bilirubinuria. Conjugated hyperbilirubinaemia without any abnormality of other liver function tests, as in the Dubin-Johnson syndrome (p. 499), is accompanied by bilirubinuria but is rare.

Hyperbilirubinaemia in hepatobiliary disease is predominantly conjugated, bilirubinuria is present, and other tests of liver function are almost always abnormal. The plasma bilirubin in parenchymal liver disease varies widely depending on the severity of the disease and its activity. Very high concentrations occur most frequently in biliary tract obstruction, with sustained high levels in malignant disease and a tendency to fluctuating levels where obstruction is caused by gallstones. The plasma bilirubin reflects the depth of jaundice and repeated estimations may be useful in following the progress of disease.

Urine tests

Simple, sensitive and inexpensive dip-stick tests for bilirubin and urobilinogen in the urine are available. Bilirubin is not found in the urine of normal persons as virtually all the plasma bilirubin is unconjugated and bound to albumin. Thus, absence of bilirubinuria in a jaundiced patient points to unconjugated hyperbilirubinaemia (above), while bilirubinuria implies a conjugated hyperbilirubinaemia and points to hepatobiliary disease. Increased amounts of urobilinogen are found in the urine in haemolytic diseases and with any cause of hepatic dysfunction, and no urobilinogen is found in the urine in complete biliary obstruction. In practice urine urobilinogen tests are of no value in liver disease.

Enzymes

Liver cells contain many enzymes which may be released into the blood during pathological processes. Measurement of their activity in the blood may give evidence of hepatobiliary disease. In practice, maximal information is obtained by measuring the activity of relatively few enzymes. None of the enzymes is specific to the liver and alternative origins should be considered, particularly where abnormalities have been found incidentally in patients with no clinical evidence of liver disease.

Aminotransferases

Alanine aminotransferase (ALT), a cytoplasmic enzyme, and aspartate aminotransferase (AST), present both in cytoplasm and mitochondria, are the two important aminotransferases. Normal plasma contains low activities of both enzymes, the source of which is unknown. Neither enzyme is specific to the liver, but ALT occurs in much higher concentration in the liver than elsewhere and consequently increased serum ALT activity reflects hepatic damage more specifically. ALT and AST are liberated into the blood whenever liver cells are damaged and increased plasma enzyme activity is a sensitive index of hepatic damage. Plasma ALT and AST activity test the integrity of liver cells. The highest activities are caused by any acute liver damage, but they

have no prognostic significance in acute or chronic liver disease.

In viral hepatitis there is greatly increased activity even in the prodromal phase, and maximal levels of 10 to 100 times the normal value are usually reached early in the jaundiced phase, after which activity falls rapidly. Equally high activity occurs in acute hepatic damage due to drugs, in acute circulatory failure, and in exacerbations of chronic active hepatitis. Most patients (80%) with infectious mononucleosis or cytomegaloviral infection have an acute hepatitis with serum aminotransferase activity raised 2 to 10 times, but few develop jaundice. Hepatic damage due to paracetamol produces particularly high activities of 100 to 500 times the normal value. Plasma aminotransferase activity in alcoholic hepatitis is usually increased less than fivefold. Patients with cirrhosis generally show only modest elevations of serum aminotransferase. In obstructive jaundice, activity may rise up to fivefold, but greater increases are unusual unless cholangitis is present.

Alkaline phosphatase

This enzyme is situated principally in the canalicular and sinusoidal membranes of liver cells. Blood normally contains alkaline phosphatase derived mainly from bone and liver, and in pregnancy additional activity of placental origin is found. About a fifth of people have plasma alkaline phosphatase of intestinal origin and its activity may increase after meals. When hepatocytes are damaged little alkaline phosphatase is liberated into the blood, most probably coming from cells which are killed. Consequently, plasma alkaline phosphatase activity does not usually rise more than two-fold in acute or chronic hepatocellular disease. In biliary tract obstruction at any level new alkaline phosphatase is synthesised in the hepatocyte membrane, much of which escapes into the blood. A greatly increased plasma alkaline phosphatase activity is, therefore, the main biochemical indicator of biliary obstruction though it provides no information about the site of that obstruction. The alkaline phosphatase activity has no prognostic significance in liver disease.

Sometimes a raised plasma alkaline phosphatase activity is found incidentally and is the sole abnormality. Hepatobiliary disease may be present, but it is important to ensure that the alkaline phosphatase does not have an extrahepatic origin before investigating the liver further. This may be done by finding increased plasma activities of enzymes more specific for the liver, such as γ-glutamyl transferase, or by electrophoretic separation of the isoenzymes of alkaline phosphatase. Increased osteoblastic activity from bone is the main alternative origin of a raised plasma alkaline phosphatase and occurs normally in adolescents when it may increase about two- to threefold. Other causes include Paget's disease, rickets,

Table 8.2 Relation of plasma aminotransferase and alkaline phosphatase activity in patients with jaundice due to acute viral hepatitis and biliary obstruction

Enzyme combination		Diagnostic likelihood	
Aminotransferase	Alkaline phosphatase	Viral hepatitis	Biliary obstruction
$> \times 6$	$< \times 2.5$	90%	10%
$< \times 6$	$> \times 2.5$	10%	80%
Other combinations		No clear separation	

Table 8.3 Drugs causing hepatic microsomal enzyme induction and increased plasma glutamyl transferase activity

Barbiturates	Glutethimide
Carbamazepine	Griseofulvin
Diphenylhydantoin	Meprobamate
Ethanol	Primidone
Glucocorticoids	Rifampicin

hyperparathyroidism, and metastatic tumour in bone. Myelomatosis is not associated with much bone repair and the plasma alkaline phosphatase is not usually raised. During the third trimester of pregnancy, alkaline phosphatase of placental origin may increase the serum activity two- to three-fold. Intestinal alkaline phosphatase is increased in about a quarter of patients with cirrhosis and it is occasionally the predominant form.

Enzyme combinations

Serum aminotransferase and alkaline phosphatase activities should be considered relative to one another. Large increases of aminotransferase activity and small increases of alkaline phosphatase activity favour hepatocellular damage; small increases of aminotransferase activity and large increases of alkaline phosphatase activity favour biliary obstruction (Table 8.2). It is important that these patterns do not separate the two diagnostic groups absolutely and other combinations give much poorer separation.

Gamma-glutamyl transferase (γ-GT)

This is a microsomal enzyme which is distributed widely in body tissues. Increased plasma γ-GT activity is a sensitive index of liver abnormality. The highest activities occur in biliary obstruction but marked increases also occur in acute parenchymal damage from any cause. Gamma-GT measurements give little information in patients with liver disease beyond that provided by transferase and alkaline phosphatase measurements. Plasma γ-GT activity is also increased by microsomal enzyme-inducing agents such as alcohol and various drugs (Table 8.3). Increased γ-GT activity is used to detect and follow alcohol abuse in patients with little or no other abnormality of liver function provided they are not taking enzyme-inducing drugs. Increased γ-GT activity due to alcohol implies prolonged intake of more than about 60 g alcohol daily; unfortunately, normal γ-GT activity does not exclude prolonged intake above that level.

Plasma proteins

Albumin

This is synthesised solely in the liver. In chronic liver disease, especially cirrhosis, the plasma albumin concentration is frequently low. Impaired albumin synthesis can be the cause but other factors such as malnutrition, fever and the dilutional effect of fluid retention with ascites can be important. Low plasma albumin concentrations usually detect patients with more severe liver damage, and a falling concentration is a bad prognostic sign especially when there is no ascites. Albumin has a long half-life in the blood (20–26 days) and changes in concentration occur slowly. Thus, even in severe acute hepatitis, the plasma albumin remains normal unless the illness continues for many weeks.

Globulins

It is characteristic of chronic liver disease that hyperglobulinaemia occurs in addition to hypoalbuminaemia, and once established it tends to persist. It may also be found irrespective of changes in the plasma albumin concentration in prolonged viral hepatitis or chronic active hepatitis. The causes of hyperglobulinaemia are not fully understood; increases in gammaglobulins are prominent and probably reflect an increased activity of the immune system, to which many factors may contribute (p. 487). In those with hypoalbuminaemia it may represent a response to a reduced colloid osmotic pressure in the plasma. Individual plasma immunoglobulins are variably increased, IgG mainly in autoimmune hepatitis and cryptogenic cirrhosis, IgA mainly in alcoholic liver disease, and IgM in primary biliary cirrhosis. Variations, however, are so frequent that Ig measurements are of no diagnostic value in liver disease.

Plasma protein electrophoresis

The commonest changes in the electrophoretic pattern of the plasma proteins in cirrhosis are a decreased albumin and an increased gammaglobulin peak but this is not of diagnostic value.

Coagulation factors

The liver synthesises all the coagulation factors, and requires vitamin K to activate factors II, VII, IX and X.

Reduced plasma concentrations of coagulation factors occur in liver damage, which is most readily recognised by prolongation of the prothrombin time. The prothrombin time depends on factors I, II, V, VII and X, and it prolongs when the plasma concentration of any of these factors falls below 30% of normal. This occurs in severe liver damage and in prolonged biliary obstruction which reduces vitamin K absorption. The prothrombin time can therefore be used as a liver function test provided that vitamin K is given first (above). Furthermore, as the normal half-lives of these factors in the blood are short (5–72 hours), prothrombin time changes occur relatively quickly when liver damage occurs, allowing the test to be used in acute and chronic liver disease. The prothrombin time is a most valuable prognostic guide in any acute or fulminant hepatitis. An increased prothrombin time indicates severe liver damage, and an increasing value indicates a progressively worse prognosis.

OTHER BIOCHEMICAL INDICES

Biochemical tests are of value in identifying the nature of hepatic disease or its cause.

Ferritin

The serum ferritin concentration is important in the diagnosis of haemochromatosis as it reflects the total body iron. The serum ferritin concentration is almost always above 1000 μg/l in symptomatic haemochromatosis; a normal serum ferritin excludes haemochromatosis as the cause of established chronic liver disease and serum ferritin measurements are used to assess the results of venesection therapy. The serum ferritin, however, cannot establish a diagnosis of haemochromatosis on its own because alcoholic liver disease is associated with increased concentrations which may exceed 1000 μg/l.

Iron binding capacity saturation

The iron saturation of the plasma iron binding capacity exceeds 60% in haemochromatosis. The serum ferritin is now generally preferred in diagnosing haemochromatosis, but iron binding capacity saturation remains useful in detecting iron overload in the relatives of patients.

Caeruloplasmin

This is a copper-containing globulin produced by the liver. The serum caeruloplasmin concentration in Wilson's disease is low and may be undetectable. Concentrations in the low normal range occur rarely, particularly during active disease, in the terminal stages, or during pregnancy or oestrogen (oral contraceptives)

therapy. Low serum concentrations also occur in fulminant hepatic failure, in any advanced and severe chronic liver disease, in protein-losing enteropathy, and malabsorption. Increased serum concentrations occur in pregnancy, when oestrogens are taken, in a wide variety of inflammatory and neoplastic diseases including acute and chronic hepatitis, and in any form of biliary obstruction.

Copper

Concentrations of copper in the liver are very high in Wilson's disease and in any condition associated with chronic cholestasis such as primary biliary cirrhosis. This excess of copper cannot be shown reliably histologically, especially in Wilson's disease, and has to be measured chemically. The serum copper concentration in Wilson's disease is low (unless fulminant hepatic failure occurs, when it is very high) and the urinary copper excretion is high. Wilson's disease can also be diagnosed by showing failure of incorporation of radioactive copper (^{64}Cu) into caeruloplasmin, but this is rarely required and is difficult to do because ^{64}Cu has a very short half-life.

Alpha$_1$-antitrypsin

This is an α_1-globulin produced by the liver which comprises 90% of the α_1-globulin peak seen on serum electrophoresis. It is a component of the protease inhibitor (Pi) system which inhibits the activity of protease enzymes. Its production is inherited through a system of co-dominant alleles each determining the synthesis of a form of α_1-antitrypsin named in accordance with its electrophoretic behaviour. The main forms of α_1-antitrypsin are PiM (medium), PiS (slow) and PiZ (very slow). PiMM is the normal phenotype giving normal serum α_1-antitrypsin concentrations, while the phenotype PiZZ gives low serum α_1-antitrypsin concentrations and is associated with liver disease (p. 530) and pulmonary disease (p. 334).

Alpha-fetoprotein

This is made mainly by the fetal liver, production falling to low levels after birth. The reappearance of substantial serum concentrations in adult life and increasing concentrations in chronic liver disease suggest strongly that a hepatocellular carcinoma has developed. Some increase in serum α-fetoprotein occurs in about 90% of patients with hepatocellular carcinoma, but moderate increases can occur in several other conditions (Table 8.4).

Bromsulphthalein (BSP) clearance

Estimation of BSP clearance from the blood is now only used in the diagnosis of the rare Dubin–Johnson syndrome (p. 499).

Table 8.4 Diseases associated with increased serum α-fetoprotein concentration

Adults	Children
Neoplastic	**Neoplastic**
Hepatocellular carcinoma[1]	Hepatoblastoma[1]
Other carcinomas (very rare)	Gonadal teratoblastoma[1]
Stomach, pancreas, gallbladder,	
bile duct, lungs	**Non-neoplastic**
	Biliary atresia
Non-neoplastic	Neonatal hepatitis
Viral hepatitis	Indian childhood cirrhosis
Chronic hepatitis (esp. CAH)	Tyrosinosis
Cirrhosis	Ataxia telangiectasia
Pregnancy	
Neural tube defects[2], fetal distress	

[1] α-Fetoprotein frequently and greatly increased.
[2] α-Fetoprotein also increased in amniotic fluid.

Table 8.5 Interpretation of main investigations used in the serological diagnosis of hepatitis B virus infection

Interpretation	HBsAg	Anti-HBc		Anti-HBs
		IgM	IgG	
Incubation period	+	+	−	−
Acute hepatitis				
Early	+	+	−	−
Established	+	+	+	−
Established (occasional)	−	+	+	−
Convalescence* (3–6 months)	±		+	±
(6–9 months)	−		+	+
Post-infection				
>1 year	−	−	+	+
Uncertain	−	−	+	−
Chronic infection				
Usual	+		+	−
Occasional	−	−	+	−
Immunisation without infection	−	−	−	+

Note: + = positive; − = negative; ± = present at low titre or absent.
HBsAg: surface antigen; Anti-HBc: antibody to core antigen;
Anti-HBs: antibody to surface antigen.
* Very variable.

SEROLOGICAL TESTS

Hepatitis A virus antigens and antibodies

Only one antigen has been found associated with the hepatitis A virus (HAV), and individuals infected with the HAV make an antibody to this antigen (anti-HAV). Anti-HAV is important in diagnosis as the HAV is only present in the blood transiently during the incubation period, excretion in the stools occurs for only 7–14 days after the onset of the clinical illness and the virus cannot be grown readily. Anti-HAV of IgM type, indicating a primary immune response, is already present in the blood at the onset of the clinical illness and is diagnostic of an acute HAV infection. Titres of this antibody fall to low levels within about 3 months of recovery. Anti-HAV of IgG type is of no diagnostic value as HAV infection is common and this antibody persists for years after infection, but it can be used to measure the prevalence of HAV infection and its presence indicates immunity to HAV.

Hepatitis B virus antigens and antibodies

The hepatitis B virus (HBV) contains several antigens to which infected persons can make immune responses (Fig. 8.5); these antigens and their antibodies are important in identifying HBV infection (Table 8.5).

(1) Acute infection

The hepatitis B surface antigen (HBsAg) is a reliable marker of HBV infection, and a negative test for the HBsAg makes HBV infection very unlikely but not impossible (Fig. 8.5). It appears in the blood late in the incubation period and before the prodromal phase of acute type B hepatitis; it may be present for only a few days, disappearing even before jaundice has developed, but it usually lasts for 3–4 weeks and may persist for up to 5 months. It should therefore be sought as soon as possible in acute hepatitis. Antibody to HBsAg (anti-HBs) usually appears after about 3–6 months and persists for many years or perhaps permanently. Anti-HBs implies either that infection has occurred at some time (in which case anti-HBc (below) is usually also present) or that the individual has been vaccinated (in which case anti-HBc is not present).

The hepatitis B core antigen (HBcAg) is not found in the blood, but antibody to it (anti-HBc) appears early in the illness and rapidly reaches a high titre which then subsides gradually and persists. Anti-HBc is initially of IgM type and IgG antibody appears later. Anti-HBc (IgM) can sometimes reveal an acute HBV infection when the HBsAg has disappeared and before anti-HBs has developed (Fig. 8.5). The hepatitis B e antigen (HBeAg) appears only transiently at the outset of the illness and is followed by the production of antibody (anti-HBe). The HBeAg reflects active replication of the virus in the liver.

(2) Chronic infection

Chronic HBV infection (p. 523) is marked by the presence of the HBsAg and anti-HBc (IgG) in the blood. Rarely, anti-HBc (IgG) alone is the sole evidence of chronic infection. Usually, the HBeAg or anti-HBe is also present; the HBeAg indicates continued active replication of the virus in the liver while anti-HBe implies that replication is occurring at a much lower level or that viral DNA has become integrated into host hepatocyte DNA. Polymerase chain reactions (PCR) can show

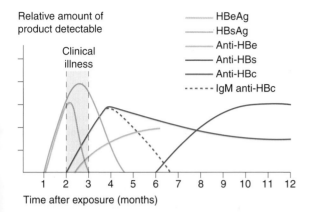

Relative amount of product detectable

—— HBeAg
—— HBsAg
—— Anti-HBe
—— Anti-HBs
—— Anti-HBc
----- IgM anti-HBc

Clinical illness

Time after exposure (months)

Fig. 8.5   Serological responses to hepatitis B virus infection. (HBsAG = hepatitis B surface antigen; anti-HBs = antibody to HBsAg; HBeAg = hepatitis B e antigen; anti-HBe = antibody to HBeAg; anti-HBc = antibody to hepatitis B core antigen.)

HBV-DNA in the blood, implying that viral replication is occurring. This is rarely needed for diagnosis but can be useful in selecting for and measuring response to therapy.

Hepatitis C virus antibodies

The hepatitis C virus (HCV) contains several antigens giving rise to antibodies in infected individuals and these are used in diagnosis. Initially, diagnosis depended on identifying antibody to a single viral antigen (C100), but this test gave false-positive reactions, especially in conditions such as autoimmune hepatitis associated with hyperglobulinaemia, and false-negative reactions. Current laboratory diagnosis depends on identifying antibodies to several viral antigens, in initial screening and subsequent confirmatory tests. These tests generally identify chronic HCV infections as the diagnostic antibodies appear irregularly in the blood during the first three months of illness. Polymerase chain reactions (PCR) can show HCV-RNA in the blood, but they are not used routinely for diagnosis. They can be used where antibody tests give equivocal results and in selecting for and measuring response to therapy.

Hepatitis D antigen and antibody

The hepatitis D virus (HDV) contains a single antigen to which infected individuals make an antibody (anti-HDV). Delta antigen appears in the blood only transiently, and in practice diagnosis depends on detecting anti-HDV. Simultaneous infection with the hepatitis B virus and the HDV followed by full recovery is associated with the appearance of low titres of anti-HDV of IgM type within a few days of the onset of the illness. This antibody generally disappears within about 2 months

but persists in a few patients. Superinfection of patients with chronic hepatitis B virus infection leads to the production of high titres of anti-HDV, initially IgM and later IgG. Such patients may then develop chronic infection with both viruses, in which case anti-HDV titres plateau at high levels.

Hepatitis E virus antibody

Individuals infected with the hepatitis E virus (HEV) produce anti-HEV which can be used in diagnosis. Assays for the serological identification of HEV infection should become available generally in the near future.

Other viruses

Cytomegalovirus and the Epstein–Barr virus (infectious mononucleosis) are occasional causes of acute hepatitis, and infection can be detected by serological tests.

Autoantibodies

Three autoantibodies in the blood are important in liver disease: antinuclear antibody, antismooth muscle antibody and antimitochondrial antibody. These autoantibodies are all heterogenous and can be found in apparently healthy people, particularly in women and in older people. Antinuclear antibodies occur in about 5% of healthy people and antismooth muscle antibody in 1.5%, but antimitochondrial antibody is rare, being found in about 0.01%. Autoantibody titres in such healthy people are usually low. Antinuclear and antimitochondrial antibodies also occur in connective tissue diseases and in autoimmune diseases, including various thyroid disorders and pernicious anaemia, while antismooth muscle antibody has been reported in infectious mononucleosis and in a variety of malignant diseases.

In liver disease, antismooth muscle antibody and to a lesser extent antinuclear antibody may occur transiently and at low titre in acute viral hepatitis. The autoantibodies are, however, more important in chronic liver disease where they are present for long periods and at relatively high titres (Table 8.6). They are found par-

Table 8.6   Approximate occurrence of antinuclear (ANA), antismooth muscle (SMA) and antimitochondrial (AMA) antibodies in chronic liver diseases not associated with chronic hepatitis virus infection

	Autoantibodies		
Disease	**ANA (%)**	**SMA (%)**	**AMA (%)**
Autoimmune hepatitis	80	70	15
Primary biliary cirrhosis	25	35	95
Cryptogenic cirrhosis	40	30	15

Note: Patients with AMA frequently have cholestatic liver function tests and may have primary biliary cirrhosis (see text).

ticularly in autoimmune hepatitis, cryptogenic cirrhosis and primary biliary cirrhosis, and until recently they were not thought to have any diagnostic specificity. However, the antimitochondrial antibody detected in most clinical laboratories is now known to be very strongly associated with primary biliary cirrhosis, and patients with connective tissue or autoimmune diseases found to have this antibody usually prove to have primary biliary cirrhosis as well. Antimitochondrial antibody found in a patient with cholestasis is of particular value in indicating the presence of primary biliary cirrhosis. Antimitochondrial antibody occurs in primary biliary cirrhosis in 95% or more of patients and in less than 1% of those with large bile duct obstruction. A rare form of chronic active hepatitis is associated with liver-kidney microsomal (LKM) antibodies, and in this condition other autoantibodies are not usually found.

None of these autoantibodies damages liver tissue, and they are therefore unlikely to have aetiological importance.

IMAGING

Imaging determines the site and general nature of structural lesions in the liver and biliary tree. Ultrasound has emerged as the most generally useful method. It can identify and localise disease but often cannot make specific diagnoses, which require further investigations as outlined in Figure 8.6.

Ultrasonography

This requires a skilled operator but is safe and comfortable for the patient and can be repeated. It detects gall-stones down to 5 mm diameter with great accuracy, and reveals gallbladder tumours and thickening due to cholecystitis (Fig. 8.7). It is the most important initial investigation in obstructive jaundice as dilation of the bile ducts implies mechanical obstruction in a large duct, and it may be possible to determine the site of the obstruction and sometimes its causes (Fig. 8.8). Normal bile ducts in a patient with obvious jaundice make a mechanical cause unlikely. Ultrasound can also be used to identify focal liver diseases including tumours, abscesses and cysts, provided they are more than about 2 cm in diameter and have echogenic characteristics sufficiently different from normal liver tissue. Fine-gauge needles can be used to obtain tissue from such lesions (p. 497). Diffuse parenchymal diseases such as fatty change and cirrhosis are more difficult to distinguish, and normal appearances do not exclude significant liver disease. Colour Doppler ultrasound now allows blood flow in the hepatic artery, portal vein and hepatic veins to be investigated in conditions such as portal hypertension, the Budd–Chiari syndrome, and venous invasion by tumours. It can also detect hepatic artery occlusion following liver transplantation.

Abdominal radiographs

A plain radiograph shows about 20% of gallstones, and can show the soft tissue mass of an inflamed gallbladder or gas in the biliary tree when a biliary-enteric fistula is present. Calcification in the gallbladder wall occurs in 'porcelain' gallbladder, in the pancreas usually reflects chronic pancreatitis and in the liver occurs occasionally in lesions such as cysts, tumours or areas of infarction.

Varices in the oesophagus and stomach can be dem-

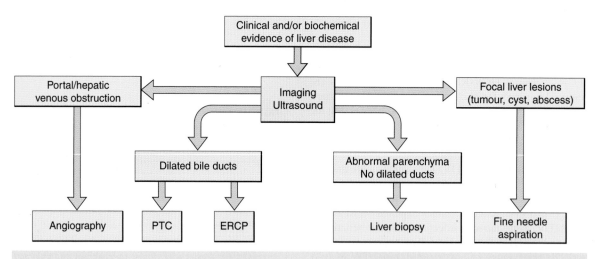

Fig. 8.6 Investigative procedures in liver disease. Suggested sequence for identifying structural lesions in the liver and biliary tract. ERCP = endoscopic retrograde cholangiopancreatography; PTC = percutaneous transhepatic cholangiography.

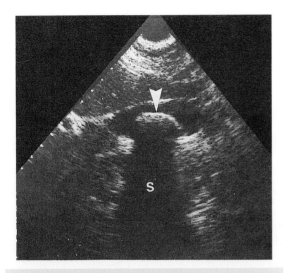

Fig. 8.7 Ultrasound of the gallbladder showing stone in the gallbladder. Stone (arrow) with acoustic shadow (S).

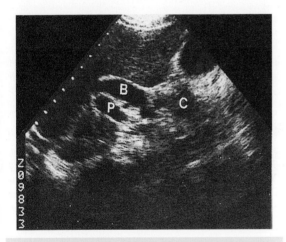

Fig. 8.8 Carcinoma of the pancreas (C) with dilated common bile duct (**B**). The portal vein (**P**) is posterior to the bile duct.

onstrated by barium swallow and meal examination. They establish the presence of portal hypertension.

Computed tomography (CT)

This can be used for the same purposes as ultrasound and has about the same sensitivity in detecting disease. CT can detect smaller focal lesions in the liver than ultrasonography, especially when done as CT portography in which contrast material is injected into the splenic or superior mesenteric artery. It is also useful in identifying the sites of focal lesions in the liver and is therefore particularly useful when surgery is planned. CT is also sensitive in detecting dilated bile ducts in

biliary obstruction and in demonstrating the cause. It is less useful in diffuse parenchymal disease.

Magnetic resonance imaging (MRI)

MRI continues to improve, especially in detecting focal liver lesions, but its place relative to ultrasonography and CT remains to be agreed.

Radionuclide imaging

Technetium (^{99m}Tc) sulphur colloid, which is taken up by the monocyte-macrophage system, is used to image the liver and spleen. It can detect focal liver lesions, diffuse liver disease and portal hypertension but is much less used for these purposes than previously. Cholescintigraphy using ^{99m}Tc-labelled imidodiacetic acid derivatives can be useful in showing cystic duct obstruction in patients with acute cholecystitis, and in common bile duct obstruction and biliary dyskinesia.

Cholecystography

This is now less used than ultrasonography but it is effective in demonstrating gallbladder function and disease. Iodine-containing compounds are given orally which are excreted in the bile and concentrated in the gallbladder which then becomes radio-opaque. Hyperbilirubinaemia greater than 35 μmol/1 (2 mg/dl) interferes with biliary excretion of the contrast agent sufficiently to prevent gallbladder visualisation. Non-opaque gallstones and adenomas show as filling defects in the opacified gallbladder. Adenomyomatosis is shown better by cholecystography than by any other method. Failure of the gallbladder to opacify is frequent in gallbladder disease, and the gallbladder is then called 'non-functioning'. This is usually due to cystic duct occlusion by a gallstone, but failure to take the tablets, vomiting, gastric outflow obstruction, diarrhoea or occasionally intestinal malabsorption will also result in failure to opacify the gallbladder. Normal gallbladders fail to opacify for unknown causes in 20% of cases, and when this occurs the test should be repeated with contrast given on two consecutive days. If under these circumstances the gallbladder fails to opacify there is virtual certainty that it is diseased.

Endoscopic retrograde cholangiopancreatography (ERCP)

This allows direct examination of the papilla of Vater, where lesions such as ampullary carcinomas can be seen and biopsied, and radiological examination of the biliary tree and pancreatic duct by injection of contrast into these systems (Fig. 8.9). It is valuable for determining the nature of cholestasis of unknown cause and for investigating pain which may be of biliary or pancreatic origin. The procedure is also used to carry out pap-

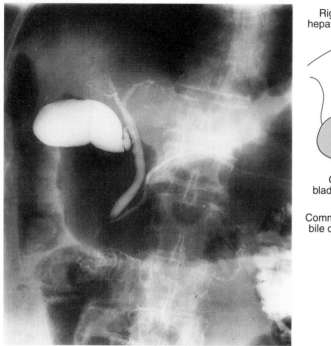

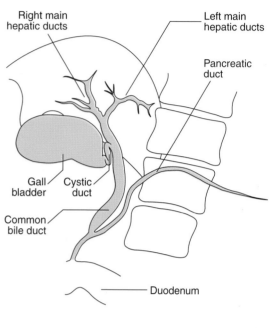

Right main hepatic ducts

Left main hepatic ducts

Pancreatic duct

Gall bladder

Cystic duct

Common bile duct

Duodenum

Fig. 8.9 **ERCP** showing normal biliary and pancreatic duct system.

illotomy at the papilla of Vater which allows stones to be removed from the common bile duct with balloon catheters or wire baskets. This can be done urgently in patients with cholangitis or pancreatitis due to gallstones who are not responding to therapy. Stents can be passed through malignant strictures to allow biliary drainage, and benign biliary strictures can be dilated. Complications of ERCP include pancreatitis in about 1–3% of cases and cholangitis which can be prevented by broad-spectrum antibiotics such as cefotaxime (1 g 8-hourly i.v.) when large duct biliary obstruction is found. Complications of papillotomy include bleeding and duodenal perforation.

Cholangiography

Percutaneous transhepatic cholangiography (PTC)

This involves injecting contrast material directly into an intrahepatic bile duct. Excellent delineation of the biliary tract is obtained, but the technique is less useful than ERCP as the pancreatic duct cannot be examined and stones cannot be removed from the biliary tract. Stents can be passed through malignant strictures, particularly those in the hepatic hilum which are not easily treated by ERCP. Complications are uncommon, but bleeding and bile leakage from the liver can occur. Accordingly, blood coagulation should be checked as for liver biopsy

before the procedure and facilities for surgery should be available.

Operative cholangiography

This should be carried out during operations on the biliary tract by injecting contrast into the cystic duct or the common bile duct.

T-tube cholangiography

This is carried out when a T-tube has been left in the common bile duct at choledochotomy. When stones are found in the common bile duct the T-tube can be left in place for 8–12 weeks to allow its track to mature after which the stones can be removed through the track with a wire (Burhenne) basket.

Arteriography

Hepatic arteriography is most useful for localising focal liver lesions, particularly tumours, and is essential in planning hepatic surgery. Hepatocellular carcinomas are usually highly vascular in contrast to metastatic tumours which usually show low vascularity. Highly vascular metastatic tumours occur occasionally and include renal, thyroid, carcinoid, islet-cell and chorion carcinomas, and sarcomas.

Venography

Portal venography

This is most useful in investigating portal hypertension of unknown cause. It is also essential prior to portal-systemic shunt surgery, though such surgery is now done infrequently. Portal venography is performed most safely by studying the venous phase following superior mes-enteric arteriography. Spleno-portography and trans-hepatic portography are more invasive and are much less used. Digital vascular imaging (DVI) can be used to examine the portal vein but the quality of the imaging is variable.

Hepatic venography

This is most important in the diagnosis of the Budd–Chiari syndrome (p. 532) and undertaken by passing a catheter into the hepatic veins via the inferior vena cava.

Interventional radiography

This is used increasingly in the management of hepa-tobiliary disease. Procedures include aspiration and drainage of focal liver lesions, plugging of biopsy tracks where coagulation is impaired, placement of biliary stents and the transjugular insertion of intrahepatic portal systemic stent shunts (TIPSS).

ENDOSCOPY

Upper gastrointestinal endoscopy is superior to barium examination in the diagnosis of oesophageal and gastric varices but small varices cannot be differentiated easily from mucosal folds. Endoscopy is the only means of diagnosing the congestive gastropathy of portal hyper-tension. Choledochoscopy is useful for identifying com-mon bile duct stones at operation.

ABDOMINAL PARACENTESIS

Analysis of ascites provides useful information. The fluid in cirrhosis is clear, the protein content usually below 30 g/l, and in the absence of infection there are less than 250 polymorphonuclear leucocytes/mm^3. Blood-stained ascites is usually due to malignant disease, and milky (chylous) ascites to obstruction of the cisterna chyli. Ascitic protein concentrations above 30 g/l occur most often in peritoneal infection, especially tuberculosis, peritoneal tumour, hepatic venous obstruction and ascites associated with pancreatic disease. The serum-ascites albumin gradient has been used to improve the dif-ferentiation of ascitic transudates and exudates but has not yet been used widely. The gradient in cirrhotic ascites is usually 1.5 or more. Amylase activity is high in ascites caused by pancreatitis. Infections, such as spon-taneous bacterial peritonitis (p. 508), can be identified by ascites polymorphonuclear leucocyte counts above 250/mm^3 and by bacteriological examination. Ascites cytology can show malignant cells, but negative exam-inations do not exclude malignant disease.

LIVER BIOPSY

This is performed with a special needle, usually through an intercostal space, using local analgesia. It requires a cooperative patient who will stop breathing when the biopsy is taken. The haemostatic mechanisms must be intact as indicated by a prothrombin time not more than 4 seconds longer than the control value and a platelet count not less than 100×10^9/l (100 000/mm^3). The pati-ent remains in bed for 24 hours after the procedure, regular pulse and blood pressure measurements must be recorded, and blood for transfusion (2 units) should be available. The main complications are abdominal and/or shoulder pain, bleeding and, rarely, biliary peritonitis which usually occurs when there is obstruction of a large bile duct. Liver biopsy is a relatively safe procedure but should never be undertaken lightly as the mortality rate is about 0.05%.

Liver biopsies can be carried out in patients with defective haemostasis if this can be corrected with fresh frozen plasma and platelets or if the biopsy is obtained by the transjugular route or percutaneously under ultra-sound control with subsequent plugging of the needle track with gelfoam.

Biopsy yields only a small sample of liver and conse-quently the best results are obtained in patients with diffuse liver disease. The procedure is essential in the diagnosis of chronic hepatitis and in separating the per-sistent, aggressive and lobular forms. It can also be impor-tant in establishing a diagnosis of cirrhosis in which it may indicate a cause such as alcohol abuse or haemo-chromatosis. Other investigations are now preferred in cholestasis (p. 501), as the histological differentiation of obstruction of a large bile duct from other liver diseases is sometimes difficult and there is an increased risk of biliary peritonitis following biopsy in cholestasis. Biopsy is not usually required in acute hepatitis for the diagnosis can normally be made on other grounds but it may be needed in atypical cases. Focal disease, particularly malignancy, is only diagnosed accurately if the site of the disease in the liver is first identified by some other method such as ultrasound or laparoscopy. Operative liver biopsy may sometimes be valuable, as in the staging of lymphoma.

LIVER ASPIRATION

This technique using fine-bore needles (20–22 gauge) usually guided by ultrasound has become the initial method of choice for investigating focal liver lesions such as tumours, abscesses and cysts. This can be done with minimal discomfort or risk provided the haemostatic mechanisms are satisfactory. Aspirated material can be examined cytologically, histologically and bacteriologically.

LAPAROSCOPY

Modern laparoscopes of relatively small size can now be used under sedation and local analgesia. They provide an excellent view of the anterior and superior surfaces of the liver as well as some of its inferior aspects and the gallbladder. The spleen, the prominent blood vessels of portal hypertension and evidence of peritoneal disease may also be seen. Biopsies can be taken directly from diseased areas, which is valuable in focal disorders, especially malignant disease. The main relative contra-indications are haemostatic abnormalities, marked ascites and previous surgery which may have caused adhesions.

PORTAL PRESSURE

This can be measured directly by passing needles or catheters into the spleen, the portal vein or the hepatic parenchyma, but these methods are invasive and rarely used. The pressure recorded by a catheter wedged in a hepatic vein (wedged hepatic venous pressure) reflects the portal venous pressure via the hepatic sinusoids, and this less disturbing procedure is most widely used for measuring the portal venous pressure. The portal venous pressure is calculated as the difference between the wedged hepatic venous pressure and the free hepatic venous pressure and is normally 3–5 mmHg.

MAJOR MANIFESTATIONS OF LIVER DISEASE

JAUNDICE

Jaundice refers to the yellow appearance of the skin, sclerae and mucous membranes resulting from an increased bilirubin concentration in the body fluids. It is detectable when the plasma bilirubin exceeds 50 μmol/l (3 mg/dl). Internal tissues and body fluids are coloured yellow but not the brain as bilirubin does not cross the blood–brain barrier other than in the immediate neonatal period. Pathological mechanisms giving rise to jaundice are listed in the information box.

MECHANISMS PRODUCING JAUNDICE

- Haemolysis
- Impaired hepatic bilirubin transport
- Hepatocellular damage
- Cholestasis (impaired bile flow)

HAEMOLYTIC JAUNDICE

This results from increased destruction of red blood cells, or their precursors in the marrow, causing increased bilirubin production (p. 790). Jaundice due to haemolysis is usually mild because a healthy liver can excrete a bilirubin load 6 times greater than normal before unconjugated bilirubin accumulates in the plasma. Exceptions to this occur in the newborn when the hepatic bilirubin transport mechanism is immature and in patients with liver disease.

Clinical features

These are detailed elsewhere (p. 790). There are no stigmata of liver disease other than jaundice. Increased excretion of bilirubin and hence stercobilinogen leads to normal coloured or dark stools, and increased uro-bilinogen excretion causes the urine to turn dark on standing as urobilin is formed. Pallor due to anaemia and splenomegaly due to excessive reticuloendothelial activity are usually present.

Investigations

The plasma bilirubin is usually less than 100 μmol/l (6 mg/dl) and the liver function tests are otherwise normal. There is no bilirubinuria because the hyperbilirubinaemia is dominantly unconjugated. Evidence of haemolytic anaemia is also present.

CONGENITAL NON-HAEMOLYTIC HYPERBILIRUBINAEMIA

Gilbert's syndrome is the only common form of congenital non-haemolytic hyperbilirubinaemia. All other forms are very rare (Table 8.7). In adults they have an excellent prognosis, need no treatment, and are clinically important only because they may be mistaken for more serious liver disease.

Table 8.7 Congenital non-haemolytic hyperbilirubinaemia

Syndrome	Inheritance	Age of presentation	Hyperbilirubinaemia Type	Hyperbilirubinaemia Severity	Bilirubinuria	Liver Defect(s)	Liver Histology	Cholecystography	Bromsulphthalein excretion	Prognosis	Treatment
GILBERT'S	Autosomal dominant	Young adult (any)	Unconjugated	Mild	No	Glucuronyl transferase reduced Occasional mild haemolysis Defective bilirubin uptake	Normal	Normal	Normal	Normal life span	None Phenobarbitone occasionally
CRIGLER–NAJJAR —Type I	Autosomal recessive	Neonate	Unconjugated	Very severe	No	Glucuronyl transferase absent	Normal	—	—	Rapid death (kernicterus)	None
—Type II	Autosomal dominant	Neonate	Unconjugated	Severe	No	Glucuronyl transferase greatly reduced	Normal	—	—	Can survive to adulthood	Phenobarbitone Ultraviolet light Liver transplant
DUBIN–JOHNSON	Autosomal recessive	Any	Conjugated	Mild	Yes	Canalicular excretion of organic anions (e.g. bilirubin, cholecystographic contrast agents) reduced	Black deposits (melanin)	Gallbladder not visualised	Normal at 45 min Secondary rise at 120 min	Normal life span	None
ROTOR	Autosomal dominant	Any	Conjugated	Mild	Yes	Defective bilirubin uptake Reduced intrahepatic binding	Normal	Gallbladder not visualised	Abnormal at 45 min No secondary rise at 120 min	Normal life span	None

GILBERT'S SYNDROME

This common benign condition is usually recognised first in adolescents or young adults. It is more common in men (male:female ratio 4:1) and occurs in about 5% of the population.

Aetiology

The aetiology is varied but it can be inherited as an autosomal dominant. The main cause of the unconjugated hyperbilirubinaemia is a deficiency of hepatic glucuronyl transferase; in some patients uptake of unconjugated bilirubin from the plasma may be impaired; in others mild haemolysis not detectable by conventional laboratory tests is present.

Clinical features

Gilbert's syndrome generally presents as mild jaundice, occasionally noted after viral hepatitis from which there has been a complete recovery, or is found incidentally. Many patients have no symptoms; others suffer episodes of malaise, anorexia and upper abdominal pain, the last occasionally severe, with increases in the jaundice. These episodes may be related to infection, fatigue or fasting. Physical examination shows mild jaundice but is otherwise normal.

Investigations

Investigations show hyperbilirubinaemia, generally below 100 μmol/1 (6 mg/dl), with no abnormality of other liver function tests. Estimations of unconjugated bilirubin are unreliable when the plasma bilirubin is below 70 μmol/1 and are generally unnecessary as failure to find bilirubin in the urine points to unconjugated hyperbilirubinaemia (p. 489). The peripheral blood count, reticulocyte count and plasma haptoglobin concentration are normal, giving no evidence of overt haemolysis. Liver biopsy is normal and should be performed only if there is clinical or biochemical evidence suggesting liver disease.

Management

No treatment is necessary.

HEPATOCELLULAR JAUNDICE

Hepatocellular jaundice results from inability of the liver to transport bilirubin into the bile as a result of liver cell damage. Bilirubin transport across the hepatocytes may be impaired at any point between uptake of unconjugated bilirubin into the cells and transport of conjugated bilirubin into the canaliculi. In addition, swelling of cells and oedema resulting from the disease itself may cause obstruction of the biliary canaliculi. In hepato-

cellular jaundice the concentrations in the blood of both unconjugated and conjugated bilirubin increase, perhaps because of the variable way in which bilirubin transport is disturbed.

Acute parenchymal liver diseases, usually due to the hepatitis viruses or to drugs, are common causes. Prolonged alcohol abuse and chronic hepatitis or cirrhosis irrespective of cause also cause hepatocellular jaundice. The severity of jaundice, the other clinical features and the investigation and treatment vary with the underlying disease and are considered later in this chapter.

CHOLESTATIC JAUNDICE

Cholestasis is a failure of bile flow, and its cause may lie anywhere between the hepatocyte and the duodenum. The causes are listed in the information box (p. 501).

Jaundice becomes progressively severe in unrelieved cholestasis because conjugated bilirubin is unable to enter the bile canaliculi and passes back into the blood, and also because there is a failure of clearance of unconjugated bilirubin arriving at the liver cells.

Aetiology

Cholestasis may be due to failure of the hepatocytes to generate bile flow, to obstruction to bile flow in the bile ducts in the portal tracts, or to obstruction to bile flow in the extrahepatic bile ducts between the porta hepatis and the papilla of Vater. Causes of cholestasis can operate at more than one of these levels, and those confined to the extrahepatic bile ducts may be amenable to surgical correction.

Clinical features

Clinical features in cholestatic jaundice include those due to cholestasis itself and to the development of cholangitis consequent on biliary obstruction. These features are listed in the information box opposite.

Jaundice is very variable; it may be static or fluctuate, and if it is prolonged and severe it can give the skin a greenish appearance. The stools are pale or clay-coloured due to deficiency of pigments derived from bilirubin and to steatorrhoea consequent on bile salt deficiency. The urine is dark from the renal excretion of conjugated bilirubin. Some patients have generalised pruritus and accessible parts of the body may show scratch marks. Lipid deposits can develop in the skin in prolonged cholestatic jaundice. Most of these are xanthelasmas on the eyelids but occasionally xanthomas also occur. Prolonged cholestasis can cause marked malabsorption leading to weight loss, severe steatorrhoea, a haemorrhagic tendency due to vitamin K deficiency, and hepatic osteodystrophy which may be associated with calcium and vitamin D deficiency. Eventually clinical

CAUSES OF CHOLESTASIS

Common causes

- Hepatocytic (canalicular) cholestasis
  Alcohol
  Drugs

- Biliary obstruction
  Choledocholithiasis
  Carcinoma (pancreas, bile duct, hepatic
    metastases)
  Primary biliary cirrhosis
  Primary sclerosing cholangitis

Other causes

- Hepatocytic (canalicular) cholestasis
  Viral hepatitis
  Chronic active hepatitis
  Cirrhosis
  Severe bacterial infections
  Postoperative
  Hodgkin's lymphoma
  Pregnancy
  Idiopathic recurrent cholestasis

- Biliary obstruction
  Cystic fibrosis (tenacious secretions)
  Parasites

- Carcinoma
  Peripapillary carcinoma (pancreas, bile duct,
    duodenum)

- Benign tumours
  Periampullary adenoma
  Biliary papilloma

- Metastatic tumours
  Lymph nodes (e.g. in porta hepatis)

- Strictures
  Trauma (usually surgical)
  Stones

- Biliary cirrhosis (secondary)
  Choledochal cyst
  Pancreatitis
  Duodenal ulcer

CLINICAL FEATURES IN CHOLESTATIC JAUNDICE

Cholestasis

Early features	Late features
• Jaundice	• Xanthelasma and
• Dark urine	xanthomas
• Pale stools	• Malabsorption:
• Pruritus	Weight loss
	Steatorrhoea
	Hepatic osteodystrophy
	Bleeding tendency

Cholangitis

- Fever
- Rigors
- Pain
- Hepatic abscess

and biochemical evidence of biliary cirrhosis and hepatocellular failure occur. Cholangitis due to infection in biliary obstruction causes fever with or without rigors, and coincident pain and hepatic tenderness may indicate the development of a hepatic abscess. Clinical features in cholestatic jaundice also include those which point to a likely cause for the condition (Table 8.8). None of these features is pathognomonic of a particular cause, but each is more likely in some diseases than in others.

Investigations

Investigations in individual patients are determined by the clinical findings, but where there is no obvious cause for cholestasis initial efforts are directed to identifying a large duct biliary obstruction (Fig. 8.6). Ultrasonography should be carried out in all cases, and tests for the antimitochondrial antibody (p. 493) should be performed. ERCP is the best investigation if the biliary tract is dilated, particularly when the dilatation extends to the lower common bile duct, and PTC is used only if ERCP is unavailable. ERCP may also be appropriate when ultrasonography does not show dilated bile ducts, if there are no clinical clues to the cause of cholestasis or if a condition such as sclerosing cholangitis which does not necessarily cause biliary dilatation is suspected, as when ulcerative colitis is also present. Liver biopsy would be preferred if evidence of liver disease such as spider telangiectasias was present.

Management

This depends on the underlying cause of the cholestasis.

UNUSUAL FORMS OF CHOLESTASIS

Cholestasis of pregnancy

This is probably caused by an inherited susceptibility of the patient's liver cells to oestrogens; the condition is sometimes precipitated by oral contraceptives. Pruritus is the dominant symptom and jaundice occurs in about a half of patients. Itching almost always starts in the third trimester of pregnancy and remits within about 2 weeks of delivery. Pruritus can be relieved with cholestyramine (p. 531). No harm comes to the fetus, but the condition tends to recur in subsequent pregnancies.

Benign recurrent intrahepatic cholestasis

This is a rare condition in which episodes of cholestasis lasting from 1–6 months occur starting in adolescence or early adult life. Genetic factors are probably important as more than one family member may be affected. Episodes start with pruritus, and painless jaundice develops later. Liver function tests show the pattern of cholestasis (p. 490), and liver biopsy shows cholestasis during an epi-

Table 8.8 Underlying causes of cholestatic jaundice related to clinical features

Clinical feature	Causes
Jaundice	
Static or increasing	Carcinoma
Fluctuating	Stone
	Stricture
	Pancreatitis
	Choledochal cyst
Abdominal pain	Stone
	Pancreatitis
	Choledochal cyst
Cholangitis	Stone
	Stricture
	Choledochal cyst
Abdominal scar	Stone
	Stricture
Irregular hepatomegaly	Hepatic carcinoma
Palpable gallbladder	Carcinoma below cystic duct (usually pancreas)
Abdominal mass	Carcinoma
	Pancreatitis (cyst)
	Choledochal cyst
Occult blood in stools	Papillary tumour

Note: Each of the diseases listed here can give rise to almost any of the clinical features shown. The more likely causes of each clinical feature are given.

sode but is normal between episodes. Treatment is required to relieve pruritus and the long-term prognosis is good.

PORTAL HYPERTENSION

Portal hypertension is a condition characterised by prolonged elevation of the portal venous pressure (normally 2–5 mmHg). Patients developing clinical features or complications of portal hypertension usually have portal venous pressures above 12 mmHg.

Aetiology and pathogenesis

Portal venous pressure is determined by the portal blood flow and by the portal vascular resistance. Increased vascular resistance is usually the main factor producing portal hypertension, irrespective of its cause, and consequently the causes of portal hypertension are classified in accordance with the main sites of obstruction to blood flow in the portal venous system. These causes are listed in the information box.

Extrahepatic portal vein obstruction is frequently the cause of portal hypertension in childhood and

adolescence, while **cirrhosis** causes 90% or more of portal hypertension in adults in most countries. Schistosomiasis is the most common cause of portal hypertension in the world but it is infrequent outside endemic areas. Increased portal vascular resistance leads to a gradual reduction in the flow of portal blood to the liver and simultaneously to the development of collateral vessels allowing portal blood to bypass the liver and enter the systemic circulation directly. Increased portal blood flow contributes to portal hypertension but is not the dominant factor. Collateral vessel formation is widespread but occurs particularly in the gastrointestinal tract, especially the oesophagus, stomach and rectum, in the anterior abdominal wall, and in the renal, lumbar, ovarian and testicular vasculature. Virtually all the portal blood normally flows through the liver, but as collateral vessel formation progresses a half or more, and occasionally almost all, can be shunted directly to the systemic circulation.

CAUSES OF PORTAL HYPERTENSION ACCORDING TO SITE OF PORTAL VENOUS OBSTRUCTION

Common causes
- Extrahepatic—sepsis (umbilical, portal pyaemia)
  —unknown (50–75%)
- Intrahepatic presinusoidal—schistosomiasis
- Intrahepatic parenchymal —cirrhosis

Other causes
- Extrahepatic
  Umbilical vein transfusion
  Thrombosis
    Thrombotic diseases
    Oral contraceptives
    Pregnancy
    Secondary (cirrhosis)
  Abdominal trauma
  Biliary surgery
  Malignant disease
    Pancreas
    Liver
  Pancreatitis
  Congenital

- Intrahepatic presinusoidal
  Myeloproliferative/lymphoproliferative disease
  Congenital hepatic fibrosis
  Drugs
  Vinyl chloride
  Sarcoidosis
  Idiopathic

- Intrahepatic parenchymal
  Budd–Chiari syndrome
  Veno-occlusive disease
  Cystic liver disease
  Partial nodular transformation of the liver
  Secondary malignant disease

Clinical features

The clinical features of portal hypertension result principally from portal venous congestion and from collateral vessel formation. **Splenomegaly** is a cardinal finding, and a diagnosis of portal hypertension is unlikely when splenomegaly cannot be shown clinically, on an abdominal radiograph or by ultrasonography. The spleen is rarely enlarged more than 5 cm below the left costal margin in adults, but much more marked splenomegaly can occur in childhood and adolescence. **Hypersplenism** is common and thrombocytopenia is the most common feature. Platelet counts are usually around $100 \times 10^9/1$, and counts below $50 \times 10^9/1$ are rare. Leucopenia occurs occasionally, but anaemia can hardly ever be attributed to hypersplenism. **Collateral vessels** may be visible on the anterior abdominal wall and occasionally several radiate from the umbilicus to form a caput medusae. Rarely, a large umbilical collateral vessel has a blood flow sufficient to give a venous hum on auscultation (Cruveilhier–Baumgarten syndrome). The most important collateral vessels occur in the oesophagus and stomach, where they can cause severe bleeding (p. 502). Rectal varices also cause bleeding and are often mistaken for haemorrhoids, which are no more common in portal hypertension than in the general population. **Fetor hepaticus** results from portasystemic shunting of blood which allows mercaptans to pass directly to the lungs.

Investigations

Radiological and endoscopic examination of the upper gastrointestinal tract can show varices which establishes the presence of portal hypertension but not its cause (Fig. 8.10). Imaging, particularly ultrasonography, can show features of portal hypertension, such as splenomegaly and collateral vessels, and sometimes the cause such as liver disease or portal vein thrombosis. Portal venography (Fig. 8.11) demonstrates the site and often the cause of portal venous obstruction and is performed prior to surgical therapy. Portal venous pressure measurements are rarely needed but can be used to confirm portal hypertension and to differentiate sinusoidal and presinusoidal forms. These investigative methods are considered elsewhere (p. 497).

Complications

These are listed in the information box.

Gastrointestinal bleeding from varices or from congestive gastropathy is the main complication. Hypersplenism is rarely sufficiently severe to be clinically significant and portal hypertension is only one factor contributing to ascites (p. 506), to renal failure (p. 508) and to hepatic encephalopathy (p. 508).

COMPLICATIONS OF PORTAL HYPERTENSION

- Variceal bleeding
  Oesophageal, gastric, other (rare)
- Congestive gastropathy
- Hypersplenism
- Ascites
- Renal failure
- Hepatic encephalopathy

VARICEAL BLEEDING

Variceal bleeding occurs from oesophageal varices within 3–5 cm of the oesophagogastric junction or from gastric varices. Large varices, endoscopic variceal stigma such as red spots and red stripes, high portal pressure and liver failure are general factors predisposing to bleeding, and drugs capable of causing mucosal erosion, such as salicylates and other non-steroidal anti-inflammatory drugs, can precipitate bleeding. Variceal bleeding is often severe, and recurrent bleeding usually occurs if preventive treatment is not given. Bleeding from other varices is comparatively uncommon and usually occurs from rectal varices or varices on intestinal stomas.

Management of acute variceal bleeding

The first priority in acute bleeding from oesophageal varices is to restore the circulation with blood and plasma because shock reduces liver blood flow and causes significant deterioration of liver function. Oesophageal or gastric varices should be confirmed as the source of bleeding as soon as acute bleeding has been controlled because about 20% of patients with varices are bleeding from some other lesion, especially acute gastric erosions. Several treatments are available to stop acute variceal bleeding and to prevent its recurring and these are listed in the information box below.

Reduction of portal venous pressure

Pharmacological reduction of portal pressure is less important than sclerotherapy or banding and is not always used. All the drugs are relatively expensive, and octreotide is probably the drug of choice currently.

(1) Vasopressin

This constricts the splanchnic arterioles and reduces portal pressure and portal blood flow. It is best given by intravenous infusion 0.4 Unit/minute until bleeding stops or for 24 hours, and then 0.2 Unit/minute for a further 24 hours. Vasoconstriction also occurs generally and can cause angina, arrhythmia and even myocardial infarction. Nitroglycerin should be given transdermally or intravenously to combat these effects, but vasopressin

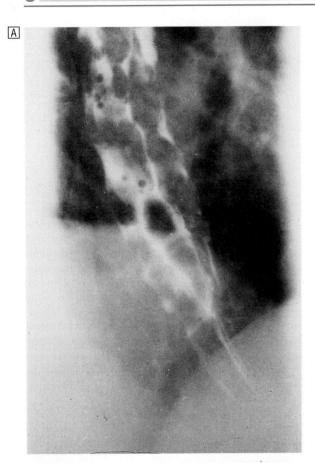

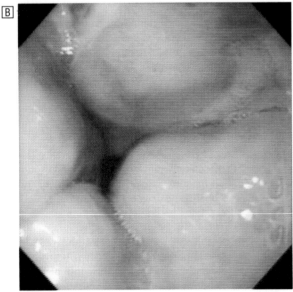

Fig. 8.10 Oesophageal varices. [A] Barium swallow.
[B] Endoscopic view showing four large varices encroaching on the lumen.

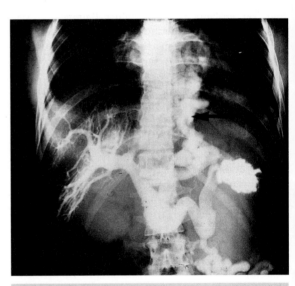

Fig. 8.11 Splenoportal venogram showing oesophageal varices (arrow), mesenteric collaterals and attenuated venous pattern in the cirrhotic liver.

should not be used in patients with ischaemic heart disease.

(2) Terlipressin

This is an alternative to vasopressin with certain advantages. Terlipressin itself is not active, but vasopressin is released from it over several hours in amounts sufficient to reduce the portal pressure without producing systemic, including cardiac, effects. It is given in a dose of 2 mg intravenously every 6 hours until bleeding stops and then 1 mg every 6 hours for a further 24 hours.

(3) Somatostatin

Octreotide, the synthetic form of somatostatin, reduces the portal pressure and can stop variceal bleeding. It is given in a dose of 50 μg intravenously followed by an infusion of 50 μg hourly.

Local measures

The measures used to control acute variceal bleeding include sclerotherapy, banding, balloon tamponade and oesophageal transection. Emergency portasystemic shunt surgery has a mortality of 50% or more and is virtually never used.

(1) Sclerotherapy

This is the most important initial treatment and is undertaken if possible at the time of diagnostic endoscopy. It stops variceal bleeding in 80% of patients and can be repeated if bleeding recurs. Active bleeding at endoscopy may make sclerotherapy hazardous, and in such circumstances bleeding should be controlled by balloon tamponade prior to sclerotherapy.

(2) Banding

This recently developed technique can be used to stop variceal bleeding but it is less easy to apply than sclerotherapy in acute bleeding.

(3) Balloon tamponade

This is effected with a Sengstaken–Blakemore tube possessing two balloons which exert pressure respectively in the fundus of the stomach and in the lower oesophagus. Current modifications such as the Minnesota tube incorporate sufficient lumens to allow material to be aspirated from the stomach and from the oesophagus above the oesophageal balloon. The tube should be passed through the mouth and its presence in the stomach should be checked by auscultating the upper abdomen while injecting air into the stomach and by radiology. Gentle traction is used to maintain pressure on the varices. The gastric balloon only should be inflated initially as this alone will usually control bleeding, and if the oesophageal balloon needs to be used it should be deflated for about 10 minutes every 3 hours to avoid oesophageal mucosal damage. Balloon tamponade will almost always stop oesophageal and gastric fundal variceal bleeding, but it only allows time for the use of more definitive therapy.

(4) Transjugular intrahepatic portasystemic stent shunting (TIPSS)

This technique, described below, can be used for acute bleeding not responding to sclerotherapy or banding.

(5) Oesophageal transection

Transection of the varices can be performed relatively easily with a stapling gun though it carries some risk of subsequent oesophageal stenosis. The operation is used when bleeding cannot be controlled by the other therapies described.

Prevention of recurrent bleeding

Recurrent variceal bleeding is the rule rather than the exception in patients who have had bleeding from oesophageal varices, and treatment to prevent this is needed.

Sclerotherapy

This is the most widely used method for preventing recurrent oesophageal variceal bleeding. Varices are injected with a sclerosing agent as soon as practicable after bleeding, and injections are repeated every 1–2 weeks thereafter until the varices are obliterated. Regular follow-up is necessary to allow treatment of any recurrence of varices. The treatment is not free of risk as injections can cause transient chest or abdominal pain, fever, transient dysphagia and occasionally oesophageal perforation. Oesophageal strictures may develop. However, mortality is low, even those with poor liver function can be treated, and recurrent bleeding is largely prevented. Prolongation of life has been claimed but this remains to be proven.

Banding

This is a recently developed technique in which varices are sucked into an endoscope accessory allowing them to be occluded with a tight rubber band. The occluded varix subsequently sloughs with variceal obliteration. The technique promises to be more effective than sclerotherapy with fewer side-effects.

Transjugular intrahepatic portasystemic stent shunting (TIPSS)

This is a recently described technique in which a stent is placed between the portal vein and the hepatic vein in the liver to provide a portasystemic shunt to reduce portal pressure. The procedure is carried out under radiological control via the internal jugular vein; prior patency of the portal vein must be determined angiographically, coagulation deficiencies may require fresh frozen plasma and antibiotic cover is provided. Successful shunt placement stops and prevents variceal bleeding. Further bleeding necessitates investigation and treatment of shunt occlusion, and hepatic encephalopathy requires that the shunt be reduced. The long-term value of the technique remains to be assessed fully.

Portasystemic shunt surgery

This was previously the treatment of choice because such shunts effectively prevent bleeding provided the shunt remains patent. However, follow-up of patients showed that they often suffered troublesome hepatic encephalopathy, and survival was not prolonged as death from liver failure occurred. In practice, portasystemic shunts are reserved for patients in whom other treatments have not been successful and are offered only to those with good liver function.

Propranolol

Propranolol (80–160 mg/day) reduces the portal venous pressure in portal hypertension and has been used to prevent recurrent variceal bleeding; however, it has not yet been accepted generally in treatment.

Prophylaxis of initial variceal bleeding

Portasystemic shunts, sclerotherapy and propranolol have all been used to try to prevent initial bleeding from varices. Propranolol alone has given beneficial results and can be used to prevent initial variceal bleeding in a dose of 80–160 mg daily.

CONGESTIVE GASTROPATHY

Long-standing portal hypertension causes chronic gastric congestion recognisable at endoscopy as multiple areas of punctate erythema. These areas may become eroded causing bleeding from multiple sites. Acute bleeding can occur, but repeated minor bleeding causing recurrent iron-deficiency anaemia is more common. Anaemia may be prevented by oral iron supplements but repeated blood transfusions often become necessary. Reduction of the portal pressure using propranolol 80–160 mg/d is the best initial treatment, and if this is ineffective a TIPSS procedure can be done. Congestive gastropathy is often restricted to the gastric antrum, but few patients are fit enough to undergo antrectomy.

ASCITES

Ascites refers to the accumulation of free fluid in the peritoneal cavity. Cirrhosis is a common cause of ascites, but there are many other causes to be considered even in a patient with chronic liver disease. The main causes of ascites are shown in the information box.

Clinical features

Ascites causes abdominal distension with fullness in the flanks, shifting dullness on percussion, and a fluid thrill when a lot of ascites is present. These signs do not appear

---

CAUSES OF ASCITES

Common causes
- Malignant disease
  hepatic, peritoneal
- Cardiac failure
- Hepatic cirrhosis

Other causes
- Hypoproteinaemia
  Nephrotic syndrome, protein-losing enteropathy, malnutrition
- Hepatic venous occlusion
  Budd–Chiari syndrome, veno-occlusive disease
- Infection
  Tuberculosis, spontaneous bacterial peritonitis
- Pancreatitis
- Lymphatic obstruction
  Chylous ascites
- Rare
  Meig's syndrome, vasculitis, hypothyroidism, renal dialysis

---

until the ascites volume exceeds a litre even in thin patients, and much larger volumes can be hard to detect in the obese. Associated features consequent on ascites include distortion or evertion of the umbilicus, herniae, abdominal striae, divarication of the recti and occasionally meralgia paraesthetica and scrotal oedema. Pleural effusions can be found in about 10% of patients, usually on the right side. Most are small and found on chest radiographs, but occasionally massive hydrothorax occurs. Pleural effusions, particularly on the left side, should not be assumed to be due to the ascites.

Investigations

Ultrasonography is the best means of confirming ascites, demonstrating ascites in the obese, or detecting small amounts. Abdominal radiographs can show ascites, but they are insensitive and non-specific. Paracentesis reveals ascites but is most useful in obtaining ascitic fluid for analysis, if necessary under ultrasonic guidance. The appearance of the ascites can point to the underlying cause (Table 8.9). The ascites protein concentration and

Table 8.9 Appearances and causes of ascites

Cause	Appearance
Cirrhosis	Clear, straw-coloured or light green
Malignant disease	Bloody
Infection	Cloudy
Biliary communication	Heavy bile staining
Lymphatic obstruction	Milky white (chylous)

Note: Milky white chylomicrons pass into supernatant on centrifugation.

the serum-ascites albumin gradient are used to separate ascites due to transudation from ascites due to exudation (p. 497). Ascites protein concentrations below 25 g/l or serum-ascites albumin gradients above 1.5 are usually found in ascites due to cirrhosis. Ascites amylase activity above 1000 U/l identifies pancreatic ascites, and low ascites glucose concentrations suggest malignant disease or tuberculosis. Cytological examination can reveal malignant cells, and polymorpho-nuclear leucocyte counts above 250/mm³ strongly suggest infection. Laparoscopy can also be valuable in detecting peritoneal disease.

Diagnosis

Ascites is caused by malignant disease, cirrhosis or cardiac failure in the great majority of patients, but the presence of cirrhosis does not necessarily mean that this is the cause of the ascites. This is particularly so when liver function is good or when there is no evidence of portal hypertension, and in such patients a complication of cirrhosis, such as hepatocellular carcinoma or portal vein thrombosis, should be sought or an independent cause of ascites considered. Ascites with a protein concentration above 25 g/l raises the possibility of infection, especially tuberculosis, malignancy, hepatic venous obstruction, pancreatic ascites or rarely hypothyroidism.

ASCITES DUE TO CIRRHOSIS

Pathogenesis

Liver failure and portal hypertension in cirrhosis cause general sodium and water retention in the body with localisation of fluid in the peritoneum owing to the high venous pressure in the mesenteric circulation. The means whereby this occurs are unknown, and two general theories have been put forward. One explanation postulates a loss of fluid into the peritoneum as ascites develops with renal retention of sodium and water to compensate for this ('underfilling theory'), while the other postulates a primary renal retention of sodium and water with eventual overspill of fluid into the peritoneum ('overflow theory'). The mechanisms for sodium retention remain poorly understood but include activation of the renin-angiotensin system with secondary aldosteronism, increased sympathetic nervous activity, alteration of atrial natriuretic hormone secretion and altered activity of the kallikrein-kinin system.

Management

Successful treatment of ascites relieves discomfort but does not prolong life, and if over-vigorous can produce serious disorders of fluid and electrolyte balance, and as a consequence hepatic encephalopathy (information box

p. 509). Treatment aims to reduce body sodium and water by restricting intake, promoting urine output, and if necessary removing ascites directly. The rate of loss of sodium and water is most easily measured by regular weighing, and as no more than 900 ml can be mobilised from the peritoneum daily, the body weight should not fall by more than 1 kg daily if fluid depletion in the rest of the body is to be avoided.

Sodium and water

Restriction of dietary sodium intake is essential to achieving negative sodium balance in patients with ascites. Restriction to 40 mmol/d initially may be adequate, but restriction to 20 mmol/d is necessary in more severe ascites and requires close dietetic supervision. Drugs containing relatively large amounts of sodium and drugs promoting sodium retention such as non-steroidal analgesic agents must be avoided. Restriction of water intake to 0.5–1.0 l/d is necessary only if the plasma sodium falls below 125 mmol/l. A few patients will have a satisfactory diuresis on this treatment alone.

Diuretic drugs

Most patients require diuretic drugs in addition to sodium restriction. Spironolactone (100–400 mg/d) is the drug of choice for long-term therapy because it is a powerful aldosterone antagonist, but unfortunately it can cause painful gynaecomastia. Some patients will also require powerful loop diuretics, though these can cause fluid, electrolyte and renal function disorders. Diuresis is improved if patients are at bed rest while the diuretics are acting, perhaps because renal blood flow increases in the horizontal position.

Paracentesis

Paracentesis of 3–5 l over 1–2 hours has always been used for immediate relief of cardiorespiratory distress due to gross ascites, but it has previously been regarded as a hazardous treatment for ascites itself. Paracentesis to dryness or the removal of 3–5 l daily is now recognised as a safe treatment provided the circulation is supported by giving a colloid such as plasma or Haemaccel as required and can be used as an initial therapy or when other treatments fail.

LeVeen shunt

The LeVeen shunt is a long tube with a non-return valve running subcutaneously from the peritoneum to the internal jugular vein in the neck which allows ascitic fluid to pass directly to the systemic circulation. It can be very effective in ascites resistant to other treatment, but complications, including infection, superior vena caval thrombosis, pulmonary oedema, bleeding from oesophageal varices and disseminated intravascular coagulopathy, limit its use.

Transjugular intrahepatic portasystemic stent shunting (TIPSS)

This technique (p. 505) has been developed to treat bleeding varices but can relieve resistant ascites in patients who are not terminally ill.

Prognosis

Ascites is a serious development in cirrhosis as only 10–20% of patients survive 5 years from its appearance. The outlook is not universally bad, however, and is best in those with well-maintained liver function and where the response to therapy is good. The prognosis is also better where a treatable cause for the underlying cirrhosis is present (p. 520) or where a precipitating cause for ascites such as excess salt intake is found.

SPONTANEOUS BACTERIAL PERITONITIS (SBP)

Patients with cirrhosis are very susceptible to infection of ascitic fluid (SBP) as part of their general susceptibility to infection. SBP usually starts suddenly with abdominal pain, rebound pain, absent bowel sounds and fever in a patient with obvious features of cirrhosis and ascites. Hepatic encephalopathy also occurs, and in about a third of patients encephalopathy and fever are the main features because abdominal signs are mild or absent. Paracentesis may show cloudy fluid, and an ascites neutrophil count above 250/mm^3 confirms infection. The source of infection cannot usually be determined but most organisms obtained on ascites and blood culture are of enteric origin and *E. coli* is the organism isolated most frequently. SBP needs to be differentiated from other intra-abdominal emergencies, and the finding of multiple organisms on culture should arouse suspicion of a perforated viscus. Treatment is started immediately with a broad spectrum of antibiotics such as cefotaxime (1 g i.v. 8-hourly) and metronidazole (1 g rectally 8-hourly). The prognosis is poor, and most patients die in spite of vigorous treatment. Recurrence of SBP is common and recurrences may be reduced by norfloxacin.

RENAL FAILURE

Renal failure consequent on liver failure can occur in cirrhosis. The kidneys themselves are intrinsically normal and renal failure is thought to result from altered systemic blood flow including diminished renal blood flow. The condition is called **functional renal failure** of cirrhosis or the **hepatorenal syndrome**. It occurs in advanced cirrhosis, almost always with ascites, and uraemia is characterised by the absence of proteinuria or abnormal urinary sediment, a urine sodium excretion below 10 mmol/d, and a urine/plasma osmolality ratio greater than 1.5. It is important to exclude hypovolaemia by measuring the central venous pressure and giving colloidal solutions such as plasma protein solution or salt-poor albumin to maintain the pressure at 0–5 cm of water and to ensure the best possible renal blood flow by giving low-dose dopamine (1–2 μ/kg/min) and thereafter using diuretic drugs. Uraemia and endogenous protein breakdown should be limited by restricting protein intake to 20 g/d and giving 300 g of carbohydrate/d. Recovery depends ultimately on improvement of liver function but in chronic liver disease this seldom occurs. Accordingly, the prognosis is very poor unless liver transplantation can be carried out.

HEPATIC (PORTASYSTEMIC) ENCEPHALOPATHY

Hepatic encephalopathy is a neuropsychiatric syndrome caused by liver disease. It occurs most often in patients with cirrhosis but is also seen in more acute form in fulminant hepatic failure.

Aetiology

Hepatic encephalopathy is generally regarded as due to a biochemical disturbance of brain function because it is reversible and rarely shows marked pathological changes in the brain. Liver failure and shunting of portal blood past the liver directly to the systemic circulation are the two general factors underlying hepatic encephalopathy and the balance between them varies in different patients. Some degree of liver failure, however, is a constant factor, as portasystemic shunting of blood rarely causes encephalopathy if the liver is normal. Little is known of the biochemical neurotoxins causing encephalopathy, but they are thought to be nitrogenous substances produced mainly in the gut, at least in part by bacterial action, which are normally metabolised by the healthy liver so that they do not enter the systemic circulation. Ammonia has long been considered an important factor and much recent interest has centred on the false neurotransmitter gamma-aminobutyric acid; both are produced in the intestine. Additional putative substances include other false neurotransmitters such as octopamine, amino acids, mercaptans and fatty acids. Some factors precipitate hepatic encephalopathy by increasing the availability of these substances; in addition the brain in cirrhosis may be sensitised to other factors such as drugs able to precipitate hepatic encephalopathy. (See the information box below.)

Disruption of the function of the blood-brain barrier is more a feature of fulminant hepatic failure where it leads to cerebral oedema.

Pathology

Chronic or recurrent hepatic encephalopathy causes marked hypertrophy and hyperplasia of cerebral astrocytes and to a lesser extent oligodendrocytes especially in the cerebral cortex. More severe changes are very rare, but neuronal degeneration and demyelination occur in rare instances of chronic hepatic encephalopathy.

Clinical features

The clinical features include changes of intellect, personality, emotions and consciousness with or without neurological signs, and when an episode develops acutely a precipitating factor may be found such as one of those listed in the information box (above). The earliest features are very mild, but as the condition becomes more severe, apathy, inability to concentrate, confusion, disorientation, drowsiness, slurring of speech and eventually coma develop. Convulsions sometimes occur. Examination usually shows a flapping tremor (asterixis), inability to perform simple mental arithmetic or draw objects such as stars, and, as the condition progresses, hyper-reflexia and bilateral extensor plantar responses. Hepatic encephalopathy should not be diagnosed when focal neurological signs are found, though these do occur rarely. Fetor hepaticus is usually present but is more a sign of liver failure and portasystemic shunting than of hepatic encephalopathy. Rarely, chronic hepatic encephalopathy gives rise to variable combinations of cerebellar dysfunction, Parkinsonian syndromes, spastic paraplegia and dementia.

Investigations

The diagnosis can usually be made clinically, but when doubt exists an electroencephalogram shows diffuse slowing of the normal alpha waves with eventual development of delta waves. The arterial ammonia is usually increased but this investigation is of little or no value as increased concentrations occur in the absence of hepatic encephalopathy.

Differential diagnosis

Hepatic encephalopathy needs to be differentiated mainly from other causes of confusion and coma unassociated with lateralising neurological signs. Head injury leading to **subdural haematoma** with headache and fluctuating consciousness is particularly important, and where this possibility exists computed tomography of the head should be carried out. **Drunkenness** can also be deceptive, but the plasma ethanol generally exceeds 30 mmol/l in the drunk and 50 mmol/l in the very drunk or comatose. Alcoholic patients with **delirium tremens** are usually alert rather than drowsy and are nervous, tremulous, confused and hallucinating, while those with **Wernicke's encephalopathy** are disorientated and show marked loss of recent memory capacity, confabulation, ophthalmoplegia and ataxia of the limbs. Young patients with liver disease and neuropsychiatric features may have **Wilson's disease. Primary psychiatric diseases** may need to be considered, and **hypoglycaemia** should be excluded when an encephalopathy has had an acute onset.

Management

Episodes of encephalopathy are common in cirrhosis and are usually readily reversed until the terminal stages occur. The principles are to treat or remove precipitating causes (see information box), to reduce or eliminate protein intake, and to suppress production of neurotoxins by bacteria in the bowel. **Dietary protein** is eliminated or reduced below 20 g/d and glucose (300 g/d) is given orally or parenterally in severe cases. As encephalopathy improves, dietary protein is increased by 10–20 g/d on alternate days to an intake of 40–60 g/d which is usually the limit in cirrhotic patients. **Lactulose** (15–30 ml 3 times daily) is a disaccharide which is taken orally and reaches the colon intact to be metabolised by colonic bacteria. The dose is increased gradually until the bowels are moving twice daily. It produces an osmotic laxative effect, reduces the pH of the colonic content thereby limiting colonic ammonia absorption, and promotes the incorporation of nitrogen into bacteria. **Lactitol** is a rather more palatable alternative to lactulose with a less explosive action on the bowels. **Neomycin** (1–4 g/4–6-hourly) is an antibiotic which acts by reducing the bowel flora. It can be used in addition to or as an alternative to lactulose if diarrhoea becomes troublesome. Neomycin is poorly absorbed from the bowel but sufficient gains access to the body to contraindicate its use when uraemia is present; it is less desirable than lactulose for long-term use. Ototoxicity is the main deleterious effect.

FULMINANT HEPATIC FAILURE

Fulminant hepatic failure is a rare syndrome in which hepatic encephalopathy, characterised by mental changes progressing from confusion to stupor and coma, results from sudden severe impairment of hepatic function. The syndrome is defined further as occurring within 8 weeks of onset of the precipitating illness, in the absence of evidence of pre-existing liver disease, to distinguish it from those instances in which hepatic encephalopathy represents a deterioration in chronic liver disease.

Aetiology

Any cause of acute liver damage can produce fulminant hepatic failure providing it is sufficiently severe (see information box p. 512). Acute viral hepatitis is the commonest cause, drugs (p. 517) being the next most frequent. Paracetamol, a very safe drug in therapeutic doses, is highly hepatotoxic in overdose (p. 518) and is a particularly important cause of fulminant hepatic failure in the UK. Otherwise fulminant liver failure occurs occasionally in pregnancy, in Wilson's disease, following shock or from poisons such as amanita phalloides, and rarely in extensive malignant disease in the liver.

Reye's syndrome

This is a rare acute encephalopathy in which cerebral oedema and severe fatty degeneration of the liver develop after an infectious illness such as influenza or chickenpox which has often been treated with aspirin. It occurs primarily in children and adolescents, but adults are affected occasionally.

Pathology

Extensive parenchymal necrosis is the most common lesion (p. 512). In fatal cases, less than 30% of the liver cells appear viable histologically and often few such cells are seen. Severe fatty degeneration is characteristic of fulminant hepatic failure caused by drugs such as tetracycline, pregnancy and Reye's syndrome.

Clinical features

Cerebral disturbance (encephalopathy) is the cardinal manifestation of fulminant hepatic failure. Its causes are uncertain (p. 508), but cerebral oedema is a particularly important factor. The earliest features are reduced alertness and poor concentration progressing through behavioural abnormalities such as restlessness, aggressive outbursts and mania, to drowsiness and coma. Confusion, disorientation, inversion of sleep rhythm, slurred speech, yawning, hiccoughing and convulsions may occur. A flapping 'hepatic' tremor (asterixis) of the extended hands is characteristic. Cerebral oedema is likely when unequal or abnormally reacting pupils, fixed pupils with spontaneous respiration, hypertensive episodes, hyperventilation, profuse sweating, local or general myoclonus, focal fits or decerebrate posturing is present. Papilloedema does not occur or is a late sign.

More general symptoms include weakness, nausea and vomiting. Right hypochondrial pain is only an occasional feature. Examination shows jaundice which develops rapidly and is usually deep in fatal cases. Jaundice is not seen in Reye's syndrome, and death occasionally occurs before it develops in other causes of fulminant hepatic failure. Fetor hepaticus, a sweet musty odour to the breath, may be present (p. 503). The liver may be enlarged initially but later becomes impalpable; disappearance of hepatic dullness on percussion indicates much shrinkage and a bad prognosis. Splenomegaly is uncommon and never prominent. Ascites and oedema occur in patients surviving a week or more and may be a consequence of fluid therapy. Other features are related to the development of complications which are considered below in the management of the condition.

Investigations

The plasma bilirubin reflects the degree of jaundice. Plasma aminotransferase activity is high initially but falls as liver damage progresses. Activity is particularly high after paracetamol overdose, reaching 100 to 500 times the normal activity. The prothrombin time rapidly becomes prolonged as coagulation factor synthesis fails; this is the laboratory test of greatest prognostic value and it should be measured twice daily. A progressive and marked prolongation carries a poor prognosis. Plasma albumin concentration remains normal unless the course is prolonged. Alkaline phosphatase activity is variable. White blood cell counts vary, leucocytosis occurring even in the absence of infection. The urine contains protein, bilirubin and urobilinogen.

Liver biopsy is contraindicated because of the severe haemostatic deficiency and because it rarely gives information required for management. Viral causes are sought serologically. Wilson's disease should always be considered (p. 529).

Complications

Life-threatening complications, some amenable to conservative therapy, can arise during management. They are listed in the information box.

Management

There is no specific treatment, but certain measures should be instituted as soon as a prolonging prothrombin time indicates severe liver damage or encephalopathy occurs. There should be close observation (see information box) in a high dependency or intensive care unit

so that complications can be corrected promptly. The patient's life is sustained in the hope that hepatic regeneration will take place or that liver transplantation can be undertaken.

Encephalopathy

Encephalopathy should be minimised by stopping all nitrogen intake and avoiding sedative drugs. Lactulose and neomycin, used in the encephalopathy of chronic liver disease, are of doubtful value and are not used. Restlessness and excitement can be treated with the smallest possible dose of a short-acting benzodiazepine such as midazolam, but such patients are often managed best by ventilation. The benzodiazepine antagonist flumazenil should be available if midazolam is used.

Cerebral oedema

This is a frequent cause of death and is difficult to diagnose as it often develops rapidly and rarely causes papilloedema. It can present as a sudden respiratory arrest. The appearance of the clinical features given in the information box (left) indicates the need for treatment. Mannitol 20% (1 g/kg body weight) should be infused intravenously over half an hour, and the dose repeated if the clinical signs are not reversed. Most patients need two doses (range 1–4) for any one episode of cerebral oedema. Mannitol is contraindicated in renal failure, and thiopentone can be used as alternative treatment. Intracranial pressure can be monitored but the placement of an intracranial pressure sensor is best done in an intensive care unit.

Nutrition

Calories are provided as glucose (300 g/d) either orally or into a large central vein as a 10–20% solution. The blood glucose should be measured 2-hourly in the severe phase because potentially fatal hypoglycaemia often occurs; its treatment may require large amounts of glucose. Estimations can be made simply by using dipstick tests, but checks using laboratory methods should also be made. Capillary blood is used for BM stix tests, and precautions to avoid infection, particularly wearing gloves, should be taken in obtaining samples. Fluid and electrolyte therapy depends on maintenance of accurate fluid balance records and on daily measurements of plasma urea, creatinine, sodium, potassium and bicarbonate. Saline is used cautiously to avoid sodium overload, and treatment is made easier by knowledge of the 24-hour urine sodium output. Potassium deficiency, which occurs readily, should be corrected.

Circulatory function

Patients have poor vasomotor control, and correction of abnormalities by intravenous infusion of fluid, colloid and blood requires regular recording of pulse, blood pressure, hourly urine output, and central venous pressure. N-acetycysteine (150 mg/kg then 10 mg/kg hourly) is given currently as its use has been reported to improve survival. The reasons for this are unknown but may include improved peripheral circulatory function.

Respiratory function

Respiratory failure requires early assisted ventilation.

Haemorrhage

Impaired haemostasis, due mainly to failure of coagulation factor production, can result in bleeding from any site. Bruising and purpura are common. Gastrointestinal bleeding from gastric erosions is frequent and can be prevented by H_2 receptor-blocking drugs (cimetidine 50 mg i.v. hourly or ranitidine 50 mg i.v. over 2 hours every 8 hours).

Infection

This is common and serious. As fever and leucocytosis may result solely from the liver disease itself, they are no guide and regular blood, urine and throat cultures and chest radiographs should be undertaken. Prophylactic antibiotics should not be used. If infection is strongly suspected, broad-spectrum antibiotics such as cefotaxime and augmentin may be given intravenously once specimens have been taken for culture.

Renal failure

This can develop and may require haemofiltration or dialysis.

Transplantation

Liver transplantation is indicated in patients with progressive liver failure (p. 535).

Prognosis

Encephalopathy identifies the development of fulminant hepatic failure, and worsening encephalopathy is associated with a worsening prognosis. Two-thirds of patients with minor signs survive, but only 10% with coma. Other important adverse prognostic factors include age under 10 years or over 40 years, hepatic damage due to non-A, non-B, non-C hepatitis or a drug, and jaundice for more than a week before the onset of encephalopathy. Adverse laboratory features include increasing prothrombin time, increasing plasma bilirubin, and uraemia

---

FURTHER READING

Grose R D, Hayes P C 1992 Review article: The pathophysiology and pharmacological treatment of portal hypertension. Alimentary Pharmacology and Therapeutics 6: 521–540

Lee W M 1993 Acute liver failure. New England Journal of Medicine 329: 1862–1872

Le Moine O, Adler M, Bourgeois Delhaye M et al 1992 Factors related to early mortality in cirrhotic patients bleeding from varices and treated by urgent sclerotherapy. Gut 33: 1381–1385

Record C O 1991 Neurochemistry of hepatic encephalopathy. Gut 32: 1261–1263

Runyon B A 1994 Care of patients with ascites. New England Journal of Medicine 330: 337–342

(p. 535). Those who recover from fulminant hepatic failure usually regain normal hepatic structure and function.

ACUTE PARENCHYMAL LIVER DISEASE

In acute parenchymal liver disease (acute hepatitis) there is sudden widespread liver damage in which variable numbers of hepatocytes undergo necrosis. These episodes are due mainly to hepatitis viruses or drugs. The causes are listed in the information box.

CAUSES OF ACUTE PARENCHYMAL LIVER DAMAGE

- **Viral infections**
  Hepatitis A virus
  Hepatitis B virus
  Hepatitis C virus
  Hepatitis D virus
  Non-A, non-B, non-C viruses
  Cytomegalovirus
  Epstein–Barr virus
  Herpes simplex virus
  Yellow fever virus

- **Post-viral infection**
  Reye's syndrome (aspirin association)

- **Non-viral infections**
  Leptospirae (usually *icterohaemorrhagiae*)
  Toxoplasma gondii
  Coxiella burneti

- **Drugs**
  See page 517

- **Poisons**
  Mushrooms (*Amanita phalloides*)
  Carbon tetrachloride

- **Metabolic**
  Wilson's disease
  Fatty change of pregnancy

- **Ischaemic**
  Shock
  Severe cardiac failure or tamponade
  Budd–Chiari syndrome

Pathology

The pathology in acute parenchymal liver damage depends on the cause of the damage. Lesions in acute virus hepatitis and in most instances of acute damage due to drugs are similar. Cell damage throughout the liver is the dominant abnormality particularly in centrilobular areas, though individual lobules are variably affected. Damaged hepatocytes have a swollen granular appearance, while dead ones become shrunken and deeply stained, sometimes losing their nuclei to form eosinophilic bodies. These bodies, originally described in yellow fever (Councilman bodies), are strong indicators of acute hepatitis. The lobules may be infiltrated with mononuclear cells. Polymorphonuclear leucocytes and fatty change are not seen. The portal tracts are enlarged and contain a predominantly mononuclear cell infiltrate. More severe damage is accompanied by collapse of the reticulin framework particularly between the central veins and portal tracts which become linked to one another; this is known as bridging or subacute hepatic necrosis. Very severe damage results in destruction of whole lobules (massive necrosis) and is the lesion underlying most instances of fulminant hepatic failure. Cholestasis is occasionally prominent. Less commonly, the main histological abnormality is fatty change. This occurs in damage due to carbon tetrachloride, tetracycline and a number of other toxins. Rarely, severe fatty degeneration of the liver is encountered in pregnancy or as a metabolic disturbance in Reye's syndrome in children (p. 510). Alcohol also causes fatty change but is not a cause of acute parenchymal liver damage (p. 527).

Differential diagnosis

Most patients with acute parenchymal liver disease are suffering from **viral hepatitis** which may be suggested by previous contact with a jaundiced person, travel to areas where viral hepatitis is endemic, parenteral drug abuse, a history of transfusion with blood or blood products or other exposure to blood. **Drug-induced hepatitis** must always be considered and enquiry should include drugs and herbal remedies taken by the patient (p. 517). **Wilson's disease** should be thought of in young patients who have had recurrent acute hepatitis of unknown cause or where haemolysis is present (p. 529), and **fatty liver of pregnancy** considered in the third trimester of pregnancy (above). Hepatic damage due to **circulatory causes** is recognised from associated shock, cardiac failure or tamponade. **Weil's disease** (p. 137) may cause severe jaundice and in contrast to viral hepatitis there is a polymorphonuclear leucocytosis and protein, blood and casts are found in the urine. The diagnosis is made by demonstrating a rise in specific antibodies, and leptospires may be isolated from the blood or urine. The development of **cholestatic hepatitis** can cause confusion with other causes of cholestasis, especially obstruction of a major bile duct. Features of an acute hepatitis at the onset of the illness, absence of features common in biliary obstruction (information box, p. 501), high plasma transaminase activity, a negative antimitochondrial test and lack of biliary dilatation on ultrasonography favour cholestatic hepatitis, but liver biopsy may be required.

VIRAL HEPATITIS

Viral hepatitis is almost always caused by one or other of the hepatitis viruses; hepatitis due to other viruses accounts for only about 1–2% of cases. All these viruses give rise to illnesses which are similar in their clinical and pathological features and which are frequently anicteric or asymptomatic. The information box on page 512 lists the causes.

Aetiology, epidemiology and prevention

Viral hepatitis is caused by four main agents (Table 8.10).

HEPATITIS A VIRUS

The hepatitis A virus (HAV) belongs to the picornavirus group of enteroviruses and it can be cultured though this is only done for research purposes. HAV is highly infectious, is spread by the faecal-oral route, and the sources in the community are persons incubating or suffering from the disease. Infected persons excrete viruses in the faeces for about 2–3 weeks before the onset of illness and for up to 2 weeks thereafter. Children are most commonly affected and conditions of overcrowding and poor sanitation facilitate spread. In occasional outbreaks water, milk and shellfish have been the vehicles of transmission. Though faeces is the usual source, a transient viraemia in the incubation period occasionally allows infection to be spread by blood and by homosexual activity, especially in men. A chronic carrier state, analogous to that for hepatitis B virus, does not occur.

Infection in the community is prevented best by improving social conditions, especially overcrowded and unhygienic situations. Individuals can be given substantial protection from infection by active immunisation with an inactivated virus vaccine (Havrix). Immediate protection can be provided by immune serum globulin if this is given soon after exposure to the virus. This can be considered for those at particular risk such as close contacts, the elderly, those with other major disease and perhaps pregnant women. Prevention can be effective in an outbreak of hepatitis, for example in a school or nursery, as injection of those at risk prevents secondary spread, for example to families. Persons travelling to endemic areas are protected best by vaccine, but where time is limited vaccine and immune serum globulin can be injected in separate sites to provide immediate and longer term protection. The protective effect of immune serum globulin is attributed to its anti-HAV content and those with anti-HAV in the blood are protected naturally.

Table 8.10   Features of the main hepatitis viruses

	A	B	C	D	E
Virus					
Group	Enterovirus	Hepadna	Flavivirus	Incomplete virus	—
Nucleic acid	RNA	DNA	RNA	RNA	RNA
Size (diameter)	27 nm	42 nm	30–38 nm	35 nm	27 nm
Incubation (weeks)	2–4	4–20	2–26	6–9	3–8
Spread					
Faeces	Yes	No	No	No	Yes
Blood	Uncommon	Yes	Yes	Yes	No
Saliva[1]	Yes	Yes	Yes	—	?
Sexual	Uncommon	Yes	Uncommon	Yes	?
Vertical	No	Yes	Uncommon	Yes	No
Chronic infection	No	Yes (5–10%)	Yes (> 50%)	Yes	?
Prevention					
Active	Vaccine	Vaccine	No	Prevented by prevention	No
Passive	Immune serum globulin	Hyperimmune serum globulin	No	of hepatitis B virus infection	No

[1] All body fluids are potentially infectious, though some (e.g. urine) are lowly infectious.

HEPATITIS B VIRUS

The hepatitis B virus (HBV) is the only hepadna virus causing infection in humans. It cannot yet be grown but can be transmitted to certain primates, such as the chimpanzee, in which it replicates. It comprises a capsule and a core containing DNA and a DNA polymerase enzyme. The virus and an excess of its capsular material circulate in the blood, where it can be identified (p. 492). Humans are the only source of infection. Individuals incubating or suffering from acute hepatitis are highly infectious for at least as long as the HBsAg is in the blood. Asymptomatic individuals and some patients with chronic liver disease have chronic infections and may carry the virus for life. These individuals are most infectious when markers of continuing viral replication such as HBeAg, viral DNA or DNA polymerase are present in the blood, and are least infectious when they are absent and anti-HBe is present.

Blood is the main source of infection and spread may follow transfusion of infected blood or blood products or injections with contaminated needles, a mode of spread most common among parenteral drug abusers who share needles. Blood and blood products used for transfusion are no longer a major source of infection provided that donor blood is tested for the virus, and less than 10% of all post-transfusion hepatitis is now attributable to the HBV. Only products such as albumin solutions and gammaglobulin which are pasteurised are wholly free of risk. Tattooing or acupuncture can also spread this disease if inadequately sterilised needles are used.

HBV can also cause sporadic infections which cannot be attributed to parenteral modes of spread. The means of non-parenteral transmission are uncertain, but the discovery of the HBsAg or viral DNA in body fluids such as saliva, urine, semen and vaginal secretions suggests many mechanisms. Close personal contact seems necessary for transmission of infection, and sexual intercourse, especially in male homosexuals, is an important route. The virus may be spread from mother to child; transmission at or soon after birth seems more likely than transplacental spread.

A recombinant hepatitis B vaccine containing HBsAg is available (Engerix) capable of producing active immunisation in 95% of normal individuals. The vaccine gives a high degree of protection and should be used particularly in those at special risk of infection who are not already immune as evidenced by anti-HBs in the blood. Those at special risk of infection are listed in the information box. The vaccine is ineffective in those already infected by the HBV.

Type B hepatitis can be prevented or minimised by the intramuscular injection of hyperimmune serum globulin prepared from blood containing anti-HBs. This should be given within 24 hours, or at most a week, of exposure to infected blood in circumstances likely to cause infection; these include accidental needle puncture, gross personal contamination with infected blood, oral ingestion or contamination of mucous membranes, or exposure to infected blood in the presence of cuts and grazes. Vaccine can be given together with hyperimmune globulin (active-passive immunisation).

HEPATITIS C VIRUS

The hepatitis C virus (HCV) is an RNA-containing flavivirus which cannot yet be grown but which can infect

AT RISK GROUPS MERITING HEPATITIS B VACCINATION IN LOWLY ENDEMIC AREAS

- **Parenteral drug abusers**
- **Homosexuals (male)**
- **Close contacts of infected individuals**
  Newborn of infected mothers
  Regular sexual partners
- **Patients on chronic haemodialysis**
- **Medical/nursing personnel**
  Dentists
  Surgeons/obstetricians
  Accident and emergency departments
  Intensive care
  Liver units
  Endoscopy units
  Oncology units
- **Laboratory staff handling blood**

primates such as the chimpanzee. Humans seem to be the sole source of infection, and inoculation with blood or blood products is the best recognised mode of transmission. HCV caused over 90% of post-transfusion hepatitis before serological tests allowed the screening of blood donors, and accounted for the high incidence of chronic hepatitis in haemophiliac patients. Screening of blood donors and heat treatment of coagulation factor concentrates should prevent infection of haemophiliacs in future. Parenteral drug abusers continue to be at high risk of HCV infection. Sporadic HCV infection also occurs but the modes of transmission are unknown. Sexual and vertical spread may occur but are probably uncommon. Neither active nor passive protection is available.

HEPATITIS D VIRUS

The hepatitis D virus (HDV) is an RNA-containing defective virus which has no independent existence; it requires the hepatitis B virus for replication and has the same sources and modes of spread as that virus. It can infect individuals simultaneously with the hepatitis B virus, or it can superinfect those who are already chronic carriers of the hepatitis B virus. Simultaneous infections give rise to acute hepatitis which is often severe but which is limited by recovery from the hepatitis B virus infection. Infections in individuals who are chronic carriers of the hepatitis B virus can cause acute infection with spontaneous recovery, and occasionally simultaneous cessation of the chronic hepatitis B virus infection occurs. Chronic infection with the hepatitis B virus and the HDV can also occur, and this frequently causes progressive chronic hepatitis and eventually cirrhosis.

HDV has been reported recently in the absence of HBV following liver transplantation, and how the HDV maintains itself in such instances is unknown.

HDV has a world-wide distribution but is endemic in parts of the Mediterranean basin, Africa and South America. It is transmitted mainly by close personal contact, occasionally by vertical transmission from mothers who also carry the hepatitis B virus in endemic areas, and by parenteral drug abuse outside endemic areas.

HEPATITIS E VIRUS

The HEV is an RNA-containing virus which is excreted in the stools and spreads by the faecal-oral route. It is found in countries where sanitation is poor and it is liable to cause large epidemics of water-borne hepatitis. Occasional cases in developed countries have occurred in persons who have visited endemic areas. Neither active nor passive protection is available.

NON-A, NON-B, NON-C HEPATITIS VIRUSES

Non-A, non-B (NANB) hepatitis was the term used previously to describe hepatitis thought to be due to a virus but not HAV or HBV. HCV and HEV are the main hepatitis viruses to emerge from this group. Further such virus(es) do exist, but the hepatitis viruses described above now account for the majority of hepatitis virus infections.

OTHER VIRUSES

Cytomegalovirus and Epstein–Barr virus infection causes abnormal liver function tests in most patients, and occasionally icteric hepatitis occurs. Herpes simplex is a rare cause of hepatitis in adults most of whom are immunocompromised, and yellow fever virus causes hepatitis in parts of the world where it is endemic.

Clinical features

Prodromal symptoms usually precede the development of jaundice by a few days to 2 weeks. They are the common manifestations of an acute infectious disease and include chills, headache and malaise. Gastrointestinal symptoms may be prominent; anorexia and distaste for cigarettes are frequent, and nausea, vomiting and diarrhoea may follow. A steady upper abdominal pain, occasionally severe, occurs as a result of stretching of the peritoneum over the enlarged liver. Initially physical signs are scanty; the liver is usually tender though not readily palpable, enlarged cervical lymph nodes may be found, and splenomegaly may occur, particularly in children. Patients with hepatitis B virus infection often have arthralgia during the prodrome, and occasionally a 'serum sickness syndrome' with skin rashes (including urticaria) and polyarthritis occurs.

Dark urine and a yellow tint to the sclerae herald the onset of jaundice. As obstruction to the biliary canaliculi develops, the jaundice deepens, the stools become paler, the urine darker, and the liver more easily palpable. At this time the appetite often improves and gastrointestinal symptoms diminish in intensity. Thereafter the jaundice usually recedes, the stools and urine regain their normal colour, the liver enlargement regresses, and in the course of 3–6 weeks the majority of patients recover.

Mild illnesses may run an anicteric course recognised by known contact with a definite case or by the association of vague gastrointestinal complaints or malaise with bilirubinuria and biochemical evidence of hepatic dysfunction.

Investigations

A plasma aminotransferase activity exceeding 400 U/l, even before jaundice develops, is the most striking abnormality. The plasma bilirubin reflects the severity of the jaundice, the alkaline phosphatase activity rarely exceeds 250 units/l unless marked cholestasis develops, and the albumin concentration is normal. Prolongation of the prothrombin time is a reliable indication of severe liver damage, and changes in the prothrombin time are a good guide to prognosis. Bilirubinuria is an early finding, occurring in the prodromal phase and usually continuing into the convalescent period. Mild proteinuria may be present. The white cell count is normal or low in uncomplicated cases, sometimes with a relative lymphocytosis; this is of some value in differentiation from Weil's disease (p. 137). Serological tests can identify hepatitis A, hepatitis B, cytomegalovirus and Epstein–Barr infection but are unreliable in acute hepatitis C infection. Tests for hepatitis E should soon be available generally. Differential diagnosis is discussed on page 513.

Complications

Many can occur but in practice serious complications are uncommon. The complications are listed in the information box.

Fatalities are rare and are attributable to the development of **fulminant hepatic failure** (p. 510). Return of symptoms and signs of acute hepatitis during recovery are characteristic of **relapsing hepatitis** and occur in 5–15% of patients. Asymptomatic 'biochemical' relapses with increases of plasma aminotransferase activity are even more common. Relapsing hepatitis does not imply a worse prognosis, because it resolves spontaneously. **Cholestatic viral hepatitis** can develop from the onset or during the course of the illness, with

---

COMPLICATIONS OF ACUTE VIRAL HEPATITIS

- Fulminant hepatic failure
- Relapsing hepatitis
   Biochemical
   Clinical
- Cholestatic hepatitis
- Posthepatitis syndrome
- Hyperbilirubinaemia (Gilbert's syndrome)*
- Aplastic anaemia
- Connective tissue disease
- Renal failure
- Henoch–Schönlein purpura
- Papular acrodermatitis
- Chronic hepatitis
- Cirrhosis (hepatitis B, C and D viruses)
- Hepatocellular carcinoma

*Gilbert's syndrome may be brought to light by follow-up of viral hepatitis.

---

more severe jaundice of a clinically and biochemically obstructive type which may follow a prolonged course. Liver biopsy shows the features of hepatitis with prominent cholestasis and no evidence of chronic liver damage. This cholestatic illness may continue for many months but the prognosis is good.

Debility for 2–3 months is common following clinical and biochemical recovery. Sometimes, particularly in anxious patients, there may be prolonged malaise, anorexia, nausea and right hypochondrial discomfort without clinical or biochemical evidence of liver disease. This syndrome, which may be exacerbated by too frequent clinical and biochemical assessment, is known as the **posthepatitis syndrome** and is not due to liver disease.

Chronic hepatitis and **cirrhosis** develop when chronic hepatitis B virus infection occurs, with or without hepatitis D virus superinfection or hepatitis C virus infection. These chronic viral infections predispose to hepatocellular carcinoma. **Unconjugated hyperbilirubinaemia** is sometimes found after acute viral hepatitis. Most instances are probably due to pre-existing Gilbert's syndrome but occasional cases can be attributed to the viral infection.

Systemic complications are rare and include **aplastic anaemia**. This seems most common after HCV and HEV virus infection and may not become apparent for up to a year after the hepatic illness. Other complications are mostly related to hepatitis B virus infection and include **connective tissue disease**, particularly polyarteritis nodosa, and **renal damage** such as glomerulonephritis. **Henoch–Schönlein purpura** and **papular acrodermatitis** have been reported in children.

Management

There is no specific treatment for acute viral hepatitis. Only more severely affected patients require care in hospital so that developing fulminant hepatic failure can be detected at an early stage. The posthepatitis syndrome is treated by reassurance.

Bed-rest

When symptoms are marked, bed-rest should be advised, the patient rising to the toilet if desired. Thereafter younger patients may be up and about, taking care only to avoid exhaustion. For those in whom the risks of hepatitis are greater, bed-rest should be continued until symptoms and signs have disappeared and liver function tests have returned substantially towards normal. These patients include those over 50 years, the pregnant, and patients with other major disease.

Diet

A nutritious diet containing 2000–3000 kcal daily is given. This is often not tolerated initially owing to anorexia and nausea, in which case a light diet supplemented by fruit drinks and glucose is usually acceptable. The content of the diet is dictated largely by the patient's wishes; however, a good protein intake should be encouraged. If vomiting is severe, intravenous fluid and glucose may be required.

Drugs

Drugs should be avoided especially in severe hepatitis because many are metabolised in the liver. This applies especially to sedative and hypnotic agents. Alcohol must be avoided during the illness but can be taken once clinical and biochemical recovery have occurred.

Oral contraceptives may be resumed after clinical and biochemical recovery.

Prognosis

The overall mortality of acute viral hepatitis is about 0.5%. Very few otherwise well patients under 40 years old die, but mortality reaches about 3% in patients over 60 years. Mortality may be much higher in patients with other serious diseases, such as carcinomas or lymphomas, or chronic liver disease. Hepatitis E virus infections can also cause a high mortality in pregnant women.

DRUGS, TOXINS AND THE LIVER

The liver is the main organ in which drugs are metabolised and consequently is important in determining the effects of drugs in the body. Liver disease may alter the capacity of the liver to metabolise drugs and unexpected toxicity may occur when patients with liver disease are given drugs in normal doses. Drugs themselves can damage the liver and there is increasing recognition of the many forms of hepatic damage attributable to drugs.

HEPATIC DRUG METABOLISM

Hepatic drug metabolism involves the conversion of fat-soluble (non-polar) drugs into water-soluble (polar) metabolites which can be excreted in the bile if they are relatively large molecules or in the urine if they are relatively small. This conversion is mediated by a group of mixed-function oxidase enzymes, the best known of which is cytochrome P_{450} located in the smooth endoplasmic reticulum of the liver cells. Drugs which are already highly polar undergo little or no metabolic change. Two types of reaction take place during hepatic drug metabolism:

Type I reactions

Type I reactions mainly involve oxidation or reduction and provide drugs with sites suitable for subsequent Type II reactions. Type I reactions usually increase drug polarity. They have very variable effects on pharmacological activity, as they can produce or reduce drug activity or leave it unchanged.

Type II reactions

Type II reactions involve conjugation, usually with glucuronide, sulphate or glutathione, and lead to the production of highly polar metabolites with no pharmacological activity. These metabolites are excreted in the bile or urine. The rate at which drugs are metabolised by the mixed function oxidase enzymes varies in relation to **genetic factors, nutritional factors, induction or inhibition of the enzymes**, and the **number of drugs** given simultaneously. Drug metabolism varies considerably between individuals mainly because of genetic factors. Nutritional factors are important as malnutrition reduces enzyme activity and reduces the rate of drug metabolism. Certain factors, especially drugs, can increase enzyme activity (enzyme induction) or inhibit enzyme activity in the liver, and they can alter the rate of drug metabolism significantly (Table 8.11). Drugs metabolised by these enzymes compete with one another for enzyme sites, and the rate of metabolism of an individual drug is reduced when another drug is given simultaneously.

Other factors

Factors other than hepatic enzyme activity affect drug metabolism by the liver, the most important of these being **hepatic blood flow**. The ability of the liver to extract drugs from the blood as it flows through the

Table 8.11 Drugs increasing or decreasing mixed-function oxidase enzyme activity in the liver

Increased activity (Enzyme induction)	Decreased activity
Alcohol (ethanol)	Cimetidine
Barbiturates	Isoniazid
Carbamazepine	Ketoconazol
Diphenylhydantoin	Propoxyphene
Ethanol	
Griseofulvin	
Primidone	
Rifampicin	

Table 8.12 Factors indicating the need for caution in drug therapy in patients with liver disease

Clinical	Investigation
Jaundice	Hypoalbuminaemia
Ascites	Prolonged prothrombin time
Encephalopathy	Oesophageal varices
Fetor hepaticus	
Palpable spleen	
Malnutrition	

sinusoids varies considerably. Some drugs are so highly extracted that liver blood flow is the dominant factor determining the rate of their elimination from the blood. These drugs are said to have a high first-pass clearance by the liver, and their rate of metabolism is greatly reduced by any reduction in hepatic blood flow or diversion of blood through or past the liver. This effect is most striking for highly extracted drugs given by mouth, for all drugs absorbed from the intestine normally flow to the liver in the portal vein. The rate of removal from the blood of lowly extracted drugs is dependent mainly on the rate of their metabolism in the liver cells. Other factors affecting the rate of removal of a drug from the blood includes its **volume of distribution** in the body and the extent of its **binding to plasma proteins** as these in turn partly determine its availability to the liver cells.

DRUG THERAPY IN LIVER DISEASE

Drug therapy is particularly likely to produce undesirable effects in liver disease because of impaired hepatic metabolism and because portasystemic shunting of blood diverts drugs away from the liver when portal hypertension is present. There is no way of predicting which patients will suffer undesirable effects, and over-caution can easily deprive patients of useful therapy. Rather, certain general principles should be observed. Drugs should only be used where they are clearly indicated, smaller than usual doses should be given initially, frequency of administration should be determined from effects, and particular care should be exercised in patients with poor liver function, signs of portal hypertension or a previous portasystemic shunt operation (Table 8.12). Particular precautions in patients with varices (p. 503), ascites (p. 507) or encephalopathy (p. 509) are given elsewhere.

HEPATOTOXICITY OF DRUGS

Liver damage due to drugs is so common that the possibility should be considered whenever liver damage occurs rather than trying to remember lists of hepatotoxic drugs. Acute liver damage due to drugs is well recognised but other forms of hepatotoxicity have become recognised increasingly in recent years. These manifestations are listed in the information box below.

MANIFESTATIONS OF DRUG HEPATOTOXICITY

- **Acute hepatic damage**
  Acute hepatitis
  Cholestatic hepatitis
  Cholestasis

- **Abnormal liver function tests**

- **Hepatic fibrosis**

- **Chronic hepatitis**

- **Cirrhosis**

- **Hepatic vascular damage**
  Sinusoidal dilatation/peliosis hepatis
  Budd–Chiari syndrome
  Veno-occlusive disease
  Hepatoportal sclerosis

- **Neoplasia**
  Adenoma
  Hepatocellular carcinoma
  Haemangloma/haemangiosarcoma

Acute hepatic damage

Acute hepatic damage is the best recognised form of drug-induced liver injury. Such damage may be **dose-related and predictable**, or it may be **unrelated to dose and unpredictable or idiosyncratic**. Predictable drug hepatotoxicity is mediated biochemically, though its occurrence and severity can be modified by factors affecting the drug metabolising enzymes such as alcohol (Table 8.11) or nutritional status.

Paracetamol in therapeutic doses is mainly conjugated to produce glucuronide and sulphate, but a small amount is metabolised to potentially toxic intermediates which are conjugated with glutathione to form mercapturic acid which is not toxic. Paracetamol in large doses produces toxic intermediates in amounts sufficient to deplete glutathione stores and damage the liver.

Alcoholic individuals can suffer increased liver damage because alcohol increases the activity of the drug-metabolising enzymes.

Unpredictable or idiosyncratic drug hepatotoxicity has usually been attributed to immunological injury and may be associated with autoantibody production as in major forms of halothane hepatitis. However, in most patients evidence for immunological injury is scanty or indirect, and unpredictable drug hepatotoxicity is increasingly being attributed to biochemical mechanisms, for example in minor forms of halothane hepatitis and in isoniazid hepatitis. The clinical features usually develop within about 3 months of starting treatment. Jaundice is often present and the illness is usually indistinguishable from acute viral hepatitis. Cholestatic features (p. 501) can be prominent with certain drugs and biliary obstruction may be suspected particularly where this is associated with upper abdominal pain as in erythromycin toxicity. Liver function tests show high transaminase activity reflecting hepatitis, and variably increased alkaline phosphatase activity reflecting cholestasis. A few drugs cause almost pure cholestasis. Diagnosis depends on relating the illness to taking the offending drug and on excluding other causes for the illness. Procedure for diagnosis is listed in the information box below.

THE DIAGNOSIS OF ACUTE DRUG-INDUCED LIVER DISEASE

- Consider the possibility of a drug
- Tabulate drugs taken
  Prescribed by doctor
  Self-administered
- Relate drugs to the onset of the illness
- Look for pre-existing liver disease
  Clinical examination
  Previous liver investigations
- Consider alternative causes
  Viral hepatitis—serological tests
  Biliary disease—ultrasound
  　　　　　　—cholecystogram
- Observe the effects of stopping the suspected drugs
- Liver biopsy
  Suspected pre-existing liver disease
  Failure to improve
- Challenge tests with drugs—never (hardly ever)

Abnormal liver function tests

Abnormal liver function tests are usually found incidentally and, even when due to a drug, may resolve in spite of continued therapy. The need to withdraw a drug suspected of causing abnormal liver function tests depends on the severity of the abnormalities, whether or not they become worse, and the importance of the drug to the patient.

Chronic liver disease

Drugs can cause chronic hepatitis, hepatic fibrosis and cirrhosis, and this should be suspected whenever chronic liver disease develops in a patient receiving long-term drug therapy. Recognition of drug-induced chronic liver disease depends on excluding other known causes of liver disease and is usually not helped by liver biopsy, as the histological abnormalities caused by drugs are variable and non-specific. Indeed, the histological features can mimic those of more common forms of liver disease, for example amiodarone causes appearances indistinguishable from alcoholic damage. Clinical and biochemical evidence of disease may not occur until liver damage is very advanced as with methotrexate, which causes hepatic fibrosis; patients receiving long-term treatment with methotrexate require occasional liver biopsy. Recognition of drug-induced chronic liver disease is important because drug withdrawal leads to improvement and full recovery occurs, provided that cirrhosis has not developed.

Hepatic vascular damage

This is an uncommon form of liver damage usually caused by oestrogens, androgens, anabolic agents or drugs used in the chemotherapy of neoplastic disease. Oral contraceptives occasionally cause hepatic vein thrombosis, and chemotherapeutic agents can cause occlusion of the central hepatic veins giving rise to features identical to the Budd–Chiari syndrome and veno-occlusive disease (p. 532). Peliosis hepatis (blood-filled cysts) and sinusoidal dilatation are usually asymptomatic but can cause intraperitoneal bleeding or portal hypertension, and damage to portal veins in the terminal portal tracts can cause portal hypertension.

Neoplastic changes

Oestrogens, androgens and anabolic agents occasionally cause neoplastic changes. Oral contraceptives have been associated with development of hepatic adenomas, and the other agents may induce malignant tumours.

HEPATIC TOXINS

Alcohol is the most common environmental hepatotoxin (p. 526). Others include the amatoxins in mushrooms (usually *A. phalloides*) which can cause fulminant hepatic failure, pyrollizidine alkaloids in several plants used to make teas which are associated with veno-occlusive disease (p. 532), aflatoxins in fungi which can cause acute liver damage and possibly hepatocellular carcinoma, and occasionally material used in herbal remedies. Industrial hepatotoxins rarely cause liver damage if proper precautions are taken. They include carbon tetrachloride, which causes liver failure due to fatty change, and vinyl chloride, which induces periportal fibrosis and portal hypertension, and rarely hepatic tumours.

FURTHER READING

Catterall A P, Murray-Lyon I M 1992 Strategies for hepatitis B immunisation. Gut 33: 576–579

Finlayson N D C 1994 Drugs and the liver. Medicine International 22: 455–459

Lau J Y N, Wright T L 1993 Molecular virology and pathogenesis of hepatitis B. Lancet 342: 1335–1340

Lee W 1993 Review article: Drug-induced hepatotoxicity. Alimentary Pharmacology and Therapeutics 7: 477–485

Rizzetto M (ed.) 1991 Hepatitis C. European Journal of Gastroenterology and Hepatology 3: 569–606

Wright T L, Lau J Y N 1993 Clinical aspects of hepatitis B infection. Lancet 342: 1340–1344

CHRONIC PARENCHYMAL LIVER DISEASE

Chronic hepatitis and cirrhosis are the two main forms of chronic parenchymal liver disease. They are closely related because some forms of chronic hepatitis progress to cirrhosis.

Aetiology

There are numerous causes of chronic parenchymal liver disease and these are listed in the information box. The most common are alcohol, hepatitis B virus and hepatitis C virus infection, autoimmune hepatitis and primary biliary cirrhosis. No cause can be found in 30% of patients (cryptogenic cirrhosis). Haemochromatosis accounts for about 5% of patients; all other causes are rare.

Alcohol

The mechanism whereby alcohol damages the liver is unknown, but it is now accepted as a direct liver toxin in man (p. 526).

Infection

Chronic hepatitis B virus infection is an important cause of chronic liver disease though its incidence shows marked geographic variation. Failure to recover from hepatitis B virus infection is probably due to a deficient immune response, and the severity of subsequent chronic liver disease is related to the activity of viral replication in the liver. Superinfection with the hepatitis D virus increases the chances of progressive chronic hepatitis in such patients. The hepatitis C virus is also

CAUSES OF CHRONIC LIVER DISEASE

- **Infection**
  Hepatitis B virus
  Hepatitis C virus
  Hepatitis D virus
- **Toxins**
  Alcohol
  Drugs
- **Biliary obstruction**
  Primary biliary cirrhosis
  Primary sclerosing cholangitis
  Secondary biliary cirrhosis
      Stricture, stone, neoplasm
- **Metabolic diseases**
  Haemochromatosis
      Primary or secondary
  Wilson's disease
  Alpha$_1$-antitrypsin deficiency
- **Fibrocystic disease**
- **Nutritional**
  Intestinal bypass surgery (obesity)
- **Hepatic congestion**
  Budd–Chiari syndrome
  Veno-occlusive disease
  Cardiac failure
- **Unknown cause**
  Autoimmune hepatitis
  Cryptogenic cirrhosis

an important cause of chronic liver disease. The hepatitis A virus does not cause chronic liver disease.

Immunological factors

Some patients with chronic liver disease of unknown cause have abnormal serum autoantibodies (p. 493). Though the autoantibodies themselves are not cytotoxic, their presence suggests that liver damage may be produced by abnormal immune mechanisms. Lymphocytes sensitised to liver cells are currently favoured as the mediators of liver damage.

Metabolic disorders

These include the excess hepatic deposition of iron in haemochromatosis and of copper in Wilson's disease. Alpha$_1$-antitrypsin deficiency may cause chronic liver disease in children or in adults, but most other metabolic conditions involving the liver manifest themselves first in childhood, e.g. glycogen storage disease and fibrocystic disease (cystic fibrosis).

Drugs

Chronic hepatitis and cirrhosis occur in some patients on long-term drug treatment (p. 519).

Cholestasis

Prolonged obstruction anywhere in the biliary system can cause cirrhosis. In primary biliary cirrhosis there is obstruction from damage to interlobular bile ducts. Cirrhosis from large-duct obstruction may occur with biliary strictures or in sclerosing cholangitis but not with neoplastic lesions because survival is too short.

Congestion

Prolonged hepatic congestion can eventually cause cirrhosis. This is rare as death usually occurs before cirrhosis develops. Congestion may be due to hepatic venous outflow obstruction (p. 532) or chronic heart failure.

Malnutrition

Malnutrition is probably not primarily responsible for cirrhosis though it often occurs secondarily in patients with cirrhosis. Permanent liver damage is not found in marasmus or kwashiorkor but malnutrition may be important in cirrhosis following intestinal bypass surgery for gross obesity.

Pathology

Chronic hepatitis

Three main types of chronic hepatitis are recognised histologically. Persistent hepatitis predominantly affects the portal tracts, aggressive hepatitis affects the portal tracts and the parenchyma, and lobular hepatitis predominantly affects the parenchyma. These histological appearances are not related to particular causes of liver disease, but in general persistent hepatitis is mild, aggressive hepatitis is more severe and progressive, and lobular hepatitis is often relapsing.

Persistent hepatitis

There is an infiltration of chronic inflammatory cells confined to the portal tracts which may be expanded or show short fibrous septa extending into the parenchyma. Changes in the hepatocytes are absent or slight, and usually comprise small foci of liver cell necrosis with inflammatory cell infiltration (spotty necrosis). Lobular architecture is normal and cirrhosis rarely develops.

Aggressive hepatitis

In this form of chronic hepatitis both the portal tracts and the parenchyma are involved, lobular architecture becomes distorted, and cirrhosis often develops. The portal tract infiltration of mononuclear cells extends irregularly into the surrounding parenchyma and the swollen liver cells become isolated in the inflammatory cell infiltrate. This process of hepatocyte destruction, called 'piecemeal necrosis', leads to septum formation linking portal tracts and central veins. The ensuing disruption of lobular architecture is accompanied by the development of regenerative nodules and eventually cirrhosis. Changes in the rest of the parenchyma are variable and resemble persistent hepatitis. These changes do not occur diffusely and may be more advanced in some areas than others.

Lobular hepatitis

In this the histological features are identical to those of acute viral hepatitis.

Cirrhosis

The changes in cirrhosis affect the whole liver but not necessarily every lobule. They include gradually progressive widespread death of liver cells associated with inflammation and fibrosis leading to loss of the normal lobular liver architecture. Destruction of the liver architecture causes distortion and loss of the normal hepatic vasculature with the formation of portal-systemic vascular shunts, and in the formation of nodules rather than lobules as surviving hepatocytes proliferate. The evolution of cirrhosis is gradual and progressive, and consequently cirrhotic livers have an infinitely variable appearance limiting the usefulness of anatomical classifications. The current anatomical classification includes **micronodular cirrhosis**, characterised by regular connective tissue septa, regenerative nodules approximating in size to the original lobules (1 mm in diameter) and involvement of every lobule, and **macronodular cirrhosis** in which the connective tissue septa vary in thickness and the nodules show marked differences in size with large ones containing histologically normal lobules. Micronodular cirrhosis tends to evolve gradually into macronodular cirrhosis, and intermediated mixed forms are seen.

CHRONIC HEPATITIS

Gradually resolving acute hepatitis must not be confused with chronic hepatitis. There is no certain way to avoid this either by clinical assessment or investigation, including liver biopsy, during the first 6 months of the illness. Accordingly, a diagnosis of chronic hepatitis should only be made firmly once liver disease has been present on clinical or other grounds for at least 6 months and a liver biopsy has then been done. Furthermore, the main chronic hepatitis syndromes are not clearly separated from one another, and patients with intermediate illnesses are encountered (Fig. 8.12).

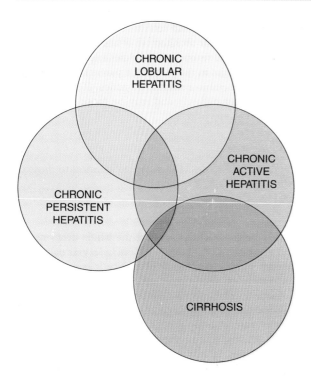

Fig. 8.12 Relationship between chronic hepatitis and cirrhosis.

CHRONIC PERSISTENT HEPATITIS (CPH)

Chronic persistent hepatitis is a mild illness comprising fatigue, poor appetite, fatty food intolerance and upper abdominal discomfort, especially over the liver. The condition may be asymptomatic and recognised only because of a previous episode of acute hepatitis or because of biochemical tests undertaken for other reasons. Examination is usually normal but may show slight hepatomegaly. There are no features of chronic liver disease.

The plasma bilirubin is normal or slightly raised, the plasma aminotransferase is raised variably, and the alkaline phosphatase is normal. Plasma albumin and globulin concentrations are normal. One or other of the causes of chronic liver disease may be present, but autoantibodies are not found in the blood. Liver biopsy shows persistent hepatitis (above).

Differentiation should be made from the post-hepatitis syndrome (p. 516), Gilbert's syndrome (p. 500), and from sclerosing cholangitis associated with ulcerative colitis or Crohn's disease (p. 544). The prognosis is usually excellent. The patient should be reassured, and no treatment is required. Patients should be kept under occasional review as progression to cirrhosis occurs rarely.

AUTOIMMUNE HEPATITIS

This form of chronic hepatitis occurs most often in women, particularly in the second and third decades of life, and it produces the most florid manifestation of disease, though mild forms are being found increasingly.

Clinical features

The onset is usually insidious with fatigue, anorexia and jaundice. In about a quarter of patients the onset is acute, resembling viral hepatitis, but normal resolution does not occur. Other features include fever, arthralgia and epistaxis. Amenorrhoea is the rule.

On examination, the general health is at first good. Jaundice is mild to moderate or occasionally absent, but signs of chronic liver disease, especially spider telangiectasia and hepatosplenomegaly, are usually present. Sometimes a 'Cushingoid' face with acne, hirsutism and pink cutaneous striae, especially on the thighs and abdomen, are present. Bruises may be seen.

Though liver disease usually dominates the clinical syndrome, many **associated conditions** occur in florid autoimmune hepatitis emphasising its essentially systemic nature. These include migrating polyarthritis, a variety of rashes, most non-specific but including inflammatory papules and urticaria, lymphadenopathy, thyroid disorders such as Hashimoto's thyroiditis, thyrotoxicosis and myxoedema, Coombs-positive haemolytic anaemia, pleurisy, transient pulmonary infiltrates, ulcerative colitis and glomerulonephritis. Some patients have Sjögren's syndrome (p. 919).

Investigations

Liver function tests vary with the activity of the disease. Active inflammation is reflected by the plasma aminotransferase activity, and the severity of liver damage by the plasma albumin concentration and the prothrombin time. Aminotransferase activity is often increased more than 10 times in relapses of florid disease, and hypoalbuminaemia and marked hyperglobulinaemia are common. Hyperglobulinaemia is due mainly to marked increases of IgG. The plasma bilirubin reflects the degree of jaundice but usually does not exceed 100 μmol/l (6 mg/dl). The plasma alkaline phosphatase activity reflects the degree of intrahepatic cholestasis. Antinuclear antibodies are found in half the patients, smooth muscle antibodies in two-thirds, and antimitochondrial antibodies in 15%. Liver biopsy shows aggressive hepatitis with or without cirrhosis.

Differential diagnosis

Differentiation from acute viral hepatitis can be impossible when autoimmune hepatitis presents with an acute exacerbation. An acute hepatitis showing unremitting activity (plasma aminotransferase activity increased at least ten-fold, or increased at least five-fold with plasma gammaglobulin increased at least twice for at least 10 weeks) is likely to be due to autoimmune hepatitis, but the diagnosis cannot be considered certain until a liver biopsy is examined at least 6 months after the onset.

Management

Treatment with corticosteroids is life-saving in autoimmune hepatitis particularly during exacerbations of active symptomatic disease. Initially, prednisolone 30 mg/d is given orally and the dose reduced gradually as the patient and liver function tests improve. Maintenance therapy is required for at least 2 years after liver function tests have become normal, and withdrawal of treatment should not be considered unless a liver biopsy is also normal. Side-effects from prednisolone are uncommon at a maintenance dose of 10 mg/d or less; azathioprine 50–100 mg/d orally may be added to the therapy to allow the dose of prednisolone to be reduced to this level. Treatment reduces the 5-year mortality to about 10%. Corticosteroids are less important in asymptomatic autoimmune hepatitis with mild biochemical and histological activity.

Prognosis

The disease occurs in exacerbations and remissions, and most patients eventually develop cirrhosis and its complications (p. 524). Hepatocellular carcinoma is uncommon. About a half of patients with symptoms die of liver failure within 5 years if no treatment is given, but this falls to about 10% with therapy.

CHRONIC HEPATITIS DUE TO HEPATITIS B AND C VIRUS INFECTION

This form of chronic hepatitis occurs most often in men over 30 years of age. It may come to attention when an episode of acute viral hepatitis fails to resolve, but more often there is no history of an acute episode and the disease is found by chance or when features of cirrhosis develop.

Clinical features

Symptoms are usually non-specific and examination often reveals little of note. Hepatomegaly is the most common abnormality, jaundice is slight or absent, and fewer than a third of patients have spider telangiectasia or splenomegaly at presentation. Systemic features other than arthralgia are uncommon.

Investigations

These show moderate increases of plasma bilirubin and aminotransferase activity and minor increases of alkaline phosphatase. Hypoalbuminaemia occurs with more advanced liver damage, and hyperglobulinaemia is not marked. Serology shows evidence of hepatitis B or C virus infection (p. 492). Patients with hepatitis B virus infection may have a hepatitis D virus superinfection. Autoantibody tests give negative results. Liver biopsy shows aggressive hepatitis with or without cirrhosis. Hepatocytes containing HBsAg may have a ground glass appearance on H&E stains, and special stains can be used to demonstrate hepatitis B virus antigens.

Prognosis

The progression of the disease is slow but usually relentless, particularly in patients with evidence of active hepatitis B replication (e.g. HBeAg) or combined hepatitis B and D virus infections, leading eventually to cirrhosis. Hepatocellular carcinoma is liable to develop in the long term.

Management

Interferon is the only drug of use in chronic hepatitis B and hepatitis C virus infection. Treatment in hepatitis B virus infection occasionally eliminates the virus, but more often causes loss of HBeAg and appearance of anti-HBe which is associated with diminished viral replication and reduced hepatic inflammatory activity. Patients with relatively recent infections and with evidence of active viral replication (p. 492) respond to treatment best. Treatment in hepatitis C virus infection often returns liver function tests to normal but a half of patients relapse even after treatment for up to a year.

CHRONIC HEPATITIS DUE TO OTHER CAUSES

These forms of chronic hepatitis can be due to a variety of causes, or no cause can be found in which case they are often assumed to be due to as yet unrecognised hepatitis virus infection. The clinical and biochemical features vary considerably. It is important to detect disease due to drugs, which usually remits on withdrawal of the drug, and to Wilson's disease, which requires specific treatment (p. 529).

CHRONIC LOBULAR HEPATITIS (CLH)

Chronic lobular hepatitis is an uncommon condition in which relapses and remissions of acute hepatitis occur over a period exceeding 6 months. The illness is initially indistinguishable from acute viral hepatitis in about half the patients and is initially insidious in the other half. Jaundice and hepatomegaly can be found in relapses but signs of chronic liver disease (below) are rare. Liver function tests show the features of an acute hepatitis and about half the patients have hyperglobulinaemia though hypoalbuminaemia is rare. The disease is associated with hepatitis B virus or hepatitis C virus infection in some patients and with antinuclear, smooth muscle and anti-mitochondrial antibodies in others. Liver biopsy shows the features of acute viral hepatitis. Most patients need no treatment, but those with active disease and auto-antibodies respond well to corticosteroids as for auto-immune hepatitis. The prognosis is good as progression to cirrhosis does not occur.

CIRRHOSIS OF THE LIVER

Hepatic cirrhosis can occur at any age and often causes prolonged morbidity. It manifests itself particularly in younger adults and is an important cause of premature death.

Clinical features

These vary greatly and include any combination of the manifestations described below. None is related specifically to particular causes of cirrhosis though florid spider telangiectasia, gynaecomastia and parotid enlargement are more common in alcoholic cirrhosis, and pigmentation is most striking in haemochromatosis and in cirrhosis associated with prolonged cholestasis. Autopsy experience shows that cirrhosis may be entirely asymptomatic, and in life it may be found incidentally at surgery or with minimal features such as isolated hepatomegaly. Frequent complaints include weakness, fatigue, muscle cramps, weight loss and non-specific digestive symptoms such as anorexia, nausea, vomiting, upper abdominal discomfort and gaseous abdominal distension. Otherwise, clinical features are due mainly to hepatic insufficiency and portal hypertension. They are listed in the information box.

Hepatomegaly is common in cirrhosis, but progressive hepatocyte destruction and fibrosis reduce liver size as the disease progresses. The liver is often hard, irregular and painless. Jaundice is usually mild when it appears first and is due primarily to failure to excrete bilirubin. Mild haemolysis occurs in cirrhosis but is not important in the development of jaundice. Ascites results from inadequate sodium and water excretion (p. 507). Jaundice and ascites are signs of advanced liver damage and are late signs of cirrhosis. Cirrhosis is associated with an increased peripheral blood circulation and a reduced visceral circulation which becomes more marked as the disease progresses. Palmar erythema is a consequence of these changes and it can be seen early in the disease,

---

CLINICAL FEATURES OF HEPATIC CIRRHOSIS

- **Hepatomegaly**
- **Jaundice**
- **Ascites**
- **Circulatory changes**
  Spider telangiectasia, palmar erythema, cyanosis
- **Endocrine changes**
  Loss of libido, hair loss
  Men: gynaecomastia, testicular atrophy, impotence
  Women: breast atrophy, irregular menses, amenorrhoea
- **Haemorrhagic tendency**
  Bruises, purpura, epistaxis, menorrhagia
- **Portal hypertension**
  Splenomegaly, collateral vessels, variceal bleeding, fetor hepaticus
- **Hepatic (portasystemic) encephalopathy**
- **Other features**
  Pigmentation, digital clubbing, low-grade fever

---

but it is of limited diagnostic value as it occurs in any condition associated with a hyperdynamic circulation as well as in some normal people. Spider telangiectasia are due to associated arteriolar changes and comprise a central arteriole, from which small vessels radiate and which occasionally raises the skin surface (Fig. 8.13). They vary in size from 1–2 mm to 1–2 cm in diameter, they are usually found only on the parts of the body above the nipples, and they can occur early in the disease. One or two small spider telangiectasia can be found in about 2% of healthy people and they can occur transiently in greater numbers in the third trimester of pregnancy, but otherwise they are strong indicators of

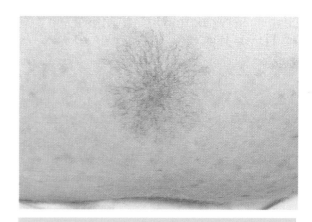

Fig. 8.13 Large spider telangiectasia with central arteriole and radiating capillaries in a patient with hepatic cirrhosis.

liver disease. Pulmonary arteriovenous shunts also develop leading to hypoxaemia and eventually to central cyanosis, but this is a late feature. Endocrine changes are noticed more readily in men who show loss of male hair distribution and testicular atrophy. Gynaecomastia is infrequent and occurs most often in alcoholic liver disease, but can also be due to drugs such as spironolactone. Easy bruising becomes more frequent as cirrhosis advances and epistaxis is common, sometimes severe, and can mimic upper gastrointestinal bleeding if much blood is swallowed. Splenomegaly, collateral vessels and fetor hepaticus are features of portal hypertension, which occurs in more advanced disease (p. 503). Haemorrhoids are often said to be more common in portal hypertension but there is no evidence for this. Evidence of hepatic encephalopathy also becomes increasingly common with advancing disease (p. 509). Nonspecific features of chronic liver disease include pigmentation, clubbing of the fingers and toes and low-grade fever. Dupuytren's contracture is traditionally associated with cirrhosis, especially that due to alcohol, but the evidence for the association is weak.

Investigations

Biochemical investigations are used to assess the activity and severity of liver disease (p. 488). The plasma transaminase reflects the activity of the disease which is usually low in established cirrhosis. Transaminase activity can be much higher during the evolution of cirrhosis, particularly that caused by autoimmune hepatitis (p. 522). The plasma alkaline phosphatase reflects the severity of cholestasis and is highest in biliary forms of cirrhosis. The plasma bilirubin and albumin concentrations and the vitamin K corrected prothrombin time reflect the severity of liver damage. All these tests may be normal in patients with well-compensated inactive disease (p. 488). Biochemical and serological tests are also used to determine the nature of the disease causing the cirrhosis (p. 488). Imaging is required for assessing the structural effects of the disease on the liver and is particularly useful in identifying complications such as hepatocellular carcinoma, portal hypertension and ascites (p. 494). Liver biopsy establishes the diagnosis of cirrhosis (Fig. 8.14). and may show the cause, but it is only needed when clinical observation and less invasive investigations have not established the diagnosis.

Differential diagnosis

This is listed in the information box.

Complications

Cirrhosis is associated with the development of several important complications which have serious effects on

DIFFERENTIAL DIAGNOSIS OF CIRRHOSIS RELATED TO PRESENTATIONS

Hepatomegaly
- Focal lesions
  Carcinoma
     Primary (cirrhosis)
     Secondary
  Other malignant disease
  Abscess
  Cysts
- Infiltration
  Myeloproliferative diseases
  Lymphoproliferative diseases
  Sarcoidosis
  Amyloidosis
- Congestion
  Cardiac failure
  Constrictive pericarditis
  Budd–Chiari syndrome
  Veno-occlusive disease
- Tropical
  Malaria
  Schistosomiasis
  Kala azar

Splenomegaly
- Portal hypertension (cirrhosis)
- Myeloproliferative disease
- Lymphoproliferative disease

Jaundice (p. 498)

Gastrointestinal bleeding (p. 503)

Ascites (p. 507)

Encephalopathy (p. 508)

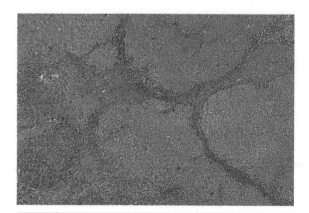

Fig. 8.14 Histology of cirrhotic liver revealing regeneration nodules surrounded by dense connective tissue.

the prognosis of the disease. These complications are listed in the information box below.

COMPLICATIONS OF HEPATIC CIRRHOSIS

- Portal hypertension
- Ascites
- Hepatic (portasystemic) encephalopathy
- Renal failure
- Infection
- Hepatocellular carcinoma

Infection

Cirrhosis predisposes to bacterial infection, and this susceptibility increases as the disease progresses. Several factors contribute, including poor nutrition, alcohol abuse and cellular and humoral immune deficiencies caused by cirrhosis itself. *Infection should be suspected in any patient whose condition deteriorates for no obvious reason,* and while infections can occur anywhere, *bacteraemia, spontaneous bacterial peritonitis* (p. 508) *and infection with unusual or occasionally multiple organisms is common.*

Management

No treatment can reverse cirrhosis or even ensure that no further progression occurs, but medical therapy can promote improved general health and alleviate symptoms. The main objectives are to detect treatable causes, to prevent and correct malnutrition, to manage chronic cholestasis (p. 531) and to treat complications (see information box above).

Aetiological factors

Treatable conditions such as alcohol abuse, drug ingestion, haemochromatosis and Wilson's disease should always be sought. Relief of biliary obstruction will prevent secondary biliary cirrhosis.

Nutrition

In the absence of encephalopathy or ascites, a high energy (3000 kcal/d), protein-rich (80–100 g/d) diet should be advised. Fat intake need not be restricted where cholestasis is not a feature. Alcohol must be forbidden. When a good diet is taken, vitamins and other supplements are not required.

Drug therapy

Patients with cirrhosis are liable to develop toxic reactions to drugs owing to their unpredictable ability to metabolise drugs, and drugs are used with special care (p. 518).

Liver transplantation

Liver transplantation should be considered in all patients with chronic liver disease who develop liver failure (p. 534).

Prognosis

The overall prognosis in cirrhosis is poor because many patients present with advanced disease or serious complications carrying a high mortality (see information box left). Overall, only 25% of patients survive 5 years from diagnosis, but where liver function is good 50% survive for 5 years and 25% for up to 10 years. The prognosis is more favourable where the cause of cirrhosis can be corrected, as in alcohol abuse, haemochromatosis and Wilson's disease.

Laboratory tests give only a rough guide to prognosis in individual patients. Deteriorating liver function as evidenced by jaundice, ascites or encephalopathy indicates a poor prognosis unless a treatable cause such as infection is found. Increasing plasma bilirubin, falling plasma albumin, marked hypoalbuminaemia (below 25 g/l), marked hyponatraemia (below 120 mmol/l) not due to diuretic therapy, and a prolonged prothrombin time are all bad prognostic signs. The course of cirrhosis is uncertain, as unforeseen complications may lead to death unexpectedly.

ALCOHOLIC (ETHANOLIC) LIVER DISEASE

In Western societies alcohol is the most common cause of liver disease.

Metabolism

Alcohol is metabolised almost exclusively in the liver. It is first converted to acetaldehyde, mainly by the mitochondrial enzyme alcohol dehydrogenase but also by the mixed-function oxidase enzymes of the smooth endoplasmic reticulum (p. 517). Alcohol is a powerful inducer of the mixed-function oxidases, increasing their activity and thereby increasing ability to metabolise alcohol and many drugs metabolised by these enzymes. Acetaldehyde is converted in turn to acetate by acetaldehyde dehydrogenase, and acetate is metabolised by the Krebs cycle enzymes.

Pathogenesis

The hepatic lesions of alcoholic liver disease (below) are attributable directly to alcohol. The risk of developing alcoholic liver disease is related directly to the amount of alcohol of any kind ingested and becomes apparent at daily intakes above 30 g (3 units) in men and 20 g (2 units) in women. More than five years of drinking

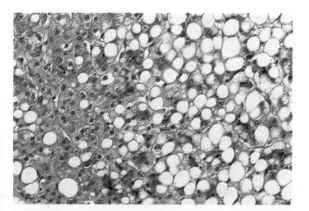

Fig. 8.15 Histology of alcoholic fatty liver. The fatty change (steatosis) is evident as fat globules within the cytoplasm of the liver cells.

and usually more than ten years is required to produce alcoholic cirrhosis, and a steady daily intake is more hazardous than intermittent drinking.

The mechanisms whereby alcohol produces individual liver lesions are poorly understood. Fatty change is attributed to an increased production and decreased use of fatty acids in the liver cells following the conversion of alcohol to acetaldehyde by alcohol dehydrogenase. The development of alcoholic hepatitis, fibrosis and cirrhosis is much more obscure. Biochemical mechanisms involving the production of toxic metabolites, called adducts, during the conversion of acetaldehyde to acetate and immune reaction to liver cells altered by alcohol may be involved in these forms of liver damage.

Pathology

Alcohol causes several different lesions in the liver which can occur together in any combination.

Fatty change

This is the most common lesion and may affect from a few to almost all hepatocytes (Fig. 8.15). It is regarded as readily reversible when alcohol is withdrawn, but it nevertheless reflects a severe metabolic derangement.

Alcoholic hepatitis

This is much more common than the severe clinical illness also called alcoholic hepatitis and is characterised by foci of necrotic hepatocytes infiltrated and surrounded by polymorphonuclear leucocytes. Related hepatocytes may be pale and swollen, and some contain dense eosinophilic masses called Mallory's hyaline. Alcoholic hepatitis is often a precursor of cirrhosis.

Mallory's hyaline

This is not pathognomonic of alcohol abuse as it occurs in other liver diseases such as primary biliary cirrhosis, Wilson's disease and liver damage due to some drugs such as amiodarone.

Central hyaline sclerosis

This is characterised by fibrosis around central veins and is a sign of severe alcohol abuse. It is often a prelude to cirrhosis and portal hypertension.

Cirrhosis

This is usually initially micronodular (p. 521), often with active inflammation in fibrous septae and marked pericellular fibrosis, and later becomes macronodular.

Siderosis

Mild siderosis is common in alcoholic liver disease. More severe siderosis should lead to consideration of associated haemochromatosis.

Clinical features

Alcoholic liver disease manifests as a clinical spectrum ranging from non-specific symptoms with few or no physical abnormalities to advanced cirrhosis. The ready availability of laboratory investigations can also reveal alcoholic liver damage in patients with other diseases or in asymptomatic people undergoing medical examination. This spectrum is often divided into four syndromes, but in reality these overlap considerably and the various pathological changes can coexist in the same liver. The clinical syndromes are listed in the information box below.

CLINICAL SYNDROMES OF ALCOHOLIC LIVER DISEASE

- **Fatty liver**
  Nonspecific symptoms
  Hepatomegaly
- **Hepatitis**
  Severe illness
  Malnutrition
  Jaundice
  Hepatomegaly
  Ascites
  Encephalopathy
- **Cholestasis**
  Jaundice
  Abdominal pain
  Hepatomegaly (often tender)
- **Cirrhosis**

Investigations

Investigations aim to establish alcohol abuse, exclude alternative causes of liver disease, and assess the severity of liver damage. The clinical history from the patient, relatives and friends is most important in establishing alcohol abuse, its duration and its severity. Biological markers of alcohol abuse suggest and support the history of alcohol abuse, and the most universally used of these are peripheral blood macrocytosis in the absence of anaemia and increased plasma γ-glutamyl transferase (p. 490). Absence of these markers does not exclude alcohol abuse. Unexplained rib fractures on a chest X-ray are also associated with alcohol abuse. Investigation of the extent of liver damage (p. 488) and possible alternative causes are given elsewhere (p. 520).

Management

Cessation of alcohol intake is the most important treatment and without this all other therapies are of limited value. Lifelong abstinence is the best advice and is essential for those with more severe liver damage. Good nutrition is also important and feeding via a fine-bore nasogastric tube may be needed in severely ill patients. Treatment for complications such as encephalopathy (p. 509), ascites (p. 507) and variceal bleeding (p. 503) may be required.

Prognosis

The single most important prognostic factor is the patient's ability to **stop drinking alcohol**. General health and longevity are improved when this occurs irrespective of the form of alcoholic liver disease. Alcoholic fatty liver has a generally good prognosis and usually disappears after about 3 months of abstinence. Alcoholic hepatitis has a significantly worse prognosis because about a third of patients die in the acute episode if liver function is poor as evidenced by a prothrombin time sufficiently prolonged to preclude liver biopsy. Patients may progress to cirrhosis after recovery, particularly if drinking continues. Alcoholic cirrhosis often presents with a serious complication such as variceal bleeding or ascites, and only about a half of patients survive 5 years from presentation. Most who survive the initial illness and who become abstinent survive beyond 5 years.

HAEMOCHROMATOSIS

Haemochromatosis is a condition in which the total body iron is increased with the excess iron deposited in and damaging several organs including the liver. It may be primary or secondary to other diseases.

Hereditary (primary) haemochromatosis

This is a disease in which the total body iron reaches 20–60 g (normal 4 g). Iron is deposited widely in the body. The important organs involved are the liver, pancreatic islets, endocrine glands and heart. In the liver,

iron deposition occurs first in the periportal hepatocytes, extending later to all hepatocytes. The gradual development of fibrous septa leads to the formation of irregular nodules, and finally regeneration results in macronodular cirrhosis. An excess of liver iron can occur in alcoholic cirrhosis but this is mild by comparison with haemochromatosis (p. 527).

Aetiology

Hereditary haemochromatosis is caused by an increased absorption of dietary iron. This inability to limit iron absorption is inherited as an autosomal recessive associated with the HLA-B3, B7 and B14 histocompatibility antigens. Homozygotes alone develop the disease, but other factors must also be important as at least 90% of patients are male. Iron loss in menstruation and pregnancy may protect females.

Clinical features

The disease usually presents in men aged 40 years or over with manifestations of hepatic cirrhosis (p. 524), especially hepatomegaly, diabetes mellitus or heart failure. Leaden-grey skin pigmentation due to excess melanin occurs especially in exposed parts, axillae, groins and genitalia, hence the term 'bronzed diabetes'. Impotence, loss of libido, testicular atrophy and arthritis with chondrocalcinosis due to calcium pyrophosphate deposition are also common. Increasingly, early clinical features are being recognised, particularly tiredness, fatigue and arthropathy.

Investigations

The serum ferritin is greatly increased and the plasma iron is increased with a highly saturated plasma iron binding capacity (p. 491). Computed tomography may show features suggesting excess hepatic iron. The diagnosis is confirmed by liver biopsy which shows heavy iron deposition and hepatic fibrosis which may have progressed to cirrhosis. The iron content of the liver can be measured directly.

Management

Treatment is by weekly venesection of 500 ml (250 mg iron) until the serum iron is normal; this may take 2 years or more. Thereafter venesection is continued as required to keep the serum ferritin normal. Other therapy includes that for cirrhosis and diabetes mellitus. Other first-degree family members should be investigated by measurement of the serum ferritin and plasma iron binding capacity saturation and any with asymptomatic disease treated.

Prognosis

Hereditary haemochromatosis has a good prognosis compared with other forms of cirrhosis, as three-quarters of patients are alive 5 years after the diagnosis. This is probably because liver function is usually well preserved at diagnosis and improves with therapy. Hepatocellular carcinoma is the main cause of death occurring in about a third with cirrhosis irrespective of therapy.

Secondary haemochromatosis

Many conditions, including chronic haemolytic disorders, sideroblastic anaemia, other conditions requiring multiple blood transfusion (generally over 50 l), porphyria cutanea tarda, dietary iron overload (p. 560) and occasionally alcoholic cirrhosis, are associated with widespread secondary siderosis. The features are similar to haemochromatosis, but the history and clinical findings point to the true diagnosis. Some patients are heterozygotes for the primary haemochromatosis gene and this may contribute to the development of iron overload.

WILSON'S DISEASE (HEPATO-LENTICULAR DEGENERATION)

This is a rare but important condition in which the total body copper is increased with excess copper deposited in and damaging several organs.

Aetiology and pathology

Wilson's disease is inherited as an autosomal recessive disorder leading to abnormal copper metabolism. Normally, dietary copper is absorbed from the stomach and proximal small intestine and is rapidly taken into the liver where it is stored and incorporated into caeruloplasmin which is secreted into the blood. The accumulation of excessive copper in the body is ultimately prevented by its excretion, the most important route being via the bile. The precise nature of the metabolic defect in Wilson's disease is unknown, but it results in a failure of biliary copper excretion causing accumulation in the body. There is almost always a failure of synthesis of caeruloplasmin also, though some 5% of patients with Wilson's disease have a normal plasma caeruloplasmin concentration. The amount of copper in the body at birth is normal, but thereafter it increases steadily and the organs most affected are the liver, the basal ganglia of the brain, the eyes, the kidneys and the skeleton.

Clinical features

Symptoms usually arise between the ages of 5 and 30 years. Hepatic disease occurs predominantly in child-

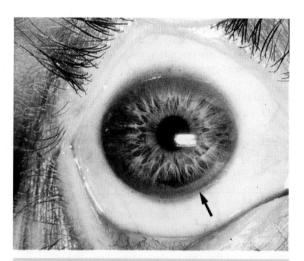

Fig. 8.16 Kayser–Fleischer rings at the junction of the cornea and sclera (arrow) in a patient with Wilson's disease.

hood and early adolescence, while neurological damage causes basal ganglion syndromes and dementia in later adolescence. These manifestations can occur alone or simultaneously. Other manifestations include haemolysis, renal tubular damage and osteoporosis, but these are virtually never presenting features.

Kayser–Fleischer rings

These are the most important single clinical clue to the diagnosis and they can be seen in most patients presenting in or after adolescence albeit sometimes only by slit-lamp examination. Appearances indistinguishable from Kayser–Fleischer rings are found rarely in other forms of chronic hepatitis and cirrhosis. Kayser–Fleischer rings are characterised by greenish-brown discolouration of the corneal margin appearing first at the upper periphery (Fig. 8.16). They eventually disappear with treatment.

Liver disease

This can manifest in many ways which are not specific. Episodes of acute hepatitis which are sometimes recurrent can occur, especially in children, and may progress to fulminant hepatic failure. Chronic persistent hepatitis and chronic active hepatitis can also develop, and eventually cirrhosis with liver failure and portal hypertension. Recurrent acute hepatitis of unknown cause, especially accompanied by haemolysis, or chronic liver disease of unknown cause in a patient under 40 years old suggests Wilson's disease.

Neurological disease

Clinical features include a variety of extrapyramidal features, particularly tremor, choreoathetosis, dystonia, parkinsonism and dementia.

Investigations

A low serum caeruloplasmin (p. 491) is the best single laboratory clue to the diagnosis. However, advanced liver failure from any cause can reduce the serum caeruloplasmin, and occasionally the serum caeruloplasmin is normal in Wilson's disease. Other features of a disordered copper metabolism should therefore be sought; these include a low serum copper concentration, a high urine copper excretion, and a very high hepatic copper content (p. 491). Patients with Wilson's disease fail to incorporate radioactive copper into caeruloplasmin, but this test is almost never needed.

Management

The copper-binding agent penicillamine is the drug of choice in Wilson's disease. The dose given must be sufficient to produce cupriuresis and most patients require 1.5 g/d (range 1–4 g). The dose can be reduced once the disease is in remission, but treatment must continue for life and care must be taken to ensure that reaccumulation of copper does not occur. Young women should continue to take the drug during pregnancy. Serious toxic effects of penicillamine are rare in Wilson's disease. If they do occur, trientine dihydrochloride (1.2–2.4 g/d) is the next drug of choice. Liver transplantation may be needed for fulminant hepatic failure and for advanced cirrhosis with liver failure.

Prognosis

The prognosis of Wilson's disease is excellent provided treatment is started before there is irreversible damage; the long-term complication of hepatocellular carcinoma does not occur as it does in haemochromatosis. Siblings of patients with Wilson's disease must be investigated and treatment should be given to any who have the disease even if it is asymptomatic.

ALPHA₁-ANTITRYPSIN DEFICIENCY

Alpha$_1$-antitrypsin (A1AT) is an α_1-globulin protease inhibitor (Pi) produced by the liver (p. 491). Several forms of A1AT are produced, and one of these (PiZ) cannot be secreted into the blood by the liver cells owing to its chemical structure. Homozygous individuals (PiZZ) have low plasma A1AT concentrations, though globules containing A1AT are found in the liver, and this form of A1AT deficiency is associated with hepatic and pulmonary (p. 334) disease. Liver disease includes cholestatic jaundice in the neonatal period (neonatal

hepatitis) which can resolve spontaneously, chronic hepatitis and cirrhosis in adults, and in the long term the development of hepatocellular carcinoma. There are no clinical features distinguishing liver disease due to A1AT deficiency from other causes of liver disease, and the diagnosis is made from the low plasma A1AT concentration and the PiZZ phenotype. A1AT-containing globules can be demonstrated in the liver but this is not necessary for making the diagnosis. Occasionally patients with liver disease and minor reductions of plasma A1AT concentrations have A1AT phenotypes other than PiZZ, such as PiMZ or PiSZ, but the relation of these to the cause of the liver disease is uncertain. No treatment other than that for any chronic liver disease is available and the patients are advised strongly to abandon cigarette smoking.

BILIARY CIRRHOSIS

Biliary cirrhosis results from prolonged obstruction anywhere between the small interlobular bile ducts and the papilla of Vater.

PRIMARY BILIARY CIRRHOSIS

This disease affects predominantly women who usually present clinically in middle age. The ready availability of diagnostic tests has shown that it is a relatively common form of cirrhosis.

Aetiology and pathology

The cause of primary biliary cirrhosis is unknown but immune reactions causing liver damage are suspected. Autoantibodies and immune complexes are found in the blood, cellular immunity is impaired, and abnormal cellular immune reactions have been described. The primary pathological lesion is a chronic granulomatous inflammation damaging and destroying the interlobular bile ducts, and progressive inflammatory damage with fibrosis spreading from the portal tracts to the liver parenchyma which eventually leads to cirrhosis and its complications (p. 524).

Clinical features

Nonspecific symptoms such as tiredness, fatigue and arthralgia are common and may precede diagnosis for a long time. Pruritus is the commonest initial complaint pointing to hepatobiliary disease and it may precede jaundice by months or years. Bile acids have been suggested as the cause of pruritus but this remains unproved. Jaundice is occasionally a presenting feature but pruritus is usually also present. Although there may be abdominal discomfort, the abdominal pain, fever and rigors which are often a feature of large bile duct obstruction do not occur. Diarrhoea from malabsorption of fat, and pain and tingling in the hands and feet due to lipid infiltration of peripheral nerves, occasionally occur. Bone pain or fractures because of osteomalacia from malabsorption or osteoporosis (hepatic osteodystrophy) can be prominent and distressing features in advanced disease.

Initially patients are well nourished but considerable weight loss can occur as the disease progresses. Scratch marks may be found. Jaundice is only prominent late in the disease and can become intense. Xanthomatous deposits occur in a minority especially around the eyes, in the hand creases and over the elbows, knees and buttocks. Hepatomegaly is virtually constant, and splenomegaly becomes increasingly common as portal hypertension develops. The complications of liver failure and portal hypertension arise as the disease progresses (p. 502).

Associated diseases

Autoimmune and connective tissue diseases occur with increased frequency in primary biliary cirrhosis, particularly the sicca syndrome (p. 919) and thyroid diseases. Hypothyroidism should always be considered in patients with fatigue.

Asymptomatic disease

Asymptomatic primary biliary cirrhosis has become recognised increasingly owing to the ready availability of liver function tests and autoantibody tests. This condition is found particularly in patients with the associated diseases mentioned above.

Investigations

Liver function tests show the pattern of cholestasis (p. 500). The antimitochondrial antibody is present in over 95% of patients, and when it is absent histological evidence for the diagnosis is needed and cholangiography by endoscopic retrograde cholangiopancreatography (ERCP, p. 495) is required to exclude other biliary disease. The antinuclear and smooth muscle antibodies may be present, and autoantibodies found in associated diseases may also be found. Ultrasound examination shows no sign of biliary obstruction (p. 494), and liver biopsy is required only in doubtful cases.

Management

No specific therapy is available. Corticosteroids, azathioprine and penicillamine have all been tried, but none is effective and all may have serious adverse effects.

Ursodeoxycholic acid is under trial currently and has the advantage of fewer side-effects.

Transplantation (p. 534) should always be considered once liver failure has developed. Treatment may be needed for the consequences of cholestasis, particularly for pruritus, malabsorption and cholangitis.

Pruritus

This is the main symptom demanding relief. It is achieved best with the anion-binding resin cholestyramine, which reduces the bile acids in the body by binding them in the intestine and increasing their excretion in the stool. A dose of 4–16 g/d orally is used. The powder is mixed in orange juice and the main dose (8 g) is taken with breakfast when maximal duodenal bile acid concentrations occur. Cholestyramine may bind other drugs in the gut (e.g. anticoagulants) which should therefore be taken one hour before the binding agent.

Cholestyramine is sometimes ineffective, especially in complete biliary obstruction. Terfenadine, an antihistamine, rifampicin, or ultraviolet light may help in such patients. Methyltestosterone (25 mg/d sublingually) or, for women, norethandrolone (10 mg 8-hourly) may also be effective, though both reversibly increase cholestasis at the canalicular membrane and jaundice worsens.

Malabsorption

Prolonged cholestasis is associated with steatorrhoea and malabsorption of fat-soluble vitamins and calcium. Steatorrhoea can be reduced by limiting fat intake to 40 g/d. Monthly injections of vitamin K_1 (10 mg), vitamin D (calciferol 1 mg/d; alfacalcidol 1 μg/d orally) and calcium supplements should also be given, the last as effervescent calcium gluconate (2–4 g/d). The effervescent preparation, however, contains much sodium and, where there is fluid retention, calcium gluconate alone should be used.

SECONDARY BILIARY CIRRHOSIS

This develops after prolonged large duct biliary obstruction due to gallstones, bile duct strictures and sclerosing cholangitis (p. 501). Carcinomas rarely cause secondary biliary cirrhosis as survival is limited. There is chronic cholestasis with episodes of ascending cholangitis or even liver abscess (p. 535). Digital clubbing is common and xanthomas and bone pain may develop. Cirrhosis, ascites and portal hypertension are late features. Cholangitis requires treatment with antibiotics, which can be given continuously if attacks occur frequently.

HEPATIC VENOUS OUTFLOW OBSTRUCTION

Obstruction to hepatic venous blood flow can occur in the small central hepatic veins, in the large hepatic veins, in the inferior vena cava or in the heart. The clinical features depend on the cause and on the speed with which obstruction develops, but congestive hepatomegaly and ascites are features in all patients.

VENO-OCCLUSIVE DISEASE

Widespread occlusion of central hepatic veins is the characteristic of this condition. Pyrollizidine alkaloids in Senecio and Heliotropium plants used to make teas are the best known causes, but cytotoxic drugs and hepatic irradiation are increasingly recognised causes. The clinical features, investigation and management of veno-occlusive disease are similar to the Budd–Chiari syndrome (below).

BUDD–CHIARI SYNDROME

Aetiology and pathology

This is an uncommon condition in which obstruction occurs in the larger hepatic veins and sometimes the inferior vena cava. The cause cannot be found in about a half of patients. In the others, thrombosis may be due to haematological diseases including primary pro-liferative polycythaemia, paroxysmal nocturnal hae-moglobinuria and antithrombin III, protein C and protein S, deficiencies. Pregnancy and oral contra-ceptives, obstruction due to tumours, particularly car-cinomas of the liver, kidneys or adrenals, congenital venous webs and occasionally inferior vena caval stenosis are the main other causes. Hepatic congestion, mainly in the centrilobular areas, is the main consequence initially; centrilobular fibrosis develops later and eventually cir-rhosis in those who survive long enough.

Clinical features

Sudden venous occlusion causes the rapid development of upper abdominal pain which is often severe, marked ascites and occasionally fulminant hepatic failure. More gradual occlusion causes gross ascites and often upper abdominal discomfort. Hepatomegaly, often with ten-derness over the liver, is almost always present. Peri-pheral oedema occurs only when there is inferior vena cava obstruction. Features of cirrhosis and portal hyper-tension develop in those who survive long enough.

Investigations

Liver function tests vary considerably depending on the presentation and can show the features of acute hepatitis (p. 490) when the onset is rapid. Ascitic fluid analysis typically shows a protein concentration above 25 g/l in the early stages but is often lower later in the disease. Ultrasound examination may reveal obliteration of the hepatic veins and reversed flow in the portal vein. Iso-tope imaging may show preservation of the caudate lobe, as it often has a separate venous drainage not involved in the disease. Hepatic venography shows occlusion of the hepatic veins and any inferior vena cava involvement, and liver biopsy demonstrates centrilobular congestion with fibrosis depending upon the duration of the illness.

Management

Predisposing causes should be removed or treated as far as possible, and where recent thrombosis is suspected treatment with streptokinase followed by heparin and oral anticoagulation are considered. Ascites is treated medically initially but often has limited success, in which case a LeVeen shunt (p. 507) or a portal-systemic shunt can be used. Direct surgical treatment of the venous obstruction is rarely possible but occasionally a web can be resected or an inferior caval stenosis dilated. Pro-gressive liver failure is an indication for liver trans-plantation.

Prognosis

The prognosis is generally poor, particularly when the onset is sudden; a third to two-thirds of patients die within a year and few live more than 5 years. Some patients survive to develop cirrhosis.

CARDIAC DISEASE

Hepatic damage due primarily to congestion is always present in cardiac failure from any cause, but the clinical features are usually dominated by the cardiac disease. Occasionally the hepatic features are more prominent.

Acute hepatitis

Rapidly developing cardiac failure sometimes causes a syndrome suggesting an acute hepatitis. This occurs most often following myocardial infarction, decom-pensation of any chronic myocardial disease or cor pul-monale, or rapidly developing cardiac tamponade. The patient is generally very ill with an enlarged tender liver, with or without jaundice, and liver function tests show-ing an acute hepatitis. The correct diagnosis is made by recognising that the cardiac output is low, the jugular venous pressure is high, and that other signs of cardiac disease are present.

Ascites

Cardiac failure sometimes causes hepatomegaly and ascites disproportionate to the degree of peripheral oedema, and hence can mimic ascites due to liver disease. A high ascites protein concentration may suggest hepatic venous outflow obstruction. Constrictive pericarditis (p. 311) is particularly likely to mislead, as a normal heart size points away from heart disease. A raised jugular venous pressure is the most important single clue to the diagnosis. Rarely, long-standing cardiac failure and hepatic congestion cause cardiac cirrhosis, and this is suggested by hard irregular hepatomegaly or a palpable spleen due to portal hypertension.

Management

The treatment of these patients is that of the underlying causative disease.

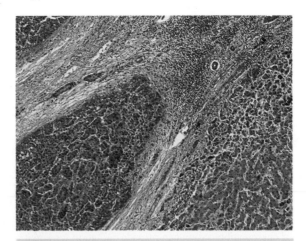

Fig. 8.17 Histology of hepatocellular carcinoma (left) arising within cirrhotic liver (right).

FURTHER READING

Blendis L M 1992 Review article: The treatment of alcoholic liver disease. Alimentary Pharmacology and Therapeutics 6: 541–548

Day C, Bassendine M F 1992 Genetic predisposition to alcoholic liver disease. Gut 33: 1444–1447

Edwards C Q, Kushner J P 1993 Screening for hemochromatosis. New England Journal of Medicine 328: 1616–1620

Mistry P, Seymour C A 1992 Primary biliary cirrhosis—from Thomas Addison to the 1990s. Quarterly Journal of Medicine 299: 185–196

Stremmel W, Riedel H D, Niederau C, Strohmeyer G 1993 Pathogenesis of genetic haemochromatosis (Review). European Journal of Clinical Investigation 23: 321–329

Yarze J C, Martin P, Munoz S J, Friedman L S 1992 Wilson's disease: current status. American Journal of Medicine 92: 643–654

TUMOURS OF THE LIVER

HEPATOCELLULAR CARCINOMA (HEPATOMA)

Hepatocellular carcinoma is the principal primary malignant liver tumour. Its incidence shows great geographic variation, being common in Africa and South East Asia but rare in temperate climates.

Aetiology

Chronic hepatitis B virus infection has emerged as the most important cause world-wide and chronic carriers of the virus have a much increased risk of the disease (p. 523). Chronic hepatitis C virus infection is also an important cause though the risk may not be so high as for hepatitis B virus. Aflatoxin contamination of foods may be important in tropical countries (p. 519). Cirrhosis and male sex are the main factors related to hepatocellular carcinoma in temperate climates. Cirrhosis is present in 80% of cases and may be of any type, but hepatocellular carcinoma appears most commonly in haemochromatosis and alcoholic cirrhosis, dominantly male diseases, and rarely in primary biliary cirrhosis, which mainly affects women. Other aetiological factors include exposure to toxins such as thorotrast and arsenic which usually produce angiosarcomas but which may also cause hepatocellular carcinomas. Oestrogens, androgens and anabolic steroids may cause adenomas or, rarely, hepatocellular carcinomas.

Pathology

Macroscopically, the tumour may comprise a single mass or multiple nodules or occasionally be diffusely invasive. Microscopically, the tumour is made up of trabeculae of well-differentiated cells resembling hepatocytes (Fig. 8.17). Bile secretion by tumour cells may be seen and is diagnostic. Intravascular invasion and growth is often a feature and may occur into the portal vein or the inferior vena cava. Spread is mainly to regional lymph nodes, the lungs and bones. Deterioration in a patient with cirrhosis should always lead to suspicion of hepatocellular carcinoma.

Clinical features

These include weakness, anorexia, weight loss, fever, abdominal pain, a large irregular liver or an abdominal mass, and ascites. Hepatocellular carcinomas are vascular and a bruit may be heard over the liver or intra-abdominal bleeding may occur.

Investigations

Metabolic abnormalities include polycythaemia, hyper-calcaemia, hypoglycaemia and porphyria cutanea tarda. Liver function tests give variable non-specific results. A greatly increased or rising serum α-fetoprotein is virtually diagnostic (p. 491). Imaging usually reveals one or more filling defects, laparoscopy may reveal the tumour and the diagnosis can be confirmed by liver aspiration or biopsy.

Management

Surgical removal requires a tumour confined to one lobe in the absence of cirrhosis and is rarely feasible, but the possibility should always be considered. Embolisation or chemoembolisation can provide palliation for hepatic pain. Chemotherapy has been disappointing. Liver transplantation can be considered for small tumours (p. 535).

Prognosis

The outlook is very poor. Surgery alone gives prolonged survival, but only about 10% of patients are suitable for this therapy. Few patients survive beyond a year.

FIBROLAMELLAR HEPATOCELLULAR CARCINOMA

This rare variant differs from other hepatocellular carcinomas in that it occurs in young adults, equally in males and females, and is not associated with cirrhosis or hepatitis B or C virus infection. It usually presents with pain due to bleeding into the tumour, which may later cause intrahepatic calcification, or intraperitoneally. The serum α-fetoprotein is usually normal, and biopsy shows large polygonal malignant hepatocytes in a dense fibrous tissue stroma. Two-thirds of tumours are resectable and transplantation is worthwhile where there is no spread beyond the liver. Two-thirds of patients survive beyond 5 years.

OTHER PRIMARY MALIGNANT TUMOURS

These are rare but include haemangioendothelial sarcomas and cholangiocarcinoma (p. 544).

SECONDARY MALIGNANT TUMOURS

These are common and usually originate from carcinomas in the bronchus, breast, abdomen or pelvis. They may be single or multiple. Peritoneal dissemination frequently results in ascites.

Clinical features

The primary neoplasm is asymptomatic in about half the patients. Hepatomegaly may suggest cirrhosis, but splenomegaly is rare. There is usually rapid liver enlargement with fever, weight loss and jaundice.

Investigations

A raised alkaline phosphatase activity is the commonest biochemical abnormality but the liver function tests may be normal. Ascitic fluid has a high protein content and may be blood-stained, and cytology sometimes reveals malignant cells. Imaging (p. 494) usually reveals filling defects, laparoscopy may reveal the tumour and the diagnosis can be confirmed by liver aspiration or biopsy.

Management

Every effort should be made to detect resectable secondary tumours, as improvements in the techniques of hepatic resection now probably improve survival and give the best palliation, particularly for relatively slow-growing tumours such as colonic carcinomas. Patients with hormone-producing tumours, such as gastrinomas, insulinomas and glucagonomas, and lymphomas may benefit from chemotherapy. Unfortunately, palliative treatment to relieve pain is all that is available for most patients and this may include embolisation of the tumour masses.

BENIGN TUMOURS

Hepatic adenomas are rare vascular tumours which may present as an abdominal mass or with abdominal pain or intraperitoneal bleeding. They are more common in women and may be caused by oral contraceptives, androgens and anabolic steroids. Haemangiomas are the commonest benign liver tumours but they rarely cause symptoms.

LIVER TRANSPLANTATION

Liver transplantation is essentially a treatment for liver failure for which there is no other medical therapy. The number of liver transplantations carried out worldwide continues to rise steadily, but important constraints on future increases include the high cost of the treatment and the limited availability of donor livers. The main indications for liver transplantation are shown in Figure 8.18.

Chronic liver disease

Chronic liver disease accounts for about three-quarters of liver transplantations. Primary biliary cirrhosis is the

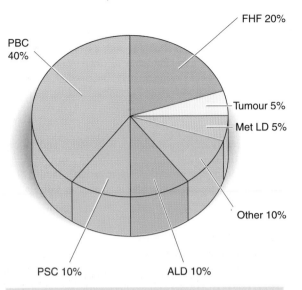

Fig. 8.18 Indications for liver transplant. ALD = Alcoholic liver disease; FHF = Fulminant hepatic failure; Met LD = Metabolic liver disease; Other = Other liver diseases; PBC = Primary biliary cirrhosis; PSC = Primary sclerosing cholangitis.

underlying disease in about a half of cases and primary sclerosing cholangitis has become increasingly important. Transplantation for alcoholic cirrhosis is done much more frequently, but most centres require that patients first demonstrate a capacity for abstinence. Rarer indications include metabolic diseases such as alpha$_1$-antitrypsin deficiency. Signs of liver failure pointing to the need for transplantation include sustained or increased jaundice (bilirubin > 100 μmol/l in cholestatic diseases such as primary biliary cirrhosis), ascites not responding readily to medical therapy, developing malnutrition and hypoalbuminaemia (< 30 g/l). Fatigue and lethargy affecting the quality of life, intractable itching in cholestatic disease, and recurrent variceal bleeding in spite of therapy are additional indications. The main contraindications are sepsis, HIV infection, hepatitis B viral infection with active replication, extrahepatic malignancy, alcohol or other substance abuse and marked cardiorespiratory or renal dysfunction not attributable to hepatic disease. Survival at one year after transplantation is about 80%, and the prognosis thereafter is good.

Fulminant hepatic failure

Fulminant hepatic failure is an increasing indication for transplantation. It should be reserved for patients whose chances of survival otherwise are very poor as patients who recover on conservative therapy regain normal liver structure and function. Such patients include those with

any three of the following: disease due to non-A, non-B hepatitis or an idiosyncratic drug reaction, age < 10 years or > 40 years, jaundice for > 1 week before onset of encephalopathy, plasma bilirubin > 300 μmol/l or a prothrombin time > 50 secs. Paracetamol overdose is an important cause of fulminant hepatic failure in the UK and transplantation is advised for patients who become acidotic (arterial pH > 7.3) or where the prothrombin time is > 100 secs and the plasma creatinine > 300 μmol/l. Patients with fulminant hepatic failure should be referred to a transplant centre once a steadily increasing prothrombin time shows worsening liver function and before severe encephalopathy occurs.

Tumours

Liver transplantation has not proved as successful for hepatobiliary carcinomas as had been hoped owing to early recurrence in the liver graft or in the lungs. Hepatocellular carcinomas are best treated by resection and should be < 3 cm in diameter for transplantation. Cholangiocarcinomas are rarely suitable for transplantation.

FURTHER READING

Elias E 1993 Liver transplantation. Journal of the Royal College of Physicians of London 27: 224–232
Shorrock C, Neuberger J 1993 The changing face of liver transplantation. Gut 34: 295–298

OTHER LIVER DISEASE

LIVER ABSCESS

Liver abscesses are either pyogenic or amoebic; the two have similar clinical features.

PYOGENIC ABSCESS

Pyogenic liver abscesses are uncommon but important because they are potentially curable, inevitably fatal if untreated, and readily overlooked.

Aetiology and pathology

Infection can reach the liver in several ways, as is shown in the information box (p. 536). Abscesses are most common in older patients and usually result from ascending infection due to biliary obstruction (cholangitis), whereas abscesses in young adults consequent on suppurative appendicitis, which were previously most common, are now rare. Immunocompromised patients are particularly likely to develop liver abscesses.

Abscesses vary greatly in size, single lesions are more common in the right liver, and multiple abscesses are usually due to infection in biliary obstruction. Many bacteria can cause liver abscesses. *E. coli* and various streptococci are the most common organisms, anaerobes including streptococci and *Bacteroides* can often be found, and several organisms are present in a third of patients.

SOURCES OF BACTERIAL INFECTION OF THE LIVER

- Biliary obstruction (cholangitis)
- Haematogenous
  Portal vein (mesenteric infections)
  Hepatic artery (bacteraemia)
- Direct extension
- Trauma
  Penetrating or non-penetrating
- Infection of liver tumour or cyst

Clinical features

Patients are generally ill with fever, sometimes rigors, and weight loss. Abdominal pain is the commonest symptom and is usually in the right upper quadrant sometimes with radiation to the right shoulder. The pain may be pleuritic. Hepatomegaly is found in more than half the patients and tenderness can usually be elicited by gentle percussion over the organ. Mild jaundice may be present and is severe only when large abscesses cause biliary obstruction. Abnormalities are present at the base of the right lung in about a quarter of patients. Atypical presentations are common and explain the frequency with which the diagnosis is made only at autopsy. This includes particularly patients with gradually developing illnesses which may not include abdominal pain, with pyrexia of unknown cause, and with clinical features pointing to an underlying cause such as colonic diverticular disease or to metastatic abscesses.

Investigations

Liver imaging is the most revealing investigation and shows 90% or more of symptomatic abscesses. Needle aspiration at ultrasound examination confirms the diagnosis and provides pus for culture. A leucocytosis is frequent, plasma alkaline phosphatase activity is usually increased, and the serum albumin is often low. The chest radiograph may show a raised right diaphragm and collapse or effusion at the base of the right lung. Blood culture should always be done as it may reveal the causative organism.

Management

This includes antibiotics and drainage of the abscess. Pending the results of culture of blood and pus from the abscess, treatment should commence with a combination such as ampicillin, gentamicin and metronidazole. Aspiration or drainage with a catheter placed in the abscess under the guidance of ultrasound is carried out, and surgical drainage may be needed for those which fail to respond.

Prognosis

The mortality of liver abscesses is 20–40% and failure to make the diagnosis is the commonest cause of death because untreated abscesses are invariably fatal. Older patients and those with multiple abscesses also have a higher mortality.

AMOEBIC ABSCESSES

Amoebic liver abscesses occur particularly in endemic areas, but they can occur anywhere in the world. Amoebic infections are considered elsewhere (p. 154).

HEPATIC NODULES

Liver diseases characterised primarily by hepatic nodules which are not neoplastic are rare, and three types are usually recognised. Neoplastic nodules such as adenomas and the nodules occurring in cirrhosis are not included with these diseases.

NODULAR REGENERATIVE HYPERPLASIA OF THE LIVER

This disease is characterised by small hepatocyte nodules throughout the liver unassociated with fibrosis. It occurs in older people and has been associated with many conditions such as connective tissue disease and haematological diseases and with immunosuppressive and corticosteroid drugs. The condition usually presents as an abdominal mass or occasionally because of portal hypertension. Diagnosis is made by liver biopsy. Liver function is good and the prognosis is very favourable, but hepatocellular carcinoma occurs occasionally.

FOCAL NODULAR HYPERPLASIA OF THE LIVER

This usually takes the form of a single subcapsular liver nodule, yellow-brown in colour and with central fibrosis. It is almost always asymptomatic and found by chance, but intraperitoneal bleeding is a rare complication.

PARTIAL NODULAR TRANSFORMATION OF THE LIVER

Nodules in this condition are restricted to the perihilar region of the liver where they can cause portal hypertension. The rest of the liver is normal and liver function is excellent. The diagnosis can be made finally only by pathological examination of the liver as needle liver biopsy is normal.

FIBROPOLYCYSTIC DISEASE

Fibropolycystic diseases of the liver and biliary system constitute a heterogeneous group of rare disorders, some of which are inherited. They are not distinct entities as combined lesions occur.

ADULT HEPATORENAL POLYCYSTIC DISEASE

The kidneys are the organs predominantly affected in this condition, which is inherited as an autosomal dominant (p. 659). Hepatic cysts which do not communicate with the biliary system are present in over half the patients with renal cysts. Hepatic cysts can occur alone and cysts are also found in other organs. Cerebrovascular aneurysms sometimes develop too.

Hepatic cysts are often discovered by chance because complications are rare, but these include pain or jaundice from cyst enlargement, haemorrhage into cysts, or cyst infection. Portal hypertension and bleeding from varices are very rare.

Diagnosis is made best by ultrasonography. Resection of a large cyst or groups of cysts is only required if symptoms are troublesome, and the prognosis is excellent as liver function is good. Cholangiocarcinoma is a rare complication.

CONGENITAL HEPATIC FIBROSIS

This is characterised by broad bands of fibrous tissue linking the portal tracts in the liver, abnormalities of the interlobular bile ducts, and sometimes a lack of portal venules. The renal tubules may show cystic dilatation (medullary sponge kidney, p. 660), and eventually renal cysts may develop. The condition can be inherited as an autosomal recessive. Liver involvement causes portal hypertension with splenomegaly and bleeding from oesophageal varices that usually presents in adolescence or in early adult life. The prognosis is good because liver function remains good. Treatment is required for variceal bleeding (p. 503) and occasionally cholangitis (p. 543). Patients can present during childhood with renal failure if the kidneys are severely affected.

CHOLEDOCHAL CYSTS

This term applies to cysts anywhere in the biliary tree (Fig 8.19). The great majority cause diffuse dilatation of the common bile duct (Type I), but others take the

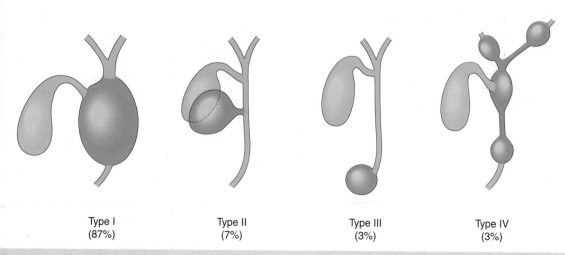

Type I	Type II	Type III	Type IV
(87%)	(7%)	(3%)	(3%)

Fig. 8.19   Classification and frequency of choledochal cysts. Reproduced with permission from Shearman D J C, Finlayson N D C 1989. Diseases of the Gastrointestinal Tract and Liver. Churchill Livingstone, Edinburgh.

form of biliary diverticula (Type II), dilatation of the intraduodenal bile duct (Type III) and multiple biliary cysts (Type IV). The last type merges with Caroli's syndrome (see below). Recurrent jaundice, recurrent abdominal pain and an abdominal mass are typical but these occur in only a minority of patients. Prolonged biliary obstruction predisposes to cholangitis, liver abscess and eventually biliary cirrhosis, and there is an increased incidence of cholangiocarcinoma. Excision is the treatment of choice if this is possible, otherwise a biliary bypass operation is performed.

CAROLI'S SYNDROME

This is very rare and is characterised by segmental saccular dilatations of the intrahepatic biliary tree. The whole liver is usually affected, and extrahepatic biliary dilatation occurs in about a quarter of patients. Recurrent attacks of cholangitis (p. 501) occur and may cause hepatic abscesses. Complications include biliary stones and cholangiocarcinoma. Antibiotics are required for episodes of cholangitis, and occasionally localised disease can be treated by segmental liver resection.

OTHER HEPATIC CYSTS

Non-parasitic cysts
Most non-parasitic liver cysts are congenital in origin and the majority are solitary. They rarely communicate with the biliary tree. They are usually asymptomatic but can cause abdominal pain, nausea or vomiting if cysts become big enough, and they may be palpable. Jaundice occasionally results from biliary compression, and infection, haemorrhage and rupture are other rare complications.

Other non-parasitic hepatic cysts include traumatic and neoplastic cysts.

Parasitic cysts
These cysts are caused by *Echinococcus granulosus* infection (p. 170). They have an outer layer derived from the host, an intermediate laminated layer, and an inner germinal layer. They can be single or multiple. Chronic cysts become calcified. The cysts may be asymptomatic or may cause abdominal pain or a mass. There is a peripheral blood eosinophilia, radiographs may show calcification, imaging shows the cyst(s), and serological tests are positive. Rupture or secondary infection of cysts can occur, and other organs may be involved. Surgical removal of the intact cyst after sterilisation with alcohol or formalin is necessary.

GALLBLADDER AND OTHER BILIARY DISEASES

GALLSTONES

Gallstone formation is the commonest disorder of the biliary tree and it is unusual for the gallbladder to be diseased in the absence of gallstones.

Pathology
Gallstones are conveniently classified into cholesterol or pigment stones. Cholesterol stones are the commonest type of gallstone encountered in industrialised countries whereas pigment stones are found more frequently in developing countries. In the Western world about 75% of stones are of the cholesterol variety, the remainder being pigment stones. Gallstones also contain varying quantities of calcium salts including calcium bilirubinate, carbonate, phosphate and palmitate, which determine the degree of radio-opacity.

Epidemiology
The prevalence of gallstones is uncertain because 80–90% of gallstones are asymptomatic. The disease affects 7% of males and 15% of females aged 18–65 years with an overall prevalence of 11%. In those under 40 years there is a 3:1 female preponderance whereas in the elderly the sex ratio is about equal. Gallstones are common in North America, Europe and Australia and are less frequent in India, the Far East and Africa. Thus the prevalence in American Pima Indians is 80% whereas in African countries it is around 14%. In developed countries the incidence of symptomatic gallstones appears to be increasing and they occur at an earlier age.

The most important risk factors for cholesterol gallstones are racial, increased age, female sex, obesity and increased parity. Other causes are diabetes mellitus and parenteral nutrition (see Table 8.13). There has been much debate over the role of diet in cholesterol gallstone disease and an increase of cholesterol, fat, calories, refined carbohydrate or lack of dietary fibres have all been blamed. At present the best data support an association between simple refined sugar in the diet and gallstones. There is a negative association between a moderate alcohol intake (2–3 units daily) and gallstones.

Table 8.13 Risk factors and mechanisms for cholesterol gallstones

Factor	Mechanism
Age	↑ Cholesterol secretion
Female	↑ Cholesterol secretion
Pregnancy	↑ Cholesterol secretion ↓ Bile salt secretion Impaired gallbladder motility
Obesity	↑ Cholesterol secretion
Rapid weight loss	↑ Cholesterol secretion
Racial	↑ Cholesterol secretion
Gallbladder stasis Brief fast TPN therapy* Spinal cord injury	Impaired gallbladder emptying

* TPN: Total Parenteral Nutrition

Table 8.14 Composition and risk factors for pigment stones

	Black	Brown
Composition	• polymerised calcium bilirubinates+++ • mucin glycoprotein++ • calcium phosphate • calcium carbonate • cholesterol	• calcium bilirubinate crystals+++ • mucin glycoprotein++ • cholesterol++ • calcium palmitate/stearate++
Risk	• haemolysis • age • hepatic cirrhosis • ileal resection/disease	• infected bile • stasis

+++ major component
++ lesser component
+ minor component

Aetiology

Cholesterol gallstones

Cholesterol is held in solution in bile by its association with bile acids and phospholipids in the form of micelles and vesicles; biliary lipoproteins may also have a role in solubilising cholesterol. In gallstone disease the liver produces bile which contains an excess of cholesterol either because there is a relative reduction in the quantity of bile salts or a relative increase in the amount of cholesterol. Such bile which is supersaturated with cholesterol is termed 'lithogenic'. Defective bile salt synthesis, excessive intestinal loss of bile salts, over-sensitive bile salt feedback, excessive cholesterol secretion and abnormal gallbladder function have all been implicated in the formation of saturated bile.

The most important factor is hepatic hypersecretion of cholesterol, which is found in all of the common epidemiological associations of gallstones. Factors influencing biliary lipid composition are shown in Table 8.13.

Cholesterol-phospholipid vesicles are present in human hepatic and gallbladder bile, and function as a second carrier for cholesterol. Under certain conditions such vesicles provide the cholesterol which will be the source of crystal deposition, growth and stone formation. Factors stabilising the vesicles, and factors which are responsible for precipitation of cholesterol from these vesicles, are probably critical in the formation of gallstones.

Factors initiating crystallisation of cholesterol in bile (nucleation factors) are also important, as patients with cholesterol gallstones have gallbladder bile which forms cholesterol crystals more rapidly than equally saturated bile from patients who do not form gallstones. Both nucleating factors (mucus, calcium fatty acids, other proteins) and antinucleating factors (apolipoproteins) have been described.

Pigment stones

Comparatively little is known about the mechanism of formation of pigment stones. The brown crumbly pigment stone is almost certainly the consequence of infection in the biliary tree. These are commonly found in the Far East where infection of the biliary tree allows bacterial beta-glucuronidase to hydrolyse conjugated bilirubin to its free form which then precipitates as calcium bilirubinate. The mechanism of black pigment gallstone formation in the Western world is not satisfactorily explained. Haemolysis does play a role in some circumstances, for example the increased prevalence of calcium bilirubinate stones in cirrhosis is related to an underlying haemolytic tendency and ileal disease or resection may be a cause (Table 8.14).

Biliary sludge

The term 'biliary sludge' describes bile which is in a gel form that contains numerous crystals or microspheroliths of calcium bilirubinate granules and cholesterol crystals as well as glycoproteins. It is an essential precursor to the formation of gallstones in the majority of patients. Biliary sludge is formed frequently under normal conditions, but then either dissolves or is cleared by the gallbladder and only in about 15% of patients does it persist to form cholesterol stones.

Natural history

The great majority of gallstones are asymptomatic and remain so. Only about 10% of those with gallstones develop clinical evidence of gallstone disease. Why this should be is not adequately explained. It is clear however that patients do not die because of the presence of gallstones, and the risk of major complications from gallstone disease is low. The great majority of patients with gallstones never require a cholecystectomy.

Clinical features

Symptomatic gallstones manifest either as biliary pain or as a consequence of developing cholecystitis. If a gallstone becomes acutely impacted in the cystic duct the patient will experience pain. The term 'biliary colic' is a misnomer because the pain does not rhythmically increase and decrease in intensity as in colic experienced in intestinal and renal disease. Instead the pain is of sudden onset and is sustained for about 2 hours; its continuation for more than 6 hours suggests that a complication such as cholecystitis or pancreatitis has developed. Pain is felt in the epigastrium (70% of patients) or right upper quadrant (20% of patients) radiating to the interscapular region or the tip of the right scapula, but other sites include the left upper quadrant, the epigastrium and the lower chest, and in these positions it can be confused with intrathoracic disease, oesophagitis, myocardial infarction or dissecting aneurysm.

Fatty food intolerance, dyspepsia and flatulence are not symptoms of gallstones. 'Gallstone dyspepsia' is a misnomer and not an indication of cholecystectomy.

Investigations

A plain abdominal radiograph will demonstrate calcified gallstones in 20% of patients. Ultrasonography is the method of choice to diagnose gallstones (Fig. 8.7, p. 495) but oral cholecystography is also a useful technique, as is computed tomography.

Complications

Occlusion of the cystic duct for any prolonged period of time will result in acute cholecystitis. Other complications include chronic cholecystitis, and hydrops of the gallbladder, in which there is slow distension of the gallbladder from continuous secretion of mucus. If this material becomes infected an empyema develops. Calcium may be secreted into the lumen of the hydropic gallbladder causing limey bile and if calcium salts are precipitated in the gallbladder wall the radiological appearance of 'porcelain' gallbladder results.

Gallstones will migrate to the common bile duct in 10–20% of patients and cause biliary colic, but choledocholithiasis may be asymptomatic. Rarely, fistulas develop between the gallbladder and the duodenum or colon or stomach, and a fistulous tract may arise between the common bile duct and adjacent organs. Air will be seen in the biliary tree on plain abdominal radiographs. If a stone larger than 2.5 cm in diameter has migrated into the gut it may impact either at the terminal ileum or occasionally in the duodenum or sigmoid colon. The resultant intestinal obstruction may be followed by 'gallstone ileus'.

Cancer of the gallbladder is rare, although it is recognised more frequently in an ageing population and in a 'porcelain' gallbladder. In over 95% of patients with gallbladder cancer there are accompanying gallstones. Cancer is usually undiagnosed until a cholecystectomy is performed for gallstone disease.

Management

The management of gallstones depends on whether they are causing symptoms. Asymptomatic gallstones found incidentally are not usually treated because the majority will never give symptoms. Symptomatic gallstones are best treated surgically (p. 541), but they can also be dissolved, fragmented in the gallbladder or removed from the common bile duct mechanically (see the information box below). Medical dissolution of gallstones can be achieved by oral administration of the naturally-occurring bile acids chenodeoxycholic acid and ursodeoxycholic acid. Radiolucent gallstones in a gallbladder that opacifies on oral cholecystography, stones not larger than 15 mm in diameter, moderate obesity and non-acute symptoms are the features which suggest that drug therapy may be useful. Success can be expected in between 70 and 75% of patients by careful selection of those who are not obese. Non-responders are probably patients who have radiolucent pigment stones which do not respond to chenodeoxycholic or ursodeoxycholic acid.

TREATMENT OF GALLSTONES

- Cholecystectomy—open or laparoscopic
- Bile acids—chenodeoxycholic or ursodeoxycholic
- Contact dissolution
- Lithotripsy
- Endoscopic sphincterotomy

The dose of chenodeoxycholic acid is 12 mg/kg daily but because it may be associated with mildly disturbed liver function tests and diarrhoea, it is being replaced by ursodeoxycholic acid, which is given in a dose of 8–12 mg/kg daily. Another popular regimen is a combination of chenodeoxycholic acid and ursodeoxycholic acid daily each in a dose of 8 mg/kg. Medication is given best as a single bedtime dose. Extracorporeal shock wave lithotripsy using shock waves generated by a variety of techniques has been introduced, with the advantage of being non-invasive and safe, but at present it is expensive. A course of bile salt therapy is necessary following lithotripsy to dissolve the gallstone fragments within the gallbladder. As in the case of oral bile salt therapy, only

30% of all patients with gallbladder disease are suitable for lithotripsy. Contact dissolution therapy with methyl terbutyl ether is available in some centres. All therapeutic regimens which retain the gallbladder have a 50% recurrence of stones after 5 years. The management of gallbladder pain is given below.

CHOLECYSTITIS

ACUTE CHOLECYSTITIS

Aetiology and pathology

Acute cholecystitis is almost always associated with obstruction of the gallbladder neck or cystic duct by a gallstone. Occasionally obstruction may be by mucus, a worm or a tumour. In 10% of patients no obstruction can be identified and the term 'acute acalculous cholecystitis' is used. The pathogenesis is unclear, but possibly the initial inflammation is chemically induced. This follows gallbladder mucosal damage which releases phospholipase, converting biliary lecithin to lysolecithin, a recognised mucosal toxin. At the time of surgery approximately 50% of cultures of the gallbladder contents are sterile.

Clinical features

The cardinal feature is pain in the right upper quadrant but also in the epigastrium, the right shoulder tip or interscapular region. It usually lasts for more than an hour but differentiation between gallstone-induced gallbladder pain and acute cholecystitis may be difficult and features suggesting cholecystitis include severe and prolonged pain, fever and leucocytosis.

Examination shows right hypochondrial tenderness, rigidity worse on inspiration (Murphy's sign), and a gallbladder mass may be palpable. Fever is present and rigors may occur. Leucocytosis is common except in the elderly patient where the signs of inflammation may not be marked. Jaundice occurs in 20–25% of patients even though there are no stones in the common bile duct, and may represent oedematous pressure on the common hepatic duct. Minor increases of plasma transaminase and amylase activity may be encountered.

If the patient is untreated the inflammation may resolve only to recur. On the other hand the inflammation may progress to an empyema or perforation and peritonitis.

Acute cholecystitis in elderly people is a particular hazard as the disease tends to be severe, may have few localising clinical signs and a high frequency of empyema and perforation (p. 542). The mortality rate in elderly patients may reach about 10%.

Differential diagnosis

This is from other causes of severe upper abdominal pain, including perforated peptic ulcer, acute pancreatitis and a retrocaecal appendicitis. Myocardial infarction and a right basal pneumonia should always be considered. Occasionally there may be confusion with renal colic, herpes zoster, epidemic myalgia, pleurisy and acute intermittent porphyria.

Investigations

Plain radiographs of the abdomen and chest may show gallstones and detect perforation of a viscus, fistulation of a gallstone into the intestine (p. 540) and pneumonia. Ultrasonography detects gallstones and gallbladder thickening due to cholecystitis, and cholescintigraphy if available shows cystic duct obstruction. The plasma amylase should be measured to detect pancreatitis (Ch. 7) which may be a complication of gallstones. The peripheral blood count often shows a leucocytosis.

Management

This consists of bed-rest, relief of pain, antibiotics and maintenance of fluid balance. Severe pain is relieved using morphine 10–15 mg intramuscularly and increased tone of the choledochal sphincter may be minimised by the concurrent use of atropine 0.6 mg intramuscularly. Less severe pain can be relieved by pethidine 100 mg or pentazocine 30 mg intramuscularly or diclofenac 75–150 mg orally daily in divided doses or a once-daily intramuscular injection of 75 mg. Effective relief of pain may require repeated doses of analgesic every 2–3 hours. Nasogastric aspiration is required only when there is persistent vomiting, in which case fluid must be given intravenously. Systemic antibiotics are required in the elderly, patients with jaundice, and those who are febrile. A cephalosporin such as cefuroxime, 750 mg intramuscularly or intravenously 6-hourly or 8-hourly is the antibiotic of choice, and metronidazole (1 g 8-hourly by suppository) is usually added in severely ill patients.

Surgical treatment

Patients with acute cholecystitis require cholecystectomy. Two options are available: early cholecystectomy or delayed (interval) cholecystectomy. Early cholecystectomy, in which the patient is operated on within 2 or 3 days of the diagnosis, is now accepted as the mortality is no higher than for the interval operation, readmission to hospital is not needed and recurrent acute cholecystitis before operation is prevented. The older interval approach entails treating the patient medically in hospital for 10–15 days, after which the patient is discharged to be readmitted 2–3 months later for an elective cholecystectomy. There is an increasing trend from open cholecystectomy to minimal access (laparoscopic) cholecystectomy. All patients undergoing surgery should receive a single dose of cefuroxime of 750 mg intramuscularly.

Emergency surgical intervention is occasionally required if the patient's condition deteriorates, if there is generalised peritonitis, an inflammatory mass in the right hypochondrium, gas present in the gallbladder wall or lumen, or evidence of intestinal obstruction.

ACUTE ACALCULOUS CHOLECYSTITIS

This condition occurs in between 8 and 10% of patients with cholecystitis, presents in the same way as acute calculous cholecystitis, and is treated identically. It can occur following trauma and after surgical operations.

ACUTE EMPHYSEMATOUS CHOLECYSTITIS

This is a severe, fulminant form of cholecystitis that is caused by a mixed infection including gas-forming organisms. Elderly males and patients with diabetes mellitus are at particular risk. The condition manifests with marked pain, shock and a rapid deterioration in the clinical condition of the patient. Gas may be recognised radiologically in the gallbladder lumen or its wall, or in the bile ducts. Urgent cholecystectomy is required once the patient's clinical condition has been stabilised, but the mortality exceeds 20%.

POSTCHOLECYSTECTOMY SYNDROME

Symptoms following cholecystectomy occur in 12–68% of patients depending on how the condition is defined, how actively symptoms are sought, and the indications for cholecystectomy. When cholecystectomy is performed for acute calculous cholecystitis at least 70% of patients remain symptom-free. Postcholecystectomy symptoms occur most frequently in women, in patients who have a history longer than 5 years prior to cholecystectomy, and in patients in whom the operation was undertaken for non-calculous gallbladder disease. The information box summarises some of the more common causes of postcholecystectomy symptoms.

The usual complaints include right upper quadrant pain, flatulence, fatty foods intolerance, and occasionally jaundice and cholangitis. Liver function tests may be abnormal and sometimes show cholestasis. Ultrasonography is used to detect biliary obstruction, and retrograde cholangiopancreatography is usually needed. Other investigations which may be required include barium studies of the gastrointestinal tract, pancreatic function tests, cholescintigraphy and a liver biopsy. If all of

---

CAUSES OF POSTCHOLECYSTECTOMY SYMPTOMS

Immediate post-surgical
- Biliary injury
- Bleeding
- Biliary peritonitis
- Abscess
- Fistula

Biliary
- Common bile duct stones
- Benign stricture
- Tumour
- Cystic duct stump syndrome
- Papillary disorders
    Dysfunction, stenosis

Extrabiliary
- Flatulent dyspepsia
- Peptic ulcer
- Pancreatic disease
- Gastro-oesophageal reflux
- Irritable bowel syndrome
- Functional abdominal pain

---

these tests are unhelpful the question of a functional illness should be considered.

Management depends on demonstrating a cause. Frequently no intra-abdominal disease is found and the patient is managed with advice regarding a low fat diet, the use of antacid preparations, and treatment for the irritable bowel syndrome (Chapter 7) depending on the nature of the symptoms which the patient is presenting.

CHRONIC CHOLECYSTITIS

Chronic inflammation of the gallbladder is almost invariably associated with gallstones. The condition may be asymptomatic. The usual symptoms are those of recurrent attacks of upper abdominal pain, often at night and following a heavy meal. The clinical features are similar to those of acute calculous cholecystitis but milder. The patient may recover spontaneously or following analgesia and antibiotics; if untreated the symptoms recur. Patients are advised to undergo a cholecystectomy.

CHOLEDOCHOLITHIASIS

Stones in the common bile duct occur in 10–15% of patients with gallstones. These secondary stones account for more than 80% of common bile duct stones, migrate from the gallbladder, and are similar in appearance and chemical composition to the stones found there. Primary bile duct stones may develop many years after a cholecystectomy and represent the accumulation of biliary sludge consequent upon dysfunction of the sphincter of Oddi. In Far Eastern countries where bile duct infection is common, primary common bile duct stones are thought to follow bacterial infection in the biliary tree secondary to parasitic infections with *Clonorchis sinensis*, *Ascaris lumbricoides* or *Fasciola hepatica*. A stone in the common bile duct can cause partial or complete bile duct obstruction which may be complicated by stricture, secondary bacterial infection, cholangitis, liver abscess and septicaemia.

Clinical features

Choledocholithiasis may be asymptomatic or manifest as recurrent abdominal pain with or without jaundice. The pain is usually in the right upper quadrant and fever, pruritus and dark urine may be present. Painless jaundice is uncommon. Physical examination may show the scar of a previous cholecystectomy; if the gallbladder is present it is usually small, fibrotic and impalpable.

Investigations

Liver function tests show a cholestatic pattern and bilirubinuria is present. Occasionally these tests are normal. If cholangitis is present the patient will have a leukocytosis. The most convenient method of demonstrating obstruction to the common bile duct is by ultrasonography which will demonstrate dilated extra- and intrahepatic bile ducts together with gallstones, but it is not always successful in indicating the cause of the obstruction. Endoscopic retrograde cholangiography has the advantage that not only can a diagnosis be made of obstruction and its cause, but common bile duct stones can be removed. Percutaneous transhepatic cholangiography may also be used but it is less satisfactory.

Management

Patients require stone removal either surgically or by endoscopic sphincterotomy. Cholangitis requires intravenous fluids and broad-spectrum antibiotics such as cefuroxime and metronidazole. Blood cultures should be taken before the antibiotics are administered.

Biliary drainage and the removal of the gallstones can be achieved either at choledochotomy or using endoscopic techniques. Following endoscopic retrograde cholangiography a sphincterotomy is performed and the stones removed or left to pass spontaneously. Increasingly this technique is used as the first approach for the removal of stones, particularly in patients over the age of 60 years. Endoscopic sphincterotomy and stone extraction is successful in over 90% of patients and has a low morbidity and mortality. Less commonly used techniques include solvent infusions via a T-tube or a nasobiliary catheter, and extracorporeal lithotripsy.

Surgical treatment of choledocholithiasis is performed less frequently because of the higher morbidity and mortality compared with an endoscopic sphincterotomy. Before exploring the common bile duct an accurate diagnosis of choledocholithiasis should be confirmed by intraoperative cholangiography or choledochoscopy. If gallstones are found a supraduodenal exploration is undertaken and following removal of the stones a T-tube is inserted into the common bile duct. Once the stones have been removed steps should be taken to ensure that complete clearance of the biliary tree has been achieved and again choledochoscopy or cholangiography will be required.

RECURRENT PYOGENIC CHOLANGITIS (ASIATIC CHOLANGIOHEPATITIS)

This disease occurs in Hong Kong, Korea and Southeast Asia. Biliary sludge, calcium bilirubinate concretions and stones accumulate in the intrahepatic bile ducts with secondary bacterial infection. The patients present with recurrent attacks of upper abdominal pain, fever and evidence of cholestatic jaundice. Investigation of the biliary tree demonstrates that both the intra- and extrahepatic portions are filled with soft biliary mud. Eventually the liver becomes scarred and liver abscess develops. The condition is difficult to manage and requires drainage of the biliary tract with extraction of stones, antibiotics and, in certain patients, partial resection of damaged areas of the liver.

TUMOURS OF THE GALLBLADDER AND BILE DUCT

CARCINOMA OF THE GALLBLADDER

This is a rare tumour occurring more often in females and is usually encountered above the age of 70. More than 90% of such tumours are adenocarcinomas; the remainder are anaplastic or rarely squamous tumours. Gallstones are usually present and may be important in the aetiology of the tumour.

The condition is usually diagnosed at surgery for gallstone disease. Occasionally it may manifest as repeated attacks of biliary pain and later persistent jaundice and weight loss. A gallbladder mass may be palpable in the right hypochondrium. Liver function tests show cholestasis, and gallbladder calcification may be found on radiograph. The tumour may be diagnosed on ultrasonography. The treatment is surgical excision but it has frequently extended beyond the wall of the gallbladder into the liver and surrounding tissues and palliative management is usually all that can be offered. Survival is generally short.

CHOLANGIOCARCINOMA

This uncommon tumour arises anywhere in the biliary tree from the small intrahepatic bile ducts to the papilla of Vater. The majority are adenocarcinomas and three morphological variants are described—papillary, nodular or the diffuse variety where the duct wall is thickened over an extensive area. The last type of lesion is difficult to differentiate from sclerosing cholangitis.

The cause of cholangiocarcinoma is unknown but it is associated with gallstones or ulcerative colitis and the disease may present either some years after procto-colectomy or as a presenting feature with ulcerative colitis only being discovered subsequently.

The cancer is classified into three anatomical areas: the upper third comprising the common hepatic duct and the confluence of hepatic ducts, the middle third and the lower third between the upper border of the duodenum and the papilla of Vater. Tumours in the upper third have the worst prognosis and are the most difficult to treat. These tumours usually arise at the junction of the right and left hepatic ducts and are difficult to diagnose.

The patient presents with jaundice which may be intermittent. Half the patients have upper abdominal pain and weight loss. Presentation with recurrent jaundice following an inappropriate cholecystectomy should not occur if intraoperative cholangiography is performed at the time of cholecystectomy. The diagnosis is made by endoscopic cholangiography or percutaneous trans-hepatic cholangiography. Cholangiocarcinomas can occasionally be excised surgically, but most patients are treated by inserting drainage stents across the tumour at endoscopic or transhepatic cholangiography.

CARCINOMA AT THE PAPILLA OF VATER

Nearly 40% of all adenocarcinomas of the small intestine arise in relationship to the papilla of Vater and present with pain, anaemia, vomiting and weight loss. Jaundice may be intermittent or persistent. Diagnosis is made by duodenal endoscopy and biopsy of the tumour. Ampullary carcinoma must be differentiated from carcinoma of the head of the pancreas and a cholangiocarcinoma because both these conditions have a worse prognosis.

Curative surgical treatment can be undertaken by pancreaticoduodenectomy or a segmental resection and the five-year survival may be as high as 50%. When this is impossible a palliative bypass or intubation is performed.

BENIGN GALLBLADDER TUMOURS

These are uncommon and usually found incidentally at operation or autopsy. Cholesterol polyps, sometimes associated with cholesterolosis, papillomas, and adenomas are the main types.

MISCELLANEOUS BILIARY DISORDERS

PRIMARY SCLEROSING CHOLANGITIS

In this increasingly diagnosed disease there is fibrotic obliteration of the intra- or extrahepatic bile duct system, which may be primary or secondary in type. Primary sclerosing cholangitis has no known cause but is often associated with ulcerative colitis and occasionally with retroperitoneal fibrosis or a variety of autoimmune disorders. There is an association between primary sclerosing cholangitis and the HLA haplotypes B8, DR2 and DR3. In secondary cholangitis there is an underlying disorder of the biliary tree causing the fibrotic state, for example retained bile duct stones or strictures following surgery.

Clinical features
The patient presents with jaundice which may be fluctuating, intermittent fever, pruritus and right upper quadrant pain. Eventually jaundice is constant. Other features include anorexia, weight loss and rarely bleeding from oesophageal varices. The illness lasts for 5–15 years with the patient finally succumbing to liver failure with or without infection.

Investigations
Liver function tests demonstrate cholestasis with elevation of the serum bilirubin and alkaline phosphatase. The prothrombin time may be prolonged. Perinuclear antineutrophil cytoplasmic antibodies (p-ANCA, p. 647) have recently been found with this disease, especially where it is associated with ulcerative colitis. Ultrasonography may not show biliary abnormality as the thickened fibrotic ducts are not dilated, and diagnosis is best made by endoscopic retrograde cholangiography which typically shows narrowed, irregular obstruction and 'beading' of the extra- and intrahepatic bile ducts. The disease may affect the whole of the biliary system or may be confined to the extra- or intrahepatic portion of the bile ducts. The diagnosis may also be made by a percutaneous transhepatic cholangiogram. At liver biopsy a typical whorled appearance of bile ducts may be seen. Bile duct tissue obtained at laparotomy may demonstrate the characteristic lymphocytic cell

infiltrate with plasma cells and giant cells. The main differential diagnosis is from a cholangiocarcinoma.

Management

There is no specific treatment; but antibiotics are needed during episodes of cholangitis. Corticosteroids and other immunosuppressive drugs are of no value. Biliary drainage may be attempted which can be either extrabiliary using a T-tube, or by placing silicone stents in the common bile duct. Liver transplantation is the only effective therapy in patients with advanced disease.

BILIARY MOTOR DISORDERS

There are patients with right upper quadrant discomfort who do not have gallstones and the term biliary dyskinesia has been introduced to describe the condition of some of these patients. The dyskinetic disorder may affect either the gallbladder or the sphincter of Oddi. Patients complain of either recurrent epigastric or right upper quadrant pain.

The diagnosis is established by showing the absence of gallstones and undertaking tests to demonstrate that contraction of the gallbladder is associated with pain or the papilla is stenosed. Endoscopic retrograde cholangiopancreatography, endoscopic manometry, intraoperative manometry and radiomanometry are all used in an attempt to define this disorder more clearly. Identification of biliary dyskinesia remains difficult and the treatment is uncertain. Some of these patients are being treated with a sphincterotomy at the time of endoscopic assessment of the condition.

CHOLESTEROLOSIS OF THE GALLBLADDER

In this condition lipid deposits in the submucosa and epithelium appear as multiple yellow spots on the pink mucosa—'strawberry gallbladder'. The condition is asymptomatic but may occasionally present with right upper quadrant pain. Radiologically the features are those of small fixed filling defects on cholecystography or ultrasonography and the radiologist can usually differentiate between gallstones and cholesterolosis. The condition is usually diagnosed at cholecystectomy; if the diagnosis is made radiologically, cholecystectomy is indicated.

ADENOMYOMATOSIS OF THE GALLBLADDER

In this condition there is hyperplasia of the muscle and mucosa of the gallbladder. The projection of pouches of mucous membrane through weak points in the muscle coat produces 'Rokitansky–Aschoff' sinuses. There is much disagreement over whether adenomyomatosis is a cause of right upper quadrant pain and other gastrointestinal symptoms. It may be diagnosed by oral cholecystography when a halo or ring of opacified diverticula can be seen around the gallbladder. Other appearances include deformity of the body of the gallbladder or marked irregularity of the outline. Then gallstones may be present. Localised adenomyomatosis in the region of the gallbladder fundus causes the appearance of a 'phygian cap'. Most patients are treated by cholecystectomy although in the absence of gallstones other diseases in the upper gastrointestinal tract must be excluded.

CHOLEDOCHAL CYST

This condition is considered on page 537.

FURTHER READING

Chapman R W 1991 Aetiology and natural history of primary sclerosing cholangitis:—a decade of progress? Gut 32: 1433–1435
Davidson B R 1993 Progress in determining the nature of bile duct strictures. Gut. 34: 725–726
Johnston D E, Kaplan M M 1993 Pathogenesis and treatment of gallstones. New England Journal of Medicine 328: 412–421
La Mont J T, Clancy M C 1992 Cholesterol gallstone formation. Progress in Liver Disease 10: 165–191
Sachmann M (ed.) 1992 Diagnosis and management of biliary stones. Clinical Gastroenterology 6: 635–822. Baillière Tindall, London
Toouli J 1989 What is sphincter of Oddi dysfunction? Gut 30: 753–761

A. S. Truswell

9

Nutritional factors in disease

No medical history is complete without enquiring about the patient's food and drink intake. What people eat is one of the major environmental influences that affect health and can sooner or later contribute to disease. Lack of food or of essential nutrients in food also leads to disease.

The word nutrition comes from the Latin '*nutrire*' which means to breast feed or nurse and from the time of Hippocrates diet has been a primary part of the management of sick people. Modern physicians can in addition use purified nutrients and parenteral formulas and they advise healthy people about prudent eating to reduce the risk of degenerative diseases.

HISTORICAL AND GEOGRAPHICAL PERSPECTIVE

The food supply and the major nutritional problems are distinctive in societies at different stages of technical development (Table 9.1). The foods and nutritional disorders in Britain are similar to those in, say, Germany or New Zealand; they have the nutritional pattern of affluent countries. In India, Egypt and Kenya on the other hand, the nutrition situation for all but a privileged few is that of urban slum dwellers or peasant agriculturalists. The nutritional disorders that doctors have to diagnose, treat and prevent are very different and fairly predictable at these three stages of technical development. Very few doctors work with nomadic pastoralists (another stage in Table 9.1) and the hunter-gatherer's way of life has almost disappeared. But our incomplete information about what hunter-gatherers ate is one source of ideas about healthy diets for modern people. For at least 99% of the time homo sapiens has been evolving from his primate precursors, he and she were hunter-gatherers. There has not been time for full genetic adaptation to the diets that humans have been eating since agriculture started 10 000 years ago.

Which nutritional disorders are common depends on where and with whom one is working, but the study of human nutrition has grown because some workers have taken a global view. Our understanding of protein deficiency and of dietary fibre originated in Africa; human zinc deficiency was first described in the Middle East and selenium deficiency in China. We first learned about the role of very long chain unsaturated fatty acids from medical studies on the Inuit people of Greenland. On the other hand some 'Western diseases' like diabetes mellitus are now increasingly occurring in tropical countries.

Nutrition and different medical specialties

Like immune reactions and infections, nutrition can affect any organ of the body or several at once. Different parts of the whole field of human nutrition are used regularly by different specialists. Cardiologists are interested in dietary fats and plasma cholesterol, nephrologists in protein deficiency and in potassium excess, gastroenterologists in multiple deficiencies from malabsorption, in dietary fibre and in hypersensitivity to wheat and milk, neurologists are interested in alcohol excess and thiamin deficiency, haematologists in deficiencies of iron, folate and vitamin B_{12}, psychiatrists

---

Table 9.1 Nutrition at five stages of technical development

Stage	People and their food	Characteristic nutritional disorders
Hunter-gatherers (HG)	Our ancestors till 10 000 years ago or less. Few contemporary HGs left, e.g. Kung Bushmen. Collect wide range of veg foods; also eat meat (lean if terrestrial) and fish. No salt, alcohol, milk (other than mother's), little cereal or sugar (wild honey)	Lean (no obesity) Malnutrition unlikely No coronary disease, hypertension; no dental caries or alcoholism
Pastoralists	Follow their grazing animals where adequate pasture, e.g. Lapps, Tibetans, Mongols, Tuareg, Fulani, Masai. Diet high in animal foods and milk	Least studied of all groups Some groups are tall Persistence of adult intestinal lactase
Peasant agriculturalists	Nearly all rural people in developing world and in industrial countries till this century. Tend to rely on one crop which yields best. Vulnerable to crop disease, crop toxin and to drought. Seasonal shortages. Milling and refining cereals increases risk of malnutrition	Famine in areas with unreliable rainfall Malnutrition from lack of some nutrient(s) in stable food, e.g. kwashiorkor, pellagra, beriberi Mycotoxins. Hypertension but no coronary disease
Urban slum and periurban shanty	The poor masses in and round the rapidly growing cities of today's developing countries. In 19th century similar situation in London, New York, etc. Loss of food traditions, no home gardens, mothers often have to work, poor food hygiene, food expensive	Children most vulnerable; not breast fed; gastroenteritis and marasmus Rickets in high latitudes Alcoholism. Adults may be obese Hypertension but not coronary disease
Affluent societies	Favourite food year round. High fat diet. Processed, convenience and take-away food. Tower of Babel of nutritional breakthroughs, scares and advice. Alternative and unorthodox advice. 'Health foods.' Many take vitamin tablets	Malnutrition confined to hospital patients and the elderly disabled. Coronary heart disease common. 'Nutritional hypochondriasis' Hypersensitivity to foods apparently common Obesity unfashionable but difficult to avoid—Anorexia nervosa

in anorexia nervosa, geriatricians in the effects of drugs on nutritional status and general practitioners in dietary advice for pregnancy and middle age and in infant feeding. Consequently some nutritional disorders are dealt with in this chapter; others have their main description elsewhere in the book.

USES OF NUTRITIONAL KNOWLEDGE IN CLINICAL MEDICINE

Primary nutritional diseases

Some diseases result primarily from disturbed nutrition—the major deficiency diseases and obesity. These are described in this chapter.

Deficiency diseases seldom present in pure form. More often than not they are secondary to some other illness. Even where food is short, not all the members of a community are equally affected. Individuals with some physical or mental abnormality usually show clinical manifestations first. Young children and disabled adults are the most vulnerable.

When malnutrition occurs it is unlikely to involve only one nutrient. Even if the clinical features suggest a single deficiency, biochemical tests usually reveal depletion of other nutrients. Treatment should therefore not be confined to large intakes of the nutrient whose deficiency is indicated by the clinical signs. Furthermore, malnourished patients are liable to complications, especially certain infections which may be the presenting illness or may occur in modified form because malnutrition has suppressed some of their characteristic signs. Thus complications of malnutrition must be looked for and treated. Much of the skill in diagnosing patients with malnutrition is being aware of and disentangling predisposing illnesses, other associated malnutrition and complicating diseases.

Secondary nutritional depletion

In developed countries, patients in hospital for long periods with a serious illness are very likely to develop some degree of nutritional depletion such as protein-calorie malnutrition and/or other deficiencies, e.g. of folate, potassium or iron. It is important to monitor patients' nutrition and provide appropriate support because nutritionally-depleted patients are weaker and have impaired wound healing and reduced resistance to infection. The principles of nutritional diagnosis and management for hospital patients are summarised in this chapter (pp. 574–578).

Dietary modification as treatment

Some diseases, notably coeliac disease, hepatic encephalopathy and phenylketonuria, are not caused by disturbed nutrition, but for each of them a specific modification of the usual diet is the principal treatment, which may be life saving. In other conditions, e.g. chronic renal failure, diabetes mellitus and mild hypertension, the appropriate diet is useful treatment, alternative or complementary to drugs (see information box below). In other chapters therapeutic diets are outlined under the diseases concerned, but space does not allow extensive detail; the reader is referred to a textbook of nutrition and dietetics (p. 584).

NON-PHARMACOLOGICAL MANAGEMENT OF HYPERTENSION

- Reduce sodium intake to 50–100 mmol/day
- Reduce body weight if patient overweight
- Restrict alcohol intake
- Ensure a good dietary potassium intake
- Regular appropriate exercise

Therapeutic diets

Therapeutic diets ask patients to make one or more of the following changes: reduce or (virtually) eliminate one or more components, increase one or more components, change the consistency of the diet, or change the feeding pattern. These are all changes to the patient's usual diet (which of course varies somewhat from day to day) or in comparison with a theoretical 'normal' or average diet for the country, culture, age and sex.

The prescription for a diet should state the nature of the modification(s), the degree of each modification, the planned duration of these, and any compensation for essential nutrients reduced as a result of the modifications.

The degree of the modification is as important as the dose in pharmacotherapy. People talk loosely about a 'low salt' diet, for example, but its sodium intake can range from 25 to 100 mmol/day, compared with a usual British sodium intake of over 150 mmol/day. Likewise with proteins, a protein-restricted diet may vary from 20 to 50 g/day compared with the standard of 70 g/day or more.

Dietary advice in the prevention of chronic degenerative diseases

Evidence is accumulating that the habitual diet is one of the multiple causative factors in many chronic degenerative diseases (e.g. coronary heart disease, hypertension, diabetes mellitus, cirrhosis of the liver, gallstones, urinary tract stones, dental caries and diverticular disease) and even in some carcinomas (e.g. stomach, liver and large bowel). These diseases take a long time to develop; exactly which dietary components are involved, and how closely, needs discussion and is often controversial. Modifications of a Western diet to reduce the risk of coronary heart disease are set out in the information box.

Elsewhere in this book the role of diet is mentioned briefly in the paragraphs on aetiology of the different diseases.

CLASSIFICATION OF NUTRITIONAL DISORDERS

These disorders are listed in the information box.

Nutrients can be subdivided into four groups as shown in the information box below.

Table 9.2 Size of adult requirements for different essential nutrients

Adult daily requirement in foods	Essential nutrients for man
g amounts	
1 kg (1 l)	Water
50–100 g	Available carbohydrate
c. 50 g	Protein (8–10 essential amino acids)
1–5 g	Na, Cl, K, essential fatty acids
c. 1 g	Ca, P
mg amounts	
300 mg	Mg
c. 50 mg	Vit C
c. 15 mg	Niacin, vit E, Fe, Zn
5–10 mg	Pantothenate, Mn
1–2 mg	Vit A, thiamin, riboflavin, vit B_6, F, Cu
μg amounts	
200 μg	Folate, Mo
c. 100 μg	Biotin, I, Se
2–10 μg	Vit B_{12}, vit D, vit K, Cr

Figures are approximate, in places rounded to fit with others on a line. The range of requirements for different nutrients is about 10^9. In addition sulphur is required in the form of the amino acids, methionine and cysteine; cobalt is required in the form of vitamin B_{12}.

In this chapter the nutritional diseases will be described under these headings and obesity will be considered on page 578.

Adult requirements for essential nutrients are given in Table 9.2.

ENERGY-YIELDING NUTRIENTS

CARBOHYDRATES

These usually provide a major part of the energy in a normal diet (4 kcal/g). No individual carbohydrate is an essential nutrient in the sense that the body needs it but cannot make it for itself from other nutrients. If the available carbohydrate intake is less than 100 g per day ketosis is likely to occur. Sugars are found in fruits, milk (lactose) and some vegetables. Starches are mostly found in cereals and root vegetables and legumes. Most forms of dietary fibre are polysaccharides too but these cannot be digested in the small intestine. The major carbohydrates in food are listed in the box below.

Sugars

Sugars are classified by the U.K. Department of Health as intrinsic (naturally incorporated in the cellular structure of fruits, milk, etc.) or extrinsic sugar (extracted, refined, concentrated, for example beet or cane sucrose). Intrinsic sugars and the foods that contain them are healthy foods and no threat to health.

Extrinsic sugars are one of the factors that can contribute to the development of dental caries. Apart from this and the possibility of contribution to obesity, the Department's expert panel concludes that moderate consumption of extrinsic sugars, particularly sucrose, plays no direct causal role in the development of cardiovascular disease or diabetes and has no specific effect on behaviour or psychological function.

Starches

Starches in cereal foods (wheat, rice), root foods (potatoes, cassava) and legumes are the nutrients which provide the largest proportion of calories in most diets round the world unless they are unusually high in fat or sugar. Although all starches are polymers of glucose, linked by the same 1–4 glycosidic linkages, they do not all behave in the same way when they are eaten.

Some starches are digested promptly by salivary followed by pancreatic amylase and produce a steep rise in blood glucose. Other starches are more slowly digested, either because they are protected in the structure of the food, or because of the crystal structure or because the molecule is unbranched (amylose). After ingestion the blood glucose rise is flatter and lower. The **glycaemic index** (see information box) quantifies the effect of different carbohydrates on the blood glucose after a test meal. A small percentage of dietary starch, more in some foods than others, may completely escape digestion in the small intestine and pass unchanged into the large intestine, where it is fermented by the resident bacteria. This **resistant starch** thus behaves in much the same way as dietary fibre. The presence of resistant starch in a food can be demonstrated in people with an ileostomy.

DIETARY FIBRE

Dietary fibre is the natural packing of plant foods. It can be defined as those parts of food which are not digested by human enzymes. The principal classes of dietary fibre are cellulose, hemicelluloses, lignins, pectins and gums.

These are all polysaccharides (i.e. carbohydrates) except lignin, which occurs with cellulose in the structure of plants. Pectins and gums are viscous, not fibrous.

Some types of dietary fibre, notably the hemicellulose of wheat, increase the water-holding capacity of colonic contents and the bulk of the faeces. They relieve simple constipation, appear to prevent diverticulosis and may reduce the risk of cancer of the colon. Other, viscous indigestible polysaccharides like pectin and guar gum have more effect in the upper gastrointestinal tract. They tend to slow gastric emptying, contribute to satiety, may flatten the glucose tolerance curve and reduce plasma cholesterol concentration.

Dietary fibre is in fact partly digested in the large intestine, by resident bacterial flora, not endogenous enzymes, with flatus formation, and a small quantity of volatile fatty acids is absorbed through the colonic mucosa. There are as yet no official recommended intakes for fibre because analyses for the different types in foods are not complete, but the present average intakes of about 15 to 20 g/day in affluent countries are thought to be too low.

FATS

With their high calorie value (9 kcal/g) fats are useful to people with a large energy expenditure. On the other hand they are an insidious cause of obesity for sedentary people. Saturated fats, especially those containing myristic (14:0) and palmitic (16:0) acids increase plasma low-density lipoproteins and total cholesterol. Monounsaturated fatty acids contain one double bond, e.g. oleic acid (18:1 ω9). Polyunsaturated fatty acids, with two or more double bonds, are in two main groups, depending on the distance of their first double bond, counting from the methyl (ω) end of the molecule. The principal polyunsaturated fatty acid in plant seed oils is linoleic acid (18:2 ω6). This and its elongated ω6 derivatives γ-linolenic acid (18:3 ω6) and arachidonic acid (20:4 ω6) are the essential fatty acids (EFAs), pre-

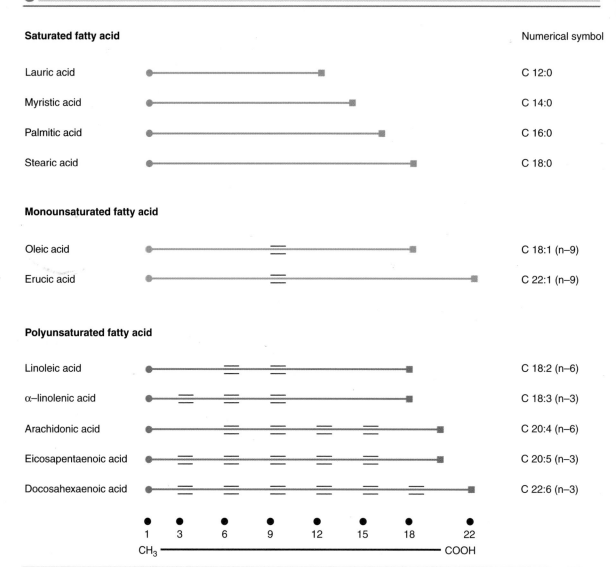

Saturated fatty acid   Numerical symbol

Lauric acid   C 12:0

Myristic acid   C 14:0

Palmitic acid   C 16:0

Stearic acid   C 18:0

Monounsaturated fatty acid

Oleic acid   C 18:1 (n–9)

Erucic acid   C 22:1 (n–9)

Polyunsaturated fatty acid

Linoleic acid   C 18:2 (n–6)

α–linolenic acid   C 18:3 (n–3)

Arachidonic acid   C 20:4 (n–6)

Eicosapentaenoic acid   C 20:5 (n–3)

Docosahexaenoic acid   C 22:6 (n–3)

1   3   6   9   12   15   18   22

CH_3 —————————————————————— COOH

Fig. 9.1   Schematic representation of the most important fatty acids in foods. Double bonds are indicated = and their positions shown in relation to the methyl (–CH_3) and acid (–COOH) ends. The alternative terminology for n − 3 is omega − 3 (ω − 3).

cursors of prostaglandins and eicosanoids and part of the structure of lipid membranes in all cells.

Essential fatty acid deficiency

This is rare in man but it has been reported in patients fed solely by vein (total parenteral nutrition) for long periods without fat emulsions. If sufficient glucose and amino acids are given (providing energy needs) they inhibit free fatty acid mobilisation from adipose tissue (where there is usually a moderate store of linoleic acid) and tissues in the rest of the body become depleted.

There is a scaly dermatitis and the diagnosis can be confirmed biochemically by an increased ratio of eicosatrienoic acid (20:3 ω9) to arachidonic in plasma lipids.

The ω3 series of polyunsaturated fatty acids, e.g. eicosapentaenoic (20:5 ω3) and docosahexaenoic (22:6 ω3) occur in fish oils. They are inhibitors of thrombosis and appear to act by competitively antagonising thromboxane A_2 formation. Purified fish body oils, e.g. 'Maxepa', are one of the treatment options which may reduce the tendency to thrombosis, for instance in people with coronary heart disease. They lower raised plasma triglycerides.

PROTEINS

These are made up of some 20 different amino acids, of which nine are essential for normal synthesis of the different proteins in the body and for maintaining nitrogen balance in adults. These **essential (or indispensable) amino acids** are listed in the information box below.

ESSENTIAL, OR INDISPENSABLE, AMINO ACIDS
(in approximate ascending order of size of requirement)

- Tryptophan
- Histidine
- Methionine+cysteine
- Threonine
- Isoleucine
- Valine
- Phenylalanine+tyrosine
- Lysine
- Leucine

Arginine is also needed in infants. Methionine can substitute for cysteine and phenylalanine for tyrosine but not vice versa. The term 'indispensable' is preferred to the older term 'essential' because dispensable (non-essential) amino acids (glycine, alanine, etc.) as well as indispensable amino acids (as above) are all essential at the cellular level. 'Indispensable' is used to mean required in the diet. The dispensable amino acids can be synthesised in the body by transamination provided there is a sufficient supply of amino groups.

The nutritive value of different proteins depends on the relative proportions of essential amino acids they contain. Proteins of animal origin, particularly from eggs, milk and meat, are generally of higher nutritive value than the proteins of vegetable origin which are deficient in one or more of the essential amino acids. However it is possible to have a diet of mixed vegetable proteins with high nutritive value if the principle of **complementation** is used. Cereals such as wheat, for example, contain about 10% protein and are relatively deficient in lysine. Legumes contain around 20% of protein which is relatively deficient in methionine. If two parts of wheat are mixed (or eaten) with one part of legume, a food results which contains 13% protein of high nutritive value. This happens because cereals contain enough methionine and legumes enough lysine to supplement the other component of the mixture.

The usual recommendation for an adequate protein intake is 10% of the total calories, i.e. about 65 g per day for the average adult. The minimum requirement is around 40 g of protein of good biological value.

Energy requirements

The largest component of energy expenditure is the basal metabolic rate (BMR). This increases with lean body mass (which is related to weight and height); it declines with age and is less in women than men. Extra energy is required for growth, pregnancy and lactation, for muscular activity and for pyrexia. There is considerable variation of energy expended between individuals of the same size, age, sex and activity. Adaptation occurs to an inadequate energy intake and to a lesser degree to superfluous energy intake. Approximate daily energy requirements are listed in the information box below.

DAILY ENERGY REQUIREMENTS

Apyrexial males in bed in industrial countries	2000 kcal	(8.4 MJ)
Male office workers in industrial countries	2700 kcal	(11.3 MJ)
Subsistence farmers in developing countries	2800 kcal	(11.7 MJ)
Men doing heavy work	3500 kcal	(14.6 MJ)
Apyrexial females in bed in industrial countries	1600 kcal	(6.7 MJ)
Healthy housewives in industrial countries	2000 kcal	(8.4 MJ)
Rural women in developing countries	2250 kcal	(9.4 MJ)

Individuals in Britain, including children, need somewhere around 2500 kcal (10.5 MJ) per day. The food moving into consumption has to provide more to allow for wastage, pets, tourists, etc. This gross value, around 3000 kcal, is easier to estimate at a national level. It is this higher figure that is discussed in the press and parliament and often confused with average physiological requirements.

There are two units in use for energy: kilocalories and kilo-joules (1 kcal = 4.184 kJ). Though both are metric, joules are SI units and are preferred in Europe for scientific usage. For a day's energy intake it is more convenient to use megajoules (MJ): 1 MJ = 1000 kJ.

FURTHER READING

Department of Health 1989 Committee on Medical Aspects of Food Policy: Dietary Sugars and Human Disease. Report of the Panel on Dietary Sugars. HM Stationery Office, London

Eaton S B, Konner M 1985 Paleolithic nutrition. A consideration of its nature and current implications. New England Journal of Medicine 312: 283–289

Schweizer T F, Edwards C A (eds.) 1992 Dietary fibre–a component of food. Springer-Verlag, Berlin

Truswell A S 1992 Glycaemic index of foods. European Journal of Clinical Nutrition 46, suppl. 2: S91–S101

World Health Organization 1985 Report of a Joint FAO/WHO/UNU Expert Consultation, Energy and Protein Requirements. Technical Report Service 724. WHO, Geneva

PROTEIN-ENERGY MALNUTRITION

PROTEIN-ENERGY MALNUTRITION (PEM) IN ADULTS

The predominant form of protein-energy malnutrition in adults is undernutrition, i.e. the result of a sustained negative energy (calorie) balance. This may be due to insufficient food supply in famine, or where food is available, to anorexia, increased energy requirements or increased energy losses. Energy to maintain life is drawn primarily from the adipose tissue, which in normally fed adults is a reserve of 450 MJ (108 000 kcal). Body fat is lost and muscles waste but at a slower rate. Gross features of visceral protein deficiency (see kwashiorkor p. 557) are rare in starvation; they are seen in some cases of hospital malnutrition (p. 574) in whom there is excessive turnover or excessive loss (for example in burns) of body protein. Depletion of electrolytes—sodium, potassium and magnesium—is common, often from diarrhoea.

Aetiology

The main causes of undernutrition and starvation are listed in the box below.

CAUSES OF UNDERNUTRITION

- Insufficient food
- Persistent regurgitation or vomiting
- Anorexia
- Malabsorption, e.g. small intestine disease
- Increased BMR, e.g. thyrotoxicosis, prolonged infections
- Loss of calories in urine, e.g. glycosuria in diabetes mellitus
- Cachexia in some cases of cancer

Starvation is severe undernutrition from a prolonged inadequacy of food intake. What follows here describes the features of severe undernutrition seen in adults and older children. In infants and pre-school children a similar process (marasmus) is described on page 556.

Clinical features

Adults lose weight and older children stop growing. The symptoms include craving for food, thirst, weakness, feeling cold, nocturia, amenorrhoea and impotence.

The face at first looks younger but later becomes old, withered and expressionless. The skin is lax, pale and dry and may show pigmented patches. Hair becomes thinned or lost except in adolescents. The extremities are cold and cyanosed and there may be pressure sores. Subcutaneous fat disappears, skin turgor is lost, and muscles waste. The arm circumference is subnormal. Oedema may be present in famine victims without hypoalbuminaemia ('famine oedema'). Body temperature is subnormal. The pulse is slow, blood pressure low and the heart small. The abdomen is distended and diarrhoea is common. Tendon jerks are diminished. Psychologically, starving people lose initiative; they are apathetic, depressed and introverted but become aggressive if food is nearby.

Under-nourished individuals are susceptible to infections. With respiratory muscles weakened by wasting, bronchopneumonia carries an increased mortality. Starving groups in famines have often had high mortalities from epidemics, e.g. typhus or cholera. The usual signs of infection may not appear. In advanced starvation patients become completely inactive and may assume a flexed, fetal position. Death comes quietly and often quite suddenly in the last stage of starvation. The very old are most vulnerable. All the organs are atrophied at necropsy except the brain which tends to maintain its weight.

Investigations

The only possible investigation in a famine is to measure the body weight, estimate the patient's height and grade the severity of undernutrition (see Table 9.3). Body mass index (BMI) is weight (kg)/(height^2) in metres.

Where other investigations are possible, plasma free fatty acids are found to be increased; there is ketosis and possibly a mild metabolic acidosis. Plasma glucose is low but albumin concentration is often normal. Insulin secretion is diminished, glucagon and cortisol tend to increase, reverse T3 replaces normal triiodothyronine. The resting metabolic rate falls, partly because of reduced lean body mass. The urine has a fixed specific gravity and creatinine excretion becomes low. There may be a mild anaemia, leucopenia and thrombocytopenia. The ESR is normal unless there is infection. Tests of delayed skin sensitivity, for example to tuberculin, are falsely negative. The ECG shows sinus brachycardia and low voltage.

Management

Whether in a famine or dealing with wasting secondary to disease, people or patients need to be graded (Table 9.3).

People with mild starvation are in no danger; those with moderate starvation need extra feeding. People who are severely underweight need hospital type care. 1500 to 2000 kcal/day will prevent the downward progress of undernutrition.

Table 9.3   Severity of undernutrition
- Mild undernutrition: weight for height 90% down to 81% of standard (BMI 20 to 18)
- Moderate undernutrition: weight for height 80% down to 71% of standard (BMI 18 to 16)
- Severe undernutrition: weight for height ≤70% of standard (BMI <16)

| Height (m) | Weight (kg) | |
	80% of standard* (BMI = 18)	70% of standard (BMI = 15.7)
1.45	38	33
1.48	39.5	34.5
1.50	40.5	35
1.52	41.5	36
1.54	42.5	37
1.56	44	38.5
1.58	45	39
1.60	46	40
1.62	47	41
1.64	48.5	42
1.66	49.5	43
1.68	50.5	44
1.70	52	45.5
1.72	53	47
1.74	54.5	48
1.76	56	49
1.78	57	50
1.80	58	51
1.82	60	52
1.84	61	53.5
1.86	62	54
1.88	63.5	55.5
1.90	65	57

*Standard weight = W/H^2 BMI = 22.5.

In severe starvation there is atrophy of the intestinal epithelium and of the exocrine pancreas, and bile is dilute. When food becomes available, it should be given in small amounts at first. Food should be bland and preferably similar to the usual staple meal, for example a cereal with some sugar, milk powder and oil. Salt should be restricted and a micronutrient supplement may be desirable, e.g. potassium, magnesium, multivitamins. During refeeding a weight gain of 5% body weight per month indicates satisfactory progress.

Circumstances and resources are different in every famine. The problems are mainly non-medical, e.g. organising transport and repair of trucks and shelters or coordinating relief from different organisations, reconciling international workers with local politicians and administrators, arranging security of food stores, ensuring that food is distributed on the basis of need and trying to procure the right food and appropriate medical supplies. Lastly, plans must be made for the future; for example, agricultural workers will be needed with enough strength to plough and plant the next crop when the rains return.

PROTEIN-ENERGY MALNUTRITION IN YOUNG CHILDREN

Classification and epidemiology

Severe protein-energy malnutrition (PEM or protein-calorie malnutrition) in early childhood is a spectrum of disease. At one end there is **kwashiorkor** in which the essential feature is deficiency of protein with relatively adequate energy intake. At the other end is **nutritional marasmus** which is total inanition of the infant, usually under one year of age, and which is due to a severe and prolonged restriction of all food, i.e. energy sources and other nutrients in addition to protein. In the middle of the spectrum is **marasmic kwashiorkor** in which there are clinical features of both disorders.

Some children adapt to prolonged energy and/or protein shortage by **nutritional dwarfism**. The most prevalent of all the varieties is **mild to moderate PEM** or the underweight child (Table 9.4). Children with one form of PEM can shift to another form. Thus a child with mild to moderate PEM may develop kwashiorkor after an infection. Such a child, when treated, loses oedema and may look marasmic. In marasmus there is a major loss of muscle, the body's main mass of protein, as well as the loss of fat; in kwashiorkor anorexia is characteristic and leads to inadequate secondary energy intake. For reasons like these, marasmus, kwashiorkor and milder forms are grouped together as protein-energy malnutrition.

The prevalence of PEM in its various forms is high in India and S.E. Asia, in most parts of Africa and the Middle East, in the Caribbean islands and in South and Central America. PEM is the most important dietary deficiency disease in the world. Severe forms affect around 2% and mild to moderate PEM affects around 20% (and in many places more) young children in developing countries.

Table 9.4   Classification of PEM in young children

	Body weight as percentage of international standard	Oedema	Deficit in weight for length
Kwashiorkor	80–60	+	+
Marasmic kwashiorkor	<60	+	++
Marasmus	<60	0	++
Nutritional dwarfing	<60	0	minimal
Underweight child	80–60	0	+

For international standard weights see Table 9.5.

NUTRITIONAL MARASMUS

Aetiology

This is the commoner form of severe protein-energy malnutrition. It is the childhood version of starvation. It occurs most commonly in the second six months of life. The cause is a diet very low in calories and incidentally in protein and other essential nutrients. Typically the child was weaned early and fed with dilute cows' milk formulae. This is a disease of infants of poor mothers in the cities of developing countries. The mother may have to go out to work and leave her baby with its grandmother, older sister or a neighbour. She has difficulty paying for the feeds and has neither the kitchen equipment nor the knowledge to prepare them without bacterial contamination. Poor hygiene leads to gastroenteritis and a vicious cycle develops. Diarrhoea leads to poor appetite and the depletion leads to intestinal atrophy and more susceptibility to diarrhoea.

Clinical features

The child is very thin with no subcutaneous fat, and looks wizened and shrunken; its muscles are severely wasted (Fig. 9.2). The head is large for the body, the ribs stand out, the abdomen may be distended (with gas), the limbs look like sticks and the buttocks are baggy. Diarrhoea is usual. In contrast to kwashiorkor,

Table 9.5 Reference or standard weights. Weight for age: birth to 5 years.[1] Sexes combined[2]

Age (months)	Weight (kg) Standard	80% Std	60% Std	Age (months)	Weight (kg) Standard	80% Std	60% Std
0	3.25	2.6	1.95	31	13.45	10.8	8.1
1	4.15	3.3	2.5	32	13.65	10.9	8.2
2	4.95	4.0	3.0	33	13.85	11.1	8.3
3	5.7	4.6	3.4	34	14.05	11.2	8.4
4	6.35	5.1	3.8	35	14.15	11.3	8.5
5	7.0	5.6	4.2	36	14.35	11.5	8.6
6	7.5	6.0	4.5	37	14.55	11.6	8.7
7	8.0	6.4	4.8	38	14.7	11.8	8.8
8	8.5	6.8	5.1	39	14.9	11.9	8.9
9	8.9	7.1	5.3	40	15.05	12.0	9.0
10	9.2	7.4	5.5	41	15.2	12.2	9.1
11	9.55	7.6	5.7	42	15.4	12.3	9.2
12	9.85	7.9	5.9	43	15.5	12.4	9.3
13	10.1	8.1	6.1	44	15.7	12.6	9.4
14	10.35	8.3	6.2	45	15.85	12.7	9.5
15	10.55	8.4	6.3	46	16.05	12.8	9.6
16	10.75	8.6	6.45	47	16.15	12.9	9.7
17	10.95	8.8	6.6	48	16.35	13.1	9.8
18	11.15	8.9	6.7	49	16.5	13.2	9.9
19	11.35	9.1	6.8	50	16.6	13.3	10.0
20	11.5	9.2	6.9	51	16.8	13.4	10.1
21	11.7	9.4	7.0	52	16.95	13.6	10.2
22	11.85	9.5	7.1	53	17.1	13.7	10.3
23	12.05	9.6	7.2	54	17.25	13.8	10.4
24	12.25	9.8	7.35	55	17.45	14.0	10.5
25	12.25	9.8	7.35	56	17.55	14.1	10.5
26	12.45	10.0	7.47	57	17.7	14.2	10.6
27	12.65	10.1	7.6	58	17.85	14.3	10.7
28	12.85	10.3	7.7	59	18.0	14.4	10.8
29	13.05	10.4	7.8	60	18.2	14.6	10.9
30	13.25	10.6	7.95				

[1]Based on: A growth chart for international use in maternal and child health care 1978. WHO, Geneva.
[2]On average boys are 0.3 kg heavier and girls 0.3 kg lighter than the mean standard but the differences are smaller than this in the first 2 months and 0.4–0.5 kg from 50–60 months.

Grossly underweight

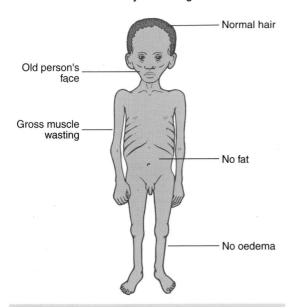

Normal hair

Old person's face

Gross muscle wasting

No fat

No oedema

Fig. 9.2 Marasmus.

there is no oedema and skin and hair changes are mild or absent. The child is not usually anorexic. Weight is reduced below 60% of standard (Table 9.5). Although the child has not been growing, weight is reduced more than length.

A search must be made for chronic infection like tuberculosis or other major disease (cardiac, renal, intestinal) that could produce secondary marasmus. Dehydration frequently occurs from diarrhoea or vomiting. There may be associated deficiencies of vitamins, such as vitamin A causing xerophthalmia, and of inorganic nutrients such as potassium and magnesium. Associated infections are shown in the box below.

Management

Severe PEM, whether kwashiorkor or marasmus, is dealt with in three phases.

INFECTIONS ASSOCIATED WITH PEM

Patients with marasmus, kwashiorkor and starvation have increased susceptibility to:
- Gastroenteritis and Gram-negative septicaemia
- Respiratory infections
- Certain viral diseases, especially measles and herpes simplex
- Tuberculosis
- Streptococcal and staphylococcal skin infections
- Helminthic infestations

Resuscitation

This consists of correction of dehydration, electrolyte disturbances, acidosis, hypoglycaemia and hypothermia and also treatment for infections.

Initiation of cure

This consists of refeeding, gradually working up the calories to 150 kcal/kg per day with protein about 1.5 g/kg per day. The major units with research experience of PEM have each evolved somewhat different dietary formulas, depending on local availability and preferences for weaning foods. They are usually based on dried skimmed milk mixed with some flour or sugar and some oil and given 5–6 times a day. Because of anorexia, children often have to be handfed, preferably in the lap of their mother or a nurse they know. Potassium, magnesium and a multi-vitamin mixture are also needed.

Nutritional rehabilitation

After about 3 weeks the child should be obviously better. If there was oedema this will have cleared, any skin lesions are healing and diarrhoea has ceased. The child is stronger, mentally bright and has a good appetite but is still underweight for his or her age. During this stage of rehabilitation and catch-up growth, the child should be looked after in a convalescent home or by the mother who should have been educated about nutrition and helped to obtain extra food. The diet should be based on nutritious combinations of local, familiar foods.

KWASHIORKOR

Aetiology

The name comes from Ghana where the condition was first described by Cicely Williams in 1933. This form of malnutrition occurs most often in the second year of life when the child is weaned from the breast on to a diet low in protein such as cassava, plantain or yam or to a cereal that has been refined and diluted. There is little milk, and custom, sometimes reinforced by taboos, determines that the limited foods of animal origin are given to the men of the family, or the small amount of protein-rich food is in a sauce made with hot peppers or spices and unsuitable for young children. If the customary diet of a population is limited in protein and in calories to around the levels of minimum requirements, a child may be in moderate health until the protein requirements are increased by an infection. Gastroenteritis, measles and malaria are all notorious precipitants of kwashiorkor.

Pathogenesis

The major pathological feature of kwashiorkor is fairly acute depletion of protein in the viscera, liver, pancreas and gut. The classical theory of the pathogenesis is that carbohydrate intake is relatively adequate so that insulin secretion is maintained. This favours movement of amino acids into muscles for protein synthesis so that with diminished amino acid supply from inadequate dietary protein the liver is depleted and cannot synthesise plasma albumin or low (and very low) density lipoproteins. These two dysfunctions lead respectively to hypoalbuminaemic oedema and fatty liver with low plasma lipids. Associated potassium depletion may contribute to the oedema. The hypothesis has been proposed recently that free radical damage plays a role in the pathogenesis of kwashiorkor.

Clinical features

The child is not very thin. There is oedema which tends to be generalised. The child is miserable and apathetic and has a characteristic mewing cry. The skin shows symmetrical changes, maximally in the napkin (diaper) area. At first it is pigmented and thickened as if varnished, then it cracks and leads to denuded areas of shallow ulceration (Fig. 9.3). In moderate cases the areas of dermatosis resemble crazy paving; when severe the desquamated area can look as if the child has been burnt (Fig. 9.4). The hair alters in colour from black to blond, reddish or grey; it becomes thin and sparse. Mucosal changes, such as angular stomatitis, may be seen. Anorexia is present and diarrhoea is common. The liver may be palpable. The characteristic laboratory finding is a very low plasma albumin concentration.

Prognosis

Severe PEM has a mortality around 20% even in well-equipped hospitals. Most deaths occur in the first 10 days. Follow-up needle biopsies have shown that the fatty liver of acute kwashiorkor resolves quickly and does not go on to cirrhosis. Physical growth of the brain is retarded in children who suffer severe PEM in the first two years of life (usually marasmus). There is circumstantial evidence that intelligence may be impaired,

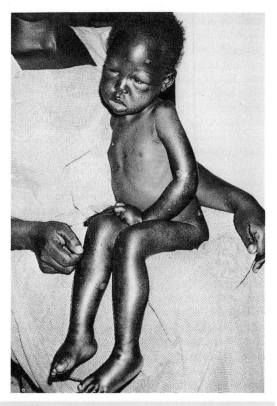

Fig. 9.3 A child with kwashiorkor. Showing oedema of face, feet and hands, and skin lesions.

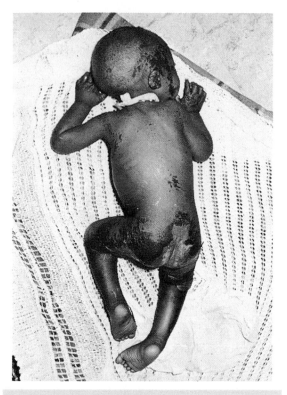

Fig. 9.4 A child with kwashiorkor. Showing pigmented lesions especially over the buttocks, thighs, side of head and backs of hands.

particularly if the child goes home to a poor environment.

MILD TO MODERATE PEM (THE UNDERWEIGHT CHILD)

For every florid case of kwashiorkor or marasmus there are likely to be 7 or 10 in the community with mild to moderate PEM. The situation is like an iceberg; there is more malnutrition below the surface than is recognisable on clinical inspection. Even the mothers themselves do not notice most of these cases because their children are similar in size and vitality to many others of the same age in the neighbourhood. Most children with subclinical PEM can, however, be detected by their weight for age, which is less than 80% of the international standard (Table 9.5). In parts of many developing countries surveys may show that up to 50% of children under five are underweight. Because scales are difficult to carry, a convenient screen test for mild to moderate malnutrition is to measure the mid-upper arm circumference with a simple piece of tape. From 12 to 60 months of age the

normal arm circumference stays the same for 4 years. Over 13.5 cm is a normal circumference (coloured green on the tape), 12.5 to 13.5 cm suggests mild malnutrition (coloured amber) and under 12.5 indicates probable malnutrition (red part of the tape).

In areas where kwashiorkor is the predominant florid form of PEM, subclinical cases have reduced plasma albumin ('pre-kwashiorkor'). Sometimes a child is seen who has adapted to chronic inadequate feeding by reduced linear growth but who looks like a normal child a year or two younger. This is known as **nutritional dwarfism**.

The great importance of mild to moderate PEM is that these children are growing up smaller than their potential and they are very susceptible to gastroenteritis and respiratory infections, which in turn can precipitate frank malnutrition. Mild to moderate PEM is probably the major underlying reason why the 1 to 4-year mortality in a developing country can be 30 to 40 times higher than in Europe or North America. Official statistics record most of these deaths as due simply to infections.

Prevention

Preventive measures for kwashiorkor and marasmus are listed in the table below.

Table 9.6   UNICEF's inexpensive measures to prevent PEM

Mnemonic GOBI

G for growth monitoring. The mother keeps the simple growth chart—the Road to Health card—in a cellophane envelope and brings the child to a clinic regularly for weighing and advice

O for oral rehydration. The UNICEF formula (NaCl 3.5 g, NaHCO$_3$ 2.5 g, KCl 1.5 g, glucose 20 g or sucrose 40 g and clean water to a litre) is saving many lives from gastroenteritis

B for breast feeding. This is a matter of life and death in a poor community with no facilities for hygiene. Additional food—which should be prepared from locally available foods—is not usually needed until 6 months of age

I for immunisation. For a few dollars a child can be protected against measles, diphtheria, pertussis, tetanus, tuberculosis and poliomyelitis. In a rational world the money for this could be taken from a small part of the 1,000 billion dollars spent on armaments each year

---

FURTHER READING

Harrison G A (ed.) 1988 Famine. Oxford University Press, Oxford
Suskind R M, Lewinter-Suskind L (eds) 1990 The malnourished child. Nestlé Nutrition; Raven Press, New York
Waterlow J C 1992 Protein energy malnutrition. Edward Arnold, London

---

WATER, ELECTROLYTES AND MINERALS

Sixteen or more inorganic elements are essential for man, as they are for other animals; deficiency disease is known for each, due to inadequate diet or from excessive losses. The elements are sodium (p. 591), potassium (p. 591), chloride, magnesium (p. 601), calcium, phosphorus, iron, iodine, zinc, copper, chromium, selenium, manganese and molybdenum. Fluoride appears to be essential for rats and optimal intakes reduce dental caries in man. Cobalt is physiologically active only in the form of vitamin B$_{12}$ and sulphur is required in the form of the amino acids methionine and cysteine.

Boron is being investigated at present to determine if it is an essential trace nutrient for man. In addition tin, vanadium, nickel and silicon have been shown, by artificial isolator systems, to be essential for animals. Human deficiency disease is not known for any of these minor trace elements.

The normal distribution of water and electrolytes, sodium, potassium and chloride in the body and the disturbances which result when their intake or output is diminished or increased are discussed in detail on pages 586 to 609.

ELEMENTS OF IMPORTANCE IN HUMAN NUTRITION

Calcium

The body of an adult normally contains about 1200 g of calcium. At least 99% of this is present in the skeleton, where calcium salts (chiefly hydroxyapatite), held in a cellular matrix, provide the hard structure of the bones and teeth. The dietary sources are listed below.

DIETARY SOURCES OF CALCIUM

- Milks, cheeses, yoghurt and their products
- Fish eaten with bone, e.g., sardines, pilchards
- Some shellfish
- Some nuts, e.g. almonds, peanuts
- Some vegetables, e.g. chick peas, beans
- Bread (if fortified), and egg

Absorption

In adults around 70% of the calcium in food is excreted in faeces; during growth the efficiency of absorption is greater. Calcium absorption may be impaired either by lack of vitamin D, by any condition causing small intestinal hurry, by the combination of calcium with excess fatty acids to form insoluble soaps in steatorrhoea, or by foods containing oxalate (e.g. spinach) or phytate (whole grain cereals) which can form insoluble salts with calcium.

Recommended intakes of calcium

The amount of calcium which has to be added to the bones to produce the final adult amount averages 180 mg/day from 0 to 18 years but reaches 400 mg/day at the peak of adolescent growth. Since calcium absorption is inefficient the reference nutrient intake in Britain is 350 mg (1–3 years) to 550 mg (7–10 years) for children and 800 (female) or 1000 (male) mg in adolescents. Expert opinion is divided on the safe minimum intake in adults. WHO recommended 500 mg/day because in many parts of Africa and Asia children develop and adults maintain healthy bones on this intake or lower. The USA recommends 800 mg for adults, and 1000 mg have been advised (in Australia) for post-menopausal women. These figures are based on calcium balances. It appears that calcium is handled less economically by people in developed countries. Possible explanations include less skin synthesis of vitamin D from sunshine and increased obligatory urinary calcium because of high animal protein and sodium intakes. In pregnancy and lactation extra calcium is needed—1200 mg per day

Calcium is the most obvious and persistent of the micro-nutrients, the fifth most abundant element, and the most abundant cation in the body, yet it is more difficult to measure adequacy of intake for calcium than for other nutrients. Any reduction of absorbed calcium does not show in the plasma concentration, which is immediately reset by increased parathyroid secretion and formation of 1,25 dihydroxy-vitamin D, probably because any change of ionised plasma concentration would disturb neuromuscular irritability and blood coagulation. The most likely cause of reduced plasma calcium is low plasma albumin, with reduced protein-bound calcium. Likewise intracellular plasma concentration, which affects activities of many enzymes, is also tightly controlled. If calcium intake is inadequate, therefore a little less will go into the bones in children or a little will be removed from the bones in adults. Small changes in total bone calcium can be measured only as research procedures at present using dual energy X-ray absorptiometry.

The two major questions about calcium nutrition are:

1. Will a high intake during the growing phase of life contribute to taller adult height or heavier bones? If so, how much is optimal?
2. Will a high intake from about 45 years onwards delay the onset of osteoporosis (p. 931)?

Phosphorus

This is used by the body in the form of phosphates which are present in many biochemical compounds and so in all unrefined plant and animal foods and in milk. Dietary deficiency is rare. Usual dietary intakes are rather higher than for calcium, about 1.5 g/day. Total body phosphorus is about 700 g, most being in the bones.

Phosphate deficiency occurs in premature infants fed on human milk, in patients with renal tubular phosphate loss, from prolonged high dosage of aluminium hydroxide antacids, sometimes when alcoholics are re-fed with high carbohydrate foods, and in patients on total parenteral nutrition if not enough phosphate is provided. The features of deficiency are hypophosphataemia (subnormal plasma inorganic phosphorus) and muscle weakness (from deficiency of ATP).

Iron

A good mixed diet with average amounts of meat and vegetables contains about 12–15 mg of iron. Cheap, monotonous high carbohydrate diets based on refined wheat flour contain much less. Foods rich in iron are listed in the information box below.

There is no physiological mechanism for secretion of

DIETARY SOURCES OF IRON

- **Haem iron**
  Muscle meat (red more than white), organ meat (e.g. liver), fish and shellfish

- **Non-haem iron**
  Oatmeal, legumes (peas, beans), nuts, dried fruit, wholemeal bread, iron-fortified cereal foods, red wine, chocolate. Foods rich in vitamin C in the same meal enhance iron absorption

---

iron so maintenance of its homeostasis depends on iron absorption. Normally body iron loss from desquamated surface cells adds up to about 1 mg daily. Assuming 15% absorption, about 8 mg are therefore required in the diet daily in men, but if there is any bleeding this brings with it much more loss of iron. Blood is the tissue richest in iron; 1 ml contains 0.5 mg of iron so that a regular blood loss of only 2 ml/day doubles the iron requirement. At menstruation 30 mg of iron is usually lost, and considerably more in a few women. For this reason premenopausal women require about twice as much iron as men, about 15 mg/day.

An account of iron metabolism and of the measures for the prevention and treatment of iron deficiency anaemia is given on page 782 onwards. This is one of the most important nutritional causes of ill-health in Britain and other prosperous countries.

Siderosis

Dietary iron overload is seen in South African Black men who cook and brew beer in iron pots. They may ingest as much as 100 mg of iron per day. Iron accumulates in the liver and when severe can lead to cirrhosis. A similar condition has been described in other countries following excessive indulgence in cheap wines which can contain 30 mg of iron per litre.

Haemochromatosis

This is caused by inherited increased absorption of iron. A similar condition can result from chronic haemolysis.

Iodine

This is present in the sea, in seafoods and in trace amounts in soil and water over most of the land and in foods grown there. Iodine is however lacking in the highest mountainous areas of the world, e.g. the Alps, Himalayas, Rockies, Andes and the mountains of central America and and Papua New Guinea. About 400 million people living in these areas are estimated to have an inadequate iodine intake. About half of them show endemic goitre.

When visible goitres are found in 10% or more of the

adolescents this indicates that the whole community has very low urinary iodine, e.g. <30 μg per 1 g creatinine. Where most women have endemic goitre, 1% or more of the babies are born with cretinism and the other 'normal' people in the community show a higher prevalence than usual of deafness, slowed reflexes and poor learning. The adult requirement for iodine is about 100 μg/day.

Endemic goitre has now almost disappeared from most of the low iodine regions of Europe and North America due to the use of iodised salt and inter-regional trade of foods. In remote mountainous parts of the developing world without roads, shops and a cash economy, iodised salt will not reach enough people and the best way of preventing cretinism is by injecting all women of child-bearing age with 1–2 ml of iodised poppyseed oil every 5 years. This contains 475 to 950 mg of iodine.

Elimination of iodine deficiency disorders (IDD) is a public health priority for WHO.

Fluoride

The regular presence of fluoride in minute amounts in human bones and teeth and its influence on the prevention of dental caries justifies its inclusion as an element of importance in human nutrition.

Most adults ingest between 1 and 3 mg of fluoride daily. The chief source is usually drinking water, which, if it contains 1 part per million (p.p.m.) of fluoride, will supply 1–2 mg/day. Soft waters usually contain no fluoride, whilst very hard waters may contain over 10 p.p.m.

Compared with that in water, the fluoride in foodstuffs is of little importance. Very few contain more than 1 p.p.m.; the exceptions are sea-fish, which may contain 5–10 p.p.m., and tea. In Britain, Australia and China, where people drink tea frequently, the adult intake from this source may be as much as 3 mg daily.

Use of fluoride in the prevention of dental caries

Epidemiological studies in many parts of the world established that where the natural water supply contains fluoride in amounts of 1 p.p.m. or more, the incidence of dental caries is lower than in comparable areas where the water contains only traces of the element.

The benefit of fluoride is greatest when it is taken before the permanent teeth erupt, while their enamel is being laid down. Traces of fluoride incorporated in the surface enamel increase its resistance to acid attack.

The deliberate addition of traces of fluoride (at 1 p.p.m.) to those public water supplies which are deficient is now a widespread practice throughout North America, where about 100 million people are now drinking fluoridated water. In at least 30 other countries similar projects have been started. In Britain regrettably some local authorities are not yet adding fluoride to their water supplies in those areas in which the element is lacking. But even here some fluoride reaches people's mouths in toothpaste.

Fluorosis

In parts of the world where the water fluoride is high (over 3–5 p.p.m.) mottling of the teeth is common. The enamel loses its lustre and becomes rough, pigmented and pitted. The effect is purely cosmetic; fluorotic teeth are resistant to caries and not usually associated with any evidence of skeletal fluorosis, or impairment of health.

Chronic fluoride poisoning

This occurs in several localities in India, China, Argentina, East and South Africa, where the water supply contains over 10 p.p.m. fluoride. Fluorine poisoning has also occurred as an industrial hazard among workers handling fluorine-containing minerals such as cryolite (sodium aluminium fluoride), used in smelting aluminium. The main clinical features are in the skeleton which shows increased density of bone, especially of the spine, pelvis and limbs, and calcification of ligaments and tendinous insertions of muscles.

Zinc

Although human deficiency was not clearly established before 1972, zinc is emerging as a nutrient of clinical importance. Zinc is an essential component of many enzymes including carbonic anhydrase, alcohol dehydrogenase, alkaline phosphatase, lactic dehydrogenase, superoxide dismutase and pancreatic carboxypeptidases, and appears to help stabilise RNA and DNA and to be part of several transcription factors. In PEM, associated zinc deficiency causes thymic atrophy, and zinc supplements may accelerate the healing of skin lesions. Causes of low plasma zinc are listed in the information box below. However, low plasma zinc is not a reliable sign of zinc depletion.

CAUSES FOR NEGATIVE ZINC BALANCE AND LOW PLASMA ZINC IN ADULTS

- Intestinal disease
- Chronic alcoholism
- Anorexia nervosa
- Diabetes mellitus
- Nephrotic syndrome
- Burns
- Haemodialysis
- Chronic febrile illnesses

Acute zinc deficiency has been reported in patients receiving prolonged intravenous alimentation without added zinc. Diarrhoea, mental apathy, a moist eczematoid dermatitis especially round the mouth, and loss of hair were accompanied by a very low plasma zinc concentration and all responded to administration of zinc.

Chronic deficiency has been described in association with dwarfism and hypogonadism in the Middle East.

The recommended daily intake is 7 mg for women and 9.5 mg for men. The best dietary sources are listed in the information box below.

DIETARY SOURCES OF ZINC

- Oysters (very high), wheat bran
- Liver, beef, lamb, other meats
- Wholemeal wheat flour and bread, oatmeal
- Sardines, crab, breakfast cereals
- Nuts, legumes

Selenium

The content of selenium in soil varies. In some areas farm animals develop disease from too much selenium; in others they will thrive only when given a selenium supplement. In Keshan in N.E. China a cardiomyopathy was described in children in 1979. Soil and blood seleniums are very low and Keshan disease can be prevented by giving small selenium supplements. In New Zealand (South Island) and Finland, selenium intakes and plasma selenium are low but there are no clear deficiency effects. In the rest of the world a little selenium should be included in the fluid for long-term total parenteral nutrition; myopathy has occurred when it was not included. Selenium is part of the enzyme glutathione peroxidase which helps prevent hydroperoxides from accumulating in lipids of cell membranes. A second function is as part of the enzyme responsible for conversion of thyroxine to triiodothyronine in liver microsomes. Some of the functions of selenium and vitamin E overlap.

Other minerals

Sulphur is mainly supplied by the S-containing amino acids in the diet—methionine and cysteine; effects of its deficiency are therefore inseparable from those of protein. **Copper** metabolism is abnormal in Wilson's disease (p. 529). Deficiency occasionally occurs in young children; the main features are anaemia, retarded growth and skeletal rarefaction. **Chromium** facilitates the action of insulin. Deficiency has been reported in some children with PEM and as a rare complication of prolonged parenteral nutrition, presenting as hyperglycaemia.

The roles of **sodium, potassium** and **magnesium** are discussed in Chapter 10.

FURTHER READING

Hetzel B S 1989 The story of iodine deficiency. Oxford University Press, Oxford

---

THE VITAMINS

Vitamins are organic substances in food which are required in small amounts but which cannot be synthesised in adequate quantities. Twelve vitamins have, so far, been demonstrated to have clinical effects in man. (see Table 9.7).

Pantothenic acid, a major component of coenzyme A, also appears to be essential, but human deficiency disease has not been reported, perhaps because the vitamin is widely distributed in foods, as its name implies. It is routinely included in total diet preparations, e.g. fluid for total parenteral nutrition.

Deficiencies of vitamins still occur in affluent countries, e.g. of folate, thiamin and vitamins D and C. Some of these are induced by diseases or drugs. In developing countries deficiency diseases are more prevalent; vitamin A deficiency (xerophthalmia) for instance is a major cause of blindness.

Some vitamins have pharmacological actions above the intake that prevents classic deficiency disease, e.g. vitamin A is used (with precautions) for acne; nicotinic acid is a standard treatment for some types of hyperlipidaemia.

Table 9.7 Names of vitamins

	Recommended name*	Alternative name(s)	Usual pharmaceutical preparation
	Vitamin A	Retinol	Retinol ester
Vitamin B complex	Thiamin	Vitamin B_1	Thiamin HCl
	Riboflavin	Vitamin B_2	Riboflavin
	Niacin	Nicotinic acid and nicotinamide	Nicotinamide
	Vitamin B_6	Pyridoxine	Pyridoxine HCl
	Pantothenic acid		Calcium panthothenate
	Biotin		Biotin
	Folate	Folacin	Folic acid
	Vitamin B_{12}	Cobalamin	Cyanocobalamin or hydroxocobalamin
	Vitamin C	Ascorbic acid	Ascorbic acid
	Vitamin D	D_2 and D_3	(Ergo)calciferol
	Vitamin E		α-Tocopherol
	Vitamin K		Vitamin K_1

*Where there is only one substance with vitamin activity (e.g. thiamin, riboflavin) the International Union of Nutritional Sciences recommends that the chemical name be used. Where there are several compounds with vitamin activity, names like vitamin A, vitamin E, cover them all.

Taking vitamin tablets is fashionable in affluent countries and a few practitioners recommend 'megavitamin therapy' of some vitamins. Doctors therefore need to know the features of both deficiency and of overdosage of the major vitamins. Side-effects are most serious with high dosage of three vitamins: A, B_6 and D.

Factors influencing the utilisation of vitamins are listed in the box below.

FACTORS INFLUENCING UTILISATION OF VITAMINS

- Digestion and absorption
- Antivitamins, e.g. thiaminase in raw fish; drugs
- Provitamins, e.g. carotenes
- Bacteria in gut—may synthesise (e.g. vit K) or extract vitamins
- Biosynthesis in skin—vitamin D
- Interactions of nutrients, e.g. more thiamin needed if diet rich in carbohydrate or alcohol

---

VITAMIN A (RETINOL)

Retinol is a fat-soluble substance, the first vitamin to be recognised (in 1913). It has multiple functions. (1) In vision 11-cis retinaldehyde is the initial part of the photoreceptor complex in rods and cones. (2) Another form of the vitamin, retinoic acid, induces differentiation of epithelial cells by binding to specific receptors which turn on responsive genes. In vitamin A deficiency mucus-secreting cells are replaced by keratin-producing cells. (3) Vitamin A has been called the anti-infective vitamin. Deficient children suffer more severe respiratory infections and gastroenteritis and increased mortality.

On the world scale vitamin A deficiency is estimated to cause 500 000 new cases of blindness a year in young children, mostly in Asia. The World Health Organization following resolutions of the World Summit for Children (1990) is giving high priority to prevention of vitamin A deficiency and its consequences, including blindness.

Dietary sources

Retinol is found only in foods of animal origin (see information box); liver is the richest source. But about two-thirds of vitamin A intake in Britain (and total intake in vegans) comes from carotenes (chiefly β-carotene), yellow and orange pigments in the leaves of vegetables and some fruits. Because absorption of (fat-soluble) β-carotene is incomplete and its cleavage to retinol is inefficient, 6 μg of β-carotene is equivalent to 1 μg of retinol

---

DIETARY SOURCES OF RETINOL

- Liver (richest natural source)
- Milk
- Butter
- Cheese
- Egg yolk
- Fish liver oils
  (Retinol or carotene is added to margarine in Britain and other countries)

DIETARY SOURCES OF CAROTENE

- Carrots (richest source)
- Dark green leafy vegetables
- Some yellow and red fruits (apricots, melon, pumpkin)
- Red palm oil

(see Fig. 9.5). The second information box below gives dietary sources of carotene.

β-carotene is one of the few compounds of the large group of carotenoids with pro-vitamin A activity. But all the **carotenoids,** including lycopene and lutein, with or without vitamin A activity are antioxidants, vital in protecting plants from oxidative side effects of photosynthesis. In humans, epidemiological evidence suggests that they may give partial protection against several common cancers.

Healthy adults in Britain have large stores of retinol in their livers (pp. 485 and 487).

NIGHT BLINDNESS

Retin*al* (the aldehyde form) is an essential component of the pigment rhodopsin on which rod vision in dim light depends. Hence sustained retinol deficiency results in impairment of dark adaptation. Night blindness is common, as also is vitamin A deficiency, in poor people

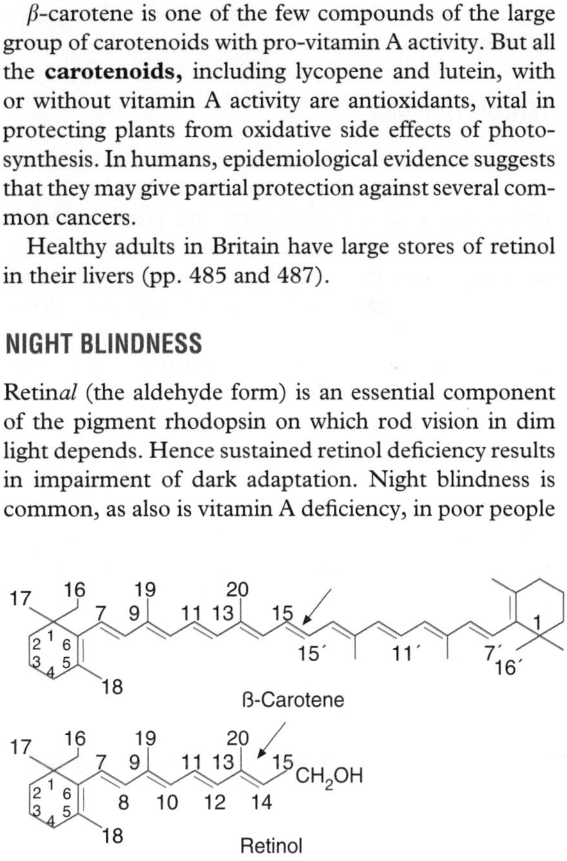

Fig. 9.5 **Formation of retinol from Beta-carotene.**

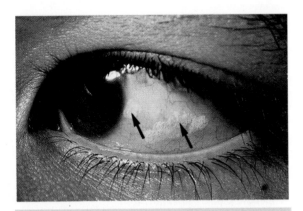

Fig. 9.6 **Bitôt's spots** showing the white triangular plaques.

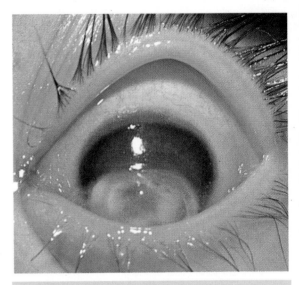

Fig. 9.7 **Keratomalacia** secondary to vitamin A deficiency. 14-month-old child with colliquative necrosis affecting the greater part of the cornea. The relative sparing of the superior aspect of the cornea is typical.

living in underdeveloped countries; it can occur in the malabsorption syndrome in affluent countries. The diagnosis of vitamin A deficiency is supported by low plasma vitamin A concentration and is confirmed by marked improvement in dark adaptation following therapeutic doses of retinol.

XEROPHTHALMIA

The earliest sign is xerosis conjunctivae—a dry, thickened and pigmented bulbar conjunctiva with a peculiar smoky appearance. Bitôt's spots are glistening white plaques of desquamated thickened conjunctival epithelium, usually triangular in shape and firmly adherent to the underlying conjunctiva (Fig. 9.6). When dryness spreads to the cornea it takes on a dull, hazy, lacklustre appearance due to keratinisation, and xerophthalmia is said to be present

In young children, xerophthalmia is almost always attributed to recent vitamin A deficiency and is usually associated with PEM. In older children and in adults its interpretation is less simple. Exposure to dust and glare may produce similar changes. They should, however, always call attention to the diet. Recognition of xerophthalmia is very important in young children because once the cornea is involved the process can rapidly progress to keratomalacia.

KERATOMALACIA

This disease causes blindness among Indians, Indonesians and other rice-eating people of Asia; it also occurs in parts of Africa, the Middle East and Latin America. In Europe and North America it is very rare. Children between the ages of 1 and 5 years are most commonly affected. It occurs only in persons who have been living for a long period on diets almost entirely devoid of vitamin A. The disease is frequently associated with PEM.

Clinical features
The earliest manifestations are night blindness and xerophthalmia. Later the cornea undergoes necrosis and ulceration (Fig. 9.7). Unless early and adequate treatment is given, there is a grave risk of blindness or death from associated diseases. Evidently vitamin A deficiency affects epithelia beyond the eye and these children have a high mortality from infections.

Management
Immediately on diagnosis a single large dose of 60 mg retinol as palmitate or acetate (200 000 i.u.) should be given orally, or if there is vomiting or severe diarrhoea 55 mg retinol palmitate by intramuscular injection. The oral dose should be repeated the next day and again prior to discharge or at a follow-up visit.

Underlying conditions such as PEM and other nutritional disorders, diarrhoea, dehydration and electrolyte imbalance and infections must be treated appropriately.

For the secondary bacterial infection, antibiotics are of value. Local treatment of the eye will be required only if disorganisation is already present, in which case the services of an ophthalmic surgeon should be obtained.

Prevention

Doctors and nurses working in the tropics, who may have been trained in Europe or North America, should make sure they are familiar with the appearances of xerophthalmia. If in doubt it is better to give a short course of vitamin A treatment.

Pregnant women should be advised to eat dark green leafy vegetables. This helps to build up stores of retinol in the fetal liver. They should also be taught to give such vegetables or locally available carotene-rich fruits to their babies. Controlled trials in Indonesia, Nepal, India and Ghana have shown that in communities where xerophthalmia occurs, single prophylactic oral doses of 60 mg retinol (200 000 i.u.) as palmitate to preschool children significantly reduce mortality from gastroenteritis and respiratory infections by about a third. In such communities a similar large dose is indicated in any child with measles.

Toxicity

Single large doses in children, as above, are well tolerated. The most serious side effect of repeated moderately high doses is teratogenicity. This is also the most serious side effect of vitamin A derivatives, retinoids used for acne and some other dermatological conditions. Acute overdose leads to nausea and headache, increased intracranial pressure, and skin desquamation. Chronic high doses can cause liver damage and hyperostosis.

THIAMIN (VITAMIN B₁)

Thiamin pyrophosphate (TPP) is an essential coenzyme for the decarboxylation of pyruvate to acetyl coenzyme A. This is the bridge between anaerobic glycolysis and the tricarboxylic acid (Krebs) cycle. TPP is also the coenzyme for transketolase in the hexose monophosphate shunt pathway and for decarboxylation of α-ketoglutarate to succinate in the Krebs cycle. Consequently when thiamin is deficient:

- the cells cannot metabolise glucose aerobically; this is likely to affect the nervous system first, since it depends entirely on glucose for its energy requirements
- there is accumulation of pyruvic acid and of lactic acid derived from it, which produce vasodilatation and increase cardiac output.

Thiamin deficiency can produce high output cardiac failure and/or peripheral neuropathy and/or encephalopathy. These occur in various combinations in wet and dry beriberi, infantile beriberi and Wernicke's encephalopathy.

- Wet beriberi: a high output cardiac failure with few ECG changes and prompt response to thiamin;
- Wernicke's encephalopathy: quiet confusion, ophthalmoplegia and ataxia. These respond to thiamin, but a memory disorder (Korsakoff's psychosis) may remain and is sometimes very persistent;
- Dry beriberi: a type of peripheral neuropathy.

Research cannot yet explain why the brain is affected in one person, the heart in another and the peripheral nerves in a third. Possibly the cardiomyopathy occurs in people who use their muscles for heavy work and so accumulate large amounts of pyruvate, producing intense vasodilatation and increasing cardiac work, while encephalopathy is the first manifestation in less active people.

High carbohydrate diets, heavy alcohol intake or intravenous glucose infusions predispose to and aggravate thiamin deficiency. The body contains only 30 mg of thiamin—30 times the adult daily requirement—and deficiency starts after about a month on a thiamin-free diet, sooner than for any other vitamin.

Dietary sources of thiamin are listed in the information box below.

DIETARY SOURCES OF THIAMIN

- Wheat germ, wholemeal wheat flour and bread
- Yeast, legumes, nuts
- Pork, duck, Marmite
- Oatmeal, fortified breakfast cereals
- White bread if flour enriched
- Cod's roe, other meats

WET BERIBERI

Aetiology

Beriberi is a nutritional disorder formerly widespread in South and East Asia. The word comes from the Sinhalese language and means 'I cannot' (said twice), signifying that the patient is too ill to do anything. Beriberi has almost disappeared from prosperous Asian countries such as Japan, Taiwan, Malaysia, Hong Kong and Singapore.

Oriental beriberi is usually caused by eating diets in which most of the calories are derived from polished, i.e. highly milled, rice. The disorder is often precipitated by infections, hard physical labour or pregnancy and lactation. In Britain and North America occasional cases of beriberi heart disease are seen, usually in alcoholics who have been consuming little but alcohol for some weeks.

Owing to a lack of thiamin, glucose is incompletely

metabolised and pyruvic and lactic acids accumulate in the tissues and body fluids. These metabolites cause dilatation of peripheral blood vessels, as in normal exercise. In beriberi this vasodilatation may be extreme, so that fluid leaks out through the capillaries, producing oedema. At the same time the blood flows rapidly through the dilated peripheral circulation. There is a high cardiac output and as the disease progresses the heart dilates because the myocardium is both overworked and unable to use glucose efficiently as an energy substrate. Serious cases can progress to low output cardiac failure ('shoshin' beriberi).

Clinical features

Oedema is the most notable feature and may develop rapidly to involve not only the legs but also the face, trunk and serous cavities. Palpitations are marked and there may be pain in the legs after walking, probably due to the accumulation of lactic acid. There is usually tachycardia and an increase in pulse pressure. The heart is enlarged and the jugular venous pressure rises.

While the circulation is well maintained, the skin is typically warm owing to the vasodilatation; as heart failure advances, the skin of the extremities can become cold and cyanotic. The mind is usually clear. Electrocardiograms often show no changes except sinus tachycardia but in some cases there are inverted T waves or conduction defects.

The best laboratory test is measurement of transketolase activity in red cells with and without added thiamin pyrophosphate (TPP) in vitro. The test requires fresh heparinised whole blood and this must be taken before thiamin treatment is started. A TPP effect above 30% is to be expected in beriberi or Wernicke's encephalopathy. Plasma pyruvate and lactic acids are elevated in acute forms of thiamin deficiency but not in the more chronic forms, and if they are increased this is not specific.

Management

Treatment must be started as soon as the diagnosis is made because fatal heart failure may occur suddenly. Complete rest is essential and 50 mg thiamin (50 times the daily requirement) should be given intramuscularly for 3 days. Thereafter 10 mg 3 times a day should be continued by mouth until convalescence is established.

The response of a patient with beriberi to thiamin is one of the most dramatic therapeutic events. Within a few hours the breathing is easier, the pulse rate slower, the extremities cooler and a rapid diuresis begins to dispose of the oedema. In a few days the size of the heart is restored to normal.

DRY BERIBERI

This is essentially a peripheral neuropathy, formerly common in South-East Asia. The nutritional background is similar to that of wet beriberi. In long-standing cases there is degeneration and demyelination of both sensory and motor nerves, resulting in severe wasting of muscles. The vagus and other autonomic nerves can also be affected. In dry beriberi the blood pyruvate level is usually normal and the transketolase test (TPP effect) may be too.

NUTRITIONAL PERIPHERAL NEUROPATHY

Deficiency of thiamin or other vitamins of the B group, niacin, vitamin B_6 and vitamin B_{12} may cause a symmetrical, mixed sensory-motor neuropathy. In alcoholics with peripheral neuropathy there are often combined deficiencies. If treated early nutritional polyneuropathy responds to a mixed diet and generous doses of the vitamin B complex.

WERNICKE'S ENCEPHALOPATHY AND KORSAKOFF'S PSYCHOSIS

Aetiology

This cerebral form of thiamin deficiency occurs in Europe, North America and Australia. It often presents acutely, usually in an alcoholic, but it is sometimes seen in people with persistent vomiting; it occurred in prisoners of war on small rations of polished rice.

Clinical features

In **Wernicke's encephalopathy** the patient is quietly confused and the most valuable clinical sign is some form of bilateral, symmetrical ophthalmoplegia. This may be in one or more than one direction and accompanied by abnormal pupillary reflexes and/or nystagmus. Ataxia is also present. The diagnosis has to be differentiated from other causes of confusion in an alcoholic, e.g. acute intoxication, head injury, drug overdose, cerebral vascular accident, etc. The oculomotor signs are an important clue. If Wernicke's encephalopathy is not treated the confusion is liable soon to progress to stupor or death. If it is treated late the residual Korsakoff's psychosis may be permanent. There is no rapid test to confirm the diagnosis. If Wernicke's encephalopathy is suspected, a heparinised whole blood sample should be taken for transketolase assay and then an injection of thiamin given.

The pathology in those who die is in the mammillary bodies, upper mid brain, hypothalamus, thalamus and parts of the cerebellar cortex. Histologically there is focal cellular necrosis, hyperaemia, petechial haemorrhages and astrocyte proliferation.

Korsakoff's psychosis. In some cases the predominant abnormality in mental function is a memory defect. Characteristically the patient is fully conscious but has a profound impairment of memory recall and new learning ability. A striking feature is a tendency to confabulate, which has been described as a falsification of memory in clear consciousness. For example if the patient is asked to describe what he did this morning (when he was lying in bed in the ward) he replies that he went to the shops, met an old friend, etc. Confabulation probably results from an inability to distinguish the temporal sequence of past events. Other cognitive functions remain intact in the Korsakoff syndrome but the memory disturbance is so profound that the patient is incapable of living independently and requires institutional care.

Amnesia also occurs in bilateral lesions of the hippocampus and hippocampal gyrus, situated on the inferomedial aspect of the temporal lobe. The clinical picture resembles that of Korsakoff's psychosis except that confabulation does not occur.

Wernicke's encephalopathy and Korsakoff's psychosis are sometimes associated with polyneuropathy and/or with superior midline cerebellar degeneration but it is surprising how uncommon these cerebral forms are in S.E. Asia and that beriberi cardiomyopathy is seldom seen with Wernicke/Korsakoff disease.

Management

Wernicke's encephalopathy should be treated without delay with 50 mg thiamin hydrochloride by slow intravenous injection followed by 50 mg intramuscularly daily for a week. Confusion, disorientation and ophthalmoplegia should respond within 2 to 3 days. Indeed this response to thiamin helps to confirm the diagnosis. The memory disorder (Korsakoff's psychosis) takes longer to improve; it may become more obvious as confusion clears and the patient's general condition improves. Some degree of memory impairment often persists.

Prevention

In Western countries the prevention of beriberi and Wernicke's encephalopathy is related to the control of alcoholism. Bread and other staple cereal foods are fortified with thiamin in most industrial countries. In a chronic alcoholic vitamin B complex tablets can at least prevent the complications of thiamin deficiency. Beriberi is much less common in Asia than it used to be.

NIACIN (nicotinic acid and nicotinamide)

Nicotinamide is an essential part of the two important pyridine nucleotides, NAD and NADP, which are hydrogen-accepting coenzymes for dehydrogenases at many steps in the pathways of glucose oxidation. NAD is also the coenzyme for alcohol dehydrogenase. Nicotinic acid is readily converted in the body into the amide. For nutritional purposes the two have equal biological activity and are considered together in foods under the generic term 'niacin'. Both are water-soluble and resistant to heat. Dietary sources are listed in the information box below.

> **DIETARY SOURCES OF NIACIN (PRE-FORMED)**
>
> - Liver, kidney
> - Meat, fish
> - Yeast (brewer's), Marmite
> - Peanuts, bran, legumes
> - Wholemeal wheat
> - Coffee

A special feature of this vitamin is that it is normally synthesised in the body in limited amounts from tryptophan, the least abundant of the essential amino acids; 60 mg of tryptophan yields 1 mg of nicotinamide. For this reason niacin equivalents in a diet are calculated by adding together the niacin plus 1/60 of the tryptophan intake (in mg). As a rule of thumb it can be assumed that tryptophan is about 1/100th of the protein intake. Therefore a protein intake of 60 g provides 10 mg $(60\,000 \times 1/100 \times 1/60$ mg$)$ of the adult daily requirement of 18 mg niacin equivalents (pre-formed niacin + that from tryptophan). Eggs and cheeses are examples of foods that contain little pre-formed niacin but provide niacin equivalents from tryptophan.

PELLAGRA

Aetiology

Pellagra is a nutritional disease due to deficiency of niacin, formerly endemic among poor peasants who subsisted chiefly on maize (American corn). The greater part of the niacin in maize is in a bound form, niacytin, which is unavailable to the consumer and, unlike other cereals, maize has an amino acid pattern relatively deficient in tryptophan. In areas where pellagra remains, e.g. in parts of Africa, the incidence is much less than formerly. In developed countries it is occasionally seen in alcoholics who have been eating poorly and in the malabsorption syndrome. In the rare inborn error of metabolism, **Hartnup disease**, tryptophan absorption is impaired and there is a pellagrous dermatitis with neurological abnormalities which respond to nicotinamide.

Clinical features

Pellagra can develop in only 8 weeks on diets very deficient in niacin and tryptophan. It has been called

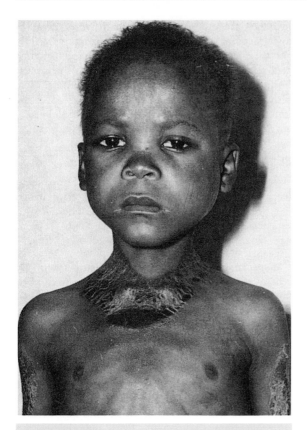

Fig. 9.8 Pellagra in a girl of 5 years. Skin lesion on the neck (Casal's collar) is pathognomonic.

the disease of the three Ds: dermatitis, diarrhoea and dementia.

Skin

The diagnosis is usually first suggested by the appearance of the skin. Characteristically, there is an erythema resembling severe sunburn, appearing symmetrically over the parts of the body exposed to sunlight and especially on the neck (Fig. 9.8). Local trauma or irritation of the skin may also determine the site of the lesion. The affected areas are well demarcated from normal skin. In acute cases the skin lesions may progress to vesiculation, cracking, exudation and crusting with ulceration and sometimes secondary infection. In chronic cases the dermatitis occurs as a roughening and thickening of the skin with a brown pigmentation. Dermatitis of the vulva, perineum and perianal area is usually present.

Alimentary tract

There may be anorexia, nausea and dysphagia. Glossitis is an early symptom and may precede the skin lesions.

The mouth is sore and often shows angular stomatitis and cheilosis (p. 414). It is probable that a non-infective inflammation extends throughout the gastrointestinal tract and accounts for the diarrhoea which is usually present.

Nervous system

In severe cases delirium is the most common mental disturbance in the acute form of the disease and dementia in the chronic form.

Biochemical tests to confirm the diagnosis are urinary N′ methylnicotinamide or red cell NAD.

Management

Nicotinamide is given in a dose of 100 mg every 6 hours by mouth, although a smaller dose is likely to be effective. The vitamin is well absorbed but can be given parenterally. The response is usually rapid; within 24 hours the erythema of the skin diminishes and the diarrhoea ceases. Often there is also striking improvement in the patient's behaviour and mental attitude.

There are likely to be associated nutritional deficiencies. A low intake of protein including tryptophan is an essential condition for development of the disease, and hypoalbuminaemia is common. Deficiencies of other B vitamins (riboflavin and vitamin B_6) are likely. Nicotinamide treatment should therefore be supplemented with a nutritious diet, high in protein. Vitamin B complex tablets should be given and iron, folic acid and vitamin B_{12} may be necessary in addition for some cases. Alcohol should be forbidden.

Prevention

In Central America the peasants eat a staple diet of maize but pellagra is unusual. This is because the traditional method of boiling the maize in lime water (dilute calcium hydroxide) before they make tortillas hydrolyses the indigestible bound niacin to free niacin. Pellagra was once endemic among the poor in the southern states of the USA. It has been eliminated by enrichment of maize meal and bread with niacin in that country since 1938.

RIBOFLAVIN

Riboflavin is a constituent of the flavoproteins which are part of the oxidation chain in the mitochondria. It is a yellow-green fluorescent compound soluble in water. Though stable to boiling in acid solution, in alkaline solution it is decomposed by heat. It is also destroyed by exposure to UV light. The requirement is 1.2 mg per day.

The dietary sources are listed in the information box below.

DISORDERS DUE TO RIBOFLAVIN DEFICIENCY

When human volunteers have been given diets very low in riboflavin, the most consistent clinical manifestations were angular stomatitis, cheilosis and nasolabial dyssebacea; these responded to the addition of pure riboflavin in the deficient diet.

Angular stomatitis

This is not specific for lack of riboflavin. Deficiencies of niacin, pyridoxine and iron can all produce it. It can follow herpes febrilis at the angle of the mouth. A common cause is ill-fitting dentures, associated with candidiasis.

Cheilosis

This is a zone of red, denuded epithelium at the line of closure of the lips. It has also occurred in experimental pure niacin deficiency. It is often associated with angular stomatitis and frequently seen in pellagra.

Nasolabial dyssebacea

This consists of enlarged follicles around the sides of the nose which are plugged with dry sebaceous material. This occurs in primates on a diet deficient only in riboflavin. It is seen in some patients with pellagra.

Other abnormalities

Vascularisation of the cornea, scrotal dermatitis, a magenta-coloured tongue and anaemia have been attributed to riboflavin deficiency but they may have alternative explanations.

Riboflavin clearly plays a vital role in cellular oxidation and there are communities and individuals who have both low dietary intakes and very low concentrations in urine or blood. Yet it is surprising that the clinical effects of riboflavin deficiency are superficial and mainly nonspecific. Features of riboflavin deficiency are most likely to be found in pellagrins and in malnourished rice-eaters in S.E. Asia. In the first situation they are overshadowed by niacin deficiency and in the second by thiamin or protein deficiency.

Management

The therapeutic dose of riboflavin is 5 mg 3 times a day by mouth. It gives the patient's urine a green fluorescence. As discussed above, other B complex vitamins should also be given.

PYRIDOXINE (VITAMIN B_6)

Pyridoxine, pyridoxal and pyridoxamine are three closely related compounds with similar physiological actions. The active form of the vitamin in man is pyridoxal 5′-phosphate, the coenzyme for a large number of different enzyme systems involved in the metabolism of the amino acids including aminotransferases. Vitamin B_6 is widely distributed in plants and animal tissues. Liver, whole grain cereals, peanuts and bananas are good sources. The requirement is related to the protein intake, 15 μg/g protein, or an average 1.4 mg/day in the UK.

DISORDERS DUE TO VITAMIN B_6 DEFICIENCY

Although a series of pathological changes in the skin, liver, blood vessels, nervous tissue and bone marrow have been produced experimentally in various animals, disorders due to deficiency of vitamin B_6 rarely occur in man, and then very seldom as a result of dietary deficiency.

A minor epidemic of convulsions in infants in the USA in the 1950s was traced to a milk formula depleted in vitamin B_6 because of a manufacturing error. In adults dermatitis, cheilosis, glossitis and angular stomatitis have been produced by means of the pyridoxine inhibitor, 4-desoxy-pyridoxine. The peripheral neuropathy associated with isoniazid therapy is due to a secondary vitamin B_6 deficiency. Certain drugs, such as isoniazid and penicillamine, act as chemical antagonists to pyridoxine. Some cases of sideroblastic anaemia respond to treatment with pyridoxine.

Biochemical features suggesting vitamin B_6 deficiency can occur in women taking oral contraceptives, and the mild depression which affects a small proportion of such women may be relieved by pyridoxine.

Toxicity

Megavitamin doses of vitamin B_6 (200 mg/day or more) taken for some weeks cause a sensory polyneuropathy.

BIOTIN

Biotin functions as coenzyme for four carboxylases involved in carbohydrate, fatty acid and amino acid metabolism. It is present in a number of different foods; the requirement is small (30–100 μg daily) and it can be synthesised by colonic bacteria. Human deficiency is rare; it has occurred in adults who have taken for long periods large amounts of raw egg-white which contain the biotin antagonist avidin, and an otherwise poor diet. It has also occurred in patients on long-term total parenteral nutrition with biotin omitted from the fluids. The clinical features include scaly dermatitis, alopecia, paraesthesia and urinary excretion of organic acids, for example propionic and 3-hydroxypropionic. A form of seborrhoeic dermatitis of infants responds to biotin.

VITAMIN B$_{12}$ AND FOLATE

These vitamins and haematological disorders due to their deficiency are discussed on page 787 and page 789.

Vitamin B$_{12}$ and the nervous system

In prolonged vitamin B$_{12}$ deficiency (causes on p. 787) there may be megaloblastic anaemia (p. 786) or neurological degeneration alone or both. In some cases the neurological disease predominates; this may be because a good intake of folate maintains erythropoiesis. Vitamin B$_{12}$, but not folate, is needed for the integrity of myelin. The biochemical basis of this is not yet settled. In severe deficiency there is insidious diffuse uneven demyelination. It may be clinically manifest as peripheral neuropathy or spinal cord degeneration affecting posterior and lateral columns ('subacute combined degeneration of the spinal cord') or there may be cerebral manifestations (resembling dementia) or optic atrophy. Plasma vitamin B$_{12}$ (before treatment) is very low, and treatment with hydroxocobalamin should produce improvement but it may be slow.

Folic acid in prevention of neural tube defects

Three major birth defects—spina bifida, anencephaly and encephalocoele—all result from imperfect closure of the neural tube which takes place 3 to 4 weeks after conception. Prevention trials, including a large multicentre prevention trial by the British Medical Research Council of recurrent neural tube defects have shown that folic acid reduces recurrence or occurrence of these deformities by about 70%, but it must be taken periconceptionally, i.e. from before conception. In a prospective study in Dublin maternity hospitals red cell folates showed lower levels in cases than in controls but not in the deficient range. Folate is directly involved in DNA and RNA synthesis and it seems that a higher level than is needed at other times in life is needed in some embryos at this critical stage of development. The UK Department of Health (1991) advises that women who have experienced a pregnancy affected by neural tube defect should take a 5 mg folic acid tablet daily from before conception and throughout the first trimester. All women in general who are planning a pregnancy should be advised to include good sources of folate in their diet (see information box).

GOOD SOURCES OF FOLATE

- Brussels sprouts
- Fortified breakfast cereals
- Spinach, asparagus, beetroot
- Orange, avocado, melon
- Potatoes, cauliflower, peas
- Marmite and Bovril
- Wholemeal bread, parsnips
- Dried beans
- Kidney

Liver is the richest source of folate but increased intakes are not advised in early pregnancy because of its high vitamin A content.

VITAMIN C (ASCORBIC ACID)

Ascorbic acid is a modified simple sugar. It is the most active reducing agent in the aqueous phase of living tissues and is easily and reversibly oxidised to dehydroascorbic acid. Its highest concentrations are in the pituitary and adrenals, the eye, and white blood cells. Presumably it has specific functions in these tissues. Stress and corticotrophin secretion lead to a loss of ascorbic acid from the adrenal cortex.

Dietary sources of vitamin C are listed in the information box below.

DIETARY SOURCES OF VITAMIN C

- Blackcurrants, guavas
- Green peppers, broccoli, cauliflower (raw)
- Oranges and other citrus fruits
- Brussels sprouts, cabbage
- Potatoes
- (Liver is the only animal food that contains it)

Ascorbic acid is very easily destroyed by heat, alkalies such as sodium bicarbonate, traces of copper or by an oxidase liberated by damage to plant tissues. Ascorbic acid is very soluble in water. For these reasons many traditional methods of cooking reduce or eliminate it from the diet. The recommended adult intake is 30–75 mg in different countries. Body stores last for about 2.5 to 3 months on a deficient diet.

SCURVY

Aetiology

In 1497 when Vasco da Gama sailed round the Cape of Good Hope, 100 out of his 160 men died of scurvy. For the next 300 years scurvy was a major factor determining the success or failure of all sea ventures even after it was recognised by Lind (1753) and by Cook (1755) that it results from the prolonged consumption of a diet devoid of fresh fruit and vegetables. Final proof and isolation of vitamin C were not possible until the guinea pig was found (1907) to provide a suitable animal model because, like man and unlike most animals, it cannot synthesise ascorbic acid from glucose.

Sporadic cases of scurvy continue to arise in infants as a result of ignorance, poverty and parental neglect and also amongst old people, especially men living alone who are not feeding themselves properly. Scurvy appears to be rare in most tropical countries but is more likely to occur in arid regions in times of drought.

Pathology

Ascorbic acid deficiency results in defective formation of collagen in connective tissue because of failure of hydroxylation of proline to hydroxyproline, the characteristic amino acid of collagen. There is in consequence delayed healing of wounds. There are also capillary haemorrhages and subnormal platelet adhesiveness (normal platelets are rich in ascorbate).

Clinical features

Adult scurvy

The pathognomonic sign is the swollen and spongy gums, particularly the papillae between the teeth, sometimes producing the appearance of 'scurvy buds'. These bleed easily. The teeth may become loose and even fall out. There is always some infection; scurvy has to be distinguished from common gingivitis. In patients without teeth the gums appear normal.

The first sign of cutaneous bleeding is often found on the lower thighs. These are perifollicular haemorrhages—tiny points of bleeding around the orifice of a hair follicle with a heaping-up of keratin-like material on the surface around the mouth of the follicle, through which a deformed 'corkscrew' hair characteristically projects. Perifollicular haemorrhages are often followed by petechial haemorrhages, independent of the hair follicles, usually first seen on the feet and ankles. Thereafter large spontaneous bruises (ecchymoses) may arise almost anywhere in the body, but usually first in the lower extremities, producing the characteristic 'woody leg'. Haemorrhage may occur into joints, into a nerve sheath, under the nails or conjunctiva or into the gastrointestinal tract; there may be epistaxis. Scurvy can present with any of these features. By the time the disease is fully developed the patient is usually anaemic.

Another characteristic of scurvy is that fresh wounds fail to heal—a possibility that the surgeon has to bear in mind. A patient with scurvy may die suddenly without warning, apparently from cardiac failure.

The dietary and social history is helpful in doubtful cases. Old, solitary people may insist that they fend very well for themselves, but careful questioning will reveal that they do not buy fresh fruit or vegetables.

Plasma ascorbate is very low or absent (Appendix Table 21.9, p. 1153); a fresh sample of plasma should be analysed because the vitamin can decompose in a few hours at warm room temperatures. If this test is done it should be *before* any vitamin C is given.

Infantile scurvy

The main clinical features are listed in the information box below.

CLINICAL FEATURES OF INFANTILE SCURVY

- Lassitude
- Anorexia
- Painful limbs
- Enlargement of costochondral junctions
- Subperiosteal haemorrhage
- Gingivitis once teeth have erupted

Management

The normal adult body contains about 1.5 g of vitamin C, so that a dose of 250 mg by mouth 3 times daily should saturate the tissues quickly. Attention should be paid to correcting the general deficiencies of the patient's former diet. If the patient is anaemic iron and sometimes folic acid are indicated. With adequate treatment no patient dies of scurvy and recovery is usually rapid and complete.

Prevention

In breast milk the vitamin C content responds to maternal intake. Cow's milk is a poor source of vitamin

C, especially when boiled. Proprietary infant formulas contain adequate amounts. Old or solitary people who will not eat fruit and vegetables should be advised to take 50 mg ascorbic acid tablets daily.

Trauma, surgery and burns, infections, smoking and certain drugs—adrenocortical steroids, aspirin, indomethacin and tetracycline—all increase the requirement for vitamin C. Consequently patients affected require more than the recommended intake.

Ascorbic acid and the common cold

It has been claimed that ascorbic acid in doses of 1–2 g daily, or even more, will prevent the common cold. If it does, this is a pharmacological and not a vitamin effect as coryza is not a manifestation of scurvy. In the largest controlled trial, in Toronto, two placebo groups were included. One of these had fewer colds than those taking 0.25, 1 or 2 g vitamin C per day prophylactically. Another 14 double-blind controlled trials found no significant preventive effect. The trials that did report benefit were smaller and less rigorously controlled. A more general reason for self medication with vitamin C supplements is the possibility that antioxidant nutrients—vitamin C and/or carotenoids and/or vitamin E—may protect against free radical damage and reduce the risk of atherosclerotic disease, some types of cancer and cataract. Though circumstantial evidence is interesting it will be some years before the results of controlled prevention trials are available.

Toxicity

Vitamin C facilitates the absorption of iron and the most important side effect of large doses is to exacerbate haemochromatosis (p. 528) or other iron storage disease, which is not a problem for the great majority of people. Oxalate is a metabolite of ascorbate; urinary oxalate is likely to increase with large intakes of vitamin C. There has been no definitive case-control study of supplement use in patients with urinary tract stones but it would be prudent for such people to avoid vitamin C medication.

VITAMIN D

The natural form, **cholecalciferol**, is a modified steroid. It is formed in the skin by the action of ultraviolet light on 7-dehydrocholesterol. **Ergocalciferol** differs chemically in having a double bond and a methyl group in the side chain. It is manufactured by the action of ultraviolet light on ergosterol, a sterol found in fungi and yeast. Although used in therapeutics, it occurs very rarely in nature.

Cholecalciferol, not itself biologically active, is

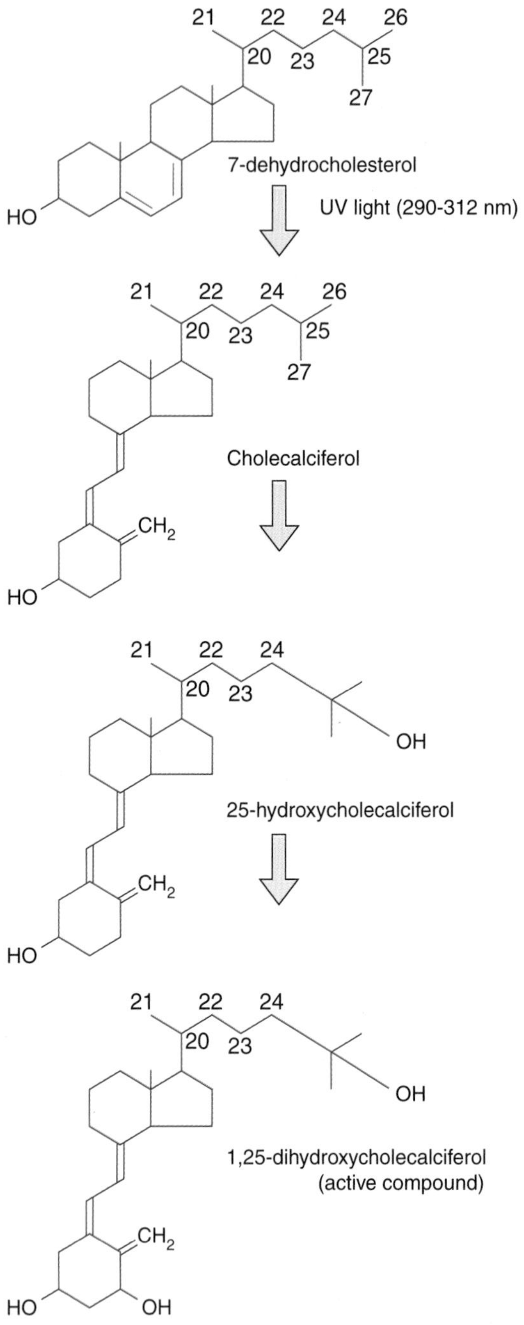

Fig. 9.9 Vitamin D pathway.

converted in the liver to 25-hydroxycholecalciferol (25-OH-D) which is further hydroxylated in the kidney, mainly to 1,25 dihydroxycholecalciferol (1,25(OH)$_2$D) (see Fig. 9.9). Most of the hydroxylated forms of vitamin D in human plasma are based on cholecalciferol derived from synthesis in the skin or from fish liver oils. A smaller proportion is based on ergocalciferol from calciferol tablets or fortified milk (e.g. in USA). They and their corresponding derivatives appear to have identical activities.

1,25(OH)₂D is many times more potent than chole-calciferol and can be regarded as a hormone. It is transported in the blood to target organs, notably gut and bone, and is regulated by a complex feedback system. At the cellular level it acts like other steroid hormones. It binds to a specific high affinity intracellular receptor which transports it to the nucleus where it stimulates production of hormone-specific mRNA which govern the transcription of several proteins. The most important is a specific transport protein in the enterocyte that increases calcium absorption. An adequate concentration of calcium is thus ensured for the formation of calcium phosphate in bone where calcium comes in contact with inorganic phosphates, liberated from organic phosphates under the influence of phosphatase produced by osteoblasts.

Alfacalcidol, 1α-hydroxycholecalciferol (1αOH-D), is a synthetic analogue which is converted into 1,25(OH)₂D in the liver without the need for hydroxylation in the kidney. It is used in treating hypocalcaemia and osteomalacia due to renal disease.

The main reasons for impaired production of 1,25(OH)₂D are:

1. deficiency of 25-OH-D due to lack of sunlight, an inadequate diet or malabsorption
2. disturbed metabolism in liver or renal disease, notably chronic renal failure
3. depression of the feedback system as in hypoparathyroidism.

Dietary sources of vitamin D

These are listed in the information box.

DIETARY SOURCES OF VITAMIN D

- Fish liver oils, e.g. cod liver oil
- Fatty fish (herring, mackerel, salmon, sardines, pilchards, tuna)
- Fortified margarine
- Infant milk formulas
- Eggs, liver

People who regularly have adequate exposure of their skin to sunlight do not normally need vitamin D in their diet. The efficiency of formation of vitamin D in the skin is reduced in old people; concentration of 7-dehydrocholesterol declines with age. Otherwise the recommended oral daily intake (WHO) for infants and children up to 5 years of age and for pregnant or lactating women is 10 μg. For older children and adults about 2.5 μg is adequate (1 μg = 40 i.u.).

RICKETS AND OSTEOMALACIA

Rickets is the characteristic result of deficiency of vitamin D in children. When the epiphyses have fused the corresponding deficiency disease is osteomalacia. Both mainly affect the bones but they differ in details. They are described in Chapter 15 (p. 927).

HYPERVITAMINOSIS D

In the case of vitamin D it is possible to have too much of a good thing. Large oral doses are toxic and cause hypercalcaemia. The symptoms include nausea, vomiting, constipation, drowsiness and signs of renal failure; metastatic calcification in the arteries, kidneys and other tissues may occur.

Since renal damage may occur before clinical signs of toxicity appear, all patients on large doses of vitamin D should have their serum calcium level checked regularly at 3-monthly intervals and if this is found to be above 2.6 mmol/l (10.5 mg/100 ml) it is an early indication of overdosage.

VITAMIN E

Alpha-tocopherol is the most potent of eight related fat-soluble substances with vitamin E activity, α, β, γ and δ (delta) tocopherol and α, β, γ and δ (delta) tocotrienol. They are absorbed with lipids, transported on plasma lipoproteins and distributed in cell membranes throughout the body. Vitamin E and carotenoids are the main fat-soluble antioxidants in the body. The vitamin E compounds exhibit steroisomerism. Natural forms are d- (or RRR) and synthetic are dl- (or racemic). The racemic form has 75% the activity of the natural form. Good sources include vegetable oils, wholegrain cereals and nuts.

Vitamin E prevents oxidation of polyunsaturated fatty acids in cell membranes by free radicals. The first feature of human deficiency is a mild haemolytic anaemia which has been described only in premature infants and in a few cases of malabsorption. Early oral administration reduces the severity of retrolental fibroplasia in premature infants given oxygen. In chronic fat malabsorption, for example in cystic fibrosis, ataxia and visual scotomas occur which respond to vitamin E.

The first action of vitamin E when it was discovered in 1922 was in preventing fetal resorption in rats.

The name comes from *tocos* (Gk) childbirth, *phero* (Gk) bring forth and *ol*, for alcohol. A popular belief that it increases sexual performance in humans could not be confirmed in controlled trials. Interest now focuses on the hypothesis that as a lipid-soluble antioxidant it may reduce atherogenesis by protecting low-density lipoprotein from oxidation. Two cross-sectional studies in Europe and two large prospective studies in the USA report negative associations of vitamin E intake with the incidence of coronary heart disease. However, association does not prove cause and effect and the results of controlled prevention trials are awaited.

Vitamin E status can be assessed by measuring plasma α-tocopherol, but as this vitamin is carried by lipoproteins, people with hyperlipidaemia can have falsely high plasma vitamin E levels. It should therefore be expressed as the ratio of vitamin E to plasma (total) lipid. For practical purposes plasma vitamin E/cholesterol+triglyceride is more convenient.

The present recommended intake of vitamin E in UK and USA is 7 to 10 mg/day in men, and 5 to 8 mg in women. If the intake of polyunsaturated fat is high, vitamin E intake should be increased. Although two other fat-soluble vitamins (A and D) are toxic in high dosage, few adverse effects of vitamin E have been reported even up to 80 times the recommended nutrient intake.

VITAMIN K

Vitamin K is the *K*oagulations–vitamin (its discovery was reported in Germany). It is required for the synthesis of an unusual amino acid, γ-carboxyglutamic (Gla). Gla residues are part of the protein molecule of four of the coagulation factors, II, VII, IX and X. The Gla residues confer on these proteins the capacity to bind to phospholipid surfaces in the presence of calcium. A few other proteins also contain Gla, notably osteocalcin, a product of the osteoblasts.

Vitamin K exists in nature in two forms. K_1 (phytomenadione or phylloquinone) is found in leafy vegetables and liver. Adequate amounts are normally supplied in the average diet and absorbed with other lipids. The requirement of vitamin K is about 80 μg/day. The second form, K_2 (menaquinone) is synthesised by bacteria in the colon; some is evidently absorbed from there and has been detected in liver.

Vitamin K has important roles in three situations. In the newborn, primary deficiency can occur because placental transfer of vitamin K is inefficient, the neonatal bowel has not yet acquired bacteria and breast milk contains little of the vitamin. Vitamin K_1 is given routinely to newborn babies to prevent **haemorrhagic disease of the newborn**. In obstructive jaundice, dietary vitamin K is not absorbed and it is very important to administer the vitamin before biliary surgery. Thirdly, warfarin and related anticoagulants (p. 840) act by antagonising vitamin K.

FURTHER READING

Bauernfeind J C 1986 Vitamin A deficiency and its control. Academic Press, Orlando

Daulane N M P, Starbuck E S, Houston R M, Church M S, Stukel T A et al 1992 Childhood mortality after a high dose of vitamin A in a high risk population. British Medical Journal 304: 207–210

Hussey G D, Klein M 1990 A randomized, controlled trial of vitamin A in children with severe measles. New England Journal of Medicine 323: 160–164

MRC Vitamins Study Research Group 1991 Prevention of neural tube defects. Results of the Medical Research Council Vitamin Study. Lancet 338: 131–137

Victor M, Adams R D, Collins G H 1989 The Wernicke–Korsakoff syndrome and related neurologic disorders due to alcoholism and malnutrition, 2nd edn. F A Davis, Philadelphia

NUTRITION OF PATIENTS IN HOSPITAL

Malnutrition does not occur only in poor children in developing countries. It affects a substantial proportion of seriously ill people in the hospitals of affluent countries. This was fully recognised only after the deficiency diseases in the Third World had been well delineated and approaches established to their management. During the 1970s it was realised that:

- some degree of malnutrition affects an important minority of patients in hospital and may be obscured by the primary illness;
- malnourished patients have a worse prognosis;
- with modern technology something can be done to maintain or improve patients' nutrition even when the gastrointestinal tract is not functioning.

Disease leads to nutritional depletion

A few patients are admitted to hospital in a malnourished state but more become nutritionally depleted in hospital. Serious illness, major operations and long stay are all associated with a greater chance of depletion partly because patients may be unable to ingest, digest or absorb their food but also because nutritional requirements and/or losses are increased in a number of diseases. The causes of nutritional depletion are listed in the box below.

CAUSES OF NUTRITIONAL DEPLETION

- Anorexia
- Unfamiliar food
- 'Nil by mouth' for hospital tests
- Failure to feed, e.g. neurological or psychological illness
- Vomiting
- Malabsorption
- Increased protein catabolism (trauma, infections)
- Increased metabolic rate (fever)
- Antagonism of nutrients by drugs
- Losses, e.g. burns, bleeding, diarrhoea, in urine

Functional consequences of nutritional depletion

These depend on the degree and type of depletion, but sooner or later malnutrition will have some or even all of the following effects:

1. reduced cellular or humoral responses to infections
2. muscular weakness, reduced ability to cough and susceptibility to bronchopneumonia
3. impaired healing of wounds (whether traumatic or surgical)
4. atrophic surface epithelium with reduced protective secretions is more easily penetrated by bacteria—especially gastrointestinal tract
5. bedsores and ulcers
6. reduced haemopoiesis
7. reduced ability to metabolise drugs
8. mental impairment
9. dehydration and its consequences
10. specific types of malnutrition, e.g. Wernicke's encephalopathy.

Controlled prospective studies show that patients with features of malnutrition have more postoperative complications, more infections, longer stay in hospital and a higher mortality. In some diseases nutritional support has been demonstrated in controlled trials to improve the outcome significantly, e.g. in inflammatory bowel disease, in burns and in patients with enterocutaneous fistulae. In other conditions clinical trials are insufficient to allow generalisations and it is sensible to assess each patient's status and, if this is subnormal, to consider the indications for the different types of nutritional support.

Patients at increased nutritional risk

Before using technical methods to work out a detailed nutritional profile, the first step is to recognise the high-risk patient. A patient in any of the categories in the information box is at increased risk of malnutrition, though it may not yet have developed.

PATIENTS AT INCREASED RISK OF HOSPITAL MALNUTRITION

- Severely underweight; weight for height <80% of standard (Table 9.4)
- Recent weight loss of 10% or more of usual body weight
- Alcoholism
- Malabsorption syndromes
- Increased metabolic rate: burns, trauma, severe infections, prolonged fever
- Increased losses, e.g. fistulae, draining wounds, renal dialysis, haemorrhage
- No food by mouth for over a week while receiving simple intravenous nutrition (glucose/electrolyte/water)
- Antinutrients or catabolic drugs, e.g. immunosuppressants, cancer chemotherapy, adrenocortical steroids
- Course of radiotherapy

SYSTEMATIC NUTRITIONAL ASSESSMENT

This consists of four components:

The dietary history

In medical use this is usually qualitative; has the patient been eating too little food, or omitted any major foods? Is an unusual diet being taken? Quantitative nutrient intake first elicits estimates of weights of all foods eaten by one of four methods—dietary history, 24 hour recall, food diary or food frequency questionnaire. By using food tables, usually in computer form, the daily intake of the major nutrients is obtained. These can then be compared against the recommended nutrient intake (dietary reference value), a more detailed version of Table 9.2. An intake just below the dietary reference value shows there is a risk of malnutrition but does not establish it because:

- the days on which food intake was estimated may have been unrepresentative;
- the physiological requirements between individuals for different nutrients range by a factor of about 2 and the dietary reference values are set to cover the requirements of nearly all healthy people;
- for some nutrients, e.g. vitamins A and B_{12}, there are considerable reserves in the body.

Clinical examination

Thinness, oedema, pallor, weakness and other signs described in this chapter may be found, but one should not wait for the classic features of deficiency disease before intervening with nutritional support in a seriously

Table 9.8 Reference standards for mid-arm circumference (mm)

	Men			Women		
		Centiles			**Centiles**	
Age	**50th**	**10th**	**5th**	**50th**	**10th**	**5th**
19–24	308	272	262	265	230	221
25–34	319	282	271	277	240	233
35–44	326	287	278	290	251	241
45–54	322	281	267	299	256	242
55–64	317	273	258	303	254	243
65–74	307	263	248	299	252	240

Figures based on a large sample of healthy US citizens from Frisancho A R 1981 American Journal of Clinical Nutrition 34: 2540–2545, and Bishop C W et al 1981 American Journal of Clinical Nutrition 34: 2530–2539.

ill patient in hospital. The primary illness may obscure or confuse signs of malnutrition.

Anthropometry

Changes of body weight reflect the water and/or energy (calorie) balance. If there is no unusual loss of water, each kilogram lost corresponds to 6000 to 7000 kcal of energy (i.e. mostly adipose tissue), unless there is increased protein catabolism when the energy value of weight lost is less. Regular weighing of patients in hospital is valuable in management but it is difficult in paralysed, deformed, and very sick patients, those nursed at strict bed rest, or with splints, fluid lines, catheters and drains. Weighing beds are scarce in most hospitals. The patient should in addition be watched for wasting of both subcutaneous fat and of muscles. If weighing is impractical these observations are more critical. Clinical estimation can be made more objective by measuring mid-arm circumference with a tape (Table 9.8). The relative contributions of fat and muscle can be calculated (mid-arm muscle circumference = arm circumference $- \pi \times$ triceps skinfold), but accurate measurement of skinfold thickness requires special calipers. Harpenden or Holtain calipers are recommended.

Laboratory investigations

These consist of:

- those that indicate the protein status
- biochemical tests for micronutrient deficiencies.

Plasma albumin concentration is the most reliable method to assess visceral protein depletion but it is also reduced (moderately) as part of the 'acute phase' reaction to trauma. Plasma transferrin and prealbumin are sometimes used as more sensitive indices of visceral and protein status but both can be influenced by other con-

ditions. Urinary nitrogen (or urea nitrogen) shows the degree of protein catabolism. A reduced total lymphocyte count indicates the possibility of impaired cell-mediated immunity of which protein depletion is one cause. Biochemical tests for vitamins and some other essential nutrients are listed in Table 9.9. As with other tests in chemical pathology there can be both false positives and negatives. Each result needs to be evaluated with critical understanding; for example serum vitamin B_{12} is increased in acute hepatitis, and alkaline phosphatase may not be elevated if rickets is accompanied by PEM.

In general when the dietary intake of a nutrient is inadequate (less than obligatory losses) the individual goes through three stages. The **first stage** is that of adaptation to the low intake. For example, urine excretion falls but there is no evidence of abnormal function or of depletion of the cells. In the **second stage** there are in addition biochemical changes indicating either impaired function, e.g. reduced red cell transketolase activity in thiamin deficiency, or cellular depletion, e.g. reduced red cell folate. But clinical manifestations of deficiency are absent or non-specific. The **third stage** is that of clinical deficiency disease.

Most clinical biochemistry laboratories provide only some of the methods as a routine but others could be set up in special circumstances or, alternatively, a laboratory specialising in nutrition research could be asked to help.

TYPES OF NUTRITIONAL DEPLETION IN HOSPITAL PATIENTS

Protein-energy malnutrition (PEM) is the most important but is not always obvious and tends to be overshadowed by the primary disease. Calories and protein cannot be given as capsules or an injection and providing enough of them parenterally is technically difficult and expensive.

As in poorly fed children, there are different forms of PEM in hospital patients. At one end of the range is **semi-starvation** seen, for example, in anorexia nervosa or obstruction of the oesophagus. There is depletion of food energy but neither increased catabolism nor increased losses of body protein. There is loss of weight, decrease of arm circumference and skinfolds and normal plasma albumin.

At the other end of the range is **hypoalbuminaemic malnutrition**, which is sometimes called 'adult kwashiorkor'. This form is to be expected in a patient with increased protein catabolism and/or losses, e.g. after burns or severe trauma, who has been receiving only intravenous glucose and water. This stimulates insulin which causes disproportional loss of visceral protein. Plasma albumin is low, there can be oedema, and cell-

Table 9.9   Biochemical methods used in diagnosing nutritional deficiencies

| Nutrient | Principal methods | | Supplementary methods |
	Indicating reduced intake	Indicating impaired function (IF) or cell depletion (CD)	
Protein	Urinary nitrogen	Plasma albumin (IF)	Fasting plasma amino acid pattern
Vitamin A	Plasma carotene	Plasma retinol	
Thiamin	Urinary thiamin	Red blood cell transketolase and TPP effect (IF)	
Riboflavin	Urinary riboflavin	Red blood cell glutathione reductase and FAD effect (IF)	
Niacin	Urinary N' methyl-nicotinamide	Red cell NAD	Fasting plasma tryptophan
Vitamin B_6	Urinary 4 pyridoxic acid and/or plasma pyridoxal phosphate	Red blood glutamic oxalacetic transaminase and PP effect (IF)	Urinary xanthurenic acid after tryptophan load
Folate	Plasma folate	Red blood cell folate (CD) (haemoglobin, packed cell volume, and bone marrow)	Urinary FIGLU after histidine load
Vitamin B_{12}	Plasma vitamin B_{12}	Elevated serum methylmalonate (haemoglobin, packed cell volume, and bone marrow)	Schilling test
Vitamin C	Plasma ascorbate	Leucocyte ascorbate (CD)	Urinary ascorbate
Vitamin D	Plasma 25-hydroxy-cholecalciferol	Raised plasma alkaline phosphatase (bone isoenzyme) (IF)	Plasma 1,25 di OH vitamin D
Vitamin E	Plasma tocopherol	Red cell haemolysis with H_2O_2 in vitro (IF)	
Vitamin K	PIVKA II	Plasma prothrombin	
Sodium	Urinary sodium	Plasma sodium	
Potassium	Urinary potassium	Plasma potassium	Total body potassium by counting ^{40}K
Iron	Plasma iron and transferrin	Plasma ferritin (CD) (haemoglobin, packed cell volume, and smear)	Stainable iron in bone marrow
Magnesium	Plasma magnesium		
Iodine	Urinary (stable) iodide	Plasma protein-bound iodide (IF), plasma thyroxine (IF)	Radioactive iodine uptake by thyroid gland
Zinc	Plasma zinc	White blood cell zinc	Hair zinc
Selenium	Plasma selenium	Plasma glutathione peroxidase	
Calcium*			Total bone mineral

FAD = flavine adenine dinucleotide.
NAD = nicotinamide adenine dinucleotide.
TPP = thiamin pyrophgosphate
FIGLU = formimino gludamic acid
PIVKA II = Protein Induced by Vitamin K Absence II
* There are no reliable simple methods for assessing calcium status.

mediated immunity is impaired so resistance to infection is reduced.

Types of **micronutrient deficiency** likely to occur in hospital are included in the information box.

NUTRITIONAL SUPPORT

Intake of vitamins and other micronutrients can be boosted by giving these in one or other pharmaceutical preparation, by mouth or by injection. When a multi-vitamin preparation is given it is important to check that it contains all the major vitamins (e.g. some omit folic acid).

As micronutrients can be provided fairly easily in hospital the main problem of nutritional support is to get water, calories and protein into the patient. There are

MICRONUTRIENT DEFICIENCY IN HOSPITAL

- Thiamin—patient starving or vomiting 3 wks if given i.v. glucose may develop Wernicke's encephalopathy
- Folate
- Vitamin B_{12} (prolonged nitrous oxide anaesthesia)
- Vitamin C—losses increased by stress; wound healing requires increased supply
- Vitamin K—from biliary obstruction, antibiotics
- Iron—from bleeding
- Zinc

four principal routes and more than one can be used together:

Oral feeding

The ordinary diet can be reinforced with calorie-dense or protein-rich supplements.

Tube (enteral) feeding

This is usually given by fine bore plastic nasogastric tubes but sometimes a gastrostomy or jejunostomy is used. Percutaneous gastrostomy is useful for long-term enteral feeding. It is more convenient for the patient and reduces the risk of aspiration. Feeding can be continuous or intermittent and there is a wide range of enteral preparations. The 'polymeric' ones are mixtures, for example, of casein, maltodextrin, oils and micronutrients. Chemically-defined, 'monomeric' or 'elemental' preparations (amino acids, glucose, oil and micronutrients) are intended for patients who cannot take whole foods, e.g. for those with inflammatory bowel disease. They are more expensive. Enteral feedings can be administered either by a bolus, over a short time, or by continuous drip. Indications for enteral nutrition are given in the information box.

INDICATIONS FOR ENTERAL NUTRITION

- Unconsciousness
- Neurological dysphagia
- Head and neck surgery
- Oesophageal obstruction
- Inflammatory bowel disease
- Short bowel syndrome
- Post-traumatic weakness
- Post-operative weakness
- Post-irradiation weakness
- Chemotherapy
- Burns
- Old age

Parenteral feeding by a peripheral vein

This is easily established and is used for supplementary calorie and/or fluid support. Glucose infusions must be at not more than 10% concentration. Higher concentrations will cause phlebitis. Since 10% glucose in 2.5 l water is 250 g glucose and provides only 1000 kcal, energy requirements cannot be achieved unless intravenous lipid emulsion is given daily.

Parenteral feeding by central venous alimentation

This allows more concentrated glucose infusions (25–35%). Although it is possible to provide all a patient's calorie needs in this way, there are disadvantages to such a high carbohydrate intake, for instance high insulin levels and essential fatty acid deficiency. It is probably best to give about 30% of energy as intravenous fat emulsion, along with glucose, amino acids and micronutrients. The day's prescription can be made up sterile in the pharmacy in a 3-litre bag container. A stable patient with intestinal failure usually requires about 2500 kcal of energy, partly from glucose/electrolyte solutions, partly from an intravenous lipid preparation, e.g. 'Intralipid' (which contains essential fatty acids) and partly from an intravenous preparation of mixed crystalline L-amino acids, e.g. 'Aminoplex', 'Synthamin' or 'Vamin N'. The amino acid infusion usually provides 10–12 g nitrogen per day. This ($\times 6.25$) is equivalent to 63–75 g of protein/day. Its pattern of essential amino acids is similar to that in egg albumin, i.e. it has a high biological value. In patients on total parenteral nutrition the minor nutrients, which are taken for granted in a diet of mixed foods by mouth, all have to be provided, i.e. all the nutrients in Table 9.2. Total parenteral nutrition costs considerably more than enteral feeding.

Indications

Total parenteral nutrition is life-saving in patients with major disease of the small intestine in which the functioning gut mass is below the amount necessary for adequate digestion and absorption of nutrients. Intestinal failure can be acute (e.g. severe inflammatory bowel disease) or chronic (e.g. massive resection of small bowel).

OBESITY

Obesity is the most common nutritional disorder in affluent societies. Its significance requires constant emphasis because it is associated with increased mortality, predisposes to the development of important diseases and diminishes the efficiency and happiness of those affected.

Obesity may be defined as a condition in which there is an excessive amount of body fat. This simple definition gives rise to two questions: how can body fat be measured, and what is 'excessive'?

All methods of measuring the fat content in the living subject are, to a greater or lesser degree, indirect. The simplest, but also the least direct, is the measurement of body weight and this is the method almost exclusively used in clinical practice. In the clinical context the 'desirable' or 'ideal' weight for height (p. 580) is that associated with the lowest mortality in actuarial terms and excessive weight is that associated with increased mortality.

Aetiology

Excess fat accumulates because there is imbalance between energy intake and expenditure. This can arise in different ways and obesity is a clinical sign with several possible causes. There is no satisfactory aetiological classification of obesity; most cases are probably multifactorial but a number of factors are known to be associated with its development.

Age

Obesity is most prevalent in middle-age, but can occur at any stage of life. Obesity in childhood and adolescence is likely to be followed by obesity in adult life.

Socio-economic

In affluent countries obesity is more common in the lower socio-economic groups. In developing countries it can occur only in the prosperous elite. Some occupations predispose to obesity, e.g. cooks and barmen, whilst jockeys, fashion models and airline pilots have to keep themselves slim. In some societies fat men are respected and fat women considered beautiful; in others they are not.

Heredity versus environment

Obesity tends to run in families. It is difficult to disentangle environmental and genetic components. A study based on the Danish Adoption Register showed a strong relation between the weight class of adoptees and their biological, not their adoptive, parents. The values for body mass index (weight in kg divided by the square of height in metres) of identical twins reared apart in a large Swedish study had an intrapair correlation coefficient of 0.68 and were only slightly lower than for identical twins reared together. Twelve pairs of identical twins in Quebec were overfed by 1000 kcal (4.2 MJ) per day 6 days a week for 100 days. The range of weight gain was from 4 to 13 kg but the similarity within each pair of twins was statistically significant. There is, however, no evidence in man of obesity produced by a single gene, as in the genetically obese strains of rodents.

On the other hand there is abundant evidence of environmental influences on overweight and obesity. Obese people are common in some communities, rare in others. In the Danish study adoptees raised in country districts were heavier than those raised in the city. In most affluent countries there has been a progressive increase in the percentage of overweight and obese people in the last 25 years.

The implication for health services of the clearer role of genetics is that efforts for prevention of obesity should be focused on those who are most vulnerable. Eighty percent of the offspring of two obese parents become obese.

Endocrine factors

An endocrine influence on body fat is seen both in normal physiological situations and in pathological states. The normal fat content of young adult women is about twice that of young men and pregnancy is characterised by an increase in body fat. Obesity in women commonly begins at puberty, during pregnancy or at the menopause. Obesity frequently, but not invariably, accompanies hypothyroidism, hypogonadism, hypopituitarism and Cushing's syndrome. However, the overwhelming majority of obese patients show no clinical evidence of an endocrine disorder. Plasma insulin and cortisol are commonly raised and growth hormone reduced in obese subjects, but these changes probably result from, rather than cause, the obesity since they disappear when weight is lost.

Obesity is also a feature of the Prader–Willi syndrome which is an uncommon condition characterised by severe congenital hypotonia, feeding difficulties and poor weight gain up to the age of two years, followed by mild mental retardation, short stature, hypogonadism, a voracious appetite and the development of obesity during childhood.

Energy balance

A very small excess of calories, if habitual, can lead eventually to a large accumulation of fat. If a person eats a slice (28 g) of bread that is not needed each day or goes by car instead of walking for 15 minutes, the daily extra 60 kcal (250 kJ) will build up over 4 years to 10 kg of fat deposited.

Social factors, such as advertising and business lunches, may contribute to overeating and some people overeat because they are unhappy. There is some evidence that in obese people eating is determined less by 'internal cues', i.e. hunger and satiety, than by external influences like the availability, appearance and taste of food or the environment in which the food is served.

Physical inactivity has an important role in the development of obesity. Affluence is commonly associated with reduced energy expenditure. It is well recognised that physical activity is less in the obese than in the lean, but this may result from, rather than cause, the obesity. Moreover, the amount of energy expended by an obese person on most tasks is likely to be greater because of the extra weight to be moved.

Many obese people believe that they do not eat more than their lean counterparts and frequently report an inability to lose weight on a low energy diet. These claims together with the failure of most dietary surveys to demonstrate a significant difference in the daily energy intake of obese and non-obese subjects have led to the hypothesis that in many instances the development of obesity is due to a metabolic defect causing reduced energy expenditure. Indirect whole body calorimetry, by measuring O_2 utilisation and CO_2 production, has shown that the basal metabolic rate and also the thermic response to food and the energy cost of standard activities are about the same in lean and obese subjects when corrected for differences in fat-free mass and total body mass. Thus it is clear that relatively mild but significant over-eating may remain undetected in nutrition surveys based on subjects' recollection or short term recorded food intake.

THE DOUBLY LABELLED WATER METHOD FOR MEASURING WHOLE BODY ENERGY EXPENDITURE

The routine is to give $^2H_2\ ^{18}O$, e.g. 10 g ^2H_2O and 200 g $H_2\ ^{18}O$; collect urine for about 10 days. The ^2H (denterium) equilibrates with the body water pool, and the ^{18}O (heavy oxygen) equilibrates with the body water and with the CO_2 and bicarbonate. The isotopes are not radioactive. The method is non-invasive. Abundance of the stable isotopes is measured in a high precision isotope ratio mass spectrometer.

Under conditions where total body water is approximately constant during the period of study the chief corrections that must be introduced are the isotope fractionation factors (^2H and ^{18}O are slightly more abundant in liquid water than in water vapour and ^{18}O is slightly more abundant in CO_2 than H_2O). When the CO_2 production per day is calculated the energy expenditure can be derived once the average respiratory quotient for the period has been (independently) estimated from the macronutrient compositon of the food.

The ^{18}O is very expensive and so is the mass spectrometer. The method can only be carried out as a research procedure in specialised centres but this is the only method that enables energy expenditure of free-living subjects to be measured over about a week.

The new non-invasive doubly labelled water technique (see information box) makes it possible to measure energy expenditure over 7 to 10 days. It is showing that while self recorded food, hence energy intake, approximates to energy expenditure in most lean people, obese people tend to record lower food energy intakes than their actual energy intakes. Since the energy expenditure is a more precise and objective measurement these food intakes must be underestimates if the subjects are not losing weight.

Drugs

The use of steroids, oral contraceptives, phenothiazines and insulin is commonly followed by weight gain, mainly because appetite is stimulated.

Clinical features

In most cases the diagnosis will be apparent from the patient's appearance but the degree of overweight or obesity should also be assessed, usually by measurement of height and weight and reference to a table such as Table 9.10. In addition, the skinfold thickness over the triceps muscle can be measured using special spring-loaded calipers. Obesity is indicated by a reading above 20 mm in a man, and above 28 mm in a woman.

This very common disorder is frequently overlooked

Table 9.10 Guidance for body weight in adults (men and women)

Height without shoes m	Approx ft in	Significantly underweight (80% of lower end of Acceptable)	Acceptable range	Obese	Grossly obese
		Weight (kg) without clothes			
1.45	4 9	34	42–53	63	84
1.48	4 10	35	44–55	66	88
1.50	4 11	36	45–56	68	90
1.52	5 0	37	46–58	69	92
1.54	5 1	38	47–59	71	95
1.56	5 1	39	49–61	73	97
1.58	5 2	40	50–62	75	100
1.60	5 3	41	51–64	77	102
1.62	5 4	42	52–66	79	105
1.64	5 5	43	43–67	81	108
1.66	5 5	44	55–69	83	110
1.68	5 6	45	56–71	85	113
1.70	5 7	46	58–72	87	116
1.72	5 8	47	59–74	89	118
1.74	5 6	48	61–76	91	121
1.76	5 9	50	62–77.5	93	124
1.78	5 10	51	63–79	95	127
1.80	5 11	52	65–81	97	130
1.82	6 0	53	66–83	99	132
1.84	6 0	54	68–85	102	136
1.86	6 1	55	69–86	104	138
1.88	6 2	57	71–88	106	141
1.90	6 3	58	72–90	108	144
1.92	6 4	59	74–92	111	147
BMI		<16	20–25	>30	>40

The body mass index (BMI) is used to define nutritional status. It is derived from the formula, weight (kg)/height (m)^2. The acceptable (normal) range is 20–25. Obesity is taken to start at a BMI of 30 and gross obesity at 40. Weights between 'acceptable' and 'obese' are classified as overweight (BMI 25.0 to 29.9). The grading of starvation is given on pages 554–555. The standards are the same for men and women.

because the doctor is preoccupied by one of its many complications or ignores it because it is so familiar.

Obesity must be distinguished from a gain in weight due to fluid retention associated with cardiac, renal or hepatic disease, bearing in mind the fact that oedema does not become manifest clinically until the extracellular fluid has increased by about 15%.

Complications

Psychological

Obese patients often have psychological difficulties, but it is difficult to distinguish between cause and effect. Depressed or anxious patients or the emotionally deprived may seek solace in food. Many obese people, especially younger adult females, are ashamed of their unattractive appearance and develop psychological and sexual problems.

Mechanical disabilities

These are listed in the information box.

MECHANICAL DISABILITIES ASSOCIATED WITH OBESITY

- Flat feet
- Osteoarthrosis of knees, hips, lumbar spine
- Abdominal hernias
- Diaphragmatic hernias
- Varicose veins
- Exertional breathlessness
- Respiratory infections
- Accidents

Metabolic disorders

Non-insulin dependent diabetes mellitus, hyperlipid-aemia (elevation of cholesterol and triglyceride), gallstones, hyperuricaemia and gout are all more common among the obese than in the general population.

Cardiovascular disorders

Obesity increases the work done by the heart, which enlarges with rising body weight. Cardiac output, stroke volume, and blood volume all increase. Hypertension is common but to get a correct brachial reading in the obese, an extra wide sphygmomanometer cuff must be used.

The contribution which obesity alone makes to the aetiology of ischaemic heart disease is complicated. There is little doubt that obesity is associated with this disease, but it is difficult to separate the contribution of obesity from that of other risk factors which may be causally associated, such as diabetes, hypertension and hyperlipidaemia. In some prospective studies a direct association has been reported between central (abdominal) obesity, with a high waist/hip ratio, and coronary disease. Special mention should also be made of physical inactivity, which may be both a cause and an effect of obesity and plays an important role in the genesis of ischaemic heart disease.

Life expectancy

Overweight is associated with an increased rate of mortality at all ages. The level of excess mortality varies more or less in proportion to the degree of obesity (see Fig. 9.10).

There is also evidence that a substantial reduction of the body weight of obese people is alone sufficient to diminish the greater death rate. In the Society of Actuaries Build and Blood Pressure Study of 1979, the mortality was reduced to near normal in those who successfully lost and maintained weight within the desirable range.

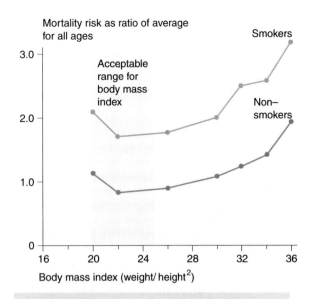

Fig. 9.10 Variations in mortality by Body Mass Index—weight (kg)/[height (m)]^2 in 750 000 men and women. Based on Lew E A, Garfinkel L 1979 Journal of Chronic Diseases 32: 563–576.

Management

Whatever the ultimate cause of obesity in the individual case the immediate cause is energy imbalance, and weight reduction can be achieved only by reducing energy intake or by increasing output, or by a combination of the two. This involves change in the individual's way of life. Thus treatment is difficult and the patient needs motivation. Rewards must be seen ahead and psychological understanding and behavioural advice are essential weapons. It is most important for success that patients should be educated and informed about their disorder and misconceptions corrected. There are no 'slimming foods' or 'slimming tablets' which do not depend on a reduced energy intake.

Long-term results are best where patients are well motivated and educated, follow a clear programme designed to provide 800 to 1600 kcal daily and are being seen and weighed regularly, every 1 to 2 weeks initially, by the same person.

It is important that obese patients should be given personal advice as to how they should reorganise their dietary and exercise habits, an agreed target weight to aim for and an indication of the rate of weight loss expected.

Success does not depend on operations, drugs, injections or other manipulations undertaken by the therapist but rather on the ability of the patient to manage the disorder himself or herself and to persist indefinitely with some restriction on dietary freedom and increase in exercise.

The physician's role is to provide advice and continuing support. Many doctors find obese people unattractive, have difficulty in sympathising with their problems and fail to establish satisfactory rapport with them. Such attitudes contribute to the frequent lack of success in treatment.

The construction of a weight-reducing diet

A weekly weight loss of 0.5 to 1 kg should be the general aim. An obese middle-aged housewife will usually lose weight satisfactorily on a diet providing 800 to 1000 kcal (3.8 to 4.2 MJ) per day. An obese man engaged in active physical work will not tolerate a diet as low as 1000 kcal per day but a satisfactory weight loss can be expected from a diet containing about 1500 kcal (6.3 MJ) per day.

Obese people seldom develop more than a trace of ketosis and never sufficient to cause symptoms as long as they consume small amounts of carbohydrate. In a diet of 1000 kcal/day, 100 g of carbohydrate is a suitable allowance, taken as foods providing complex carbohydrates and dietary fibre (such as fruits and vegetables and whole grain cereals).

Fat

Dietary fat is by far the most important contributor to adiposity of all the dietary components. First of all it provides 9 kcal per gram compared with around 4 for carbohydrates and proteins. Secondly, the use of fat in food preparation makes foods appetising and hard to stop eating. Thirdly, much of the fat in foods is invisible, e.g. in biscuits, cakes, pies, many mixed dishes. Fourthly, metabolic experiments show major differences in our handling of high intakes of fat, compared to carbohydrate or protein. Whereas carbohydrate oxidation is increased to match its intake, this does not happen after an ingested load of fat. Restriction of fat intake is, therefore the first essential in a weight-reducing diet. A 1000 kcal diet containing 100 g of carbohydrate and 50 g of protein cannot include more than 40–45 g of fat. This allowance of fat, though small, is sufficient to make the diet palatable and provide essential fatty acids.

Vitamins

The diet should contain plenty of green vegetables and fruits, since they contain few calories; while their bulk helps to fill the stomach and provide satiety, they also help to minimise the constipation common with a low food intake. Their vitamin A activity and vitamin C content will be sufficient to meet the body's needs. With meat, fish and egg and fruit and vegetables in the diet there should be enough of the other vitamins.

Minerals

The only minerals that need serious consideration are calcium and iron. Provided the diet includes 300 ml of skimmed or very low fat milk (100 kcal), there is little likelihood of a negative calcium balance developing in an adult. The supply of iron is less sure and may call for the prescription of iron supplements.

Alcoholic drinks

These are also a source of calories without essential nutrients and tend to stimulate appetite. They are best avoided, but if taken, a corresponding reduction in the diet is necessary. A 100 ml glass of dry wine or 30 ml whisky and water provide 70 kcal and half a pint of lager 80 kcal.

In different cultures dietitians can devise socially acceptable diets following the above principles. Because there are many effective weight-reducing diets—not just one—we do not print an example in this Chapter.

Failure to respond to such a diet nearly always indicates non-compliance, despite protestations to the contrary! In such cases, treatment in hospital under strict supervision for 1 to 2 weeks may be beneficial to demonstrate that the prescribed regimen is effective if carefully followed and to allow a period of intensive education.

Exercise

Increased exercise is the other, positive part of the management of obesity. Strenuous exercise is neither feasible nor advisable but most obese people are capable of moderate aerobic exercise such as walking, swimming, gardening, dancing, provided it does not exceed their cardiovascular capacity. Because of their heavy weight obese people expend more food energy than lean people doing exercise of this type. Regular daily exercise is much more valuable than episodic activity.

As well as its contribution to the desired negative energy balance, regular exercise improves the fitness of obese people and their feeling of well being, and some specialists treating obesity consider it also gives people more control over their appetite.

An hour's walk at 3 miles per hour will expend about 240 kcal above basal (or more for a heavy person). This may seem a small amount, equivalent to about 30 g of body fat, but if the daily walk becomes a habit it will add up, other things being equal, to a weight loss of 10 kg in a year. Doctors should suggest, discuss and work out with each patient an increasing programme of exercise which is within their physical capacity and which will add to the quality of life of the individual (see Table 9.11).

Table 9.11 Energy used in exercise (rounded approximate figures)

At rest (Men+10%, women − 10%	1 kcal/min
Moderate exercise For example, walking, gardening, golf	5 kcal/min
Intermediate For example, cycling, swimming, tennis	7 kcal/min
Strenuous For example, squash, jogging, hill climbing, heavy work	10 kcal/min

In SI units 1 kcal/min = 4.2 kJ/min = 70 watts

Therapeutic starvation

A period of several weeks of starvation in hospital with only water, non-caloric drinks with vitamin, mineral and protein supplements being allowed, has been recommended for very obese patients who have failed to respond to orthodox treatment.

Although the initial loss of weight may be marked, the long-term results are no more satisfactory than with other systems since many patients regain most of the weight lost when strict measures are discontinued. Such a regimen is contraindicated for older patients, especially if they have cardiovascular complications, since deaths have occasionally occurred. Ketosis may be troublesome in the early stages and hyperuricaemia, sometimes accompanied by gout, can develop.

Drug therapy

This is no substitute for a dietary regimen but has a limited use as an adjunct in carefully selected patients with refractory obesity. Some of the more effective drugs used in the past, notably amphetamine, are addictive and have been so widely abused that they should not be prescribed for the treatment of obesity.

Other amphetamine-like drugs (e.g. diethylpropion, phentermine) are no longer recommended. They are not very effective appetite suppressants and have some, though less, cerebral stimulant activity. In the UK they are subject to the prescription requirements of the Misuse of Drugs Regulations 1985.

The most useful group of drugs at present to support a weight reducing regime are the serotoninergic compounds. The first of these was dl-fenfluramine ('Ponderax'), now largely replaced by second generation drugs d-fenfluramine (dexfenfluramine) and fluoxetine. These increase satiety rather than suppress appetite and they do so by potentiating serotonin in the hypothalamus. Side effects are usually mild and include drowsiness, dry mouth, headache. Effectiveness on weight loss varies considerably between individuals. The effect lasts for only a few months. One of these drugs is best used where there is a medical need for short-term weight reduction, e.g. if obesity is associated with diabetes or hypertension.

Other potential drugs for obesity are being developed by the drug houses and actively investigated. These include: (1) β3-adrenoceptor agonists which in animals increase the metabolic rate by stimulating brown adipose tissue; (2) analogues of cholecystokinin (appetite suppressant) which persist longer in the circulation; (3) inhibitors of intestinal lipase.

These drugs must not be given to a patient with a history of psychiatric illness. Diuretics must be used with care and only if there is oedema, because potassium depletion is more likely than usual while patients are on a restricted diet.

The administration of thyroxine to euthyroid patients is not only useless but is potentially dangerous, especially if heart disease is present. It should be prescribed only if hypothyroidism coexists with obesity.

Surgical treatment

Wiring the jaws together to prevent eating has been used to treat those who have found it impossible to adhere to a low-energy diet. Although this usually results in marked loss of weight, many patients regain weight when the procedure is reversed. An alternative and fairly safe operation (though a major one) is to reduce the size of the stomach, for example by stapling, which can be undone. Small intestine bypass, aimed at inducing malabsorption, has been undertaken in some centres for the treatment of severe 'morbid' obesity but complications can be severe and sometimes fatal. It should be emphasised that surgery should be considered only for those with gross, intractable obesity.

Prognosis

It is easy for an obese person to lose up to 5 kg in weight. This accounts for the temporary success of numerous popular 'slimming cures'. How difficult it is to achieve further losses is not generally realised. The published records of seven obesity clinics in the USA showed that satisfactory results ranged only from 12 to 28% if the index of success was the loss of 12 kg or more.

Experience in many clinics has also shown that it is difficult for patients to maintain their reduced weight since this requires some restriction of energy intake on a long-term basis.

Prevention

This must depend in part on the doctor who notices when patients, be they infants, children or adults, are overweight or gaining too much weight. For this purpose alone, among the most useful information that a doctor can keep about patients is a record of body weight, measured at regular intervals. The doctor's responsibility with an overweight patient, at any time, is advisory and educational; the attention of patients must be drawn to the dangers of obesity and to the appropriate methods of correcting it.

All the health agencies available should be mustered to support a steady campaign of education and persuasion of patients and potential patients on the need to avoid obesity. The antenatal services, infant welfare clinics, school health authorities, health visitors and many others to whom the public look for advice should contribute to this educational programme. The media also play an increasingly important role.

FURTHER READING

Obesity
Lew E A, Garfinkel L 1979 Variations in mortality by weight among 750 000 men and women. Journal of Chronic Diseases 32: 563–576
Prentice A M et al 1986 High levels of energy expenditure in obese women. British Medical Journal 292: 983–987
Ravussin E, Swinburn B A 1992 Pathophysiology of obesity. Lancet 340: 404–408
Royal College of Physicians 1983 Obesity. Royal College of Physicians, London. A comprehensive report
General nutrition
Cameron M, Hofvander Y 1983 Manual on feeding infants and young children (for application in the developing areas of the world with special reference to home-made weaning foods), 3rd edn. Oxford University Press, Delhi
Garrow J S, James W P T 1994 Davidson's human nutrition and dietetics, 9th edn. Churchill Livingstone, Edinburgh
Shils M E, Olson J A, Shike M 1993 Modern nutrition in health and disease, 8th edn. Lea and Febiger, Malvern, PA
Truswell A S 1992 ABC of nutrition, 2nd edn. ABC Series, British Medical Journal, London

10

A. D. Cumming, C. P. Swainson

Disturbances in water, electrolyte and acid-base balance

Disturbances in water, electrolyte and acid-base balance are common problems encountered in general medical and surgical practice. Some are trivial, but others are associated with a high mortality and require urgent assessment and treatment. The kidneys play an important part in maintaining normal water, electrolyte and acid-base balance. Many of these disturbances occur in older patients with moderate, often undiagnosed, chronic renal failure whose homeostatic abilities are compromised.

Normal functioning of the human body requires that the concentrations of hydrogen ions and the major electrolytes, sodium, potassium, calcium, magnesium and phosphate, remain within narrow limits inside cells and outside in the interstitial fluid. Disturbances of water, electrolyte and acid-base balance occur in a wide variety of diseases described in appropriate chapters of this book. It is convenient to group many of them together in order to explain the underlying pathophysiology and provide a framework for their diagnosis and treatment.

The anatomy of the kidney and the physiology of glomerular function are described in Chapter 11.

PHYSIOLOGY OF WATER AND ELECTROLYTES

REGULATION OF WATER EXCRETION

About two-thirds of the filtered water is reabsorbed with an equivalent amount of sodium in the proximal tubules. The remainder passes through the distal nephron where its reabsorption (Fig. 10.1) is regulated by the antidiuretic hormone, arginine-vasopressin (AVP). **In the presence of AVP** the collecting duct becomes permeable to water which is then passively reabsorbed in response to the high concentrations of sodium, chloride and urea in the medullary interstitium. The urine thus becomes concentrated. **In the absence of AVP** the distal nephron is almost impermeable to water. In these circumstances tubular reabsorption of sodium chloride without water in the thick ascending limb of the loop of Henle results in formation of a dilute urine.

REGULATION OF ELECTROLYTES

This depends upon selective reabsorption and secretion of electrolytes by the renal tubules.

Sodium

In the proximal tubule, about 65% of filtered sodium is reabsorbed by a complex combination of active and passive transport. In the early proximal tubule reabsorption of sodium is coupled to that of glucose and amino acids, because their uptake by the cells requires sodium. About 90% of filtered bicarbonate is reabsorbed with sodium in the proximal tubule. Most filtered chloride is reabsorbed by a passive mechanism linked to primary active transport of sodium. About two-thirds of the filtered water is reabsorbed passively in association with the electrolytes, its movement being determined by a small transepithelial osmotic gradient.

Control of proximal tubular reabsorption of sodium and water is poorly understood. It is linked to the glomerular filtration rate (GFR) so that the fraction reabsorbed is normally constant. An increase in extracellular fluid (ECF) volume is associated with reduced reabsorption of sodium and water at this site. Among the mechanisms proposed are angiotensins, atrial natriuretic peptide, changes in physical forces operating across peritubular capillary walls, increased local release of dopamine, and other unidentified natriuretic factors.

Most of the remaining sodium and chloride is reabsorbed without water in the thick ascending limb of the loop of Henle. Sodium, chloride and potassium are taken up from the lumen into cells by a co-transport system. Sodium is then transported across the peritubular membrane by Na^+/K^+ ATPase. Potassium and chloride leave the cell by a KCl co-transporter which depends on the gradient for potassium across the peritubular membrane. The diuretic drug frusemide competes with chloride for the luminal co-transport exchanger, thus inhibiting absorption of sodium, potassium and chloride. As in the proximal tubule, reabsorption of sodium in the ascending limb is flow-dependent, the amount reabsorbed depending on the proportion of filtrate delivered to the site.

Unabsorbed sodium passes into the distal tubule, collecting tubule and collecting duct. Here the cell membrane is relatively impermeable to chloride. Much of the sodium is reabsorbed 'in exchange' for potassium and hydrogen ions, which diffuse from cell to lumen down a lumen-negative electrochemical gradient created by active sodium transport. The cells lining this part of the nephron can sustain a large concentration gradient for sodium between tubular and peritubular fluids. Thus in a sodium depleted individual the concentration of sodium in the urine can be reduced to almost zero. At this site sodium transport is stimulated by aldosterone and prostaglandins, and inhibited by atrial natriuretic peptide and kinins.

Potassium

More than 90% of filtered potassium is reabsorbed actively in the proximal tubule and in the ascending limb (see above). Urinary potassium is largely derived from cells in the distal nephron, where active absorption of

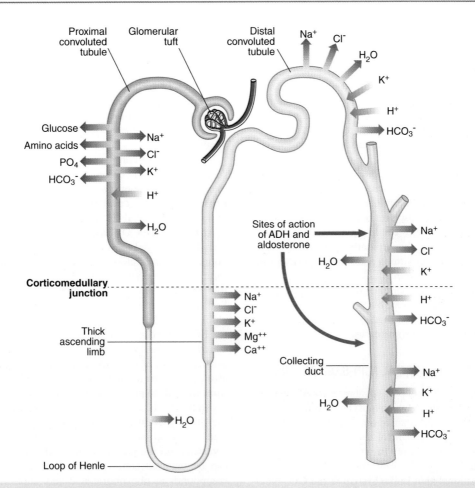

Proximal convoluted tubule

Glomerular tuft

Distal convoluted tubule

Na^+ Cl^-

H_2O

K^+

H^+

HCO_3^-

Glucose

Amino acids

PO_4

HCO_3^-

Na^+

Cl^-

K^+

H^+

H_2O

Sites of action of ADH and aldosterone

Na^+

Cl^-

H_2O

K^+

Corticomedullary junction

Na^+
Cl^-
K^+
Mg^{++}
Ca^{++}

H^+

HCO_3^-

Thick ascending limb

Collecting duct

Na^+

K^+

H_2O

H^+

HCO_3^-

H_2O

Loop of Henle

Fig. 10.1   Excretion of water and electrolytes. In the proximal tubule approximately two-thirds of filtered water is reabsorbed together with glucose, amino acids, phosphate and bicarbonate. In the thick ascending limb of the loop of Henle sodium, potassium, calcium, magnesium and chloride are reabsorbed whilst in the distal tubule sodium is reabsorbed under the influence of aldosterone with associated excretion of potassium and hydrogen ions. Water is reabsorbed from the distal nephron under the influence of AVP and the hypertonic medulla.

sodium creates a lumen-negative potential difference. An electrochemical gradient is created by active transport of potassium from the peritubular fluid into the cells, a process stimulated by aldosterone, while the intraluminal potential negative with respect to the peritubular fluid favours diffusion of potassium from cells to lumen. Factors influencing the rate of potassium excretion are in the information box.

The dual actions of the adrenocortical and antidiuretic hormones on the renal tubules play an important role in determining the total sodium, potassium and water content of the body. While the rate of secretion of vasopressin is determined mainly by changes in osmolality of the blood, it is known to increase in response to pain, stress and a reduction in ECF volume. Aldosterone secretion is increased by reduction in renal perfusion pressure and the sodium chloride concentration of the

FACTORS INCREASING K⁺ EXCRETION

- Rise in tubular cell K^+, e.g. hyperaldosteronism, alkalosis
- High urine flow rate
- Avid Na^+ reabsorption
- Excess poorly reabsorbed anions, e.g. phosphate, ketones

fluid reaching the macula densa. These stimuli increase secretion of renin by the juxtaglomerular apparatus (JGA); this in turn acts on its substrate angiotensinogen to produce the decapeptide Angiotensin I (AI). This is then acted on by angiotensin-converting enzyme (ACE) which converts AI to Angiotensin II, which stimulates synthesis of aldosterone by the adrenal cortex.

Calcium, phosphate and magnesium

Filtered calcium (that fraction not bound to plasma proteins) is reabsorbed throughout the nephron in a fashion similar to sodium; thus the rate of excretion of calcium usually varies with that of sodium. Parathyroid hormone (PTH) enhances distal tubular reabsorption of calcium, which may contribute to the development of hypercalcaemia in primary hyperparathyroidism. Vitamin D_3 may stimulate proximal tubular calcium reabsorption.

Phosphate is filtered from plasma and reabsorbed principally by the proximal tubule, normally at close to its maximum capacity, so that in most circumstances the GFR is the major determinant of urinary phosphate excretion. Tubular phosphate reabsorption is reduced by PTH, contributing to the low plasma phosphate in primary and secondary hyperparathyroidism.

Most filtered magnesium is reabsorbed, partly under the influence of PTH, in the thick ascending limb of the loop of Henle. Tubular handling of calcium, phosphate and magnesium is influenced by various drugs, including diuretics, leading to disturbed plasma concentrations and clinical sequelae in some cases.

MAINTENANCE OF NORMAL ACID-BASE BALANCE

Oxidative metabolism of proteins, fats and carbohydrate generates acid products which must be excreted to maintain body fluids within an optimal hydrogen ion concentration. Acid-base control involves **body buffers**, **lung function**, and **kidney function** (in order of speed of response).

The most important buffer system is the CO_2-bicarbonate system. Arterial blood H^+ concentration ($[H^+]$) depends on the concentrations of carbonic acid ($H_2CO_3 \approx 1.2$ mmol/l in health), CO_2 (at a partial pressure of 5.2 kPa) and bicarbonate (24 mmol/l).

This is an 'open' buffer system because the bicarbonate and CO_2 components are under physiological control, reacting to changes in hydrogen ion concentration.

$$H^+ + HCO_3^- \leftrightharpoons H_2CO_3 \leftrightharpoons H_2O + CO_2$$

(regulated by kidneys)   *(regulated by lungs)*

$[H^+]$ = dissociation constant (K) $\times [CO_2] / [HCO_3^-]$
i.e $[H^+]$ depends on the ratio of $[CO_2]$ to $[HCO_3^-]$

If H^+ ions are added to the blood (metabolic acidosis, e.g. poisoning by an acid) the equation is *pushed* to the right, and ventilation increases via stimulation of chemoreceptors, to blow off CO_2. If the $[CO_2]$ rises, as in Type II respiratory failure, the equilibrium is *pushed* to the left, increasing $[H^+]$ (respiratory acidosis). To compensate, the kidney must excrete more H^+ and

regenerate more bicarbonate to set up a new equilibrium. In contrast, if H^+ ions are lost (e.g. vomiting in pyloric stenosis), the equation is *pulled* to the left (metabolic alkalosis). To bring the $[H^+]$ back to normal, more CO_2 is needed, and $[CO_2]$ rises through reduced ventilation by the lungs. Voluntary or involuntary hyperventilation leads to a fall in $[CO_2]$, and the equation is *pulled* to the right, with a fall in $[H^+]$ (respiratory alkalosis).

The process of compensation takes time, particularly renal compensation. Therefore acute disorders are less likely to be compensated than chronic ones. Compensation may be complete (H^+ concentration restored to normal) or partial (H^+ concentration still abnormal).

Apart from the CO_2-bicarbonate system, other buffers include haemoglobin in red cells and hydroxyapatite in bone. These are 'closed' buffer systems which can be saturated. Haemoglobin in red cells is the major buffer that transfers H^+ and CO_2 from tissues to the lungs. Some CO_2 is transported reversibly bound to haemoglobin as a carbamino compound, but most is converted to H_2CO_3 since red cells are rich in carbonic anhydrase, which catalyses this reaction in either direction. Hydrogen ions from H_2CO_3 are taken up by Hb after it has given up oxygen to the tissues, while the HCO_3^- moves from red cells to plasma in exchange for chloride (chloride shift, Fig. 10.2). Most of the carbonic acid added to the blood therefore appears as HCO_3^- rather than as acid. As blood passes through the lungs the process is reversed, and the CO_2 formed is exhaled. Not all acids can be oxidised completely to CO_2 and water. Such compounds as phosphoric acid and sulphuric acid are excreted by the kidneys.

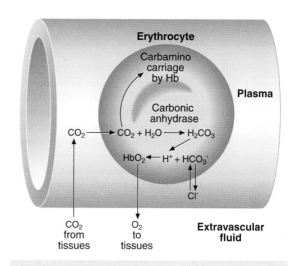

Fig. 10.2 Transport of CO_2.

The kidney is crucial in the response to changes in H^+ concentration. In proximal tubular cells, CO_2 derived from cellular metabolism or diffusion from the tubular lumen combines with water to form carbonic acid, which dissociates to H^+ and a bicarbonate ion. The H^+ ion is actively pumped into the tubular lumen, where it 'traps' filtered bicarbonate to form carbonic acid. Under the influence of carbonic anhydrase, carbonic acid in the lumen dissociates to water and CO_2, which (unlike bicarbonate) is able to back-diffuse into the tubular cell, to continue the cycle. The original intracellular bicarbonate ion is actively co-transported with sodium into the interstitium, and hence the circulation. The net effect is that for each proton excreted, one bicarbonate ion is returned to the blood, so that bicarbonate reserves are regenerated (Fig. 10.3). Filtered bicarbonate ions are reabsorbed mainly by this mechanism up to a threshold plasma concentration of 25 mmol/l. Above this level, reabsorption is incomplete and the excess is eliminated in the urine.

Active H^+ secretion continues all along the nephron. When most of the filtered bicarbonate has been reabsorbed, secreted hydrogen ions are taken up by other bases in the tubular fluid. The corresponding conjugate acids are excreted in the urine. Filtered bases, of which disodium hydrogen phosphate is the most important, accept about one third of the hydrogen ions destined for excretion (Fig. 10.3). This allows secretion of H^+ ions to continue without too high an opposing concentration gradient. The amount excreted in this way is limited by the magnitude of the hydrogen ion gradient between blood and tubular fluid which can be sustained by cells in the distal nephron. The urine pH cannot be reduced much below 4.5. Two-thirds of secreted protons are therefore accepted by the base ammonia (NH_3) formed within the tubular cell from glutamine. NH_3 enters the acid urine by non-ionic diffusion and accepts a proton to form the weak acid, NH_4^+. The luminal cell membrane is relatively impermeable to this charged particle, and it is excreted in the urine (Fig. 10.3).

In the distal tubule and collecting duct, sodium is reabsorbed in exchange for either potassium or hydrogen ions, under the influence of aldosterone. When intracellular potassium is low, H^+ is preferentially exchanged, and vice versa. Hence the observed clinical associations between hypokalaemia and alkalosis, and hyperkalaemia and acidosis (although acidosis also inhibits the Na^+/K^+ ATPase which pumps potassium into cells). Diuretics which block sodium reabsorption in the loop of Henle, by increasing the delivery of sodium to the distal tubular exchange site, cause increased loss of both H^+ ions and potassium (hypokalaemic alkalosis).

A healthy person eating a mixed diet excretes 40–80 mmol of hydrogen ion in the urine daily. When the rate of production of protons is increased (e.g. in diabetic ketoacidosis) the healthy kidney produces larger quantities of ammonia and up to 500 mmol/day of hydrogen ions may be excreted in the urine, mainly as NH_4^+. By contrast, when a diet consisting mainly of fruit and vegetables is taken, disodium hydrogen phosphate and bicarbonate are excreted and tubular secretion of ammonium ions is suppressed.

NORMAL DISTRIBUTION OF WATER AND ELECTROLYTES

Water

The body of a healthy 65 kg man contains approximately 40 litres of water distributed as shown in Figure 10.4. Water passes freely from one body compartment to another and its distribution is determined by osmotic and hydrostatic forces. In healthy individuals body water remains remarkably constant despite wide variations in intake.

Electrolytes

All electrolytes are dissolved in body water but distributed differently in the various compartments (Fig. 10.5). The effective osmolality (tonicity) of plasma and interstitial fluid is determined by the concentrations of

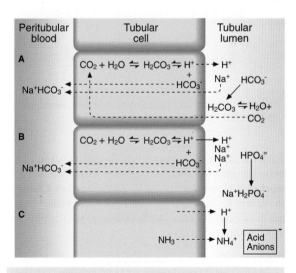

Fig. 10.3 Hydrogen ion excretion. [A] Carbonic acid is generated from CO_2 and H_2O in tubular cells. Hydrogen ions (H^+) from this acid are secreted into the tubular lumen in exchange for sodium which is reabsorbed into the blood along with bicarbonate ions liberated from the carbonic acid. [B] Some hydrogen ions are buffered by filtered disodium hydrogen phosphate in the tubular fluid forming dihydrogen sodium phosphate. [C] Other H^+ are buffered by ammonia (NH_3) to form the weak acid NH_4^+. Anions of inorganic and organic acids are excreted largely as ammonium salts.

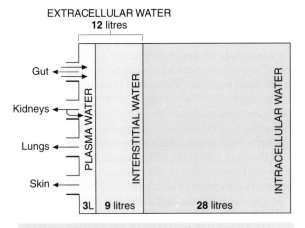

Fig. 10.4 Distribution of water in a 65 kg man. The vascular compartment is in contact with the environment at 4 portals. Net gain or loss of water and electrolytes occurs by these routes.

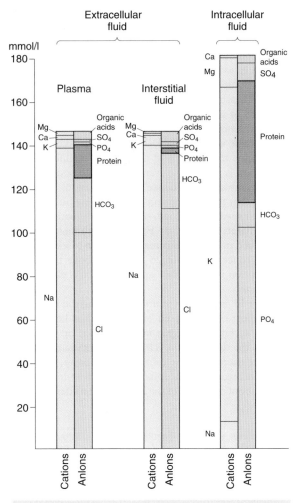

Fig. 10.5 Distribution of electrolytes in plasma, interstitial fluid and cell fluid.

sodium (Na^+) and chloride (Cl^-), while that of the intracellular fluid is determined by the concentrations of potassium (K^+), magnesium (Mg^{2+}), phosphate and sulphate. The amount of hydrogen ion $[H^+]$ in the extracellular fluid is tiny (40 nmol/l) and much can be buffered by cationic proteins such as albumin and haemoglobin.

The differences in ionic composition of cells and the interstitial fluid are essential to normal cell function. They are maintained by a number of active bidirectional pumps in both the apical and basolateral membranes, such as Na^+/K^+ ATPase.

INTERPRETATION OF LABORATORY RESULTS

Sodium

The plasma sodium concentration reflects the water added to or leaving body fluids. Hypernatraemia usually indicates primarily a lack of water and hyponatraemia an excess of water in plasma, rather than changes in sodium balance, although hyponatraemia is common after salt loss because of excessive AVP stimulating water retention.

Pseudohyponatraemia is seen with gross hyperlipidaemia. The autoanalyser measures the sodium in the whole sample and reports a low value when the true concentration in the plasma water is normal. This can be detected by observing that the plasma is lipaemic if the sample is left to stand for 10 minutes.

Potassium

Changes in the plasma K^+ concentration reflect changes in ECF K^+ quite closely, and also mirror an increase or decrease in total body K^+. However, because most of the K^+ is inside cells, changes in the **distribution** of K^+ between plasma and intracellular fluid can have a marked effect on the plasma K^+ concentration. Changes in plasma K^+ concentration therefore may reflect changes in external K^+ balance **or** changes in the distribution of K^+ within the body.

Calcium, phosphate, magnesium

Approximately 40% of plasma calcium is bound to plasma proteins, primarily albumin. This proportion is decreased by acidosis and increased by alkalosis. Thus, for example, rapid administration of sodium bicarbonate to patients with hypocalcaemia may precipitate tetany, as the ionised calcium fraction falls. Ionised calcium can be directly measured using appropriate electrodes. When the plasma albumin concentration is abnormal, the total plasma calcium concentration will be affected. An appropriately adjusted value can be calculated from the formula:

$$\text{Adjusted P}_{\text{calcium}} \text{ [mmol/l]} = \text{measured P}_{\text{calcium}} \text{ [mmol/l]} \\ + 0.02 \times (40 - \text{P}_{\text{albumin}} \text{ [g/l]})$$

Similar considerations apply to the plasma magnesium concentration. The plasma phosphate concentration may reflect changes in body phosphate balance, but acute alterations usually represent a shift between the extracellular and intracellular compartments.

Bicarbonate and chloride

The sum of bicarbonate (HCO_3^-) and chloride (Cl^-) concentrations accounts for most of the anions in plasma, with about 10–12 mmol/l from proteins and less than 10 mmol/l from a mixture of inorganic and organic salts. The plasma bicarbonate reflects acute changes in acid base balance. Reduction in plasma bicarbonate (acidaemia) may be the first clue to an acute metabolic acidosis, and an abnormal rise in plasma bicarbonate (alkalaemia) will indicate an acute or chronic alkalosis. The 'anion gap' is sometimes a useful concept when considering the cause of an acute metabolic acidosis (p. 603). The sum of the measured cations ($Na^+ + K^+$) is always slightly more than the measured anions ($HCO_3^- + Cl^-$), i.e. there is a normal anion gap of 8–14 mmol/l. If the anion gap is abnormally large it usually indicates that an exogenous acid has been added to the body, e.g. diabetic ketoacidosis, salicylate poisoning.

FURTHER READING

Burckhardt G, Greger R 1992 Principles of electrolyte transport across plasma membranes of renal tubular cells. In: Windhager E E (ed.) Handbook of Physiology. Section 8: 639–658. Oxford University Press, New York

Knepper M A, Chou C L, Layton H E 1993 How is urine concentrated in the renal inner medulla? Contributions to Nephrology 102: 144–160

Zeidel M L, Strange K, Emma F, Harris H W 1993 Mechanisms and regulation of water transport in the kidney. Seminars in Nephrology 13: 155–167

MAJOR MANIFESTATIONS OF ELECTROLYTE AND ACID-BASE DISORDERS

CLINICAL ASSESSMENT

Most patients exhibit few and subtle signs. Gross physical signs are usually associated with severe abnormalities and a correspondingly high mortality. Major electrolyte disturbances are most commonly associated with abnormalities of neurological or muscular function. A history of recent acute illness or surgery, drug ingestion or

Table 10.1 Aetiology of hyponatraemia

Low ECF	Normal ECF	High ECF
Volume depletion (e.g. by excessive diuretics, salt-losing renal disease, diarrhoea, ileostomy)	Nephrotic syndrome Hypothyroidism Diuretics, NSAIDs Post-operative pain and analgesia	Cardiac failure Renal failure SIADH (Diuretics)
Cirrhosis Adrenal failure Diabetic ketoacidosis		

ECF = Extracellular fluid volume; NSAIDs = Non-steroidal anti-inflammatory drugs; SIADH = Syndrome of inappropriate secretion of antidiuretic hormone

poisoning is always important. Careful review of fluid and weight charts may show discrepancies in intake and output.

Sodium

Clinical signs associated with hyper- or hyponatraemia are rare. **Hypernatraemia** is often accompanied by thirst, mild confusion and/or disorientation. Severe water depletion may lead to coma with marked muscle weakness and progressive signs of volume depletion, i.e. postural hypotension, tachycardia and low jugular venous pressure (JVP). **Hyponatraemia** may be associated with a mild confusional state, lassitude and sleepiness progressing to gross confusion, myoclonic jerks and generalised seizures. Serious clinical signs occur in patients in whom the plasma sodium has changed abruptly or is very low (< 110 mmol/l). This is a medical emergency, as the mortality is about 40% and the risk of neurological damage (central pontine myelinolysis) is high.

It is important to assess the **volume status** to facilitate diagnosis and rational treatment. Postural hypotension, the JVP and the presence or absence of oedema are the main clinical signs to decide whether a patient has a normal plasma volume, is volume depleted or overloaded. The more common causes of hyponatraemia are shown in Table 10.1 in relation to the assessment of volume status.

Potassium

Clinical signs of **hyperkalaemia** are rare. Patients may complain of tingling around the lips or in the fingers but are more likely to present with collapse due to a dangerous brady-arrhythmia. Thus a cardiac arrhythmia may be the first and only sign of hyperkalaemia and an irregular pulse should be checked with an ECG. Typical ECG changes are shown in Figure 10.6. Patients may also develop severe muscular weakness resulting in a flaccid paralysis and loss of tendon jerks. Abdominal distension and ileus may also be present. These patients

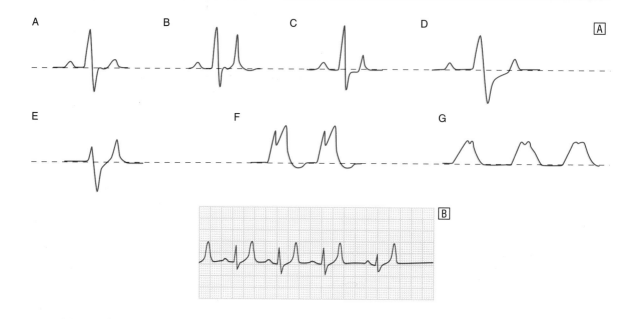

Fig. 10.6   Changes in the ECG associated with hyperkalaemia. [A] Progressive ECG changes in hyperkalaemia. **A**. Normal; **B**. Tall, peaked, symmetrical T waves, tentlike shape, narrow base; **C**. T waves of normal amplitude, but with tentlike shape and narrow base; **D**. P–R and QRS intervals lengthen; R wave and P wave decrease in height; S wave increases in depth; RS–T segment depressed. **E**, **F**. P wave may disappear; QRS may lengthen further; ventricular rhythm may become grossly irregular at this point and may give appearance of bundle branch block; **G**. QRS complexes lose angular shape and become smoother and wider; continuous sine wave; may give appearance of paroxysmal ventricular tachycardia. [B] ECG showing hyperkalaemia. The T waves are tall, peaked, tentlike and the P–R interval and QRS complexes are lengthened.

CLINICAL EVALUATION OF ACID-BASE DISTURBANCES

History
- Diabetes, liver disease, kidney disease
- Drugs (aspirin, metformin) or toxins (alcohol, methanol, antifreeze)
- Severe infection

Physical examination
- Circulation—? shock with lactic acidosis
- ECF volume—? fluid depletion or overload
- Respiration—? respiratory distress, ? type (Kussmaul's respiration in metabolic acidosis)
- Ketones on breath

Blood tests
Arterial blood gases
- H^+ concentration (36–44 nmol/l, pH 7.35–7.45)
- Partial pressure CO_2 (*PaCO$_2$*) (4.4–6.1 kPa, 1.2 mmol/l)
- Arterial bicarbonate concentration (21–27 mmol/l)
- Partial pressure O_2 (*PaO$_2$*) (12–15 kPa)
Venous blood
- Total CO_2 (measures venous bicarbonate concentration) (24–30 mmol/l)
- Urea concentration (indicates renal function) (2.5–6.6 mmol/l)
- Potassium concentration (3.3–4.7 mmol/l)

require emergency treatment, and clinical suspicion should be confirmed by an emergency plasma K^+ estimation.

Hypokalaemia may be suggested by tiredness and muscular weakness which in extreme cases can result in the patient being unable to walk or climb stairs. Neurological functions are usually normal, but tingling in the fingers, apathy, paralysis and coma may be present in extreme cases. Long-standing hypokalaemia damages renal tubular structures and results in a failure of the antidiuretic response to vasopressin (nephrogenic diabetes insipidus). Patients with hypokalaemia may therefore present with nocturia or marked polyuria and polydipsia. The ECG may be helpful (Fig. 10.7) and the development of arrhythmias on a combination of digoxin and diuretics should raise clinical suspicion.

Acid-base balance

Disturbances in acid-base balance may be accompanied by mild central nervous system dysfunction and abnormalities of respiration. Acidosis may be suggested by a marked decline in conscious level with confusion and irritability. A classic sign is Kussmaul's respiration,

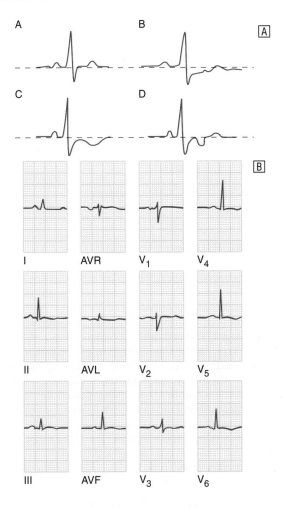

Fig. 10.7   Changes in the ECG associated with hypokalaemia. [A] Progressive ECG changes in hypokalaemia. **A**. Normal; **B**. Flattening of T wave and depression of S-T segment; **C**. S-T segment depression resembling an inverted T wave; prolongation of Q-T interval; **D**. Inverted T wave; U wave appears. These patterns are not necessarily sequential; patterns C and D are most common. [B] ECG showing effects of hypokalaemia. Sinus rhythm with normal QRS complexes. In all leads the T waves are flattened and it is difficult to measure the Q-T interval, but this is probably 0.44 seconds. U waves are present in most leads.

which is slow, deep and sighing. Clinical signs are rare in alkalosis, but severe alkalosis may be accompanied by depression of conscious level and hypoventilation. Tetany may be present because of a low ionised calcium.

In the clinical assessment of acid-base disorders, the history, particularly of chronic diseases such as diabetes or obstructive airways disease, and of recent acute illness or drug ingestion, is important. Often the cause is obvious because acid-base disturbances accompany a variety of serious acute disorders. Assessment of volume status

is also important in these patients as it will help to guide therapy.

Additional laboratory tests

A good history, clinical examination, review of the patient's illness and fluid balance charts will often suggest a likely cause of the problem. In most cases the plasma urea and creatinine will be required to assess renal function. The urinary sodium and osmolality are helpful in judging the contributions of renal sodium loss and of arginine vasopressin (AVP), especially in cases of hyponatraemia. Hyponatraemia with a high urine osmolality (AVP effect) and a low urinary sodium is an appropriate response to volume depletion. If plasma volume is thought to be normal or is increased, then a high urine osmolality indicates an inappropriate excess of AVP— the syndrome of inappropriate secretion of ADH (SIADH).

FURTHER READING

Abraham W T, Schrier R W 1994 Body fluid volume regulation and health in disease. Advances in Internal Medicine 39: 23–47
Preuss H G 1993 Fundamentals of clinical acid-base evaluation. Clinics in Laboratory Medicine 13: 103–116

MAJOR ELECTROLYTE DISORDERS

HYPERNATRAEMIA

Hypernatraemia is characteristic of primary water depletion. The water content of the body is reduced both absolutely and relative to the Na^+ content, so that the osmolar concentration of all body fluids rises.

An adult in a temperate climate loses between 0.5–1 l/day in expired air and by evaporation from the skin. This loss can be increased considerably by a rise in temperature and sweating. Water can be conserved by the kidneys up to a limit determined by renal concentrating ability (up to 1200 mosm/kg) and the amount of solutes that need to be excreted; a high solute load requires an obligatory high urine output.

The causes of water depletion (Table 10.2) are most commonly a reduced intake, and an increase in insensible loss in elderly patients with infection. Excessive loss of water in the urine due to impaired concentrating ability is much less common.

Consequences of water depletion

As water is lost from the body the ECF becomes hypertonic and the plasma $[Na^+]$ rises. Water migrates from cells to re-establish osmotic equilibrium, and intracellular dehydration develops when more than 8% of body water is lost. Renal reabsorption of Na^+ and Cl^- and excretion of K^+ increase secondary to secretion of aldosterone. Retained Na^+ and Cl^- increase ECF tonicity and facilitate transfer of water from cells. The overall loss of water is thus shared by the intracellular and extracellular compartments, so that the circulatory disturbance in water depletion is much less marked than in salt and water depletion of comparable magnitude.

CLINICAL FEATURES OF PREDOMINANT WATER DEPLETION

Mild 1–2 l in adult
- Thirst, concentrated urine

Moderate 2–4 l in adult
- Marked thirst, difficulty swallowing
- Dizziness, mild confusion/aggression and weakness
- Oliguria, concentrated urine, rising plasma urea and Na^+

Severe 4–10 l in adult
- Severe thirst
- Confusion, coma, muscle weakness
- 'Doughy' skin and tissues
- Tachycardia, low BP
- Oliguria, concentrated urine, raised plasma urea, Na^+ and Hb

---

Diagnosis

Diagnosis is made on the base of the history, clinical findings and the presence of hypernatraemia. A measurement of urine osmolality will be helpful; if this is >600 mosm/kg a renal cause is most unlikely. The urine should be tested for sugar to exclude diabetes mellitus, and renal function checked by measurement of plasma urea and creatinine concentrations. Marked polyuria of more than 3 l/day and urine osmolality of <200 mosm/kg suggests AVP-deficient diabetes insipidus or one of the renal lesions in Table 10.2.

Management

Management of water depletion in adults is given in the accompanying box. It can often be prevented by ensuring an adequate intake in ill patients and this is especially important in patients receiving enteral feeds. Fluid charts and daily weights are useful to monitor progress. It is essential that large water deficits are replaced gradually over several days to avoid rapid shift of water into cells which can cause severe disturbance of neurological function. Where there is specific cause (e.g. diabetes insipidus, diabetes mellitus, hypercalcaemia) then this requires rigorous specific therapy in addition to water replacement.

GUIDELINES FOR REPLACEMENT OF WATER DEFICIT

Mild
- Water 2 l by mouth or 5% dextrose i.v. 6–12 hours

Moderate
- 5% dextrose 2–4 l i.v. 24 hours

Severe
- 0.9% saline 1 l i.v. 1 hour
- 5% dextrose 4 l i.v. 24 hours
- 5% dextrose 2–4 l i.v. + oral water 24–48 hours

Maintenance treatment
- 5% dextrose + oral water to balance urine + insensible loss until plasma Na^+ and urea normal

---

HYPONATRAEMIA

Hyponatraemia results when the water content of the body is increased absolutely and relative to the Na^+ content, so that the osmolality of body fluids falls.

Healthy adults can drink up to 20 l/day and the kidneys will respond with a vigorous water diuresis. However, elderly patients for example, with restricted renal function, cannot respond in this way and may become hyponatraemic with much smaller volumes. Most patients regulate their intake of water through the thirst mechanism, but some mentally disturbed patients may voluntarily drink excessive fluids and as a consequence develop hyponatraemia. Patients cannot regulate their fluid intake when a proportion is given intravenously or in a tube feed.

Table 10.2 Causes of pure or predominant water depletion

Reduced intake	Water unavailable Infants, aged, apathy, depression Coma Inability to swallow, nausea Primary hypodipsia
Increased loss from skin	Fever, hyperthyroidism Hot environment
Increased loss from respiratory tract	Hyperventilation, fever High altitudes
Increased loss in urine due to marked impairment of urinary concentrating mechanism	*ADH deficiency* Diabetes insipidus *Renal tubular unresponsiveness to ADH* (nephrogenic diabetes insipidus) Hypercalcaemia, K^+ depletion Chronic interstitial nephritis Amyloidosis, obstructive uropathy Medullary cystic disease *Solute diuresis* Diabetes mellitus Enteral or parenteral feeds with high solute concentration Infant feeds wrongly made up

Table 10.3   Causes of hyponatraemia

Pathogenesis		Clinical condition	Extracellular fluid volume
Increased total body water	1. Impaired water excretion	SIADH Adrenocortical failure Hypothyroidism Hypopituitarism Psychogenic polydipsia	Slightly increased; no oedema
	2. Excess water intake		
Relative increase in extracellular water	Shift of water from cells	Uncontrolled diabetes mellitus Mannitol	Normal or slightly reduced
Reduction in total body sodium exceeds reduction in total body water	1. Severe untreated Na$^+$ and water depletion 2. Na$^+$ and water depletion treated by water replacement (e.g. 5% dextrose)	Any cause of mixed Na$^+$ and water depletion (Table 10.4)	Reduced
Increase in total body water exceeds increase in total body sodium	Retention of Na$^+$ associated with impaired water excretion	Cardiac failure Liver failure Nephrotic syndrome Cirrhosis Renal failure Diuretics	Increased—often oedema

A number of disease processes and drugs interfere with normal water excretion. Hyponatraemia can also be caused where water is transferred out from cells because of a sudden rise in plasma osmolality. This may occur in uncontrolled diabetes mellitus with hyperglycaemia or following the administration of an osmotic diuretic, e.g. mannitol. The causes of hyponatraemia are shown in Table 10.3.

The most common pathogenesis of hyponatraemia is **mixed salt and water depletion**, where the loss of salt from the body exceeds the reduction in total body water, often because patients continue to drink and to absorb water in the early stages of these illnesses. Major causes are given in Table 10.4. These are generally associated with a clinical history and clinical evidence of volume depletion. Hyponatraemia in these patients is maintained by excessive AVP secretion which has been stimulated by volume depletion. The stimulus to AVP secretion, which occurs when the plasma volume is reduced by about 5%, overrides osmoreceptor mediated signals to switch off AVP production as plasma osmolality falls. The urine thus shows paradoxical concentration in the face of dilute body fluids.

The last group of conditions associated with hyponatraemia are those in which the increase in total body water exceeds a simultaneous increase in body sodium. In these conditions the retention of sodium is associated with a simultaneous inability to excrete water. This is often mediated at the kidney level by both excessive sodium retention at proximal sites and excessive inappropriate AVP secretion. Causes of the syndrome of inappropriate ADH secretion are shown in Table 10.5.

Diagnosis

Because of the large number of diagnostic possibilities in hyponatraemia, determining the cause may be difficult. Clinical assessment of plasma volume is crucial in assessing the contribution of sodium depletion or excess to the overall picture. The history, including recent drug ingestion, review of fluid balance charts and weight, followed by careful clinical examination paying attention to the conditions listed in Table 10.3, will generally identify a cause. Measurement of plasma and urinary sodium and osmolality will help to confirm sodium retention, and any effect of excessive AVP secretion, which is characterised by a high urine osmolality in face of a low plasma osmolality (inappropriate concentration of the urine).

Management will often need to be started before the results of all investigations are available. In some cases it will be necessary to await the results of endocrine investigations before coming to a definite diagnosis, but these will be uncommon.

Management

All patients are best managed by restriction of water intake, which may need to be as little as 0.5 l/day in severe cases, together with treatment of the underlying cause. In patients with severe neurological symptoms the plasma sodium should be raised more rapidly by giving 100 ml of a 3% NaCl solution intravenously over 1 hour. This can be repeated every 2–3 hours until the plasma sodium is > 120 mmol/l or the patient has shown

Table 10.4 Causes of mixed sodium and water depletion

Loss from alimentary tract	***External loss*** Vomiting Aspiration of GI contents Fistulae Diarrhoea Villous adenoma of large bowel ***Sequestration of fluid in bowel*** Ileus Intestinal obstruction

Loss in urine	***Extrarenal factors acting on kidney***
	Osmotic diuresis
	   Diabetes mellitus
	   Mannitol
	Diuretics
	Metabolic acidosis
	Adrenocortical insufficiency
	Renal disease
	Diuretic phase acute tubular necrosis
	Post obstructive diuresis
	Chronic renal insufficiency
	Proximal renal tubular acidosis
	Medullary cystic disease
	Congenital polycystic disease
	Chronic interstitial nephritis

Loss in sweat	Fever, hot environment
Loss in exudates and transudates, 'third' space losses	***Loss from body surfaces*** Burns Extensive dermatitis ***Loss into body cavities or soft tissues*** Ascites Peritonitis Acute pancreatitis Rhabdomyolysis Inferior vena cava thrombosis

Table 10.5 Conditions associated with the syndrome of inappropriate secretion of ADH (SIADH)

Neoplasm	Carcinoma of bronchus (small cell), pancreas, duodenum, ureter, bladder, prostate, lymphoma, thymoma, mesothelioma
Disorders of CNS	Meningitis, encephalitis, brain abscess, head injury, cerebral tumour, cerebral vascular accident, hydrocephalus, cerebral or cerebellar atrophy, delirium tremens, psychosis, Guillain–Barré syndrome
Non-malignant pulmonary lesions	Tuberculosis, pneumonia (bacterial, viral)
Drugs	Narcotics, phenothiazines, carbamazepine, tricyclic antidepressants, monoamine oxidase inhibitors, clofibrate, vincristine, vinblastine, cyclophosphamide*, chlorpropamide, non-steroidal anti-inflammatory drugs*
Miscellaneous	Pain, postoperative period, nausea

* Potentiate effect of ADH on collecting duct.

satisfactory clinical improvement. A loop diuretic may be required in these patients to prevent volume overload. Frequent monitoring of the plasma sodium and overall fluid balance is essential.

Transfer of water from cells

Patients with uncontrolled diabetes mellitus and hyponatraemia are treated with isotonic fluids and insulin. Where mannitol is the underlying cause, no active treatment should be necessary as it is excreted over 6–8 hours.

Mixed salt and water depletion

These patients require restoration of plasma volume, which can be achieved with NaCl 0.9% solution supplemented by plasma expanders (e.g. plasma protein solutions, colloidal starch, etc.) or sodium bicarbonate 1.26% solution when severe acidosis is also present. The JVP and blood pressure should be monitored. Acutely ill patients or those with heart disease will require a central venous pressure (CVP) line and monitoring. Intake of water should be restricted, and dextrose 5% solution should not be administered until the plasma sodium is within the normal range.

Retention of salt and water

These patients require sodium restriction (50–80 mmol/day) as well as water restriction and careful use of a loop diuretic. Where the hyponatraemia is caused by a drug then withdrawal of the drug and water restriction is usually sufficient. Hyponatraemia caused by diuretics may require volume expansion with NaCl 0.9% solution.

HYPERKALAEMIA

Principal causes of hyperkalaemia are given in Table 10.6. The aetiology in many patients is multifactorial. For example, in diabetic ketoacidosis, hyperkalaemia is relatively common because of metabolic acidosis (shift of potassium out of cells) and hypovolaemia (impaired K^+ excretion), despite an overall K^+ deficit accumulated during the period of osmotic diuresis. During treatment with insulin hyperkalaemia rapidly resolves and may be followed by a significant hypokalaemia.

Pseudo-hyperkalaemia is caused by the release of K^+ in vitro from abnormal or damaged cells, such as the abnormal white blood cells in acute leukaemia. It is also common in poorly handled blood specimens which have been left for too long at room temperature before separation and analysis.

Diagnosis

Hyperkalaemia must be suspected in the circumstances outlined in the information box and confirmed by urgent analysis. Hyperkalaemia is dangerous because cardiac arrest can occur when the plasma K^+ exceeds 7 mmol/l, and this may be the earliest and only manifestation. The blood results must be acted on immediately.

Table 10.6   Causes of hyperkalaemia

Increased intake	i.v. fluid containing K⁺, high K⁺ foods Drugs containing K⁺
Tissue breakdown	Bleeding into soft tissues, GI tract or body cavities Haemolysis, rhabdomyolysis Catabolic states
Shift of K⁺ out of cells	Tissue damage (e.g. following ischaemia, shock) Acidosis Insulin deficiency Aldosterone deficiency β-adrenoceptor antagonists ECF hypertonicity
Impaired excretion	**Renal disease** Acute renal failure Severe chronic renal failure (GFR <15 ml/min) Impaired tubular secretion K⁺ (SLE, transplanted kidney, amyloidosis, sickle cell disease) **Acute circulatory failure** **Drugs which inhibit renal K⁺ secretion** Aldosterone antagonists, triamterene, amiloride **Abnormalities of renin-angiotensin-aldosterone axis** Addison's disease, adrenal enzyme deficiencies Primary hypoaldosteronism, hyporeninaemic hypoaldosteronism, β-adrenoceptor antagonists, NSAIDs, ACE inhibitors
Pseudohyperkalaemia	Release of K⁺ in vitro from abnormal blood cells or incorrectly handled specimens

MANAGEMENT OF ACUTE HYPERKALAEMIA

- Identify and treat cause
- Inject 10 ml 10% calcium gluconate over 1 min (reduces risk of cardiac arrest)
- Inject 50 ml 50% glucose. Monitor plasma glucose; give insulin if hyperglycaemia occurs. Monitor plasma K⁺ after 20–30 mins and repeat if necessary
- Start infusion of 10–20% dextrose 500 ml 4–6 hourly (to minimise rebound ↑K⁺)
- Calcium resonium (exchange resin, binds K⁺ in exchange for calcium) may be given, 15–30 g orally
- If metabolic acidosis present—infuse sodium bicarbonate 1.26% 500 ml 6–8 hourly until plasma [HCO₃⁻] in normal range. NB: Watch for circulatory overload
- Correct volume depletion, respiratory acidosis if present
- Use haemodialysis/haemofiltration or peritoneal dialysis if the above fail

SUSPECT HYPERKALAEMIA

- Release of K⁺ from dead/injured cells, e.g. tissue damage, rhabdomyolysis, haemolysis, GI bleeding
- Rapid administration of K⁺ by mouth or intravenously
- Impaired renal excretion of K⁺, including severe renal failure, use of K⁺-sparing diuretics (spironolactone, amiloride, triamterene)
- Acidosis

Management

Hyperkalaemia should be prevented in conditions associated with oliguria (p. 615). The established case can be dealt with by the measures shown in the information box.

Recurrence of hyperkalaemia can then be prevented by dietary restriction of foods rich in K⁺ and further use of calcium resonium 15–30 g 2–3 times daily.

HYPOKALAEMIA

Most of body potassium is in cells at a concentration of about 140 mmol/l. The ECF contains less than 2% of all the potassium in the body, maintained within a narrow concentration range. The active transport mechanisms which maintain a high intracellular potassium are stimulated by insulin, beta-adrenoceptor agonists, aldosterone and alkalosis. Dietary intake of K⁺ is 60–80 mmol/day; over 85% is excreted in the urine and the remainder in stools. The maintenance of K⁺ balance depends on regulation of urinary K⁺ excretion. Potassium excretion is increased when cell K⁺ rises (in alkalosis), when urine flow is high and when there is active reabsorption of sodium mediated by increased aldosterone. When potassium intake is very low, urinary excretion falls gradually to about 5 mmol/day, but this small continuing loss, together with the daily stool loss of 8–10 mmol, results in moderate K⁺ depletion.

The causes of potassium depletion are given in Table 10.7. Most of the gastrointestinal disorders listed are associated with loss of Na⁺ and water as well as K⁺, and result in volume depletion. The increase in circulating aldosterone leads to additional loss of K⁺ in urine. A number of drugs, including most diuretics, promote potassium loss.

Diagnosis

Plasma K⁺ is low in most cases of K⁺ depletion. However, in the presence of severe ECF depletion, metabolic acidosis or deficiency of insulin or aldosterone, clinically significant K⁺ depletion may develop without a change in plasma K⁺, for example, in untreated diabetic ketoacidosis. Conversely, patients suffering from metabolic alkalosis, or who have been taking excessive insulin or beta-adrenergic agonists, may have a low plasma K⁺ despite a normal total body K⁺ because of movement of K⁺ into cells. The diagnosis depends on careful assessment of the clinical history, including drugs, and examination for gastrointestinal or renal

Table 10.7 Causes of potassium depletion

Reduced intake	Diet containing adequate calories and insufficient potassium Potassium-free intravenous fluid

Loss from alimentary tract	*External loss*
	Vomiting
	Aspiration of GI contents
	Fistulae
	Diarrhoea[1]
	  Acute
	  Chronic (laxative addicts,
	    malabsorption syndrome)
	Villous adenoma large bowel
	Ureterosigmoidostomy
	Sequestration of fluid in bowel
	Ileus
	Intestinal obstruction

Loss in urine	*Extrarenal factors acting on kidney* Primary aldosteronism[2] Bartter's syndrome Secondary aldosteronism (e.g. renovascular disease, accelerated hypertension[2], cirrhosis, cardiac failure, nephrotic syndrome) Cushing's syndrome[2] Diabetic ketoacidosis Metabolic alkalosis Chronic metabolic acidosis Drugs, e.g. diuretics, amphotericin B, corticosteroids[2], liquorice[2], carbenoxolone[2] *Renal disease* Recovery phase acute tubular necrosis Following relief urinary tract obstruction Renal tubular acidosis

[1] Considerable amounts of potassium may be lost in diarrhoea.
[2] Associated with hypertension.

disease. The urinary K^+ may be helpful, as a value of <20 mmol/day excludes renal K^+ loss, while a urinary K^+ of >30 mmol/day is strongly suggestive of a renal cause.

Management

Potassium depletion can be treated by giving a K^+ salt orally or intravenously. The former route is preferable as it is less potentially hazardous. Oral KCl (1 g = 13.4 mmol K^+) is satisfactory unless a metabolic acidosis is present. These preparations may cause gastrointestinal irritation; oesophageal and small bowel erosions and strictures are uncommon complications. A diet rich in K^+, i.e. containing fruit and fruit juices, coffee, milk and animal protein, is helpful.

In ill patients and those with marked clinical features, intravenous KCl is needed. Associated salt and water deficiency should be treated first and intravenous administration of potassium avoided until urine output is established. 80–100 mmol K^+/day is usually sufficient. No more than 20 mmol of K^+ should be given in any 3-hour period.

Prevention is better than cure, and strategies for prevention are shown in the information box.

PREVENTION OF POTASSIUM DEPLETION

- **Diuretics**: additional KCl 20–60 mmol/day. Plasma K^+ should be monitored. (NB: Not with potassium-sparing diuretics or patients on ACE inhibitors)
- **Corticosteroids**: some patients on high doses need potassium supplements
- **IV fluids**: most patients will need $\sim$ 60 mmol/day K^+ distributed over 24 h. The plasma K^+ should be monitored daily

---

SODIUM AND WATER EXCESS

In health the total body Na^+ is kept within narrow limits despite considerable day-to-day variation in intake.

Aetiology

Accumulation of Na^+ occurs when renal excretion fails to keep pace with the amount ingested. Since Na^+ retention is accompanied by retention of an approximately iso-osmotic amount of water, the volume of the ECF is increased but ECF Na^+ concentration is not materially altered. Generalised oedema due to accumulation of fluid in the interstitial spaces is the clinical consequence of expansion of the ECF, and becomes evident when the ECF volume is increased by about 15%.

Accumulation of generalised oedema requires:

1. a change in the forces acting upon the microcirculation which determine distribution of water and electrolytes between intravascular and interstitial fluid;
2. renal retention of Na^+ and water in the face of increased body Na^+ and expansion of the ECF.

The sequence of events depends on the underlying disease and its stage of development (Fig. 10.8). The simplest pattern is seen in patients with minimal lesion nephropathy (p. 644) in which heavy proteinuria coexists with a normal or raised GFR. Loss of water and electrolytes from plasma into the interstitial space results in underfilling of the vascular bed and stimulation of intravascular receptors. This leads to appropriate activation of mechanisms designed to maintain plasma volume, all of which increase renal Na^+ reabsorption. As a consequence of the disturbance of the physical forces acting across the capillary walls, the retained Na^+ and water accumulates primarily in the interstitium.

In patients with acute nephritis, or nephrotic patients in whom GFR is low, the plasma volume appears to be normal or increased; the stimulus to increased Na^+

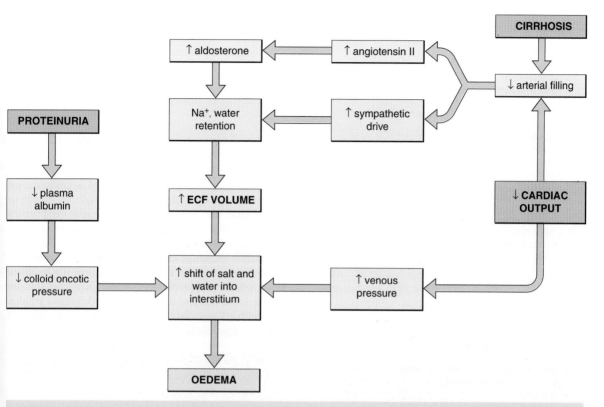

Fig. 10.8 The main forces acting to increase renal sodium and water reabsorption are shown for proteinuria, heart failure and cirrhosis.

reabsorption, as yet unknown, appears to be a property of the kidney itself.

Sodium retention in congestive cardiac failure is probably initiated by stimulation of intra-arterial receptors by the reduced arterial blood flow, resulting from a fall in cardiac output. An increase in both pulmonary and systemic venous pressure leads to sequestration of retained Na^+ and water in the interstitial spaces of both circuits; this further reduces effective arterial flow. The problem is compounded by loss of the normal natriuretic response to atrial dilatation. Atrial natriuretic peptide concentrations in plasma are raised, but the kidney apparently fails to respond.

In hepatic cirrhosis, gross distortion of intrahepatic architecture gives rise to obstruction to hepatic venous outflow, to portal hypertension and to the development of portasystemic shunts (p. 521). Receptors within the hepatic circulation are thought to respond to increased hepatic venous pressure, and to initiate Na^+ retention via sympathetic hepato-renal reflexes. There may also be relative underfilling of the vascular system, due to dilatation of the systemic circulation and to sequestration of fluid in the peritoneal cavity; this may further

stimulate renal sodium retention through neuro-endocrine mechanisms, such as renin-angiotensin-aldosterone activation.

Knowledge of this subject is incomplete and changing rapidly, but clearly in all these disorders, stimuli arising from an underperfused section of the vascular tree are important in initiating and maintaining renal Na^+ retention despite increased total body Na^+. Conditions associated with generalised oedema are shown in the information box.

Clinical features

These depend to some extent on the distribution of retained fluid and are described under the various diseases.

Management

The principles of management are simple and are shown in the information box.

Diuretic therapy

Drugs which block Na^+ reabsorption also increase urinary volume, because reabsorption of water in the nephron is passive and depends on Na^+ reabsorption.

CONDITIONS ASSOCIATED WITH GENERALISED OEDEMA

- Cardiac failure
- Nephrotic syndrome
- Acute nephritic syndrome
- Acute oliguric renal failure; advanced chronic renal failure (GFR <15 ml/min)
- Hepatic cirrhosis, acute liver failure, hepatic vein thrombosis
- Protein-losing enteropathy
- Starvation
- Thiamine deficiency
- Premenstrual fluid retention
- Pregnancy
- Acute anaphylaxis
- Drugs which cause sodium retention—
  antihypertensives (calcium channel blockers, vasodilators)
  corticosteroids
  NSAIDs
  oestrogens
  liquorice, carbenoxolone

MANAGEMENT OF OEDEMA

- Restrict dietary sodium to 100 mmol/day ('no added salt') or 50 mmol in severe cases
- Diuretics
- Specific treatment directed at the cause, e.g. ACE inhibitor in heart failure, corticosteroids in minimal change nephropathy

---

Table 10.8 provides information about commonly used diuretics. The choice of drugs depends upon the severity of the oedema and whether or not the patient is resistant to the effects of diuretics. Mild cases, e.g. ankle oedema in an elderly person with cardiac failure, usually respond to a combination of moderate salt restriction and benzothiadiazine diuretic. Hydrochlorothiazide 50–100 mg/day or bendrofluazide 5–10 mg/day may be given or, if a slower and more prolonged diuresis is desired, chlorthalidone 50 mg/day can be used. More severe cases should receive a high potency diuretic—oral frusemide 40–120 mg/day or bumetanide 1–3 mg/day, with a diet containing about 100 mmol/day Na^+. Intravenous frusemide, 20–40 mg, is valuable in treating acute pulmonary oedema. Intravenous ethacrynic acid should be avoided because of ototoxicity. Causes of resistance to the effects of diuretics are given in the information box.

Patients with chronic renal failure often respond to large doses of oral frusemide (250 mg–1 g) or bumetanide (5 mg). If this fails a combination of one of these diuretics with metolazone (5–10 mg) or bendrofluazide

---

CAUSES OF DIURETIC RESISTANCE

- Reduced renal function
- Volume depletion and secondary hyperaldosteronism
- Profound hypoproteinaemia

(10 mg) may succeed, since these drugs act synergistically. In patients with resistant oedema due to cirrhosis or severe cardiac failure whose renal function is not compromised, a combination of spironolactone (100–200 mg) or amiloride (20 mg) with frusemide or bumetanide may induce diuresis. These lower potency drugs are poor diuretics alone, but are of value when combined with a loop diuretic, as they inhibit Na^+ reabsorption in exchange for K^+ or H^+ in the distal nephron. Since they reduce K^+ excretion they must not be given along with K^+ supplements, nor used when renal function is impaired, lest dangerous hyperkalaemia results. When severe hypoproteinaemia is present, addition of salt-poor albumin to the regime usually induces diuresis.

Adverse effects of diuretic therapy on water and electrolyte balance

(1) Potassium depletion

High and medium potency diuretics, which deliver an increased amount of Na^+ to the distal nephron, induce K^+ depletion (p. 591), especially when given repeatedly over long periods and when combined with a low Na^+ diet. Symptoms of K^+ deficiency may arise before satisfactory loss of oedema has been achieved and are then superimposed upon clinical features of Na^+ and water accumulation. This is liable to occur during the treatment of severe heart failure (p. 218) and may be responsible for development of digitalis toxicity before the heart failure has been controlled. In hepatic disease with ascites and oedema, K^+ depletion may aggravate or precipitate hepatic encephalopathy.

Prophylactic administration of K^+ is essential when diuretics are given frequently. Potassium chloride 3–4 g/day in divided doses is given, usually as slow release or effervescent tablets.

(2) Metabolic alkalosis (see p. 605)

(3) Sodium depletion and reduced blood volume

Overtreatment with diuretics results in Na^+ and water depletion. This may occur when high potency drugs are given over prolonged periods without adequate supervision. The clinical features of Na^+ and water depletion are described on page 594.

Patients with severe oedema resistant to therapy

Table: 10.8 Commonly used diuretic drugs

Class	Drugs	Principal sites of action in nephron	Extrarenal actions	Principal side-effects of the group	Individual side-effects
HIGH POTENCY DIURETICS	Frusemide	1 Inhibition reabsorption NaCl thick ascending limb loop of Henle 2 Minor inhibition reabsorption NaCl proximal tubule 3 Increase renal blood flow	Increase venous capacitance	Postural hypotension, K^+ depletion, Mg^{++} depletion, alkalosis, hyperuricaemia, hyperglycaemia, hypersensitivity (rash, myelosuppression, hepatic dysfunction, interstitial nephritis)	Ototoxic
	Bumetanide	As above			Myalgia
	Ethacrynic acid	As above			Ototoxic
MEDIUM POTENCY DIURETICS	Benzothiadiazines (thiazides)	1 Inhibition reabsorption NaCl early distal tubule (diluting site) 2 Inhibition reabsorption NaCl proximal tubule 3 Some inhibit reabsorption $NaHCO_3$ in proximal and distal tubules (minor)	Antihypertensive	K^+ depletion, alkalosis, hyponatraemia, hyperuricaemia, hyperglycaemia, hyperlipidaemia, hypersensitivity (rash, myelosuppression, acute pancreatitis, hepatic dysfunction, interstitial nephritis)	
	Metolazone	As above 1 and 2			
LOW POTENCY DIURETICS	Acetazolamide	Inhibits reabsorption $NaHCO_3$ in proximal and distal tubule	Decreased rate of formation aqueous humour		K^+ depletion, acidosis, drowsiness, hypersensitivity (rash, myelosuppression, interstitial nephritis), renal stones
K^+-SPARING LOW POTENCY DIURETICS	Spironolactone	Aldosterone antagonist inhibits aldosterone sensitive Na^+/K^+ exchange in collecting tubule	Gynaecomastia		Hyperkalaemia, acidosis
	Triamterene	Inhibits reabsorption Na^+ in collecting tubule, thus indirectly inhibits K^+ secretion at that site			Hyperkalaemia, acidosis, formation renal stones containing triamterene, acute renal failure when given with indomethacin
	Amiloride	As triamterene			Hyperkalaemia, acidosis

sometimes develop clinical features of reduced blood volume while still oedematous. In these cases hypotension, tachycardia and a raised blood urea are often associated with a low plasma $[Na^+]$. Such patients usually suffer from advanced cardiac, hepatic or renal disease associated with hypoproteinaemia. Persistent attempts to reduce the oedema usually lead to further deterioration. Diuretics should be withheld temporarily and a more liberal salt intake permitted. Cautious infusion of 25–100 g plasma protein solution or 20–40 g salt-poor albumin over a period of 3 or 4 hours to increase the blood volume may help. Signs of circulatory overload are an indication to stop the infusion.

(4) Hyponatraemia

Patients with severe oedema may develop hyponatraemia because they are unable to excrete water normally (Table 10.3). This is exacerbated by the use of thiazides or metolazone which interfere with urinary dilution. The clinical features associated with hyponatraemia and its management are discussed on pages 594–5.

CALCIUM, PHOSPHATE AND MAGNESIUM

Calcium metabolism in health and disease is discussed in Chapter 9 (p. 559).

HYPOPHOSPHATAEMIA

Most body phosphate (80%) is in the bony skeleton, and around 20% in cells, predominantly muscle. Phosphate molecules are critical to many biochemical processes, including cell energetics (ATP), intracellular signalling (cAMP), and nucleic acid synthesis. A body deficit of phosphate therefore has widespread effects. In the presence of a plasma phosphate less than 0.4 mmol/l (normal range 0.8–1.4 mmol/l), widespread cell dysfunction and death occurs. Rapid changes in plasma phosphate usually reflect redistribution from plasma to cells. In this respect, phosphate behaves similarly to potassium, and enters cells in association with insulin-stimulated carbohydrate metabolism. In clinical situations where carbohydrate is administered acutely, with a background of impaired nutrition and a total body phosphate deficit, severe hypophosphataemia may ensue, with the consequences shown in the information box below. This is referred to as the nutritional recovery syndrome. Alkalosis also stimulates a shift into cells. Causes of hypophosphataemia are shown in Table 10.9.

CONSEQUENCES OF HYPOPHOSPHATAEMIA AND PHOSPHATE DEPLETION

- Muscle pain and weakness, increased plasma creatine kinase
- Respiratory muscle weakness
- Cardiac arrhythmias
- Neuroencephalopathy—confusion, convulsions, coma
- Haemolysis
- Hypercalciuria, hypermagnesuria

Table 10.9 Causes of reduced plasma phosphate concentration

Hyperparathyroidism (by increased urinary excretion)
Primary
Secondary, e.g. Vitamin D deficiency/osteomalacia
　　　　　　　Malabsorption
　　　　　　　Familial hypophosphataemic rickets

Increased carbohydrate metabolism and insulin action (by shift into cells)
Intravenous glucose infusions
Insulin infusion
Treatment of diabetic ketoacidosis
Parenteral nutrition
Nutritional recovery syndrome

Alkalosis (by shift into cells)
Metabolic, e.g. bicarbonate infusion
Respiratory, e.g. artificial hyperventilation

Reduced oral absorption of phosphate
Oral phosphate binding agents, e.g. aluminium hydroxide
Starvation (only minor reduction because of ↓ carbohydrate metabolism)
Chronic alcoholism, alcohol withdrawal

Phosphate removal
Haemodialysis
Peritoneal dialysis

Extracellular fluid volume expansion

NB: HYPOPHOSPHATAEMIA IS OFTEN MULTIFACTORIAL IN ORIGIN.

Management

In many cases, and particularly if there is no prior body phosphate depletion, hypophosphataemia is transient and of no clinical significance. The duration and severity should be taken into account when deciding on treatment. Sustained values of < 0.4 mmol/l require therapy. Oral treatment is preferred. Milk is a good source (up to 2 l/day), or oral supplements such as Phosphate-Sandoz (16 mmol phosphate, 20 mmol sodium, 3 mmol potassium per tablet), one 3 to 6 times daily. Intravenous therapy should be given with care, and in general should not exceed 18 mmol/24 h of a mixed phosphate solution. Plasma concentrations of calcium, phosphate, potassium and magnesium must be closely monitored during treatment.

HYPERPHOSPHATAEMIA

This is most commonly seen in acute or chronic renal failure, or in states of massive cell necrosis, such as acute rhabdomyolysis, acute haemolysis, or in neoplastic disease treated by chemotherapy (tumour lysis syndrome). Sustained hyperphosphataemia is associated with a risk of metastatic calcification, secondary stimulation of the parathyroid glands, and symptoms such as pruritus. Treatment with oral phosphate binders and/or dialysis may be required (see Ch. 11, Diseases of the Kidney).

MAGNESIUM DEFICIENCY AND EXCESS

Disorders of magnesium metabolism are occasionally responsible for otherwise puzzling clinical features.

Aetiology of magnesium depletion

The important causes of magnesium depletion are shown in Table 10.10.

Clinical features of magnesium depletion

These are predominantly neuromuscular, with tremor and choreiform movements. Depression, confusion, agitation, epileptic fits and hallucinations also occur. The diagnosis can be confirmed by finding a plasma magnesium concentration of less than 0.7 mmol/l. Since most magnesium is intracellular, a body deficit may still rarely be present with a normal plasma concentration.

Bartter's syndrome is an uncommon renal tubular disorder characterised by severe hypokalaemia and, usually, hypomagnesaemia. In contrast to primary hyperaldosteronism, blood pressure is normal. Nonsteroidal anti-inflammatory drugs may reduce, but seldom abolish, the need for regular oral potassium chloride supplements and intermittent intravenous magnesium supplementation.

Table 10.10   Causes of magnesium depletion

Reduced intake	Protein-energy malnutrition (PEM)
	Prolonged administration of Mg^{++}-free intravenous fluids
Loss from GI tract	Vomiting
	Chronic diarrhoea (malabsorption, laxative abuse)
	Fistulae; aspiration of GI contents
Losses in urine	***Extrarenal factors acting on the kidney***
	Drugs, e.g. loop diuretics, gentamicin, cis-platinum
	Ketoacidosis
	Chronic alcoholism
	Hyperparathyroidism
	Primary or secondary aldosteronism
	Renal disease
	Bartter's syndrome
	Post-obstructive diuresis
	Diuretic phase of acute tubular necrosis
	Renal tubular acidosis
Miscellaneous	Acute pancreatitis
	Excessive lactation

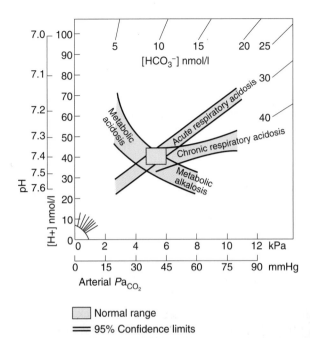

☐ Normal range

═══ 95% Confidence limits

Fig. 10.9   Diagram showing changes in blood [H$^+$], $PaCO_2$ and plasma [HCO$_3^-$] in stable compensated acid-base disorders. The rectangle indicates limits of normal reference ranges for [H$^+$] and $PaCO_2$. The bands represent 95% confidence limits of single disturbances in human blood in vivo. When the point obtained by plotting [H$^+$] against $PaCO_2$ does not fall within one of the labelled bands, compensation is incomplete or a mixed disorder is present (Flenley D 1971 Lancet 1: 1921).

Management

Magnesium is very poorly absorbed orally, and oral supplements are of little value. The condition is best treated by giving 30–50 mmol magnesium chloride intravenously in a litre of isotonic saline or 5% dextrose over 12–24 hours. Thereafter 15–20 mmol magnesium should be infused daily until plasma Mg^{++} is normal. When renal function is impaired the amount of magnesium should be halved.

Magnesium excess

This mainly occurs in acute or chronic renal failure, and may contribute to the central nervous system disturbance associated with severe uraemia. Treatment is that of the underlying condition.

relationship between [H$^+$] and $PaCO_2$ in stable acid-base disorders is well-defined; diagrams such as Figure 10.9 are sometimes helpful in defining the nature and extent of the disturbance.

The **anion gap** represents those negative ions not

ACID-BASE DISORDERS

There are four main types of disturbance of hydrogen ion concentration since **acidosis** and **alkalosis** may be either **respiratory** or **metabolic** in origin. These may be **pure** or **mixed** disorders, and their effects are eventually modified by compensatory changes (p. 588). Changes in arterial blood [H$^+$], $PaCO_2$ and plasma [HCO$_3^-$] in acid-base disturbances are shown in Table 10.11.

METABOLIC ACIDOSIS

Metabolic acidosis is characterised by a reduction in plasma bicarbonate and a consequent rise in [H$^+$]. The $PaCO_2$ is reduced secondarily by hyperventilation, which mitigates the rise in [H$^+$] (Table 10.11). The

Table 10.11   Changes in arterial blood [H$^+$], $PaCO_2$ and plasma [HCO$_3^-$] in acid-base disturbances

Disorder	[H$^+$]	$PaCO_2$	[HCO$_3^-$]
Metabolic acidosis			
Acute	↑	→	↓
Compensated (by ↑ ventilation)	↗ or →	↓	↓
Metabolic alkalosis			
Acute	↓	→	↑
Compensated (by ↓ ventilation)	↘ or →	↑	↑
Respiratory acidosis			
Acute (duration—hours)	↑	↑	→
Compensated (duration—days) (by renal retention of HCO$_3^-$)	↗ or →	↑	↑
Respiratory alkalosis			
Acute	↓	↓	→
Compensated (by ↑ renal excretion of HCO$_3^-$)	↘ or →	↓	↓

DISTURBANCES WHICH GIVE RISE TO METABOLIC ACIDOSIS

- Overproduction of acids other than H_2CO_3
- Ingestion of acids or potential acids
- Failure to excrete acids other than H_2CO_3 at a rate equal to their generation
- Loss of the base bicarbonate in urine or from the GI tract

CAUSES OF LACTIC ACIDOSIS

Group A
- Shock from any cause (septic shock most common)
- Respiratory failure
- Poisoning with cyanide or carbon monoxide
- Severe anaemia

Group B
- Diabetes mellitus
- Hepatic failure
- Severe infection
- Drugs (biguanides such as metformin, salicylates, isoniazid, sorbitol)
- Toxins (ethanol, methanol)
- Congenital enzyme defects

normally measured in clinical practice. These include phosphate and sulphate, lactate, ketoacids and albumin. A convenient formula is:

$$\text{Anion Gap} = \text{plasma } Na^+ - (Cl^- + HCO_3^-)$$

Values in health range from 8 to 14 mmol/l. In some types of metabolic acidosis, reduced bicarbonate in plasma is accompanied by an increase in plasma chloride, leading to a normal anion gap. Where excessive acid is added to the plasma, either by disordered metabolism or by addition of exogenous acid, or there is failure of acid excretion, the anion gap is increased. This should prompt attempts to identify the abnormal anion(s) and correct the underlying problem (Table 10.12). A low anion gap is occasionally seen in multiple myeloma, in lithium poisoning and in severe hypercalcaemia or hypermagnesaemia.

Aetiology

The physiological disturbances which give rise to metabolic acidosis are shown in the information box, and conditions in which these develop are listed in Table 10.12. In most situations, metabolic acidosis is accompanied by sodium and water depletion, and the aetiology of this is also indicated in Table 10.12.

Lactic acidosis occurs when the rate of production of lactic acid from pyruvate in muscle, skin, brain and erythrocytes exceeds the rate of removal by liver and kidney. As indicated by the equation,

$$[\text{lactate}] = K[\text{NADH}]/[\text{NAD}] \times [\text{pyruvate}] \times [H^+]$$

lactate production increases when oxidative metabolism is reduced, glycolysis increased, and [pyruvate] and [NADH] rise. Causes of lactic acidosis are shown below. Those in Group A are associated with hypotension and/or severe tissue hypoxia. Disorders in Group B are not, but are associated with impaired mitochondrial respiration and increased lactate production.

Diabetic ketoacidosis is discussed on page 748. In chronic renal failure, the most important factor limiting H^+ excretion is reduced production of NH_4^+ by the diminished mass of tubules. Failure either to conserve

or to regenerate bicarbonate characterises proximal and distal renal tubular acidosis respectively (pp. 661–662).

Clinical features

The most obvious clinical consequence is stimulation of respiration by the raised $[H^+]$. In severe cases, respirations become deep and sighing (Kussmaul's respiration). When the $[H^+]$ exceeds 70 nmol/l, myocardial function is compromised, cardiac output falls, and this, in conjunction with peripheral vasodilatation, results in a fall in blood pressure. Such patients are frequently confused or drowsy.

In many cases the clinical picture is determined by the underlying disorder and the presence of concomitant Na^+ and water depletion.

Management

The cause of acidosis should be identified and treated whenever possible. Treatment of ketoacidosis and lactic acidosis results in metabolism of the accumulated acids to CO_2 and water, a process which regenerates bicarbonate. Any associated sodium and water depletion should be corrected using intravenous isotonic sodium chloride solution. This neutral solution might be expected to have relatively little influence on the acidity of body fluids. However, provided kidney function is normal, it will usually correct a metabolic acidosis of moderate severity. Adequately perfused kidneys will generate HCO_3^- and retain this along with the infused sodium, rejecting the chloride in the urine.

In the presence of renal disease, or of markedly reduced renal function due to the sodium and water depletion, renal generation of bicarbonate is impaired. Approximately 30% of the total requirement for sodium and water should then be given as isotonic (1.26%) sodium bicarbonate. Blood $[H^+]$ and $[HCO_3^-]$ should be monitored, and infusion of sodium bicarbonate stopped when $[H^+]$ is normal.

Table 10.12 Causes of metabolic acidosis

Mechanism	Clinical disorders	Accumulating acid	Anion gap[1]	Cause of associated Na⁺ depletion
ADDITION OF EXCESSIVE ACID TO PLASMA				
1 Disorders of intermediary metabolism	Ketoacidosis	Acetoacetic β hydroxybutyric	Increased	Loss in urine with anion of abnormal acid
	Lactic acidosis	Lactic	Increased	Loss in urine with anion of abnormal acid
2 Addition of exogenous substances	Methanol poisoning	Formic	Increased	Loss in urine with anion of abnormal acid
	Ethylene glycol poisoning	Glycolic, oxalic	Increased	Loss in urine with anion of abnormal acid
	Salicylate poisoning[2]	Various organic	Increased	Loss in urine with anion of abnormal acid
FAILURE TO EXCRETE ACID AT A NORMAL RATE				
1 Inadequate renal NH₄⁺ production	Chronic renal failure	Sulphuric, phosphoric etc. produced by metabolism	Increased	Impaired renal Na⁺ conservation
2 Inability to maintain [H⁺] gradient between blood and urine	Distal renal tubular acidosis	Hydrochloric	Normal	Reduced Na⁺/H⁺ exchange in distal tubule
3 Oliguria	Acute renal failure	Sulphuric, phosphoric etc. produced by metabolism	Increased	Usually absent
LOSS OF BICARBONATE				
1 In urine	Proximal renal tubular acidosis	Hydrochloric	Normal	Reduced Na⁺/H⁺ exchange in proximal tubule
	Carbonic anhydrase inhibitors	Hydrochloric	Normal	Reduced Na⁺/H⁺ exchange throughout nephron
2 From GI tract	Diarrhoea, fistulae	Hydrochloric	Normal	Loss of Na⁺ in GI secretions
	Ureterosigmoidostomy	Hydrochloric	Normal	Loss of Na⁺ in GI secretions

[1] Anion gap = plasma $[Na^+] - ([Cl^-]+[HCO_3^-])$ normal 8–14 mmol/l.
[2] Especially in children; in adults respiratory alkalosis usually predominates.

In cardiogenic shock or after cardiac arrest, acidosis develops without sodium depletion. Treatment with i.v. sodium bicarbonate is usually unnecessary. Treatment of diabetic ketoacidosis and of lactic acidosis in diabetes is described on pages 749–751. In chronic renal failure, oral sodium bicarbonate supplements may be required on a long-term basis.

METABOLIC ALKALOSIS

Metabolic alkalosis, which is less common than metabolic acidosis, is characterised by an increase in plasma bicarbonate, a fall in blood [H⁺], and a small compensatory rise in $PaCO_2$ (Fig. 10.9 and Table 10.11). In health, when plasma HCO_3^- rises above normal, the filtered load of HCO_3^- exceeds the tubular reabsorptive capacity, so that urinary excretion of HCO_3^- increases rapidly. It is therefore very difficult to produce metabolic alkalosis in the presence of normal renal function.

Irrespective of how it is induced, metabolic alkalosis can only be sustained if certain conditions are present, as shown in the information box.

Commonly several factors contribute to the devel-

CASE EXAMPLE 10.1

A 32-year-old man is admitted very ill. He had been drinking with friends, but had not been seen for some hours. On admission he is barely conscious and breathing heavily.

Arterial blood gases
[H⁺] **98** nmol/l $PaCO_2$ **2.7** kPa HCO_3^- **6** mmol/l
PaO_2 **13** kPa
a. What is the likely diagnosis?
b. How would you confirm it?
c. What treatment would you give?

ANSWERS
a. Severe acute **metabolic acidosis**, due to poisoning—his drink had probably been 'spiked' with methanol, which is metabolised to formic acid. Low $PaCO_2$ reflects partial respiratory compensation.
b. Blood and urine to laboratory for toxicology analysis—measurement of lactate, methanol, ethylene glycol.
c. Give intravenous 1.26% sodium bicarbonate to restore safe [H⁺] (≈ 70 nmol/l) over 12–24 hours. Give intravenous fluids to establish a diuresis, to facilitate renal excretion of methanol and formic acid. If blood methanol level high, give oral ethanol to competitively slow metabolism of methanol. Consider haemodialysis if any evidence of renal failure.

CONDITIONS IN WHICH METABOLIC ALKALOSIS CAN BE SUSTAINED

Reduced filtered bicarbonate
- Very low glomerular filtration rate
- Low plasma bicarbonate

Increased proportion of filtered sodium reabsorbed with bicarbonate
- Strong stimulus to reabsorb sodium (i.e. hypovolaemia), particularly in the presence of a low plasma chloride, and thus reduced filtered chloride
- Increased secretion of H^+ by renal tubular cells:
  Increased delivery of sodium to the distal nephron (e.g. by loop diuretics)
  High $PaCO_2$ (e.g. chronic respiratory failure)
  Tubular cell K^+ depletion
  Increased mineralocorticoid activity

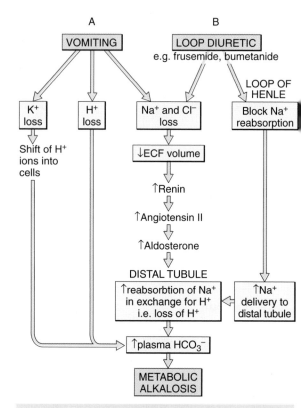

Fig. 10.10 Simplified scheme showing pathogenesis of metabolic alkalosis. Metabolic alkalosis due to [A] loss of gastric contents and [B] use of loop diuretics.

Table 10.13 Commonest causes of metabolic alkalosis

Underlying mechanism	Clinical condition
Loss of Na^+, Cl^-, H^+ and water (ECF depletion)	Vomiting or aspiration gastric contents Congenital chloridorrhoea[1] Administration of diuretics (benzothiadiazines, frusemide, bumetanide)
Potassium depletion	See Table 10.7[2]
Excessive mineralocorticoid activity	Primary aldosteronism, Cushing's syndrome Bartter's syndrome, Adrenal enzyme defects, Secondary aldosteronism Administration of liquorice, carbenoxolone
Administration of exogenous alkali	Oral or i.v. HCO_3^-, citrate[3] Administration of gluconate, acetate, lactate

[1] A rare disorder associated with loss H^+ and Cl^- in diarrhoeal stools.
[2] Alkalosis is uncommon in K^+ depletion due to primary renal disease.
[3] Present in transfused blood.

opment of metabolic alkalosis. It is convenient to consider an initiation phase, in which plasma $[HCO_3^-]$ increases, and a maintenance phase during which the raised plasma $[HCO_3^-]$ is sustained because of altered renal function.

Aetiology

Important causes are shown in Table 10.13. When H^+ ions are secreted into the gastric lumen, bicarbonate from parietal cells is added to the blood; this is subsequently neutralised by reabsorption of the secreted H^+ in the small bowel. Loss of H^+ in vomitus or because of gastric aspiration therefore initiates metabolic alkalosis. The disturbance is sustained because loss of sodium, chloride, water and potassium in the gastric secretions gives rise to extracellular fluid depletion, hypochloraemia and a potassium deficit. All of these enhance the renal reabsorption of sodium in exchange for H^+ (Fig. 10.10).

Prolonged use of loop diuretics results in a selective loss of sodium chloride and water from ECF, and therefore initiates a raised plasma bicarbonate. This is sustained because the drugs, by reducing tubular sodium reabsorption in the loop of Henle, deliver increased amounts of sodium to the distal nephron. Here, secondary aldosteronism stimulates reabsorption of sodium, and because of accompanying tubular cell K^+ depletion, this is preferentially in exchange for secretion of H^+ ions, which perpetuates the alkalosis (Fig. 10.10).

In potassium deficiency, the alkalosis is initiated by shift of H^+ from ECF into cells, and maintained by enhanced secretion of protons by the K^+-depleted distal tubular cells. In conditions where there is an excess of mineralocorticoid, such as primary aldosteronism, alkalosis is initiated and sustained by corticosteroid-stimulated reabsorption of sodium in exchange for H^+ in the distal nephron. Potassium is also lost, which further stimulates renal Na^+/H^+ exchange.

In the presence of a reduced GFR, or any factor which enhances bicarbonate reabsorption (see information box), administration of exogenous base (e.g. some antacid preparations) will cause alkalosis.

Consequences of metabolic alkalosis

The compensatory increase in $PaCO_2$, which partially restores the ECF H^+ concentration towards normal, actually stimulates H^+ secretion by the kidney, and thus bicarbonate reabsorption. The urine therefore often remains acidic.

Clinical features

Alkalosis rarely causes specific clinical symptoms. Acute alkalosis may cause tetany, either spontaneous or induced by Trousseau's manoeuvre (p. 705). This is due primarily to the acute fall in plasma ionised calcium (p. 590), although enhanced release of acetylcholine is another cause of increased neuromuscular excitability. Apathy, confusion and drowsiness may occur in severe cases, although this is often multifactorial. Severe long-standing alkalosis may be associated with reduced renal function and uraemia.

Management

In patients without renal disease, restoration of the ECF volume and the plasma chloride and potassium concentrations will remove the stimulus to renal H^+ secretion, and allow renal excretion of the excess bicarbonate. In patients who have lost gastric contents, e.g. in pyloric outlet obstruction, this should be done with isotonic (0.9%) sodium chloride solution (3–6 litres per 24 hours) and sufficient KCl to restore the K^+ deficit (40–60 mmol/day). Patients who require continuous aspiration of gastric contents in preparation for surgery should have the volume of aspirate replaced by intravenous infusion of an equal amount of isotonic (0.9%) sodium chloride solution containing KCl (20 mmol/l).

Alkalosis associated with K^+ deficiency is corrected by sufficient KCl to restore body K^+ to normal (p. 598). Diuretic-induced alkalosis can be difficult to correct. If possible the diuretic should be stopped for a few days and the intake of sodium chloride increased. If this is not possible (e.g. in severe cardiac failure) or ineffective, the carbonic anhydrase inhibitor acetazolamide (500–1000 mg/daily) should be substituted for the diuretic for a few days to induce excretion of bicarbonate. Any K^+ deficit must be corrected. When alkalosis is due to mineralocorticoid excess, the underlying disorder must be treated. Restriction of dietary sodium and correction of K^+ deficiency with KCl mitigates the alkalosis.

CASE EXAMPLE 10.2

A 44-year-old lady with a long history of indigestion begins to vomit at home. She becomes unwell after 4 days and is admitted to hospital because of marked muscle weakness.

Arterial blood gases
H^+ **28** nmol/l $PaCO_2$ **6.5** kPa HCO_3^- **40** mmol/l
PaO_2 **10.1** kPa Plasma potassium 2.1 mmol/l
a. What is the likely diagnosis?
b. What treatment would you give?

ANSWERS
a. **Metabolic alkalosis**, due to pyloric stenosis, due to chronic duodenal ulcer. Vomiting has caused loss of potassium, H^+, sodium and chloride. There is a total body deficit of sodium, which stimulates tubular sodium reabsorption in the distal tubule (which can only be in exchange for either H^+ or K^+). The kidney therefore cannot conserve H^+ or K^+. Also, because of chloride deficit, more bicarbonate is reabsorbed than normal.
b. Isotonic (0.9%) sodium chloride solution, 3–6 litres per day, to correct associated sodium chloride deficit. This removes the stimulus to sodium reabsorption and allows the kidney to conserve H^+ and K^+. Some intravenous K^+ will also be necessary (40–60 mmol/day). Surgery will be required to correct pyloric stenosis.

RESPIRATORY ACIDOSIS

This arises when the effective alveolar ventilation fails to keep pace with the rate of CO_2 production. As a result, $PaCO_2$, blood $[HCO_3^-]$ and $[H^+]$ all rise.

The kidney responds by increased H^+ secretion, so that the urine becomes acid, bicarbonate is added to the blood, and the blood $[H_2CO_3]$ is partially restored. The distinction between respiratory acidosis and metabolic alkalosis can usually be made from knowledge of the cause of the disturbance, and the fact that characteristically the $[H^+]$ is raised in respiratory acidosis and reduced in metabolic alkalosis (Table 10.11).

Aetiology and clinical features of respiratory acidosis are described on page 588.

CASE EXAMPLE 10.3

A 56-year-old man, who has smoked heavily for many years, develops a worsening cough with purulent sputum, and is admitted to hospital because of difficulty in breathing. He is drowsy and cyanosed.

Arterial blood gases

H^+ **65** nmol/l $PaCO_2$ **9.5** kPa HCO_3^- **28** mmol/l
PaO_2 **6.2** kPa
a. What is the likely diagnosis?
b. What treatment would you give?

ANSWERS

a. Acute **respiratory acidosis**, due to an infective exacerbation of obstructive pulmonary disease.

If his respiratory failure became **chronic**, with a persistent rise in $PaCO_2$, the kidney would compensate by retaining bicarbonate, e.g.

H^+ **43** nmol/l $PaCO_2$ **8.5** kPa HCO_3^- **38** mmol/l
PaO_2 **8.1** kPa

b. Try to improve respiratory function—nebulised bronchodilators, physiotherapy, antibiotics, controlled low-flow oxygen (e.g. 28%).

CASE EXAMPLE 10.4

A 13-year-old schoolboy is brought to the Casualty Department having become acutely unwell in the Headmaster's office. He is alert and agitated, the respiratory rate is 35/min, and he complains of tingling in his hands.

Arterial blood gases

H^+ **29** nmol/l $PaCO_2$ **2.8** kPa HCO_3^- **22** mmol/l
PaO_2 **16** kPa
a. What is the likely diagnosis?
b. What treatment would you give?

ANSWERS

a. Acute **respiratory alkalosis**, due to hyperventilation induced by anxiety. The tingling is due to a fall in plasma ionised calcium caused by the alkalosis.
b. Calm him down by reassurance and discussion, persuade him to breathe slowly.

RESPIRATORY ALKALOSIS

This occurs when there is excessive loss of CO_2 due to over-ventilation of the lungs. $PaCO_2$ and $[H^+]$ fall. The low $PaCO_2$ results in reduced renal Na^+/H^+ exchange, loss of bicarbonate in the urine, and a fall in plasma bicarbonate which mitigates the fall in blood $[H^+]$. The more common causes of respiratory alkalosis are shown in the information box.

CAUSES OF RESPIRATORY ALKALOSIS

- Hysterical overbreathing
- Assisted ventilation, if excessive
- Lobar pneumonia
- Pulmonary embolism
- Meningitis, encephalitis
- Salicylate poisoning
- Hepatic failure

MIXED ACID-BASE DISORDERS

Particularly in very ill patients, there may be both metabolic and respiratory factors contributing to an acid-base disturbance. The most common pattern is a mixed metabolic and respiratory acidosis (see example). Nomograms such as Figure 10.9 are often useful to clarify such complex cases. Management involves the treatments outlined above for each element of the disturbance.

FURTHER READING

Arieff A I 1993 Management of hypernatraemia. British Medical Journal 307: 305–308
Latta K, Hisano S, Chan J C 1993 Perturbations in potassium balance. Clinics in Laboratory Medicine 13: 149–156

CASE EXAMPLE 10.5

A 64-year-old man develops a chest infection and goes to bed. He is given antibiotics by his GP, but fails to improve. 48 hours later he is admitted to hospital. He is semiconscious, has a blood pressure of 80/40 mmHg and feels cold to the touch.

Arterial blood gases

H^+ **75** nmol/l $PaCO_2$ **5.8** kPa HCO_3^- **14** mmol/l
PaO_2 **8** kPa

a. What is the acid-base disturbance?
b. Other than chest infection/pneumonia, what else could he be suffering from?
c. What other tests would you perform?
d. What treatment would you give?

ANSWERS

a. **Mixed metabolic and respiratory acidosis**—although the $PaCO_2$ is within normal limits, it should be much lower for this degree of acidosis if it were purely metabolic.
b. **Septicaemia**, leading to lactic acidosis and renal failure; respiratory failure due to pneumonia; he could also have diabetes mellitus with ketoacidosis. If he is on metformin for Type II diabetes, lactic acidosis becomes even more likely.
c. **Plasma urea, electrolytes**:
    urea 25.4 mmol/l (renal failure)
    K^+ 6.5 mmol/l ($\downarrow$ excretion due to renal failure; shift out of cells due to acidosis)
    glucose 33 mmol/l (indicates uncontrolled diabetes)
    blood lactate 11 mmol/l (high—indicates lactic acidosis)
d. Intravenous insulin to control diabetic ketoacidosis; i.v. fluids (0.9% NaCl, 5% dextrose) to correct hypovolaemia and restore renal function; i.v. bicarbonate only if acidosis does not respond to these measures. Antibiotics, chest physiotherapy.

A. M. Davison, A. D. Cumming, C. P. Swainson

11

Diseases of the kidney and genito-urinary system

Diseases of the kidney and genito-urinary system are of interest and importance for a variety of reasons. The clinical manifestations of renal disease are largely determined by the part of the kidney involved, and can be explained by the disruption to normal physiological processes. For example, disorders of the medulla are frequently associated with increased urine volume due to interference with the medullary concentrating ability, whereas glomerular diseases usually are accompanied by reduced renal function and hypertension, due to impairment of glomerular filtration and stimulation of the renin-angiotensin-aldosterone system. An understanding of basic renal physiology is of great help in appreciating renal pathophysiology.

Renal disease is influenced by social, economic and geographical factors. It is recognised that, as with other systems, there have been significant changes in disease patterns due to improved public health measures and improved nutrition. For instance, post-streptococcal glomerulonephritis is now uncommon in developed countries and is currently mostly found associated with skin infections in developing countries. Similarly, childhood bladder stone has virtually disappeared from developed countries, but is common due to inadequate nutrition in children in developing countries. Interestingly, in contrast, nephrolithiasis seems to be precipitated by a Western lifestyle and has an increased incidence in affluent countries. Other conditions are important because of their prevalence; symptomatic urinary tract infection occurs in about 50% of women at some time whereas in men it is uncommon before the sixth decade.

Renal failure is of significance due to the fact that the kidney is the only organ for which an artificial device can successfully replace function for prolonged periods. In patients with acute reversible renal failure, the artificial kidney has played a central role in maintaining adequate homeostasis for long enough to enable the patient's own kidneys to recover and return to normal. This latter event is the reason why intensive management of such patients can be justified—few other intensive care situations are followed by a return to normality of the involved organ.

In the past thirty years the artificial kidney has been increasingly used to maintain the life of patients with chronic irreversible renal failure, such that in the United Kingdom, for example, many patients currently receive regular dialysis. This has of course brought its own problems, such as cost—£22 000/patient/year at 1993 prices. It has also been accompanied by the emergence of conditions related to prolonging life by such artificial means. Dialysis-related encephalopathy, a disabling dementia, was eventually traced to cerebral accumulation of aluminium contaminating the water used to prepare dialysis

fluid. Similarly, β2-microglobulin (β2-M) amyloidosis results from the prolonged accumulation of β2-M in tissues as a consequence of the inability of the artificial kidney to remove an adequate amount. These two conditions would never have been recognised but for the fact that patients with end stage renal failure can now be kept alive for many years by dialysis.

Transplantation has also brought major benefits to patients with end stage renal failure. The transplanted kidney, unlike the artificial kidney, replaces endocrine as well as excretory function. This allows for a return of erythropoiesis by the secretion of erythropoietin, and a return to normal calcium metabolism by the hydroxylation of cholecalciferol. However, transplantation requires continued immunosuppression with the associated risk of opportunistic infections and malignancy. In addition, the demand for kidneys to transplant far outweighs the supply of available organs and this raises difficult ethical questions of who should be transplanted. One solution has been to transplant from living persons, but this has resulted in the growth, in certain countries, of commercialisation in organ donation. Whilst it is easy to condemn such practice in the developed countries it is difficult to take such a stance in countries where cadaver organs are unavailable.

The spectrum of renal medicine thus ranges from the management of common non-life-threatening conditions such as cystitis to the use of expensive advanced technology to replace renal function. In recent years there have been many significant advances in the management of renal disease, but there remains a need for further development, particularly in the management of glomerular diseases and systemic diseases such as diabetic nephropathy.

ANATOMY, PHYSIOLOGY AND INVESTIGATION

Each kidney contains approximately one million nephrons. A schematic structure is illustrated in Figure 11.1. The blood supply of the kidneys is relatively large, about one-quarter of the cardiac output at rest, i.e. 1300 ml per minute, and subject to considerable physiological variation. The afferent arterioles, which give rise to the glomerular capillaries, arise from intralobular branches of the renal artery. Emerging from the glomeruli, the capillaries unite to form the efferent arterioles which supply blood to proximal and distal convoluted tubules in the cortex. The medulla is supplied by arterioles arising from glomeruli in the deeper regions of the cortex, and directly by branches from the arcuate arteries. For a short distance the afferent arterioles and distal con-

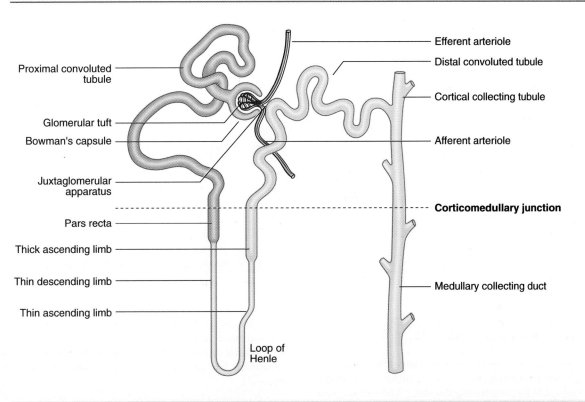

Fig. 11.1 Nephron with long loop of Henle (deep nephron). The afferent arteriole enters the glomerulus and divides into capillary loops and leaves at the efferent arteriole. From the glomerulus the proximal convoluted tubule descends to the corticomedullary junction where it becomes the loop of Henle with a thin descending limb and an ascending limb, the upper third of which is thick. The nephron then progresses on to the distal convoluted tubule and then to the collecting tubule which passes through the medulla to open at the tip of the papilla.

voluted tubules are in contact (Fig. 11.1). At this point the tubular cells become tall and columnar, forming the macula densa, and the wall of the arteriole is thickened by myoepithelial cells which contain large secretory granules of renin. These structures, together with the agranular lacis cells which lie between the glomerular hilum and the macula densa, constitute the juxta-glomerular apparatus (JGA) (Fig. 11.2) which is intimately concerned in extracellular fluid volume regulation, blood pressure control and potassium balance.

Glomerular filtration is the process whereby water and solutes pass across the glomerular membrane by bulk flow or diffusion. The mean filtration pressure, about 10 mmHg, results in production of filtrate identical in its composition with plasma, except that it normally contains no fat and very little protein.

The filtrate thus formed passes through the tubule, and is modified according to the needs of the body by selective reabsorption and tubular secretion. The glomerular filtration rate (GFR) remains remarkably constant

FACTORS INFLUENCING GLOMERULAR FILTRATION RATE

- Permeability of glomerular membrane
- Surface area of glomerular membrane
- Blood flow through glomerular capillaries
- Mean filtration pressure

Mean filtration pressure $= [mCHP - mPCOP] - [mTHP - TCOP]$
Where $mCHP$ = mean capillary hydrostatic pressure
$mPCOP$ = mean plasma colloid osmotic pressure
$mTHP$ = mean tubular hydrostatic pressure
$TCOP$ = tubular colloid osmotic pressure

over a range of values of renal perfusion pressure and renal blood flow. This depends mainly on alterations in the relative tone of afferent and efferent arterioles, brought about in part by release of renin from the JGA in response to changes in the delivery of solute to the macula densa (tubulo-glomerular feedback).

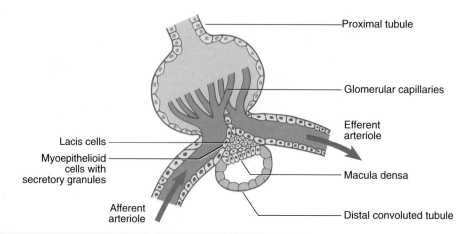

Fig. 11.2 Juxtaglomerular apparatus. The juxtaglomerular apparatus consists of special myoepithelioid cells which arise from the afferent arteriole, and lacis cells together with the macula densa which consists of columnar cells of the distal convoluted tubule.

FUNCTIONS OF THE KIDNEYS

In health the volume and composition of the body fluids vary within narrow limits. The kidneys are largely responsible for maintaining this state. The various functions of the kidneys are considered further in Chapter 10.

Retention of substances vital to body economy

Glucose is normally reabsorbed so completely by the proximal tubules that none can be detected in urine by clinical tests. Amino acids are reabsorbed in the proximal tubule, where several specific transport mechanisms exist. Most filtered phosphate is reabsorbed in the proximal tubule, by processes linked to reabsorption of sodium and water, inhibited by parathyroid hormone and increased by Vitamin D. In health only a small amount of protein reaches the fluid in Bowman's capsule. The volume of glomerular filtrate, however, is so great that if this small amount were not reabsorbed, more than 3 g of protein would be excreted in the urine in 24 hours. In health up to 150 mg protein daily may be excreted in the urine.

Excretion of waste metabolic products

The end products of metabolism, especially those of protein, are excreted in the urine. Excretion of urea depends mainly on the GFR, but a certain amount is reabsorbed by diffusion down concentration gradients produced by water reabsorption. Thus the proportion excreted increases during water diuresis. Creatinine is excreted mainly by filtration, though a small amount is secreted. Proximal tubular reabsorption of filtered uric acid is linked to that of sodium and water, and is therefore increased in extracellular fluid volume depletion. In the distal nephron, uric acid is both secreted and reabsorbed, and certain drugs compete with it for these processes.

Hormonal and metabolic functions

The JGA secretes renin in response to a number of stimuli:

- reduced afferent arteriolar pressure
- increased sympathetic activity
- changes in composition of fluid reaching the macula densa.

The sequence shown in Figure 12.20 (p. 706) then takes place. Angiotensin II plays an important part in regulating the intrarenal circulation by constricting the glomerular efferent arteriole, stimulates aldosterone secretion by the adrenal cortex, and causes systemic vasoconstriction. This may be the sequence of events whereby renal ischaemia produces hypertension.

The kidney is the main source of erythropoietin (see p. 777) and hydroxylates 25-hydroxycholecalciferol to form 1,25-dihydroxycholecalciferol (see p. 572). Two vasodilator prostaglandins (PGE_2 and PGI_2), both concerned with the control of the renal circulation, are produced by mesangial cells in the glomeruli and interstitial cells in the medulla. The kidney also secretes glandular kallikrein, an enzyme which generates vasodilator peptides, bradykinin and kallidin, from kininogen precursors. These may influence renal blood flow and sodium and water excretion, but their precise function is not yet known.

INVESTIGATION OF RENAL DISEASE

In many patients suffering from renal disease, symptoms and signs are not referred to the anatomical site of the kidneys. Clinical features commonly arise from abnormalities in the chemical composition of the body or from hypertension, anaemia, or metabolic bone disease. Their origin may be suspected only after detection of urinary abnormalities. Thus the importance of routine examination of the urine cannot be over-emphasised.

EXAMINATION OF THE URINE

Urine volume
In health in temperate climates the 24-hour urine output usually varies from 800 to 2500 ml. The ability to concentrate urine is limited, and on a normal diet a minimum volume of about 500 ml is needed to excrete the urinary solutes, mainly urea and electrolytes. **Oliguria** is the failure to produce enough urine to enable solute to be excreted in adequate amounts, and the 'milieu interieur' (internal environment) to be preserved. If the renal concentrating power is seriously reduced or the solute load greatly increased, e.g. in severe infections or after trauma, a daily output of 2–3 litres of urine may be insufficient.

Oliguria develops when renal blood flow and/or GFR are reduced, e.g. reduced blood volume, septicaemia, cardiac failure, acute glomerulonephritis, acute tubular necrosis. In these circumstances urine flow may cease—**anuria**. Anuria more commonly indicates obstruction of the outflow from both kidneys (or from a sole functioning kidney) or deprivation of all functioning renal tissue of its blood supply. Anuria should be distinguished from **urinary retention**, in which distension of the bladder will be found on examination, and confirmed if necessary by catheterisation. **Polyuria** is a persistent increase in urinary output. It must be distinguished from frequency of micturition, in which there is frequent passage of small volumes of urine without an increase in total daily volume. Polyuria may be due to an increased osmotic load, disturbances of the concentrating mechanism, certain drugs or excessive water intake.

Urine concentration
This can be tested by measuring the osmolality of a specimen of urine obtained after water deprivation or administration of vasopressin. Urine osmolality (Uosm) is determined by the number of particles of solute per kilogram water. The ability to concentrate urine is best determined by measuring Uosm after 8 hours of water

CAUSES OF POLYURIA

- **Osmotic**
  e.g. hyperglycaemia, chronic renal failure
- **Disturbance of concentrating mechanism**
  Diabetes insipidus, e.g. trauma, pituitary tumours, idiopathic
- **Nephrogenic diabetes insipidus**, e.g. congenital, hypercalcaemia, obstructive uropathy, papillary necrosis
- **Drugs**
  e.g. diuretics, lithium
- **Excessive water intake**

deprivation, when it should reach 800 mOsm/kg (see appendix, p. 668).

The water deprivation test procedure is potentially dangerous when renal concentrating ability is impaired (e.g. diabetes insipidus) and hence patients should be weighed at the start of the test and at intervals throughout. If the patient loses more than 3% of their body weight then the test should be stopped.

Urine dilution
A number of conditions interfere with urinary dilution and normal water excretion (Table 10.4, p. 597). Occasionally, it is desirable to test these functions by the administration of a water load (see appendix to this chapter, p. 668).

Urine pH and acid excretion
In health urinary pH ranges from about 4.3 to 8.0. A pH greater than 8 nearly always indicates urinary tract infection with an organism which splits urea to form ammonia. In certain circumstances the ability to excrete hydrogen ions is depressed. This may be due to failure to form a very acid urine, or inability to excrete a sufficient quantity of ammonium ion (NH_4^+). This can be tested by a urinary acidification test (see appendix to this chapter, p. 668).

BLOOD ANALYSIS

Determination of the plasma creatinine gives a useful indication of the degree of renal failure. The blood urea, which is more readily affected by dietary protein, tissue breakdown and hydration, is a less reliable guide to overall renal function. Neither plasma creatinine nor blood urea increases to greater than the accepted normal maximum until renal function is reduced by at least 50%.

The diminishing capacity to excrete hydrogen ions results in metabolic acidosis, the severity of which may be estimated by measurement of arterial [H$^+$], [HCO$_3$$^-$], and $PaCO_2$.

Estimations of plasma sodium, potassium, calcium, phosphate and protein concentrations are of value in certain circumstances. For example, in chronic renal failure, metabolic acidosis is frequently accompanied by hyponatraemia, hyperkalaemia, hypocalcaemia, and hyperphosphataemia.

Renal clearance

Glomerular function is best studied by measuring renal clearance, where clearance **C = UV/P**, U and P being the urinary and plasma concentrations of any substance and V the volume of urine formed per minute. If a substance in plasma passes freely through the glomerular filter and is neither absorbed nor excreted by the tubules, the quantity excreted in urine (UV) is identical with the amount filtered by the glomeruli; the clearance of such a substance therefore equals the rate of glomerular filtration (GFR).

The polysaccharide, inulin, appears to be excreted in this way and its clearance is used to estimate GFR, which for the average adult is about 120 ml/min. A similar value is obtained using the clearance of ^{51}Cr-EDTA, and here a single injection technique is possible. In clinical practice the clearance of creatinine, which approximates to that of inulin, is usually measured by collecting a 24-hour urine sample and withdrawing a sample of blood at the end of the collection. In declining renal function, some creatinine may be secreted by tubules, and this may result in an overestimate of GFR.

IMAGING

A plain radiograph of the abdomen detects opaque calculi or calcification within the renal tract (Fig. 11.3). When the kidneys are outlined by perirenal fat it can give an indication of their shape, size and position, but this information is best obtained by ultrasound or intravenous urography.

Renal ultrasound

This is the method of choice for assessing overall renal size and cortical thickness and distinguishing solid tumours from cysts. It is an excellent screening test for polycystic kidney disease. In investigation of suspected malignant renal tumours ultrasound can give additional information by detecting extension of tumour to renal veins, vena cava, lymph nodes or liver. It can demonstrate dilation of the renal pelvis and ureters, which may indicate urinary tract obstruction (Fig. 11.4). It can also be used to assess residual urine in the bladder after micturition, the presence of which may indicate incomplete bladder emptying and bladder neck obstruction.

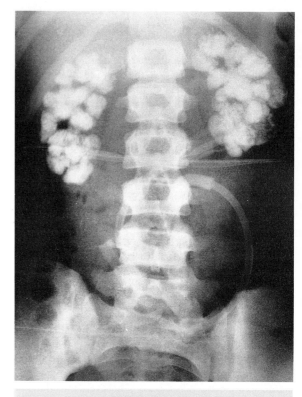

Fig. 11.3 Nephrocalcinosis. Bilateral nephrocalcinosis in a patient with primary hyperoxaluria. This demonstrates the size and position of the kidneys, which have widespread calcinosis of the cortex and medulla. This patient was in terminal renal failure and receiving continuous ambulatory peritoneal dialysis (note CAPD catheter in situ).

Perinephric abscess or haematoma can be demonstrated. Calculi are usually detected but very small stones may be missed. Cyst puncture, renal biopsy and

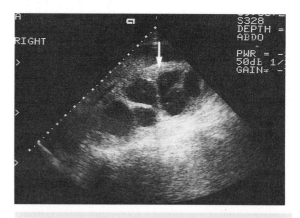

Fig. 11.4 Renal ultrasound examination—chronic urinary tract obstruction. The dilated pelvi-calyceal system is apparent, with thinning of the surrounding renal cortex (arrow).

antegrade pyelography are best done under ultrasound screening. It is quick, inexpensive and harmless, and portable equipment is available to investigate seriously ill patients.

Intravenous urography (IVU)

This is carried out by intravenous injection of an organic iodine-containing contrast compound. Approximately one third of the contrast is excreted, largely by glomerular filtration, within the first hour. It is used, often in association with tomography, to demonstrate the size, shape and position of the kidneys and to study the outflow tract. Following injection, films are taken at timed intervals. There is first an increase in the radiographic density of renal substance (nephrogram) as contrast is concentrated in the tubules, and this shows the size and shape of the kidneys. Within a few minutes contrast is excreted into the calyceal system, pelvis and ureters, which are best demonstrated within the first 20 minutes.

In the adult, healthy kidneys usually measure 11–14 cm in length, bi-polar diameter being similar in length to that of three lumbar vertebrae. Renal cortical thickness can be assessed and any focal or generalised cortical defect seen, e.g. scars of chronic pyelonephritis. In significant unilateral renal artery stenosis, early films show a delay on the stenotic side in the nephrogram, which subsequently becomes more dense and persists longer compared with the normal side. This is also apparent on angiography (Fig. 11.5). Thus in hypertensive patients it is useful to obtain early films to detect this difference. Abnormalities of the papillae, e.g. papillary necrosis, may be seen, and the appearance of the pelvi-calyceal

system, ureters and bladder will show any structural abnormality or partial or complete obstruction. Clubbed calyces and slow excretion are common in chronic obstruction. Severe obstruction may result in distention of the pelvis, thinning of the cortex, and extravasation of contrast into extrarenal tissue. In renal tuberculosis calcification and cavitation are common. Adult polycystic disease causes bilateral renal enlargement and the calyces are stretched and spidery. Calculi may be localised.

Excretion urography is not without risk. A few patients may react to the contrast agent. In those with known atopy, diabetes mellitus or renal insufficiency and any with a history of adverse reaction to contrast agents, a special low osmolar contrast medium should be used if the procedure is essential. Formerly, all patients were dehydrated before IVU to increase the concentration of dye in the kidney and collecting systems. In some (diabetic patients, small children, and those with myeloma or renal failure) this resulted in significant renal impairment. Use of tomography and of modern contrast agents, which can be given in large doses, has made water deprivation unnecessary in these patients.

Micturating cystourethrography (MCU)

MCU is used to diagnose vesico-ureteric reflux and to assess its severity (Fig. 11.6). Using a catheter the bladder is filled with contrast medium and while the patient voids fluoroscopic screening is carried out and films taken. MCU is used, in combination with urodynamic studies, in assessment of disordered bladder emptying and urethral abnormalities.

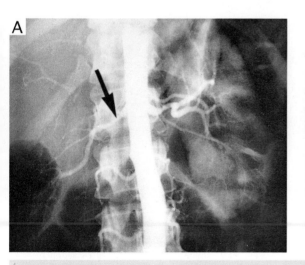
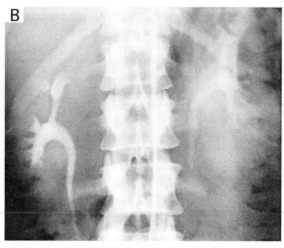

Fig. 11.5 Renal artery stenosis. Ⓐ Angiography demonstrating an irregular calibre of both renal arteries, more marked on the right (arrowed) due to fibromuscular hyperplasia. Note that the nephrogram on the left has appeared before the right kidney is visible. Ⓑ Excretory phase of the same arteriogram indicating more dense dye on the right side due to increased concentration of urine as a compensation for the arterial stenosis.

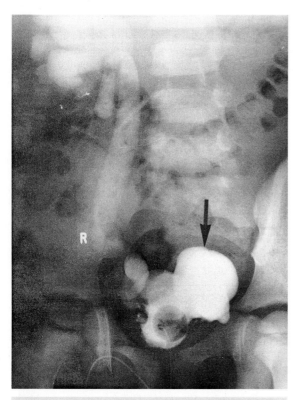

Fig. 11.6 Vesico-ureteric reflux. Gross reflux of dye from the bladder to widely distended ureter and pelvi-calyceal system in a child with reflux nephropathy. The bladder also contains a large diverticulum (arrow). The filling defect in the bladder is the balloon of the Foley catheter through which the dye was instilled to the bladder.

Cystoscopy and retrograde pyelography

These investigations are used mainly to investigate lesions of the ureter and renal pelvis and define the cause of ureteric obstruction. Cystoscopy allows direct inspection of the bladder and ureteric orifices. Contrast medium is then injected under screening control into ureteric catheters inserted during cystoscopy. Antibiotic cover is essential when the urine contains organisms.

Antegrade pyelography

This requires percutaneous insertion of a fine catheter into the pelvi-calyceal system under radiograph or ultrasound control. Injection of contrast allows detailed examination of the pelvi-calyceal system and ureters and localisation of any obstruction. The procedure can be extended to allow percutaneous drainage (nephrostomy) of an obstructed system, which will frequently result in recovery of renal function.

Renal arteriography

This is used to demonstrate the anatomy of the renal arterial system and is valuable when investigating renal artery stenosis, arteriovenous malformation, and persistent bleeding after trauma. It has been largely superseded by ultrasonography and computed tomography when investigating renal masses. Following percutaneous catheterisation of the femoral artery the catheter tip is advanced and contrast injected first into the aorta and then into the renal arteries (Fig. 11.7).

Arteriography can be extended (1) to carry out balloon angioplasty to dilate the artery in patients with arterial

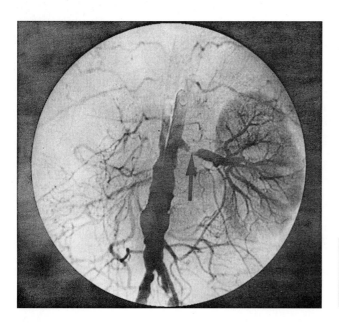

Fig. 11.7 Digital subtraction arteriogram showing renal artery stenosis. The angiogram demonstrates an absent right renal artery, with stenosis (arrowed) of left renal artery. The dye has passed the stenosis and the developing nephrogram can be seen.

stenosis, (2) to perform arterial embolisation in patients with inoperable renal carcinoma who have haemorrhage or intractable pain, or (3) to perform arterial embolisation in patients bleeding from the kidney after trauma, or occasionally after renal biopsy.

Renal vein sampling and venography

The renal veins can be catheterised via the femoral vein and blood taken to measure renin. This may be of value in assessing the haemodynamic significance of a renal artery stenosis. Venography will demonstrate renal vein thrombosis and invasion by tumour (Fig. 11.8).

Computed tomography

This is less widely available than ultrasound, but is particularly helpful in diagnosis of masses in the kidney and in perirenal and retroperitoneal tissues (Fig. 11.9). The information obtained can be increased by use of contrast agents. Extension of renal tumours to perirenal tissue, retroperitoneal nodes, liver and thorax can be identified. It is of value in assessing the extent of renal trauma, particularly when vascular damage is suspected, and in demonstrating radio-opaque stones.

Radionuclide studies (DMSA, DTPA)

These studies require the injection of gamma ray-emitting radiopharmaceuticals which are taken up and excreted by the kidney, a process which can be monitored by a computer-linked gamma camera. In this way function of individual kidneys can be assessed.

Renography

Diethylenetriamine penta-acetic acid labelled with technetium (^{99m}Tc-DTPA) is excreted by glomerular filtration. Following injection of DTPA, computer analysis of uptake and excretion (Fig. 11.10(a)) can be used to provide information about arterial perfusion of each kidney. In renal artery stenosis transit time is prolonged, peak activity delayed, and excretion reduced (Fig. 11.10(b)). In obstruction of the outflow tract, persistence of nuclide in the renal pelvis is shown by prolongation of phase 2 and absence of phase 3 of renogram (Fig. 11.10(c)). Poor renal function is indicated by curve of low amplitude. The technique can help in distinguishing poor perfusion from tubular necrosis, but it is not diagnostic.

Diuretic renography

This may be used to distinguish a dilated outflow tract from urinary tract obstruction with increased pressure in the calyceal system (Fig. 11.11). The diuretic is given during the course of the renogram and if genuine obstruction is not present, activity drains away.

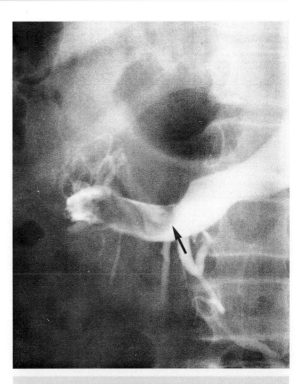

Fig. 11.8 Renal venography. Contrast injected into the renal vein demonstrates renal vein thrombosis (arrow).

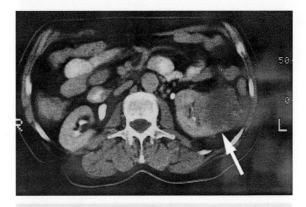

Fig. 11.9 CT of the abdomen. The left kidney contains a large tumour (arrow) which is extending laterally through the capsule. Compare with the normal right kidney.

Renal imaging

Dimercaptosuccinic acid labelled with technetium (^{99m}Tc-DMSA) is filtered by glomeruli and partially bound to proximal tubular cells. Following intravenous injection, images of the renal cortex can be obtained using a gamma camera (Fig. 11.12). These allow comparison of the two kidneys as they show the shape, size and function of each. This is a sensitive method of

Radioactivity
(counts)

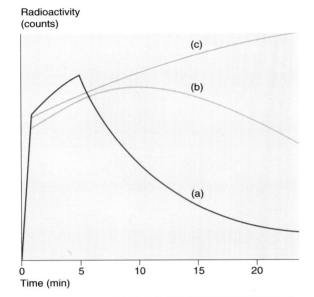

Time (min)

Fig. 11.10 Isotope renogram. (a) Normal renogram showing three classical phases. (b) Renogram pattern in renal artery stenosis showing prolonged transit time, delayed peak and reduced excretion. (c) Renogram pattern in complete obstruction showing absent phase III and a fall in the slope of phase II, indicating deteriorating renal function.

RENOGRAM 5MBQ TC99M MAG3

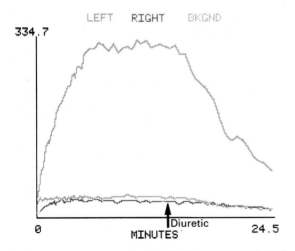

Fig. 11.11 Isotope renogram showing a non-functioning right kidney (red tracing). The left kidney drains slowly (green tracing) but responds promptly to injection of a diuretic, indicating that functional obstruction is not present.

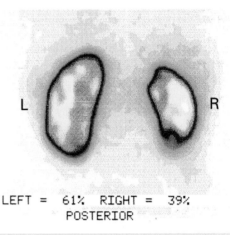

LEFT = 61% RIGHT = 39%
POSTERIOR

Fig. 11.12 DMSA isotope scan showing a posterior view of a normal left kidney and a small right kidney with evidence of cortical scarring at upper and lower poles and which contributes only 39% of total renal function.

demonstrating early cortical scarring. It is possible to assess the relative contribution of each kidney to total function.

RENAL BIOPSY: INDICATIONS AND CONTRAINDICATIONS

General indications
- To determine the nature of the renal disease
- To document the natural history of a disease
- To establish the response to therapy

Specific indications
- Adult nephrotic syndrome
- Persistent proteinuria > 1 g/24 hours
- Adult acute nephritic syndrome
- Persistent microscopic or macroscopic haematuria (disordered haemostasis excluded)
- Systemic diseases with renal involvement
- Chronic renal failure with normal or near normal sized kidneys
- Unexplained acute renal failure
- Occasionally where documentation of specific renal disease is required for insurance or occupational purposes
- Childhood nephrotic syndrome, if significant haematuria present or unresponsive to corticosteroid therapy
- Childhood acute nephritic syndrome, if significant urinary abnormalities persist for longer than 12 months or renal functional impairment present

Contraindications to renal biopsy
- Disordered coagulation
- Thrombocytopenia
- Uncontrolled hypertension
- Solitary kidney (except in transplanted kidneys)
- Small contracted kidneys, i.e. less than 60% of expected bipolar length

RENAL BIOPSY

This technique has increased greatly our understanding of renal disease and, in particular, knowledge of glomerulonephritis. To obtain the maximum information from this invasive investigation, it is important to examine the tissue obtained by light and electron microscopy and by immunohistological techniques.

RENAL BIOPSY: COMPLICATIONS

- **Pain**, usually mild
- **Bleeding**, usually mild but may be considerable and produce clot colic
- **Perirenal bleeding**, may cause hypertension
- **Arteriovenous anastomosis**, rarely clinically significant
- **Infection**, more common where significant haematuria has developed

---

FURTHER READING

Carlson J A, Harrington J T 1992 Laboratory evaluation of renal function. In: Schrier R W, Gottschalk C W (eds) Diseases of the kidney. Little, Brown, Boston
Davies J 1993 How to build a kidney. Seminars in Cell Biology 4: 213–219
Johnston C I et al 1993 Intrarenal renin-angiotensin system in renal physiology and pathophysiology. Kidney International Supplement 42: S59–63
Murer H et al 1994 Regulation of proximal tubular Na/H exchange: a tissue culture approach. Kidney International Supplement 44: S23–31

MAJOR MANIFESTATIONS OF RENAL DISEASE

ABNORMAL CONSTITUENTS OF URINE

PROTEINURIA

Protein in the urine, detectable by dipstix, usually indicates the presence of renal disease. Its magnitude bears little relation to overall renal function. Significant proteinuria does not occur in disease of the lower urinary tract, though small amounts can be detected in severe urinary tract infection or obvious haematuria. Minor degrees of proteinuria are usually found in chronic interstitial disease of the kidney, in the course of febrile illness and in heart failure. Large amounts of protein (3 g/day or more) invariably indicate glomerular disease. The most accurate way to assess the magnitude of proteinuria is to measure the amount of protein in urine collected over a 24-hour period. When this is impractical an assessment of the total urinary protein excretion can be obtained by calculating the urine protein/creatinine ratio. As this has a diurnal variation it is best to obtain the urine sample for analysis at mid morning. The most commonly used screening tests for detecting proteinuria is the 'stix' test. The 'stix' test uses a paper strip impregnated with bromophenol blue dye, which in the presence of protein at a suitable pH (pH3) will change colour to blue. As the strip has a yellow background this colour change is observed as green, the intensity of which is approximately proportional to the concentration of protein in the urine. The change is pH dependent and a highly alkaline urine (pH > 8) will induce colour change. The test must be performed on fresh urine and the lower limit of detection is in the range 50–100 mg/l. It is particularly sensitive for albumin, but has a low sensitivity for other proteins such as globulins and Bence–Jones protein.

If this screening test is positive, then laboratory examination to detect the degree and type of proteinuria should be undertaken. The great bulk of urinary protein is albumin, and larger molecular weight plasma proteins are present in only small amounts. The pattern of proteinuria can be determined and an index of **selectivity** assessed. In highly selective proteinuria, the larger molecular weight proteins are virtually absent; in nonselective proteinuria they are found in significant amounts. The degree of selectivity is an indication of the amount of glomerular damage and helps predict the response to corticosteroid therapy. Highly selective proteinuria, most commonly found in minimal lesion nephropathy, is usually responsive (see p. 644).

Asymptomatic proteinuria

Asymptomatic proteinuria is defined as the chance detection of proteinuria during routine urine testing, frequently in young people who are undergoing medical examination for employment or insurance purposes. The proteinuria may be orthostatic (see below) or exercise-induced, when it is usually benign. Renal biopsy is indicated if the proteinuria exceeds 1 g daily, if there is associated hypertension, haematuria, impaired renal function, or when the underlying renal disease has to be clearly defined for employment, insurance or any other purpose.

Postural (orthostatic) proteinuria

In a number of apparently healthy persons, usually children or adolescents, small amounts of protein are excreted in relation to assuming the erect posture but without demonstrable renal disease. In such patients urine formed in recumbency is free from protein so that the specimen voided immediately on rising is normal. Urine formed during day-time activities or after vigorous exercise contains protein. Tests of renal function show no abnormality and further investigations are not justified unless required to obtain employment or for insurance purposes. Follow-up studies of such patients indicate that the condition is benign.

Microalbuminuria

Microalbuminuria is a term used to indicate an increase in urinary albumin excretion which is not manifest by an increase in urinary protein detected by conventional methods, and indicates an albumin excretion rate of approximately 20–200 μg/min. As urinary albumin varies with posture and exercise, it is important to collect the urine under very standard conditions; short-term (2 hours) during rest, overnight (approximately 8 hours), or an early morning sample. For screening purposes an early-morning urine specimen is adequate, and if the albumin/creatinine ratio is found to be greater than 3.5 mg/mmol, then a timed overnight sample should be obtained for estimation of the albumin excretion rate. Methods are now available for the rapid detection of urinary albumin by immunoassay, and these are very specific. Interpretation of results is, however, difficult as albumin excretion will increase with exercise, hypertension, cardiac failure, urinary tract infection, and also after drinking large amounts of fluid. Nonetheless it is a particularly useful test for the detection of early diabetic nephropathy. Incipient diabetic nephropathy is suspected when microalbuminuria is detected in two of three samples collected over a six-month period in patients in whom other causes of an increased urinary albumin excretion have been excluded. Overt diabetic nephropathy is indicated by finding a urinary albumin excretion of greater than 200 μg/min in two of three samples collected at an interval of six months.

Bence–Jones proteinuria

Many patients suffering from one of the monoclonal gammopathies (p. 821) excrete immunoglobulin light chains (Bence–Jones protein) in their urine. These proteins are not detected by dipstix and can best be identified by immunoelectrophoresis of urine.

HAEMATURIA

Blood is found in the urine (haematuria) in a wide variety of clinical conditions and may indicate serious disease of the urinary tract. The appearance of the urine varies with the amount of blood. When traces are present it appears normal; with larger amounts the urine appears smoky, bright red or reddish brown. Microscopic examination of the urine should be performed, as the presence

Table 11.1 Causes of haematuria

KIDNEY	URETER
Glomerulonephritis	Neoplasia
Primary	Stone
Mesangial proliferative	
Endocapillary	**BLADDER**
Mesangiocapillary	Neoplasia
IgA nephropathy	Cystitis
Secondary	Stone
Systemic lupus erythematosus	Trauma
Polyarteritis	Schistosomiasis
Subacute bacterial endocarditis	
Cryoglobulinaemia	**PROSTATE**
	Prostatitis
Other glomerular disease	Neoplasia
Benign familial haematuria	
Loin pain haematuria syndrome	**URETHRA**
Alport's syndrome	Urethritis
Fabry's disease	Trauma
Interstitial disease	**DISORDERS OF**
Severe acute pyelonephritis	**HAEMOSTASIS**
Papillary necrosis (diabetes	
mellitus, analgesic nephropathy,	
sickle cell disease)	
Neoplastic (primary, secondary)	
Arteriovenous abnormalities	
Cystic disease	
Adult polycystic disease,	
medullary cystic disease	
Solitary cyst	
Stone disease	
Trauma	

of red cell casts indicates a glomerular lesion. Red cells which are deformed and crenated indicate upper tract bleeding, whereas those with a normal morphology tend to indicate ureteric, bladder, prostatic or urethral bleeding.

Haematuria may indicate blood loss from anywhere in the urinary tract from the glomerulus to the urethra (Table 11.1).

CONDITIONS WHICH MAY MIMIC HAEMATURIA

- **Haemoglobinuria**: urine gives a positive chemical test for haemoglobin, but no red cells are detectable

- **Myoglobinuria**: no red cells are seen, but chemical tests for haemoglobin are positive. Myoglobin can be distinguished by spectrometry

- **Acute intermittent porphyria**: fresh urine appears normal, but on standing for some hours a dark red colour develops

  Beetroot, senna, dyes used to colour sweets, and phenolphthalein may also mimic haematuria

PUS CELLS AND BACTERIA

Pus cells may be found in the urinary sediment in inflammation of any part of the urinary tract. Their presence usually indicates bacterial infection, but they are found in the absence of bacteria in acute glomerulonephritis, interstitial nephritis and polycystic disease. Bacteria may be seen under the microscope, but urine must be cultured if infection is suspected. In obtaining the specimen for culture it is best to avoid catheterisation. A mid stream specimen (MSU) should be obtained from both male and female patients and cultured within 2 hours. Suprapubic aspiration of the bladder is easily performed, without local anaesthetic, when the bladder is full. This is a useful technique for obtaining an uncontaminated sample of urine, particularly from small children. Quantitative culture of the urine should be performed; bacterial counts of more than 10^5/ml indicate significant infection in a properly obtained MSU. The presence of any bacteria in suprapubic aspirate must be considered significant.

CASTS

Casts are microscopic cylindrical structures found in the urinary sediment (Fig. 11.13). They are formed in renal tubules by coagulation of protein. Red cells, polymorphs or epithelial cells may be impressed upon this matrix, producing erythrocyte, leucocyte and epithelial casts respectively. All such casts are found in acute glomerulonephritis and in other diseases in which there is glomerular inflammation. Leucocyte casts appear during acute urinary infections. Granular casts are formed by degeneration of the impressed cells. Epithelial and granular casts are indicative of inflammation and degeneration of the renal tubules. Hyaline casts consist of coagulated protein without cellular elements. They are found in chronic glomerulonephritis, and occasionally in small numbers in normal urine, especially after vigorous exercise.

CLINICAL SYNDROMES

ACUTE GLOMERULONEPHRITIS SYNDROME

This clinical syndrome is characterised by the sudden onset of haematuria, proteinuria, oliguria and hypertension. Not all features may be present simultaneously. In some cases the condition develops 7–20 days after a streptococcal infection (Group A beta-haemolytic *Streptococcus* of types 1, 2, 4, 12, 18, 25, 49, 55, 57 and 60 have been implicated) or other infection (*Staphylococcus*, *Pneumococcus* and *Salmonella* have been described). The infection may be minor or pass unnoticed. There is no relationship between severity of infection and the probability of developing acute nephritis.

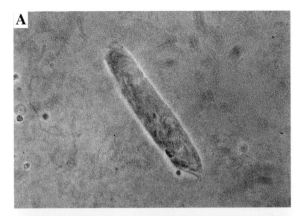

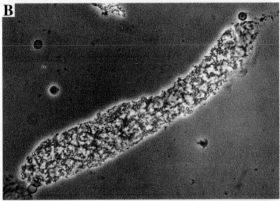

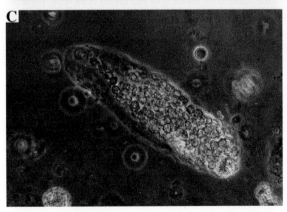

Fig. 11.13 Urinary casts. Ⓐ hyaline cast; Ⓑ granular cast; Ⓒ red cell cast. Casts are demonstrated using phase contrast microscopy.

Clinical features

Characteristically the urine is slightly discoloured with a smoky appearance, but occasionally it is red. Proteinuria is usually non-selective and seldom exceeds 3 g/day. Microscopic examination of the urinary deposit reveals red cells, leucocytes, epithelial cells and granular casts. Erythrocyte casts are characteristic and are formed in the tubules by binding of red blood cells with Tamm–Horsfall mucoprotein. In the early stages, the urine is concentrated. The GFR is usually transiently reduced and serum creatinine and blood urea increased. During the acute phase, there is evidence of complement activation by the classical pathway. Acute phase proteins may be increased. In favourable cases complete recovery occurs. This is likely in the majority of children. The acute manifestations lessen in the course of 3 to 4 days, and the temperature, pulse and blood pressure return to normal. Diuresis occurs, and oedema, haematuria and the number of casts in the urine diminish. Small amounts of blood and protein may persist in the urine for weeks or months.

Management

Patients should be advised to rest until the acute phase of the illness has resolved. Any underlying infection, particularly a streptococcal throat infection, should be treated as appropriate. Previously, long-term antibiotic therapy was given, but this is no longer considered necessary. If there is renal functional impairment, this should be managed by dietary and fluid control, as detailed later in this chapter (pp. 628–631). Dialysis may be required transiently. Oedema requires diuretic therapy, and hypertension should be controlled to maintain a blood pressure within the normal range.

NEPHROTIC SYNDROME

The nephrotic syndrome is characterised by heavy proteinuria, hypoproteinaemia and generalised oedema. Normally, only a small amount of protein crosses the glomerular capillary wall, and this is reabsorbed in the proximal tubules. When the permeability of the glomerular capillary wall is increased by glomerular inflammation, change in surface charge and alteration in pore size, the amount of protein presented to the tubules exceeds their reabsorptive capacity and protein spills over into the urine. Protein reabsorbed by the tubules is catabolised, and therefore the net loss of protein is always greater than can be accounted for by the measured urinary loss. If the loss of protein exceeds the rate of hepatic synthesis, hypoproteinaemia will ensue. This reduces the plasma colloid osmotic pressure. As a result there is accumulation of fluid in the extravascular space, due to a reduction in the return of extravascular extracellular fluid to the vascular space. Hypovolaemia then leads to stimulation of the renin-angiotensin-aldosterone system and other mechanisms causing increased tubular reabsorption of sodium, and to an increase in AVP secretion resulting in increased water reabsorption. Not all patients have a reduced plasma volume, suggesting that there may be other intrarenal mechanisms, such as redistribution of intrarenal blood flow, to account for sodium and water retention. However, conservation of sodium and water by the kidney, in the presence of a low plasma colloid osmotic pressure, results in further accumulation of fluid in the interstitial spaces (see p. 598, Ch. 10). The plasma albumin and the total plasma proteins are greatly reduced. Lipoproteins and other proteins such as fibrinogen and other coagulation factors are increased, while antithrombin 3 is lost in the urine. This may help to account for the increased incidence of atherosclerosis and thrombosis in patients with the nephrotic syndrome. Plasma cholesterol is usually increased and the plasma may look milky due to an increase in fat and lipoproteins.

Clinical features

Patients present with gradually increasing generalised oedema which first involves subcutaneous tissue and later serous sacs. The face is characteristically pale and puffy. General health may remain good, but eventually is progressively impaired, with increased liability to infection of the oedematous tissues or serous cavities. Protein malnutrition may occur. The course and prognosis depends on the underlying renal lesion, which can only be determined by renal biopsy.

Management

This is directed at relief of oedema. Patients should be advised to take a 'no added salt' diet (80–100 mmol sodium). A high protein intake should no longer be advised. Increasing the plasma protein concentration will increase the amount of protein filtered by the glomerulus and therefore lost by catabolism and excretion. Moreover, in patients whose renal function is already impaired, there is evidence that an increased intake of protein is associated with hyperfiltration in the remaining nephrons, which may result in glomerulosclerosis and renal failure.

Diuretics are of great value when controlling oedema (see p. 599, Ch. 10). When oedema is mild, satisfactory diuresis may be obtained by using drugs acting on the early distal tubule, e.g. bendrofluazide 5–10 mg daily. They have the advantage of inducing a fairly gentle diuresis, so may be useful in patients who are working. In moderate oedema it is frequently necessary to start treatment with a loop diuretic, e.g. frusemide 80–120 mg daily, bumetanide 2–3 mg daily. These have the disadvantage that they induce a large diuresis rapidly, and some patients find that this renders them housebound for up to 4 hours after taking the drug. In severe oedema, a combination of drugs is frequently required because when there is a strong stimulus to retain sodium, it is essential to block sodium reabsorption at more than one site in the nephron. Frusemide inhibits reabsorption of sodium in the ascending limb of the loop of Henle, thereby delivering more sodium to the distal nephron. When there is marked secondary aldosteronism, much of this sodium will be reabsorbed in the collecting duct. Only when distally-acting agents such as spironolactone 100–200 mg/day or amiloride 5–10 mg daily have been added will effective diuresis occur. In a few patients, combined diuretic therapy with 3 drugs acting at different sites, e.g. frusemide, metolazone and spironolactone, is required. In patients who are profoundly oedematous, it may be necessary to give intravenous salt-poor albumin (20 g in 100 ml in 1 hour with frusemide 40 mg intravenously) to increase the plasma colloid osmotic pressure temporarily. When an oedema-free state has been achieved, patients can frequently maintain this on a much smaller dose of diuretic.

GLOMERULAR LESIONS RESULTING IN NEPHROTIC SYNDROME

- **Primary glomerulonephritis (GN)**
  Minimal change nephropathy
  Focal segmental glomerulosclerosis
  Membranous GN
  Proliferative GN—mesangial proliferative, focal proliferative
  Mesangiocapillary GN

- **Associated with systemic disease**
  Systemic lupus erythematosus
  Polyarteritis nodosa; microscopic polyarteritis; Wegener's granulomatosis
  Amyloidosis
  Diabetes mellitus

- **Associated with infection**
  Bacterial endocarditis
  Malaria
  Hepatitis B
  Syphilis

- **Associated with tumours**
  Carcinoma
  Hodgkin's disease
  Chronic lymphatic leukaemia

- **Associated with drugs***
  Penicillamine
  Captopril
  Gold, mercury
  Trimethadione, phenindione
  Heroin (contaminated)

* Many more have been reported, frequently as single cases

RECURRENT HAEMATURIA

Painless recurrent haematuria is most commonly confused with the acute glomerulonephritis syndrome. In recurrent haematuria, however, there is no latent period between the associated infection and appearance of macroscopic haematuria. In most patients, there are repeated episodes of frank haematuria usually appearing within 1 or 2 days of the development of a mucosal inflammatory illness. The macroscopic haematuria usually lasts for 2–3 days, and between episodes microscopic haematuria can often be detected. Proteinuria rarely exceeds 2 g/day. Hypertension and oliguria are uncommon. Recurrent haematuria occurs most commonly in young adults, and is most frequently associated with IgA nephropathy (see p. 639).

Recurrent haematuria is also a feature of the 'loin pain—haematuria syndrome'. This consists of episodes of recurrent haematuria associated with unilateral or bilateral loin pain. In some patients the haematuria is solely microscopic. It occurs most commonly in young adult women. On biopsy there may be slight mesangial cell increase, and deposition of the third component of complement (C3) may be seen in arterioles. The aetiology and pathogenesis are unknown. No treatment other than symptomatic measures is indicated. There is a risk of progressively increasing analgesic intake, which must be avoided. The condition does not cause renal failure.

HYPERTENSION

In some patients the finding of hypertension is the first indication of glomerular disease. In the absence of a typical acute glomerulonephritis syndrome this usually indicates long-standing glomerulonephritis and, not uncommonly, there is associated impairment of renal function.

ACUTE RENAL FAILURE

Acute renal failure (ARF) is characterised by an acute and usually reversible deterioration of renal function, which develops over a period of days or weeks, and results in uraemia. A marked reduction in urine volume is usual, but not invariable. Clinical features are determined by the underlying condition and by the rapidly developing uraemia, and patients may present complex problems of diagnosis and management. Many of the disorders giving rise to acute renal failure carry a high mortality, but if the patient survives, renal function usually returns to normal or near normal.

ACUTE RENAL FAILURE DUE TO PRERENAL DISORDER

Pathogenesis
The kidneys receive approximately 25% of the cardiac output at rest. If cardiac output is reduced, regional vasoconstriction occurs, limiting the blood flow to organs other than the heart and brain. Initially skin blood flow is diminished. This is followed by reduction in perfusion of the gastrointestinal tract and muscles. When the renal blood supply is restricted, glomerular filtration is reduced by selective cortical vasoconstriction, and oliguria results.

CLASSIFICATION OF ACUTE RENAL FAILURE

- **Prerenal ARF**: the kidneys are inadequately perfused and the GFR greatly diminished. This may be due to cardiac failure, vascular disease limiting renal blood flow, or underfilling of the vascular bed due to haemorrhage, severe fluid depletion or vasodilatation resulting from sepsis.
- **Renal** causes of ARF include diseases of the renal arterioles such as vasculitis or microangiopathic haemolytic states; rapidly progressive (crescentic) glomerulonephritis; injury to tubular cells (acute tubular necrosis) by toxins or ischaemia; intraluminal obstruction of nephrons from precipitation of crystals or protein; and acute interstitial nephritis due to infections or drug reactions.
- **Postrenal ARF** is caused by obstruction of the urinary tract at any point in its course.

Prompt identification of the cause of prerenal or postrenal ARF and institution of appropriate treatment will often restore renal function. The longer the period of inadequate perfusion or obstruction, the more likely it is that actual damage to kidney tissue will occur.

PRERENAL ACUTE RENAL FAILURE: THE MOST IMPORTANT CAUSES

- **Reduced circulation blood volume**
  Haemorrhage from any cause, including complications of pregnancy, trauma and gastrointestinal bleeding
  Loss of plasma as in burns and crushing injuries

  Sodium and water depletion:
  —from the gastrointestinal tract in severe vomiting, diarrhoea, acute intestinal obstruction, paralytic ileus, pancreatitis, fistulae
  —in urine due to excessive treatment with diuretics, diabetic ketoacidosis
  —from the skin due to sweating
- **Reduction of cardiac output and myocardial failure** (cardiogenic shock), or an **increase in the size of the vascular bed** (septicaemia)
- **Intravascular haemolysis**
- **Rhabdomyolysis** (breakdown of skeletal muscle), due to the toxic effects on the kidney of released globins
- **Diseases of the major renal vessels** which result in renal underperfusion—e.g. thrombosis of the arteries, occlusive embolus of the aorta or renal arteries, or aortic aneurysm.

Clinical features
Patients often present with marked reduction of blood pressure and signs of inadequate peripheral perfusion. However, renal vasoconstriction and prerenal ARF may occur in the absence of systemic hypotension. The cause of the circulatory disturbance is usually obvious, but

significant concealed blood loss can occur into the gastrointestinal tract, following trauma (particularly where there are fractures of the pelvis or femur) and into the uterus in concealed accidental haemorrhage. It is also difficult to assess the magnitude of the loss of intravascular fluid into tissues after crush injuries or in severe inflammatory dermatoses.

Management

The cause of the disorder must be established and corrected. When hypovolaemia or septicaemia is present, the circulation must be restored as rapidly as possible, by replacing blood, plasma or sodium and water as indicated and by judicious use of inotropic drugs. It is often necessary to monitor central venous or pulmonary wedge pressure to determine the rate of administration of fluid and/or inotropes. In severe cases with circulatory failure, more sophisticated monitoring is necessary to enable the cardiac output and systemic vascular resistance to be calculated.

Prognosis

Provided treatment is instituted early, restitution of renal blood flow is usually accompanied by a return of renal function. If oliguria persists in spite of restoration of the circulation to normal, then the structural changes of acute tubular necrosis (below) are likely to have developed. In a few cases, particularly those complicated by disseminated intravascular coagulation (p. 837), irreversible cortical necrosis may occur.

ACUTE RENAL FAILURE DUE TO INTRINSIC RENAL DISEASE

The most common intrinsic renal cause of acute renal failure is **acute tubular necrosis**. This is usually due to acute ischaemia, the effects of toxic agents such as drugs (p. 663) or bacterial endotoxins.

In addition, ARF sometimes develops in conditions which affect the intrarenal arteries and arterioles, such as vasculitis, accelerated hypertension and disseminated intravascular coagulation. A number of glomerular diseases also produce acute deterioration in renal function, particularly those which run a rapid course, such as crescentic nephritis or focal necrotising proliferative glomerulonephritis. Acute tubulo-interstitial nephritis (p. 631), often due to drugs, may cause ARF.

ACUTE TUBULAR NECROSIS

There are two varieties of acute tubular necrosis—the more common ischaemic type, and a type caused by toxins, either chemical or bacterial. Although the aetiology of acute ischaemic tubular necrosis varies, the common factor in all cases is a diminution in the supply of oxygen and essential nutrients to the metabolically active tubular cells. This results in reduction and subsequent cessation of cell function and patchy necrosis. Fortunately, tubular cells have the capacity to regenerate and to reform the basement membrane. Thus, providing the patient can be kept alive during the regeneration phase, kidney function usually returns to near normal values.

Pathogenesis

The initial insult causes disruption of the cell membrane, leading to intracellular anoxia and consequently to a rapid influx of calcium ions. This disturbs mitochondrial respiration, leading to anaerobic glycolysis and intracellular acidosis. If this process continues it causes denaturation of intracellular protein, lysosomal disruption and cell death. Small focal breaks in the tubular basement membrane then develop, and tubular contents escape into the interstitial tissue.

During shock, renal blood flow is greatly reduced. Measurements made during the established phase of acute renal failure (oliguric phase) indicate that when the circulation is restored in shocked patients, renal blood flow remains about 20% of normal. During the oliguric phase there is significant selective reduction in cortical blood flow. This is due in part to interstitial oedema, and in part to swelling of the endothelial cells of glomeruli and peritubular capillaries, resulting in an increase in vascular resistance. Cortical blood flow may be further reduced by local and systemic vasoconstrictors such as thromboxane, vasopressin, noradrenaline and angiotensin II. The effects of some of these are probably counter-balanced by the action of intrarenal vasodilator prostaglandins.

It is likely that all these mechanisms have some part to play in the pathogenesis of the oliguric phase, although their relative importance may vary depending on the nature of the primary insult.

After a period of about 10–20 days, renal function returns. There is often a transient diuretic phase during which the urine output increases rapidly and remains excessive for several days before returning to normal. This is due in part to dissipation of the normal medullary concentration gradient during the period of oliguria. Maintenance of the medullary gradient depends not only on tubular transport, but also on the continued delivery of filtrate to the ascending limb of the loop of Henle. Both factors are disturbed during the acute phase of ARF. The medullary concentration gradient is gradually 'washed out', and is not re-established until glomerular filtration and tubular function are at least partly restored. Not all patients exhibit the diuretic phase, which is to some extent dependent on the severity of the renal damage and the rate of recovery.

Pathology

The appearances depend on the stage of the illness. In established cases, the kidneys may be enlarged and the cortex paler than normal. Histologically the glomeruli appear relatively normal, although on electron microscopy there may be endothelial cell swelling and some fibrin deposition. The most obvious abnormality is the presence of scattered breaks in tubular basement membranes, sometimes associated with visible necrosis of associated tubular cells. Actual tubular cell necrosis is surprisingly insignificant, but many tubules are lined by swollen vacuolated cells. Late in the disorder, tubular epithelial cells appear flattened, and during the regenerative phase there may be evidence of mitotic activity. There is frequently interstitial oedema and infiltration with macrophages, plasma cells and a few polymorphs. In cases where the condition has been caused by drugs, the interstitial inflammatory infiltrate is more marked, and constitutes an acute tubulo-interstitial nephritis (p. 631).

Clinical features

These reflect the causal condition, together with features of rapidly developing uraemia. In many patients, there is an obvious underlying cause such as trauma or septicaemia. In the majority of patients the urine volume is reduced to between 50 and 500 ml daily. Anuria is rare (urine volume less than 50 ml daily), and often indicates acute urinary tract obstruction. In about 20% of cases the urine volume is normal or increased, but the quality is very poor due to a low GFR and a gross reduction of tubular function. Thus excretion is inadequate despite an apparently good urine output, the plasma urea and creatinine increase, and the clinical picture of uraemia develops. The rate at which the plasma urea and creatinine increase is determined by the rate of tissue breakdown. In patients who are suffering from severe infections or who have undergone major surgery or trauma, the daily increment in plasma urea usually exceeds 5 mmol/l.

Disturbances of water, electrolyte and acid-base balance arise as a consequence of loss of kidney function. Hyperkalaemia is common, particularly when there is massive tissue breakdown, haemolysis or metabolic acidosis. Since it predisposes to ventricular arrhythmias, it must be promptly controlled. Patients may present with dilutional hyponatraemia, having received inappropriate amounts of intravenous fluid, such as 5% dextrose, or having continued to drink freely despite oliguria. Metabolic acidosis develops unless there has been excessive vomiting or aspiration of gastric contents. Hypocalcaemia, due to reduced renal production of 1,25-dihydroxycholecalciferol, is common.

At first the patient may feel well, but after some days, features of uraemia appear. Initially these are anorexia, nausea and vomiting. Apathy is followed by mental confusion, and later muscular twitching, fits, drowsiness, coma and bleeding episodes occur. The respiratory rate is often increased, due to acidosis, pulmonary oedema or respiratory infection. Pulmonary oedema may result from administration of excessive amounts of fluids. There is also evidence that pulmonary capillary permeability is increased in uraemia, and in those patients who have had circulatory failure, damage to pulmonary capillaries also predisposes to the development of pulmonary oedema (adult respiratory distress syndrome, see p. 388). Anaemia, which is common, may be due to excessive blood loss, haemolysis or decreased erythropoiesis. Many patients have an increased bleeding tendency due to disordered platelet function and disturbances of the coagulation cascade. Gastrointestinal haemorrhage may occur, often late in the illness, from mucosal erosions throughout the length of the gastrointestinal tract. Severe infections often complicate the course of ARF because humoral and cellular immune mechanisms are depressed by uraemia.

Management

The principles are as follows:

Emergency resuscitative measures

Hyperkalaemia (plasma $K^+ > 6$ mmol/l) must be counter-acted and corrected to prevent life-threatening cardiac arrhythmia (see p. 596, Ch. 10). An ECG monitor should be connected, and reliable intravenous access in a large vein established. Calcium gluconate (10 ml 10%) should be given intravenously for its membrane-stabilising effect. Rapid reduction of plasma K^+ can be achieved by intravenous glucose (50 ml 50% dextrose). It is not necessary to add insulin unless the patient is known to have diabetes mellitus or becomes hyperglycaemic, and if insulin is given (12 units rapid acting insulin intravenously), a watch must be kept for subsequent hypoglycaemia. Correction of acidosis with intravenous sodium bicarbonate will also reduce the plasma potassium. Exchange resins (e.g. calcium resonium 30 g) can be given orally and/or rectally. Their action is somewhat delayed, and they are thus of use primarily as prophylaxis. The plasma potassium should be rechecked after approximately 30 minutes, and it may be necessary to repeat the above measures. Once the plasma potassium is less than 6 mmol/l, an infusion of 20% dextrose (30 ml/h) should be maintained to promote continued shift of potassium into cells and prevent rebound hyperkalaemia. Dialysis will be required as definitive treatment in many cases (see below).

The circulating blood volume must be corrected by prompt transfusion with appropriate fluids. This often requires monitoring of central venous or pulmonary wedge pressure. Patients who present with severe pulmonary oedema usually require haemodialysis or peritoneal dialysis to remove sodium and water.

Determination of the cause of ARF

In many cases the underlying cause is obvious. When this is not the case a wide range of investigations, including renal biopsy, may be needed to establish the diagnosis.

General management of the oliguric phase

In established acute renal failure, the main aims are to control fluid and electrolyte balance, maintain nutrition, control the disordered chemistry and protect the patient from infection. Patients with severe acute renal failure are seriously ill and require skilled nursing. Particular attention must be paid to the care of the skin and the mouth, and to preventing infection of in-dwelling intravascular lines. Plasma urea, creatinine and electrolytes should be estimated, and cultures of blood, urine and wounds carried out regularly. Great care must be exercised in the use of drugs (see p. 664). In many cases some form of dialysis will be required.

(i) **Fluid and electrolyte balance**. Following initial resuscitation, the patient should be maintained on a daily fluid intake which equals the urine output, plus an additional 500 ml to balance the difference between insensible loss and water of oxidation. Febrile patients require an increased allowance. As no electrolytes are lost, the intake of these substances should be minimal. Should abnormal losses of fluid occur, as in diarrhoea, additional fluid and electrolytes will be required. If possible the patient should be weighed daily. Large changes in body weight, or the development of either oedema or signs of water and electrolyte depletion, indicate the need for a reappraisal of water and electrolyte intake.

(ii) **Protein and energy**. In patients in whom it is hoped to avoid dialysis, dietary protein is restricted to about 40 g/day. Attempts are made to suppress endogenous protein catabolism to a minimum, by giving as much energy as possible in the form of fat and carbohydrate. For this purpose, a diet restricted in protein and electrolyte content may be supplemented by preparations containing glucose polymers. Patients treated by dialysis may have a more liberal intake of nitrogen (70 g protein daily, 10–12 g nitrogen).

In some patients who cannot maintain an adequate calorie intake, liquid feeding via a nasogastric tube may be helpful. In the presence of severe vomiting, or if bowel integrity or function are disrupted, enteral intake should be stopped and parenteral nutrition given. In hypercatabolic patients it may be necessary to resort to parenteral nutrition in order to maintain a suitable intake of energy and nitrogen. This may involve giving a greater volume than would be required to maintain fluid balance, and consequently more frequent dialysis or haemofiltration may be necessary.

Recovery phase

After approximately 7–20 days, renal function returns. In a number of patients a diuretic phase develops, when the urine output is frequently 3–5 litres daily. This usually persists for 3–4 days. During this time the concentration of blood urea tends to remain constant, whereas the creatinine may fall slowly. Sufficient fluid must be given to replace the loss of water in the urine. Intravenous fluids are frequently required. Supplements of sodium chloride and sodium bicarbonate may be needed during the diuretic phase, to compensate for increased urinary loss. Potassium chloride may also be required. After a few days the urine volume returns to normal as the concentrating mechanism is restored. This is associated with a gradual return of the ability to conserve sodium and potassium and regenerate bicarbonate. The blood urea and serum creatinine return to normal and the patient can resume a normal diet.

Prognosis

The high mortality from acute tubular necrosis has been greatly reduced by the measures described above. Prog-

DIALYSIS TREATMENT—INDICATIONS, OPTIONS, TECHNIQUES

INDICATIONS FOR RENAL REPLACEMENT THERAPY IN ARF INCLUDE:

- **Increased plasma urea or creatinine concentration**. In general, a plasma urea greater than 30 mmol/l and creatinine greater than 600 μmol/l are undesirable, but much depends on factors such as the rate of biochemical deterioration and the risks of dialysis for the patient involved.
- **Hyperkalaemia**. While this can usually be controlled by medical measures as above in the short term, dialysis is often required for definitive control.
- **Fluid overload** not controlled by fluid restriction and diuretics.
- **Uraemic pericarditis** (uncommon in ARF).

THE PRINCIPAL OPTIONS FOR RENAL REPLACEMENT ARE:

- Haemodialysis
- Continuous arterio-venous or veno-venous haemofiltration
- Peritoneal dialysis

INTERMITTENT TECHNIQUES

HAEMODIALYSIS

Although continuous haemofiltration techniques as outlined below are being used increasingly in the management of ARF, haemodialysis (HD) is still the principal treatment modality in most renal units.

(i) Vascular access

It is necessary to maintain an extra-corporeal circulation for HD. Two principal techniques are used:

- **double-lumen catheters placed in major veins**. Veins accessed include the internal jugular, subclavian, and the femoral. Lifespan of these catheters is often limited, due to thrombosis or infection.
- **Scribner shunts**. These consist of teflon tips and siliconised rubber tubing placed to connect an artery and a vein, at the ankle or wrist. The tubing is then separated for connection to the dialyser.

(ii) Anticoagulation

Haemodialysis machines are equipped to infuse **heparin** at a rate sufficient to prevent clotting of the extracorporeal circuit. The efficiency of anticoagulation is monitored by the Activated Clotting Time (ACT). It has been claimed that the use of **prostacyclin** for anticoagulation is associated with less risk of bleeding on dialysis, and many units use this in selected patients.

(iii) Dialysis prescription

Most patients can be treated by 3–4 hours of haemodialysis, either daily in catabolic patients, or on alternate days. Dialysis regimes are adjusted to maintain a pre-dialysis urea concentration less than 30 mmol/l, adequate control of potassium and phosphate, and normal ECF volume status.

HAEMOFILTRATION

This technique involves the rapid removal and replacement of 12–20 litres of plasma ultrafiltrate over 3–4 hours, using an artificial membrane with a very high ultrafiltration capacity, on a daily or alternate-day basis. The fluid removed is replaced by haemofiltration fluid (e.g. Haemafiltrasol). It is claimed that this technique induces less circulatory instability than haemodialysis.

CONTINUOUS TECHNIQUES

HAEMOFILTRATION

This includes **continuous veno-venous haemofiltration (CVVH)** and **continuous arterio-venous haemofiltration (CAVH)**. These systems cause less haemodynamic disturbance than conventional haemodialysis.

CVVH is pump-driven, allowing a reliable extracorporeal circulation. Most patients are controlled by removal and replacement of 1 litre of filtrate per hour.

In **CAVH** the circuit is driven by the arteriovenous pressure difference. Poor filtration rates and clotting of the filter may result from low arterial pressure and/or elevated central venous pressure.

PERITONEAL DIALYSIS

This has been supplanted in most centres by the techniques outlined above. It is less efficient than haemodialysis, and seldom achieves good biochemical control in catabolic patients. It is not feasible after recent abdominal surgery, but can be useful in patients with cardiovascular instability, e.g. after cardiac surgery. A trocar and cannula system is used for acute peritoneal access, and 500 ml volumes of peritoneal dialysis fluid (e.g. Dineal) are infused and drained cyclically. Flow can be regulated manually or by an automatic cycler. Cloudy effluent indicates the development of peritonitis, in which case the catheter should be removed immediately.

nosis depends on the speed and efficiency with which these are put into operation, on the prompt recognition and effective treatment of complications, and on the nature and severity of the causal disorder. In cases of uncomplicated acute renal failure, such as those due to simple haemorrhage or drugs, the mortality is now negligible even when dialysis is required. In severe renal failure, complicated by serious infection and functional failure of multiple organs, mortality is still 50–70%. The outcome is determined by the severity of the underlying disorder and by complications, rather than by the renal failure itself.

Other causes of intrinsic acute renal failure

When acute renal failure arises as a result of renal disease other than acute tubular necrosis, the clinical picture is that of the underlying condition, with features of acute uraemia. Frequently the diagnosis is not immediately obvious and renal biopsy must be performed to define the nature of the pathology. Management is along the

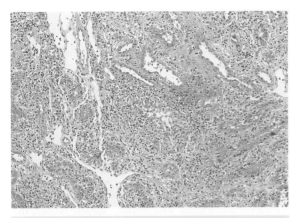

Fig. 11.14 Interstitial nephritis. Widespread interstitial infiltrate of inflammatory cells producing considerable destruction of normal architecture.

lines already discussed, but in addition specific treatment of the underlying renal disease may be required. Thus corticosteroids, immunosuppressive drugs and rarely plasma exchange may be of value in acute renal failure due to vasculitis and crescentic glomerulonephritis (p. 642). Control of blood pressure is critical when acute renal failure is due to accelerated hypertension (p. 269).

Acute tubulo-interstitial nephritis is a well-recognised cause of acute renal failure. It results most commonly from hypersensitivity to drugs such as penicillin, ampicillin, sulphonamides or rifampicin. Other manifestations of hypersensitivity, such as fever, arthralgia, rashes, marrow depression, eosinophilia and disturbance of liver function, may be present. Renal biopsy usually shows an acute tubulo-interstitial nephritis associated with inflammatory cells, including eosinophils (Fig. 11.14). Most cases resolve if the drug is discontinued.

ACUTE RENAL FAILURE DUE TO POSTRENAL DISEASE

Acute renal failure may result from obstruction at any point in the urinary tract (p. 655). In the presence of two functioning kidneys, ureteric obstruction causes uraemia only when it is bilateral. The diagnosis may be suggested by a history of previous urinary symptoms, such as loin pain, haematuria, renal colic, nocturia or difficulty in micturition. Often the onset is clinically silent, and the cause of obstruction discovered only after appropriate investigation. In contrast to the oliguria associated with tubular necrosis, anuria is common, and suggests an obstructive cause.

In patients with anuria, ultrasound examination of both kidneys and ureters should be done as soon as possible. When pelvic or ureteric dilatation is found, percutaneous nephrostomy can be undertaken to decompress the urinary system (p. 656). Dialysis can thereby usually be avoided. Antegrade pyelography may reveal the cause of the obstruction. Alternatively, cystoscopy and retrograde pyelography can be done.

In a number of instances obstruction is caused by a malignant pelvic tumour, such as carcinoma of the cervix or of the recto-sigmoid junction, which may be palpable on rectal or vaginal examination. Unfortunately the disease is often so advanced that active intervention is inadvisable.

When the obstruction has been relieved and the blood chemistry has returned to near normal, the underlying cause must be defined and treated (p. 656).

CHRONIC RENAL FAILURE

Chronic renal failure is irreversible deterioration in renal function. The ensuing impairment of the excretory, metabolic and endocrine functions of the kidney leads to the development of the clinical syndrome of uraemia.

CLINICAL FEATURES OF URAEMIA

- Anaemia
- Metabolic bone disease (renal osteodystrophy)
- Neuropathy
- Myopathy
- Endocrine abnormalities
- Hypertension and atherosclerosis
- Acidosis
- Susceptibility to infection

These patients usually have bilateral small kidneys. A presumptive diagnosis of progressive glomerulonephritis is made on the basis of significant proteinuria, haematuria and hypertension in the absence of any other obvious cause of renal failure. Renal biopsy is usually inadvisable because of the risk of bleeding, the difficulty in determining the precise histology in small contracted kidneys, and the fact that treatment is unlikely to improve renal function significantly.

The social and economic consequences of chronic renal failure are considerable. In Britain approximately 70 new patients per million of the adult population are accepted for long-term dialysis treatment each year. Introduction of dialysis and transplantation has transformed the outlook for such patients, and these techniques must be regarded as among the most significant medical advances of this century.

Aetiology

Chronic renal failure may be caused by any condition which destroys the normal structure and function of the

Table 11.2   Aetiology of chronic renal failure

Congenital and inherited diseases
Polycystic kidney disease (infantile
  or adult)
Alport's syndrome
Congenital hypoplasia
	Interstitial disease
	Chronic infective interstitial
	  nephritis (chronic
	  pyelonephritis)
	Vesico-ureteric reflux
	Tuberculosis

Vascular disease Arteriosclerosis Vasculitis (PAN, SLE, scleroderma)	Analgesic nephropathy Nephrocalcinosis Schistosomiasis Unknown origin

Glomerular disease
Proliferative GN
Crescentic GN
Membranous GN
Mesangiocapillary GN
Glomerulosclerosis
Secondary GN
  (PAN, SLE, amyloidosis,
  diabetic glomerulosclerosis)
	Obstructive uropathy
	Calculus
	Retroperitoneal fibrosis
	Prostatic hypertrophy
	Pelvic tumours
	Other causes (see Table 11.5)

SIGNS AND SYMPTOMS OF URAEMIA

- Vague ill-health
- Generalised weakness and lack of energy
- Breathlessness on exertion
- Anorexia
- Nausea and vomiting, particularly in mornings
- Disordered intestinal motility
- Headaches
- Visual disturbances
- Pruritus
- Pallor
- Pigmentation
- Loss of libido

kidney (Table 11.2). In many patients the condition progresses insidiously over a number of years and frequently it is impossible to determine the nature of the underlying renal disease.

Pathogenesis

Disturbances in water, electrolyte and acid-base balance undoubtedly contribute to the clinical picture in patients with chronic renal failure, but the exact pathogenesis of the clinical syndrome of uraemia is unknown. Almost any substance present in abnormal concentration in the plasma has been suspected of being an 'uraemic toxin'. It is most likely that the syndrome is caused by accumulation in body fluids of a number of substances, among which must be included phosphate, parathyroid hormone, urea, creatinine, guanidine, phenols and indoles.

Clinical features

In the early stages of the disease, the patient may be asymptomatic and the existence of renal insufficiency may be revealed by discovery of proteinuria, anaemia, hypertension or a raised blood urea during routine examination. When renal function deteriorates slowly it is not uncommon for patients to remain asymptomatic until the GFR is 15 ml/min or less. Subsequently, because of the widespread effects of progressive renal failure, symptoms and signs are referable to almost every system and many patients present with complaints which at first sight may not suggest their renal origin.

None of these symptoms alone is indicative of underlying renal disease, but the occurrence of more than one should suggest the possibility of renal failure. The rate of progression to end-stage renal failure is very variable but inevitably as the disease advances, renal function deteriorates and uraemia increases, the patient looks

more ill and the anaemia becomes more severe. With the exception of those who develop cardiac failure, the patients are usually not only free from oedema, but may exhibit signs of water and sodium depletion. The skin and tongue are dry and the blood pressure may decline from its previous high value. Acidosis contributes to the breathlessness, and respirations are deep (Kussmaul's respiration). Later, hiccoughs, pruritus, muscular twitching, fits, drowsiness and coma ensue.

Anaemia

Anaemia is common and to some extent reflects the severity of uraemia. Several factors contribute, including (1) a reduced dietary intake of iron and other haematinics due to anorexia and dietary restrictions, (2) impaired intestinal absorption of iron, (3) diminished erythropoiesis due to toxic effects of uraemia on marrow precursor cells, (4) reduced red cell survival and (5) increased blood loss due to capillary fragility and poor platelet function. Plasma erythropoietin is usually within the normal range and thus inappropriately low for the degree of anaemia. In patients with polycystic kidneys, anaemia is less severe—possibly because the large kidneys produce more erythropoietin.

Management involves correction of any iron and vitamin deficiency. Some patients will respond to oral iron supplements, and body iron stores (serum iron, iron-binding capacity, and ferritin) should be checked before additional treatment is considered. Human recombinant erythropoietin has been shown to be effective in correcting anaemia. It is usually given to patients with end-stage chronic renal failure who have haemoglobin concentrations of less than 8 g/dl, or who are symptomatic of anaemia. The best route of administration is now thought to be by subcutaneous injection. A starting dose of 50 U/kg twice weekly is usual, and the dose is titrated to achieve an increase in haemoglobin concentration of not more than 2 g/dl per month, with a target figure of around 10 g/dl. The treatment is expensive, and should be reserved for patients likely to benefit in terms of mobility and quality of life. Complications of treatment include an increase in blood pressure, which in a few cases has been associated with hypertensive encephalopathy. Initiation or adjustment of antihypertensive medication is often necessary. There is also an increase in blood coagulability, and a particular watch must be kept for thrombosis of the arterio-venous fistulae used for haemodialysis.

Renal osteodystrophy

This metabolic bone disease which accompanies uraemia consists of a mixture of osteomalacia, hyperparathyroid bone disease (osteitis fibrosa) (Fig. 11.15), osteoporosis and osteosclerosis. Osteomalacia results from diminished activity of the renal 1-hydroxylase enzyme, with consequent failure to convert cholecalciferol to its active metabolite 1,25-dihydroxycholecalciferol. A deficiency of the latter leads to diminished intestinal absorption of calcium, hypocalcaemia and reduction in the calcification of osteoid. Osteitis fibrosa results from secondary hyperparathyroidism. The parathyroid glands are stimulated by the low plasma calcium, and also by hyperphosphataemia. In some patients tertiary or autonomous

hyperparathyroidism develops. Osteoporosis occurs in many patients, possibly related to mild malnutrition. Osteosclerosis is seen mainly in the sacral area, at the base of the skull and in the vertebrae; the cause of this unusual reaction is not known.

Generalised myopathy

Generalised myopathy is due to a combination of poor nutrition, hyperparathyroidism, vitamin D deficiency and disorders of electrolyte metabolism. Muscle cramps and the 'restless leg syndrome' are common.

Neuropathy

There is a demyelination of medullated fibres, the longer fibres being involved earlier. Sensory neuropathy may cause paraesthesiae and motor neuropathy may present as foot drop. Development of uraemic autonomic neuropathy may in part explain development of disorders of gastrointestinal motility and postural hypotension in the absence of sodium and water depletion. Clinical manifestations of neuropathy appear very late in the course

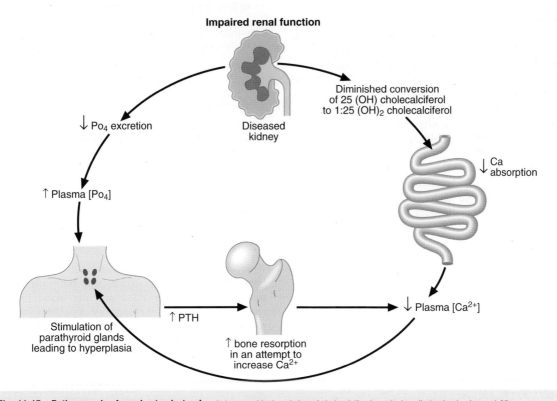

Fig. 11.15   Pathogenesis of renal osteodystrophy. A decreased hydroxylation of cholecalciferol results in a diminution in plasma 1,25-dihydroxycholecalciferol. The effect of this is to reduce intestinal absorption of calcium resulting in a reduction in the plasma calcium with a consequent stimulation of the parathyroid glands to increase PTH secretion. The increased PTH has an effect on bone by causing increased osteoclastic activity with consequent bone resorption. In addition, the diminished 1,25-dihydroxycholecalciferol results in impaired mineralisation of bone. The net result is bone which exhibits increased osteoclastic activity and increased osteoid as a consequence of decreased mineralisation.

of chronic renal failure. They improve, and may, indeed resolve, when dialysis is started.

Endocrine function

A number of hormonal abnormalities may be present in the female. Amenorrhoea is common. In both sexes there is loss of libido presumably due to the associated hyperprolactinaemia (p. 683). Thyroid function is diminished, although clinical hypothyroidism is uncommon. Uraemia is frequently mistaken for hypothyroidism.

Cardiovascular disorders

Hypertension develops in approximately 80% of patients with chronic renal failure. It must be controlled, as it causes further vascular damage, thus increasing renal failure. Atherosclerosis is common due to abnormalities of lipid and carbohydrate metabolism, and may be accelerated by hypertension. Vascular calcification may develop, and be sufficiently severe to cause inadequate perfusion of the limbs. Pericarditis is very common in untreated end-stage renal failure.

Acidosis

Declining renal function is associated with metabolic acidosis (p. 615) which is commonly asymptomatic. Nevertheless, wherever possible, the plasma bicarbonate should be maintained above 18 mmol/l by giving sodium bicarbonate supplements. The dose can only be determined by clinical trial, but it is appropriate to commence with 1 g 8-hourly and increase as required up to a total of 12–15 g daily. The dose may be limited by the adverse effect of the sodium, which may induce hypertension and/or oedema. In such patients it is worth considering calcium carbonate (up to 9 g daily) as an alternative. Sustained acidosis results in protons being buffered in bone, thereby aggravating the uraemic osteodystrophy.

Infection

Both cellular and humoral immunity are impaired, and thus there is increased susceptibility to infection. Urinary tract infections are very common and must be treated promptly, as they may lead to further destruction of functioning renal tissue.

Management

The management of chronic renal failure falls into three distinct parts:

- Investigations to determine the nature of the underlying renal disease and to detect any reversible factors which are exacerbating the uraemic state (see information box).

- Measures designed to limit adverse effects of loss of renal function and, when possible, to prevent further renal damage.
- In patients with progressive destruction of renal tissue, there comes a point when supportive measures in the form of either dialysis or transplantation are required.

When the patient first presents, a detailed history and physical examination are required, with particular attention being paid to the cardiovascular and genito-urinary systems. It is important to consider all possible underlying causes, and both family history and drug history are important. Wherever possible, the nature of the underlying disease should be determined by undertaking appropriate biochemical, radiological and biopsy investigations. The degree of functional impairment should be assessed and the extent of any systemic complications documented. In every case a search must be made for reversible factors, correction of which will result in improved renal function.

REVERSIBLE FACTORS IN URAEMIA

- Hypertension
- Urinary tract infection
- Urinary tract obstruction
- Reduced renal perfusion:
  bilateral renal artery stenosis
  sodium and water depletion
  haemorrhage
  cardiogenic shock
- Septicaemia
- Infections which increase urea production
- Nephrotoxic medications

In patients with established irreversible renal failure a number of measures can be undertaken which will reduce symptoms and may slow the progression to terminal renal failure.

Hypertension and cardiac failure

Hypertension must be controlled, but over-zealous treatment must be avoided and the blood pressure reduced gradually. In the majority of patients, the best results are obtained by maintaining the diastolic pressure in the region of 90 mmHg. Cardiac failure should be treated along the usual lines, great care being taken to modify the dose of any drugs used (p. 664).

Diet

When the serum creatinine consistently exceeds 300 μmol/l, dietary protein should be restricted in the adult to approximately 40 g daily, with an adequate intake of carbohydrate (250 g) and fat (60 g) to provide an energy value of at least 1700 kcal. It is not advisable to reduce the dietary protein intake further except in those patients who are unsuitable for long-term dialysis, who should receive 20 g/d.

Fluid

The daily intake will depend on the nature of the underlying disease. Because of the impaired concentrating power, a large volume of urine, about 2.5 l/d, is needed to excrete end-products of metabolism, and a fluid intake of 3 l/d is desirable. Fluid restriction is necessary only when the GFR is less than 5 ml/min or cardiac failure is present. Patients with cystic disease, obstructive uropathy or rare tubular lesions who have marked polyuria will require additional fluid.

Electrolytes

In the absence of oedema, cardiac failure or hypertension, sodium restriction is contraindicated. Excessive loss of sodium in the urine (salt-losing nephropathy) occurs in some forms of renal failure but not in chronic glomerular disease. Patients with salt-losing nephropathy readily become depleted of sodium and water, particularly if they are vomiting. When this occurs, fluid and electrolytes must be given intravenously. The volume and nature of the fluid required depends on the severity of the sodium and water depletion (p. 596) and the degree of acidosis (p. 603). Thereafter oral supplements of sodium chloride and sodium bicarbonate are usually required (p. 596). Generally in patients with glomerular diseases and/or hypertension, a diet containing about 80–100 mmol of sodium per day ('no added salt' diet) should be prescribed. When the creatinine clearance has fallen to less than 10 ml/min, potassium restriction is often required, and is achieved by advising the patient to avoid high potassium foods (e.g. bananas, tomatoes, coffee, chocolate, etc.).

Osteodystrophy

The plasma calcium and phosphate concentrations should be kept as near to normal as possible. Hypocalcaemia can be corrected by giving 0.25–1 μg/d of 1α hydroxycholecalciferol, a synthetic analogue of vitamin D. The plasma calcium must be monitored regularly and the dose adjusted to avoid hypercalcaemia. Hyperphosphataemia is common, and the plasma phosphate can be reduced by the dietary restriction of foods with a high phosphate content (milk, cheese, eggs) and the use of phosphate-binding drugs such as calcium carbonate 500 mg with each meal. Aluminium hydroxide also has a phosphate-binding effect (aluminium hydroxide capsules [Alucap] 300–600 mg before each meal). To prevent aluminium toxicity, the dose of aluminium hydroxide should be kept to a minimum and should only

be administered immediately before meals. Hyperparathyroid bone disease responds well to such measures, but in severe osteitis fibrosa, parathyroidectomy is usually indicated. Osteomalacia is frequently resistant, presumably because of some other inhibitory factors acting on the bone calcification site. The osteoporotic and osteosclerotic components of renal osteodystrophy have no satisfactory treatment.

Replacement of renal function

The excretory function of the kidney can be partially replaced by dialysis. This technique, however, does not replace the endocrine and metabolic functions, which can only be achieved by successful renal transplantation. The best results are obtained by an integrated approach to management, using the most appropriate form of therapy—haemodialysis, continuous ambulatory peritoneal dialysis or transplantation—for the patient, depending on the clinical circumstances present.

Haemodialysis

The introduction of regular intermittent haemodialysis has prolonged the lives of many patients with chronic renal failure. Haemodialysis should be started when, despite adequate medical treatment, the symptoms of uraemia have become troublesome, preferably before the patient has developed serious consequences of uraemia. An arteriovenous fistula should be formed, usually in the forearm, when the serum creatinine is consistently in excess of 600 μmol/l so that there will be time for this to develop prior to being required. Due to the increased blood pressure in the veins from the fistula, there is distension and thickening of the vein wall (arterialisation) which allows the repetitive insertion of needles for vascular access for haemodialysis. Once the patient is symptomatic, usually with a creatinine in the region of 1000 μmol/l, regular haemodialysis is commenced. Haemodialysis is usually carried out for 3–5 hours 3 times weekly, and some patients are trained to carry out their treatment at home. Most patients notice a gradual reduction of their uraemic symptoms during the first 6 weeks of treatment. Serum creatinine and blood urea do not return to normal. Anaemia, although improved, persists, and osteodystrophy may progress. Nevertheless, many patients lead relatively normal and active lives, and prolonged survival in excess of 20 years is now regularly reported.

Continuous ambulatory peritoneal dialysis

Continuous ambulatory peritoneal dialysis (CAPD) is a form of long-term dialysis involving insertion of a permanent intraperitoneal catheter into the abdominal cavity. Normally 2 litres of sterile isotonic dialysis fluid are introduced and left for a period of approximately

6 hours. The fluid is then drained and fresh dialysis fluid introduced. This cycle is repeated 4 times daily, during which time the patient is fully mobile and able to undertake normal daily tasks. It is particularly useful in young children, in elderly patients with cardiovascular instability and in patients with diabetes mellitus. Its long-term use may be limited by episodes of peritonitis, but many patients have now been treated for periods in excess of 10 years without serious complications.

Renal transplantation

This offers the possibility of restoring normal kidney function and thereby correcting the many metabolic abnormalities of uraemia. The graft is usually taken from a cadaver donor or from a sibling or a parent. ABO (blood group) compatibility is essential, and it is customary to select donor kidneys on the basis of HLA (Human Leucocyte Antigen) compatibility. Results of transplantation have improved significantly in the past few years. The 3-year graft survival is now in the region of 70–80%, while 3-year patient survival is approximately 90%.

Long-term immunosuppressive therapy is required. Many therapeutic regimens have been used, but the most common involves a combination of prednisolone and cyclosporin A. Prednisolone is commenced at a dose of 60 mg daily, reducing over 10 days to 30 mg daily and eventually after approximately 3–4 months to 10–15 mg daily. Immediately post-transplant, cyclosporin is commenced at a dose of 10 mg/kg daily in two divided doses 12 hours apart. The dose is gradually reduced in the following 3 months to 3–6 mg/kg daily. There is concern about the long-term nephrotoxicity of cyclosporin, and some centres routinely convert patients to therapy with prednisolone and azathioprine 6 months post-transplant. Azathioprine is usually given in a dose of 2 mg/kg daily, but this may require reduction if there is any evidence of marrow suppression.

Immunosuppression is associated with an increased incidence of infections, particularly opportunistic infections, and a greatly increased incidence of malignant neoplasms, especially of skin. Approximately 50% of patients will have some skin malignancy by 15 years post-transplant. Nonetheless, transplantation does offer the best hope of complete rehabilitation and is the most cost-effective of all the options.

Prognosis

Unless some form of supportive therapy such as dialysis or transplantation is available, chronic renal failure is eventually fatal. When the serum creatinine persistently exceeds 300 μmol/l there is usually progressive deterioration in renal function, irrespective of aetiology. The rate of deterioration is very variable from patient to

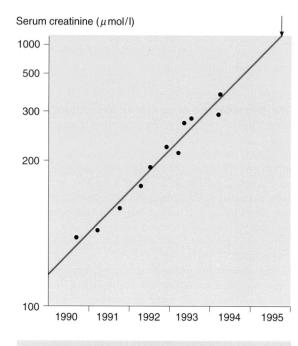

Fig. 11.16 Logarithmic plot of serum creatinine against time in progressive renal failure. Serial plasma creatinine estimations demonstrating a steady deterioration in renal function over a four-year period and projecting forward to indicate that a serum creatinine of 1000 μmol/l is likely to be achieved in mid 1995. At this point renal replacement therapy is likely to be required.

patient. This is in part related to the aetiology and to development of hypertension, but it is relatively constant for any particular patient. A plot of the logarithm of the serum creatinine concentration against time allows the physician to determine when the serum creatinine will reach a value in the region of 1000 μmol/l and dialysis will be required. Such a plot will also detect any unexpected worsening of the renal failure (Fig. 11.16).

Information about the long-term prognosis for patients on dialysis or following transplantation is limited because these techniques have been available only for the past 30 years, and technology is changing rapidly. Nevertheless, dialysis and transplantation can be considered as highly effective forms of treatment, with a 5-year survival of approximately 80% for home haemodialysis, 65% with a transplanted kidney, 55% for hospital haemodialysis and 45% for CAPD. These figures are not directly comparable because of patient selection and the fact that many older patients and those with systemic disease (e.g. diabetes mellitus) are treated by CAPD. However, they can be used as a guide and indicate how the outlook of end-stage renal disease is very much better than in many other potentially fatal diseases.

FURTHER READING

Cameron J S 1990 Proteinuria and progression in human glomerular diseases. American Journal of Nephrology 10, Suppl 1: 81–87

Carome M A et al 1992 Nephrotic syndrome in adults. A diagnostic and management challenge. Postgraduate Medicine 92: 209–215

England B K, Mitch W E 1993 Toxins versus abnormal cell metabolism in the pathophysiology of chronic renal failure. Contributions to Nephrology 102: 48–58

Guignard J P et al 1993 Acute renal failure. Critical Care Medicine 21 (9 Suppl): S349–351

Mehta R L 1994 Therapeutic alternatives to renal replacement for critically ill patients in acute renal failure. Seminars in Nephrology. 14: 64–82

GLOMERULAR DISEASES

The term glomerulonephritis signifies glomerular inflammation, and can be considered as primary when the major problem appears to start in the glomerulus, and secondary when involvement is part of a systemic disease (Table 11.3). This distinction, while convenient, is somewhat artificial, as primary glomerulonephritis may well have systemic effects, and it is not uncommon in certain systemic diseases for the glomerular involvement to be the initial clinical feature.

The classification of glomerulonephritis was in the past confused because glomerular diseases were identified by clinical presentation. The introduction of percutaneous renal biopsy provided a detailed histological

Table 11.3 Glomerular diseases

PRIMARY

Minimal change nephropathy
Proliferative glomerulonephritis
  Mesangial
  Diffuse endocapillary
  Focal
  IgA nephropathy
  Mesangiocapillary Type I (subendothelial)
                    Type II (dense deposit)
  Crescentic (Goodpasture's syndrome)
  Membranous glomerulonephritis
  Focal segmental glomerulosclerosis

SECONDARY

Common	Uncommon
Systemic lupus erythematosus	Pre-eclampsia
Polyarteritis (nodosa and	Eclampsia
microscopic)	Malignancy associated
Diabetes mellitus	Cryoglobulinaemia
Amyloidosis	Sarcoidosis
Henoch–Schönlein purpura	Rheumatoid arthritis
Malarial nephropathy	Scleroderma
(in tropical countries)	Haemolytic uraemic syndrome
Paraproteinaemia	Cytomegalovirus nephropathy
Wegener's granulomatosis	AIDS nephropathy

classification which has been further expanded following development of immunohistological techniques and electron microscopy. It is now recognised that there is poor correlation between the clinical presentation and the histological appearance. Only a few patients can be diagnosed accurately on clinical presentation. In addition, in different types of glomerular diseases, the clinical features are present to a variable extent and not all will be present in all patients.

CLINICAL FEATURES OF GLOMERULONEPHRITIS

- Proteinuria
- Haematuria
- Hypertension
- Impairment of renal function

Pathogenesis

In the majority of patients with glomerulonephritis there is clear histological evidence of inflammation; in others, such as minimal change nephropathy, there is no obvious evidence of an inflammatory process. In some circumstances, the causative factors are known and the pathogenesis understood; in others we are ignorant of both. Experimental models of glomerular disease have been very useful in furthering the understanding of the pathogenesis of glomerulonephritis (Fig. 11.17).

PATHOGENESIS OF GLOMERULONEPHRITIS

- Binding of antibodies directed against specific glomerular basement membrane antigens (anti-GBM disease)
- 'Trapping' of circulating small soluble immune complexes in the glomerular capillary wall
- 'In situ' formation of immune complexes in the glomerular capillary wall and/or mesangium from circulating antibody and 'fixed' or planted antigen
- The action of 'primed' T cells in association with circulating macrophages

When an antigen excites antibody formation there is normally an excess of antibody, and the complexes so formed are large, insoluble and readily removed, mainly by Kupffer cells and splenic macrophages. When the complexes are relatively small and soluble, they may circulate for long periods and eventually become deposited in glomerular capillary walls. This situation usually occurs where there is a modified immune response and relative antigen excess or antigen–antibody equivalence. It is possible therefore that patients who

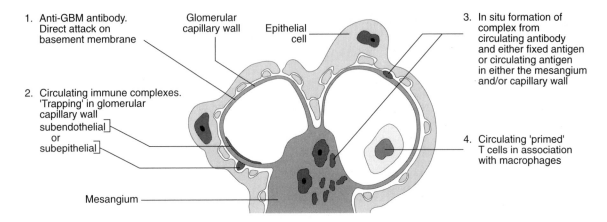

1. Anti-GBM antibody. Direct attack on basement membrane

Glomerular capillary wall

Epithelial cell

3. In situ formation of complex from circulating antibody and either fixed antigen or circulating antigen in either the mesangium and/or capillary wall

2. Circulating immune complexes. 'Trapping' in glomerular capillary wall
subendothelial
  or
subepithelial

4. Circulating 'primed' T cells in association with macrophages

Mesangium

Fig. 11.17   Pathogenesis of glomerulonephritis.

develop immune complex glomerulonephritis suffer from some minor defect of their immune system restricting antibody production, resulting in the formation of abnormal complexes. The site of deposition within the glomerulus depends on the size, solubility and electrical charge of the particles, and upon the electrical charge of the capillary basement membrane. Following interaction of antigen and antibody an inflammatory response develops.

In a number of instances of glomerulonephritis the causal antigen is known, but it has become apparent that no single agent produces a uniform glomerular response. Furthermore, even in well-defined forms of glomerulonephritis the rate of progression of the disease varies greatly from patient to patient. It is possible that the glomerular response to a specific insult is genetically determined, a theory supported by the fact that a number of forms of glomerulonephritis are associated with particular HLA types, e.g. HLA Bw35 and DR4 in IgA nephropathy, HLA B12 and DRw7 in minimal change nephropathy. In addition, in some patients the HLA type may give some indication of prognosis, e.g. HLA B8 and DRw3 are associated with a poor prognosis in membranous glomerulonephritis. It is likely that most glomerulonephritis results from some environmental factor, such as viral or bacterial antigens, acting in a susceptible patient who is relatively immuno-incompetent due to inherited or acquired factors.

'PRIMARY' GLOMERULONEPHRITIS

In a number of clinical syndromes the glomerulus is primarily involved in the disease process. Renal biopsy identifies three main histological types: proliferative, membranous, and minimal change lesions. The majority of cases of glomerulonephritis belong to the proliferative group (> 70%) which can be further subdivided according to certain histological appearances (Table 11.3). This classification is a useful working structure but many of these histological patterns may also be found in other conditions, e.g. in systemic lupus erythematosus there may be either a proliferative or membranous glomerular lesion.

PROLIFERATIVE GLOMERULONEPHRITIS

In proliferative glomerulonephritis there is a varying degree of proliferation of mesangial, epithelial and sometimes endothelial cells associated, in the acute phase of the process, with infiltration of polymorphonuclear leucocytes, and monocytes.

Aetiology

It may occur following an infection, e.g. post-streptococcal or post-viral glomerulonephritis. However, in the majority of cases it is not possible to identify the antigen which has stimulated the development of antibody and subsequently of immune complex formation. Numerous infections are associated with glomerulonephritis, and although the streptococcus has been widely implicated, its incidence in Europe has declined significantly. It is still, however, common in developing countries where the site of infection is usually the skin.

Pathology

Histologically two main groups can be identified, although these may represent a continuous spectrum rather than distinct entities:

- Severe proliferative changes (diffuse endocapillary proliferative glomerulonephritis) in which there is a marked increase of mesangial cells associated with variable infiltration with polymorphonuclear leucocytes and macrophages (Fig. 11.18). On immunofluorescence microscopy, immunoglobulins, complement and fibrin can usually be identified in the capillary walls and/or mesangium indicating the inflammatory nature of the condition. On electron microscopy subepithelial immune complex deposits ('humps') may be observed on the basement membrane. Frequently electron-dense deposits can be observed within the mesangium. In some patients capsular adhesions and small crescents may be seen in a few glomeruli.
- Mild to moderate cellular proliferation (mesangial proliferative glomerulonephritis) in which there is a less marked mesangial cell increase associated with a variable increase in mesangial matrix. On immunofluorescence microscopy, immunoglobulins may be detected within the mesangium in association with complement. There is variable inflammatory cell infiltrate and the appearances are of a relatively benign condition.

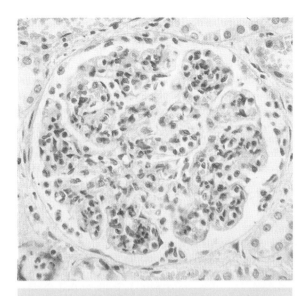

Fig. 11.18 **Proliferative glomerulonephritis.** A 'solid' looking glomerular tuft in which there is an infiltration of polymorphonuclear leucocytes and a proliferation of mesangial cells with associated endothelial cell swelling and loss of capillary lumina.

Clinical features

Proliferative glomerulonephritis occurs at any age and in either sex. It presents in many different ways, most commonly as acute glomerulonephritis or nephrotic syndrome. In the majority of patients unselective proteinuria is present, and may be sufficient to cause the nephrotic syndrome (i.e. greater than 3.5 g/day in adult patients). Haematuria is universal and the presence of red cell casts is diagnostic of glomerular bleeding. In the majority of patients renal function is normal, but some develop significant impairment of function and a small proportion proceed to chronic renal failure. During the early or acute phase of the illness, particularly if post-infective, there may be evidence of complement activation (a reduction in C3 and C4 indicating 'classical' pathway activation of complement). In many patients, however, investigations are undertaken at a 'late' stage in the illness when complement abnormalities have frequently returned to normal. The plasma albumin will be reduced depending on the degree of proteinuria. Serum creatinine and blood urea will be increased depending on the extent of the renal functional impairment.

Management

No specific therapy has yet been developed for this condition and treatment is therefore entirely symptomatic. A search should be made for any underlying infection and appropriate treatment instituted. Antihypertensive therapy should be introduced as required to maintain a normal blood pressure; beta antagonists (e.g. atenolol 50–100 mg daily), calcium channel blockers (e.g. nifedipine 30–60 mg daily) and ACE inhibitors (e.g. enalapril 5–10 mg daily) are particularly useful. Diuretic therapy should be introduced if peripheral oedema is manifest; loop diuretics (frusemide, bumetanide) are usually required.

Prognosis

The natural history is variable and depends upon the severity of the glomerular lesion, the degree of renal impairment at the onset and the presence of hypertension.

FACTORS INDICATING A POOR PROGNOSIS IN PROLIFERATIVE GLOMERULONEPHRITIS

- Age: older patients more frequently progress to renal failure
- Nephrotic range proteinuria
- Hypertension
- Impaired renal function at time of presentation
- Histology showing sclerosis in glomeruli or marked interstitial fibrosis

IgA NEPHROPATHY

IgA nephropathy can be considered as a variant of proliferative glomerulonephritis in which the predominant immunoglobulin deposited, mainly in the mesangium, is IgA. It was first described more than 20 years ago by Berger and co-workers from Paris. It has been subsequently reported in many countries, although the incidence varies considerably. It is prevalent in Japan where it accounts for 30–40% of primary glomerulonephritis, and also in Southern Europe where it accounts for 20–35%. In Britain and North America it is detected in approximately 10% of renal biopsies. The geographical differences may be accounted for by different biopsy practice, but in view of the known association with HLA Bw35 and DR4 it is possible that population genetics are important.

Aetiology

The pathogenesis is unknown but in view of the close association between the episodes of macroscopic haematuria and mucosal infections, it is possible that mucosal IgA plays some part. It is likely that there is mesangial deposition of IgA immune complexes or aggregates of IgA secreted by lymphocytes in mucosal tissues in response to stimulation by bacterial or viral antigens. A number of patients have chronic liver disease, in which there is possibly inadequate clearing of intestinally-derived IgA complexes.

Pathology

On light microscopy there is diffuse and mild mesangial proliferative glomerulonephritis or focal segmental mesangial proliferation. Commonly, mesangial IgA deposition (Fig. 11.19) is associated with complement (C3) and IgG and IgM. The diffuse increase in mesangial matrix may progress to focal glomerulosclerosis (below).

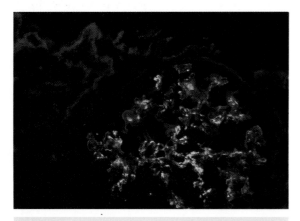

Fig. 11.19 IgA nephropathy. An immunofluorescence preparation demonstrating the deposition of IgA predominantly in the mesangium with small amounts also present in capillary walls.

Clinical features

IgA nephropathy most commonly presents as recurrent haematuria in young adult males, although it can occur at any age. In the majority of patients the episodes of macroscopic haematuria are closely associated with mucosal infections, usually of the upper respiratory tract.

Between episodes of macroscopic haematuria, microscopic haematuria is common. In a small proportion of patients the haematuria is associated with loin pain. Minor proteinuria is common but approximately 20% of patients develop nephrotic syndrome. The majority of patients (80%) are normotensive but older patients most commonly present with hypertension or chronic renal failure.

Management

No specific therapies, such as corticosteroids or immunosuppression, have been shown to affect the natural history of this condition, although in patients with nephrotic syndrome or a rapidly progressing course, corticosteroids may be of some value. As the episodes of macroscopic haematuria are associated with upper respiratory tract infections, long-term antibiotic therapy and/or tonsillectomy have been advocated, but have not been shown to be of value.

Prognosis

It usually follows a benign course and after an interval of 5–10 years many patients become asymptomatic. 25% of patients may develop some renal functional impairment and, in Britain, about 10% eventually require chronic dialysis. Features which indicate a poor prognosis are proteinuria in excess of 3.5 g daily, hypertension, older age of onset, and the appearance of focal glomerulosclerosis on biopsy. IgA nephropathy can recur in transplanted kidneys.

MESANGIOCAPILLARY GLOMERULONEPHRITIS

Mesangiocapillary glomerulonephritis (MCGN) is a variant of proliferative glomerulonephritis, in which there are marked changes in the mesangium, proliferation and expansion of matrix, associated with thickening of the glomerular capillary walls. Thickening is due to subendothelial deposition of the products of inflammation (**Type I or subendothelial type**) or the deposition of immune material within the basement membrane (**Type II or 'dense deposit' type**).

Aetiology

The pathogenesis is unclear. In some instances Type I apparently follows upper respiratory tract infections, or is associated with bacterial endocarditis or an infected

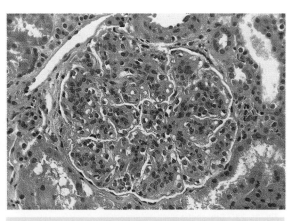

Fig. 11.20   Mesangiocapillary glomerulonephritis type I.
A glomerulus showing widespread proliferation of mesangial cells with increase in mesangial matrix displacing the capillary lumina to the periphery of the lobules.

ventriculo-atrial shunt. The activation of complement would suggest that it is immune-mediated, and circulating complexes have been reported. In Type II there is a **nephritic factor**, an IgG autoantibody which activates complement by the alternate pathway, i.e. at C3. It is likely that the consequent low C3 predisposes to glomerular disease. In some patients it is known that the hypocomplementaemia precedes the glomerular lesion.

The stimulus to production of nephritic factor is unknown.

Pathology

The glomeruli in MCGN show a marked enlargement of mesangial tissue, due both to cellular proliferation and to a disproportionately large increase in matrix. This gives the glomeruli a lobular appearance. The capillary lumen is often diminished and may be displaced to the periphery of the lobule. Electron microscopy reveals two main subgroups. In Type I, large subendothelial deposits are present and the mesangial cytoplasm extends from the mesangium to the capillary wall. There is the formation of a new layer of basement membrane-like material on the luminal side giving the appearance of a double contour (Fig. 11.20). In Type II the capillary wall is thickened due to the deposition of electron-dense linear deposits in the lamina densa of the basement membrane (Fig. 11.21). Similar deposits can be found in Bowman's capsule and tubular membrane.

Clinical features

The two types have many clinical similarities. They most commonly present between the ages of 15 and 25 years and there is slight female preponderance. The clinical presentation is usually with an acute glomerulonephritis syndrome, although some may present with recurrent

Dense intramembranous deposits

Ⓐ
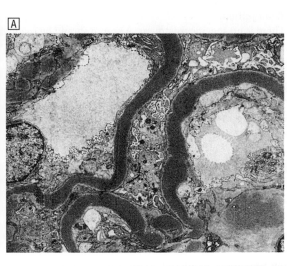

Ⓑ
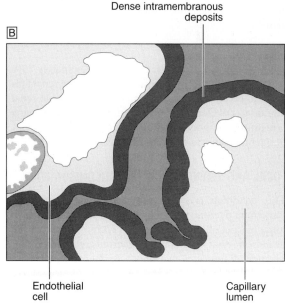

Endothelial
cell

Capillary
lumen

Fig. 11.21   Mesangiocapillary glomerulonephritis type II. Ⓐ Dense intramembranous deposits within the glomerular capillary walls.
Ⓑ Drawing indicating main features.

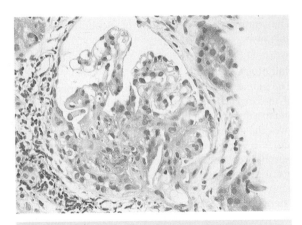

Fig. 11.22 Focal and segmental glomerulonephritis. One glomerulus showing segmental proliferation in the lower part, with normal capillary loops in the upper part.

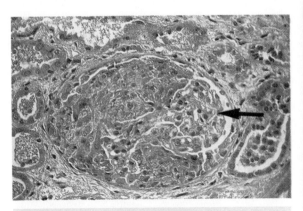

Fig. 11.23 Crescentic glomerulonephritis. One glomerulus showing a large circumferential crescent surrounding the compressed glomerular tuft (arrow).

haematuria and a few with nephrotic syndrome. Hypertension and impaired renal function are frequently present at diagnosis. Many have hypocomplementaemia. In Type I this is due to classical pathway activation whereas in Type II the alternate pathway is involved due to the presence of nephritic factor.

Management

There is no specific treatment for either type. A number of regimens have been suggested, including corticosteroids, immunosuppressive drugs, anticoagulants and antiplatelet drugs. None has been shown to be of definite value.

Prognosis

In both types the prognosis is poor, approximately 75% of patients eventually progressing to end-stage renal failure. However, a number of patients retain stable renal function. Development of hypertension or increasing proteinuria are poor prognostic signs. Type II MCGN frequently recurs in transplanted kidneys.

FOCAL AND SEGMENTAL GLOMERULONEPHRITIS

This condition is characterised by proliferative and sometimes necrotic changes which occur in segments of some but not all glomeruli (Fig. 11.22). 'Focal' is used to indicate that only some glomeruli are affected and 'segmental' indicates that only a segment of the glomerulus is involved.

Aetiology

It is frequently associated with systemic disease such as Henoch–Schönlein purpura, microscopic polyarteritis, Wegener's granulomatosis and bacterial endocarditis.

The aetiology in cases not associated with other systemic disease is unknown.

Clinical features

The most common presenting feature is haematuria or acute glomerulonephritis syndrome. The condition occurs most commonly in young adults and there is often hypertension and impairment of renal function. Complement studies are usually normal unless there is an associated systemic disease such as systemic lupus erythematosus.

Management

There is no specific treatment. A search should be made for underlying systemic disease which might be amenable to therapy.

Prognosis

The prognosis is generally good and only a small minority progress to renal impairment. In patients with an underlying systemic disease this determines the outlook.

CRESCENTIC GLOMERULONEPHRITIS (IDIOPATHIC)

In this form of glomerulonephritis the most striking feature is the presence of large cellular epithelial crescents occurring in 70% or more of glomeruli. These large crescents are associated with glomerular ischaemia, and the remaining glomerular tuft usually shows no proliferation and is frequently distorted (Fig. 11.23).

Aetiology

The pathogenesis is unknown. It is likely that the initiating event is immunologically mediated, and that there is rupture of the capillary basement membrane with subsequent leakage of fibrinogen into Bowman's space. This acts as a stimulus to the parietal epithelial cells to divide and thereby form crescents. Monocytes and neutrophils accumulate in Bowman's space. There is no association with any specific agent, although many patients appear to have had a preceding viral illness.

Clinical features

Clinically, crescentic glomerulonephritis occurs most commonly in adults and presents as acute glomerulonephritis or acute renal failure. Renal failure is common, hypertension usually mild, and proteinuria minor. There is usually a fairly rapid clinical course with development of severe functional impairment.

Management

There is no universally successful treatment for this condition. High-dose prednisolone (1 mg/kg daily), pulse methylprednisolone (1 g intravenously daily for 3 days), cyclophosphamide (2 mg/kg daily) and plasma exchange have all been advocated, and are effective in restoring renal function in some cases.

Prognosis

In the majority of patients renal function deteriorates very rapidly and haemodialysis is often required early in the illness. Although a number of patients respond to immunosuppressive therapy, the majority will develop irreversible renal failure.

GOODPASTURE'S SYNDROME

This is a variety of proliferative glomerulonephritis in which there is a circulating antibody directed against antigens of the glomerular capillary basement membrane.

Aetiology

The pathogenesis is unknown, but in some patients the onset appears to follow viral infection of the respiratory tract. The capillary wall is severely disrupted, and fibrinogen passes through to the urinary space to stimulate formation of epithelial crescents. The result is usually a crescentic glomerulonephritis of a type known clinically as Goodpasture's syndrome.

Pathology

On biopsy the appearances are those of crescentic glomerulonephritis. Immunofluorescence microscopy reveals a linear deposition of IgG along glomerular capillary walls (Fig. 11.24).

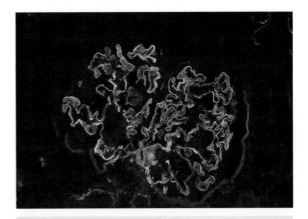

Fig. 11.24 Goodpasture's syndrome. Linear immunofluorescence to IgG on glomerular capillary walls in a patient with Goodpasture's syndrome.

Clinical features

Clinically the syndrome usually presents as acute renal failure and occurs most commonly in young adult males and during springtime. There is cross-reactivity between the glomerular basement membrane and pulmonary basement membrane. Some patients therefore have associated intrapulmonary haemorrhage and may present with haemoptysis. In such patients the chest radiograph reveals pulmonary infiltration and there may be significant impairment of lung function. In the majority of patients irreversible renal failure develops rapidly.

Management

The diagnosis should be established as early as possible, since plasma exchange combined with immunosuppression is highly effective in patients who still retain renal function. There is no general agreement but most would suggest pulse methylprednisolone (1 g intravenously on 3 consecutive days) followed by high-dose corticosteroids (prednisolone 1 mg/kg daily) for 4–6 weeks, with a subsequent cautious and gradual reduction in dose. Many advocate the addition of either cyclophosphamide (2 mg/kg daily) or azathioprine (2 mg/kg daily), but there are no good clinical trials to support this view.

Prognosis

The prognosis for renal function is poor. When oliguria develops there may not be any recovery of renal function even with intensive therapy. Intrapulmonary haemorrhage carries a poor prognosis for survival and may occur in these patients in association with any intercurrent febrile illness.

MEMBRANOUS GLOMERULONEPHRITIS

In membranous glomerulonephritis the glomerular capillary basement membrane is uniformly thickened and there is no significant proliferation of cells, although there may be a minor mesangial cell increase.

Aetiology

Membranous glomerulonephritis is found in association with a number of conditions. The pathogenesis is most likely the in situ formation of immune complexes, due to the presence of circulating antigen becoming deposited in the basement membrane and subsequent reaction with a circulating low avidity antibody.

CONDITIONS ASSOCIATED WITH MEMBRANOUS NEPHROPATHY

Infections
- Malaria
- Syphilis
- Hepatitis B

Drugs
- Gold
- Mercury
- Penicillamine
- Captopril

Malignancy
- Carcinoma (lung, breast, gastrointestinal)
- Lymphoma

Systemic disease
- SLE

Pathology

On light microscopy there is a diffuse regular thickening of the capillary basement membrane of all glomeruli, which on electron microscopy reveals numerous small subepithelial electron-dense deposits (Fig. 11.25). On immunofluorescence microscopy these deposits contain immunoglobulins and complement. In some cases, where there is an underlying predisposing cause, relevant antigens may be detected, e.g. tumour antigens.

Clinical features

Most patients present with nephrotic syndrome, although some are detected because of asymptomatic proteinuria. Membranous glomerulonephritis is most common in middle age and in males. Proteinuria usually exceeds 3.5 g/day and is non-selective. Hypertension occurs in approximately one-third of patients and renal failure develops in approximately 50%. It is important to search for any underlying condition, particularly a malignant tumour.

Management

A number of therapeutic regimens have been reported to be beneficial in treatment, including high-dose alternate day corticosteroid therapy, immunosuppressive drugs, chlorambucil, antiplatelet agents and anticoagulants. As in any condition where a wide variety of different regimens is advocated, it is likely that none is universally successful. Therapy should only be introduced after investigation and diagnosis in a nephrology centre. In view of the fact that only 50% of patients will progress to renal failure, it is best to reserve therapy for those with documented deterioration. Blood pressure must be controlled and oedema treated.

Prognosis

Approximately 50% of patients develop impaired renal function, while 25% have complete remission. Patients who present with a severe nephrotic syndrome, chronic renal failure, hypertension, male patients, and older patients appear to have an increased risk of progressive renal failure. The presence of HLA B8 or DRw3 is associated with a poor prognosis.

MINIMAL CHANGE NEPHROPATHY

Minimal change nephropathy is so called because on light microscopy no significant abnormalities are present. It is best to use the term nephropathy instead of glomerulonephritis as in this condition there is no evidence of any underlying inflammation.

Aetiology

A number of patients are atopic. The pathogenesis is unknown, but it is thought to be immunologically related because of the universal satisfactory response to corticosteroid therapy and because relapses are frequently associated with intercurrent infections. It is likely that the condition results from many different stimuli which can induce increased suppressor T cell activity. There is an association with HLA B12 and DRw7.

Pathology

In minimal change nephropathy the morphological changes are minor and in many the renal biopsy appears normal on light microscopy. In some however there is a very slight proliferation of mesangial cells. On electron microscopy there is usually a moderate to marked loss of epithelial pedicel structure (Fig. 11.26). This appears to be a nonspecific change and may be a reflection of the heavy proteinuria.

Clinical features

The lesion occurs most commonly in children between 3 and 15 years, less commonly in adults. It usually presents as a nephrotic syndrome associated with selective proteinuria (see p. 621). Hypoproteinaemia is common and there is frequently a compensatory increase in β-2

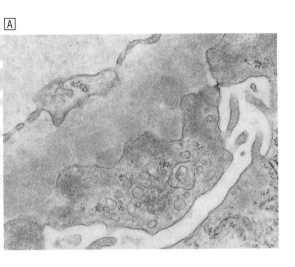

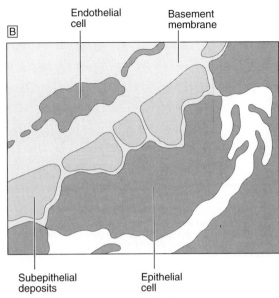

Fig. 11.25 Membranous glomerulonephritis. A An electron micrograph from a patient with membranous glomerulonephritis showing subepithelial deposits on the outer aspect of the glomerular capillary wall basement membrane. B Drawing indicating main features.

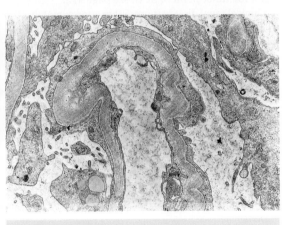

Fig. 11.26 Minimal change nephropathy showing relatively normal endothelial cell and basement membrane with smearing of the epithelial cells on the outer surface of the capillary walls (electron microscopy ×20 000).

treatment consists of therapy to control oedema. Diuretics may have to be combined with infusions of salt-poor albumin. Specific treatment is with corticosteroids. These are most commonly given as prednisolone 60 mg/m^2 orally, once daily for 4 weeks or until proteinuria disappears. When the urine has been free from protein for 2 weeks, the prednisolone dose should be gradually reduced to zero over 4 weeks. Some 30% of patients will have a relapse within 3 years. For those who have frequent relapses and require repeated courses of corticosteroids, the use of alternate day prednisolone therapy may reduce the incidence of steroid toxicity. For patients who have frequent relapses or develop unacceptable corticosteroid side-effects, cyclophosphamide may be of value. This is usually given in a dose of 2 mg/kg daily and continued for 2 weeks after remission, or withdrawn after 6 weeks if no beneficial effect is obtained.

globulins and cholesterol. Haematuria and hypertension are rare. Renal function is usually normal although where there is significant hypovolaemia, pre-renal acute renal failure may develop.

Management

In children the diagnosis can be made without renal biopsy by finding selective proteinuria in the absence of haematuria, impaired renal function or hypertension. In adults diagnostic biopsy is required. Symptomatic

Prognosis

Minimal change nephropathy characteristically has a remitting and relapsing course. In time a number of patients undergo spontaneous remission, but corticosteroid therapy is indicated because of the complications of chronic hypovolaemia and the risk of infections in patients who are grossly oedematous. Relapses occurring many years later are recognised, but even in the long term there does not seem to be any deterioration of renal function.

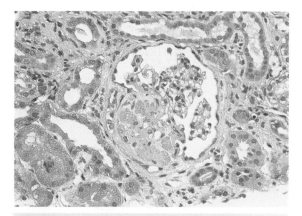

Fig. 11.27 Focal and segmental glomerulosclerosis.
Sclerosis is present to the lower left side of the glomerulus whilst in the remainder there is little abnormality apart from slight mesangial expansion.

FOCAL AND SEGMENTAL GLOMERULOSCLEROSIS

The term 'glomerulosclerosis' refers to partial or total replacement of a glomerulus by hyaline material, which in most cases is excess mesangial matrix. In some circumstances this appears to develop in glomeruli which are chronically ischaemic, whereas in other cases it seems to result from a previous focal proliferative glomerulonephritis. There is however a separate entity, focal glomerulosclerosis, in which there is no underlying condition to account for the sclerosis, which is typically focal and segmental (Fig. 11.27). The aetiology of this form of glomerulosclerosis is unknown.

Pathology

Unlike other forms of glomerulonephritis, focal glomerulosclerosis appears initially to affect the juxtamedullary glomeruli. In these glomeruli there is an increase in mesangial matrix which gradually expands to destroy the surrounding lobule, until global sclerosis occurs. In time similar lesions appear in glomeruli throughout the cortex. The pathogenesis is unknown.

Clinical features

In focal glomerulosclerosis, the patient presents with the nephrotic syndrome and in the early stage the condition may be clinically indistinguishable from minimal change nephropathy. Later haematuria, hypertension and renal failure are common. It occurs at any age, but is most common in children and young adults.

Management

There is no specific treatment. Hypertension and oedema require to be controlled. Treatment for renal failure should be introduced as required. Regular follow-up is mandatory in view of the frequent progression to renal failure. Unfortunately recurrence in transplanted kidneys is well recognised.

RENAL INVOLVEMENT IN SYSTEMIC DISEASES

Certain systemic diseases, e.g. systemic lupus erythematosus, vasculitis, amyloidosis and diabetes mellitus are frequently accompanied by significant renal involvement. Most of these diseases involve small blood vessels or capillaries, and the vascular structure of the kidney makes it particularly vulnerable. In many patients, the systemic manifestations will be apparent before any renal abnormality is found, but in a small number the presenting features arise from renal involvement, the more widespread systemic manifestations becoming apparent later. Once renal involvement is manifest, the prognosis worsens significantly.

Systemic lupus erythematosus

For a full description of SLE, see page 912.

Clinical renal disease is present in approximately 40% of patients at presentation and this incidence increases with time. However, even at initial presentation there is evidence of renal involvement in almost all patients who undergo renal biopsy. The renal lesion is due to deposition of immune complexes containing DNA and anti-DNA antibodies, and the inflammatory response which results.

Clinically, proteinuria is the most common sign of renal involvement, which may be asymptomatic or sufficient to produce a nephrotic syndrome. Haematuria is also common but usually microscopic. Hypertension occurs in approximately 20% of patients. Acute or chronic renal failure may develop.

Renal pathology

Most commonly there is a diffuse proliferative glomerulonephritis, which may vary in severity from mild proliferation to necrosis and crescent formation. Some 20% of patients show focal glomerulonephritis. In 15% the appearances are those of membranous glomerulonephritis. Wire loop lesions in the capillary walls are highly suggestive of SLE. Haematoxylin bodies (disordered nuclei of cells damaged by autoantibodies) are specific to SLE.

Management

The management of SLE is fully discussed on page 915. The detection of clinical renal involvement indicates a worse prognosis and requires more regular clinical supervision and renal biopsy. The mainstay of treatment has been corticosteroids, but the dose required to achieve satisfactory control is very variable and can only be determined by trial and error. The initial dose should be prednisolone 60 mg/day. If disease activity is controlled, a reduction to 40 mg/day should be made after 4–6 weeks, followed by a 10 mg/day reduction in daily dose after a further 2–6 weeks, until the daily dose is 20 mg. Thereafter reductions should be in 2.5 mg decrements. Patients who do not achieve satisfactory remission with corticosteroids alone should have azathioprine 2 mg/kg daily added, and in very severe cases plasma exchange may be required. Cycles of bolus intravenous cyclophosphamide (5–10 mg/kg) for up to 2 years may be necessary in some patients. There have been recent anecdotal reports of the value of cyclosporin (p. 636), but as yet there is no consensus as to the use of this treatment. Although none of these regimens have been evaluated in randomised controlled trials of sufficient size, those that include an immunosuppressive drug appear to provide better long-term control. Disease activity can be followed by regular estimation of anti-DNA antibodies and plasma complement (C3 and C4).

Prognosis

The prognosis of SLE is variable and to some extent depends upon the type and severity of renal involvement. In patients whose renal biopsy reveals normal histology or only minor changes, the prognosis is good. Focal glomerulonephritis usually has a relatively benign course with a 5-year survival of approximately 65%. Patients with a membranous lesion also have a good prognosis. Those patients with diffuse proliferative changes, particularly when crescents or necrosis are present, have a poor prognosis.

VASCULITIS

This is a syndrome complex due to inflammation of blood vessels, frequently associated with necrosis. It may affect arteries, capillaries or veins alone or in combination. The inflammation usually leads to a reduction in lumen with consequent ischaemia. There is no satisfactory classification because the clinical and pathological manifestations frequently overlap, therefore the various syndromes represent a spectrum rather than distinct entities. (See page 921 for detailed description of this group of diseases.) Vasculitis may exist as a primary condition, or may complicate an underlying disease due to immune stimulation or drug therapy. Renal involvement is common in polyarteritis nodosa and Wegener's granulomatosis, is variable in microscopic polyarteritis

and Henoch–Schönlein purpura, and uncommon in other forms of vasculitis.

Polyarteritis

In **polyarteritis nodosa** (p. 921) haematuria is a feature, and in some patients loin pain develops due to areas of renal infarction. **Microscopic polyarteritis** is a multisystem inflammation of capillaries. Renal involvement is variable, consisting of either focal or segmental proliferative glomerulonephritis, with or without fibrinoid necrosis, or crescentic glomerulonephritis. Hypertension is less common than in the nodosa form. The clinical presentation is usually as acute glomerulonephritis or acute renal failure. Treatment is with corticosteroids, but in both forms the prognosis is poor, renal failure being the most common cause of death.

Wegener's granulomatosis

This is a vasculitis characterised by granulomatous lesions in the upper respiratory tract and lungs (see p. 922), associated with fibrinoid necrosis of blood vessels and a focal necrotising glomerulonephritis often with glomerular crescents. Frequently patients present with nasal symptoms. Renal manifestations tend to occur late. The condition usually responds to prednisolone and cyclophosphamide (2 mg/kg/day) which may have to be given on a long-term basis.

Anti-neutrophil cytoplasmic antibody test (ANCA)

These recently discovered autoantibodies are proving useful in the diagnosis of vasculitic disorders. They are abnormal antibodies, detected in the serum of most patients with vasculitis, which are directed against components of the cytoplasm of normal neutrophils (Fig. 11.28). They can be detected by immunofluorescence or by solid-phase immunoassays. Two patterns can be distinguished. The cytoplasmic, or c-ANCA, which is usually due to antibodies against proteinase-3, is usually positive in Wegener's granulomatosis. The perinuclear, or p-ANCA, often represents antibodies against myeloperoxidase. It is usually positive in microscopic polyarteritis, and sometimes in other forms of vasculitis. The antibodies sometimes, but not always, disappear with treatment of the disease. Persistent high titres are often associated with clinical relapse.

Henoch–Schönlein purpura

This may involve the kidneys, and cause either asymptomatic proteinuria, haematuria, acute glomerulonephritis, nephrotic syndrome or acute renal failure. Children are more commonly affected than adults, and in them the prognosis is good, whereas approximately 50% of adults progress to renal failure.

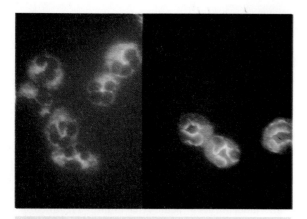

Fig. 11.28 Anti-neutrophil cytoplasmic antibodies (ANCA). The patient's serum is incubated with normal neutrophils; binding of ANCA to components of the neutrophils is detected by a secondary fluorescein-labelled anti-IgG antibody. The left panel shows diffuse staining of the cytoplasm; 'c-ANCA' is found in Wegener's granulomatosis, and is usually directed against Proteinase 3. The right panel shows peri-nuclear staining; this 'p-ANCA' is common in microscopic polyarteritis, and is often directed against myeloperoxidase.

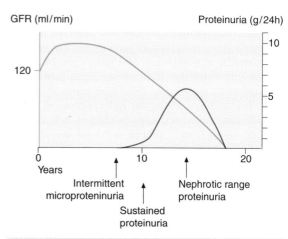

Fig. 11.29 Natural history of diabetic nephropathy. In the first few years of insulin-dependent diabetes mellitus there is hyperfiltration which declines fairly steadily to return to a normal value at approximately 10 years. At this time intermittent microproteinuria is noted frequently in association with exercise. After about 10 years there is sustained proteinuria and by approximately 14 years it has reached the nephrotic range. Renal function continues to decline with end stage being reached at approximately 16 years.

Amyloidosis

Because of a reduction in the incidence of chronic suppurative lesions in the Western world, there is now approximately an even distribution of primary and secondary forms in patients with renal amyloidosis. When the kidney is involved, the extracellular deposits of fibrils and protein damage glomerular capillaries and cause proteinuria. In 30% of patients this is sufficient to cause nephrotic syndrome. Renal amyloidosis may cause proximal or distal renal tubular acidosis, or nephrogenic diabetes insipidus. Renal impairment is common. There is no satisfactory treatment. Approximately 50% of patients will progress to terminal renal failure within 6 months of renal involvement becoming manifest.

Diabetic nephropathy

Diabetic nephropathy occurs in both type I and type II diabetes mellitus (see p. 759). The natural history of nephropathy in type I is shown in Figure 11.29. Renal involvement appears more common in type I (Fig. 11.30) but this may be due to the long natural history and the fact that patients with type II are much older when the illness becomes clinically apparent. It is unknown why some patients develop clinically apparent renal involvement with microangiopathy while others seem to remain unaffected.

At present there is much interest in the role of diabetic control and the renal complications of diabetes mellitus. The early hyperfiltration can be abolished with very strict blood glucose control, but whether this will prevent progression of the renal lesions is, as yet, not known. Once microalbuminuria appears, this too can be controlled by maintaining the blood glucose within normal limits. Later in the natural history, however, once persistent proteinuria is manifest, the role of glucose control in the prevention of progression is not clear. At this late stage, control of blood pressure is of prime importance, and there is some evidence that angiotensin-converting enzyme inhibitors, such as captopril 25 mg 12-hourly,

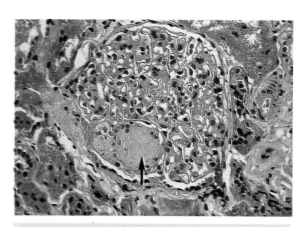

Fig. 11.30 Diabetes mellitus. Nodular diabetic glomerulosclerosis. There is thickening of basement membranes and mesangial expansion, and a Kimmelstein-Wilson nodule (arrow).

or enalapril 5–20 mg daily, may have a more beneficial effect than other hypotensive drugs.

The renal lesions of diabetes mellitus are only one manifestation of a widespread microangiopathy. Patients with renal failure frequently have clinical evidence of retinopathy, neuropathy and other system involvement. These are discussed in detail on pages 752–759.

FURTHER READING

Couser W G 1993 Pathogenesis of glomerulonephritis. Kidney International Suppl 42: S19–S26
Glassock R J 1992 Treatment of immunologically mediated glomerular disease. Kidney International Suppl 38: S121–S126
Ponticelli C, Passerini P 1994. Treatment of the nephrotic syndrome associated with primary glomerulonephritis. Kidney International 46: 595–604

INFECTIONS OF THE KIDNEY AND URINARY TRACT

The urinary tract, like the respiratory and digestive tracts, ends on the body surface and therefore can never be sterile throughout its length. However, when the tract is anatomically and physiologically normal, and local and systemic defence mechanisms intact, organisms are confined to the lower end of the urethra. Urinary tract infection (UTI) is associated with multiplication of organisms in the urinary tract, and is defined by the presence of more than 100 000 organisms per ml in a midstream sample of urine (MSU). Such infections are much more common in women, cause considerable morbidity, and account for 1.2% of all consultations in general practice. In an undetermined minority, destruction of renal parenchyma and severe chronic renal failure ensue.

CLINICAL PRESENTATION OF URINARY TRACT INFECTION

- Asymptomatic bacteriuria
- Symptomatic acute urethritis and cystitis
- Acute prostatitis
- Acute pyelonephritis
- Septicaemia (usually Gram-negative bacteria)

Community surveys suggest that the prevalence of urinary tract infection in women is about 3% at the age of 20, increasing by about 1% in each subsequent decade. About 50% of women suffer symptoms of urinary tract infection sometime during their adult lives. In males such infections are uncommon except in the first year of life and in those over 60, in whom urinary tract obstruction due to prostatic hypertrophy is relatively common.

INFECTIONS OF THE LOWER URINARY TRACT

Pathogenesis

Urinary tract infections may be uncomplicated or complicated; the latter may result in permanent renal damage, the former rarely if ever do so. Uncomplicated infections are almost invariably due to a single strain of organism.

URINARY TRACT INFECTION: UNCOMPLICATED AND COMPLICATED

Uncomplicated
- Anatomically and physiologically normal urinary tract, normal renal function and no associated disorder which impairs defence mechanism

Complicated
- Abnormal urinary tract, e.g. obstruction (Table 11.5), calculi, vesico-ureteric reflux, neurological abnormality, indwelling catheter, chronic prostatitis, cystic kidney, analgesic nephropathy, renal scarring
- Impaired renal function
- Associated disorder which impairs defence mechanisms (e.g. diabetes mellitus, immunosuppressive therapy)

In domiciliary practice *E. coli* derived from the faecal reservoir account for about 75% of infections, the remainder being due to Proteus, Pseudomonas species, streptococci or *Staphylococcus epidermidis*. In hospital a greater proportion of infections are due to organisms such as Klebsiella or streptococci, but faecal *E. coli* still predominate. The differences between the groups are mainly due to the frequency of complicated infections and the high risk of cross infection with virulent organisms in hospital patients. Certain strains of *E. coli* appear well adapted to invade the urinary tract, possibly because they possess surface fimbriae which allow them to adhere to surface receptors on the urothelium. Haematogenous infections do occur, but particularly in women most are ascending infections originating in the lower urinary tract. The first stage is colonisation of the periurethral zone with pathogenic faecal organisms. The urothelium of susceptible persons may have more surface receptors to which adherent strains of *E. coli* become attached. Colonisation is also facilitated by tissue damage from previous UTI, by infections of the genital tract or perineal skin, by inadequate perineal hygiene and possibly by use of disinfectants, deodorants and certain toilet preparations. Ascent of organisms into the bladder is facilitated in women by the short urethra and absence of bactericidal prostatic secretions. Sexual intercourse causes minor urethral trauma and forces introital bacteria into the bladder. Instrumentation of the bladder readily introduces organisms. Urine is a good culture medium, and multiplication of organisms introduced into the bladder depends on the size of the inoculum and virulence of the bacteria. Factors which limit the multiplication of organisms in the urinary tract are shown below.

FACTORS WHICH LIMIT MULTIPLICATION OF ORGANISMS IN THE URINARY TRACT

- A high rate of urine flow
- Regular complete bladder emptying
- Urinary glycosaminoglycans (Tamm–Horsfall mucoprotein) which may bind to *E. coli* thus preventing their attachment to urothelium
- Mucosal defences: thin surface layer of glycosaminoglycans, secretions of IgA and IgG, mucosal phagocytosis and other unknown factors

---

Residual urine left after voiding interferes with mucosal defence mechanisms; thus patients with obstruction below the bladder, gynaecological abnormalities, pelvic floor weakness or neurological problems are susceptible to infection. In those with ureteric reflux (p. 653) urine expelled into the ureters during voiding returns to the bladder when it relaxes. Injury to the mucosa and the presence of a foreign body in the bladder also depress vesical defence mechanisms.

Clinical features

There is often an abrupt onset of frequency of micturition and dysuria. Scalding pain is felt in the urethra during micturition, while cystitis may give rise to suprapubic pain during and for a few moments after voiding. After the bladder has been emptied there may be an intense desire to pass more urine due to spasm of its inflamed wall. Systemic symptoms are usually slight. Suprapubic tenderness is often present and the urine may have an unpleasant odour and appear cloudy. Gross haematuria occasionally occurs. The diagnosis depends on:

- The characteristic clinical features
- Demonstration of more than 10^5/ml organisms in an MSU or any organisms in urine from suprapubic aspirations.

Pyuria is common but not invariable. Children, men and those women with recurrent infection or signs of acute pyelonephritis must be more fully investigated.

INVESTIGATIONS IN PATIENTS WITH ACUTE URINARY TRACT INFECTION

Investigation	Indications
• Quantitative culture of MSU or urine obtained by suprapubic aspiration	All patients
• Microscopic examination of urine for red blood cells, white blood cells, and casts	All patients
• Examination of urine for blood, protein, glucose (dipstix)	All patients
• Measurement 24 hr urine protein excretion or urinary protein/creatinine ratio	When dipstix protein ++ or more
• Full blood count	Adults with acute pyelonephritis, prostatitis; children, infants
• Blood urea, creatinine, electrolytes	Acute pyelonephritis; recurrent UTI; children, infants
• Creatinine clearance	Acute pyelonephritis; recurrent UTI; children, infants
• Blood culture	Rigors, high fever, or evidence septicaemia
• Pelvic examination	Women with recurrent UTI
• Rectal examination	Men (to examine prostate)
• Intravenous urography (IVU) including film of bladder after voiding, to identify physiological and anatomical abnormalities	Infants, children. Men after single UTI. Women who (1) have acute pyelonephritis, (2) have recurrent UTI after urinary tract treatment, (3) have had UTI or covert bacteriuria in pregnancy (IVU 6/52 after delivery)
• Renal ultrasonography	Alternative to IVU to identify obstruction, cysts, calculi
• Micturating cysto-urethrography (MCU) to identify and quantify vesico-ureteric reflux and disturbed bladder emptying	Infants, children with abnormal IVU. Any patient thought to have disturbance of bladder emptying
• Cystoscopy	Patients with chronic haematuria. Patients with suspected bladder lesion

Management

Table 11.4 shows antibiotic regimens for treatment of UTI in adults. Ideally results of urine culture should be available before starting specific therapy, but if the patient is in acute discomfort an MSU should be sent for culture and treatment started while awaiting the result. Since infection is usually due to *E. coli*, initial use of trimethoprim or amoxycillin is rational. The antibiotic

Table 11.4 Antibiotic regimens for treatment of urinary tract infections in adults[1]

| Drug | Treatment of presumed urinary tract infection | | Treatment of presumed pyelonephritis | | Treatment of acute prostatitis | | Prophylactic or suppressive therapy |
	Dose	Duration course	Dose	Duration course	Dose	Duration course	Dose
Trimethoprim	300 mg daily	3 days	300 mg daily	7 days	200 mg/12-hourly	4–6 weeks	100 mg/night
Ampicillin or Amoxycillin	250 mg 8-hourly	3 days	250–500 mg 8-hourly oral	7 days			250 mg/night
Tobramycin[2]			3 mg/kg i.v. 3 mg/kg i.v. daily	Loading dose 7 days			
Cefuroxime			250 mg 12-hourly oral or 750 mg 6–8-hourly i.v.	7 days To start treatment in seriously ill patient			
Ciprofloxacin	250–500 mg 12-hourly	3 days	250–500 mg 12-hourly oral or 100 mg 12-hourly i.v.		250 mg/12-hourly	4–6 weeks	
Cephalexin							250 mg/night
Erythromycin					250 mg/6-hourly	4–6 weeks	

[1] Modification of dosage is necessary when renal function is impaired.
[2] As determined by plasma [creatinine] and [tobramycin]. Given in divided doses.

can be changed if a resistant organism is identified or the response is unsatisfactory. Symptomatic relief usually occurs within 48 hours and the course need not exceed 5 days. A fluid intake of at least 2 litres/day ensures regular voiding and reduces renal medullary tonicity. Urine culture should be repeated on the seventh day after the end of the antibiotic course.

Failure to eradicate an organism or re-appearance of the same organism in the urine within a few days of stopping treatment suggests that one of the complications listed in the information box on page 649 is present. Investigations should be undertaken to diagnose the underlying problem, which should then be eradicated by appropriate treatment. Failing this, after completion of a further therapeutic course of antibiotics, suppressive therapy must be instituted to try to prevent recurrent symptoms, septicaemia and further renal damage (Table 11.4). The urine is cultured at regular intervals and the drug changed as required.

Re-infection with another organism, or with the same organism after an interval of at least 2 weeks, is much more common than failure to eradicate the initial infection, particularly in sexually active women. Opinions differ as to when to investigate the urinary tract. Some perform intravenous urography after the second episode, others restrict investigation to patients who develop acute pyelonephritis, haematuria or septicaemia. In women with recurrent infections the defences of the lower urinary tract may be inadequate, and simple measures may prevent recurrence. If these fail, freedom from attacks may be achieved by taking a single nightly dose of a suitable antibiotic after voiding and before going to bed (Table 11.4).

PROPHYLACTIC MEASURES TO BE ADOPTED BY WOMEN WITH RECURRENT URINARY INFECTIONS

- Fluid intake of at least 2 litres/day
- Regular emptying of bladder (3 hr intervals by day and before retiring)
- Ensure complete emptying of bladder
- Double micturition if reflux present. (The patient should be advised, particularly before retiring for the night, to empty the bladder and then attempt to empty the bladder a second time approximately 10–15 minutes later)
- Emptying bladder before and after intercourse
- Application of 0.5% cetrimide cream to periurethral area before intercourse

This regime is started after completion of curative course of treatment and continued for several months

COVERT OR ASYMPTOMATIC BACTERIURIA

This is defined as more than 10^5/ml organisms in the MSU of apparently healthy asymptomatic patients. Surveys indicate that approximately 1% of children under the age of 1, about 1% of schoolgirls, 0.03% of schoolboys and men, about 3% of non-pregnant adult women and 5% of pregnant women have covert bacteriuria. There is no evidence that this condition causes chronic interstitial nephritis (chronic pyelonephritis) in non-pregnant adults with normal urinary tracts. When it occurs in infants, pregnant women or in an abnormal urinary tract, investigation (information box on p. 650) and treatment (Table 11.4) are required. Any structural abnormality of the urinary tract should be corrected if possible.

URETHRAL SYNDROME

Some patients, usually female, have symptoms suggestive of urethritis and cystitis but no bacteria are cultured from the urine. Possible explanations include infection with organisms not readily cultured by ordinary methods (e.g. chlamydia, certain anaerobes), allergy to toilet preparations or disinfectants, urethral congestion related to sexual intercourse and post-menopausal atrophic vaginitis. Antibiotics are not indicated.

ACUTE PROSTATITIS

This is often accompanied by perineal pain and considerable systemic disturbance. The prostate is usually very tender. The diagnosis is confirmed by a positive culture from urine or from urethral discharge obtained after prostatic massage. The treatment of choice is trimethoprim or erythromycin, which penetrate prostatic secretions. A 4–6 week course is required (Table 11.4).

INFECTIONS OF THE UPPER URINARY TRACT

The proportion of patients with cystitis or covert bacteriuria in whom the kidney is involved is unknown, but a figure of 50% has been suggested. Clinically, it is impossible to distinguish with certainty those with renal infection and there is no reliable test suitable for general clinical use.

Pathogenesis

Bacterial infection of the renal parenchyma is usually due to ascent of organisms by the ureter, although in a few cases it is blood-borne. About 75% of infections are due to *E. coli*, the remainder to Proteus species, Klebsiella, staphylococci or streptococci. Commonly one or more complicating factors are present (information box, p. 649) but in adult women and infants infection, possibly due to a virulent organism, can occur in the absence of such factors. Stasis within the tract compromises its defences, and renal cysts or medullary scars due to previous inflammation facilitate establishment of bacteria because they obstruct groups of nephrons. Very few organisms are required to infect the medulla. Once infection is established there, eradication

is difficult because low blood flow, high osmolality and high concentrations of H^+ and ammonia interfere with mobilisation of leucocytes and phagocytosis. The high osmolality probably favours conversion of bacteria to antibiotic resistant L-forms.

ACUTE PYELONEPHRITIS

Pathology

The renal pelvis is acutely inflamed and there is often coincident cystitis. Small cortical abscesses and linear streaks of pus in the medulla are often evident. Histological examination shows focal infiltration of renal tissue by polymorphonuclear leucocytes and many polymorphs in tubular lumina.

Clinical features

There is commonly sudden onset of pain in one or both loins, radiating to the iliac fossae and suprapubic area. In some cases, particularly in children, pain is confined to the epigastrium or iliac fossae. About 30% of patients have dysuria, strangury and frequent passage of small amounts of scalding, cloudy urine due to associated cystitis. In most cases the temperature rises rapidly to 38–40°C with general manifestations of fever. Rigors and vomiting may occur and occasionally septicaemia and hypotension supervene. Tenderness and guarding are usually present in the renal angle and lumbar region. Characteristically there is a leucocytosis. Microscopic examination of urine reveals numerous pus cells and organisms, some red cells and epithelial cells.

Acute pyelonephritis in infants and children often presents as fever without localising symptoms. The initial feature may be a convulsion but apathy, abdominal distension and diarrhoea sometimes occur. In the febrile child the urine should always be examined for pus cells and organisms. Acute necrotising papillitis very rarely follows a severe attack of acute pyelonephritis. Fragments of renal papillae may then be excreted in the urine and can be identified histologically. This complication, which may lead to acute renal failure, is liable to occur in patients with diabetes mellitus, paraplegia or analgesic addiction.

Differential diagnosis

Acute pyelonephritis should be distinguished from acute appendicitis, salpingitis, cholecystitis and diverticulitis, in which pus and organisms are not present in the urine. Less commonly it may be mimicked by perinephric abscess due to infection by *Staph. aureus*. In this condition there is marked pain and tenderness in the renal region, and often bulging of the loin on the affected side. The patient is usually extremely ill, with fever, leucocytosis, and a positive blood culture. Urinary symptoms are absent, and the urine contains neither pus nor organisms. An untreated perinephric abscess may eventually discharge in the loin or groin.

Management

The information box on page 650 shows the necessary investigations. Diagnosis depends on the clinical features and results of urine culture. Intravenous urography or ultrasound should be performed without delay if there is clinical suspicion of obstruction or septicaemia; if not, an IVU should be done 4 to 6 weeks after recovery. When abnormalities of the urinary tract are found, further investigations and treatment are usually necessary. Antibiotic regimens for adults are shown in Table 11.4. It is often necessary to start treatment without knowing the organism or its sensitivity and to change the drug if necessary when these become available. In most cases oral trimethoprim, ampicillin or amoxycillin, all active against *E. coli*, can be used. Severe or septicaemic cases require intravenous therapy using an aminoglycoside such as tobramycin, a cephalosporin such as cefuroxime, or ciprofloxacin. Urine culture should be repeated during the course and 7 and 21 days after treatment. Any abnormality of the urinary tract should, if possible, be corrected.

REFLUX NEPHROPATHY (CHRONIC PYELONEPHRITIS)

This is a chronic interstitial nephritis resulting from urinary tract infection associated with vesico-ureteric reflux in early life. The morphological changes in the kidney are not entirely diagnostic, but the most important feature is the presence of coarse scars, most commonly in the upper pole, each of which is associated with contraction of the related papilla and dilatation of the corresponding calyx. These features can be identified by IVU or radionuclide scanning or on examination of the kidney at operation or autopsy. Histological features are not significantly different from those of chronic ischaemia or non-infective chronic tubulointerstitial nephritis (p. 663). The incidence of reflux nephropathy is not known. About 20% of patients in Europe requiring treatment for end-stage renal disease are said to have renal scarring, but the precise diagnostic criteria used are variable, so there is doubt about the accuracy of the figures.

Pathogenesis

In the absence of urinary tract abnormalities, acute pyelonephritis in patients over the age of 5 rarely leads to serious chronic renal disease. Possibly the most important predisposing factor is the presence of severe vesico-ureteric reflux (VUR) in children. Reflux of urine

from the bladder into the ureter during voiding is normally prevented because the ureter passes through the vesical wall obliquely and is therefore occluded during contraction of the bladder. Abnormalities of the intramural ureter allow reflux to occur and organisms from the bladder may then reach the kidney. VUR may be unilateral or bilateral, and its severity varies. In mild cases small amounts of urine pass a short distance up the ureter during voiding, returning to the bladder after cessation of micturition to form residual urine. In severe cases reflux occurs up the entire length of the ureter (Fig. 11.6); this results in a rise in intrapelvic pressure, the orifices of the compound renal papillae are forced open and urine refluxes into the renal parenchyma as far as the cortex. VUR is commonly congenital, but can be due to obstructive lesions at the bladder neck. It is thought that it usually occurs in utero, and that the scars of reflux nephropathy form during the first year of life. In young children with recurrent UTI the scars are found in 8–13%, and VUR is usually demonstrable on the side of the scarred kidney. Reflux diminishes as the child grows, and usually disappears. It is rarely demonstrable in an adult with a scarred kidney due to infection in childhood. Intrarenal reflux in young children interferes with renal growth. When UTI occurs in the presence of obstruction or stasis, whatever the cause, permanent damage may result in any age group.

In pregnant women permanent damage may result from UTI. The hormonal changes of pregnancy cause reduced ureteric motility and ureteric dilatation and may also facilitate establishment of infection in the renal parenchyma. About 5% of pregnant women have covert bacteriuria, and if no antibiotics are given, acute pyelonephritis occurs in up to 40% of such cases; hence the importance of treating asymptomatic bacteriuria in pregnancy.

When scarring has occurred, destruction of renal tissue usually continues despite the absence of recurrent infections. Why this happens is not known. Possible explanations include damage to remaining functioning glomeruli by progressive ischaemia resulting from lesions of blood vessels sustained during acute infections, or survival of bacterial variants in the hypertonic medullary tissue.

Pathology

The changes, which are not diagnostic, may be unilateral or bilateral and of any grade of severity. The fully developed case usually shows gross scarring of the kidneys, which may be much reduced in size with narrowing of the cortex and medulla. Renal scars are juxtaposed to dilated calyces. Histologically there is patchy fibrosis with chronic inflammatory cell infiltration, tubular atrophy, periglomerular fibrosis and eventual disappearance of nephrons. The arteries and arterioles may show sclerosis and narrowing. In patients who develop heavy proteinuria and hypertension, renal biopsies have shown focal glomerulosclerosis (see p. 646).

Clinical features

In many cases no symptoms arise directly from the renal lesions, and the patient consults the doctor because of lassitude, vague ill-health or symptoms of uraemia. Discovery of hypertension or proteinuria on routine examination may be the first indication of the disease. Symptoms arising from the urinary tract may also be present and include frequency of micturition, dysuria and aching lumbar pain. Occasionally weakness and fainting result from salt loss in the urine. Pyuria and low level proteinuria are common, but not invariable.

A number of women present with hypertension or proteinuria in pregnancy. In some families a positive family history is obtained with an autosomal dominant pattern of inheritance.

Investigations

The IVU shows the diagnostic features. The kidneys are reduced in size and there is localised contraction of the renal substance associated with clubbing of the adjacent calyces (Fig. 11.31). Culture of the urine is mandatory. When infection is present *E. coli* is the most common organism. Other agents include Proteus, *Pseudomonas aeruginosa* and staphylococci. Investigations such as rectal and vaginal examination, cystoscopy and urography are performed to identify any abnormality causing obstruction to the flow of urine. A micturating renogram or cystourethrogram will disclose vesico-ureteric reflux. Renal function should be assessed by estimation of the blood urea and creatinine, plasma electrolytes and creatinine clearance. It may be necessary to assess urinary acidification or renal sodium conservation. Women who present with hypertension of pregnancy should be investigated 2–3 months after delivery and their children should be screened for infection and reflux.

Management

Chronic infection is difficult to eradicate. Attempts should be made to correct abnormalities of the urinary tract, including malformations, and to remove calculi. An antibiotic to which the organism is sensitive should be given for 7 days. If the infection is not eradicated, suppressive therapy may be required for months (Table 11.4), the antibiotic being changed in response to the changing pattern and sensitivity of the organisms. Simple measures outlined in the information box (p. 651) should be adopted. Control of hypertension is essential and may delay the onset of uraemia. When pyonephrosis develops or renal infection is unilateral, nephrectomy

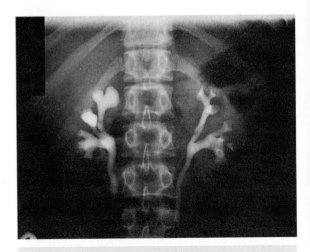

Fig. 11.31 Chronic pyelonephritis. Intravenous urogram revealing clubbing of the calyces particularly marked in the upper right pole. The appearances on the left are virtually normal.

may be indicated. Rarely, hypertension is cured by the removal of the diseased kidney. The role of surgery in correction of VUR is limited because childhood reflux tends to disappear spontaneously.

Patients who lose excessive amounts of sodium in the urine develop extracellular fluid depletion which exacerbates their uraemia. These patients benefit from taking 5–10 g/day (85–170 mmol/day) of sodium chloride by mouth. It is usual to start with 3–4 g/day and increase the dose as required. The limit for additional salt is set by development of systemic or pulmonary oedema, or aggravation of hypertension. Sodium bicarbonate may be substituted in part for sodium chloride when acidosis is severe (see p. 596, Ch. 10). Severe renal impairment is treated as indicated on page 633.

Prognosis

The course is usually long and punctuated by acute exacerbations. Infection is difficult to eradicate even when underlying abnormalities are relieved, and in elderly, diabetic or paraplegic patients a fulminating infection may be the terminal event. Pyonephrosis may occur, especially in the presence of renal calculi. It is characterised by persistent lumbar pain, intermittent pyrexia, rigors, emaciation, pyuria, and if both kidneys are involved, uraemia. One or both kidneys may become palpable.

RENAL TUBERCULOSIS

Tuberculosis of the kidney is invariably secondary to tuberculosis elsewhere (see p. 366) and occurs as a result of blood-borne infection. The initial lesion develops in the renal cortex, and if untreated, may ulcerate into the pelvis, with consequent involvement of the bladder, epididymis, seminal vesicles and prostate. The disease tends to occur in young people, and may manifest itself with recurrent haematuria and dysuria due to secondary involvement of the bladder. In addition, the general features of tuberculosis, i.e. malaise, fever, lassitude and weight loss, may be present. Chronic renal failure may result from destruction of kidney tissue, or be due to obstruction of the urinary tract when lesions heal by fibrosis. Culture of the urine by ordinary methods may be sterile in spite of pyuria, and indeed sterile pyuria is an indication to perform special cultures for tubercle bacilli. The extent of the infection with regard to the lower urinary tract should be ascertained by cystoscopic examination.

FURTHER READING

Stamm W E, Hooton T M 1993 Management of urinary tract infections in adults. New England Journal of Medicine 329: 1328–1334

OBSTRUCTION OF THE URINARY TRACT

Obstruction to the flow of urine from the kidney is a common disorder. It causes stasis and an increase in pressure above the obstruction, which in turn predispose to infection, stone formation and renal failure. Obstruction may occur at any level, but is most common at the pelvi-ureteric junction, at the bladder neck or in the urethra (Fig. 11.32). Obstruction at the pelvi-ureteric junction causes hydronephrosis. Obstruction of the ureter causes hydroureter and subsequently hydronephrosis. Obstruction of the bladder neck or urethra distends the bladder, causes hypertrophy of its muscle (seen on cystoscopic examination as trabeculation) and subsequently leads to hydroureter and hydronephrosis. If obstruction is unrelieved, slowly progressive destruction of renal tissue occurs. Superimposed infection often results in rapid deterioration of renal function.

Aetiology

Obstruction may be due to a structural lesion, or to a congenital neuromuscular defect which prevents the contraction wave, and thus the flow of urine (Table 11.5).

Clinical features

These vary with the cause and site of the lesion. When the obstruction is above the bladder, renal colic may occur, especially if the onset is sudden. More commonly

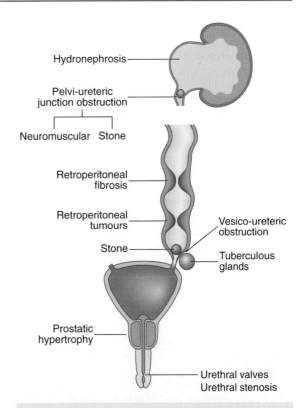

Fig. 11.32 Obstruction of the urinary tract. Obstruction to the urinary tract can arise at the pelviureteric junction, in the ureter, at the vesico-ureteric junction, at bladder outflow and also in the urethra.

Table 11.5	Important causes of urinary tract obstruction
Structural	
Lumen	Stone, blood clot, caseous or necrotic debris, sloughed papilla
Wall	Tumour Fibrosis following trauma, stone, instrumentation, surgery or infection (TB, schistosomiasis, gonorrhoea) Congenital bladder neck obstruction Urethral valves
External	Aberrant renal artery crossing upper ureter Retroperitoneal tumour Retroperitoneal fibrosis (idiopathic, leaking aortic aneurysm, drug-induced, neoplastic) Prostatic enlargement Phimosis Accidental ligation of ureter at operation
Functional	Congenital neuromuscular defects (pelvi-ureteric junction, ureter, bladder neck)

the obstruction is gradual, and aching pain in the loins, sometimes aggravated by drinking, develops. Superimposed infection causes malaise, fever, dysuria and sometimes septicaemia. Haematuria is common. In partial obstruction, transmission of the increased hydrostatic pressure to the kidney interferes with the counter-current concentrating mechanism and, paradoxically, may result in polyuria. Occasionally a hydronephrotic kidney is palpable. Sometimes the patient presents with anuria and acute renal failure (see above). Intermittent anuria suggests a diagnosis of stone or retroperitoneal fibrosis. Obstruction below the bladder causes difficulty in micturition. The urinary stream is thin in calibre and poor in force. Complete urinary retention may occur with consequent distension of the bladder, which may be visible and palpable as a swelling of the lower abdomen. Anuria or overflow incontinence may ensue. In the latter event, catheterisation reveals the presence of residual urine in the bladder after the patient has voided. Infection is extremely common.

Investigations

Rectal or vaginal examination should be carried out to detect prostatic enlargement or pelvic tumour.

Ultrasound examination will detect dilatation of the renal pelvis and upper ureter (Fig. 11.4). It is particularly valuable when acute renal failure is present (p. 631). In cases with renal failure, it can be combined with percutaneous nephrostomy to relieve the obstruction, followed by antegrade pyelography to identify the site of the lesion.

Intravenous urography can also be used to diagnose obstruction; when obstruction is present, both nephrogram and pyelogram are delayed, dilatation of the outflow system is seen, and the site of obstruction can often be identified. A post-voiding film should be performed to detect bladder abnormalities.

Neither ultrasound nor IVU can distinguish a distended urinary tract in which there is no resistance to flow (e.g. after pregnancy) from genuine urinary tract obstruction. However, this distinction can often be made by a diuretic renogram (Fig. 11.11). Cystoscopy, retrograde pyelography, urethrography and cystometry may be required to define lesions in the bladder, urethra or lower ureter, and for removal of stones or debris from the ureter or bladder. Culture of urine and, if the patient is systemically unwell, of blood should be carried out. Assessment of renal function is essential.

Management

The ultimate objective is to remove the source of obstruction, but in order to preserve renal function, relieve symptoms and treat infection, temporary drainage of the urinary tract may be required. Obstruction of the bladder neck or urethra should be relieved using a urethral or, rarely, a suprapubic catheter. Obstruction of the upper urinary tract can be treated by insertion of a catheter into the renal pelvis under ultrasound guidance (percutaneous nephrostomy).

Relief of obstruction may be followed by a massive diuresis (post-obstructive diuresis) due to impaired tubular function, loss of the medullary concentration gradient, and the diuretic effect of retained solute and water. In this situation, electrolyte losses must be replaced intravenously. When obstruction is incomplete, or is due to stones or debris which are likely to be passed spontaneously, temporary drainage is rarely necessary unless infection supervenes. Antibiotics are required to treat severe infection or to cover surgical procedures. Dialysis may be necessary before surgery.

Once the underlying lesion has been identified and renal function assessed, definitive treatment is often possible, e.g. removal of stone, transurethral resection of the prostate. When obstruction is irremediable, the ureters may be anastomosed to an isolated loop of ileum opening on to the abdominal wall (ileal conduit). Alternatively, in-dwelling stents may be left in one or both ureters, and changed at regular intervals (usually 6-monthly) to prevent infection.

Patients who have undergone treatment for urinary tract obstruction should thereafter have periodic assessment of renal function. Unilateral nephrectomy may be indicated because of persistent infection and, occasionally, hypertension due to renin production in the damaged kidney. When both kidneys are permanently damaged, treatment for chronic renal failure is required (p. 631).

FURTHER READING

Barton D P J et al 1992 Percutaneous nephrostomy and ureteral stenting in gynaecological malignancies. Obstetrics and Gynaecology 80: 805–811

URINARY TRACT CALCULI AND NEPHROCALCINOSIS

Aetiology

Urinary calculi consist of aggregates of crystals and small amounts of proteins and glycoprotein, but their genesis is poorly understood. Different types of stone occur in different parts of the world, and dietary factors probably play a part in determining the varying patterns. In Britain, stones in which the crystalline component consists of calcium oxalate are the most common (39% of calculi in one survey). In this study, 14% of stones contained both calcium oxalate and calcium phosphate, 13% calcium phosphate alone, and 15% contained magnesium ammonium phosphate. Small numbers of cystine stones and uric acid stones were found.

In developing countries, bladder stones are common, particularly in children. In industrialised countries the incidence of childhood bladder stone is low, and renal stones in adults are more common. One survey found that 4% of the population has stones in the urinary tract, but prevalence varies in different areas. It is surprising that stones and nephrocalcinosis are not more common, since some of the constituents are present in urine in concentrations which exceed their maximum solubility in water. However, urine contains glycosaminoglycans, pyrophosphate and citrate which, by forming complexes, may keep otherwise insoluble salts in solution.

Certain conditions are frequently associated with stone formation.

CONDITIONS FREQUENTLY ASSOCIATED WITH STONE FORMATION

Acquired disorders
- Obstruction of urinary tract → Formation of phosphate stones
- Infection of urinary tract → Formation of phosphate stones
- Climate or occupation giving rise to excessive sweating → Formation of stones due to high concentration of constituents in reduced urine volume, resulting in precipitation
- Hypercalciuria → Formation of calcium oxalate stones
- Hyperoxaluria → Formation of calcium oxalate stones

Inherited disorders
- Cystinuria → Formation of cystine stones
- Xanthinuria → Formation of xanthine stones
- Gout, myeloproliferative disorders → Formation of uric acid stones
- Medullary sponge kidney

CONDITIONS ASSOCIATED WITH HYPERCALCIURIA AND HYPEROXALURIA

Hypercalciuria
- High dietary intake calcium (dairy produce)
- Hyperparathyroidism
- Vitamin D poisoning
- Sarcoidosis
- Cushing's syndrome
- Myelomatosis
- Renal tubular acidosis
- Prolonged immobilisation
- Idiopathic hypercalciuria
  (a) excessive absorption of calcium from gut
  (b) reduced renal tubular absorption of filtered calcium

Hyperoxaluria
- High dietary intake oxalate (fruit and vegetables)
- Increased absorption of oxalate from gut:
  (a) ileal disease
  (b) low calcium diet

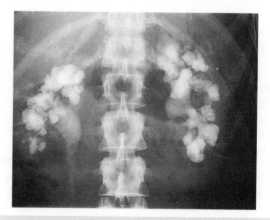

Fig. 11.33   Intravenous pyelogram showing bilateral staghorn calculi in both kidneys. Some dye is being excreted by right kidney with little function on the left.

The pH of urine influences the formation of stones. An alkaline urine tends to increase precipitation of calcium phosphate, and may be responsible for calcium phosphate stones in patients with renal tubular acidosis. Solubility of uric acid and cystine is reduced in acid urine. Today in prosperous countries most calculi occur in healthy young men in whom investigations reveal no clear cause for stone formation. Multiple aetiological factors are probably present in such cases, and it is likely that an alteration in the relative proportions of crystalloids and glycosaminoglycans in the urine is of particular importance.

Pathology

Urinary concretions vary greatly in size. There may be particles like sand anywhere in the urinary tract, or large round stones in the bladder. Staghorn calculi fill the whole renal pelvis and branch into the calyces (Fig. 11.33); they are usually associated with pyelonephritis. Deposits of calcium may be present throughout the renal parenchyma, giving rise to nephrocalcinosis (Fig. 11.3, p. 616). This is especially liable to occur in chronic pyelonephritis, renal tubular acidosis, hyperparathyroidism, vitamin D intoxication and healed renal tuberculosis.

Clinical features

These vary according to the size, shape and position of the stone, and the nature of any underlying condition. Renal calculi or nephrocalcinosis may be present for years without giving rise to symptoms, and may be discovered during radiological examination for another disorder. More commonly, patients present with pain, recurrent urinary infection or clinical features of urinary tract obstruction. The most common complaint arising from renal calculi is intermittent dull pain in the loin or back, increased by movement. Protein, red cells or leucocytes may appear in the urine.

When a stone becomes impacted in the ureter, an attack of **renal colic** develops. The patient is suddenly aware of pain in the loin, which soon radiates round the flank to the groin and often into the testis or labium, in the sensory distribution of the first lumbar nerve. The pain steadily increases in intensity to reach a maximum in a few minutes. The patient is restless, and generally tries unsuccessfully to obtain relief by changing position and by pacing the room. There is pallor, sweating and often vomiting, and the patient may groan in agony. Frequency, dysuria and haematuria may occur. The intense pain usually subsides within 2 hours, but may continue unabated for hours or days. The pain is usually constant during attacks, though slight fluctuations in severity may occur. Contrary to general belief, attacks rarely consist of intermittent severe pains coming and going every few minutes.

Investigations

The diagnosis of renal colic is usually easily made from the history and by finding red cells in the urine. Any patient suspected of having stones should have radiographs of the urinary tract. If there is doubt about the cause of pain an IVU during an attack may help. When the pain is due to a stone in the ureter, the radiograph shows a dense renal shadow and appearance of dye in the renal pelvis is delayed (Fig. 11.34). Subsequently the site of obstruction may be visible.

Appropriate investigations should be undertaken to discover any underlying disorder (Table 11.6).

Management

The immediate treatment of loin pain or renal colic is bed rest, application of warmth to the site of pain, and administration of analgesia, e.g. diclofenac suppository (100 mg). In severe cases, pethidine (100 mg), morphine (10–20 mg), and antispasmodic drugs, e.g. atropine sulphate (0.8 or 1.2 mg) may be given intramuscularly. If possible the patient should drink 2 litres of fluid daily. Small stones, less than 0.5 cm in diameter, are usually passed naturally, but larger stones may require active intervention. Immediate action is required if anuria, bilateral hydronephrosis, or significant infection such as pyonephrosis develops (p. 654).

Attempts to dissolve calculi have failed, but in some centres a lithotriptor is available. Using this apparatus, many calculi can be fragmented, in vivo, by shock waves, generated under water, focused on the stone, and

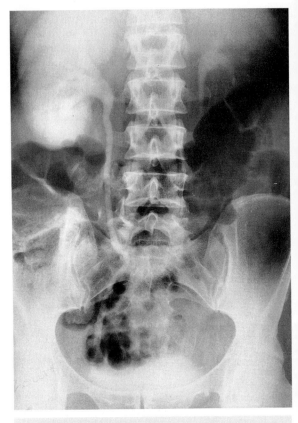

Fig. 11.34 Unilateral obstruction. Intravenous urogram of a patient with a stone (not visible) at the lower end of the right ureter. This film taken two hours post-injection demonstrates persistence of dye in the right kidney, pelvi-calyceal system, and ureter whereas only a small amount of dye is visible in the left pelvi-calyceal system.

INDICATIONS FOR INTERVENTION IN RENAL CALCULI

- The patient is anuric*
- The ureter or pelvi-ureteric junction is obstructed, totally* or partially, by a stone unlikely to pass spontaneously or one which has not moved for several weeks
- Infection is present*
- The patient has intolerable or recurrent pain

*Indications for urgent intervention

applied to the body surface. The fragments are then passed in the urine. This technique requires free drainage of the tract below the stones.

Stones in the renal pelvis can be removed by open operation, or endoscopically via a percutaneous nephrostomy, or fragmented using the lithotriptor. Ureteric stones can be removed endoscopically via the bladder or

Table 11.6   Investigation of patients with renal calculi

Investigation of urinary tract	Examination urine for protein, r.b.c, w.b.c.	Indicates abnormality of urinary tract
	Quantitative culture MSU	Urinary infection
	Plain film abdomen	Shows opaque calculi, nephrocalcinosis
	IVU	Shows calculi, obstruction, abnormalities urinary tract, e.g. medullary sponge kidney
Investigation of renal function	Blood urea, plasma creatinine	
	Creatinine clearance	
Investigation to determine underlying cause	Chemical analysis calculus	Provides information as to what investigations to pursue
	Plasma calcium, phosphate	Hypercalcaemia
	Plasma PTH	If hypercalcaemia present, to investigate possible hyperparathyroidism
	24 h urine calcium ($\times$ 2)	Hypercalciuria
	Plasma urate	In patients with urate stones or calcium stones
	24 h urine urate ($\times$ 2)	
	24 h urine cystine ($\times$ 2)	In patients with cystine stones
	24 h urine oxalate ($\times$ 2)	Hyperoxaluria
	Acidification of urine (p. 668)	Distal renal tubular acidosis

a percutaneous nephrostomy, or can be pushed up into the renal pelvis, and then removed through a nephrostomy or disintegrated by lithotripsy. Bladder stones are removed or fragmented during cystoscopy. Rarely cystotomy is needed to remove large stones. Antibiotic cover should be given for stone removal.

A daily urine output of at least 2 litres is advisable in all patients with stone disease. Fluid intake should therefore be about 3 litres per day—more if the climate or the patient's occupation causes much sweating. Suitable measures should be instituted to correct any known cause of stone formation. Preparations containing vitamin D must be avoided.

In idiopathic hypercalciuria due to excessive absorption of calcium, the intake of high calcium foods (milk and cheese) and of oxalate should be reduced. In idiopathic hypercalciuria of renal origin, bendrofluazide 5 mg/day reduces urinary calcium excretion by about 30%. An alternative is to use sodium cellulose phosphate (5 g sachet with meals). Each 5 g dose will bind approximately 350 mg of calcium.

In patients with recurrent oxalate stones, foods rich in oxalate, such as rhubarb and spinach, should be avoided. Persons who have passed several uric acid or urate stones benefit from allopurinol, 100–300 mg/day, depending on renal function. Allopurinol also has a place in treating calcium oxalate stone disease, to which urates may contribute by acting as a nidus for stone formation.

Phosphate-containing calculi are formed only in alkaline urine; hence acidifying the urine by giving ammonium chloride may be effective. In contrast, cystine and urate stones may be prevented, or sometimes dissolved, by giving sufficient sodium bicarbonate to make the urine persistently alkaline, and ensuring a high urine output of 2–4 litres daily. When these measures fail or are unacceptable to the patient, treatment with penicillamine, a chelating agent, in a dose of 1–1.5 g/day may be tried. This drug can cause membranous glomerulonephritis or Goodpasture's syndrome, both of which eventually recover when penicillamine is stopped, and a number of other unpleasant side-effects including fever, disturbances of taste, and blood dyscrasias.

FURTHER READING

Whitfield H N 1992 Modern management of urinary tract stones. In: Raine A E G (ed.) Advanced renal medicine. Oxford University Press, Oxford.

CONGENITAL ABNORMALITIES OF THE KIDNEYS

Anomalies of the urinary tract affect more than 10% of infants and, if not immediately lethal, may lead to complications in later life. About 1 in 500 infants is born with only one kidney. Although usually compatible with normal life, this is often associated with other abnormalities.

POLYCYSTIC KIDNEY DISEASE

This genetically-determined abnormality of renal structure may be associated with other congenital abnormalities, such as polycystic liver disease (p. 537). Infantile polycystic kidney disease is very rare, inherited as an autosomal recessive and usually fatal in the first year of life. Adult polycystic kidney disease (APKD) affects approximately 80/100 000 of the general population. It is inherited as an autosomal dominant trait, males and females being equally affected. Data obtained using recombinant DNA techniques and genetic linkage analysis have located the APKD gene on the distal short arm of chromosome 16.

Pathology

Small cysts, present in infancy, subsequently enlarge at a variable rate. In fully developed APKD the kidneys are asymmetrically enlarged and contain numerous cysts. These vary in size and are surrounded by a variable amount of parenchyma which often shows extensive fibrosis and arteriolosclerosis.

Clinical features

Affected subjects may be asymptomatic until late in life. After the age of 20 there is often an insidious onset of hypertension, which may or may not be associated with deterioration of renal function. Common clinical features are shown in the information box.

ADULT POLYCYSTIC KIDNEY DISEASE: COMMON CLINICAL FEATURES

- Vague discomfort in loin or abdomen due to increasing mass of renal tissue
- Acute loin pain or renal colic due to haemorrhage into a cyst
- Hypertension
- Haematuria
- Urinary tract infection
- Uraemia

Often one or both kidneys can be palpated, and the surface may be nodular. In addition to polycystic disease, other diseases in which the kidneys may be palpably enlarged are hydronephrosis or pyonephrosis, solitary cyst, renal carcinoma, other renal tumours, and renal amyloid. It should be remembered, however, that in some normal people the right kidney, and occasionally the lower pole of the left kidney, may be felt on clinical examination. This is particularly true in slim women. On the other hand, pathologically enlarged kidneys are not always palpable, particularly in obese people.

About one-third of patients with APKD have hepatic cysts, but disturbance of liver function is rare. Berry aneurysms of cerebral vessels are an associated feature, and about 10% of patients have a subarachnoid haemorrhage. The outlook is better than is generally appreciated. Although there is a gradual reduction in renal function, almost 50% of patients never require chronic dialysis.

Investigations

The diagnosis is made on the basis of clinical findings, family history and ultrasound, which is a sensitive method for demonstrating cysts (Fig. 11.35). Now that the gene defect responsible for APKD has been identified it is possible to make a specific genetic diagnosis.

Management

Control of blood pressure is vital, since uncontrolled hypertension accelerates the development of renal failure. Urinary infections must be treated promptly. Patients with impaired ability to conserve sodium ('salt wasters') require supplements of sodium chloride and sodium bicarbonate. When renal function is severely compromised, the regime for management of chronic renal failure must be instituted (see p. 631).

Screening and counselling

Screening by ultrasound can be used to detect asymptomatic cases of APKD amongst relatives of patients. Screening and counselling should be offered to those over 18 years. Ultrasound is much less reliable in the 10–18 age group, who in any case have difficulty understanding the implications of a positive diagnosis. A diagnosis made in early adult life allows regular monitoring of blood pressure and renal function, and permits genetic counselling to be given before most patients start their family. It does, however, have implications for life insurance, mortgages and employment, and not everyone offered screening will accept it. Now that the gene defect has been discovered, specific genetic testing will be used both for screening and for antenatal diagnosis.

MEDULLARY CYSTIC DISEASE

Cysts predominantly in the renal medulla are found in two different conditions. In **medullary sponge kidney**

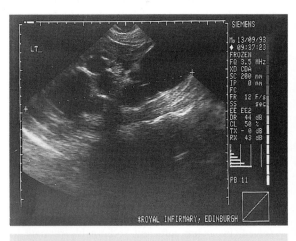

Fig. 11.35 Renal ultrasound—adult polycystic kidney disease. Numerous cysts of varying size are seen replacing most of the renal substance.

the cysts are confined to the papillary collecting ducts. Affected patients, usually adults, present with pain, haematuria, stone formation, or urinary infection. The diagnosis is made by IVU. Contrast medium is seen to fill dilated or cystic tubules, which are sometimes calcified. The prognosis is generally good.

In **medullary cystic disease** small cortical cysts are also present, and these lead to progressive destruction of the nephron. This condition, characterised by thirst and polyuria (due to nephrogenic diabetes insipidus), occurs in younger patients, and there is often a family history. Sometimes affected patients are 'salt wasters', which aggravates the degree of renal failure. Even when treated appropriately, serious renal failure is usual.

DEFECTS OF TUBULAR FUNCTION

Renal glycosuria is a benign defect of tubular reabsorption of glucose, usually inherited as an autosomal recessive. Glucose appears in the urine in the presence of a normal blood glucose concentration.

Cystinuria is a rare condition in which reabsorption of filtered cystine, ornithine, arginine and lysine is defective. The high concentration of cystine in urine leads to cystine stone formation (p. 657). Other uncommon tubular disorders include **vitamin D resistant rickets**, in which reabsorption of filtered phosphate is reduced; **nephrogenic diabetes insipidus**, in which the tubules are resistant to the effects of vasopressin; and the **Fanconi syndrome** (p. 662).

RENAL TUBULAR ACIDOSIS (RTA)

RTA (see Table 11.7) results from a failure of *either* reabsorption of bicarbonate in the proximal tubule *or* acidification of the urine in the distal tubule. There may be little or no overall reduction in renal function.

Distal renal tubular acidosis (classical or type 1)

In this condition the ability to form a very acid urine is lost, and the urine pH cannot be reduced to less than 5.3 even in the presence of severe systemic acidosis. This defect is demonstrated by the ammonium chloride test (see Appendix, p. 668), and is due to failure of the collecting ducts to secrete hydrogen ions or to sustain the gradient for hydrogen ions between the luminal fluid and the tubular cell. Two types have been described. In **complete RTA** there is persistent hyperchloraemic acidosis. In the **incomplete** form, the plasma bicarbonate is normal, but the urine pH does not fall to less than 5.3 after ammonium chloride.

The management consists of determining and dealing

Distal RTA (type 1)	Proximal RTA (type 2)
Table 11.7 Causes of renal tubular acidosis	

Table 11.7 Causes of renal tubular acidosis

Distal RTA (type 1)	Proximal RTA (type 2)
Primary	
Familial autosomal dominant	Sporadic familial
Secondary	
Renal diseases	
Pyelonephritis	Nephrotic syndrome
Medullary sponge kidney	Transplanted kidney
Hydronephrosis	
Sickle cell disease	
Transplanted kidney	
Drugs	
Lithium	Tetracycline (outdated)
Amphotericin	Carbonic anhydrase inhibitors
Dysproteinaemias	
Amyloidosis	Amyloidosis
Hyperglobulinaemia	
Cryoglobulinaemia	
Disordered calcium metabolism	
Vitamin D intoxication	Cystinosis
Hyperparathyroidism	Tyrosinosis
Immunologically mediated	**Heavy metals**
Chronic active hepatitis	Cadmium
Primary biliary cirrhosis	Lead
Sjögren's syndrome	Copper
SLE	Mercury

CLINICAL FEATURES OF DISTAL (TYPE 1) RENAL TUBULAR ACIDOSIS

- Anorexia, fatigue
- Osteomalacia, due to buffering retained H^+ in bone, with associated muscle weakness
- Hypercalciuria, hyperphosphaturia, recurrent renal calculi, nephrocalcinosis
- Loss of excessive amounts of sodium in urine (diminished Na^+/H^+ exchange in collecting ducts)
- Extracellular fluid volume depletion
- Loss of excessive amounts of potassium in urine (reflecting activation of the renin-angiotensin-aldosterone axis)

Young children present with failure to thrive, polyuria, thirst, constipation.

with the underlying cause where possible (Table 11.7). Bicarbonate supplements should be given in a dose sufficient to keep the plasma bicarbonate in excess of 18 mmol/l. Large doses may be required, starting with a dose of 1 g of sodium bicarbonate 8-hourly and increasing the dose until the desired plasma bicarbonate is achieved, and there are no signs of sodium depletion (p. 591). When hypokalaemia is present, a mixture of sodium and potassium bicarbonate should be given. Initially about half of the total bicarbonate supplement is given as the potassium salt. The proportion of potassium bicarbonate is determined by regular monitoring of plasma potassium. Patients with severe osteomalacia may require 1α-hydroxycholecalciferol (Alfacalcidol). The starting dose is 0.5 μg daily for adults. The plasma calcium must be checked regularly and the dose adjusted appropriately.

Proximal renal tubular acidosis (type 2)

This may occur as an isolated defect (primary proximal RTA). More commonly, there are multiple defects in proximal tubular function, and patients have glycosuria, aminoaciduria, phosphaturia and uricosuria (Fanconi syndrome). Proximal tubular sodium/hydrogen exchange is impaired, resulting in decreased bicarbonate reabsorption, large losses of bicarbonate in the urine, and a marked reduction in plasma bicarbonate. Once the plasma bicarbonate has fallen to about 12 mmol/l, the reduced filtered load can be reabsorbed by the proximal tubular cells, and the amount of bicarbonate reaching the distal tubular is negligible. In these circumstances, it is possible to show that the collecting duct cells can secrete hydrogen ions against a gradient, so that the urine pH falls below 5.3. There is frequently associated hyperchloraemia, potassium depletion and hypocalcaemia. Distinction of proximal and distal RTA requires special tests not considered here.

Any underlying cause should be treated (Table 11.7). The plasma bicarbonate should be maintained greater than 18 mmol/l with appropriate supplements of sodium bicarbonate. Very large amounts of bicarbonate are needed, and it is recommended that the starting dose should be 1 mmol/kg daily. A 500 mg sodium bicarbonate capsule provides 6 mmol of bicarbonate. In those patients with hypokalaemia, a proportion of the dose, determined by monitoring plasma potassium, is given as potassium bicarbonate. Where necessary, calcium supplements and 1α-hydroxycholecalciferol are given.

FURTHER READING

Fick G M, Gabow P A 1994 Hereditary and acquired cystic disease of the kidney. Kidney International 46: 951–964

DRUGS AND THE KIDNEY

DRUG-INDUCED RENAL DISEASE

The susceptibility of the kidney to damage by drugs stems from the fact that it is the route of excretion of many water soluble compounds, including drugs and their metabolites. These are delivered in large amounts to the kidney, which receives 25% of the cardiac output. Drugs such as cephalosporins may reach high concentrations in the renal cortex as a result of proximal tubular transport mechanisms. Others, such as aspirin, are concentrated in the medulla by the operation of the counter-current system. Renal damage can arise during treatment with a large number of drugs, and a variety of lesions may result. An accurate drug history is therefore essential in all patients, particularly those with unexplained impairment of renal function. Table 11.8 gives some indication of the range of lesions, the drugs known to cause them and the ways in which patients may present. Drug-induced acute renal failure is usually reversible, but a few patients fail to recover full renal function.

ANALGESIC NEPHROPATHY

Renal papillary necrosis and chronic interstitial nephritis due to long continued ingestion of analgesic drugs accounts for between 5 and 17% of end-stage renal disease in European countries. In animals, lesions can be induced with almost any non-steroidal anti-inflammatory drug (NSAID). In man, mixtures containing aspirin and phenacetin were historically important, but probably all NSAIDs can induce the lesion if taken regularly, even in small doses. Dehydration, which reduces medullary blood flow and results in concentration of the drugs in the renal medulla, is an important contributory factor.

Pathology

Diffuse interstitial fibrosis and tubular atrophy develop. Acute papillary necrosis is common, and is probably the initial lesion in most cases. A recognised complication is development of carcinoma of the renal pelvis.

Clinical features

Most patients are women who suffer from anxiety or who have personality problems. Other patients may have taken analgesic preparations for many years for headaches, rheumatoid arthritis or osteoarthrosis. Asymptomatic disease may be disclosed when abnormalities of blood or urine are found during medical examination. Patients with moderate renal impairment present with malaise, thirst and polyuria due to impaired urinary concentration, or recurrent urinary infection. Approximately 60% of patients are hypertensive. Renal damage is predominantly tubular, and failure to conserve sodium and renal tubular acidosis are common. Renal colic or ureteric obstruction and acute renal failure may be caused by passage of fragments of necrotic papillae, which can be recognised by microscopic examination of the urine. Acute renal failure may also follow urinary

Table 11.8 **Drug-induced renal disease**

Pathological lesion	Clinical presentation	Drugs which give rise to the lesion
Drug induced (toxic) tubular necrosis	Proteinuria Abnormalities of urinary sediment Varying degrees of renal impairment including acute renal failure and oliguria	Aminoglycosides[1] Cephalosporins Iodine contrast media Paracetamol overdose Amphotericin Cisplatinum
Acute ischaemic tubular necrosis	Hypotension Reduced renal perfusion Pre-renal failure Acute renal failure $\pm$ oliguria	1. Antihypertensive drugs, ACE inhibitors 2. Drugs inducing volume depletion (diuretics, drugs causing severe diarrhoea/vomiting) 3. NSAIDs by reducing intrarenal vasodilator prostaglandins
Acute tubulo-interstitial nephritis	Proteinuria, microscopic haematuria Varying degrees of renal impairment including acute renal failure and oliguria Arthralgia Rash Fever Eosinophilia Marrow suppression	Penicillins Sulphonamides Cephalosporins Rifampicin[2] Allopurinol Fibrates Azathioprine Cimetidine NSAIDs[3] Frusemide
Hypersensitivity vasculitis	Proteinuria Micro- or macroscopic haematuria Varying degrees of renal impairment including acute renal failure and oliguria Other manifestations of vasculitis, e.g. rash, fever, eosinophilia, arthralgia	Sulphonamides Penicillins Rifampicin Isoniazid Procainamide
Intravascular coagulation	Acute or subacute renal failure Manifestations of DIC, e.g. coagulation disturbances, vascular lesions in other organs, thrombocytopenia, fragmentation of r.b.c.	Oral contraceptives Oestrogens
Glomerulonephritis	Proteinuria Nephrotic syndrome Acute renal failure Chronic renal failure	Penicillamine[4] Gold Captopril NSAIDs

Disturbance of tubular function	Failure of concentration
	
	Failure to excrete water
	Renal tubular acidosis
	  Distal
	  Proximal
	
	Potassium loss
	
	Magnesium loss
		Lithium
		Demeclocycline
		Methoxyfluorane
		(see p. 594)
		Amphotericin B, lithium
		Outdated tetracyclines
		Cyclosporin A
		Amphotericin B
		Carbenicillin (large dose)
		Gentamicin
		Cisplatinum

Obstruction Retroperitoneal fibrosis	Intermittent urinary tract obstruction Impaired renal function Acute renal failure Chronic renal failure	Methysergide Practolol
Crystals	Acute oliguric renal failure	Uric acid crystals—chemotherapy for malignancy Crystals of drug—sulphonamides
Papillary necrosis and chronic interstitial nephritis	'Analgesic nephropathy syndrome'	Compound analgesics (e.g. aspirin/phenacetin/codeine, aspirin/paracetamol, etc.) Aspirin, phenacetin, indomethacin, naproxen, possibly other NSAID

[1] Combination of aminoglycosides with cephalosporin or frusemide particularly likely to induce lesion.
[2] Particularly likely if given intermittently.
[3] This lesion often associated with heavy proteinuria, suggestive of accompanying glomerular lesion.
[4] May cause Goodpasture's syndrome.

infection or a sudden increase in the intake of analgesics. Many cases present with established chronic renal failure. Analgesic nephropathy may be part of a widespread syndrome associated with analgesic abuse, which includes peptic ulceration, anaemia, skin pigmentation and premature ageing.

Investigations

Apart from the history of drug ingestion, the diagnosis can sometimes be made on the basis of radiological findings and biochemical evidence of tubular dysfunction. The appearance of the papillae on IVU or retrograde pyelography is often characteristic. The contrast medium appears as a small tract within the papillary substance; later the papillae may separate, giving a ring shadow. Urine usually contains red cells and sterile pyuria is common. Proteinuria rarely exceeds 1 g/24 hours at presentation, but tends to increase as renal failure develops.

Management

Provided that analgesic preparations are withdrawn, there is a reasonable prospect of some recovery of function; otherwise irreversible renal failure develops. Treatment consists of withdrawing the drug, maintaining a fluid intake of 2 to 3 litres per day, treating hypertension and when necessary providing supplements of sodium chloride and sodium bicarbonate to restore ECF volume and correct metabolic acidosis. Regular follow-up is essential. When renal function is severely impaired the regimen for management of chronic renal failure should be instituted (p. 633).

USE OF DRUGS IN PATIENTS WITH IMPAIRED RENAL FUNCTION

Adverse reactions to drugs are significantly more common when renal function is impaired, because urinary excretion of many drugs and their active water soluble metabolites is reduced, leading to increased plasma concentrations. Moreover, uraemia is associated with alterations in distribution of drugs throughout body fluids, reduced binding of drugs by plasma albumin and changes in their metabolism. The dose of many commonly used drugs must therefore be reduced in renal failure, e.g. cephalosporins, cotrimoxazole, aminoglycosides, digoxin, opiates. The following principles should be observed when treating patients with impaired renal function.

USE OF DRUGS WITH IMPAIRED RENAL FUNCTION

- No drug should be given unless specifically indicated
- The least toxic alternative must be chosen
- The British National Formulary or other reference should be consulted to determine:
  (a) recommended dose for degree of renal impairment (use creatinine clearance as indication of degree of impairment)
  (b) adverse effects of drug
- The patient must be observed regularly for signs of adverse effects and the drug stopped or the dose reduced if these develop
- Measurement of plasma drug concentration may be helpful in monitoring dosing schedule

---

FURTHER READING

Cleland J G F 1993 Renal function in heart failure—the effect of ACE inhibitors. In: Cleland J G F (ed.) Clinician's guide to ACE inhibition. Churchill Livingstone, Edinburgh

Whelton A, Hamilton C W 1991 Non-steroidal anti-inflammatory drugs: effects on kidney function. Journal of Clinical Pharmacology 31: 588–598

TUMOURS OF THE KIDNEY AND GENITO-URINARY TRACT

RENAL CARCINOMA

Between 1 and 2% of malignant tumours arise in the kidney. Renal adenocarcinoma, the most common, occurs most frequently in adult men. Occasionally the affected kidney contains multiple tumours, or both kidneys are involved.

Pathology

The tumour, which is composed of large cells with clear cytoplasm, arises from proximal tubular epithelium. The cut surface appears yellow, and large tumours contain haemorrhagic or cystic areas. Local spread is by penetration of the renal capsule and invasion of renal veins. Spread to the opposite kidney occurs via the veins. The tumour is vascular, and metastasises to regional lymph nodes, bone, lung and liver.

Clinical features

Haematuria is the most common presenting symptom. About 20% of patients present late with haematuria, pain in the loin or renal colic and a palpable mass in the flank. In 30%, changes due to systemic effects of tumour metabolites are the first indication of disease (Table 11.9). These effects resolve after nephrectomy and must

Table 11.9 Syndrome associated with renal carcinoma

Findings	Per cent of patients with renal tumour with this finding	Explanation
Raised ESR	55	Changes in serum proteins associated with many tumours
Hypertension	37	Secretion of renin by tumour
Anaemia	36	Depression of erythropoiesis plus or minus haematuria
Weight loss	34	Tumour products depress appetite
Pyrexia	17	Circulating pyrogens
Abnormal liver function	14	This may disappear after nephrectomy
Raised alkaline phosphatase	9	Secreted by tumour?
Hypercalcaemia	5	Parathyroid hormone-like peptide secretion by tumour
Polycythaemia	4	Erythropoietin secretion
Neuromyopathy	3	Tumour-associated antibodies to nerve tissue
Amyloidosis	2	Possibly associated with immunological reactions to the tumour

(Adapted from Boulton Jones et al 1982.)

not be attributed to metastases. Approximately 30% of patients present with established metastases.

Investigations

Investigations are designed:

- To demonstrate the presence of a solid tumour and to make a specific histological or cytological diagnosis
- To determine the extent of spread of the tumour: (a) local (b) to nodes and (c) haematogenous.

IVU with nephrotomography usually shows a renal mass with splaying and distortion of the collecting system. In the great majority of patients, ultrasound (U/S) will distinguish a tumour from a simple cyst. Cyst fluid or tumour cells can be aspirated under U/S control and the cytology examined. The size of the tumour can be assessed from the IVU and U/S. CT scanning is of value in determining spread through the renal capsule (Fig. 9). Invasion of the renal vein and vena cava can usually be shown by U/S, although occasionally pre-operative venography is required. Spread to lymph nodes can be assessed by CT scanning, and haematogenous metastases detected by chest radiograph, CT scanning and radionuclide bone scanning.

Management

Early surgery affords the only real prospect of cure. The treatment of choice is removal of the affected kidney, en bloc, within the perinephric fascia. Simultaneous removal of the adrenal gland and regional lymph nodes is performed. The 5-year survival for tumours confined to the kidney is 60–75%. For all grades of tumour it is approximately 30%.

Partial nephrectomy may be performed for carcinoma of a solitary kidney or tumour involving both kidneys. If all renal tissue must be removed, chronic dialysis is instituted. Treatment of advanced disease is unsat-

isfactory. Nephrectomy or arterial embolisation of the kidney may be necessary for loin pain or haematuria. Radiotherapy often relieves pain due to metastases, and progesterone-like hormones may slow the advance of metastatic disease. Neither radiotherapy, chemotherapy, hormonal therapy nor immunotherapy have been shown to alter the course of advanced disease significantly.

NEPHROBLASTOMA (WILM'S TUMOUR)

This is the second most common malignant tumour of the kidney. It presents in the first decade, and often in the first year of life, most commonly as an abdominal mass. Haematuria tends to occur late in the disease. The tumour is radiosensitive, and responds to chemotherapy (p. 855). The best hope of cure is early diagnosis.

TUMOURS OF THE RENAL PELVIS, URETER AND BLADDER

These are histologically similar to each other, being usually transitional cell carcinomas. They spread locally by direct invasion, and also by implantation to other parts of the urinary tract. While some are benign, e.g. papillomas, all urinary tract tumours are liable to recur, even after apparently adequate treatment. The bladder is by far the most common site. Epidemiological studies have shown that males are more often affected, and that this tumour is particularly likely to develop in patients who work in industries such as dyeing and printing, where there may be exposure to aniline, in areas endemic for urinary schistosomiasis, in heavy smokers and as a complication of analgesic nephropathy.

Clinical features

Painless haematuria is commonly the sole presenting symptom. Unexplained frequency, dysuria or symptoms due to urinary tract obstruction also occur. The features of urinary infection may be superimposed.

Investigations

Patients with haematuria should have an IVU. Carcinoma in the renal pelvis appears as an abnormality on the urogram. If the IVU is normal, cystoscopy is performed, unless the patient is young and the haematuria obviously associated with urinary infection. In such a case the patient should be followed up, and cystoscopy carried out if haematuria persists. Biopsy of suspicious lesions can be performed at cystoscopy. Urinary cytology may be helpful. Local spread from tumours of the renal pelvis is apparent on CT scanning. Local spread of bladder tumours is assessed by bimanual examination under anaesthesia, from appearances at cystoscopy, and from the histology. Spread to lymph nodes is assessed by CT scanning, and metastasis elsewhere by chest radiograph, bone scan and liver function tests.

Management

Renal pelvic and ureteric tumours are treated by nephroureterectomy. Radiotherapy and chemotherapy are of little value. These patients may develop bladder tumours later, and therefore require regular follow-up by cystoscopy. Localised, well-differentiated bladder tumours (approximately 60% of such tumours) are treated by diathermy. Cystoscopy and IVU should be performed at yearly intervals thereafter to detect recurrence. Treatment of histologically malignant tumours or those which have spread beyond the bladder mucosa is unsatisfactory. Extensive superficial tumour can be treated by intravesical chemotherapy, and locally invasive lesions with radiotherapy. If this fails or the patient has severe bladder symptoms, total cystectomy and transplantation of the ureters into an ileal conduit may be required. Systemic methotrexate and cis-platinum have been used to treat metastases but results are poor. Analgesics and palliative radiotherapy are used to relieve pain. The 5-year survival of patients with superficial well-differentiated lesions is 90%, whilst in those with invasive, poorly differentiated tumours it is 30%.

PROSTATIC CARCINOMA

Adenocarcinoma of the prostate accounts for 70% of all cancers in men and causes 19 deaths/100 000 males annually in the UK, mostly in men over 50. Autopsy reports indicate that many men over 80 have latent foci of prostatic cancer.

Clinical features

The lesion may be found incidentally on examination of tissue removed during transurethral resection for supposedly benign prostatic hypertrophy. It may also present with symptoms of urethral obstruction similar to those of the benign condition. Local spread causes pain, incontinence and sometimes acute renal failure due to involvement of the lower ends of both ureters. Patients may present with bone pain due to metastases. On examination per rectum, the prostate is hard and the median furrow often obliterated. Spread of tumour is often associated with increased serum prostate-specific antigen (PSA) which acts as a tumour marker.

Investigations

The diagnosis depends on the clinical findings and examination of biopsy material. Local invasion is assessed by bimanual examination under anaesthesia and by U/S. Screening for metastasis includes measurement of serum prostate-specific antigen, bone scan, radiographs of bones and chest, and liver function tests.

Management

When asymptomatic disease is discovered incidentally, it may be best to defer treatment until symptoms develop, particularly in older men. Nevertheless, radical prostatectomy, pelvic radiotherapy and hormonal treatment designed to deprive the tumour of androgens have been advocated for these cases. When symptoms or evidence of local spread are present, radiotherapy or androgen deprivation is indicated. The latter can be achieved by administration of oestrogens or gonadotrophin-releasing hormone analogues, or by orchidectomy. Stilboestrol has a useful palliative action. The dose should be restricted to 1–3 mg/day by mouth, as larger doses, in addition to their feminising effects, are associated with increased risk of cardiovascular complications. Alternatively a gonadotrophin-releasing hormone analogue such as buserelin can be given by subcutaneous injection as 500 µg 8-hourly for 7 days. Thereafter 100 µg doses delivered by a metered nasal spray are instilled into the nostrils 6 times daily. During the early days of therapy tumour growth may increase. Cyproterone acetate, which blocks the effect of androgens on target tissue, can be used as a second line drug; 100 mg orally 8-hourly. Transurethral resection may be required to relieve obstruction. Metastatic disease can be treated by androgen deprivation or palliative radiotherapy, or if these measures fail, hypophysectomy. Trials of chemotherapy are in progress.

BENIGN PROSTATIC HYPERTROPHY

This is most commonly found in men over 60, and may be associated with diminished androgen secretion.

Histologically, the inner zone of the gland undergoes hyperplasia and hypertrophy, and there is an increase in fibromuscular stroma. The enlarged prostate obstructs the outflow of urine by compressing, displacing, distorting and elongating the prostatic urethra, with the effects on bladder and renal function referred to on page 655. Clinical features are those of progressive obstruction to urinary flow. Acute urinary retention may arise if the gland suddenly increases in size because of superimposed infection or congestion, or if cardiac failure develops in the elderly. In this situation the patient has a sudden desire to micturate but is unable to do so, and the bladder becomes tense and tender. Chronic retention may pass unnoticed for some time, but there is a gradual increase in the volume of urine which remains in the bladder after micturition. Haematuria due to urethral bleeding may also occur and may be the presenting symptom. On rectal examination the prostate may feel large, elastic and uniform in consistency. When the median lobe alone is affected the prostate feels normal and the condition can be recognised only by cystoscopy. α-adrenoceptor antagonists may provide symptomatic relief. Transurethral resection of prostatic tissue is the treatment of choice to relieve the outflow obstruction.

TESTICULAR TUMOURS

These are the most common form of malignant disease in men aged 25–34 years. The lesion may be a seminoma arising from spermatogonia, a teratoma from toti-potential germ cells, or a combined tumour. These tumours occur in fit young men and should nowadays be regarded as curable. Early diagnosis and appropriate specialist treatment is essential.

Clinical features
A seminoma presents as a painless, often uniform, rapid enlargement of the testis. A teratoma causes more nodular changes and may secrete chorionic gonadotrophin producing gynaecomastia. The tumour may be overlooked if obscured by a hydrocoele or if the examination is inadequate. Some cases present with metastases.

Investigations
Spread to regional lymph nodes can be demonstrated by CT scanning. Screening for metastases should include chest radiograph and liver function tests.

Management
The tumour should be removed using the inguinal approach. Histology gives some idea of prognosis. A seminoma confined to the testicle or with metastasis below the diaphragm is treated by radiotherapy, to which it is very sensitive. More widespread seminoma requires chemotherapy; this is the treatment of choice for teratoma. The usual agents are cisplatinum and bleomycin. Circulating tumour markers (alpha-fetoprotein, human chorionic gonadotrophin and lactic dehydrogenase) are of help in assessing response to treatment and for monitoring patients in remission.

FURTHER READING

Mevorach R A et al 1992 Renal cell carcinoma. Incidental diagnosis and natural history: review of 235 cases. Urology 39: 519–522

Chapter appendix overleaf.

APPENDIX

WATER DEPRIVATION TEST

- No coffee, tea or smoking on test day
- Free fluids until start of test
- Light breakfast
- No fluids for 8 hours after 0830
- Weigh patient at start and after 5 and 8 hours
- Stop test if patient loses more than 3% of body weight
- Measure Uosm after 8 hours—should reach 800 mOsm/kg

If there is a failure to concentrate urine normally then consider giving exogenous desmopressin (DDAVP, 2 μg intramuscularly) and then collecting urine hourly for a further 4 hours. In patients with ADH-deficient diabetes insipidus the urine osmolality will then increase. This does not occur in polyuria due to primary renal lesions (nephrogenic diabetes insipidus). Measurement of plasma osmolality (Posm) at the start and the end of the test is valuable. Patients with psychogenic polydipsia usually have a low plasma osmolality, whereas those with diabetes insipidus have an elevated value. After water deprivation the plasma osmolality rises and a value greater than 300 mOsm/kg is usually diagnostic of diabetes insipidus

TEST OF URINARY DILUTING ABILITY

The subject should drink 1000 ml water in 20 min. Urine is collected at hourly intervals for 4 hours.

Result:
At least 750 ml of urine should be excreted in the 4 hours. The osmolality of one sample should be less than 100 mOsm/ kg

Note: Inadvisable in patients with adrenal insufficiency; invalidated by pain or anxiety which stimulates release of vasopressin

URINARY ACIDIFICATION TEST

Give oral ammonium chloride, 0.1 g/kg in gelatine capsules (it may be necessary also to give an anti-emetic). Collect urine hourly for 8 hours into container holding a small quantity of liquid paraffin to prevent exposure to air. Measure urine pH, total titratable acid, and total NH_4^+ in each sample. During test the patient may eat normally and should drink 200 ml hourly.
Failure to reduce the urine pH below 5.3 is characteristic of distal renal tubular acidosis (p. 661). In chronic renal failure the urine pH often falls below 5.3, but this disorder is characterised by a reduced rate of NH_4^+ excretion (less than 30 μmol/min after ammonium chloride)

C. R. W. Edwards, J. D. Baird, B. M. Frier,
J. Shepherd, A. D. Toft

12

Endocrine and metabolic diseases, including diabetes mellitus

Endocrinology is the biological science concerned with the synthesis, secretion and action of hormones. These are defined as chemical messengers which coordinate the activities of different cells in multicellular organisms. The body thus has two major control systems which allow specialised tissues to function in an integrated way: the nervous system and the endocrine system.

Classically the nervous system depends on electrochemical signals passing via specific nervous pathways and the endocrine system on hormones being released into the circulation and acting at a site distant from that of secretion (ορμῶν: to stir up). However, it is becoming increasingly obvious that the situation is much more complex. Thus many hormones are now known to be neurotransmitters. In addition it is clear that the hormones may act on adjacent cells (paracrine system) or even back on the cell of origin (autocrine system) and that many have an inhibitory rather than stimulatory role. It is not surprising that this sophisticated system is associated with a large number of congenital and acquired abnormalities. Most of these endocrine diseases can be classified on the basis of being associated either with hormonal excess or deficiency (Table 12.1). Specific examples of this classification are given in the information box.

CLASSIFICATION OF ENDOCRINE DISEASE ON A FUNCTIONAL BASIS

Hormonal excess	Example
• Primary gland overproduction	Adrenal tumour→cortisol→ Cushing's syndrome
• Secondary to excess production of trophic substance	Thyroid stimulating antibody→thyroxine→ thyrotoxicosis

Hormonal deficiency	
• Primary gland failure	Adrenal antibodies→adrenal failure→Addison's disease
• Secondary to lack of stimulation by a trophic hormone	Pituitary disease→loss of ACTH secretion→cortisol deficiency
• Target organ resistance	Defective aldosterone receptor→ pseudohypoaldosteronism

---

The commonest endocrine diseases are those involving the thyroid gland and that resulting from either an absolute or relative lack of insulin (diabetes mellitus). The prevalence of these conditions varies greatly in different parts of the world (Table 12.2).

The World Health Organization statistics indicate that endocrine diseases are a relatively rare cause of death (1–5%). However, they are an important cause of morbidity. Modern methods have resulted in earlier diagnosis and more effective therapy. The treatment of

some conditions such as hypothyroidism is very satisfactory and results in return of normal function. For others, such as diabetes mellitus, however, current therapy is far from optimal.

THE HYPOTHALAMUS AND THE PITUITARY GLAND

ANATOMY AND PHYSIOLOGY

The pituitary gland is enclosed in the sella turcica, bridged over by the diaphragma sellae, with the sphenoidal air sinuses below, and the optic chiasma above (Fig. 12.1). The cavernous sinuses are lateral to the pituitary fossa and contain the 3rd, 4th and 6th cranial nerves. The gland is composed of two lobes, anterior and posterior, and is connected to the hypothalamus by the infundibular stalk which has portal vessels (Fig. 12.2) carrying blood from the median eminence of the hypothalamus to the anterior lobe and nerve fibres to the posterior lobe.

The anterior lobe

This consists of three main types of cell as identified by conventional staining: chromophobe, acidophil and basophil. Classic descriptions of pituitary tumours suggest that acidophil tumours are associated with growth hormone or prolactin excess and basophil with adrenocorticotrophic hormone hypersecretion. However, many chromophobe tumours are associated with similar hormonal excess. Thus immunohistochemistry using specific antisera against the pituitary hormones is more valuable in identifying the hormone(s) secreted by specific pituitary cells.

There are seven pituitary hormones, four of which act on target endocrine glands while the other three act primarily on target tissues. The functions of the anterior pituitary are shown in Table 12.3.

Each of these hormones is controlled by a substance produced in the hypothalamus and released into the portal blood. These hormones or factors may either stimulate or inhibit anterior pituitary hormone secretion (Fig. 12.3). Hypothalamic function is in turn dependent on a wide variety of stimuli of nervous, metabolic, physical or hormonal origin, in particular feedback control by hormones produced by the target glands (thyroid, adrenal cortex and gonads).

Thyroid stimulating hormone (TSH)

The hypothalamic tripeptide TRH releases TSH (thyroid stimulating hormone) from the anterior pituitary. In its turn TSH stimulates the thyroid gland to produce

Table 12.1   Diseases of the endocrine system

	Hormonal excess	Hormonal deficiency	Hormonal resistance
Hypothalamus	? Cushing's disease	Isolated releasing hormone deficiencies for LH, TSH, GH, ACTH	
Pituitary	Acromegaly Cushing's disease Prolactinoma	Hypopituitarism Diabetes insipidus	Nephrogenic diabetes insipidus Laron dwarfism
Gonads	Tumours	Klinefelter's syndrome Turner's syndrome Menopause Autoimmune gonadal failure	Androgen resistance syndromes (e.g. testicular feminisation)
Thyroid	Hyperthyroidism	Hypothyroidism	Thyroid hormone resistance
Adrenals	Cushing's syndrome Conn's syndrome Phaeochromocytoma	Addison's disease	Glucocorticoid resistance Pseudohypoaldosteronism
Parathyroids	Hyperparathyroidism	Hypoparathyroidism	Pseudohypoparathyroidism
Pancreas	Insulinoma Glucagonoma	Diabetes mellitus	Insulin resistance syndromes

Table 12.2   Prevalence of the commonest endocrine diseases

Disease	Area	% of population
Thyroid dysfunction (Goitre)	Endemic goitre area (e.g. Himalayas) Non-endemic goitre area (e.g. UK)	>10% 4% of women aged 20–30
Diabetes mellitus	Industrialised countries Native Americans Australian Aborigines	1.5–2% >15%

the thyroid hormones, thyroxine (T_4) and triiodothyronine (T_3). These then exert a negative feedback control on TRH and TSH secretion. Even though T_4 is a prohormone which is then converted to the biologically active T_3, the pituitary secretion of TSH is more affected by circulating T_4. This is because of rapid deiodination of T_4 to T_3 by the pituitary.

Table 12.3   Functions of anterior pituitary hormones

Function	Hormone	Abbreviation
Growth	Growth hormone	GH
Thyroid activity	Thyroid stimulating hormone	TSH
Sexual activity and fertility	Luteinising hormone Follicle stimulating hormone	LH FSH
Lactation	Prolactin	PRL
Adrenal glucocorticoid production	Adrenocorticotrophic hormone	ACTH
Skin pigmentation	Adrenocorticotrophic hormone +β-lipotrophin	ACTH β-LPH

Luteinising hormone (LH) and follicle stimulating hormone (FSH)

The gonadotrophin-releasing hormone GnRH is a decapeptide and acts on the pituitary to release both luteinising hormone (LH) and follicle stimulating hormone (FSH). These are glycoprotein hormones with molecular weights of about 30 000 Daltons. They have structural similarity with TSH and human chorionic gonadotrophin (hCG) in that they all share a common α subunit but have a variable β subunit.

Despite the fact that there is only one releasing hormone, LH and FSH can be secreted independently. This depends on the feedback of gonadal steroids (and a polypeptide, inhibin) on the pituitary. These modulate the response to the releasing hormone.

Male: FSH stimulates Sertoli cells in the seminiferous tubules to secrete androgen-binding protein (ABP), transferrin, plasminogen activator and inhibin. LH stimulates interstitial (Leydig) cells to produce testosterone. Some oestradiol is also produced. Both FSH and LH are necessary for spermatogenesis. hCG will also stimulate interstitial cells and is used to test the ability of the testis to produce testosterone.

Female: FSH produces growth and development of ovarian follicles during the first 14 days of the menstrual cycle (the follicular phase). This leads to a gradual increase in oestradiol (E2) production. This increasing E2 level initially suppresses FSH secretion (negative feedback) but then results in increased LH secretion (positive feedback). This is due to an increase in both the frequency and amplitude of GnRH pulses. The mid-cycle peak of LH (the LH surge) induces ovulation. After release of the ovum the follicle differentiates into a

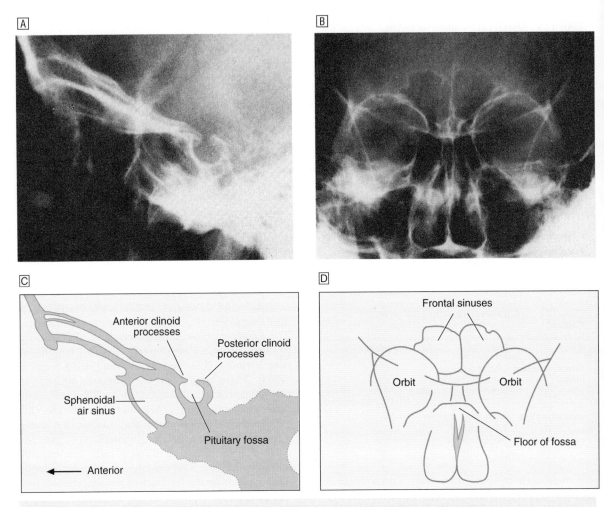

A B C D

Anterior clinoid
processes

Posterior clinoid
processes

Sphenoidal
air sinus

Pituitary fossa

Anterior

Frontal sinuses

Orbit

Orbit

Floor of fossa

Fig. 12.1 **Plain skull radiographs and diagrams showing anatomy of normal pituitary fossa.** A, C Lateral view.
B, D Postero-anterior view.

corpus luteum which secretes progesterone. The second
half of the cycle is known as the luteal phase.

Gonadotrophin-releasing hormone (GnRH)

GnRH is secreted in a pulsatile manner in both males
and females leading to pulses of gonadotrophin
secretion. This pattern of secretion is critical. Continuous administration of GnRH down-regulates receptors on the pituitary gonadotrophs and therefore
paradoxically inhibits gonadotrophin secretion. Thus
long-acting analogues of GnRH are being used in the
treatment of hormone-dependent prostate and breast
cancer and may have a role as contraceptives.
Conversely, pulsatile administration of GnRH via a

portable pump is proving to be an important way of
treating certain types of hypogonadotrophic hypogonadism.

In addition to steroid feedback, endogenous opiates
also appear to play a role in determining LH pulse frequency. Thus the opiate antagonist naloxone increases
the frequency in patients with hypothalamic amenorrhoea such as that associated with excessive exercise.

Inhibin

This is a glycoprotein hormone secreted by the ovary
and testis. Its major role is thought to be to act on the
pituitary to suppress FSH release. It consists of an α and
β subunit. Two forms of the β subunit have been isolated

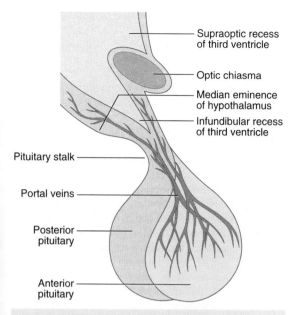

Supraoptic recess of third ventricle

Optic chiasma

Median eminence of hypothalamus

Infundibular recess of third ventricle

Pituitary stalk

Portal veins

Posterior pituitary

Anterior pituitary

Fig. 12.2 Anatomical relationships of human pituitary.

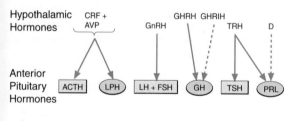

Hypothalamic Hormones

CRF + AVP

GnRH

GHRH GHRIH

TRH

D

Anterior Pituitary Hormones

ACTH LPH LH + FSH GH TSH PRL

acting on

glands or tissues

Hypothalamic hormone stimulating anterior pituitary (———►)

Hypothalamic hormone inhibiting anterior pituitary (- - - -►)

Fig. 12.3 The principal direct relationships between the hypothalamus and the anterior pituitary. Hypothalamic hormones: CRF Corticotrophin-releasing factor; AVP Arginine vasopressin; GnRH Gonadotrophin-releasing hormone; GHRH Growth hormone-releasing hormone; GHRIH Growth hormone release inhibitory hormone (somatostatin); TRH Thyrotrophin-releasing hormone; D Dopamine (prolactin release inhibitory factor).

(β-A and β-B). Inhibin A is a heterodimer of α and β-A. Inhibin B consists of α and β-B. Recently the homodimer of the β-subunit (i.e. 2 β-A subunits) (Activin) has been isolated. Interestingly this stimulates FSH release. It is clear that the control of LH and FSH secretion is much more complex than previously thought.

Growth hormone (GH)

GH is controlled by a dual system, namely growth hormone-releasing hormone (GHRH) and an inhibitory hormone (GHRIH or somatostatin). GHRH was first identified from a pancreatic tumour in a patient with acromegaly and has been shown to be the same as that present in the hypothalamus. It circulates in both a 40 and an N-terminally extended 44 amino acid form. The pulsatile release of growth hormone appears to be due to stimulation by GHRH and loss of inhibition by somatostatin. This is a tetradecapeptide which has many other actions, apart from its effect on growth hormone. These are shown in the information box below.

SOMATOSTATIN

Somatostatin inhibits release of:
- GH
- Gastrin
- TSH
- Glucagon
- Gastric acid
- Insulin
- Pancreatic enzymes

Sites of production:
- Hypothalamus
- Gastrointestinal tract
- Delta cells of pancreas

The major effects of GH are mediated via an insulin-like growth factor (IGF-I) (original name somatomedin C). This polypeptide circulates in the blood bound to a specific carrier protein. The liver is a major source of IGF-I production.

Prolactin (PRL)

PRL secretion differs from that of other anterior pituitary hormones in that it is under predominantly inhibitory control. The inhibitory factor is dopamine which is secreted by the hypothalamus into the portal system. Thus cutting the pituitary stalk leads to an elevation of prolactin secretion but inhibits the secretion of all the other anterior pituitary hormones. Administration of TRH stimulates prolactin as well as TSH release but there is little evidence that TRH normally controls prolactin release. Vasoactive intestinal polypeptide (VIP) will also release prolactin but like TRH its physiological role is unknown.

Corticotrophin (ACTH)

The secretion of adrenocorticotrophic hormone (ACTH) is under the control of corticotrophin-releasing factor (CRF), a 41 amino acid peptide identified in 1981. In addition the hypothalamus produces arginine vasopressin (AVP) and both CRF and AVP act synergistically to release ACTH.

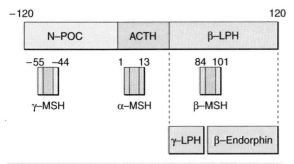

Fig. 12.4 ACTH/LPH precursor, pro-opiocortin (POC). The hatched areas represent the common core MSH sequence within different molecules. β-LPH is further broken down to γ-LPH and β-endorphin.

ACTH is secreted as part of the large precursor molecule, pro-opiocortin, and is cleaved from the N- and C-terminal parts prior to release from the pituitary corticotroph (Fig. 12.4). The control of ACTH secretion is shown in the information box.

CONTROL OF ACTH SECRETION

ACTH release is affected by:
- Circadian rhythm—highest level on waking in morning, lowest level on going to bed at night
- Stress—dominant control, e.g. trauma, pain, fever, hypoglycaemia
- Negative feedback—lowering cortisol levels, e.g. with enzyme inhibitor metyrapone or in primary adrenal failure, stimulates CRF and hence ACTH

β-Lipotrophin (β-LPH)

β-melanocyte stimulating hormone (β-MSH) is now known to be an artefact created by extracting the pituitary under harsh conditions. The β-MSH amino acid sequence is contained within β-lipotrophin (LPH) which is the C-terminal part of the ACTH precursor molecule, pro-opiocortin. This core sequence is also present within ACTH (α-MSH) and in the N-terminal part of pro-opiocortin (γ-MSH) (Fig. 12.4). Thus there are several molecules derived from pro-opiocortin which may function as melanocyte stimulating hormones and cause pigmentation of the skin and mucous membranes by increasing melanin synthesis in the melanocytes. However, the pigmenting activity of LPH is low and ACTH is probably the most important pigmenting hormone.

The C-terminal part of β-LPH (61–91) is β-endorphin, one of the endogenous substances with morphine-like actions. The first five amino acids of β-endorphin are the same as those of the pentapeptide opioid, met-enkephalin. Current evidence suggests, however, that metenkephalin is not derived from β-endorphin but from another precursor molecule.

The posterior lobe

The posterior lobe (neurohypophysis) contains neural fibres which emanate from the supraoptic and paraventricular nuclei of the hypothalamus.

Hormones of the posterior lobe

The neurohypophysis secretes two hormones, arginine vasopressin (AVP)—here referred to as vasopressin—and oxytocin, together with their specific binding proteins (neurophysins). The principal action of vasopressin is to increase the reabsorption of water by the renal tubules and because of this action it is also known as the antidiuretic hormone (ADH). The secretion of vasopressin is controlled by three main mechanisms. A rise in plasma osmolality stimulates vasopressin release which in turn results in water retention to preserve homeostasis. A fall of about 15% in plasma volume without any change in osmolality can also stimulate vasopressin secretion by activating volume receptors in the thorax. In addition the central nervous system also can play a role. Pain, for example, produces an antidiuresis.

The role of oxytocin in the male is unknown. In the female it has traditionally been thought to be important in parturition and the expression of milk from the breast but its role in parturition has been questioned.

INVESTIGATION OF PITUITARY FUNCTION

All the protein and peptide hormones of the pituitary gland can be measured in body fluids by radioimmunoassay, and access to a laboratory with a full range of these assays is critical for the proper evaluation of pituitary function. Approximate adult reference values for hormone concentrations in the plasma are given on page 1152. In addition the hypothalamic hormones, TRH, GnRH, CRF and GHRH, have been synthesised and can be used clinically to stimulate the release of the appropriate pituitary hormones. In most tests the pituitary hormone itself is measured (e.g. GH, prolactin) but in the case of ACTH it is cheaper and easier to measure cortisol as a marker of ACTH secretion. The exception is when primary adrenal disease is suspected when both ACTH and cortisol should be measured.

One of the fundamental principles of the investigation of endocrine disorders is that if high levels of a hormone are suspected then an appropriate suppression test should be used. Conversely if there is hormone deficiency a stimulation test is normally required. Thus in assessing the increased production of growth hormone in acromegaly a **glucose tolerance test** is performed with measurement of growth hormone at half-hourly intervals for 2 hours along with measurement of blood glucose. Under physiological conditions growth hormone secretion is promptly suppressed by a rise in the blood glucose while there is either absent suppression or a paradoxical rise in patients with pituitary tumours secreting growth hormone (Fig. 12.5).

Basal function of anterior pituitary

Assessment of this should include measuring plasma:

08.00 h	cortisol
	prolactin
	thyroxine
In the male	testosterone
In the female	oestradiol
In the post-menopausal female	LH/FSH

Assessment of GH secretion

In normal subjects sampled during the day growth hormone levels are commonly undetectable. In suspected hypopituitarism, therefore, some form of dynamic function test is necessary to distinguish normal from abnormal growth hormone secretion (see the information box).

TESTS OF GROWTH HORMONE SECRETION

- Post-exercise
- 1 hour after going to sleep — Physiological
- Frequent sampling during sleep

- Insulin-induced hypoglycaemia
- Clonidine — Pharmacological
- Arginine
- Glucagon

Of these the insulin tolerance test remains the gold standard. It has the additional advantage that it stimulates the secretion of ACTH and hence cortisol. Prolactin is also released.

GH response to GHRH is of value in distinguishing patients who lack the releasing hormone (the usual cause of isolated GH deficiency).

ACTH

If the basal plasma cortisol is normal (>180 nmol/l) then this indicates that basal ACTH secretion is normal. However, it does not mean that the patient can respond normally to stress (e.g. surgery). To determine whether or not the stress response is normal further dynamic function testing is usually necessary (the exception is a patient with 08.00 h plasma cortisol >550 nmol/l).

INSULIN TOLERANCE TEST

Use:
- Assessment of hypothalamic-pituitary-adrenal axis
- Assessment of growth hormone deficiency

Contraindications:
- Ischaemic heart disease
- Epilepsy
- Severe hypopituitarism (0800 h plasma cortisol <180 nmol/l)

Dose:
- 0.15 U/kg body weight soluble insulin intravenously

Aim:
- To produce adequate hypoglycaemia (signs of neuroglycopenia—tachycardia and sweating—with blood glucose less than 2.2 mmol/l: 40 mg/100 ml)

Blood samples:
- 0, 30, 45, 60, 90, 120 minutes for blood glucose, plasma cortisol and growth hormone

Results:
- Normal subjects GH > 20 mU/l
- Normal subjects cortisol > 550 nmol/l

The best simple, safe screening test is that giving synacthen (β1-24 tetracosactrin, ACTH).

ACTH STIMULATION TEST

Use:
- Diagnosis of primary or secondary adrenal insufficiency

Dose:
- 250 μg tetracosactrin (Synacthen) by intramuscular injection

Blood samples:
- 0, 30, 60 minutes for plasma cortisol

Results:
- Normal subjects plasma cortisol > 550 nmol/l

If plasma cortisol after ACTH is less than 550 nmol/l then an insulin hypoglycaemia test should carried out as some patients will respond normally to insulin (and stress) and yet have a subnormal response to synacthen. In patients in whom hypoglycaemia is contraindicated (see above) then other tests such as that giving glucagon can be performed. However, this is a less reliable index of the ability of the hypothalamic-pituitary-adrenal axis to respond to stress.

ACTH/cortisol response to CRF is of little value in determining stress responsiveness but is helpful in distinguishing pituitary-dependent Cushing's disease (exaggerated ACTH/cortisol response) from the ectopic ACTH syndrome (no response) (p. 708).

TSH, prolactin

The ability of the pituitary to secrete TSH and prolactin can be tested by giving TRH. It should be stressed that the value of this test is limited. In secondary hypothyroidism (i.e. due to hypothalamic or pituitary disease) a normal TSH response may be found and the diagnosis is made on the thyroxine level and not the TSH response to TRH. In primary hypothyroidism there will be an exaggerated TSH response to TRH but the diagnosis can be made on the basis of the elevated basal TSH.

The prolactin response to TRH may be absent in postpartum pituitary necrosis (Sheehan's syndrome). It is blunted in patients with prolactinomas. However, the overlap with other causes of hyperprolactinaemia is such that the prolactin response to TRH has little discriminatory value in the individual patient. The basal prolactin level is much more valuable.

LH and FSH

The pulsatile release of LH and FSH makes it difficult to assess the results of single blood samples with the exception of those from the post-menopausal patient. Here, one would expect the values of LH and FSH to be high, reflecting ovarian failure. If, however, they are not then this suggests hypothalamic or pituitary disease.

The ability of the pituitary to synthesise and release LH and FSH can be tested by giving GnRH. Patients with GnRH deficiency may respond to the pulsatile administration of GnRH.

To test the ability of the hypothalamus to produce GnRH the LH and FSH response to the anti-oestrogen

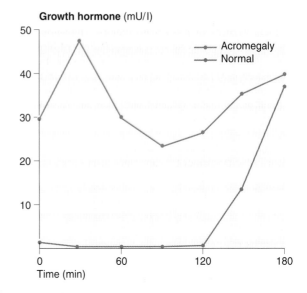

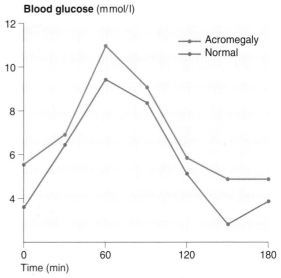

Fig. 12.5   Oral glucose tolerance tests in a normal subject and a patient with acromegaly with measurement of blood glucose and plasma growth hormone.

THYROTROPHIN-RELEASING HORMONE (TRH) TEST

Use:
- Diagnosis of primary and secondary hypothyroidism
- Diagnosis of hyperthyroidism
- Diagnosis of prolactin deficiency/excess

Dose:
- 200 μg thyrotrophin-releasing hormone intravenously

Side effects:
- May produce flushing, nausea, tingling in anterior urethra

Blood samples:
- 0, 20, 60 minutes for TSH (and/or prolactin)

Results:
- Normal subjects show a rise of TSH which is maximal at 20 minutes and then falls. A flat response is found in thyrotoxicosis, patients on pharmacological doses of glucocorticoids and some patients with hypothalamic/pituitary disease. In primary hypothyroidism the basal TSH is elevated and there is an exaggerated TSH response (peak greater than 20 mU/l). In hypothalamic disease 60 minutes TSH may be greater than 20 minutes

---

clomiphene citrate is measured. Clomiphene (3 mg/kg/d, maximum dose 150 mg/d) is given for 10 days with serial measurements of LH and FSH.

POSTERIOR PITUITARY FUNCTION

This is considered in the section on diabetes insipidus (p. 684).

SYNDROMES DUE TO ANTERIOR PITUITARY HYPOSECRETION

HYPOPITUITARISM

Aetiology

The causes of hypopituitarism are best classified on the basis of whether the lesion is in the hypothalamus or pituitary.

CAUSES OF HYPOPITUITARISM

Site of lesion	Common deficiencies/causes	Rare deficiencies/causes
HYPOTHALAMUS		
(a) Congenital	GnRH (Kallmann's syndrome)	TRH
	GHRH	CRF
(b) Acquired	Craniopharyngioma	Sarcoidosis
	Head injury	Tuberculosis
	Surgery	Histiocytosis-X
	Radiotherapy	Tumour: primary or secondary
PITUITARY	Pituitary tumour	2° tumour
	Surgery	Post-partum necrosis
	Radiotherapy	Autoimmune
	Head injury	Haemorrhage (apoplexy)
		Haemochromatosis

Clinical features

These depend on the underlying lesion. In the congenital defects of the hypothalamus where there is an isolated failure of production of a releasing hormone (e.g. GnRH) then, apart from the failure of LH and FSH production and hence of gonadal steroids, the rest of hypothalamic-pituitary function is normal. There is, however, in this case an important associated abnormality, anosmia, which often points to the diagnosis.

With progressive lesions of the pituitary such as a gradually expanding non-functioning pituitary tumour there is a characteristic sequence of loss of pituitary hormone secretion. GH secretion is often the earliest to be lost but this produces few obvious symptoms in the adult. Next LH secretion becomes impaired with, in the male, loss of libido and impotence and, in the female, oligomenorrhoea or amenorrhoea. Later in the male there may be gynaecomastia and decreased frequency of shaving. In both sexes axillary and pubic hair eventually become sparse or even absent. The skin becomes characteristically finer and more wrinkled. FSH secretion tends to be lost later than LH.

The next hormone to be lost is usually ACTH and thus cortisol resulting in symptoms of adrenal insufficiency. In contrast to primary adrenal insufficiency zona glomerulosa function is not lost and hence angiotensin II-induced aldosterone secretion maintains normal plasma electrolytes. In some patients, however, there may be a dilutional hyponatraemia. Cortisol is required for normal water handling by the kidney. In contrast to the pigmentation of Addison's disease a striking degree of pallor is usually present principally because of lack of melanin in the skin.

Finally TSH secretion is lost with consequent secondary hypothyroidism. This further contributes to the apathy and cold intolerance. In contrast to primary hypothyroidism frank myxoedema is not seen.

Untreated severe hypopituitarism eventually results in **coma**. This may follow some mild infection or injury. Several factors may contribute to this (Table 12.4). Investigation is detailed on page 674.

Management

The aim should be to provide adequate substitution therapy according to the deficiencies demonstrated.

Table 12.4	Coma in patient with hypopituitarism	
Possible cause	**Measure**	**Aetiology**
Hypoglycaemia	Blood glucose (low)	lack of GH → ↑sensitivity to insulin
Water intoxication	Electrolytes (Na$^+$, K$^+$ and urea all decreased)	Cortisol required for excretion of water load
Hypothermia	Rectal temperature (may be <32°C)	Hypothyroidism

Table 12.5 Sex hormone replacement therapy in males

Preparation	Dose	Route of administration	Frequency	Comment
Depot testosterone esters (Sustanon)	250–500 mg	Intramuscular injection	Every 2–4 weeks	Monitor on basis of symptoms + packed cell vol (every 6–12 months)
Testosterone undecanoate	80–120 mg	Oral	12 hourly	May produce variable blood levels
Testosterone implant	600–800 mg	Subcutaneous	Every 3–6 mnths	Probably best method for obtaining normal blood levels

Cortisol replacement

This should be started if there is ACTH deficiency. In someone who is not critically ill cortisol should be given by mouth, 20 mg on waking and 10 mg at 18.00 h. The precise dose may need to be adjusted for the individual patient. Excess weight gain usually indicates over-replacement whilst persistent lethargy may be due to an inadequate dose. Measurement of plasma cortisol levels during the day—a cortisol day curve—may be helpful in assessing the requisite dose. As indicated above, mineralocorticoid replacement is not required.

Thyroid hormone replacement

If this is required then thyroxine 0.1–0.15 mg once daily should be given. It is dangerous to give thyroid replacement to patients with adrenal insufficiency without first giving glucocorticoid therapy.

Sex hormone replacement

This is indicated if there is gonadotrophin deficiency to restore normal sexual function and to prevent osteoporosis. Male sex hormone replacement is shown in Table 12.5.

In **premenopausal females** the treatment is cyclical oestrogen therapy (e.g. ethinyloestradiol 20–30 μg daily for 3 weeks) with a progestogen such as medroxyprogesterone acetate (5 mg daily) for days 14–21.

Patients requiring **fertility** will usually need to be given gonadotrophin therapy. In the **postpubertal male** it is usual to give human chorionic gonadotrophin (hCG) (3000 IU intramuscularly weekly) to stimulate testosterone production by the interstitial cells for the first 6 months and then hCG weekly together with FSH (usually as pergonal, human menopausal gonadotrophin, which contains equal amounts of LH and FSH) 75 IU intramuscularly 3 times per week. This combination should be continued for 9–12 months. If there is a hypothalamic cause for the hypopituitarism then pulsatile GnRH therapy with a portable infusion pump may be effective (1–10 μg/pulse every 60–90 minutes).

In the **female** requiring fertility the same principles obtain. If there is gonadotrophin deficiency then both hCG and LH/FSH have to be given. The precise dose of FSH required to induce follicular development has to

be very carefully monitored by serial measurements of urinary or plasma oestradiol. If the oestrogen response is satisfactory then hCG is given to induce ovulation. An excessive oestrogen response indicates hyperstimulation—hCG should then not be given. To do so may result in multiple ovulation with production of ovarian cysts. As with the male, if the problem is GnRH deficiency then pulsatile therapy may be given. This is much less likely to produce multiple ovulation.

GROWTH HORMONE DEFICIENCY

In children hyposecretion of GH causes short stature. This is usually due to an inability to secrete GHRH rather than a primary pituitary abnormality. The next most common cause would be a craniopharyngioma.

In children with short stature it is essential that accurate records of height and weight are kept and entered on a percentile chart. Single measurements are of less value than serial estimates. With the latter the growth velocity can be plotted. If a child is below the 3rd centile or has measurements which cross the centile lines then careful serial measurements are necessary. If growth velocity is below the 25th centile or above the 75th centile then the child should be referred to a specialist growth clinic. The parental heights should be noted. There is a clear relationship between the mid-parental height and the expected height of the child—95% of normal children will be within 8.5 cm of the mid-parental height.

Differential diagnosis of short stature

Short stature may be due to a large number of different reasons, both endocrine and non-endocrine. The presenting growth velocity may be normal or impaired as shown in the information box.

Investigations

The tests used to assess GH secretion are detailed on page 675.

Management

GH therapy is indicated in children with documented GH deficiency and impaired growth (biosynthetic GH 24 Units/m^2 per week divided into daily bedtime sub-

DIFFERENTIAL DIAGNOSIS OF SHORT STATURE

Impaired growth velocity
- **Endocrine**
  Isolated GH deficiency
  Panhypopituitarism
  Primary hypothyroidism
  Cushing's syndrome
  Pseudohypoparathyroidism
- **Abnormal body proportions**
  Short limbs for spine (e.g. achondroplasia)
  Short limbs and very short spine (e.g.
  mucopolysaccharidoses)
- **Other conditions**
  Chromosome abnormalities (e.g. Turner's)
  Malabsorption (coeliac, Crohn's, colitis)
  Systemic illness (asthma, heart, renal disease)
  Malnutrition
  Psychosocial deprivation

Normal growth velocity on presentation
- **Prior problem affecting growth but no longer active**
  Intra-uterine growth retardation
  Congenital heart disease
- **Constitutional short stature**
  Normal bone age
- **Physiological growth delay**
  Retarded bone age

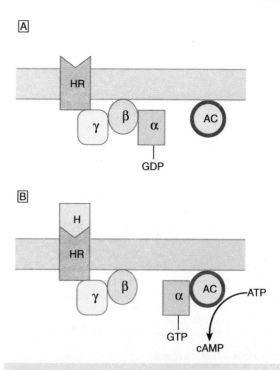

Fig. 12.6   Role of G-proteins in transducing the effect of hormone binding to a cell surface receptor leading to activation of adenylyl cyclase. HR: hormone receptor; H: hormone; α, β, γ: G-protein subunits; GDP: guanosine diphosphate; GTP: guanosine triphosphate; AC: adenylyl cyclase; ATP: adenosine triphosphate; cAMP: cyclic adenosine monophosphate.

cutaneous injections). Patients with other causes of short stature such as Turner's syndrome may benefit from GH therapy. In the case of a normal short child the role of GH treatment is not yet clear and is being examined in a series of clinical trials.

TUMOURS OF THE PITUITARY GLAND

Aetiology

Some of the factors leading to the development of pituitary tumours and autonomous hypersecretion of hormones are now starting to be understood. These tumours are monoclonal and thus arise from a somatic mutation in a single cell. In up to 40% of growth hormone-secreting pituitary tumours there is a mutation in the gene for the α subunit of the adenylyl cyclase stimulatory G-protein (G_S) which is then converted into an oncogene. The G-proteins belong to a family of GTP-binding proteins which are located on the cytosolic side of the plasma membrane and play a key role in the transduction of the signal for many hormones which bind to cell surface receptors (Fig. 12.6). When bound to guanosine triphosphate (GTP) the complex stimulates the production of cyclic-AMP. G_S consists of an α, β and γ subunit. The nucleotide (GTP or GDP) binding site is on the α-subunit. Binding of the hormone to the receptor causes displacement of bound GDP by GTP.

This dissociates the $\beta\gamma$-dimer and α-GTP complex, thus allowing the interaction of the α-GTP complex with adenylyl cyclase. This then increases the production of cyclic-AMP. Mutation of the α-subunit of G_S leads to constitutive activation of adenylyl cyclase (i.e. the cell produces its product, in this case growth hormone, without the pituitary being stimulated by growth hormone-releasing hormone). Similar mutations have been found in some thyroid adenomas and in the McCune–Albright syndrome (polyostotic fibrous dysplasia, skin pigmentation, precocious puberty) and a variety of other hormonal excess syndromes.

The pathology of tumours is shown in the information box overleaf.

GH hypersecretion is usually due to an acidophil (or a mixed acidophil and chromophobe) macroadenoma. Very rarely it may result from ectopic production of GHRH (e.g. by pancreatic tumour).

Excess secretion of ACTH and of β-lipotrophin is usually associated with a microadenoma (75% cases) of basophil (or mixed basophil and chromophobe) cells (Cushing's disease). There is usually little or no enlargement of the pituitary fossa. If, however, the Cushing's is treated by bilateral adrenalectomy with no definitive treatment for the pituitary, then Nelson's syndrome may develop (hyperpigmentation associated with aggressive pituitary tumour).

PATHOLOGY OF TUMOURS OF THE PITUITARY GLAND

Pituitary tumours may be:
- Macroadenomas >10 mm diameter
- Microadenomas <10 mm diameter

The large tumours may:
- Produce hypofunction by pressure on surrounding normal pituitary tissue (see Clinical features)
- Involve adjacent structures
  Dura—headache
  Optic chiasma, nerve or tract—visual field loss
  Cavernous sinus—IIIrd, IVth, or VIth nerve palsy
- Prevent prolactin inhibitory factor, dopamine, from reaching pituitary lactotroph—disconnection hyperprolactinaemia

Both micro- and macroadenomas may be functional or non-functional. The functional tumours may secrete:
- GH—Acromegaly/gigantism
- Prolactin—Galactorrhoea/menstrual dysfunction/impotence
- ACTH—Cushing's disease
- TSH—Hyperthyroidism

There may also be mixed tumours secreting more than one hormone, e.g. GH and prolactin

---

Prolactin-secreting tumours are the most common of the pituitary adenomas. They may be acidophil (densely granulated) or more commonly chromophobe (sparsely granulated). It is important to understand that the conventional classification of pituitary tumours based on the staining characteristics of the cells may be misleading. Thus many tumours with hormone secretion have little stored hormone and hence are chromophobe. For this reason the increased sensitivity of immunohistochemistry is useful in characterising these tumours. Specific antibodies against the pituitary hormones can then be used to localise hormones.

Craniopharyngiomas are tumours, usually cystic, developing in cell rests of Rathke's pouch, and may be located within the sella turcica, or commonly in the suprasellar space, where they frequently calcify. In either situation their clinical presentation is likely to be due to pressure on adjacent structures, e.g. the visual pathways.

Primary carcinoma of the pituitary gland is rare, but a metastatic tumour from a primary in the breast, lung, kidney or elsewhere may occur in the hypothalamus and reduce pituitary function. Other tumours, for example pinealoma, ependymoma or meningioma, may occasionally be associated with some disturbance of the pituitary or hypothalamus. Conditions such as sarcoidosis or syphilis may mimic pituitary tumours.

Clinical features

These vary, depending on the type of lesion in the pituitary gland and the effect of that lesion on surrounding structures. Enlarging tumours of the gland may present with signs attributable to increased output of hormones or to failure of secretion. Some tumours secreting hormones compress the remaining pituitary tissue, so that there may be failure of some functions of the gland in the presence of an excess of others. Headache is the most constant but least specific symptom.

Involvement of an optic nerve, the optic chiasma, or an optic tract leads to impaired visual fields. Bitemporal hemianopia is the most characteristic finding associated with pressure upon the chiasma. Optic atrophy may be apparent on ophthalmoscopy. Diplopia and strabismus may follow pressure on the third, fourth or sixth cranial nerves.

Some tumours expand sufficiently to interfere with ADH secretion and so cause diabetes insipidus. Damage to the posterior pituitary per se will not normally produce diabetes insipidus as vasopressin secretion by the hypothalamus continues. Thus if there is diabetes insipidus it usually indicates that the tumour has a suprasellar extension. Tumours which expand upwards to impinge on the hypothalamus may cause obesity and disturbance of sleep, thirst, temperature control and appetite.

Investigations

Anatomy: radiological investigation

Plain radiographs of the pituitary fossa may demonstrate enlargement of the sella turcica (Fig. 12.7) and erosion of the clinoid processes. Suprasellar calcification may be seen in a craniopharyngioma. A 'double floor' of the sella (Fig. 12.8) may be present if the tumour enlarges the fossa asymmetrically.

Computed tomography (CT). This (usually with contrast enhancement) is essential for demonstrating the suprasellar and parasellar anatomy in patients with macroadenomas and may show a hypodense microadenoma.

Nuclear magnetic resonance scanning (NMR) is probably the most valuable imaging technique for pituitary lesions but is available in relatively few centres (Fig. 12.9).

Cisternography involves injecting a water soluble contrast medium by cisternal puncture. It is usually done in conjunction with CT scanning to demonstrate an empty sella (i.e one in which the pituitary fossa is no longer filled by the pituitary gland), the superior aspect of a pituitary tumour or a hypothalamic lesion.

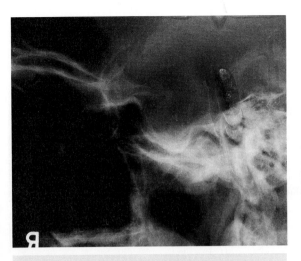

Fig. 12.7 Lateral radiograph of pituitary fossa showing gross enlargement by pituitary tumour.

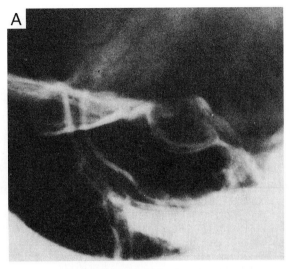

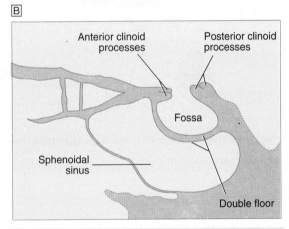

Fig. 12.8 Radiograph of pituitary fossa showing double floor secondary to asymmetrical expansion of fossa by pituitary tumour. A Lateral view. B Diagram of the same view.

Visual fields. Both central and peripheral visual fields should be plotted (i.e. not just perimetry). Classically, pressure on the optic chiasma produces a bitemporal hemianopia. However, it is important to recognise that *any type of visual field defect* may result from suprasellar extension of a pituitary tumour as the growth may involve the optic nerve (to produce unilateral loss of acuity or a scotoma), the optic chiasma, or the optic tract (homonymous hemianopia).

Function

Both anterior (p. 682) and posterior (p. 684) pituitary function need to be assessed. The latter cannot be done until the anterior pituitary function has been tested and, if there is ACTH or TSH insufficiency, the patient started on replacement therapy (cortisol and thyroxine necessary for normal water handling by the kidney).

If the clinical features suggest hormonal hypersecretion then this must be assessed as detailed below.

Management

If there is evidence of pressure on the visual pathways then urgent treatment is required. The type of treatment depends on the nature of the pituitary tumour. If this is a prolactinoma then bromocriptine should be given (p. 682) as this will shrink about 80% of these tumours and surgery can be avoided. If, however, bromocriptine is stopped then the tumour can rapidly (i.e. over a few days) re-enlarge and thus many patients are given definitive treatment with external radiotherapy (3500 rads in 33 fractions is often used).

If there is a non-functioning tumour with visual field defect then surgery is required. Almost all tumours can be decompressed by a trans-sphenoidal approach rather than the trans-frontal which has a higher morbidity and mortality. Following decompression external radiotherapy is necessary to prevent recurrence.

When there is hyperfunction of the pituitary sufficiently severe to affect the patient's welfare and prognosis, then treatment aimed at either destroying the tumour, or affecting its capacity to grow or secrete, should be considered. In Cushing's disease (pituitary-dependent Cushing's syndrome), prolactinomas and acromegaly it may be possible by trans-sphenoidal surgery to remove an adenoma selectively and leave sufficient pituitary tissue to maintain normal function. Alternatively, suppression of tumour growth and, to a less predictable extent, of secretory capacity may be

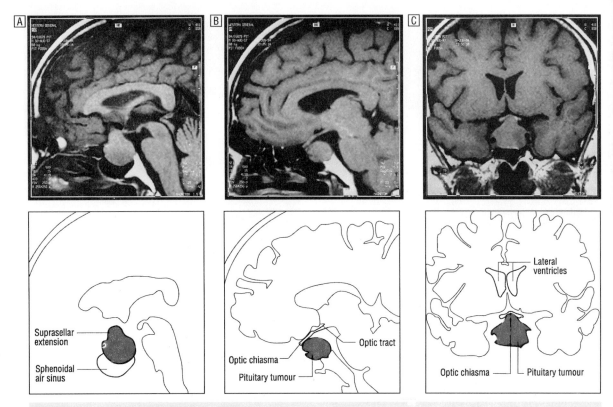

Fig. 12.9 **Magnetic resonance image of pituitary tumour showing** Ⓐ Suprasellar extension of large pituitary tumour (lateral view). Ⓑ Relationship between optic chiasma and the superior surface of the pituitary tumour (lateral view). Ⓒ Coronal view of pituitary tumour showing suprasellar extension and optic chiasma.

achieved by external radiotherapy usually with a linear accelerator. The implantation of yttrium in the pituitary fossa is an alternative form of irradiation used only in certain specialist centres. The same is true for proton beam therapy.

SYNDROMES DUE TO ANTERIOR PITUITARY HYPERSECRETION

GIGANTISM AND ACROMEGALY

Clinical features
If growth hormone hypersecretion occurs before epiphyses have fused then gigantism will result. More commonly GH excess occurs in adult life after epiphyseal closure and acromegaly ensues. If hypersecretion starts in adolescence and persists into adult life then the two conditions may be combined. The clinical features are listed in the information box.

In addition the pituitary tumour, almost invariably

the source of GH, may produce headaches, visual field defect or cranial nerve palsies (p. 680). The tumour may also affect other anterior pituitary hormone secretion. In about 30% of patients prolactin levels are elevated.

Investigations
These patients should be investigated in the same way as the patients with non-functioning pituitary tumours (p. 680). The clinical diagnosis must be confirmed by measuring GH levels during an oral glucose tolerance test (Fig. 12.5). In normal subjects GH suppresses to below 2 mU/litre. In acromegaly it does not suppress and in about 50% of patients there is a paradoxical rise. In 70% of acromegalics there is a GH rise after TRH administration. This is not found in normal subjects. The tissue effects of raised GH result in high circulating insulin-like growth factor, IGF-1.

Management
Medical. Bromocriptine, a long-acting dopamine agonist, will lower GH in about 75% of patients but only a small number of patients get levels below 10 mU/litre.

The usual dose is 20–30 mg/day in divided doses with food. This must be started at low dose, 1.25–2.5 mg/day, and then gradually increased. It may initially cause nausea, vomiting and postural hypotension especially if too large a dose is given. On maintenance therapy constipation may occur. More recently a long-acting analogue of somatostatin (octreotide) has been used with considerable success. It has to be given by sub-cutaneous injection usually 3 times daily.

Surgical. Trans-sphenoidal surgery may enable selective removal of an adenoma with cure. However, with large tumours surgical cure of GH excess is much more difficult. Surgery may, however, be required if there is a visual field defect. After decompression external radiotherapy should be given.

Radiotherapy. Conventional external radiotherapy given using a linear accelerator is an effective treatment of acromegaly in that it stops tumour growth and lowers GH levels. The problem is that GH levels fall slowly and hypopituitarism occurs in about 35% of patients. In a few centres interstitial irradiation is given by implanting rods of yttrium into the pituitary via a transnasal stereotaxic operation.

CUSHING'S DISEASE

This is dealt with in the section on Cushing's syndrome (p. 707).

HYPERPROLACTINAEMIA

Elevation of plasma prolactin levels is a common endocrine finding and may arise from a variety of causes. Even though the list is long it is usually possible to rapidly reach a presumptive diagnosis by taking a careful history, especially with regard to drug therapy. The causes are listed in the information box.

Clinical features

Hyperprolactinaemia may be associated with galactorrhoea and therefore the breasts in both sexes must be examined. Hippocrates was one of the first to observe that milk secretion was associated with decreased gonadal function. Thus in women, amenorrhoea, oligomenorrhoea, deficient luteal phase progesterone production or menorrhagia may all be associated with hyperprolactinaemia. It is important to measure prolactin in cases of unexplained infertility.

In men hyperprolactinaemia usually presents with loss of libido or impotence. Unfortunately at this stage many have a macroadenoma often with associated visual field defects.

Investigations

Plasma prolactin levels greater than 4000 mU/litre almost invariably indicate a diagnosis of prolactinoma (upper limit of normal for many assays is 360 mU/l). Because of variation with stress of venepuncture it is useful to have more than one basal prolactin level. The value of dynamic function tests of prolactin secretion and the assessment of pituitary anatomy and function are detailed on page 674.

Management

Medical. In almost all cases of hyperprolactinaemia dopamine agonist therapy with bromocriptine will lower prolactin levels, often to below normal, with return of gonadal function (regular periods with fertility in women, return of libido and potency in males). The usual dose is 2.5 mg orally 3 times daily with meals. As with acromegaly the drug must be started at a low dose, 1.25 mg daily, and gradually increased. If gonadal function does not return despite effective lowering of prolactin then there may be associated gonadotrophin deficiency or, in the female, the onset of a premature or natural menopause.

Surgical. As discussed on page 682, bromocriptine not only lowers prolactin levels but shrinks the majority of prolactin-secreting macroadenomas. Thus surgical decompression of these large tumours is not usually necessary unless they are cystic. However, micro-adenomas can be removed selectively by trans-sphenoidal surgery with a cure rate of about 80%.

Radiotherapy. External irradiation may be required as definitive treatment for some macroadenomas to prevent regrowth if bromocriptine is stopped.

Pregnancy. Prolactinomas may enlarge rapidly during pregnancy and thus these patients need careful assessment prior to becoming pregnant and supervision with assessment of prolactin levels and visual fields during pregnancy.

SYNDROMES DUE TO POSTERIOR PITUITARY HYPOSECRETION OR RENAL UNRESPONSIVENESS TO VASOPRESSIN

DIABETES INSIPIDUS (DI)

This uncommon disease is characterised by the persistent excretion of excessive quantities of dilute urine, and by constant thirst. Diabetes insipidus can be divided into:

- **Cranial DI**—deficient production of antidiuretic hormone (ADH), arginine vasopressin (AVP)
- **Nephrogenic DI**—renal tubules unresponsive to vasopressin.

Aetiology

The aetiology of cranial and nephrogenic diabetes insipidus is shown in the information boxes.

> **CAUSES OF CRANIAL DIABETES INSIPIDUS**
>
> - **Genetic defect**
>   Dominant
>   Recessive (DIDMOAD syndrome—association of DI with diabetes mellitus, optic atrophy, deafness)
> - **Hypothalamic or high stalk lesion**
>   e.g. histiocytosis-X, sarcoidosis, craniopharyngioma, pituitary tumour with suprasellar extension, basal meningitis, head injury, surgery, encephalitis
> - **Idiopathic**

If there is associated cortisol deficiency then diabetes insipidus may not be manifest until glucocorticoid replacement therapy is given.

> **CAUSES OF NEPHROGENIC DIABETES INSIPIDUS**
>
> - **Genetic defect**
>   Sex-linked recessive
>   Cystinosis
> - **Metabolic abnormality**
>   Hypokalaemia
>   Hypercalcaemia
> - **Drug therapy**
>   Lithium
>   Demethylchlortetracycline
> - **Poisoning**
>   Heavy metals

Clinical features

The most marked symptoms are polyuria and polydipsia. The patient may pass 5–20 or more litres of urine in 24 hours. This is of very low specific gravity and osmolality (less than plasma usually). In the unconscious patient or one with damage to the hypothalamic thirst centre DI is potentially lethal unless the condition is recognised and appropriate therapy given.

Investigations

The key test is that involving water deprivation to distinguish between DI and psychogenic polydipsia. If DI is suspected then the test is followed by vasopressin administration to demonstrate whether the kidney can (cranial) or cannot (nephrogenic) respond. The details of this test are given on page 667.

In cranial DI the pre-testing plasma osmolality is usually high and with fluid deprivation often exceeds 300 mOsm/kg. The urine osmolality of the DI patients is usually less than that of the plasma at the end of the test but rises when vasopressin is given, whereas in normal subjects urine osmolality after 8 hours' fluid deprivation is about 800 mOsm/kg and does not increase when vasopressin is given.

In psychogenic polydipsia the initial plasma osmolality is usually below normal and the urine osmolality fails to rise normally with water deprivation. The renal response to exogenous vasopressin is also impaired because of the effect on the kidney of long-term overhydration.

In nephrogenic DI appropriate tests include plasma electrolytes, calcium and investigation of the renal tract.

The suprasellar anatomy in patients with cranial DI needs to be assessed as indicated on page 670.

Management

For cranial DI this is usually with the long-acting analogue of vasopressin, desmopressin (DDAVP). The amount of vasopressin required to keep the patient in water balance must be determined by measuring the fluid output. Desmopressin is given intranasally; 10–20 μg once or twice daily elicits a response as effectively as vasopressin given by injection.

A variety of other drugs have been used. Chlorpropamide (125–250 mg/d), the oral hypoglycaemic agent, enhances the renal responsiveness to vasopressin. As might be anticipated hypoglycaemia can be a problem. An alternative drug with a similar action is carbamazepine (100–200 mg/d). Thiazide diuretics (e.g. bendrofluazide 5–10 mg/d) remain the only effective drug therapy for nephrogenic DI and reduce urine volume in this condition by about 50%. Plasma potassium levels need to be carefully monitored.

FURTHER READING

Chrousos G P 1992 Regulation and dysregulation of the hypothalamic-pituitary-adrenal axis. Endocrinology and Metabolism Clinics of North America 21: 833–858

Grossman A 1992 Clinical Endocrinology. Blackwell Scientific Publications, Oxford

Molitch M E 1992 Clinical manifestations of acromegaly. Endocrinology and Metabolism Clinics of North America 21: 597–614

THE THYROID GLAND

PHYSIOLOGY

The thyroid secretes predominantly thyroxine (T_4), and only a small amount of triiodothyronine (T_3); approximately 85% of T_3 is produced by mono-deiodination of T_4 in other tissues such as liver, muscle and kidney. T_4 is probably not metabolically active until converted to T_3, and may be regarded as a prohormone. T_3 and T_4 circulate in plasma almost entirely bound ($>99.9\%$) to transport proteins, mainly thyroxine-binding globulin (TBG). It is the minute fraction of unbound or free hormone which diffuses into tissues and exerts its metabolic action. It is possible to measure the concentration in plasma of total or free T_3 and T_4 but the advantage of the free hormone measurements is that they are not influenced by changes in concentration of binding proteins, e.g. in pregnancy TBG levels are increased and total T_3 and T_4 may be raised but free thyroid hormone levels are normal.

Production of T_3 and T_4 in the thyroid is stimulated by thyrotrophin (thyroid-stimulating hormone, TSH), a glycoprotein released from the thyrotroph cells of the anterior pituitary in response to the hypothalamic tripeptide, thyrotrophin-releasing hormone (TRH) (see p. 670). A circadian rhythm of TSH secretion can be demonstrated with a peak at 01.00 hours and trough at 11.00 hours, but the variation is small and does not influence the timing of blood sampling for assessment of thyroid function.

There is a negative feedback of thyroid hormones on the thyrotrophs such that in hyperthyroidism when plasma concentrations of T_3 and T_4 are raised, TSH secretion is suppressed, and in hypothyroidism due to disease of the thyroid gland, low T_3 and T_4 are associated with high circulating TSH levels. The anterior pituitary is very sensitive to minor changes in thyroid hormone levels within the normal range. Although the reference range for total T_4 is 60–150 nmol/l, a rise or fall of 20 nmol/l in an individual in whom the level is usually 100 nmol/l would on the one hand be associated with undetectable TSH and on the other hand with a raised TSH. The combination of 'normal' T_3 and T_4 and suppressed or raised TSH is known as subclinical hyperthyroidism (p. 692) or subclinical hypothyroidism (p. 696) respectively.

Non-thyroidal illness

In ill patients, e.g. in myocardial infarction or pneumonia, not only is there a decreased peripheral conversion of T_4 to T_3 but also alterations in the concentrations of binding proteins and in their affinity for thyroid hormones. In addition TSH levels may be subnormal, or may even rise into the hypothyroid range during convalescence. It follows that the biochemical assessment of thyroid function may be difficult in such patients and should not be undertaken unless there is strong clinical evidence of thyroid disease requiring urgent treatment.

HYPERTHYROIDISM

Hyperthyroidism is the clinical syndrome which results from exposure of the body tissues to excess circulating levels of free thyroid hormones. It is a common disorder with a prevalence of about 20/1000 females; males are affected 5 times less frequently.

Aetiology

It is important to identify the cause of hyperthyroidism (Table 12.6) in order to prescribe appropriate treatment. In over 90% of patients the hyperthyroidism is due to Graves' disease, multinodular goitre or an autonomously functioning solitary thyroid nodule (toxic adenoma). Excess pituitary secretion of TSH which may or may not originate from a tumour, intrinsic thyroid stimulating activity of human chorionic gonadotrophin in hydatidiform mole and choriocarcinoma, ovarian teratoma containing thyroid tissue (struma ovarii) and metastatic differentiated carcinoma of the thyroid are extremely rare causes.

Clinical features

Hyperthyroidism usually develops insidiously and most patients have had symptoms for at least 6 months before presentation. Almost every system is affected and the clinical features are listed in the information box. There is great individual variation in the dominant features; for example the initial presentation may be to a cardiologist on account of palpitations, to a dermatologist because of pruritus or to a gastrointestinal clinic with diarrhoea. Weight loss in older patients may be associated with anorexia, raising the possibility of carcinoma. Atrial fibrillation, which is seldom seen in young patients unless

Table 12.6 Causes of hyperthyroidism and their relative frequencies in a series of 2087 patients presenting to the Royal Infirmary, Edinburgh in the 10-year period 1979–1988

Cause	Frequency (%)
Graves' disease	76
Multinodular goitre	14
Autonomously functioning solitary thyroid nodule	5
Thyroiditis	
Subacute (de Quervain's)*	3
Post-partum*	0.5
Iodide-induced	
Drugs* (e.g. amiodarone)*	1
Radiographic contrast media*	—
Iodine-prophylaxis programme*	—
Extrathyroidal source of thyroid hormone excess	
Factitious hyperthyroidism*	0.2
Struma ovarii*	—
TSH-induced	
Inappropriate TSH secretion by pituitary	0.2
Choriocarcinoma and hydatidiform mole	—
Follicular carcinoma ± metastases	0.1

* These causes of hyperthyroidism are characterised by a negligible radio-iodine uptake test result.

there is severe long-standing disease, occurs in up to 50% of patients over 60 years of age and characteristically the ventricular rate is not influenced by digoxin. In children, medical attention may be sought because of behaviour disorders, deteriorating academic performance or a premature growth spurt.

GRAVES' DISEASE

Graves' disease is distinguished clinically from other forms of hyperthyroidism by the presence of diffuse thyroid enlargement, ophthalmopathy and rarely pretibial myxoedema. It can occur at any age but is unusual before puberty and most commonly affects the 30–50-year-old age group.

Pathogenesis

Graves' disease is the major immunologically mediated form of hyperthyroidism, the other being postpartum thyroiditis (p. 691). The hyperthyroidism results from the production of IgG antibodies directed against the TSH-receptors on the thyroid follicular cell which stimulate thyroid hormone production and, in the majority, goitre formation. These antibodies are termed thyroid-stimulating immunoglobulins or TSH-receptor antibodies (TRAb) and can be detected in the serum of most patients with Graves' disease. Why these antibodies are produced is not clear but there are important genetic and environmental considerations.

In Caucasians there is an association of Graves' disease with HLAB8, DR3 and DR2, and with inability to secrete the water-soluble glycoprotein form of the ABO blood group antigens coded for on chromosomes 6 and 19 respectively. Family studies show that 50% of monozygotic twins are concordant for hyperthyroidism as opposed to 5% of dizygotic twins. The trigger for the development of hyperthyroidism in genetically susceptible individuals may be infection with viruses or bacteria. Certain strains of the gut organisms *Escherichia coli* and *Yersinia enterocolitica* possess cell-membrane TSH receptors. The production of antibodies to these microbial antigens which might cross-react with the TSH receptor on the host thyroid follicular cell could result in the development of hyperthyroidism. Stress is usually dismissed as aetiologically unimportant but many experienced endocrinologists are impressed from time to time by the temporal relationship between the onset of hyperthyroidism and a major life event such as the death of a close relative.

The concentration of TRAb in the serum is presumed to fluctuate because of the natural history of Graves' disease (Fig. 12.10). The ultimate thyroid failure in some patients is thought to result from the presence of yet another immunoglobulin, a blocking antibody

CLINICAL FEATURES OF HYPERTHYROIDISM

- **Goitre**
  Diffuse ± bruit[1]
  Nodular
- **Gastrointestinal**
  Weight loss despite normal or increased appetite[2]
  Hyperdefecation[2]
  Diarrhoea and steatorrhoea
  Anorexia[3]
  Vomiting
- **Cardiorespiratory**
  Palpitations[2], sinus tachycardia, atrial fibrillation[3]
  Increased pulse pressure
  Ankle oedema in absence of cardiac failure
  Angina, cardiomyopathy and cardiac failure[3]
  Dyspnoea on exertion[2]
  Exacerbation of asthma
- **Neuromuscular**
  Nervousness, irritability, emotional lability[2], psychosis
  Tremor
  Hyper-reflexia, ill-sustained clonus
  Muscle weakness, proximal myopathy, bulbar myopathy[3]
  Periodic paralysis (predominantly Chinese)
- **Dermatological**
  Increased sweating[2], pruritus
  Palmar erythema, spider naevi
  Onycholysis
  Alopecia
  Pigmentation, vitiligo[1]
  Digital clubbing[1]
  Pretibial myxoedema[1]
- **Reproductive**
  Amenorrhoea/oligomenorrhoea
  Infertility, spontaneous abortion
  Loss of libido, impotence
- **Ocular**
  Lid retraction, lid lag[1]
  Grittiness[1], excessive lacrimation[1]
  Chemosis[1]
  Exophthalmos[1], corneal ulceration[1]
  Ophthalmoplegia[1], diplopia[1]
  Papilloedema[1], loss of visual acuity[1]
- **Other**
  Heat intolerance[2]
  Fatigue[2], apathy[3]
  Gynaecomastia
  Lymphadenopathy[1]
  Thirst

[1]Features of Graves' disease only
[2]The most common symptoms of hyperthyroidism,
  irrespective of its cause
[3]Features found particularly in elderly patients

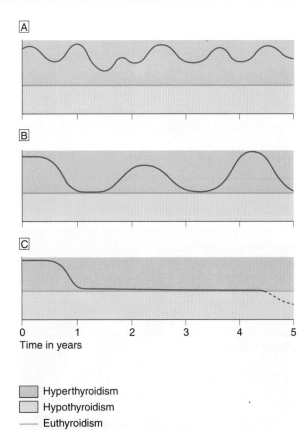

Time in years

- ▭ Hyperthyroidism
- ▭ Hypothyroidism
- —— Euthyroidism

Fig. 12.10 Natural history of the hyperthyroidism of Graves' disease. The majority (60%) of patients have either prolonged periods of hyperthyroidism of fluctuating severity **(A)**, or periods of alternating relapse and remission **(B)**. It is the minority who experience a single short-lived episode followed by prolonged remission and in some cases by the eventual onset of hypothyroidism **(C)**.

against the TSH receptor, and from tissue destruction by cytotoxic antibodies and cell-mediated immunity.

The pathogenesis of the ophthalmopathy and dermopathy is less well understood. Both are immunologically mediated but TRAb is not implicated. Within the orbit there is proliferation of fibroblasts which secrete hydrophilic glycosaminoglycans. The resulting increased interstitial fluid content combined with a chronic inflammatory cell infiltrate causes marked swelling of the extraocular muscles (Fig. 12.11) and a rise in retrobulbar pressure. The eye is displaced forwards (proptosis, exophthalmos) and in more severe cases there is optic nerve compression.

Clinical features

Goitre
The diffusely enlarged gland is usually 2–3 times the normal volume and increased blood flow may be manifest by a thrill or bruit. In some patients, particularly the elderly, no thyroid enlargement is palpable or the gland may be nodular. The largest goitres tend to occur in young men.

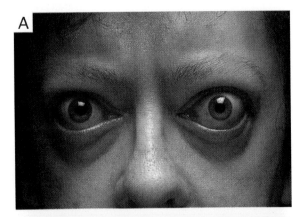

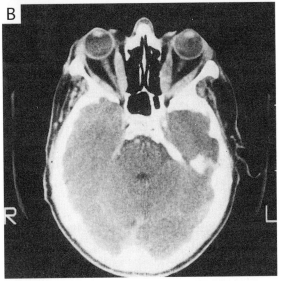

Fig. 12.11 A **Bilateral ophthalmopathy of Graves' disease** in a 42-year-old man developing two years after successful treatment of hyperthyroidism with ^{131}I. The main symptoms were those of diplopia in all directions of gaze and reduced visual acuity in the left eye. The periorbital swelling is due to retrobulbar fat prolapsing into the eyelids, and increased interstitial fluid as a result of raised intra-orbital pressure. B **Transverse CT scan of the orbits of the same patient as in A, showing the extraocular muscles enlarged to three times their normal bulk.** This is most obvious at the apex of the left orbit, causing compression of the optic nerve and reduced visual acuity.

Ophthalmopathy

This is only present in 50% of patients when first seen but may also develop after successful treatment of the hyperthyroidism of Graves' disease, or precede its development by many years (exophthalmic Graves' disease). The most frequent presenting symptoms are related to increased exposure of the cornea resulting from proptosis and lid retraction. There may be excessive lacrimation made worse by wind and bright light, and

pain may be due to conjunctivitis or corneal ulceration. In addition there may be loss of visual acuity and/or visual field resulting from corneal oedema or optic nerve compression. If the extraocular muscles are involved and do not act in concert, diplopia will result.

Pretibial myxoedema

This infiltrative dermopathy takes the form of raised pink coloured or purplish plaques on the anterior aspect of the leg extending on to the dorsum of the foot. The lesions may be itchy and the skin may have a *peau d'orange* appearance with growth of coarse hair; less commonly the face and arms may be affected.

Investigations

A clinical diagnosis can usually be made but, in view of the likely need for prolonged medical treatment or destructive therapy, it is essential to confirm the diagnosis biochemically by more than one test of thyroid function. Serum T_3 and T_4 concentrations are elevated in the majority, but T_4 is in the upper part of the normal range and T_3 raised (T_3-thyrotoxicosis) in 5% of patients, particularly those with recurrent hyperthyroidism following surgery or a course of antithyroid drugs. TSH is undetectable if a sensitive assay capable of recording values of 0.1 mU/1 or less is used. If this is not available it will be necessary to demonstrate an absent serum TSH response following the intravenous administration of 200 μg TRH. Measurement of ^{131}I uptake by the thyroid and TRAb may be of value in diagnosing Graves' disease if exophthalmos, goitre and pretibial myxoedema are not present. Other non-specific abnormalities are given in the information box below.

NON-SPECIFIC BIOCHEMICAL ABNORMALITIES IN HYPERTHYROIDISM

- **Hepatic dysfunction**
  Slightly raised concentrations of bilirubin, alanine aminotransferase and gamma-glutamyl transferase; elevated alkaline phosphatase derived from bone and liver
- **Mild hypercalcaemia (5%)**
- **Glycosuria**
  Associated diabetes mellitus
  'Lag storage' (p. 734)

Management of hyperthyroidism of Graves' disease

Table 12.7 compares the different treatments. If it were possible to predict with confidence the natural history of the hyperthyroidism in an individual patient at presentation it would be appropriate to give an antithyroid drug for 12–18 months to those in whom a single episode was anticipated and to advise destructive therapy with

^{131}I or surgery for those likely to experience recurrent disease. With the exception of young men with large goitres and those with severe hyperthyroidism such a prediction is not possible. For patients under 40 years of age many centres adopt the empirical approach of prescribing a course of carbimazole and recommending surgery if relapse occurs. Although there is no evidence that thyroid carcinoma or leukaemia is induced by ^{131}I, or that its use results in an increased frequency of congenital malformation among subsequent offspring, radioactive iodine treatment is usually reserved in the UK for patients over the age of 40.

Antithyroid drugs

The most commonly used are carbimazole and its active metabolite, methimazole (not available in the UK). Propylthiouracil is equally effective but the dose is 10 times that of carbimazole. These drugs reduce the synthesis of new thyroid hormones by inhibiting the iodination of tyrosine. Carbimazole also has an immunosuppressive action, leading to a reduction in serum TRAb concentrations, but this is not enough to influence the natural history of the hyperthyroidism significantly. The dosage is given in the information box.

CARBIMAZOLE

- **Dosage**
  0–3 weeks:
  15 mg 8-hourly
  4–8 weeks:
  10 mg 8-hourly
  Maintenance: 5–20 mg daily
- **Duration of treatment**
  18–24 months
- **Adverse effects**
  Rash 2%
  Agranulocytosis 0.2%

There is subjective improvement within 10–14 days of starting carbimazole and the patient is usually clinically and biochemically euthyroid at 3–4 weeks. The maintenance dose is determined by measurement of T$_4$ and TSH, attempting to keep both hormones within their respective reference ranges. In most patients it can be taken as a single dose and is continued for 18–24 months in the hope that during this period permanent remission will occur. Unfortunately, hyperthyroidism recurs in at least 50%, usually within 2 years of stopping treatment. Rarely, despite good drug compliance, T$_4$ and TSH levels fluctuate between those of hyperthyroidism and hypothyroidism at successive review appointments, presumably due to rapidly changing concentrations of TRAb. In such patients satisfactory control can be achieved by blocking thyroid hormone synthesis with carbimazole 10 mg 8-hourly and adding T$_4$ 150 μg daily as replacement therapy.

The adverse effects of the antithyroid drugs develop within 7–28 days of starting treatment. Agranulocytosis cannot be predicted by routine measurement of white blood cell count, and is fortunately reversible. Patients should be warned to stop the drug and contact their medical attendant immediately should a severe sore throat develop. Cross sensitivity between the antithyroid drugs is unusual and another member of the group can be substituted with good effect.

Subtotal thyroidectomy

Patients must be rendered euthyroid before operation. The antithyroid drug is stopped 2 weeks before surgery and replaced by potassium iodate 170 mg daily orally. This maintains euthyroidism in the short term by inhibiting thyroid hormone release and reduces the size and vascularity of the gland making surgery technically easier. Complications of surgery are rare (Table 12.7). One year after surgery 80% of patients are euthyroid, 15% permanently hypothyroid and 5% remain thyrotoxic. Thyroid failure within 6 months of operation may be temporary. Long-term follow-up of patients treated surgically is necessary, as the late development of hypothyroidism and recurrence of thyrotoxicosis are well-recognised.

Radioactive iodine

^{131}I acts either by destroying functioning thyroid cells or by inhibiting their ability to replicate. The variable radiosensitivity of the gland means that the choice of dose is empirical. In most centres 185–370 MBq (5–10 mCi) is given orally, the dose depending upon clinical assessment of goitre size. This regimen is effective in 75% of patients within 4–12 weeks. During the lag period symptoms can be controlled by propranolol 160 mg per day or, in more severe cases, by carbimazole 15 mg 8-hourly for 4–6 weeks starting 48 hours after radioiodine therapy. If hyperthyroidism persists at 12 weeks a further dose of ^{131}I should be employed. The disadvantage of ^{131}I treatment is that the majority of patients eventually develop hypothyroidism and long-term follow-up is therefore necessary.

β-adrenoceptor antagonists

A non-selective β-adrenoceptor antagonist, such as propranolol, will alleviate but not abolish symptoms of hyperthyroidism within 24–48 hours. The usual dose is 160 mg daily. β-adrenoceptor antagonists cannot be recommended for long-term treatment, but they are extremely useful in the short term, e.g. patients awaiting hospital consultation or following ^{131}I therapy. Propranolol alone or in combination with iodine has been used in the preparation of patients for subtotal thyroidectomy, but this treatment cannot be recommended as standard practice.

Table 12.7 Comparison of the different treatments for the hyperthyroidism of Graves' disease

Management	Indications	Contraindications	Disadvantages/complications
Antithyroid drugs, e.g. carbimazole	1st episode in patients <40 years	Hypersensitivity Breast feeding—(propylthiouracil suitable)	>50% relapse rate usually within 2 years of stopping drug
Subtotal thyroidectomy	1 Recurrent hyperthyroidism after course of antithyroid drugs in patients <40 yrs 2 Initial treatment in males with large goitres and in those with severe hyperthyroidism, i.e. total $T_3 > 9.0$ nmol/l 3 Poor drug compliance	Previous thyroid surgery Dependence upon voice, e.g. opera singer, lecturer	Transient hypocalcaemia (10%) Hypoparathyroidism (1%) Recurrent laryngeal nerve palsy[2] (1%)
Radio-iodine	1 Patients >40 yrs[1] 2 Recurrence following surgery irrespective of age 3 Other serious illness, e.g. multiple sclerosis irrespective of age	Pregnancy or planned pregnancy within 6 months of treatment	Hypothyroidism, approx. 40% in 1st year, 80% after 15 years

[1] In certain parts of the world, ^{131}I is used more liberally and prescribed for young women in the 20–40 age group.
[2] It is not only vocal cord palsy which alters the voice following thyroid surgery; the superior laryngeal nerves are frequently transected and result in minor changes in voice quality.

Management of ophthalmopathy

The majority of patients require no treatment other than reassurance. Lid retraction will usually resolve when the patient becomes euthyroid and exophthalmos usually lessens gradually over a period of 2–3 years. For those with symptomatic ophthalmopathy, methylcellulose eyedrops will counter the gritty discomfort of dry eyes and tinted glasses or side shields attached to spectacle frames will reduce the excessive lacrimation triggered by sun or wind. Corneal ulceration is an indication for lateral tarsorrhaphy or a lid lengthening procedure. Persistent diplopia can be corrected by extraocular muscle surgery but this should be delayed until the degree of diplopia is stable.

Papilloedema, loss of visual acuity or visual field defect require urgent treatment with prednisolone 60 mg daily if blindness is to be prevented. Close cooperation between endocrinologist and ophthalmologist is necessary and, if significant improvement is not evident within 7–10 days, orbital decompression is indicated.

Management of dermopathy

The pretibial myxoedema of Graves' disease rarely requires to be treated. Local injections of triamcinolone or the application of betamethasone ointment under occlusive dressings may be effective.

TOXIC MULTINODULAR GOITRE

Like Graves' disease, this form of hyperthyroidism is more common in women. The mean age of presentation is 60 years. Thyroid hormone levels are usually only slightly elevated but, as an older age group is affected, cardiovascular features such as atrial fibrillation or cardiac failure tend to predominate. Treatment is usually with a large dose of [131]I (555–1850 MBq, 15–50 mCi) as the gland is relatively resistant to radiation. Hypothyroidism is less common than after treatment of Graves' disease. If there is significant tracheal compression or retrosternal extension of the goitre, partial thyroidectomy is indicated. Long-term treatment with antithyroid drugs is not appropriate as relapse is invariable after drug withdrawal.

TOXIC ADENOMA

The presence of a toxic solitary nodule is the cause of less than 5% of all cases of hyperthyroidism. The nodule is a follicular adenoma which autonomously secretes excess thyroid hormones and inhibits endogenous TSH secretion with subsequent atrophy of the rest of the thyroid gland. The adenoma is usually greater than 3 cm in diameter. In some cases spontaneous resolution of hyperthyroidism has occurred as a result of infarction of the adenoma.

Most patients are female and over 40 years of age. Although most nodules are palpable, the diagnosis can be made with certainty only by isotope scanning. The hyperthyroidism is usually mild and in almost 50% of patients the plasma T_3 alone is elevated (T_3 thyrotoxicosis). Treatment is by hemithyroidectomy or by ^{131}I, 555–1110 MBq (15–30 mCi). Permanent hypothyroidism does not occur following surgery and is unusual after treatment with ^{131}I, since the atrophic cells surrounding the nodule will have received little or no irradiation.

HYPERTHYROIDISM ASSOCIATED WITH A LOW IODINE UPTAKE

In patients with hyperthyroidism, the thyroid uptake of ^{131}I is usually high but a low or negligible uptake of iodine occurs in some rarer causes. If the radioactive iodine uptake test is not routinely performed in patients with thyrotoxicosis who do not have obvious Graves' disease or nodular goitre, the correct diagnosis may not be made and inappropriate treatment given.

Subacute (de Quervain's) thyroiditis

Subacute thyroiditis is a virus-induced (Coxsackie, mumps, adenovirus) inflammation of the thyroid gland which results in release of colloid and its constituents into the circulation.

This form of hyperthyroidism is characterised by pain in the region of the thyroid gland which may radiate to the angle of jaw and the ears and is made worse by swallowing, coughing and movement of the neck. The thyroid is usually palpably enlarged and tender. Systemic upset is common. Affected patients are usually females aged 20–40 years.

Thyroid hormone levels are raised for 4–6 weeks until the preformed colloid is depleted. The iodine uptake is low because the damaged follicular cells are unable to trap iodine and because endogenous TSH secretion is suppressed. Low titre thyroid autoantibodies appear transiently in the serum, and the ESR is usually raised. The hyperthyroidism is followed by a period of hypothyroidism which is usually asymptomatic, and finally by full recovery of thyroid function within 4–6 months. The pain and systemic upset usually respond to simple measures such as aspirin or other non-steroidal anti-inflammatory drugs. Occasionally, however, it may be necessary to prescribe prednisolone 40 mg daily for 3–4 weeks. The hyperthyroidism is mild and treatment with propranolol, 160 mg per day, is usually adequate. Antithyroid drugs are of no benefit.

Post-partum thyroiditis

The maternal immune response which is modified during pregnancy to allow survival of the fetal homograft is enhanced after delivery and may unmask previously unrecognised subclinical autoimmune thyroid disease. Surveys have shown that transient biochemical disturbances of thyroid function, i.e. hyperthyroidism, hypothyroidism and hyperthyroidism followed by hypothyroidism, lasting a few weeks, occur in 5–10% of women within 6 months of delivery. Those affected are likely to possess antithyroid peroxidase (microsomal) antibodies in the serum in early pregnancy. Thyroid biopsy shows a lymphocytic thyroiditis. Symptoms of thyroid dysfunction are rare and there is no association

between postnatal depression and abnormal thyroid function tests. However, symptomatic hyperthyroidism presenting for the first time within 6 months of childbirth is unlikely to be due to Graves' disease, and the diagnosis of post-partum thyroiditis can be confirmed by a negligible radio-iodine uptake.

If treatment of the hyperthyroid phase is necessary, a β-adrenoceptor antagonist should be prescribed and not an antithyroid drug. Post-partum thyroiditis tends to recur after subsequent pregnancies and eventually patients progress over a period of years to permanent hypothyroidism.

A similar painless form of thyroiditis, unrelated to pregnancy, has been increasingly recognised in North America and Japan, and accounts in these countries for up to 20% of all cases of hyperthyroidism.

Iodine-induced hyperthyroidism

The administration of iodine either in prophylactic iodinisation programmes, radiographic contrast media or drugs such as the anti-arrhythmic agent, amiodarone, may result in the development of hyperthyroidism which is usually mild and self-limiting. Affected individuals are thought to have underlying thyroid autonomy or Graves' disease in remission. If it is not possible to discontinue amiodarone or substitute another drug, hyperthyroidism can be controlled with carbimazole.

Factitious hyperthyroidism

This uncommon condition occurs when an emotionally disturbed person, usually a nurse, has been taking excessive amounts of a thyroid hormone preparation, most often thyroxine. The exogenous T_4 suppresses pituitary TSH secretion and hence iodine uptake, serum thyroglobulin and release of endogenous thyroid hormones. As a result the $T_4:T_3$ ratio (approximately 30:1 in conventional hyperthyroidism) is increased to approximately 70:1 because circulating T_3 in factitious thyrotoxicosis is derived exclusively from the peripheral monodeiodination of T_4. The combination of negligible iodine uptake, high $T_4:T_3$ ratio and a low or undetectable thyroglobulin is diagnostic and has made what was often a difficult diagnosis much simpler.

SPECIAL SITUATIONS

Hyperthyroidism in pregnancy

The coexistence of pregnancy and hyperthyroidism is unusual as anovulatory cycles are common in thyrotoxic patients and autoimmune disease tends to remit during pregnancy. The hyperthyroidism is almost always caused by Graves' disease.

The hyperthyroidism is treated with carbimazole

which crosses the placenta and also treats the fetus, whose thyroid gland is exposed to the action of maternal TRAb. It is important to use the smallest dose of carbimazole (optimally less than 15 mg per day) which will maintain maternal (and presumably fetal) free hormones and TSH within their respective normal ranges in order to avoid fetal hypothyroidism and goitre.

The patient should therefore be reviewed every 4 weeks and it is a wise precaution to discontinue carbimazole 4 weeks before the expected date of delivery to avoid any possibility of fetal hypothyroidism at the time of maximum brain development. If the assay is available measurement of TRAb in the maternal serum at this stage is valuable; a high titre identifies those fetuses at particular risk of developing neonatal hyperthyroidism.

If maternal hyperthyroidism occurs after delivery and the patient wishes to continue breast feeding, propylthiouracil (p. 689) is the drug of choice as it is excreted in the milk to a much lesser extent than carbimazole.

If subtotal thyroidectomy is necessary because of poor drug compliance or hypersensitivity, it is most safely performed in the middle trimester. Radioactive iodine is absolutely contraindicated as it invariably induces fetal hypothyroidism.

Hyperthyroidism in childhood

Graves' disease is almost invariably the form of thyrotoxicosis in childhood and usually presents in the second decade. Treatment should be with carbimazole until the patient is about 18 years of age in an attempt to guarantee the important stages in the physical and educational development of the child.

Hyperthyroid crisis

This is a rare and life-threatening increase in the severity of the clinical features of hyperthyroidism. The most prominent signs are fever, agitation, confusion, tachycardia or atrial fibrillation and, in the older patient, cardiac failure. It is a medical emergency and, despite early recognition and treatment, the mortality rate is 10%. Thyrotoxic crisis is most commonly precipitated by infection in a patient with previously unrecognised or inadequately treated hyperthyroidism. It may also develop shortly after subtotal thyroidectomy in an ill-prepared patient or within a few days of ^{131}I therapy when acute irradiation damage may lead to a transient rise in serum thyroid hormone levels.

Patients should be rehydrated and given a broad spectrum antibiotic. Propranolol is rapidly effective orally (80 mg 6-hourly) or intravenously (1–5 mg 6-hourly). Sodium iopodate 500 mg per day orally will restore serum T_3 levels to normal in 48–72 hours. It is a radiographic contrast medium which not only inhibits the

release of thyroid hormones, but also reduces the conversion of T_4 to T_3 and is therefore more effective than potassium iodate or Lugol's solution. Carbimazole 15 mg 8-hourly orally inhibits the synthesis of new thyroid hormone. If the patient is unconscious or uncooperative carbimazole can be administered rectally with good effect, but no preparation is available for parenteral use.

Sodium iopodate and propranolol can be withdrawn after 10–14 days and the patient maintained on carbimazole.

Subclinical hyperthyroidism

This term is used to describe clinically euthyroid patients in whom serum thyroid hormone concentrations are normal, but usually in the upper part of the reference range, and TSH undetectable in the absence of non-thyroidal illness. Subclinical hyperthyroidism occurs most often in patients with exophthalmic Graves' disease (50%), multinodular goitre (25%) and in a variable proportion following therapy of hyperthyroidism. Although there is evidence from studies of hepatic, renal and cardiac function that such patients are probably mildly hyperthyroid, treatment is not usually instituted. There is a significant risk of overt hyperthyroidism developing and follow-up is indicated.

HYPOTHYROIDISM

PRIMARY HYPOTHYROIDISM

In primary hypothyroidism there is an intrinsic disorder of the thyroid gland, e.g. following ^{131}I therapy for Graves' disease, in which low levels of thyroid hormones are associated with raised TSH. The classification is shown in the information box below.

CLASSIFICATION OF PRIMARY HYPOTHYROIDISM

- **Spontaneous atrophic**
- **Goitrous:**
  Hashimoto's thyroiditis
  Drug-induced
  Iodine deficiency
  Dyshormonogenesis
- **Post-ablative**
- **Transient**
- **Subclinical**
- **Congenital**

Spontaneous atrophic hypothyroidism, thyroid failure following ^{131}I or surgical treatment of hyperthyroidism and the hypothyroidism of Hashimoto's thyroiditis account for over 90% of cases in those parts of the world which are not iodine deficient. The prevalence of primary hypothyroidism is 10/1000 but increases to

50/1000 if patients with subclinical hypothyroidism (normal T$_4$ raised TSH) are included. The female:male ratio is approximately 6:1.

SPONTANEOUS ATROPHIC HYPOTHYROIDISM

This form of primary hypothyroidism increases in incidence with age and, like Graves' disease and Hashimoto's thyroiditis, is an organ-specific autoimmune disorder. There is destructive lymphoid infiltration of the thyroid, ultimately leading to fibrosis and atrophy. There is also evidence for the presence of TSH-receptor antibodies which block the effects of endogenous TSH. In some patients there is a history of Graves' disease treated with antithyroid drugs 10–20 years earlier and, very occasionally, patients with this form of hypothyroidism develop Graves' disease. As with any of the immunologically-mediated thyroid disorders, patients are at risk of developing other organ-specific autoimmune conditions such as type I diabetes mellitus, pernicious anaemia and Addison's disease, and autoimmune disease is not uncommon in their first and second degree relatives.

Clinical features

These depend on the duration and severity of the hypothyroidism. In the patient in whom complete thyroid failure has developed insidiously over months or even years many of the clinical features listed in the information box are likely to be present. A consequence of prolonged hypothyroidism is the infiltration of many body tissues by the mucopolysaccharides, hyaluronic acid and chondroitin sulphate, resulting in a low-pitched voice, poor hearing, slurred speech due to a large tongue, and compression of the median nerve at the wrist. Infiltration of the dermis gives rise to non-pitting oedema or myxoedema which is most marked in the skin of the hands, feet and eyelids. The resultant periorbital puffiness is often striking and, when combined with facial pallor due to vasoconstriction and anaemia, or a lemon-yellow tint to the skin due to carotinaemia, purplish lips and malar flush, the clinical diagnosis is simple. Most cases of hypothyroidism are not so obvious, however, and unless the diagnosis is positively entertained in a middle-aged woman complaining of symptoms such as tiredness, weight gain or depression, or with the carpal tunnel syndrome, an opportunity for early treatment will be missed. On the other hand many patients are asymptomatic and thyroid failure is detected by screening during hospital admission or by routine testing of thyroid function in patients known to be at risk of developing hypothyroidism, e.g. following ^{131}I therapy of Graves' disease. It is in this group of patients

that there is often little or no subjective benefit from thyroxine replacement therapy.

CLINICAL FEATURES OF HYPOTHYROIDISM

- **General**
  Tiredness, somnolence
  Weight gain
  Cold intolerance
  Hoarseness
  Goitre
- **Cardiorespiratory**
  Bradycardia, hypertension, angina, cardiac failure*
  Xanthelasma
  Pericardial and pleural effusion*
- **Neuromuscular**
  Aches and pains, muscle stiffness
  Delayed relaxation of tendon reflexes
  Carpal tunnel syndrome, deafness
  Depression, psychosis*
  Cerebellar ataxia*
  Myotonia*
- **Haematological**
  Macrocytosis
  Anaemia
    Iron deficiency (premenopausal women)
    Normochromic
    Pernicious
- **Dermatological**
  Dry flaky skin and hair, alopecia
  Purplish lips and malar flush, carotenaemia
  Vitiligo
  Erythema ab igne (Granny's tartan)
  Myxoedema
- **Reproductive**
  Menorrhagia
  Infertility
  Galactorrhoea*, impotence*
- **Gastrointestinal**
  Constipation
  Ileus*
  Ascites*

*Rare but well-recognised features

Investigations

Serum T$_4$ is low and TSH raised, usually in excess of 20 mU/l. T$_3$ concentrations do not discriminate reliably between euthyroid and hypothyroid patients and should not be measured. Other non-specific abnormalities include elevation of the enzymes lactate dehydrogenase and creatine kinase, raised cholesterol and triglyceride levels and low serum sodium. In severe prolonged hypothyroidism the electrocardiogram (ECG) classically demonstrates sinus bradycardia with low voltage complexes and ST-T wave abnormalities.

Management

Hypothyroidism should be treated with thyroxine which is available as 25, 50 and 100 μg tablets. It is customary to start slowly and a dose of 50 μg per day should be given for 3 weeks increasing thereafter to 100 μg per day for a further 3 weeks and finally to 150 μg per day. In the elderly and in patients with ischaemic heart disease the initial dose should be 25 μg per day. Thyroxine should always be taken as a single daily dose as it has a plasma half-life of approximately 7 days. The correct dose of thyroxine is that which restores serum TSH to normal. There is some evidence that the finding of an undetectable TSH concentration indicates over-treatment even in the presence of a normal T_4, although in certain circumstances, e.g. Hashimoto's thyroiditis and differentiated thyroid carcinoma, the aim is to suppress TSH without inducing overt hyperthyroidism.

Patients feel better within 2–3 weeks. Reduction in weight and periorbital puffiness occurs quickly, but the restoration of skin and hair texture and resolution of any effusions may take 3–6 months (Fig. 12.12).

SPECIAL PROBLEMS

Ischaemic heart disease

Untreated primary hypothyroidism is associated with hyperlipidaemia but there is doubt whether, in the absence of hypertension, it leads to increased coronary atheroma. However, 5% of patients with long-standing hypothyroidism complain of angina at presentation or develop it during treatment with thyroxine. Although angina may remain unchanged in severity or paradoxically disappear with restoration of metabolic rate, exacerbation of myocardial ischaemia, infarction and sudden death are well-recognised complications, even using doses of thyroxine as low as 25 μg per day. Approximately 40% of patients with angina cannot tolerate full replacement therapy despite the use of β-adrenoceptor antagonists and vasodilators. Although there is still reluctance to operate on patients with untreated or partially treated hypothyroidism, coronary artery surgery and balloon angioplasty can safely be performed in such patients and, if successful, allow full replacement dosage of thyroxine in the majority.

Hypothyroidism in pregnancy

Until recently it was thought that the dose of thyroxine did not need to be changed during pregnancy. However, on the basis of serum TSH measurements most pregnant women with primary hypothyroidism require an increase in the dose of thyroxine of some 50 μg daily. One explanation for this phenomenon is the well-recognised increase in serum thyroxine-binding globulin concentration during pregnancy, resulting in a decrease in serum-free thyroid hormone concentrations which cannot be compensated for by thyroidal secretion. Serum TSH and free T_4 should be measured during each trimester and the dose of thyroxine adjusted to maintain a normal TSH.

Myxoedema coma

This is a rare presentation of hypothyroidism in which there is a depressed level of consciousness, usually in an elderly patient who appears myxoedematous. Body temperature may be as low as 25°C, convulsions are not uncommon and cerebrospinal fluid (CSF) pressure and protein content are raised. Mortality rate is 50% and survival depends upon early recognition and treatment of hypothyroidism and other factors contributing to the altered conscious level, e.g. drugs such as phenothiazines, cardiac failure, chest infection, dilutional hyponatraemia, hypoxaemia and hypercapnia due to hypoventilation.

Myxoedema coma is a medical emergency and treatment must begin before biochemical confirmation of the diagnosis. Thyroxine is not usually available for parenteral use and triiodothyronine is given as an intravenous bolus of 20 μg followed by 20 μg every 8 hours until there is sustained clinical improvement. In survivors there is a rise in body temperature within 24 hours and, after 48–72 hours, it is usually possible to substitute oral thyroxine in a dose of 50 μg per day. Unless it is apparent that the patient has primary hypothyroidism, e.g. thyroidectomy scar or goitre, the thyroid failure should be assumed to be secondary to hypothalamic or pituitary disease and treatment given with hydrocortisone sodium succinate 100 mg intramuscularly 8-hourly, pending the results of T_4, TSH and cortisol concentrations. Other measures include slow rewarming by wrapping the patient in a space blanket, cautious use of intravenous fluids, broad spectrum antibiotics and high-flow oxygen. Occasionally, if hypoxaemia, hypercapnia and respiratory acidosis persist assisted ventilation may be necessary.

Ensuring compliance

Patients often do not take long-term medication in the recommended dose and thyroxine is no exception (Fig. 12.12). It is, therefore, important to measure thyroid function tests every 1–2 years once the dose of thyroxine is stabilised and at each visit to reinforce the need for regular medication. In some patients in whom tablet taking is erratic, thyroxine is taken diligently or even in excess for the few days prior to a clinic visit, resulting in the seemingly anomalous combination of a high serum T_4 and high TSH.

Inappropriate thyroxine therapy

In some patients treatment with thyroxine may have been started in the past without biochemical confirmation of the diagnosis for a variety of complaints such as obesity, tiredness or alopecia and may have been given for many years to patients in whom thyroid failure could have been short-lived, e.g. post-partum thyroiditis. Thyroxine should be stopped and serum T_4 and TSH concentrations measured 4–6 weeks later. This period allows for any thyroxine-induced suppression of pituitary thyrotrophs to recover and a biochemical distinction to be made between primary and secondary hypothyroidism. If the patient is truly hypothyroid, lack of thyroxine for 4–6 weeks will be relatively easily tolerated.

GOITROUS HYPOTHYROIDISM

The following conditions are not always associated with hypothyroidism and should therefore be included in the differential diagnosis of a euthyroid patient with goitre.

Hashimoto's thyroiditis

This is the most common cause of goitrous hypothyroidism. It typically affects 20–60-year-old women who present with a small or moderately-sized diffuse goitre which is characteristically firm or rubbery in consistency. The goitre may be soft, however, and impossible to differentiate from simple goitre by palpation alone. Thyroid status depends upon the relative degrees of lymphocytic infiltration, fibrosis and follicular cell hyperplasia within the gland but 25% of patients are hypothyroid at presentation. In the remainder serum T_4 is normal and TSH normal or raised but these patients are at risk of developing overt hypothyroidism in future years. In 90% of patients with Hashimoto's thyroiditis thyroid peroxidase antibodies are present in the serum. In those under the age of 20 years the ANF may be positive.

Thyroxine therapy is indicated not only for hypothyroidism but also for goitre shrinkage. In this context the dose of thyroxine should be sufficient to suppress serum TSH to undetectable levels without inducing hyperthyroidism (usually 150 μg daily but in some patients 200 μg daily).

Drug-induced hypothyroidism

Lithium carbonate. This is widely used for the treatment of manic-depressive illness. Like iodide, lithium inhibits the release of thyroid hormones. Although the most common evidence of thyroid dysfunction is a raised serum TSH, some patients, usually those with underlying autoimmune thyroiditis, develop goitre and hypothyroidism.

Iodine. When taken for prolonged periods iodine may cause goitrous hypothyroidism in patients with under-

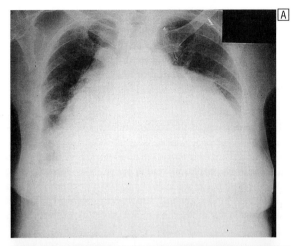

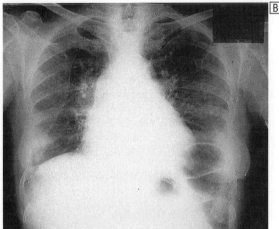

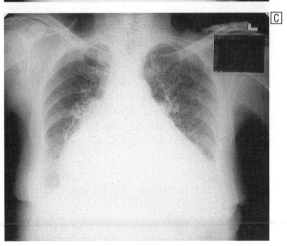

Fig. 12.12 Sequential chest radiographs in a patient with severe long-standing hypothyroidism. Ⓐ **Before treatment.** Cardiomegaly is due to a combination of dilatation and pericardial effusion. Ⓑ **After treatment with thyroxine for 9 months.** Ⓒ **Recurrence of cardiomegaly** 2–3 years after patient stopped taking thyroxine.

lying autoimmune thyroiditis. This is usually seen in those with chronic respiratory diseases given expectorants containing potassium iodide, or in patients receiving the antidysrhythmic drug, amiodarone, which contains a significant amount of iodine.

Iodine deficiency

In certain parts of the world, such as the Andes, Himalayas and central Africa, where there is dietary iodine deficiency, thyroid enlargement is common (more than 10% of the population) and is known as endemic goitre. Most patients are euthyroid and have normal or raised TSH levels. In general the more severe the iodine deficiency, the greater the incidence of hypothyroidism.

Dyshormonogenesis

Dyshormonogenesis is an unusual genetically determined defect in thyroid hormone synthesis. The mode of inheritance is autosomal recessive. Although several forms have been described, the most common results from deficiency of the intrathyroidal peroxidase enzyme. Homozygous individuals present with congenital hypothyroidism; heterozygotes present in the first two decades of life with goitre, normal thyroid hormone levels and a raised TSH. The combination of dyshormonogenetic goitre and nerve deafness is known as Pendred's syndrome.

TRANSIENT HYPOTHYROIDISM

This is often observed during the first 6 months after subtotal thyroidectomy or ^{131}I treatment of Graves' disease, in the post-thyrotoxic phase of subacute thyroiditis and in post-partum thyroiditis (Fig. 12.13). In these conditions thyroxine treatment should not be necessary as the patient is usually asymptomatic during the short period of thyroid failure. In some neonates transplacental passage of TSH-receptor blocking antibodies from a mother with autoimmune thyroid disease is a cause of hypothyroidism which, like neonatal thyrotoxicosis, is temporary.

SUBCLINICAL HYPOTHYROIDISM

Subclinical hypothyroidism is a term used to describe asymptomatic patients who are clinically euthyroid, with thyroid hormone levels at the lower end of the reference range, but raised serum TSH. It is most often encountered after ^{131}I or surgical treatment of hyperthyroidism and may persist for many years. The present consensus is that these patients are mildly hypothyroid

and failure to recognise this is a reflection of the poor discrimination of clinical examination. Thyroxine should be given in a dose of 50–150 μg daily—sufficient to restore TSH concentrations to normal.

CONGENITAL HYPOTHYROIDISM

It has long been recognised that early treatment with thyroxine is essential to prevent irreversible brain damage in children with congenital hypothyroidism. Thyroid failure, however, is difficult to diagnose clinically in the first few weeks of life. Routine screening of TSH levels in blood spot samples obtained 5–7 days after birth has revealed an incidence of approximately 1 in 3000 resulting from either thyroid agenesis, ectopic or hypoplastic glands or dyshormonogenesis. Congenital hypothyroidism is thus 6 times more common than phenylketonuria.

It is now possible to start thyroid replacement therapy within 2 weeks of birth. Developmental assessment of infants treated at this early stage has revealed no differences between cases and controls in most children.

SECONDARY HYPOTHYROIDISM

This form is much less common than primary hypothyroidism. There is atrophy of an inherently normal thyroid gland caused by failure of TSH secretion in patients with hypothalamic or anterior pituitary disease, e.g. sarcoidosis, chromophobe adenoma. There is usually deficiency of other anterior pituitary hormones and clinical evidence of hypopituitarism or, in the case of hypothalamic dysfunction, diabetes insipidus may be present. Recently there have been reports that pituitary hypothyroidism may result from an autoimmune lymphoid hypophysitis.

SIMPLE GOITRE

This is the term used to describe diffuse or multinodular enlargement of the thyroid which occurs sporadically and is of unknown aetiology. It is likely, however, that suboptimal dietary iodine intake, minor degrees of dyshormonogenesis and stimuli such as epidermal growth factor and growth-stimulating immunoglobulins are important in the development of simple goitre. Affected patients are euthyroid, usually female and often have a family history of goitre.

Simple diffuse goitre

This form of goitre usually presents between the ages of 15 and 25 years, often during pregnancy, and tends to be noticed not by the patient but by friends and relatives. Occasionally, there is a tight sensation in the neck, particularly when swallowing. The goitre is soft, symmetrical and the thyroid enlarged 2–3 times normal. There is no tenderness, lymphadenopathy or overlying bruit. Concentrations of T_3, T_4 and TSH are normal and no thyroid autoantibodies are detected in the serum. No treatment is necessary and in most cases the goitre regresses. In some, however, the unknown stimulus to thyroid enlargement persists and as a result of recurrent episodes of hyperplasia and involution during the following 10–20 years the gland becomes multinodular with areas of autonomous function (simple multinodular goitre, Fig. 12.14).

Simple multinodular goitre

Presentation is rare before middle age. The patient may have been aware of goitre for many years, perhaps slowly increasing in size. Rarely, medical advice may have been sought because of painful swelling lasting a few days caused by haemorrhage into a nodule or cyst. The goitre is nodular or lobulated on palpation and may extend retrosternally. Very large goitres may cause mediastinal compression with stridor, dysphagia and obstruction of superior vena cava. Hoarseness due to recurrent laryngeal nerve palsy can occur but is strongly suggestive of thyroid carcinoma. Serum T_3 and T_4 are normal and in the majority are associated with normal TSH. In approximately 25% thyroid hormone levels are in the upper part of their respective normal ranges and TSH is undetectable (subclinical hyperthyroidism). Radiographs of the thoracic inlet may show tracheal displacement or compression, intrathyroidal calcification and the extent of retrosternal extension.

If the goitre is small no treatment is necessary other than annual review as the natural history is progression to a toxic multinodular goitre. Partial thyroidectomy is indicated for large goitres which cause mediastinal compression or which are cosmetically unattractive. Unfortunately, recurrence 10–20 years later is not uncommon and cannot be prevented by the long-established custom of treatment with thyroxine which may serve to aggravate any associated hyperthyroidism.

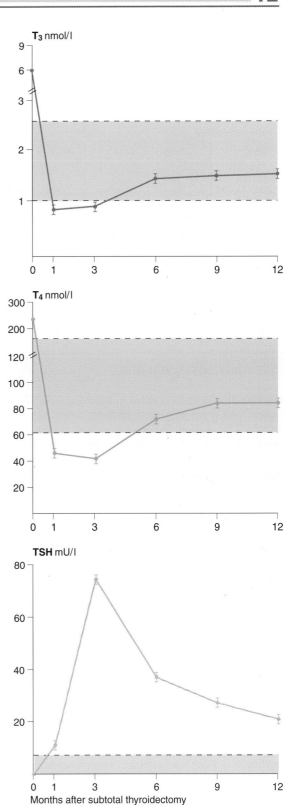

Fig. 12.13 Total T_3, T_4 and TSH levels before and after subtotal thyroidectomy in a series of patients with temporary hypothyroidism. The normal ranges are indicated by the broken lines. (Adapted from Toft et al 1978 New England Journal of Medicine 298: 643–647.)

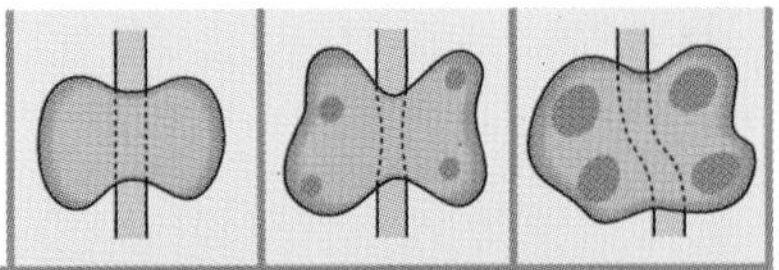

Age (year)	15–25	35–55	>55
Goitre	Diffuse	Nodular	Nodular
Tracheal compression/ deviation	No	Minimal	Yes
T_3, T_4	Normal	Normal	Raised
TSH	Normal	Normal or undetectable	Undetectable

Fig. 12.14   Natural history of simple goitre.

SOLITARY THYROID NODULE

Palpable thyroid nodules occur in approximately 5% of females and are even more commonly found at post-mortem examination. Whereas multinodular goitre is benign, solitary nodules may be malignant. In those who seek medical attention it is important therefore to determine whether the nodule is benign, e.g. cyst, colloid nodule, or malignant. With the exception of haemorrhage into a cyst when thyroid enlargement is of rapid onset and painful, or the presence of cervical lymphadenopathy which is highly suggestive of carcinoma, it is rarely possible to make this distinction on clinical grounds alone. However, a solitary nodule presenting in childhood or adolescence, particularly if there is a past history of head and neck irradiation, or presenting in the elderly, should raise the suspicion of malignancy. Very occasionally a secondary deposit from a renal, breast or lung carcinoma presents as a painful, rapidly growing solitary thyroid nodule.

Investigations

The most useful is fine-needle aspiration of the nodule. This is performed in the outpatient clinic without local anaesthetic, using a standard 21 gauge venepuncture needle and a 20 ml syringe. Aspiration may be therapeutic in the small proportion of patients in whom the swelling is a pure cyst, although recurrence on more than one occasion is an indication for surgery. Usually 2–3 aspirates are taken from the nodule. Cytological examination will differentiate benign (80%) from sus-

picious or definitely malignant nodules (20%), of which half are confirmed as cancer at surgery. The advantage of fine-needle aspiration over long-established tests such as isotope and ultrasound scanning is that a much higher proportion of patients avoid surgery. The limitation of the method is that it cannot differentiate between follicular adenoma and carcinoma.

It is important to measure serum T_3, T_4 and TSH in all patients with a solitary thyroid nodule. The finding of undetectable TSH is very suggestive of an autonomously functioning thyroid adenoma which can only be confirmed by thyroid isotope scanning, is for practical purposes always benign, and is treated with ^{131}I or surgery.

MALIGNANT TUMOURS

Primary thyroid malignancy is rare, accounting for less than 1% of all carcinomas, and has a prevalence of 25 per million. As shown in Table 12.8 it can be classified according to the cell-type of origin. With the exception of medullary carcinoma, thyroid cancer is always more common in females.

DIFFERENTIATED CARCINOMA

In most patients presentation is with a palpable solitary nodule.

Papillary carcinoma

This is the commonest of the malignant thyroid tumours and accounts for 90% of irradiation-induced thyroid cancer. It may be multifocal, and spread is to regional cervical lymph nodes. Some patients present with cervical lymphadenopathy and no apparent thyroid enlargement and the primary lesion may be less than 10 mm in diameter.

Follicular carcinoma

This is always a single encapsulated lesion. Spread to cervical lymph nodes is rare. Metastases are blood-borne and are most often found in bone, lungs and brain.

Management

This is usually by total thyroidectomy followed by a large dose of ^{131}I (3000 MBq) in order to ablate any remaining thyroid tissue, normal or malignant. Thereafter long-term treatment with thyroxine in a dose sufficient to suppress TSH (usually 150–200 μg daily) is important as there is some evidence that differentiated thyroid carcinoma may be TSH-dependent. Follow-up is by measurement of serum thyroglobulin which should be low or undetectable in patients taking a suppressive dose

Table 12.8 Malignant thyroid tumours

Origin of tumour	Type of tumour	Frequency (%)	Usual age of presentation (years)	Approximate 20-year survival (%)
Follicular cells	Differentiated carcinoma			
	Papillary	70	20–40	95
	Follicular	10	40–60	60
	Undifferentiated carcinoma			
	Anaplastic	5	>60	<1
Parafollicular C-cells	Medullary carcinoma	5–10	>40*	50
Lymphocytes	Lymphoma	5–10	>60	10

* Patients with medullary carcinoma as part of multiple endocrine neoplasia syndromes may present in childhood.

of thyroxine. A level in excess of 15 μg/l is strongly suggestive of tumour recurrence or metastases which may be detected by whole body scanning with ^{131}I and which may respond to further radio-iodine therapy.

Prognosis

Most patients have an excellent prognosis when treated appropriately. Patients under 50 years of age with papillary carcinoma can anticipate a near normal life expectancy if the tumour is less than 2 cm in diameter, confined to the thyroid and cervical nodes and of low-grade malignancy histologically. Even for patients with distant metastases at presentation the 10-year survival is approximately 40%.

ANAPLASTIC CARCINOMA AND LYMPHOMA

These two conditions are difficult to distinguish clinically but not by cytological examination of fine-needle aspiration biopsy. Patients are usually elderly women in whom there is rapid thyroid enlargement over 2–3 months. The goitre is hard and symmetrical. There is usually stridor due to tracheal compression and hoarseness due to recurrent laryngeal nerve palsy. There is no effective treatment of anaplastic carcinoma although radiotherapy may afford temporary relief of mediastinal compression. The prognosis for lymphoma which may arise from pre-existing Hashimoto's thyroiditis is better. External irradiation often produces dramatic goitre shrinkage and when combined with chemotherapy may result in survival for 5 years or more.

MEDULLARY CARCINOMA

This tumour arises from the parafollicular C-cells of the thyroid. In addition to calcitonin, the tumour may secrete serotonin, various peptides of the tachykinin family, ACTH and prostaglandins. As a consequence carcinoid syndrome and Cushing's syndrome have been described in association with medullary carcinoma.

Patients usually present in middle age with a firm thyroid mass. Cervical lymphadenopathy is common, but distant metastases are rare initially. Serum calcitonin levels are raised and are useful in monitoring response to treatment. Despite the very high levels of calcitonin found in some patients, hypocalcaemia is extremely rare.

Treatment is by total thyroidectomy with removal of affected cervical nodes. Since the C-cells do not concentrate iodine there is no role for ^{131}I therapy. Prognosis is very variable, some patients surviving 20 years or more and others less than 1 year.

Familial medullary carcinoma of thyroid and multiple endocrine neoplasia (MEN) syndromes

Rarely, medullary carcinoma of the thyroid may be familial with an autosomal dominant mode of inheritance. It may be associated with phaeochromocytoma, frequently bilateral, and occasionally parathyroid hyperplasia, a complex known as MEN IIa.

In MEN IIb the above features are accompanied by mucosal neuromas, marfanoid habitus with poor muscle development and skeletal abnormalities such as kyphosis, pectus excavatum, pes cavus and high arch palate. The facial appearance is characteristic with thick lips (Fig. 12.29), broad-based nose, everted eyelids and grossly abnormal dental enamel. Diarrhoea is common and thought to be due to disordered autonomic function.

Fifty per cent of all first-degree relatives of patients with familial medullary carcinoma of thyroid will carry the predisposing gene on chromosome 10. This gene codes for a receptor tyrosine kinase (RET). This is a family of cell surface molecules which transduce signals for cell growth and differentiation. The kinase encoded by the RET proto-oncogene is re-arranged and thus permanently switched on in familial medullary thyroid carcinoma and MEN IIa. A separate RET mutation affecting the tyrosine kinase domain is found in MEN IIb and in Hirschsprung's disease. Accurate detection of gene carriers is now possible by DNA analysis. A positive result is an indication for screening using serum calcitonin measurements whereas a negative result will save the individual from future surveillance and therefore from much anxiety.

RIEDEL'S THYROIDITIS

This is not a form of thyroid cancer but the presentation is similar and the differentiation can usually only be made by thyroid biopsy. It is an exceptionally rare condition of unknown aetiology in which there is extensive infiltration of the thyroid and surrounding structures with fibrous tissue. There may be associated mediastinal and retroperitoneal fibrosis. Presentation is with a slow growing goitre which is irregular and stony hard. There is usually tracheal and oesophageal compression necessitating partial thyroidectomy. Other recognised complications include recurrent laryngeal nerve palsy, hypoparathyroidism and eventually hypothyroidism.

> **FURTHER READING**
>
> Franklyn J A 1994 The management of hyperthyroidism. New England Journal of Medicine 330: 1731–1738
> Toft A D 1994 Thyroxine therapy. New England Journal of Medicine 331: 174–180

THE PARATHYROID GLANDS

PHYSIOLOGY

Parathyroid hormone (PTH) is a single chain polypeptide of 84 amino acids which is synthesised by the chief cells of the parathyroid glands. The important actions of PTH are on renal function, vitamin D metabolism and bone.

Renal function

PTH stimulates tubular reabsorption of calcium, but decreases reabsorption of phosphate and bicarbonate.

Vitamin D metabolism

Vitamin D_3 (cholecalciferol) is the major dietary form of vitamin D and is the form synthesised in skin exposed to ultraviolet light. Cholecalciferol is hydroxylated in the liver to give 25-hydroxycholecalciferol (25-HCC) which is the predominant circulating form of the vitamin. Further hydroxylation occurs in the kidney to give $1\alpha,25$-dihydroxycholecalciferol (1,25-DHCC) which is the most potent form of the vitamin known. It is this second hydroxylation which is stimulated by PTH. The major actions of 1,25-DHCC are to increase intestinal absorption of calcium and phosphate, and in combination with PTH, to mobilise calcium from bone.

Bone

Bone contains 99% of the total body calcium and is in dynamic equilibrium with the extracellular fluid by processes of bone resorption and deposition. The initial effect of PTH on bone is to stimulate osteolysis, returning calcium, from bone to extracellular fluid. Prolonged exposure of bone to PTH is associated with increased osteoclastic activity, extensive bone remodelling and osteoblastic repair.

Role of PTH in calcium homeostasis

This is summarised in Figure 12.15. The normal response to a fall in serum ionised calcium is an increase in circulating levels of PTH. The actions of PTH on renal handling of calcium, on vitamin D metabolism and on bone resorption combine to return serum ionised calcium to normal. Conversely, an elevation in serum ionised calcium is normally corrected by suppression of PTH secretion. Calcitonin, a peptide secreted by the parafollicular C-cells of the thyroid, may have a role in reducing serum ionised calcium in response to an acute increase by opposing the action of PTH on renal tubular reabsorption of calcium and phosphate and on bone resorption. Parathyroid disease results in failure of calcium homeostasis, the clinical features being a consequence of tissue exposure to abnormal concentrations of ionised calcium and PTH.

HYPERPARATHYROIDISM

It is customary to distinguish 3 categories of hyperparathyroidism. In primary hyperparathyroidism there is usually autonomous secretion of PTH by a single parathyroid adenoma varying in size from a few millimetres to several centimetres in diameter. The categories are shown in the information box below. Secondary hyperparathyroidism is present when there is

> **HYPERPARATHYROIDISM**
>
> | **Primary** | Serum calcium and PTH raised |
> |---|---|
> | • Single adenoma (90%) | |
> | • Multiple adenomata (4%) | |
> | • Nodular hyperplasia (5%) | |
> | • Carcinoma (1%) | |
> | **Secondary** | Serum calcium low |
> | • Chronic renal failure | PTH raised |
> | • Malabsorption | |
> | • Osteomalacia and rickets | |
> | **Tertiary** | Serum calcium and PTH raised |

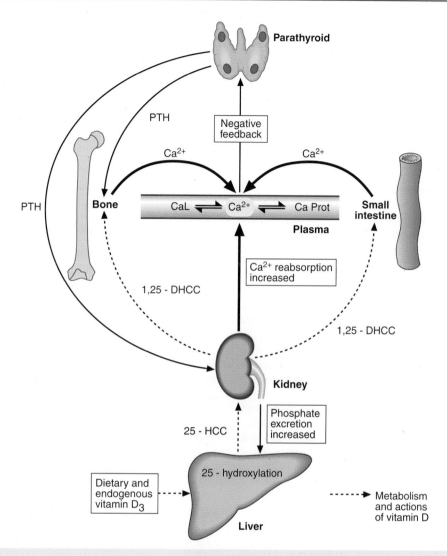

Fig. 12.15 Outline of calcium homeostasis showing response to decreased serum ionised calcium level. Calcium in serum exists as 50% ionised (Ca^{2+}), 10% non-ionised or complexed with organic ions such as citrate and phosphate (CaL) and 40% protein-bound, mainly to albumin (Ca prot). It is the ionised calcium concentration which regulates PTH and 1,25 DHCC production.

hyperplasia with increased PTH secretion in an attempt to compensate for prolonged hypocalcaemia. Its effect is to restore serum calcium levels at the expense of the skeleton.

In a very small proportion of cases of secondary hyperparathyroidism continuous stimulation of the parathyroids may result in adenoma formation and autonomous PTH secretion. This is known as tertiary hyperparathyroidism.

PRIMARY HYPERPARATHYROIDISM

This is the commonest of the parathyroid disorders with a prevalence of about 1 in 800. The current detection rate is 20–30 per 100 000 annually and reflects the increasing number of asymptomatic cases discovered as a result of biochemical profile investigations performed in the hospital population. It is 2–3 times more common in women than men and 90% of patients are over 50 years of age.

Clinical features

About 50% of patients with biochemical evidence of primary hyperparathyroidism are asymptomatic. Many others have non-specific symptoms. These include: anorexia, nausea, vomiting, constipation and weight loss; polyuria and polydipsia; weakness, tiredness and lassitude; drowsiness, poor concentration, memory loss and depression. Such vague symptoms may progress to acute hypercalcaemic crisis.

Calculus disease is a common renal manifestation, and 5% of first stone formers and 15% of recurrent stone formers have hyperparathyroidism. Nephrocalcinosis may also occur and is due to deposition of calcium salts in the renal parenchyma, particularly the medullary region and the collecting ducts. Renal function may be adversely affected as evidenced by uraemia, hypokalaemia, hyperuricaemia, hyperchloraemic acidosis and poor urine concentrating ability.

Osteitis fibrosa, in which there is increased bone resorption by osteoclasts with fibrous replacement in the lacunae, is the characteristic skeletal disorder. Cystic expansion may accompany the osteitis fibrosa. These changes may present clinically as bone pain and tenderness, fracture and deformity. Rarely, primary hyperparathyroidism may present as a local swelling, usually of the mandible, due to an isolated cyst. Chondrocalcinosis is due to deposition of calcium pyrophosphate crystals within articular cartilage. This typically affects the menisci at the knees and can result in secondary degenerative arthritis or predispose to attacks of acute pseudogout, especially following parathyroidectomy.

Other features of primary hyperparathyroidism include corneal calcification best seen by slit-lamp examination, ectopic calcification in arterial walls and soft tissues of hands, peptic ulceration, hypertension, myopathy and pruritus.

Investigations

Biochemical

The diagnosis of primary hyperparathyroidism depends upon the finding of a raised serum calcium and raised PTH (Fig. 12.16). The serum PTH concentrations in other causes of hypercalcaemia are shown in Table 12.9.

It is preferable to avoid artefactual increases in serum calcium by collecting blood under standardised conditions with the patient supine and avoiding the use of a tourniquet while withdrawing the sample. Although changes in serum calcium in response to dietary intake are small, specimens should be collected with the patient fasting. If serum albumin is low, the value for calcium should be adjusted upward by 0.1 mmol/l for each 6 g/l that the albumin is below the laboratory mean. Serum phosphate is usually low in hyperparathyroidism and chloride elevated. Serum alkaline phosphatase, an index of osteoblastic activity, may be raised depending on the degree of involvement of bone.

Table 12.9 Serum parathyroid hormone (PTH) concentrations in the different causes of hypercalcaemia grouped according to frequency of presentation

Cause of hypercalcaemia	Serum PTH concentration
Common:	
Malignancy	Low or undetectable
Primary hyperparathyroidism	Raised
Chronic renal failure (Tertiary hyperparathyroidism)	Raised
Rare:	
Sarcoidosis	Low or undetectable
Hyperthyroidism	Low or undetectable
Vitamin D intoxication	Low or undetectable
Thiazide diuretics	Low or undetectable
Very rare:	
Milk-alkali syndrome	Low or undetectable
Inadequately treated Addison's disease	Low or undetectable
Familial hypocalciuric hypercalcaemia	Variable
Lithium therapy	Variable

Apart from primary hyperparathyroidism, the most common other cause of hypercalcaemia is a malignancy. Those malignancies most frequently causing hypercalcaemia are: breast, kidney, lung, thyroid, ovary and colon. The primary is usually obvious and in 90% of cases there are radiologically evident metastases in bone. The hypercalcaemia of multiple myeloma is also caused by bone destruction. In the absence of metastases, the hypercalcaemia of malignancy is due to the production by the tumour of a PTH-related peptide, the structure of which shows considerable homology with the biologically critical NH_2 terminal region of PTH (Fig. 12.17). This is not detected by the newer PTH assays (Fig. 12.16).

Radiological

In the early stages there may be demineralisation and subperiosteal erosions may be noted in the phalanges (Fig 12.18). These are most marked on the radial side of the middle phalanx. There may also be resorption of the terminal phalanges. A 'pepper-pot' appearance may be seen on lateral radiographs of the skull (see p. 822). Cystic changes are rare. In nephrocalcinosis scattered opacities may be visible within the renal outline. There may be soft tissue calcification elsewhere.

Localisation of parathyroid tumour

In over 90% of patients an experienced surgeon will locate the adenoma without difficulty and routine preoperative localisation is not usually performed. If surgical exploration has been unsuccessful, however,

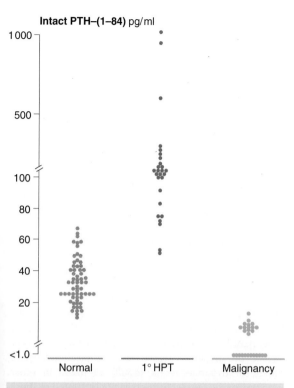

Intact PTH–(1–84) pg/ml

Fig. 12.16   Intact PTH 1–84 measurements by immuno-radiometric assay in sera from normal individuals, patients with surgically proven primary hyperparathyroidism and patients with malignancy associated hypercalcaemia. (From Nussbaum et al 1987 Clinical Chemistry 33: 1364.)

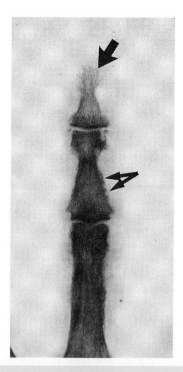

Fig. 12.18   Radiograph of subperiosteal erosions in a phalanx with terminal resorption in a patient with primary hyperparathyroidism.

ultrasonography, selective neck vein catheterisation with PTH measurements, CT scanning and subtraction imaging may prove useful. In this last technique the neck is imaged during the successive injections of two short-lived isotopes: thallium-201(^{201}Tl) (taken up by thyroid and parathyroid), followed by technetium-99m (^{99m}Tc) (taken up by thyroid only). Computer subtraction of the two images leaves a parathyroid image if an adenoma is present. Recent improvements in ultrasound technology

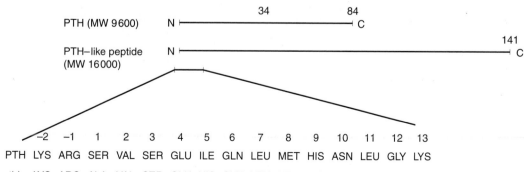

Fig. 12.17   Structures of the parathyroid hormone-related peptide and human parathyroid hormone. (From Broadus et al 1988 New England Journal of Medicine 319: 556.)

are likely to make ultrasound one of the most useful methods of localising parathyroid tumours.

Management

Apart from asymptomatic patients over the age of 65 years with serum calcium levels less than 3.0 mmol/l for whom no treatment is necessary other than review every 6–12 months, the only therapy of primary hyper-parathyroidism is surgical removal of the adenoma. At operation the surgeon ideally attempts to locate and assess all parathyroid tissue. Problems may arise from the variability in number and site of the glands, especially if some lie within the thyroid or superior mediastinum. The current management of hyperplasia is to remove all 4 glands and to transplant some of the excised tissue to the forearm. If hypercalcaemia returns part of the transplant can be removed under local anaesthetic.

Postoperative hypocalcaemia is not uncommon during the first 2 weeks while residual suppressed parathyroid tissue recovers. It is usually mild or asymptomatic and can be controlled with oral calcium supplements, e.g. 80 mmol daily. It is recognised that patients with particularly high preoperative serum calcium levels and obvious bone or renal damage are especially likely to develop prolonged symptomatic hypocalcaemia after operation, as there is a major net shift of calcium into healing bone. This hypocalcaemia can be minimised by giving 1α-hydroxycholecalciferol 2 μg daily for 48 hours before surgery and continuing for 1–2 weeks after operation. Intravenous calcium gluconate as 10 ml of 10% solution which can be given every 3–4 hours and oral calcium supplements may also be necessary.

Hypercalcaemic crisis

In recent years this condition has been increasingly recognised as a mode of presentation of primary hyper-parathyroidism, especially in the elderly. It is also a manifestation of malignant disease. The clinical features are those of dehydration and hypotension, associated with abdominal pain, vomiting, pyrexia and altered conscious level. Management is a medical emergency and is aimed at replacing fluid deficit, correcting electrolyte imbalance and lowering serum calcium levels which are usually in excess of 3.5 mmol/l. In the first 24 hours it is usually necessary to replace 4–6 litres of 0.9% saline (145 mmol/l). Any associated hypokalaemia and hypo-magnesaemia should also be corrected by intravenous supplements. In most cases intravenous fluids alone will reduce serum calcium to approximately 3.0 mmol/l. During this period of rehydration, biochemical, radiological and other investigations, such as bone marrow examination, will usually enable primary hyper-parathyroidism to be distinguished from other causes

of hypercalcaemia. In those rare instances when serum calcium concentration is greater than 4.5 mmol/l the life-threatening hypercalcaemia can be rapidly but transiently lowered by 500 ml 0.1 M neutral phosphate given intravenously over 6–8 hours. In addition to rehydration the most appropriate treatment of the hypercalcaemia of malignancy is a biphosphonate, such as sodium clodronate, which suppresses osteoclast-mediated bone resorption. If given intravenously in a dose of 300 mg daily, normocalcaemia is achieved in 3–5 days and can be maintained thereafter by 800–1600 mg twice daily orally.

FAMILIAL HYPOCALCIURIC HYPERCALCAEMIA

This is a poorly understood syndrome, inherited as an autosomal dominant in which there is increased renal tubular reabsorption of calcium with resultant low urinary calcium in the presence of hypercalcaemia. Serum PTH levels are normal or marginally elevated. Patients have few if any symptoms and it is difficult to make the distinction from primary hyperparathyroidism. Surgery of the parathyroid glands which are hyperplastic fails to correct the hypercalcaemia. In this circumstance a search for hypercalcaemia should be made in other members of the family. Surgery is not indicated in those identified as the course of the condition should be uneventful.

Association of primary hyperparathyroidism with other endocrine disorders

Hyperparathyroidism may occur, usually in the form of hyperplasia, with pancreatic islet cell tumours secreting insulin or gastrin and pituitary tumours (MEN I) or in association with medullary carcinoma of the thyroid and phaeochromocytomas (MEN II, p. 699).

HYPOPARATHYROIDISM

This unusual condition may arise from a variety of causes, but with each the clinical feature in common is tetany (see p. 705). Biochemically, a depressed concentration of calcium and a raised concentration of phosphate in serum are characteristic.

Postoperative hypoparathyroidism

The commonest cause of hypoparathyroidism is damage to the parathyroid glands or their blood supply during thyroid surgery, although this complication occurs in only 1% of thyroidectomies. Transient hypocalcaemia develops in 10% of patients 12–36 hours following subtotal thyroidectomy for Graves' disease.

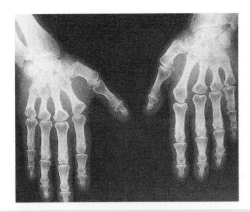

Fig. 12.19 Radiograph of hands in a patient with pseudohypoparathyroidism showing short fourth and fifth metacarpals.

Infantile hypoparathyroidism

This may be transient and associated with maternal hyperparathyroidism or calcium deficiency. It persists in thymic aplasia (Di George syndrome).

Idiopathic hypoparathyroidism

This idiopathic form may develop at any age, and is sometimes associated with autoimmune disease of the adrenal, thyroid or ovary, especially in young people. In addition to tetany other features of prolonged hypocalcaemia include grand mal epilepsy, psychosis, cataracts, calcification of basal ganglia and papilloedema. In addition there is an association with mucocutaneous candidiasis particularly affecting finger nails, mouth and oesophagus.

Pseudohypoparathyroidism

This is the term applied to a congenital variety in which there is tissue resistance to the effects of parathyroid hormone. The PTH receptor is normal but there is a defective post-receptor mechanism. Pseudohypoparathyroidism also presents with the biochemical and clinical features of hypoparathyroidism. Unlike cases of idiopathic hypoparathyroidism there is no associated mucocutaneous candidiasis, but patients may have mental retardation and characteristically there are skeletal abnormalities such as small stature and short 4th and 5th metacarpals and metatarsals (Fig. 12.19). These patients have elevated levels of serum PTH.

The term pseudo-pseudohypoparathyroidism is given to patients exhibiting the above skeletal abnormalities but in whom serum calcium concentration is normal.

Management

Commercial preparations of parathyroid hormone are unsatisfactory for the treatment of parathyroid insuf-

ficiency because they have to be given by frequent injections, and soon become ineffective because of antibody formation. In the acute phase, calcium is given intravenously as for tetany; substitution therapy for persistent hypoparathyroidism and for pseudohypoparathyroidism is provided by 1α-hydroxycholecalciferol (alfacalcidol) which is hydroxylated in the liver or 1,25-dihydroxycholecalciferol (calcitriol). The dose of these preparations is 1–3 μg daily. It is important to monitor the serum calcium level every 3–6 months once the dose has been stabilised.

TETANY

Aetiology

There is an increased excitability of peripheral nerves due either to a low serum calcium or to alkalosis in which the proportion of the serum calcium in the ionised form is decreased, although the total calcium concentration remains unaltered. Magnesium depletion should also be considered as a possible contributing factor, particularly in malabsorption. The most common cause of hypocalcaemia is a low serum concentration of albumin which does not result in tetany. The causes of tetany are listed in the information box.

CAUSES OF TETANY

- **Due to hypocalcaemia**
  Malabsorption
  Osteomalacia
  Hypoparathyroidism
  Acute pancreatitis
  Chronic renal failure*

- **Due to alkalosis**
  Repeated vomiting of gastric juice
  Excessive intake of oral alkalis
  Hyperventilation
  Primary hyperaldosteronism

*Coincident acidosis usually prevents tetany

Clinical features

In *children* a characteristic triad of carpopedal spasm, stridor and convulsions occurs, though one or more of these may be found independently of the others. The hands in carpal spasm adopt a characteristic position. The metacarpophalangeal joints are flexed, the interphalangeal joints of the fingers and thumb are extended and there is opposition of the thumb (*main d'accoucheur*). Pedal spasm is much less frequent. Stridor is caused by spasm of the glottis.

Adults complain of tingling in the hands, feet and around the mouth. Less often there is painful carpopedal spasm while stridor and fits are rare.

Latent tetany may be present when signs of overt tetany are lacking. It is best recognised by eliciting *Trousseau's sign.* Inflation of the sphygmomanometer cuff on the upper arm to more than the systolic blood pressure is followed by carpal spasm within 3 minutes. A less specific sign of hypocalcaemia is that described by Chvostek in which tapping over the branches of the facial nerve as they emerge from the parotid gland produces twitching of the facial muscles.

Management

Control of tetany

Injection of 20 ml of a 10% solution of calcium gluconate slowly into a vein will raise the serum calcium concentration immediately. An intramuscular injection of 10 ml may also be given to obtain a more prolonged effect. In severe cases of alkalotic tetany, intravenous calcium gluconate often relieves the spasm, while specific treatment of the alkalosis, which will vary with the cause, is being applied. If tetany is not relieved by giving calcium the administration of magnesium may be required.

Correction of alkalosis

In persistent vomiting, intravenous isotonic saline is the most effective treatment.

When alkalis have been given to excess their withdrawal may suffice to stop the tetany but, if not, ammonium chloride 2 g should be given 4-hourly by mouth until relief has been obtained.

The inhalation of 5% carbon dioxide in oxygen may be prescribed for the correction of the alkalosis of hyperventilation, or more simply the patient should be made to rebreathe expired air from a suitable bag. The hysterical patient should also have appropriate psychotherapy.

FURTHER READING

Burtis W J, Brady T G, Orloff J et al 1990 Immunochemical characterization of circulating parathyroid hormone-related protein in patients with humoral hypercalcaemia of cancer. New England Journal of Medicine 322: 1106–1112

THE ADRENAL GLANDS

ANATOMY AND PHYSIOLOGY OF THE ADRENAL CORTEX

Each adrenal consists of an inner medulla and an outer cortex. This is divided into three zones:

- zona glomerulosa → aldosterone (mineralocorticoid)
- zona fasciculata → cortisol (glucocorticoid)
- zona reticularis → androgens.

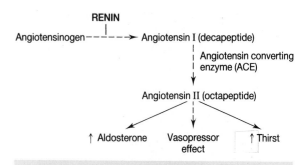

Fig. 12.20   Renin-angiotensin-aldosterone system.

Zona glomerulosa

Aldosterone, the body's most important sodium retaining hormone (**mineralocorticoid**), is produced by the outermost zone of the adrenal and is principally under the control of angiotensin II (AII). ACTH and hyperkalaemia are less important stimuli. Low salt intake stimulates aldosterone secretion by activating the renin-angiotensin system (Fig. 12.20). It also enhances the response of the zona glomerulosa to AII. High salt intake has the opposite effect. Standing levels of plasma renin activity are about double those when lying down. Factors controlling the increase of renin are thus key to understanding aldosterone secretion.

Angiotensin-converting enzyme (ACE) is present in the lung, in the circulation and in the blood vessel walls. The introduction of ACE inhibitors such as captopril or enalapril has been of major importance in the treatment of hypertension and congestive heart failure (see pp. 270 and 223).

Aldosterone acts on the distal nephron to produce sodium retention and urinary potassium loss. Thus hypokalaemia is an important clue to the possibility of hyperaldosteronism.

Zona fasciculata

Cortisol is the major product of this zone. Under most circumstances this steroid acts as a **glucocorticoid** hormone. As the name suggests such steroids have antiinsulin effects and raise blood sugar by converting amino acids from protein breakdown to glucose (gluconeogenesis). The major rate-limiting enzyme in this process is phosphoenolpyruvate carboxykinase (PEPCK). This is turned off by insulin and on by glucocorticoids. Glucocorticoids also elevate glucose levels by decreasing its peripheral uptake by tissues such as muscle.

In the circulation more than 95% of cortisol is bound to protein, principally cortisol-binding globulin (CBG). It is the free fraction which is biologically active. This readily crosses the cell membrane and binds to cyto-

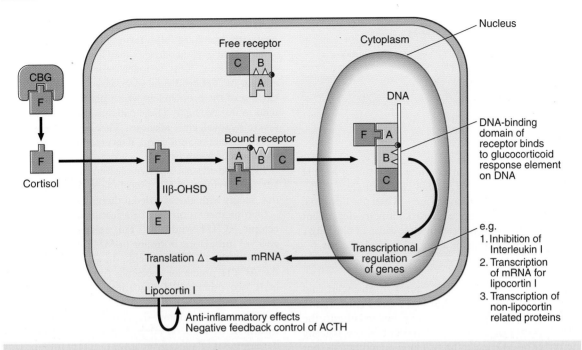

Fig. 12.21 Entry of cortisol into cell and consequent effects. (CBG: cortisol binding globulin; F: cortisol; E: cortisone; ABC: glucocorticoid receptor; 11β-OHSD: 11β-hydroxysteroid dehydrogenase.)

plasmic receptors (Fig. 12.21). These receptors have a steroid binding domain and a separate DNA binding sequence. Binding of the steroid results in the uncovering of this sequence. The bound receptor is then translocated to the nucleus where it can bind to DNA.

Glucocorticoids have a wide range of biological effects. In clinical practice they are extensively used as anti-inflammatory agents. This action results from suppression of the synthesis of some proteins such as the cytokine interleukin I and enhanced synthesis of others including lipocortin I. This 37 kd protein is produced within 30–60 minutes of the exposure of certain cells to cortisol and is rapidly transported to the cell surface where it binds to a high-affinity binding protein. This in turn produces a series of biological effects probably mainly through inhibition of the pro-inflammatory eicosanoids. It seems likely that lipocortin I production also plays an important role in the negative feedback effects of cortisol on the pituitary secretion of ACTH.

Cortisol is converted by 11β-hydroxysteroid dehydrogenase (11β-OHSD) into inactive cortisone. This conversion is used by the kidney to protect the non-specific mineralocorticoid receptor from exposure to cortisol. Loss of this protection by inhibition of 11β-OHSD by liquorice results in cortisol acting as a potent sodium-retaining steroid.

Zona reticularis

The innermost zone of the adrenal cortex produces androgens such as dehydroepiandrosterone sulphate, dehydroepiandrosterone and androstenedione. These are increased during the adrenarche which results in initial pubic hair development. The control of adrenal androgen production is unclear. Certainly ACTH plays a role. However, there may possibly be a separate androgen stimulating hormone (ASH).

HYPERFUNCTION OF THE ADRENAL GLAND

GLUCOCORTICOID EXCESS

CUSHING'S SYNDROME

Cushing's syndrome is defined as the symptoms and signs associated with prolonged inappropriate elevation of free corticosteroid levels.

Patients with Cushing's syndrome can be classified into two groups on the basis of whether the condition is ACTH-dependent or independent (Table 12.10).

Epidemiology

Cushing's syndrome of pituitary origin or associated with an adrenal tumour is four times more common

Table 12.10 Classification of Cushing's syndrome

ACTH-dependent	Non-ACTH-dependent
Iatrogenic (ACTH therapy)	Iatrogenic (e.g. prednisolone)
Pituitary-dependent bilateral adrenal hyperplasia (Cushing's disease)	Adrenal adenoma Adrenal carcinoma
Ectopic ACTH syndrome (benign or malignant non-endocrine tumour)	

in women than men. In contrast the ectopic ACTH syndrome (often due to a small cell carcinoma of the bronchus) is more common in men. When the iatrogenic and ectopic groups are excluded pituitary-dependent Cushing's disease is the commonest cause of Cushing's syndrome, accounting for about 80% of adult cases.

Clinical features

The features common to all causes of glucocorticoid excess are indicated in Table 12.11 and Figure 12.22. Weight gain is the commonest symptom and obesity the most frequent sign. The distribution of fat is classically described as centripetal (like a lemon on toothpicks) but generalised obesity may be just as common. Because of this it is useful to compare the prevalence of the symptoms and signs in patients with Cushing's syndrome with those in patients with simple obesity. When this approach is used, bruising, myopathy and hypertension are the best discriminants and thus the features to look for in an obese patient in whom Cushing's syndrome is suspected.

Glucocorticoid excess leads to collagen breakdown which results in thinning of the skin and blood vessels with resultant bruising, striae (livid stretch marks especially over the abdomen, buttocks and thighs) and a plethoric appearance. The loss of protein in muscle leads to a proximal myopathy (difficult or impossible to get up from a squatting position) and the changes in bone to osteoporosis. The latter may present with back pain from vertebral compression fractures. Other frac-

tures such as in the ribs are more common and tend to heal with exuberant callus formation.

Increased gluconeogenesis may lead to impaired glucose tolerance. This is much more common in the ectopic ACTH syndrome secondary to a small cell carcinoma of the bronchus in which plasma cortisol levels tend to be very high. These patients also usually have a severe hypokalaemic alkalosis. This hypokalaemia may inhibit insulin secretion and, if severe, produce muscular weakness or paralysis.

Increased adrenal androgen secretion (especially with adrenal carcinomas) can contribute to the hirsutism but this occurs with glucocorticoid therapy alone.

Skin pigmentation may be a feature especially of the ectopic ACTH syndrome. This relates to the α-melanocyte stimulating hormone (α-MSH) sequence which is part of the ACTH molecule. In addition, the rest of the ACTH precursor molecule (pro-opiocortin) contains two other MSH sequences (β-MSH in β-lipotrophin and γ-MSH in the N-terminal part (p. 674)). In patients with pituitary-dependent Cushing's disease, treatment by bilateral adrenalectomy may lead to the development of a locally invasive pituitary tumour with very high levels of ACTH and hyperpigmentation (Nelson's syndrome). This tumour contrasts with the microadenoma (less than 10 mm in diameter) which is found in the pituitary of about 75% of patients with Cushing's disease. Hence local symptoms related to the pituitary tumour (e.g. visual field defect) are rare in untreated Cushing's disease.

Skin infections, especially with fungi such as *Tinea versicolor*, are common. Minor trauma produces gaping skin wounds which heal poorly.

Hypertension is common. Glucocorticoids increase plasma volume. This appears not to relate to sodium retention. Cortisol also enhances vascular responsiveness to noradrenaline.

Gonadal function is frequently abnormal with oligomenorrhoea or amenorrhoea in women and impotence in men.

Growth retardation is almost invariable in children. Adults frequently present with psychiatric problems (especially depression).

Investigations

In a patient suspected of having Cushing's syndrome the investigations should be divided into two stages to answer these questions:

1. Diagnosis: Does the patient have Cushing's syndrome (Table 12.12)?
2. Differential diagnosis: What is the cause of the adrenocortical hyperfunction (Table 12.13)?

Table 12.11 Clinical features of Cushing's syndrome (after Ross & Linch, 1982)

Symptoms	Patients presenting (%)	Signs	Patients presenting (%)
Weight gain	91	Obesity	97
Menstrual irregularity	84	Plethora	94
Hirsutism	81	Moonface	88
Psychiatric	62	Hypertension	74
Backache	43	Bruising	62
Muscle weakness	29	Striae	56
		Muscle weakness	56

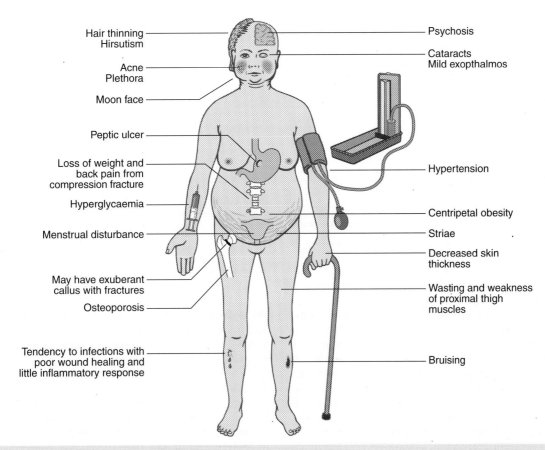

Hair thinning
Hirsutism

Acne
Plethora

Moon face

Peptic ulcer

Loss of weight and
back pain from
compression fracture

Hyperglycaemia

Menstrual disturbance

May have exuberant
callus with fractures

Osteoporosis

Tendency to infections with
poor wound healing and
little inflammatory response

Psychosis

Cataracts
Mild exopthalmos

Hypertension

Centripetal obesity

Striae

Decreased skin
thickness

Wasting and weakness
of proximal thigh
muscles

Bruising

Fig. 12.22 Cushing's syndrome: symptoms common to all causes.

Table 12.12 Does the patient have Cushing's syndrome?	
Test	**Abnormality in Cushing's syndrome**
Circadian rhythm of plasma cortisol (08.00 and 24.00 samples)	Loss of rhythm
Low dose dexamethasone suppression 1.5 mg at midnight: 09.00 plasma cortisol next day*	>180 nmol/l
0.5 mg 6-hourly for 48 hours: plasma cortisol at 48 hours	>180 nmol/l
Urinary free cortisol 24-hour or overnight excretion*	Elevated (value depends on method used)
Insulin-induced hypoglycaemia	No rise in plasma cortisol

* Useful outpatient screening tests.

Only if the answer to Question 1 is 'yes' should any further tests be performed.

In Cushing's syndrome there is a characteristic loss of the circadian rhythm of plasma cortisol (i.e. instead of cortisol levels being lowest at midnight they are about the same throughout the 24 hours). This may also be lost by stress caused from hospital admission, depression or heart failure. In Cushing's syndrome negative feedback control is abnormal and cortisol levels are not suppressed by low doses of dexamethasone. This synthetic glucocorticoid is not measured by the cortisol radio-immunoassay (this test may be invalid in patients on enzyme-inducing drugs such as phenytoin which markedly reduce dexamethasone half-life).

Urinary free cortisol is a reflection of the free (i.e. non-protein bound) cortisol in plasma and is a very useful index of increased cortisol secretion.

Insulin-induced hypoglycaemia stimulates a rise in plasma cortisol in normal and depressed subjects but not in patients with Cushing's syndrome. It is thus the only test of those listed in Table 12.12 which distinguishes patients with severe depression from those with Cushing's syndrome. As depression is common in

Table 12.13 What is the cause of Cushing's syndrome?

Test	Pituitary dependent	Ectopic ACTH	Adrenal tumour
Plasma ACTH 08.00	N or ↑	↑ or ↑↑	Undetectable
Metyrapone 750 mg 4-hourly × 6 doses: measure 11-deoxycortisol at 24.00	↑↑	↑	→↑
High dose dexamethasone 2 mg 6-hourly for 48 hours: plasma cortisol 48 hours	↓	→	→
Plasma K⁺	N	<3.5 mmol/l	N
Corticotrophin-releasing factor 1 μg/kg body weight plasma ACTH and cortisol over 3 hours	↑	→	→

N = normal; ↑ = increased; → = no change; ↑↑ = markedly increased; ↓ = suppressed.

Cushing's syndrome and patients with depression may well be obese, hypertensive and glucose intolerant it is important to be able to distinguish these two conditions.

Measurement of plasma ACTH is the key to establishing the differential diagnosis (Table 12.13). Very high levels (above 300 ng/l) suggest the ectopic ACTH syndrome and are typical of patients with small cell carcinoma of bronchus. Levels within the normal range for 08.00 h plasma ACTH (10–80 ng/l) usually indicate a pituitary source. Values between 80 and 300 ng/l may relate to either pituitary-dependent disease or the ectopic ACTH syndrome (usually from a benign tumour such as bronchial carcinoid). Techniques such as venous catheterisation with measurement of inferior petrosal sinus ACTH (i.e. draining directly from the pituitary) may be necessary to distinguish these. Other tests include giving the enzyme inhibitor metyrapone. This blocks the last step in cortisol biosynthesis (11-deoxycortisol to cortisol) and thus activates negative feedback control (Table 12.13). In addition, high-dose dexamethasone suppression, measurement of plasma potassium and the ACTH/cortisol response to corticotrophin-releasing factor are helpful in distinguishing the different causes of Cushing's syndrome.

Radiological and other investigations

Plain skull radiographs are usually normal in patients with pituitary-dependent Cushing's disease. High resolution CT scanning may be of value (Fig. 12.23A) but false positive and false negative results are not uncommon. Plain radiographs of the chest may show a bronchogenic carcinoma. If this is normal and an ectopic source of ACTH is suspected then CT scans of the anterior mediastinum and upper abdomen to include the pancreas should be done. If ACTH is undetectable, suggesting an adrenal tumour, then an adrenal scan using selenium-75-labelled cholesterol is useful in locat-

ing an adrenal adenoma. Carcinomas do not usually take up the isotope.

Management

This is essential as untreated Cushing's syndrome has a 50% 5-year mortality. Treatment of choice depends on the cause.

Adrenal tumours

Adrenal adenomas should be surgically removed via a loin approach. It may take several months for the contralateral adrenal and the hypothalamus and pituitary to recover. During this time suboptimal replacement therapy is required (0.5 mg dexamethasone in the morning). Adrenal carcinomas should also be resected if possible, the tumour bed irradiated and the patient given the adrenolytic drug o,p′DDD (usually 6–9 g/d). This may produce nausea and ataxia. Cortisol over-production can be reduced by metyrapone (start with 250 mg 8-hourly) or the more toxic aminoglutethimide (250 mg 6–8 hourly).

Cushing's disease

Trans-sphenoidal surgery with selective removal of the adenoma (found in 75% of cases) is the treatment of choice and results in cure in about 80% of patients. Recurrence is rare. If no tumour is found and the diagnosis is definitely pituitary-dependent Cushing's, then a radical hypophysectomy may be required. If the diagnosis is not certain then bilateral adrenalectomy with pituitary irradiation to prevent the development of Nelson's syndrome may be the correct treatment. External pituitary irradiation alone is of little value in adults but is surprisingly effective in children with Cushing's disease. The implantation of yttrium-90 (⁹⁰Y) (interstitial irradiation) produces good results in both adults and children. Medical treatment with drugs such as metyr-

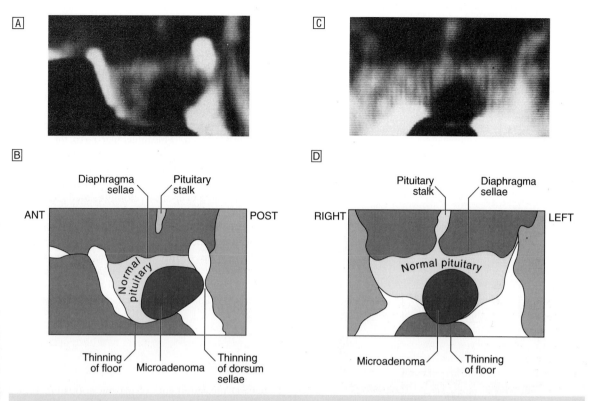

Ⓐ

Ⓒ

Ⓑ

Diaphragma
sellae   Pituitary
stalk

ANT   POST

Normal
pituitary

Microadenoma

Thinning
of floor   Thinning
of dorsum
sellae

Ⓓ

Pituitary
stalk   Diaphragma
sellae

RIGHT   LEFT

Normal pituitary

Microadenoma   Thinning
of floor

Fig. 12.23   CT scan of pituitary in patient with Cushing's disease (5 mm tumour subsequently removed by trans-sphenoidal surgery). Ⓐ, Ⓒ Lateral and coronal views. Ⓑ, Ⓓ Diagrams of the same views.

apone is usually only of value in preparing patients for surgery.

Following successful selective adenomectomy plasma cortisol should be undetectable as the ACTH-producing cells around the adenoma are suppressed. The patient should be given dexamethasone 0.5 mg in the morning and plasma cortisol measured at 08.00 hours (before dexamethasone) at 2-weekly intervals. When the level is above 180 nmol/l dexamethasone can be stopped. An insulin hypoglycaemia test should then be performed to demonstrate if the response to stress is normal. The rest of the pituitary function will also need to be assessed.

Nelson's syndrome is the association of a locally invasive pituitary tumour with very high levels of ACTH and hyperpigmentation which may occur in some patients with Cushing's disease following bilateral adrenalectomy (p. 710). It should not occur if such patients are treated with pituitary irradiation in addition to the bilateral adrenalectomy. If it does happen then surgery, radiotherapy and drugs such as the γ-aminobutyric acid inhibitor, sodium valproate, may all be necessary but are often ineffective.

Ectopic ACTH syndrome

Benign tumours causing this syndrome (e.g. bronchial carcinoid) should be removed. Malignancies such as small cell carcinoma of bronchus may initially respond to radiotherapy and chemotherapy. When they recur, then lowering cortisol levels with metyrapone or aminoglutethimide may help to control severe hypokalaemia and hyperglycaemia.

MINERALOCORTICOID EXCESS

Overproduction of aldosterone (hyperaldosteronism), the major salt-retaining hormone, may be due to a primary abnormality in the zona glomerulosa or secondary to stimulation of aldosterone secretion by angiotensin II following activation of the renin-angiotensin system (p. 706).

PRIMARY HYPERALDOSTERONISM (CONN'S SYNDROME)

Patients with this syndrome are almost invariably hypertensive and the condition is usually only discovered by

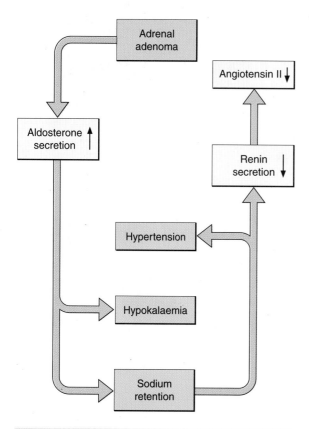

Fig. 12.24   Primary hyperaldosteronism.

detailed biochemical investigation. In the classic case, overproduction of aldosterone either by an adenoma (present in about 60% of cases) or bilateral zona glomerulosa hyperplasia is associated with hypertension and hypokalaemia (Fig. 12.24). Occasional patients may present with the symptoms of hypokalaemia (muscle weakness or even paralysis, especially in Chinese; polyuria secondary to renal tubular damage which produces nephrogenic diabetes insipidus; and occasionally tetany because of the metabolic alkalosis with low ionised calcium). Not uncommonly treatment of hypertension in such patients with a thiazide diuretic produces marked hypokalaemia. Conversely a low salt intake decreases the sodium available for sodium potassium exchange in the distal nephron and elevates plasma potassium.

The prevalence of Conn's syndrome has been the subject of considerable debate. If only hypertensive patients with hypokalaemia are investigated then less than 1% of patients with hypertension will be found to have primary hyperaldosteronism. However, recent studies in which hypertensive patients have been inves-

tigated using aldosterone/renin profiling (see below) have suggested that the prevalence is about 5%. Of these about 70% have normal plasma potassium.

In one form of primary hyperaldosteronism with zona glomerulosa hyperplasia, the aldosterone excess can be treated by giving exogenous glucocorticoid to suppress ACTH secretion. This is then referred to as glucocorticoid-responsive or dexamethasone–suppressible hyperaldosteronism. The molecular basis for this syndrome has recently been discovered. At meiosis there is normally exchange of genetic information between identical chromatids. In this condition there has been unequal crossing over of two closely related genes which are adjacent on the same chromosome. This results in a hybrid or chimeric gene (Fig. 12.25) which thus has the promoter sequence of 11β-hydroxylase (under ACTH control) and the coding sequence of aldosterone synthase (normally under dominant angiotensin II control). Thus ACTH now controls the aldosterone secretion in such patients. The condition is inherited as an autosomal dominant.

Investigations

1. Several measurements of plasma potassium should be made when patient is not taking diuretics and when the hypertension has been controlled. Blood samples should be taken without occlusion or muscular exercise of the arm and the samples separated soon after being drawn with care to avoid haemolysis. The patient should be on a normal salt intake (i.e. not low).
2. If hypokalaemia persists then plasma and/or urinary aldosterone and plasma renin activity (PRA) should be measured. In Conn's syndrome aldosterone levels will be elevated and PRA suppressed (Fig. 12.24).
3. Aldosterone/renin profiling. As indicated above, many patients with Conn's syndrome are not hypokalaemic and the diagnosis may thus be missed if this is not appreciated. Simultaneous measurement of plasma aldosterone and plasma renin activity overcomes this problem. In primary aldosteronism the ratio of aldosterone to renin will be high in comparison to that found in essential hypertension.

If possible antihypertensive drugs should be stopped for at least 2 weeks beforehand as many of these affect the renin-angiotensin system (e.g. β-adrenoceptor antagonist drugs inhibit whilst thiazide diuretics stimulate renin secretion). If this is not possible then the adrenergic neurone-blocking drug bethanidine (10 mg 8-hourly), which has minimal effect on the renin-angiotensin system, should be adopted.

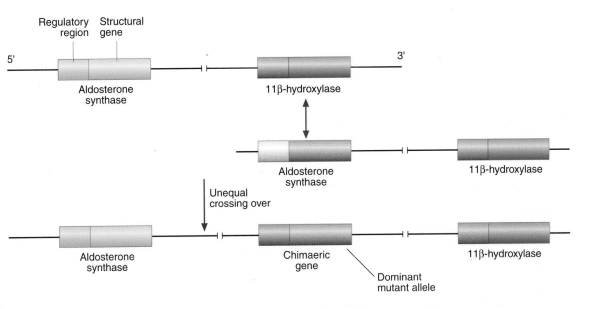

Fig. 12.25   Molecular pathogenesis of glucocorticoid-suppressible hyperaldosteronism.

Differential diagnosis

If aldosterone levels are high and renin suppressed, then further investigation is necessary to differentiate between an adenoma and hyperplasia (may be either idiopathic or glucocorticoid-suppressible). These tests are:

Aldosterone response to posture and time

This depends upon the fact that in normal subjects standing elevates plasma renin activity and hence aldosterone. In idiopathic hyperplasia the zona glomerulosa is very sensitive to angiotensin II and the small rise with standing increases aldosterone. In contrast Conn's adenoma is very responsive to ACTH as is the adrenal in glucocorticoid-suppressible hyperaldosteronism. During the course of the morning ACTH levels normally fall and hence aldosterone decreases.

Adrenal vein catheterisation

A difficult investigation to perform but necessary in some cases where other tests are equivocal. Adrenal venous cortisol levels should be measured in addition to aldosterone to demonstrate that the catheter is correctly positioned. In patients with an adenoma there is unilateral hypersecretion of aldosterone in comparison to bilateral elevation in those with hyperplasia.

Dexamethasone

This lowers plasma aldosterone transiently in Conn's adenoma patients (24–48 h) in contrast to the long-term suppression found in glucocorticoid-suppressible hyperaldosteronism.

The measurement of 18-OH-cortisol

This is valuable as this steroid is very high in patients with adenomas and glucocorticoid-suppressible hyperplasia in comparison to slight elevation in idiopathic hyperplasia.

Scanning of the adrenal with selenium-75 cholesterol

This may be helpful in demonstrating an adenoma. The test is often performed with the patient on dexamethasone to decrease uptake by the rest of the adrenal.

CT scanning

CT scanning is also of value but it is important to realise that non-functioning adrenal adenomata are present in about 20% of patients with essential hypertension.

If a patient with hypertension and hypokalaemia has suppression of both aldosterone and renin then rare enzyme defects (11β-hydroxylase, 11β-hydroxysteroid dehydrogenase or 17α-hydroxylase), excessive ingestion of liquorice or carbonoxolone, or Liddle's syndrome (renal tubular abnormality) need to be considered.

Management

The aldosterone antagonist spironolactone is valuable in treating both hypokalaemia and hypertension in Conn's syndrome. High doses (up to 400 mg/d) may be required. The blood pressure response to spironolactone correlates well with the results of removal of an adenoma by unilateral adrenalectomy (60% normotensive, 20% improved). Idiopathic hyperplasia may respond to spironolactone but often requires additional therapy for the hypertension. Surprisingly, ACE inhibitors are often of value. Up to 20% of males develop gynaecomastia on spironolactone. Amiloride (10–40 mg/d) can then be substituted.

SECONDARY HYPERALDOSTERONISM

This is a very common clinical problem resulting from excessive activity of the renin-angiotensin system (Fig. 12.26). The reasons for this can be divided into physiological and pathological.

Physiological reasons

Salt depletion either by inadequate intake or by excessive loss from the kidney or gastrointestinal tract activates the renin-angiotensin-aldosterone axis by reducing the intravascular and extracellular fluid volume which leads to renin release and also by increasing the sensitivity of the zona glomerulosa to angiotensin II. In pregnancy the natriuretic steroid progesterone is produced and higher levels of aldosterone are necessary to maintain salt balance.

Pathological reasons

In conditions such as the nephrotic syndrome, cirrhosis with ascites and congestive heart failure, there is a reduced effective intravascular volume which leads to decreased renal perfusion and hence increased renin release. Bartter's syndrome usually presents with short stature. Investigations show hypokalaemia, gross elevation of renin with less marked hyperaldosteronism, hyperplasia of the juxtaglomerular apparatus and increased urinary prostaglandin excretion.

Whereas secondary hyperaldosteronism is common in accelerated or malignant phase hypertension, it is unusual in renovascular disease unless there is a severe renal artery stenosis. Renin-secreting tumours (haemangiopericytomas) are very rare. Diuretic therapy, especially when excessive, is by far the commonest cause of secondary hyperaldosteronism.

Investigations

- The plasma electrolytes reveal hypokalaemia often associated with plasma sodium levels which are in the lower part of the reference range or subnormal.
- Plasma aldosterone and plasma renin activity are both elevated.

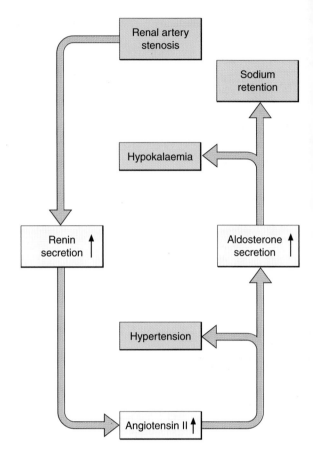

Fig. 12.26   Secondary hyperaldosteronism.

Management

This depends on the underlying cause. If this is salt depletion then intravenous saline may be required. In congestive heart failure, treatment with either spironolactone or an angiotensin-converting enzyme (ACE) inhibitor (e.g. captopril 25–50 mg 12-hourly) may produce considerable haemodynamic and electrolyte improvement. In Bartter's syndrome spironolactone often with indomethacin to inhibit prostaglandin synthesis is indicated.

With effective antihypertensive therapy plasma potassium usually returns to normal in patients with accelerated or malignant phase hypertension. Renovascular disease can be effectively treated by an ACE inhibitor but definitive therapy such as transluminal angioplasty of a stenosed renal artery needs to be considered. If diuretic therapy (e.g. with a thiazide) produces problems with hypokalaemia then a potassium-sparing drug such as amiloride, triamterene or spironolactone can be given.

HYPOFUNCTION

ADRENOCORTICAL INSUFFICIENCY

This can be divided into primary and secondary causes as shown in the information box below.

CAUSES OF ADRENOCORTICAL INSUFFICIENCY

Primary
- Addison's disease   ACTH↑
- Congenital or acquired enzyme defects   ACTH↑

Secondary
- Hypothalamic or pituitary disease   ACTH↓
- Glucocorticoid therapy   ACTH↓

PRIMARY ADRENOCORTICAL INSUFFICIENCY— ADDISON'S DISEASE

Aetiology

This is a rare condition with an estimated incidence in the developed world of 0.8 cases per 100 000 population. However, adrenal insufficiency is a well-recognised complication in patients with AIDS and may result from a variety of causes including tuberculosis, fungal and cytomegalovirus infections. Thus this figure is likely to be a significant underestimate.

Addison's classic description *Diseases of the suprarenal capsules* published in 1855 included detailed drawings of caseating adrenal tuberculosis. However, in one case in which the patient had gross vitiligo (a marker of auto-immune disease) he was unable to get an autopsy (Fig. 12.27). Most likely this patient had autoimmune adre-nalitis, now the commonest cause of primary adrenal failure. As with other autoimmune diseases this is more common in females than males (2:1). The causes are listed in the information box.

Clinical features

These result from glucocorticoid usually together with mineralocorticoid insufficiency, loss of adrenal andro-gen production and increased ACTH secretion. The clinical features are listed in the information box below.

The patient may present with an acute, chronic or acute on chronic illness. The initial symptoms are often misdiagnosed and it is the pigmentation that commonly raises the suspicion of the diagnosis.

CLINICAL FEATURES OF ADDISON'S DISEASE

- **Glucocorticoid insufficiency**
  Weight loss
  Malaise
  Weakness
  Anorexia
  Nausea
  Vomiting
  Gastrointestinal—diar-rhoea or constipation
  Postural hypotension
  Hypoglycaemia
- **Mineralocorticoid insufficiency**
  Hypotension
- **Increased ACTH secretion**
  Pigmentation
    Sun exposed areas
    Pressure areas, e.g. elbows, knees
    Palmar creases, knuckles
    Mucous membranes
    Conjunctivae
    Recent scars
- **Loss of adrenal androgen**
  Decrease body hair, esp. in female

CAUSES OF ADDISON'S DISEASE

Common
- Autoimmune:
  Sporadic
  Polyglandular deficiency type I (Addison's disease, chronic mucocutaneous candidiasis, hypoparathyroidism)
  Polyglandular deficiency type II (Addison's disease, primary hypothyroidism, primary hypogonadism, insulin-dependent diabetes mellitus, pernicious anaemia, vitiligo)
- Tuberculosis
- Bilateral adrenalectomy

Rare
- Metastatic tumour, lymphoma
- Intra-adrenal haemorrhage (Waterhouse–Fridericksen syndrome following meningococcal septicaemia)
- Amyloid
- Haemochromatosis
- Adrenal infarction or infection other than TB (esp. AIDS)

The blood pressure may be normal with the patient lying down. Hence, the pressure should also be meas-ured after standing for 1 minute. Postural hypotension is almost invariably present.

The cause of the pigmentation is probably the high circulating level of ACTH stimulating melanin pro-duction rather than the associated pro-opiocortin pep-tides (β-LPH and N-POC), even though both of these have common core MSH sequences (Fig. 12.4).

Vitiligo is present in about 10–20% (Fig. 12.27). Other autoimmune diseases which may be present are listed in the information box.

Surgery or other stress may precipitate an acute adre-

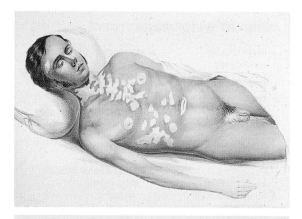

Fig. 12.27   Vitiligo in a patient with Addison's disease.

nal crisis. Alternatively such patients may take much longer than normal to recover from an illness or operation.

Investigations

Biochemical tests are essential to confirm the diagnosis of Addison's disease. The key investigations are:

ACTH stimulation test

In Addison's disease there is almost always a failure of the plasma cortisol to rise following administration of ACTH. The basal 08.00 h plasma cortisol is usually low but may be normal; in this context 'normal' is difficult to define as the level may be within the normal reference range but actually inappropriately low for a seriously ill patient.

The usual ACTH test involves giving β1-24 ACTH (i.e. the biologically active 24 out of the total 39 amino acids in the natural molecule). This is tetracosactrin (synacthen); 0.25 mg is given either intramuscularly or intravenously. Blood samples for the measurement of plasma cortisol should be taken at 0, 30 and 60 minutes. In normal subjects in response to ACTH the plasma cortisol should exceed 550 nmol/litre.

Patients with secondary adrenocortical insufficiency may also get a subnormal cortisol rise. They can be distinguished from primary adrenal failure either by measurement of ACTH (see below) or by giving depot tetracosactrin (1 mg intramuscularly daily for 3 days). In secondary insufficiency there is a progressive increase in plasma cortisol whereas in primary it is less than 700 nmol/l at 8 hours after the last injection.

If glucocorticoids have to be given prior to testing the adrenal response to ACTH, then the corticosteroid should be changed to a steroid such as dexamethasone (0.75 mg/d) which does not cross-react in the plasma cortisol radioimmunoassay.

Measurement of plasma ACTH

The simultaneous measurement of 08.00 h plasma cortisol and ACTH is the most sensitive test of primary adrenal failure. Thus even if the plasma cortisol is normal the ACTH value will be elevated (>80 ng/l).

Plasma electrolytes

The plasma sodium is usually low, the potassium high, normal or frankly elevated, and the plasma urea raised.

Blood glucose

This may be low especially in severe adrenal insufficiency.

Plasma renin activity (PRA) and aldosterone

PRA values are nearly always high with plasma aldosterone being either low or normal.

After the diagnosis has been made the specific cause must be identified. A chest radiograph should be taken to look for evidence of TB. Such patients may have adrenal calcification which may be visible on a plain abdominal radiograph or CT scan. Blood should be tested for adrenal and other organ-specific antibodies. The adrenal antigen is the 21-hydroxylase enzyme. Associated thyroid disease, pernicious anaemia and diabetes should be excluded.

Management

Patients with Addison's disease always need glucocorticoid replacement therapy and usually mineralocorticoid. **Cortisol (hydrocortisone)** is the drug of choice. In the past cortisone acetate was given but this has to be converted to cortisol by the liver and in some patients this may be impaired. Hydrocortisone 20 mg is given orally on getting up in the morning and 10 mg at 18.00 h (see p. 678 for assessment of dose); cortisone acetate 25 mg in the morning and 12.5 mg in the evening.

Fludrocortisone is the mineralocorticoid used to replace aldosterone. The usual dose is 0.05–0.1 mg daily. Adequacy of replacement can be assessed by measurement of blood pressure, plasma electrolytes and plasma renin activity.

If the Addison's disease results from tuberculosis then this will need to be appropriately treated (p. 358).

Advice to patients is given in the information box.

ADRENAL CRISIS

Patients may present in shock with severe hypotension, hyponatraemia, hyperkalaemia and, in some instances, hypoglycaemia. Muscle cramps, nausea, vomiting, diarrhoea and unexplained fever may be present. Intercurrent disease or infection may be the precipitating cause. The adrenal crisis is a medical emergency and requires intravenous hydrocortisone hemisuccinate 100 mg and intravenous fluid (normal saline and 5% dextrose if hypoglycaemia). Parenteral hydrocortisone should be continued (100 mg intramuscularly 6-hourly) until the gastrointestinal symptoms abate before starting oral therapy. The precipitating cause should be sought and, if possible, treated.

PRIMARY ADRENOCORTICAL INSUFFICIENCY—CONGENITAL ENZYME DEFECTS

Defects in the cortisol biosynthetic pathway result in activation of ACTH secretion via negative feedback control. ACTH then stimulates the production of steroids up to the enzyme block. This produces adrenal hyperplasia. The commonest enzyme defect is that of the 21-hydroxylase enzyme (Fig. 12.28). In about one-third of cases this defect affects both mineralocorticoid (aldosterone) and glucocorticoid (cortisol) production. This results in severe salt wasting which may be fatal in the first few weeks of life if untreated. In the other two-thirds mineralocorticoid secretion is not affected.

The increased ACTH drive results in high levels of 17-OH-progesterone and androgens. The latter produce clitoromegaly, accelerated growth and premature fusion of the epiphyses. In boys there may be enlargement of the penis and pubic hair development but without testicular enlargement (precocious pseudo-puberty).

Defects of all the other enzymes have been described but are much rarer. 17-hydroxylase and 11β-hydroxylase deficiency may produce hypertension due to excess mineralocorticoid production.

Investigations

High levels of plasma 17-OH-progesterone are found in 21-hydroxylase deficiency. These can be measured in blood spot samples taken in the first week of life from heel pricks for phenylketonuria testing. In the past the metabolite of 17-OH-progesterone, pregnanetriol, was measured in the urine. Specific antenatal diagnosis can now be made. Plasma electrolytes, renin activity and aldosterone should be measured. Bone age should be carefully followed.

Management

The aim is to suppress ACTH and hence adrenal androgen production by glucocorticoid therapy. Treatment of the female can be started in utero if the diagnosis is made and hence clitoromegaly prevented. Under-replacement with glucocorticoid will fail to control the initially increased growth velocity. However, excess glucocorticoid will suppress growth. It is usual to give reverse replacement therapy, i.e. larger dose of glucocorticoid just before going to bed to suppress nocturnal ACTH rise and smaller dose in the morning.

PRIMARY ADRENOCORTICAL INSUFFICIENCY—ACQUIRED ENZYME DEFECTS

Certain drugs can inhibit cortisol biosynthesis by enzyme inhibition. The most commonly used is metyrapone which blocks 11β-hydroxylase (Fig. 12.25—see p. 713).

SECONDARY ADRENOCORTICAL INSUFFICIENCY—HYPOTHALAMIC OR PITUITARY DISEASE

The clinical features, investigation and management of this condition are detailed on page 674.

Glucocorticoid therapy

The administration of supra-physiological doses of glucocorticoids may result in the suppression of the hypothalamic-pituitary-adrenal axis with eventual adrenal atrophy. In this situation if the glucocorticoid therapy is suddenly stopped and, particularly if the patient is stressed (e.g. major surgery), then adrenocortical insufficiency may result (see below for withdrawal of corticosteroids). Unlike patients with Addison's disease these patients do not have mineralocorticoid insufficiency.

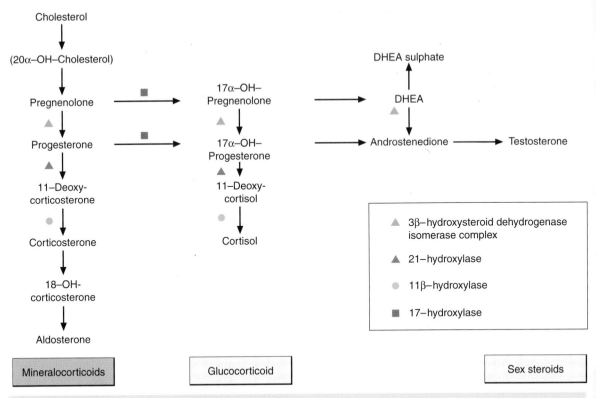

Fig. 12.28 The major pathways of synthesis of adrenal corticosteroids. (DHEA: Dehydroepiandrosterone.)

USE OF CORTICOSTEROIDS IN THE TREATMENT OF DISEASE

The anti-inflammatory actions of corticosteroids have led to their use in a wide variety of clinical conditions. The first glucocorticoid used was cortisone acetate. When given in high dose this had significant sodium retaining effects (the active metabolite cortisol can bind to type 1 mineralocorticoid and type 2 glucocorticoid receptors). This led to the synthesis of a large number of other steroids with more selective binding to the type 2 receptor (e.g. prednisolone and especially betamethasone and dexamethasone). Doses are listed in the information box below.

SIDE-EFFECTS OF CORTICOSTEROID THERAPY
(see p. 901)

The metabolic effects are identical to those found in Cushing's syndrome (p. 707). They are dose-related and hence, if possible, the dose should be kept to less than prednisolone 10 mg per day. Some patients experience marked changes in mood on high-dose glucocorticoid

EQUIVALENT DOSES OF GLUCOCORTICOIDS (ANTI-INFLAMMATORY POTENCY)

- Hydrocortisone   20 mg
- Cortisone acetate   25 mg
- Prednisolone   5 mg
- Betamethasone   0.75 mg
- Dexamethasone   0.75 mg

therapy ranging from euphoria to profound depression. Osteoporosis is a major problem of long-term, high-dose therapy. Glucose intolerance or frank diabetes mellitus may be produced. Hypertension is common.

Even though the drug is being used for its anti-inflammatory effect this may produce problems. Thus perforation may be masked and the patient show no febrile response to an infection. Gastric erosions are more common probably because of impaired prostaglandin synthesis. Hence the combination of corticosteroid with analgesic drugs such as aspirin may lead to haemorrhage from the stomach or duodenum. Latent tuberculosis may be reactivated.

Suppression of the hypothalamic-pituitary-adrenal (HPA) axis

As indicated above this may occur with high dose glucocorticoid therapy. The timing of glucocorticoid ingestion is important. Thus prednisolone 5 mg orally on going to bed will suppress ACTH secretion whereas 5 mg in the morning will have little or no effect on the HPA axis. Thus, if the condition being treated permits, the glucocorticoid should be taken as a single morning dose.

WITHDRAWAL OF CORTICOSTEROID THERAPY

If possible, corticosteroids should be withdrawn slowly unless they have only previously been given for a short period. As indicated the dose should be given in the morning as this will enhance recovery of the HPA axis. Giving ACTH to stimulate adrenal recovery is of no value as the hypothalamus remains suppressed. In a patient with a completely suppressed axis it may take months or years to recover. If the glucocorticoid-requiring condition allows, then giving dexamethasone 0.5 mg in the morning instead of the glucocorticoid will usually result in gradual recovery. This can be monitored by measuring 08.00 h plasma cortisol just before the dexamethasone dose.

When the plasma cortisol exceeds 180 nmol/l then dexamethasone can be stopped and a short synacthen test performed (p. 675). A rise of plasma cortisol to >550 nmol/l indicates that the patient will respond normally to stress and thus does not require corticosteroid cover for surgery, etc.

CATECHOLAMINE EXCESS

PHAEOCHROMOCYTOMA

This is a rare tumour of chromaffin tissue which secretes catecholamines and is responsible for less than 0.1% of cases of hypertension. The tumours are usually benign (10% malignant) and may arise from any part of the sympathetic chain. However, in over 90% of cases the tumour is found in the adrenal medulla. In multiple endocrine neoplasia (MEN) type IIa phaeochromocytoma (almost invariably involving both adrenals) is associated with medullary carcinoma of thyroid and hyperparathyroidism (usually hyperplasia). In MEN IIb the same abnormalities are associated with Marfanoid body habitus, bumpy lips and mucosal neuromas of tongue, eyelids and cornea (Fig.12.29). Both these conditions may arise spontaneously or be inherited as an autosomal dominant.

CLINICAL FEATURES OF PHAEOCHROMOCYTOMA

- Hypertension (usually paroxysmal) (often postural drop of blood pressure)
- Attacks with:
  Pallor (sometimes flushing)
  Palpitations
  Sweating
  Headache
  Anxiety (fear of death—angor animi)
- Abdominal pain, vomiting
- Constipation
- Weight loss
- Glucose intolerance

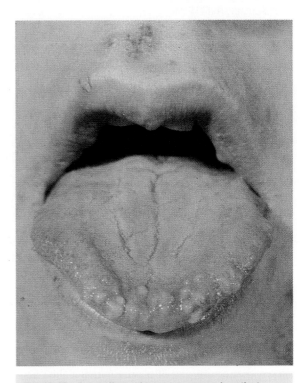

Fig. 12.29 Bumpy lips and tongue neuromas in patient with multiple endocrine neoplasia type IIb who presented with vomiting and paroxysmal hypertension, and was found to have bilateral phaeochromocytomas and medullary carcinoma of thyroid.

Clinical features

These depend on the catecholamine secretion. The clinical features are listed in the information box.

Some patients may present with a complication of the hypertension, e.g. stroke, myocardial infarction, left ventricular failure. Occasionally the patients may be hypotensive (especially dopamine-secreting tumours). Neurofibromatosis is associated with an increased incidence of phaeochromocytomas.

Investigations

The diagnosis is made on the basis of biochemical testing. Provocative tests of catecholamine release should not be used. The enzyme that synthesises adrenaline from noradrenaline is phenylethanolamine-N-methyl transferase (PNMT). This is induced by high glucocorticoid levels. Hence small adrenomedullary tumours bathed in cortisol by the centripetal blood flow of the adrenal produce the highest levels of adrenaline. Large adrenal tumours which have outgrown the normal cortical supply or extra-adrenal tumours produce almost entirely noradrenaline.

> **USUAL SCREENING TESTS FOR PHAEOCHROMOCYTOMAS**
>
> - 24-hour urine for 3-methoxy-4-hydroxymandelic acid (VMA)
>   or 24-hour metanephrines
>   or 24-hour free urinary catecholamines
>
> **Plasma noradrenaline and adrenaline should be measured in:**
> - Established or borderline cases
> - Paroxysmal hypertension
> - Renal failure

Screening tests are given in the information box above.

In some patients the diagnosis remains in doubt and a suppression test may be useful (e.g. plasma catecholamines 10 minutes after intravenous pentolinium 2.5 mg. Normal subjects' levels will suppress, unlike those with phaeochromocytoma).

Once the diagnosis has been made, then the tumour must be localised. This can be done using computed tomography (CT) scanning (Fig. 12.30). Scintigraphy using meta-iodobenzyl guanidine (MIBG) can be useful: MIBG labelled with radioactive iodine is taken up by both benign and malignant phaeochromocytomas. If the tumour cannot be localised then selective venous sampling with measurement of plasma noradrenaline may be required.

In patients with multiple endocrine neoplasia, genetic screening is greatly facilitating the investigation of relatives who may have the dominant gene (see p. 23).

Management

This requires excision of the tumour or, failing this, long-term treatment with α (and usually β) adrenoceptor blockade. Prior to surgery it is essential to give alpha-antagonist drugs such as phenoxybenzamine 10–20 mg orally 3–4 times daily preferably for a minimum of 6 weeks to allow restoration of normal plasma volume. If alpha-blockade produces a marked tachycardia then a β-antagonist drug such as propranolol (10–20 mg 3 times

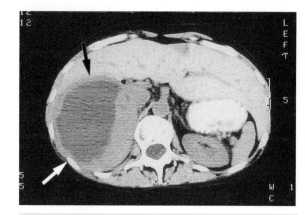

Fig. 12.30   CT scan of abdomen showing large right phaeochromocytoma.

daily) should be added. On no account should the β-antagonist be given before the α-antagonist as vasoconstriction due to unopposed α-adrenoceptor activity may occur with a further increase in blood pressure. During surgery sodium nitroprusside and the short acting α-antagonist phentolamine are very useful in controlling hypertensive episodes which may result from anaesthetic induction or tumour mobilisation. Postoperative hypotension may occur and require volume expansion and very occasionally noradrenaline. This is uncommon if the patient has been prepared with phenoxybenzamine for at least 6 weeks.

> **FURTHER READING**
>
> Bravo E L 1991 Phaeochromocytoma: new concepts in the pathophysiology, diagnosis and treatment. Kidney International 40: 554–556
> Edwards C R W 1995 Adrenocortical diseases. In: Oxford Textbook of Medicine, 3rd edn. Oxford University Press, Oxford
> Lifton R P, Dluhy R. G, Powers M et al 1992 A chimeric 11-hydroxylase/aldosterone synthase gene causes glucocorticoid-remediable aldosteronism and human hypertension. Nature 355: 262–265
> Trainer P J, Grossman A 1991 The diagnosis and differential diagnosis of Cushing's syndrome. Clinical Endocrinology 34: 317–330

SEXUAL DISORDERS

THE MALE

Male sexual disorders can be classified on the basis of hypogonadism and precocious puberty.

HYPOGONADISM

Hypogonadism is classified in the information box below.

CLASSIFICATION OF HYPOGONADISM

Secondary hypogonadism
- Hypothalamic-pituitary disease
  Hypogonadotrophic ($\downarrow$ LH $\downarrow$ FSH)

Primary testicular failure
- Hypergonadotrophic ($\uparrow$ LH $\uparrow$ FSH or $\uparrow$ FSH alone)
  Anorchia
  Klinefelter's syndrome
  Mumps orchitis—bilateral
  Tuberculosis
  Testicular tumours
  Idiopathic
  Chemotherapy/irradiation

Clinical features

These will depend on the underlying pathology. Thus in Kallmann's syndrome with isolated GnRH deficiency there is associated anosmia (p. 677). Pituitary tumours may present with symptoms of the tumour such as a visual field defect. The age of presentation is also important. If the defect is present prior to the normal onset of puberty then this will be delayed. Such a delay may be constitutional (often positive family history and short stature) or due to a variety of conditions other than hypothalamic-pituitary-gonadal disease. These conditions are listed in the information box.

OTHER CAUSES OF DELAYED PUBERTY

- Systemic disease (e.g. malnutrition, cystic fibrosis, renal failure, heart disease, malabsorption)
- Androgen receptor defect (testicular feminisation or partial defects)
- 5α-reductase deficiency
- Anorexia nervosa
- Emotional deprivation
- Excessive exercise

Failure to go into puberty results in failure of normal fusion of the epiphyses of long bones with consequent excessive height (long arms and long legs in comparison to trunk height—eunuchoid proportions). The typical eunuch is tall with a hairless face, high-pitched voice, small external genitalia and rather immature personality. Some pubic hair is usually present as the result of adrenal androgen production—adrenarche.

If the hypogonadism develops *post-pubertally* then the clinical features are usually those relating to loss of tes-

tosterone secretion. These are listed in the information box.

CLINICAL FEATURES OF HYPOGONADISM IN POST-PUBERTY

- Impotence
- Loss of libido $\Big\}$ Early symptoms
- Tiredness
- Decreased shaving
- Decreased body hair $\Big\}$ Late symptoms
- Decreased muscle power

Sudden loss of testosterone as with surgical castration may produce hot flushes and profuse sweating unless replacement therapy is given.

The loss of testosterone allows unopposed effects of oestrogen. The latter is increased when there is increased LH drive to the interstitial cells as in Klinefelter's syndrome. This leads to breast enlargement (gynaecomastia). Oestrogen secreting tumours may arise from interstitial cells and present with impotence and gynaecomastia. The tumour is often very small.

Males with hyperprolactinaemia frequently present with impotence, and occasionally with galactorrhoea. Thus the breasts should be carefully examined.

In cases of delayed puberty the extent of development should be classified using the 5 stages described by Marshall and Tanner:

- In G1 the patient is pre-pubertal
- In G2 there is testicular enlargement to 4 ml (measured using a Prader orchidometer with a series of ellipsoids of known volumes)
- In G3 there is further scrotal and testicular enlargement (8–10 ml) with increased length of penis
- G4: Length and breadth of penis increases with development of glans, testicular volume 12 ml
- G5: Genitalia adult in size and shape with testes > 15 ml.

Pubic hair is assessed in a similar manner (see the information box).

In complete androgen resistance (testicular fem-

CLASSIFICATION OF PUBIC HAIR

PH 1—no pubic hair
PH 2—sparse growth of straight, lightly pigmented hair
PH 3—hair spreads over pubes, darker, coarser, curlier
PH 4—adult in character but smaller area
PH 5—hair extends onto inner aspects of thighs and up towards umbilicus

---

inisation) the phenotype is female and the condition due to defective androgen receptors in target tissues. The testes may be found in the groins. Pubic hair is absent. Breasts develop normally and the patient may present with primary amenorrhoea.

In 5-alpha-reductase deficiency there is failure of conversion of testosterone to dihydrotestosterone. The latter is required for the development of the external genitalia. Thus these patients are usually brought up as females but have growth of the phallus at puberty. They then often change sexual orientation to that of a male.

The loss of FSH secretion leads to failure of spermatogenesis. This is also affected by LH deficiency as testosterone is required for spermatogenesis. If there is damage to testicular germ cells (e.g. by chemotherapy for malignant disease) then this can be detected by finding elevated FSH with normal LH.

Investigations

The tests for hypothalamic-pituitary dysfunction are detailed on page 674.

In primary gonadal disease plasma testosterone, LH and FSH should be measured. If there is gynaecomastia then oestradiol should also be estimated: if elevated then the source must be determined (?exogenous, ?adrenal or testicular tumour). If indicated, a karyotype should be performed. Bone age should be assessed in boys with delayed puberty.

Management

This depends on the cause. The androgen deficiency should be replaced using one of the drugs and routes indicated on page 678.

With delayed puberty there are various possibilities including intramuscular testosterone oenanthate 50–100 mg at 6-weekly intervals, hCG injections (1500 IU i.m. weekly) or pulsatile GnRH therapy.

The treatment of infertility in secondary hypogonadism is given on page 678. There is no effective therapy for infertility resulting from primary gonadal failure. However, it is important to exclude causes such as sulphasalazine therapy when the effects are reversible.

CRYPTORCHIDISM

Cryptorchidism (undescended testis) usually occurs in otherwise normal boys but may be the presenting feature of hypogonadotrophic hypogonadism. Highly retractile testes, particularly in an obese boy, may be mistaken for cryptorchidism. If the testes remain in the inguinal canal they are more liable to trauma than if situated in the scrotum. The seminiferous tubules will fail to develop in an undescended gland and, if the condition is bilateral, sterility will follow. Even in testes which remain unde-

scended into adult life the interstitial cells function normally, so that the secondary sex characteristics develop in the usual way. A course of chorionic gonadotrophin should be given at about 6 years of age. Alternatively GnRH can be given intranasally for 1–4 weeks. With inguinal testes the success rate for descent is about 40%, which is similar to that with gonadotrophin. If medical treatment is unsuccessful the testis or testes should be placed in the scrotum surgically.

In maldescent the testis takes an abnormal route and is liable to develop malignancy. Such testes should either be brought down into the scrotum or, if discovered in the adult, removed.

IMPOTENCE

Erectile dysfunction or failure (impotence) was thought to be due to psychological causes in the majority of cases. However, the incidence of this condition increases with age; vascular disease involving the internal pudendal artery or its branches is common in these patients. This alone may be the cause of the impotence or a trigger for psychological dysfunction. Impotence may also be an early symptom in diabetes mellitus, multiple sclerosis and tabes dorsalis. Endocrine causes of impotence are uncommon and there is usually an associated loss of libido.

PRECOCIOUS PUBERTY

True precocious puberty results from the premature activation of the hypothalamic-pituitary-gonadal axis and needs to be distinguished from precocious pseudopuberty associated with gonadal or adrenal tumours or congenital adrenal hyperplasia (p. 717). True precocious puberty is usually idiopathic in girls and there is frequently a positive family history. In boys it is more commonly indicative of central nervous system disease. Long-acting analogues of gonadotrophin-releasing hormone are now being used to treat precocious puberty and thus improve the adult height prognosis and avoid the physical and psychological problems.

THE FEMALE

As with the male disorders can be classified into those arising from either hypothalamic-pituitary or primary gonadal defects. The presentation is often with menstrual abnormalities such as primary or secondary amenorrhoea.

PRIMARY AMENORRHOEA

This may be due to a chromosomal abnormality, e.g. Turner's syndrome (p. 17). These patients are usually short and have features such as a webbed neck and increased carrying angle. However, some cases have none of these phenotypic features.

Unrecognised or ineffectively treated congenital adrenal hyperplasia (p. 717) may present with primary amenorrhoea. The testicular feminisation syndrome due to defective androgen receptors is usually obvious because of the lack of pubic hair and good breast development.

Any hypothalamic (e.g. craniopharyngioma) or pituitary (i.e. prolactinoma) lesion may be first manifest with failure to start menstruation. Primary autoimmune ovarian failure is a rare cause.

Structural abnormalities of the genital tract need to be excluded. It is important to recognise that any chronic systemic disease may delay the onset of menstruation.

SECONDARY AMENORRHOEA

This is a relatively common problem. The differential diagnosis is included in the information box.

SECONDARY AMENORRHOEA

- **Hypothalamic dysfunction** (see p. 670) +
  Anorexia nervosa, excessive exercise, psychogenic
- **Pituitary disease** (see p. 674)
  Especially hyperprolactinaemia
- **Ovarian dysfunction**
  Polycystic ovary syndrome
  Androgen-secreting tumours
  Autoimmune (premature menopause)
  Turner mosaic
  Menopause (see below)
- **Adrenal disease**
  Cushing's syndrome, congenital adrenal hyperplasia, androgen-secreting tumours
- **Thyroid disease**
  Hypo- and hyperthyroidism
- **Other conditions**
  Severe systemic disease, e.g. renal failure, endometrial TB

Clinical features

These will depend on the condition. If there is weight loss then this may be primary as in anorexia nervosa or secondary to an underlying disease such as TB, malignancy or hyperthyroidism. Weight gain may suggest Cushing's syndrome, hypothyroidism or, very rarely, a hypothalamic lesion. Hirsutism may indicate androgen excess. A very common cause of this is the polycystic ovary syndrome. Androgen-secreting tumours are much

rarer. They may produce virilisation, e.g. clitoromegaly, deepening of the voice, temporal recession, breast atrophy. The breasts need to be carefully examined for milk (p. 683). The presence of other autoimmune disease should raise the possibility of autoimmune ovarian failure.

Investigations

High levels of LH and FSH suggest primary ovarian failure. This may be premature, as with autoimmune ovarian failure. Elevated LH is common in the polycystic ovary syndrome together with slightly increased plasma testosterone with low levels of sex hormone-binding globulin. High levels of plasma testosterone may be due to an androgen-secreting tumour. If prolactin levels are elevated then this requires detailed investigation (p. 683). Low levels of gonadotrophins and oestradiol suggest hypothalamic or pituitary disease.

Management

This depends on the cause. Androgen excess, as in the polycystic ovary syndrome, is a common problem. The hirsutism is usually of more concern to the patient than the menstrual abnormality. In about 75% of cases hair growth improves with cyproterone acetate (anti-androgen). In pre-menopausal patients this is usually given as cyproterone acetate 50 mg 12-hourly on days 1–10 with ethinyl oestradiol 30 μg daily on days 1–21. This allows regular menstruation. In primary ovarian failure, especially if premature, oestrogen replacement will normally be required (see below).

THE MENOPAUSE

The cessation of menstruation in Western women occurs at a median age of 50.8 years. In the 5 years before there is a gradual increase in the number of anovulatory cycles. This period is referred to as the climacteric. Oestrogen secretion falls and negative feedback results in increased pituitary secretion of LH and FSH.

Clinical features

Irregular periods commonly precede the menopause and hence the exact timing of it can only be recognised in retrospect (e.g. 6 months after last period). The symptoms relate to oestrogen deficiency. In some patients they are relatively minor but in others a major problem. The symptoms are given in the information box below.

The flushes may start when the patient still has regular periods. In most patients the vasomotor symptoms gradually improve but in about one-quarter they go on for more than 5 years. They are almost invariably relieved by oestrogen therapy. Their precise cause remains unknown. They are associated with an LH

MENOPAUSAL SYMPTOMS

- **Vasomotor effects**
  Hot flushes
  Sweating
- **Psychological**
  Anxiety
  Emotional lability
  Irritability
- **Genitourinary**
  Dyspareunia ('senile
  vaginitis')
  Vaginal infections ↑
  Urgency of micturition

OESTROGEN REPLACEMENT THERAPY

- **Oral oestrogens**
  e.g. cyclical ethinyl oestradiol 0.01–0.02 mg/day for 21
  days with medroxyprogesterone acetate 5 mg daily for last
  10 days
- **Percutaneous**
  Patches with reservoir of oestradiol giving oestradiol
  25–50 μg/day. Change every 3–4 days. Add oral
  progestogen for 10 days per month
- **Topical oestradiol**
  e.g. for atrophic vaginitis 0.01% dienoestrol cream

---

pulse. The fall in oestrogen secretion is associated with increased bone resorption. There is an initial rapid loss of bone mass which is most marked in the axial skeleton (1–3% per annum for 4 years and then 0.5% per annum). This eventually results in osteoporosis with an increased incidence of vertebral compression fracture, fractured neck of femur and distal radius in comparison to the male. This is a major and apparently increasing problem with significant morbidity, mortality (17% per 30 000 women per annum in the UK with hip fractures) and enormous cost. It is not at present possible to predict with accuracy a population at risk. This depends on bone density at the time of menopause and the rate of bone loss. However, those women who smoke cigarettes appear to be at particular risk. The earlier the menopause, the greater the problem. Excessive alcohol and lack of exercise seem to be additional risk factors. Oestrogen started at the time of menopause has been shown to prevent the normal post-menopausal bone loss.

Management

Many women seek explanation and reassurance rather than treatment. In some the vasomotor symptoms may be the main problem. These may be helped by clonidine 50 μg 12-hourly but in many patients oestrogen therapy is required. This has the advantage of not only improving symptoms but also having beneficial effects on bone and soft tissues. Giving oestrogen is referred to as hormone replacement therapy (HRT). It can be given in a variety of different ways. These are included in the information box below.

Percutaneous oestrogen is a relatively new form of treatment. It has the advantage of not having the same effect on liver production of coagulation factors as oral oestrogen. Patients should not be given long-term unopposed oestrogen as this increases the risk of endometrial cancer ($\times 5$). Nausea and breast tenderness may be a problem. The blood pressure should be measured before and at 6-monthly intervals on treatment. The duration of treatment is debatable. For symptoms such as hot flushes a year may be reasonable with gradual withdrawal. For prevention of osteoporosis much longer treatment is necessary. For patients with a premature

menopause oestrogen should be given until at least age 50. A cervical smear should be taken and the breasts and pelvis examined before giving oestrogen.

FURTHER READING

Grady D, Rubin S M, Petitti D B et al 1992 Hormone therapy to prevent disease and prolong life in postmenopausal women. Annals of Internal Medicine 117: 1016–1037
Grumbach M M, Styne D M 1992 Puberty: Ontogeny, Neuroendocrinology. In: Williams Textbook of Endocrinology, 8th edn. Saunders, Philadelphia
Tolis G, Bringer J, Chrousos G P (eds) 1993 Introovarian regulators and the polycystic ovary syndrome. Annals of the New York Academy of Sciences 687: 1–304

DIABETES MELLITUS

Diabetes mellitus is a clinical syndrome characterised by hyperglycaemia due to absolute or relative deficiency of insulin. This can arise in many different ways (Table 12.14). Lack of insulin, whether absolute or relative, affects the metabolism of carbohydrate, protein, fat, water and electrolytes. Death may result from acute metabolic decompensation while long-standing metabolic derangement is frequently associated with permanent and irreversible functional and structural changes in the cells of the body, those of the vascular system being particularly susceptible. These changes lead in turn to the development of well-defined clinical entities, the so-called 'complications of diabetes' which most characteristically affect the eye, the kidney and the nervous system.

EPIDEMIOLOGY

Epidemiological study of whole populations has shown that the distribution of blood glucose concentration is unimodal with no clear division between normal and abnormal values. Diagnostic criteria are therefore arbi-

Table 12.14   Classification of diabetes mellitus

Type	Examples
A PRIMARY	
Type I Insulin-dependent diabetes mellitus (IDDM)	
Type II Non-Insulin-dependent diabetes mellitus (NIDDM)	
B SECONDARY TO OTHER PATHOLOGY	
1 Pancreatic pathology	Pancreatitis
	Haemochromatosis
	Neoplastic disease
	Pancreatectomy
	Cystic fibrosis
2 Excess endogenous production of hormonal antagonists to insulin	Growth hormone (acromegaly)
	Glucocorticoids (Cushing's syndrome)
	Thyroid hormones (hyperthyroidism)
	Catecholamines (phaeochromocytoma)
	Human placental lactogen (pregnancy)
	Glucagon (glucagonoma)
	Counterregulatory hormones (severe burns, trauma)
3 Medication with	Corticosteroids
	Thiazide diuretics
	Phenytoin
4 Liver disease	
C ASSOCIATED WITH GENETIC SYNDROMES	DIDMOAD (i.e. diabetes insipidus, diabetes mellitus, optic atrophy, nerve deafness)
	Lipoatrophy
	Muscular dystrophies
	Friedreich's dystrophies
	Down syndrome
	Klinefelter's syndrome
	Turner's syndrome

trary. Studies involving Pima Indians in Arizona and civil servants in Whitehall have demonstrated that hyperglycaemia represents an independent risk factor for the development of disease of small and large blood vessels respectively. Current diagnostic criteria for diabetes (Table 12.18, p. 734) have been selected on the basis of identifying those who have a degree of hyperglycaemia which, if untreated, has been shown to be associated with a significantly increased risk of disability and death from vascular disease, whatever the basic cause of the hyperglycaemia. The implication of these criteria is that *there is no such thing as 'mild' diabetes not requiring effective treatment.*

Diabetes is world-wide in distribution and the incidence of both types of primary diabetes, i.e. Insulin Dependent Diabetes Mellitus (IDDM) (sometimes called type I diabetes) and Non-Insulin Dependent Diabetes (NIDDM) (sometimes called type II diabetes) is rising. However, the prevalence of both varies considerably in different parts of the world. This seems to be due to differences in both genetic and environmental factors. The prevalence in Britain is between 1 and 2% but almost 50% of cases of NIDDM remain undetected. The great majority of cases seen world-wide have primary diabetes and in Europe and North America the ratio of NIDDM:IDDM is approximately 7:3.

AETIOLOGY

Although the precise aetiology is still uncertain in both main types of primary diabetes, environmental factors interact with a genetic susceptibility to determine which of those with the genetic predisposition actually develop the clinical syndrome and the timing of its onset. However, both the pattern of inheritance and the environmental factors differ in IDDM and NIDDM.

IDDM

Genetics

The inheritance of human IDDM is polygenic. It has been estimated that over 50% of the heritability is contributed by the HLA class II genes (that is the D loci on the short arm of chromosome 6) which determine immune responsiveness. Within this region the strongest association is with the DQ locus which is subdivided into alpha and beta loci. Although analysis of DNA sequences from patients with IDDM has not so far shown unique class II sequences, it has been found that susceptibility to IDDM is directly related to the amino acid at position 57 of the N-terminal B-1 domain of the

HLA-DQ beta chain. Thus almost complete resistance to the development of IDDM is conferred by inheritance of two alleles with aspartic acid at position 57 (Asp 57-positive homozygosity), while maximum susceptibility is associated with Asp 57-negative homozygosity, that is alanine, valine or serine substituted for aspartate (>80% of IDDM patients), and Asp 57 heterozygosity carries a much lower risk of developing IDDM (10% of IDDM patients). It is thought that DQ beta polymorphisms determine the specificity and extent of an autoimmune response against pancreatic islet insulin-secreting cells and are necessary, but not in themselves sufficient, for the development of IDDM. This implies either the existence of other specific IDDM-related gene(s) or involvement of more than one HLA-D gene controlling the intensity of the beta cell destructive process (which appears to be mediated by cytokines), or an important role for environmental factors in clinical expression of the disease in genetically susceptible persons. The latter hypothesis is supported by the fact that about 60% of pairs of monozygotic twins are discordant for IDDM.

OVERALL RISK OF DEVELOPING IDDM IN AN INDIVIDUAL WITH A FIRST DEGREE RELATIVE WITH IDDM

Relative with IDDM	% risk
• Identical twin	36
• HLA identical sib	12
• Non-HLA identical sib	6
• Father	6
• Mother	2

Environmental factors

Viruses

The evidence that viral infection might cause some forms of human IDDM is derived from epidemiological studies and isolated case reports. Studies in mice have shown that viruses can induce diabetes by two distinct pathogenic mechanisms: destruction of the pancreatic beta cells by direct cytolysis results from infection with the D variant of the EMC virus, Mengo virus 2T and Coxsackie B4 virus; induction of an autoimmune destructive process results from infection with reo virus type 1 and rubella. The ability of viruses to induce diabetes in mice is dependent on the genetic background of the host as well as on the genetic makeup of the virus. The induction of diabetes by infection with EMC, Mengo or Coxsackie B4 viruses can be prevented by administration of live attenuated vaccine while reo virus-induced diabetes can be prevented by immuno-suppression.

Diet

Dietary factors have been invoked as a possible explanation for the rising incidence of IDDM in Northern Europe and North America. There are no direct data relating diet after weaning to the development of IDDM in genetically susceptible children. However, two reports have provided circumstantial evidence supporting the proposition that dietary factors may at least in certain circumstances influence the development of human IDDM. Thus an unusually high incidence of IDDM in boys born in the month of October in Iceland has been linked to the high nitrosamine content of a smoked mutton traditionally consumed at Christmas. Subsequent experiments in mice suggested that this effect was mediated via the parental germ cells rather than by a direct effect on the pancreatic beta cells of the fetus. In the second report anti-gliadin antibodies were reported in 54% of children (none of whom had coeliac disease) at diagnosis of IDDM under 2 years of age. In addition, studies using the spontaneously diabetic, insulin-dependent BB rat suggest that certain components of the diet may be essential for the expression of clinical IDDM in genetically susceptible animals. Wheat and milk protein have been shown to have the strongest diabetogenic effect and are evidently capable of triggering the string of events which results ultimately in destruction of pancreatic islet insulin-secreting cells.

Recent population studies have shown that introduction of cow's milk before the age of 2–3 months is associated with the presence of antibodies to bovine serum albumin and an increased risk of developing IDDM. It is suggested that a short sequence of bovine serum albumin may cross-react with a protein (p69) which can be induced on the pancreatic islet beta cell membrane by the inflammatory mediator interferon-gamma.

Immunological factors

The information box below summarises the evidence that IDDM is a slow autoimmune disease. Detailed family studies have produced evidence that contrary to clinical impression destruction of the insulin-secreting cells in the pancreas is a slow process occurring over many years. Hyperglycaemia accompanied by the classical symptoms of diabetes occurs only when 90% of insulin-secreting cells are already destroyed. It is clear also that in both humans and animals with spontaneous insulin-dependent diabetes the immune system retains the capacity to recognise and destroy transplanted insulin-secreting cells indefinitely.

Pancreatic pathology

Three outstanding features characterise the pathological picture in the prediabetic pancreas in IDDM:

EVIDENCE THAT IDDM IS A SLOW AUTOIMMUNE DISEASE

- HLA-linked genetic predisposition
- Association with other autoimmune disorders
- Circulating islet cell cytoplasmic and surface and insulin-autoantibodies in new cases
- Mononuclear cell infiltration of pancreatic islets resulting in selective destruction of insulin-secreting cells
- Recurrence of insulitis and selective destruction of insulin-secreting cells in pancreatic grafts

- 'Insulitis', that is infiltration of the islets with mononuclear cells.
- The initial patchiness of this lesion, with, until a very late stage, lobules containing heavily infiltrated islets commonly seen immediately adjacent to unaffected lobules.
- The striking beta cell specificity of the destructive process within infiltrated islets where the glucagon and other hormone-secreting cells invariably remain intact.

Figure 12.31 shows the sequence of pancreatic events in the development of IDDM.

NIDDM

Genetics

NIDDM is not HLA-linked and there is no evidence that autoimmunity or viruses have anything to do with its development. Studies of monozygotic twins have shown that genetic factors are more important in the development of this type of diabetes than in IDDM, with concordance for NIDDM approaching 100%, but there is little information about what is inherited.

One of the most characteristic features of NIDDM is that it is commonly associated with several other disorders such as obesity, hypertension and hyperlipidaemia. It has been suggested that this cluster of conditions is a specific entity ('Syndrome X' or the 'Metabolic Syndrome') with insulin resistance being the primary defect. It seems likely that the various components of the Metabolic Syndrome represent separate polygenic items each of which is expressed at a clinical level by a 'Westernised' lifestyle so that a higher than expected proportion meet the diagnostic criteria of disease. But although NIDDM commonly occurs in subjects who are obese and insulin-resistant these two are insufficient to cause diabetes unless accompanied by impaired beta cell function. Therefore it seems likely

Hyperexpression of class I MHC antigens within islets and on vascular endothelium

Insulitis

(infiltrate contains activated macrophages, helper cytotoxic and suppressor T lymphocytes, natural killer cells, and B lymphocytes)

Intense expression of class I MHC antigens now extends to all pancreatic cells

Selective destruction of beta cells

End stage islet with no residual insulin consisting of clumps of glucagon and somatostatin secreting cells

Regression of infiltrate

Fig. 12.31 Sequence of pancreatic events in the development of IDDM.

that NIDDM represents a combination of major and minor genes affecting insulin secretion, insulin action and obesity. Although so far no specific genetic variation has been shown to be consistently linked with NIDDM, a mutation of the glucokinase gene is associated with some cases of the uncommon syndrome of Maturity Onset Diabetes in the Young (MODY).

Environmental factors

Lifestyle

Epidemiological studies of NIDDM provide evidence that over-eating, especially when combined with obesity and underactivity, is associated with the development of NIDDM. Other more direct studies have shown that middle-aged diabetic patients eat significantly more and are fatter and less active than their non-diabetic siblings. The majority of middle-aged diabetic patients are obese but only a few obese people develop diabetes. Obesity probably acts as a diabetogenic factor (through increasing resistance to the action of insulin) in those genetically predisposed to develop NIDDM.

Age

In Britain over 70% of all cases of diabetes occur after the age of 50 years. In contrast to IDDM which mainly affects younger people, NIDDM is principally a disease of the middle-aged and elderly. Thus ageing is an important risk factor for NIDDM.

Pregnancy

During normal pregnancy the level of plasma insulin is raised by the action of placental hormones, thus placing a burden on the insulin-secreting cells of the pancreatic islets. The pancreas may be unable to meet these demands in women genetically predisposed to develop both types of diabetes. The term 'gestational diabetes' refers to hyperglycaemia occurring for the first time during pregnancy (p. 760). This may or may not disappear following delivery. Repeated pregnancy may increase the likelihood of developing permanent diabetes, particularly in obese women. Long-term studies show that some 80% of women with gestational diabetes ultimately develop permanent clinical diabetes requiring treatment.

Pancreatic pathology and insulin secretion

In contrast to IDDM where at diagnosis the insulin-secreting cells have largely disappeared from the pancreas so that plasma immunoreactive insulin is either very low or undetectable, in NIDDM there is only moderate reduction in the total mass of islet tissue consistent with a measurable, though, when related to the blood glucose level, reduced concentration of insulin in plasma. There are, however, some pathological changes which are typical of NIDDM and demonstrable in most, although not all cases. The most consistent of these changes is probably deposition of amyloid which is accompanied by atrophy of the normal tissue, particularly islet epithelial cells. In more advanced lesions, the islet is more or less converted to amyloid and the reduction in the number of insulin-secreting cells is more pronounced than that of glucagon-secreting cells. Islet amyloid is not a qualitative marker of NIDDM but rather a quantitative one. Heavy deposition of amyloid in islets is rare without diabetes. Small quantities of islet amyloid are very common in elderly non-diabetic patients. Deposition of amyloid is probably not a cause of diabetes but rather reflects a pathological process which is increased in NIDDM.

Insulin resistance

Increased hepatic production of glucose and resistance to the action of insulin in muscle are invariable in both obese and non-obese patients with NIDDM.

Insulin resistance may be due to any one of three general causes: an abnormal insulin molecule, an excess-
ive amount of circulating antagonists, and target tissue defects. The last is the common cause of insulin resistance in NIDDM and seems to be the predominant abnormality in those with more severe hyperglycaemia.

PATHOPHYSIOLOGY, CLINICAL FEATURES AND DIAGNOSIS

Actions of insulin

Insulin has profound effects on the metabolism of carbohydrate, fat, protein and electrolytes (Table 12.15). These can be divided into anabolic and anticatabolic actions. The balance of these effects in the fasting and post-prandial states, and during exercise is controlled by:

1. variation in the relative circulating concentration of insulin (the only anabolic hormone) and several catabolic hormones, namely glucagon, growth hormone, cortisol, catecholamines and thyroid hormones (Table 12.16)
2. the fact that insulin exerts its anticatabolic effects at a lower concentration than that required for its anabolic actions.

During an oral glucose tolerance test (Fig. 12.32) or a mixed meal the first one-and-a-half hours are dominated by increased secretion of insulin, and both growth hormone and glucagon secretion are inhibited. Cortisol and adrenaline levels do not change significantly.

Exercise represents a special stress with a rapid

Table 12.15 Actions of insulin

Increase (anabolic effects)	Decrease (anticatabolic effects)
Carbohydrate metabolism	
Glucose transport (muscle, adipose tissue)	Gluconeogenesis
Glucose phosphorylation	Glycogenolysis
Glycogenesis	
Glycolysis	
Pyruvate dehydrogenase activity	
Pentose phosphate shunt	
Lipid metabolism	
Triglyceride synthesis	Lipolysis
Fatty acid synthesis (liver)	Lipoprotein lipase (muscle)
Lipoprotein lipase (adipose tissue) activity	Ketogenesis
	Fatty acid oxidation (liver)
Protein metabolism	
Amino acid transport	Protein degradation
Protein synthesis	
Electrolytes	
Cellular potassium uptake	

Table 12.16 Probable actions of hormones countering the effect of insulin in man

	Insulin release	Muscle glucose uptake	Hepatic gluconeogenesis	Ketogenesis	Lipolysis	Proteolysis
Catecholamines	↓	↓	↑	↑	↑	↑
Glucagon	—	—	↑	↑	—	—
Growth hormone	—	↓	—	↑	↑	↓
Glucocorticoids	—	↓	↑	↑	↑	↑
Thyroid hormones	—	—	↑	↑	↑	↑

↑ = increase; ↓ = decrease; — = no significant primary effect.

increase in the demand for metabolic fuel. At rest 90% of the energy requirements of muscle come from fatty acids and ketone bodies. In the initial stages of strenuous exercise, energy comes from oxidation of stored glycogen but, if the demand for oxygen outstrips supply, anaerobic glycolysis becomes all important. Glycogen supplies are rapidly depleted and glucose is extracted from the circulation independent of insulin. Blood glucose levels fall and secretion of insulin also decreases. Catecholamine and cortisol levels rise, stimulating lipolysis and gluconeogenesis. The increase in hepatic glucose production matches the increased extrahepatic utilisation so that glucose levels do not change markedly (Fig. 12.33). As anaerobic glycolysis continues, blood lactate concentration rises and this is recycled by the liver as new glucose.

PATHOPHYSIOLOGY

Whatever the aetiology, in all cases the hyperglycaemia of diabetes develops because of an absolute (IDDM) or relative (NIDDM) deficiency of insulin which leads to:

- Decreased anabolism
- Increased catabolism.

Figure 12.34 relates the metabolic consequences of lack of insulin to its symptoms. When the concentration of glucose in the plasma exceeds the renal threshold (that is the capacity of renal tubules to reabsorb glucose from the glomerular filtrate), glycosuria occurs. The renal threshold is approximately 10 mmol/l but there is wide individual variation. Note that the severity of the classical symptoms of diabetes, namely polyuria and polydipsia, is related directly to the degree of glycosuria. If hyperglycaemia develops slowly over many months or even years, as in NIDDM, the renal threshold for glucose rises and both glycosuria and the symptoms of diabetes are then correspondingly slight. This is one reason for the large number of undetected cases of NIDDM. Such individuals may have significant but symptomless hyperglycaemia for many years before glycosuria is noted on routine urine testing. Sometimes they eventually present with symptoms due to one or more of the complications of long-term diabetes: paraesthesiae, pain, and muscle atrophy in the legs, or impotence due to neuropathy; deterioration of vision due to retinopathy; or ulceration of the feet due to a combination of neuropathy, peripheral vascular disease and infection. Uncontrolled diabetes is associated with an increased susceptibility to infection and patients may present with skin sepsis, intractable and recurrent urinary tract infections, pulmonary tuberculosis or poor healing of a wound following surgery.

A minority of cases of diabetes first present as severe ketoacidosis, either associated with an acute infection or other illness or even without evidence of a precipitating cause. In such cases abdominal pain and vomiting may be the presenting complaints. This is more likely to occur in IDDM. Diabetic ketoacidosis must therefore be considered in the differential diagnosis of a patient who complains of acute abdominal symptoms.

Mechanisms underlying the development of ketoacidosis

The extent to which increased lipolysis occurs is proportional to the degree of insulin deficiency. If the latter is marked the normal response to feeding, namely suppression of lipolysis, may be lost and the plasma concentration of non-esterified fatty acids may remain constantly elevated. Fatty acids are taken up by the liver and degraded through 8 steps within the mitochondria of the liver cells. Each stage yields one molecule of acetyl-co-enzyme A. Normally most of these molecules enter the citric acid cycle by condensing with oxaloacetic acid but, in the absence of insulin, more is formed than can enter the citric acid cycle and acetyl-co-enzyme A is converted to aceto-acetic acid. Most of this is then reduced to beta hydroxy-butyric acid, while some is decarboxylated to acetone. These ketone bodies, when formed in small amounts, are oxidised and utilised as

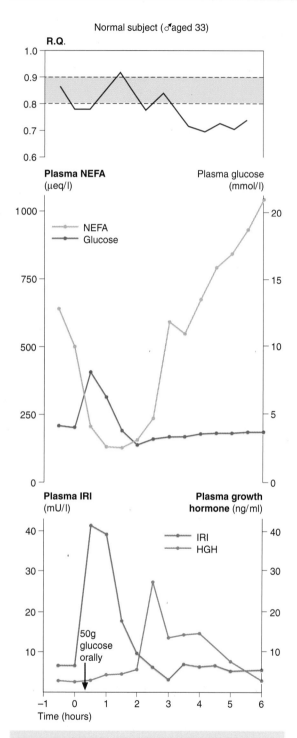

Fig. 12.32 Changes in respiratory quotient and plasma concentration of glucose, non-esterified fatty acids, immunoreactive insulin and human growth hormone following ingestion of 50 g glucose by a normal, thin young man.

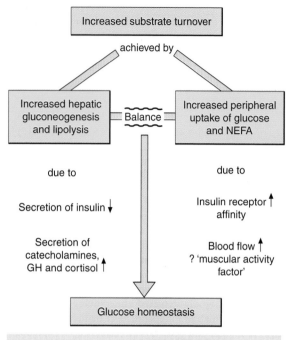

Fig. 12.33 Main features of the metabolic adaptation to moderate exercise.

metabolic fuel. However, the rate of utilisation of ketone bodies is limited. When the rate of production by the liver exceeds that of removal by the peripheral tissues then hyperketonaemia results.

Ketone bodies increase the osmolality of plasma and so also lead to withdrawal of water from cells. They are acids which dissociate almost completely at physiological pH, releasing hydrogen ions into the body fluids. The fall in pH is countered by the buffers of the blood, the most important being bicarbonate. The dissociation of carbonic acid is reduced, the ratio of bicarbonate ions to carbonic ions falls, and measurement of plasma bicarbonate will show a lower value than normal. The rise in hydrogen ion concentration in the arterial blood stimulates pulmonary ventilation so that hyperpnoea or 'air hunger' is observed clinically.

The extent to which the clinical features of dehydration and ketoacidosis are seen in the individual case will depend on such factors as the speed at which the condition develops and the extent to which the patient increases the intake of fluid as well as on the degree of insulin deficiency present. Thus when insulin deficiency is partial, as in patients with NIDDM, the anticatabolic effect of insulin may be relatively well preserved while its anabolic action is more seriously defective. In these circumstances lipolysis is not markedly accelerated and the concentration of ketone bodies in the blood remains

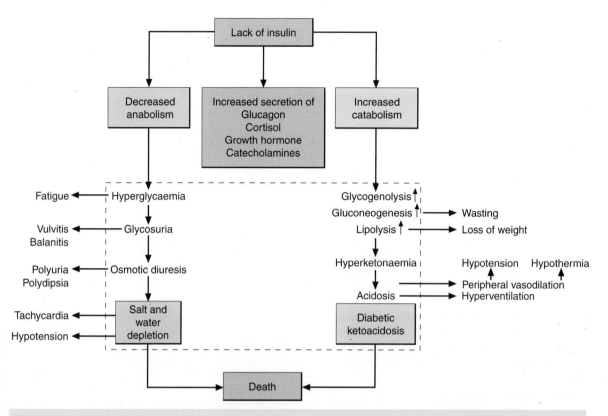

Fig. 12.34 Pathophysiological basis of the symptoms and signs of untreated or uncontrolled diabetes mellitus.

relatively normal despite severe hyperglycaemia. This state has been designated 'hyperosmolar diabetic coma'.

CLINICAL FEATURES

In Table 12.17 the classical clinical features of the two main types of diabetes are compared. While the distinction between IDDM and NIDDM is broadly true in relation to the features listed, overlap occurs particularly in age at onset of diabetes, duration of symptoms and family history. Thus some young people have a form of NIDDM designated Maturity Onset Diabetes in the Young (the MODY syndrome) while some middle-aged and elderly patients present with typical autoimmune type I IDDM.

Patients with IDDM usually show no physical signs attributable to diabetes. In the fulminating case the most striking features are those of salt and water depletion, that is a loose dry skin, a furred tongue and cracked lips, tachycardia, hypotension and reduced intraocular pressure. Breathing may be deep and sighing due to acidosis, the breath is usually fetid and the sickly sweet

Table 12.17 Comparative clinical features of IDDM and NIDDM

	IDDM	NIDDM
Age at onset	<40 years	>50 years
Duration of symptoms	Weeks	Months-years
Body weight	Normal or low	Obese
Ketonuria	Yes	No
Rapid death without treatment with insulin	Yes	No
Autoantibodies	Yes	No
Diabetic complications at diagnosis	No	10–20%
Family history of diabetes	No	Yes
Other autoimmune disease	Yes	No

smell of acetone may be apparent. Mental apathy, confusion or coma may also be present.

The physical signs present in patients with NIDDM at diagnosis depend on the mode of presentation. Pruritus vulvae or balanitis is a common presenting symptom since the external genitalia are especially prone to infection by fungi (candida) which flourish on skin and mucous membranes contaminated by glucose. Ophthalmoscopy may show the typical appearances of diabetic retinopathy. Depression or loss of the tendon reflexes at the ankles and impaired perception of vibration sensation distally in the legs indicate neuropathy. Other abnormalities of neurological examination are less common. Hypertension and signs of atherosclerosis are common and may include diminished or impalpable pulses in the feet, bruits over the carotid or femoral arteries and gangrene of the feet. Signs of water and salt depletion with associated mental changes may be seen in cases with severe hyperglycaemia.

Apart from patients with established clinical diabetes two other categories are recognised: potential and latent diabetes.

Potential diabetics are persons with a normal glucose tolerance test who have an increased risk of developing diabetes for genetic reasons, e.g. an individual who has a first-degree relative with diabetes. The information box (p. 726) shows the approximate overall risk of an individual developing IDDM when various first-degree relatives already have IDDM, while the information box below shows the risk of developing NIDDM up to the age of 80 years for siblings of probands with NIDDM subdivided according to age at onset.

RISK OF DEVELOPING NIDDM

Up to the age of 80 years for siblings of probands with NIDDM

Age at onset of NIDDM in proband	Age corrected risk of NIDDM for siblings (%)
25–44	52.9
45–54	36.5
55–64	38.4
65–80	30.7
Overall 25–80	37.9

Latent diabetics are persons in whom the glucose tolerance test is normal but who are known to have given an abnormal result under conditions imposing a burden on the islet beta cells, e.g. during pregnancy, infection or other severe stress, mental or physical, during treatment with corticosteroids, thiazide diuretics or other diabetogenic drugs, or when overweight.

Potential and latent diabetic patients usually complain of no symptoms and show no abnormality on examination. However, certain features are recognised as being characteristic of such states without necessarily implying that such individuals will progress to clinical diabetes. For example, they are predisposed to coronary and peripheral arterial disease, may show abnormal lipid patterns in response to oral contraceptives, and have an increased incidence of stillborn, abnormally large and heavy babies and babies with congenital defects.

DIAGNOSIS

When the symptoms suggest diabetes the diagnosis may be confirmed by finding glycosuria, with or without ketonuria, and a random blood glucose concentration greater than 14 mmol/l. This is shown in the information box below.

DIAGNOSIS OF DIABETES

Patient complains of symptoms suggesting diabetes
- Test urine for glucose and ketones
- Measure random blood glucose, plasma electrolytes, HbA_1. Diagnosis confirmed by random plasma glucose
  >14 mmol/l $\pm$ HbA_1 $>9.0\%$

Indications for glucose tolerance test
- Glycosuria $\pm$ ketonuria found on routine urine test
- Patient has minimal or no symptoms
- Random plasma glucose 6.0–13.0 mmol/l $\pm$ HbA_1 8–9%

Urine testing

Testing the urine for glucose is the most usual procedure for detecting diabetes, both in the consulting room and in population screening surveys. Sensitive and glucose-specific dipstick methods are available. A positive response gives a rough indication that the urinary glucose concentration exceeds 0.55–1.11 mmol/l. If possible, the test for urinary glucose should be performed on urine passed 1.5–2 hours after a main meal since this will detect more of the milder cases of diabetes than a fasting urine specimen.

The most serious disadvantage of using urinary glucose as a diagnostic or screening procedure is the individual variation in renal threshold. Thus some undoubtedly diabetic individuals will have a negative urine test whilst other non-diabetic individuals with a low renal threshold for glucose will give a positive result. Estimation of the blood glucose concentration (either in a random sample of blood or following a 75 g oral glucose load), using an accurate laboratory method rather than a side-room technique, is therefore essential in making the diagnosis (see information box above), and glycosuria, however slight, always warrants full assessment.

Clinically important amounts of ketone bodies can be recognised by the nitroprusside reaction which is conveniently carried out using tablets or test papers. Ketonuria may be found in normal people who have been fasting or exercising strenuously for long periods, who have been vomiting repeatedly or who have been eating a diet very high in fats and low in carbohydrate. Ketonuria is therefore not pathognomonic of diabetes

Venous plasma glucose mmol/l (mg/100 ml)

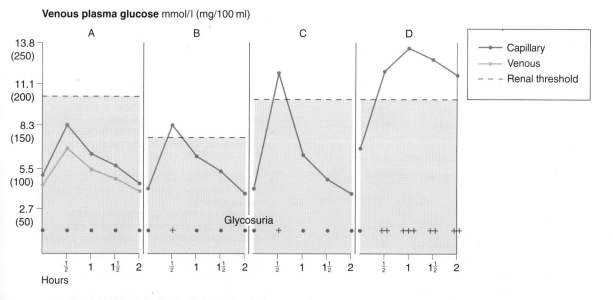

Fig. 12.35 The glucose tolerance test

Fig. 12.35   The glucose tolerance test: blood glucose curves after 75 g glucose by mouth, showing A normal curve, B normal curve but with a low renal threshold leading to renal glycosuria, C alimentary (lag storage) glycosuria and D diabetes mellitus of moderate severity.

but, if both ketonuria and glycosuria are found, the diagnosis of diabetes is practically certain.

Gestational diabetes

The term 'gestational diabetes' is used to refer to hyperglycaemia occurring for the first time during pregnancy in individuals who have an inherited predisposition to develop diabetes. Both IDDM and NIDDM are involved. The hyperglycaemia may or may not disappear following delivery. Normal pregnancy is characterised by hyperinsulinaemia in response to the production of hormonal insulin antagonists such as human placental lactogen and progesterone. A suboptimal endocrine pancreas may be unable to meet this demand. Since even minimal hyperglycaemia in pregnancy is associated with increased perinatal mortality and morbidity it is important to detect and treat these cases effectively. Detection may present problems. Glycosuria is common in normal pregnancy (due to a fall in the renal threshold for glucose secondary to an increase in the glomerular filtration rate) and in late pregnancy lactose appears in the urine. The finding of reducing substances in the urine of a pregnant woman should, however, never be lightly dismissed and in all cases the blood glucose concentration should be carefully measured (see p. 761).

The oral glucose tolerance test

The patient, who should have been taking an unrestricted carbohydrate diet for at least 3 days prior to the test, fasts overnight. Ideally out-patients should rest for at least half an hour before starting the test, and should remain seated and refrain from smoking during the test. A sample of blood is taken to measure the fasting plasma glucose level and 75 g glucose dissolved in 300 ml of water is then given by mouth. Thereafter samples of blood are collected at half-hourly intervals for at least 2 hours and their glucose content is estimated. The diagnostic criteria for diabetes mellitus and normality recommended by WHO in 1985 are shown in Table 12.18, page 734. Intermediate readings are classified as Impaired Glucose Tolerance and indicate the need for further evaluation of the patient including the history. It may be necessary to keep the patient under observation and to repeat the test at a later date. The diagnostic criteria for diabetes in pregnancy are more stringent than those recommended for non-pregnant subjects and pregnant women with impaired glucose tolerance should be referred urgently to a specialist unit for full evaluation.

Renal glycosuria

Apart from diabetes the commonest cause of glycosuria is a low renal threshold for glucose (Fig. 12.35) which commonly occurs temporarily in pregnancy and is a much more frequent cause of glycosuria than diabetes in young people. Renal glycosuria is a benign condition unrelated to diabetes and is not accompanied by the classical symptoms associated with diabetes.

Table 12.18 Diagnostic criteria for diabetes mellitus using an oral glucose (75 g) tolerance test (WHO 1985)

	Venous plasma (whole blood) glucose concentration mmol/l	
	Normal	Diabetic
Fasting	<6.1(5.6)	≥7.8 (6.7)
2 hours after glucose	<8.9 (6.7)	≥11.1 (10.0)

Note:
1. These figures refer to the concentration of glucose estimated by a specific enzymatic assay.
2. Most hospital laboratories measure the concentration of glucose in plasma samples.

Alimentary (lag storage) glycosuria

In some individuals an unusually rapid but transitory rise of blood glucose follows a meal and the concentration exceeds the normal renal threshold; during this time glucose will be present in the urine. This response to a meal or to a dose of glucose is traditionally known as a 'lag storage' blood glucose curve, although alimentary glycosuria is a better term (Fig. 12.35). It may occur in otherwise normal people or after gastric surgery when it is due to rapid gastric emptying leading to an increased rate of absorption of glucose into the blood stream. It is not uncommonly seen in patients with hyperthyroidism, peptic ulceration or hepatic disease. This type of blood glucose curve is usually regarded as benign and unrelated to diabetes: although the peak blood glucose concentration is abnormally high, the value 2 hours after oral glucose is normal.

MANAGEMENT

Three methods of treatment are available for diabetic patients: diet alone, diet and an oral hypoglycaemic drug, and diet and insulin. Approximately 50% of new cases of diabetes can be controlled adequately by diet alone, 20–30% will need an oral hypoglycaemic drug and 20–30% will require insulin. Regardless of aetiology the type of treatment required is determined by the circulating plasma immunoreactive insulin concentration (Fig. 12.36, p. 736). At a clinical level the age and weight of the patient at diagnosis are closely correlated with the plasma insulin concentration and indicate with a high degree of probability the type of treatment likely to be required (Fig. 12.37, p. 736). However, the regimen eventually adopted in each individual case is ultimately chosen by therapeutic trial.

SUMMARY OF DIAGNOSIS OF DIABETES

- Diabetes is a very common disorder—50% of cases are undiagnosed; 10–20% already have serious vascular disease at presentation. Diabetic retinopathy is the commonest cause of blindness in the UK.
- The earlier diabetes is diagnosed the easier it is to treat effectively and the greater the chance of avoiding the development of serious vascular disease.
- Testing the urine for sugar is an essential part of a routine clinical examination. The urine sample tested should preferably be passed within 2 hours of a main meal.
- All patients with glycosuria should be considered diabetic until proved otherwise on the basis of blood measurements.
- A negative urine test for sugar does not exclude diabetes. A case can be made for including *accurate* measurement of the glucose concentration in a random plasma sample as an essential component of a routine clinical examination.
- Wherever practicable, estimation of the blood glucose concentration 2 hours after 75 g glucose orally should be used as the screening test for detecting diabetes.
- HbA_1 alone is not sensitive enough to detect early, relatively mild cases of diabetes.
- Particular attention should be paid to high-risk groups such as the first-degree relatives of known diabetics, the obese, and pregnant women.

DIETARY MANAGEMENT

General principles

Dietary measures are required in the treatment of all diabetic patients to achieve the overall therapeutic goal: normal metabolism. The purposes of dietary measures are set out in the information box below.

PURPOSES OF DIETARY MEASURES IN THE MANAGEMENT OF DIABETES

Dietary measure	Purpose
Maintain daily intake of food constant from day to day in nutritional content and distribution	Allow matching of insulin/tablet regime to diet
Specify total daily energy intake	Maintain desirable body weight
Allocate proportion of energy derived from carbohydrate, protein and fat (see information box)	Avoid atherogenic diet
Reduce rate of carbohydrate absorption (see information box)	Avoid glycaemic peaks and troughs
Frequent, relatively small meals, i.e. 3 main meals and 3 between-meal snacks	Avoid glycaemic peaks and troughs

Daily energy intake

The first step in preparing any dietary regimen is to decide the individual patient's daily energy requirement. This must be estimated after considering such factors as age, sex, actual weight in relation to desirable weight, activity and occupation. An approximate range for the various groups of patients might be:

an obese middle-aged or elderly person, 1000–1600 kcal daily;
an elderly person not overweight, 1400–1800 kcal daily;
a young active person, 1800–3000 kcal daily.

The body weight should be maintained at or slightly below the ideal for the patient's height. Thus these suggested ranges for energy intake for the various groups of patients may have to be extended after considering this, e.g. young overweight patients may have to have their daily intake reduced to below 1800 kcal while elderly thin patients may require more than 1800 kcal to maintain weight.

Proportion of energy derived from proximate principles

Next the proportion of energy derived from carbohydrate, protein and fat must be allocated.

PROPORTION OF ENERGY DERIVED FROM CARBOHYDRATE, PROTEIN, FAT		
	UK national diet	Recommended diet
Carbohydrate	42%	50–60%
Protein	15%	10–15%
Fat	40%	30–35%

This information box shows the approximate ratio in the British national diet. The intake of fat is high and a large proportion of this consists of saturated fat. This type of diet is generally considered to be atherogenic and it is recommended that the percentage of calories derived from carbohydrate should be increased and that from fat reduced. Diabetic patients are peculiarly prone to develop atherosclerosis and it is therefore particularly important that the general guidelines issued to the public by nutritional organisations concerned with heart disease should be followed by diabetic patients. It is important to realise, and to explain to the individual diabetic patient, that the 'diabetic diet' is simply that which is now recommended for the population in general.

Carbohydrate and fibre

All the carbohydrate prescribed should be taken in the form of starches and other complex sugars. Simple sugars such as glucose and sucrose should generally be avoided because they may cause a sudden rise in the blood glucose concentration. The daily intake of carbohydrate ranges from 100 g (the minimum sufficient to prevent ketonuria) to a maximum of 300 g. In the latter case each of 3 main meals can provide 60 g carbohydrate, each of 3 snacks 30 g, and 30 g comes in 0.5 l milk taken in the course of the day.

Slowing the rate of carbohydrate absorption may be usefully exploited in the treatment of diabetes. The information box lists methods by which this has been achieved.

> **METHODS OF SLOWING THE RATE OF CARBOHYDRATE ABSORPTION**
>
> - Nibbling rather than gorging
> - Use of soluble fibre supplements and soluble fibre-rich foods
> - Use of foods with low glycaemic index
> - Alpha-glucosidase inhibition

Spreading the nutrient load throughout the day as 3 main meals and 3 snacks ('nibbling' as opposed to 'gorging') not only results in lower blood lipid as well as reduced blood glucose and insulin concentrations in all diabetic patients but also, in the case of those taking insulin or an oral hypoglycaemic agent, safeguards against the development of hypoglycaemia. Consumption of both soluble fibre supplements (e.g. guar, pectin, locust bean gum) and fibre-rich foods (e.g. barley, oats, legumes, beans, peas and lentils) has been associated with improved blood glucose control and lower blood lipids in both normal, diabetic and hyperlipidaemic persons. Long-term compliance is better with fibre-rich foods than with soluble fibre supplements. Classification of foods according to their acute effect on the blood glucose concentration ('glycaemic index') has been suggested as a useful means of determining the optimal carbohydrate foods for diabetic patients but is not widely used. This applies also to the use of enzyme inhibitors (anti-amylase, sucrase and maltase activity) and alpha-glucosidase inhibition with acarbose. Although their use has been shown to reduce post-prandial glucose, insulin and triglyceride concentrations, the side-effects are troublesome in some patients and the long-term effects are uncertain.

Protein

In patients with NIDDM, consumption of protein along with carbohydrate will lower the blood glucose concentration due to amino-acid stimulation of insulin secretion; this helps to compensate for the defect in glucose-mediated insulin secretion seen in so many of these patients. Protein also promotes satiety and helps

Plasma insulin (mU/l)

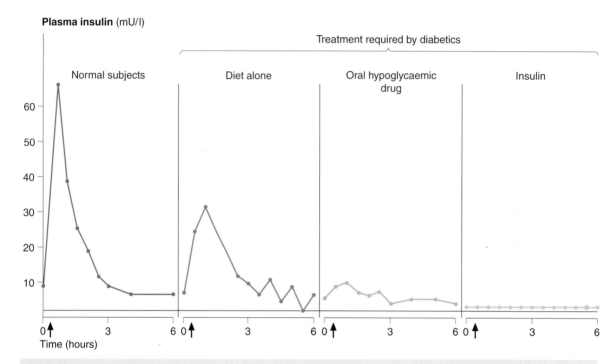

Fig. 12.36 Mean (± SEM) plasma concentration of immunoreactive insulin in the fasting state and at half-hourly intervals after 50 g glucose orally (indicated by ↑) in normal subjects and in newly diagnosed untreated diabetic patients grouped on the basis of the treatment they were subsequently found to require on clinical grounds. The solid line at the foot of the section relating to insulin secretion indicates the lower limit of sensitivity of the assay.

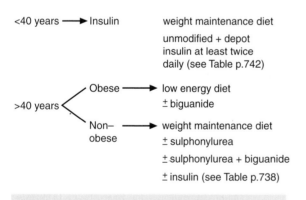

Fig. 12.37 The long-term type of treatment probably required by any individual patient can be determined by considering their age and weight at diagnosis of diabetes.

both types of diabetic patient to adhere to the carbohydrate allowance.

Fat
The total intake of fat should be reduced and the proportion of unsaturated fat increased if possible. Frying food is a traditional way of cooking for many people and they need to be made aware of other methods of cooking such as grilling, baking, poaching and steaming. Fish is particularly rich in long-chain polyunsaturated fatty acids.

Alcohol
In general, diabetic individuals should take the same precautions regarding alcohol intake as the general population. However, account must be taken of:

- the energy and sometimes the carbohydrate content of alcoholic drinks
- the fact that alcohol may potentiate the hypoglycaemic action of oral hypoglycaemic drugs and of insulin
- the tendency of alcohol to predispose towards the development of lactic acidosis in patients taking biguanides (p. 740)
- the fact that alcohol can induce a disulfiram type of reaction (p. 739) in patients taking sulphonylurea drugs.

Abstinence should be encouraged if obesity, hypertension or hypertriglyceridaemia is present.

Salt

Diabetic patients should follow the advice given to the general population, namely to reduce sodium intake to no more than 6 g daily. Further restriction of sodium intake (to less than 3 g daily) is important in the management of hypertensive diabetic patients.

Diabetic foods and sweeteners

Low calorie and sugar-free drinks are useful for patients on low calorie diets. These drinks usually contain non-nutritive sweeteners. Many 'diabetic foods' contain sorbitol or fructose which may have gastrointestinal side-effects, are relatively high in energy, may be expensive and are therefore not particularly recommended as part of the diabetic diet.

Non-nutritive sweeteners (saccharin, aspartame, sucramate and acesulphame K) are the most widely used non-nutritive sweeteners and provide means for reducing energy intake without loss of palatability.

Nutritive sweeteners, sorbitol and fructose are particularly useful in baking. They contain as many calories as sucrose and their total intake should not therefore exceed 50 g daily. Gastrointestinal side-effects do not usually occur at these quantities provided the intake is spread over the day.

Types of diabetic diets

Two basic types of diet are used in the treatment of diabetes: low energy, weight-reducing diets and weight maintenance diets. The benefits of a reduction in body weight on the metabolism of the obese patient with NIDDM are striking (Fig. 12.38). Even where the initial blood glucose concentration is high and the plasma immunoreactive insulin low, additional treatment with insulin or an oral hypoglycaemic agent can often be avoided. The benefit of weight reduction on the mortality rate of obese non-diabetic persons is well known and applies even more strikingly to obese diabetics. Management of obese people (both diabetic and non-diabetic) with a diet low in refined and high in unrefined carbohydrate and restricted in total energy content results in increased insulin sensitivity which is associated with a rapid fall in the blood glucose concentration in diabetic, obese patients. The precise mechanism of this effect is uncertain. Reduction in body weight increases this effect, and in the long run the plasma insulin concentration rises in many patients as shown in Figure 12.38.

Low energy, weight-reducing diet

Diabetics who are obese should adhere to a strict low calorie diet. The method of achieving reduction in weight is the same for obese diabetic patients as for those with simple obesity (see p. 582). A strict diet is to be

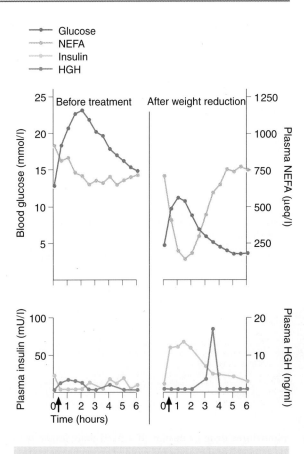

Fig. 12.38 Changes in the concentration of blood glucose and plasma non-esterified fatty acids, immunoreactive insulin, and human growth hormone following ingestion of 50 g glucose (↑) in an obese patient with NIDDM at diagnosis and after reduction in weight. Note the marked rise in plasma IRI and the restoration of the normal postprandial surge of HGH following treatment with a low energy diet.

followed only temporarily until the standard weight is reached; thereafter the diet may be increased, and if the patient is sufficiently intelligent, advice can then be given on how to avoid monotony by using a list of exchanges for diabetic diets. The administration of a sulphonylurea or insulin should be avoided if at all possible in these patients since both increase appetite and weight and intensify the total disability. Metformin has a place in the treatment of obese, non-insulin-dependent patients who remain hyperglycaemic either after losing weight or because they fail to lose weight.

Weight maintenance diet

Dietary measures are an essential part of the treatment of diabetic patients who require treatment with a sul-

Table 12.19 Basic food units used in diabetic diets

Food		Carbohydrate (g)	Protein (g)	Fat (g)	Energy (kcal)
Carbohydrate	20 g bread	10	1.5	0.3	50
Protein	30 g meat	—	7	5	70
Fat	15 g butter	—	—	15	110
Milk	585 ml	30	18	24	400

Using Atwater calorie conversion factors of 4, 4 and 9 kcal/g for carbohydrate, protein and fat respectively to calculate the energy content.

Table 12.20 Method of constructing a diabetic weight-maintenance diet

Exchanges	Carbohydrate (g)	Energy (kcal)
21 carbohydrate	210	1050
2/3 pint milk	20	260
4 protein	—	280
2 fat	—	220
Total	230	1810

1. The diet contains approximately 1800 kcal (7560 kJ) with 230 g carbohydrate, 72 g protein, 66 g fat providing 51%, 16% and 33% of calories respectively.
2. The 23 carbohydrate and 4 protein exchanges are distributed throughout the day according to the eating habits and daily routine of the patient.

phonylurea drug or insulin. If a fixed daily intake is to be achieved and monotony avoided an exchange system is necessary. The 'exchanges' or portions employed as units are arbitrary and decided mainly on the basis of the food habits of each particular country. In most parts of the world the carbohydrate unit recommended is 10 g. In the UK the staple carbohydrate food is bread and the basic carbohydrate exchange for the purposes of calculating an individual diet is 20 g bread which contains 10 g carbohydrate along with 1.5 g protein and 0.3 g fat. Table 12.19 shows the basic food units used in diabetic diets in the UK. Table 12.20 shows how a diabetic weight-maintenance diet is constructed. When this has been done the figures must be translated into practical instructions in the form of a diet book individually prepared for each patient; the book must include a comprehensive list of carbohydrate exchanges. The information box below lists examples of useful carbohydrate exchanges.

Unmeasured diets

If insulin or an oral hypoglycaemic agent is not required, marked obesity is not present or hyperglycaemia is relatively mild, it may not be necessary for the patient to follow such accurate diets as described above. Sometimes, for various reasons, it may be impracticable to do

USEFUL CARBOHYDRATE EXCHANGES

Each item on this list =
1 carbohydrate exchange = 10 g carbohydrate
- 1/2 slice bread from a large loaf
- 1 large digestive biscuit
- 2 cream crackers
- 2/3 teacup natural unsweetened orange or grapefruit juice
- 1 medium-sized eating apple or orange
- 2/3 teacup cornflakes
- 1 small potato
- 10 grapes
- 1 small banana
- 1/3 pint (200 ml) milk
- 1 teacup cooked porridge
- 1 teacup cream or tinned soup
- 1 small packet crisps
- 1 small *plain* yoghurt

so. In such cases an unmeasured diet of the type listed in the information box may be adequate.

UNMEASURED DIABETIC DIET

- **Foods to be avoided**
  Sucrose, glucose and foods high in sucrose/glucose
- **Foods to be eaten in moderation**
  Breads of all kinds, rolls, scones, biscuits, crispbreads; breakfast cereals and porridge; potatoes, peas, baked beans; all fresh and dried fruit; pasta, custard, thick soups; 'diabetic foods'; milk; meat, fish, eggs, cheese
- **Foods which can be eaten as desired**
  Green vegetables; clear soups, meat extracts, tomato or lemon juice; tea and coffee

ORAL HYPOGLYCAEMIC DRUGS

A number of compounds are effective in reducing hyperglycaemia in patients with NIDDM who are not adequately controlled by dietary measures alone and who would otherwise require treatment with insulin. These drugs fall into two categories: the sulphonylureas and the biguanides. Although their mechanism of action is different, the effect of both groups of drugs depends upon a supply of endogenous insulin and they therefore have no hypoglycaemic effect in patients with IDDM.

Sulphonylureas

Mechanism of action

The defect in insulin secretion in NIDDM appears to be selective for glucose since the response to other stimuli such as amino acids and sulphonylurea drugs is relatively normal at least in the early stage of the disease. Thus the initial effect of sulphonylurea compounds in lowering the blood glucose concentration is due to stimulation of the release of insulin from the pancreatic

Table 12.21 Sulphonylureas—comparative features

Approved name	Daily dose range (mg)	Potency	Approximate biological half-life (hours)	Special points
First generation drugs				
Acetohexamide	500–1500	Medium	5	
Chlorpropamide	100–500	Strong	36	Risk of serious hypoglycaemia particularly in the elderly
				Disulfiram-like reaction with alcohol
				Occasionally cholestatic jaundice, SIADH, exfoliative dermatitis
Tolbutamide	500–3000	Relatively weak	4	
Tolazamide	100–750	Strong	7	
Second generation drugs				
Glibenclamide	2.5–20	Strong	12	Particularly prone to induce severe hypoglycaemia, especially in the elderly
Gliclazide	40–320	Medium	10–12	
Glipizide	2.5–30	Strong	3.5	

beta cell. The long-term hypoglycaemic action, however, seems to be due to extra-pancreatic effects, particularly in reducing the hepatic release of glucose and diminishing insulin resistance.

Indications for use

Sulphonylureas are valuable in the treatment of non-obese patients with NIDDM who fail to respond to dietary measures alone.

Although sulphonylureas will lower the blood glucose concentration of obese patients with NIDDM, such patients should be treated energetically by individually prescribed and carefully designed dietary measures only in the first instance since treatment with sulphonylureas is often associated with an increase in weight which in the long run will intensify the total disability and increase insulin resistance. The latter commonly leads to secondary failure to respond to the drugs, so that ultimately treatment with insulin may be required. The diabetic dietary prescription often involves a major change in lifestyle and its effective implementation requires the skill of an experienced dietitian. Only if it is clear that dietary measures alone are insufficient should patients be started on an oral hypoglycaemic drug.

Table 12.21 lists the sulphonylureas in common use. The main differences between the individual compounds lie in their potency, length of action and cost.

Tolbutamide is the mildest and probably also the safest of the sulphonylureas. It is very well tolerated and toxic reactions are rare. Its duration of action is relatively short so that it has to be given 2 or 3 times daily. The usual maintenance dose is 250–500 mg 2 or 3 times daily. Tolbutamide is a useful drug in the elderly where the risk and the consequences of inducing hypoglycaemia are increased.

Chlorpropamide has a biological half-life of about 36 hours and an effective concentration can be maintained in the blood by a single dose at breakfast. The usual maintenance dose is between 100 and 350 mg daily; larger doses should not be used on a long-term basis since above this level there is an increased risk of toxic effects such as cholestatic jaundice, skin rash and blood dyscrasia. Facial flushing and other features of a disulfiram-like reaction occur in some patients after taking alcohol. Occasionally chlorpropamide can induce the syndrome of inappropriate antidiuretic hormone secretion (SIADH). Chlorpropamide may cause severe and prolonged hypoglycaemia (due to its long biological half-life). Care must be taken to avoid this, particularly in elderly patients, and in this group once glycosuria has been abolished and symptoms relieved the daily dose should be reduced to a minimum. Many patients requiring 250–330 mg daily initially can be maintained on a long-term basis on 50–100 mg per day.

Second generation sulphonylureas are more expensive but glipizide and gliclazide are widely used and cause few side-effects. Glibenclamide is particularly prone to induce severe hypoglycaemia in the elderly and should be avoided in those over 70 years of age.

Patients with NIDDM who fail to achieve initial control with sulphonylureas are considered 'primary treatment failures'. The incidence of primary treatment failure depends mainly on the criteria for initial selection and patient compliance with diet. Patients with 'secondary failure' are not a homogeneous group; they include some with type I IDDM who have an absolute deficiency of insulin and others with significant circulating insulin levels who are commonly obese and have failed to lose weight while supposedly taking a low energy diet. Failure to comply with the diet is the commonest cause of secondary treatment failure. With continuing follow-up 'secondary failure' affects 3–10% of patients each year.

Biguanides

The biguanides are less widely used than the sulphonylureas because of a high incidence of side-effects, particularly gastrointestinal symptoms, and because there has been a significant number of deaths from lactic acidosis in patients taking these drugs.

Mechanism of action

The mechanism of action of these compounds has not been precisely defined. They have no hypoglycaemic effect in normal people but, in the diabetic, insulin sensitivity and peripheral glucose uptake are increased. There is some evidence that they also impair glucose absorption and reduce hepatic gluconeogenesis. Although secretion of some endogenous insulin is mandatory for their hypoglycaemic action these compounds do not increase insulin secretion and hypoglycaemia does not occur in patients being treated with these drugs.

Indications for use

Some of the biguanides are associated with the development of lactic acidosis and are no longer in clinical use. However, metformin is less associated with this development and may be useful in two difficult clinical situations. Firstly, its administration is not associated with a rise in body weight and it may therefore be preferred when an obese patient with NIDDM must be treated because hyperglycaemia persists despite efforts to adhere to a diet and reduce weight. Secondly, as the hypoglycaemic effect of metformin is synergistic with that of the sulphonylurea drugs, there is a case for combining the two when sulphonylureas alone have proved inadequate. Such combined therapy should be used only when there are clear contraindications to treatment with insulin since, despite euglycaemia, the plasma concentration of intermediary metabolites (including lactate, pyruvate, alanine, glycerol and ketone bodies) is abnormal in patients treated in this way.

Metformin is given with food 2 or 3 times daily. The usual starting dose is 500 mg twice daily with a gradual increase as required to a maximum of 1 g 3 times daily. Its use is contraindicated in patients with impaired renal or hepatic function and in those who take alcohol in excess because the risk of lactic acidosis is significantly increased in such patients. Its administration should be discontinued, at least temporarily, if any other serious medical condition develops. In such circumstances treatment with insulin should be substituted.

Lactic acidosis

The increased blood lactate levels seen in patients taking biguanides seem to result from an increased flow of glucose through glycolysis combined with reduced lactate removal due, partly at least, to inhibition of gluconeogenesis. Lactic acidosis has a high mortality—

at least 50% even in specialist centres. It is further discussed on page 751.

INSULIN

Types of insulin preparation

Two main types of insulin preparation are used clinically: unmodified, rapid onset, short-acting; and modified or 'depot', delayed onset, long-acting (Table 12.22).

Unmodified insulins are clear solutions which, when injected subcutaneously, produce an effect in about 30 minutes which lasts for approximately 6 hours. Unmodified insulin is essential in new cases of diabetes with dehydration and/or ketoacidosis, in acute metabolic decompensation in established cases of diabetes (both IDDM and NIDDM) from whatever cause, in combination with depot insulins for the day-to-day management of nearly all patients with IDDM, and *in any situation where intravenous insulin is required*, e.g. in infusion pumps.

Depot insulin preparations are cloudy solutions. Their delayed and prolonged action is achieved in two main ways. In isophane preparations insulin is adsorbed on to a foreign protein, namely fish protamine, in exactly equivalent amounts, from which it is gradually released in the tissues. Although a foreign protein, protamine is virtually non-immunogenic. *As with all the complexed insulins, isophane preparations may only be used by subcutaneous injection.* Unmodified insulin mixed with isophane retains its characteristic action. Insulin zinc suspensions do not contain foreign protein. Their duration of action depends on the size and form of the insulin crystals as well as on the rate at which these crystals are dissolved and absorbed. The former is achieved by carefully controlling the conditions of precipitation; the latter is delayed by buffering with acetate and adding zinc. These insulin zinc suspensions must contain excess free zinc in solution and when mixed with unmodified insulin the zinc will blunt the onset of its action.

For many years insulin was regarded as non-antigenic. It is now known that even homologous pancreatic insulin can, in some circumstances, act as a weak antigen. The factors determining the immunogenicity of therapeutic preparations of insulin are listed in the information box.

The older preparations of insulin were strongly antigenic because they consisted usually of bovine insulin, were commonly prepared at low pH, frequently contained added protein to delay their action and always contained trace amounts of pro-insulin and other pancreatic hormones. *Care must be taken to avoid hypoglycaemia when transferring patients from the older animal to the newer human preparations.*

Table 12.22   Insulin preparations in common use

Type	Proprietary preparations	Species	Approximate duration (hours)
Unmodified Clear solutions Rapid onset Short action	Actrapid (Novo-Nordisk) Velosulin (Novo-Nordisk) Humulin S (Lilly) Hypurin Neutral (CP Pharm)	Human Human Porcine Human Bovine	6
Modified (depot) Cloudy solutions Delayed onset Prolonged action	Monotard (Novo-Nordisk) Insulatard (Novo-Nordisk) Humulin I (Lilly) Hypurin Isophane (CP Pharm)	Human Human Porcine Human Bovine	12
	Ultratard (Novo-Nordisk) Humulin Zn (Lilly) Hypurin Protamine (CP Pharm)	Human Human Bovine	24

* In Britain and the U.S.A all these insulin preparations are available
only in 100 IU/ml strength for routine clinical use. In other parts
of the world insulins are also available in 40 and 80 IU/ml strength.
Premixed insulin preparations, containing a wide range of fixed ratios
of unmodified and intermediate depot, are also available.

**FACTORS DETERMINING THE IMMUNOGENICITY OF
THERAPEUTIC PREPARATIONS OF INSULIN**

Origin
Bovine > Porcine > Human

Additives
Used to delay and prolong action; increase
immunogenicity

Purity
Older preparations contain trace amounts of pro-insulin
and other islet hormones which stimulate the formation
of antibodies cross-reacting with insulin

pH
Acidity increases immunogenicity: new preparations neutral

Management with insulin

The total daily dose of insulin, the type of insulin preparation, and the number and timing of injections required to achieve satisfactory control without undue risk of hypoglycaemia, varies widely and is established by clinical trial.

Factors determining the type and amount of insulin required in an individual case include the patient's sensitivity to the action of insulin (those thin and active are generally more sensitive than the obese) and way of life (e.g. meal pattern, occupation and hours of work, amount and timing of exercise). More insulin will be needed to cover main meals and periods of inactivity, and vice versa. Various combinations of the numerous preparations of insulin available can be tried and the time at which they are taken altered on the basis of the results of blood glucose estimations at different times of the day until good metabolic control is achieved over the whole 24-hour period. Table 12.23 shows how to adjust the dose of individual insulins in 3 commonly used regimes. The aim is to achieve preprandial blood glucose readings within the range 4–6.7 mmol/l along with a blood glucose concentration not less than 5 mmol/l at 03.00 hours. Thus if a patient on a 2 injections daily insulin regime has a persistently raised blood glucose concentration before breakfast the long-acting (cloudy) insulin preparation given before the evening meal should be increased. However, this runs the risk of nocturnal hypoglycaemia. If the blood glucose concentration prior to lunch is high, then the morning dose of short-acting (clear) insulin should be increased. Figure 12.39 (p. 743) shows an example of a patient poorly controlled by one insulin regime but well controlled by another. Other commonly used insulin regimes are shown in Table 12.23 (p. 742).

ASSESSMENT OF METABOLIC CONTROL

The aim of treatment is to achieve as near normal metabolism as is practicable. It is clear that the nearer the body weight approaches the ideal level and the closer the blood glucose concentration is kept to normal the more normal is the body's total metabolic profile and the lower the incidence of vascular disease (p. 744). The various methods of assessing blood glucose control are listed in the information box on page 742.

Semi-quantitative preprandial urine testing is the time-honoured method of assessing blood glucose control, but its limitations in this role have become increasingly apparent, not only in patients with IDDM (Fig. 12.40, p. 744) but also in NIDDM patients where a raised renal threshold for glucose (which is very common in these patients) may mask persistent hyperglycaemia. In addition, negative urine tests fail to distinguish between normal and low blood glucose levels which is a particular disadvantage since the aim of treatment is a normal blood glucose level while avoiding hypoglycaemia. Wherever possible all patients should be taught to perform blood glucose measurements at home using blood glucose test strips read either visually or with a reflectance meter (Table 12.24, p. 744). The great advantage of self-monitoring of capillary blood glucose concentration by patients is that information is immediately available and permits those well informed and motivated to make appropriate adjustments in insulin, oral hypoglycaemic agent and/or diet on a day-to-day basis. Thus the development of serious ketoacidosis can be avoided, a normal or near normal metabolism achieved without frequent and disabling hypoglycaemia

Table 12.23 Adjusting the dose of insulin

Insulin regime	Before breakfast	Before lunch	Before evening meal	At bedtime
2 INJECTIONS DAILY **Note**: Significant risk of hypoglycaemia 24.00–04.00 h (particularly in C-peptide negative patients)	↑ A+M or V+Ins or S+Iso		↑ A+M or V+Ins or S+Iso	
Blood glucose conc. indicates the effect of the insulin specified	Teatime cloudy insulin taken previous evening	Breakfast clear insulin	Breakfast cloudy insulin	Teatime clear insulin
3 INJECTIONS DAILY **Note**: Risk of nocturnal hypoglycaemia reduced	↑ A+M or V+Ins or S+Iso		↑ A or V or S	↑ M or Ins or Iso (should *not* be taken *before 23.00 h*)
Blood glucose conc. indicates the effect of the insulin specified	Bedtime cloudy insulin taken previous evening	Breakfast clear insulin	Breakfast cloudly insulin	Teatime clear insulin
4 INJECTIONS DAILY **Note**: A pen-injector can be used to deliver the clear insulin	↑ A or V or S	↑ A or V or S	↑ A or V or S	↑ M or Ins or Iso (*should not be taken before 23.00 h*)
Blood glucose conc. indicates the effect of the insulin specified	Bedtime cloudy insulin taken previous evening	Breakfast clear insulin	Lunch clear insulin	Teatime clear insulin

A = Actrapid; M = Monotard; V = Velosulin; Ins = Insulatard; S = Soluble; Iso = Isophane (see Table 12.22)

METHODS OF ASSESSING BLOOD GLUCOSE CONTROL

Urinary glucose
- Preprandial tests
- 24-hour collection

Blood glucose
- Single, random clinic measurements
- Day profile:
  - Inpatients
  - Day patients
- Capillary blood spot profiles: home-based patients
- Patient home monitoring
  - Test-strips (visual)
  - Test-strips (meters)

Glycated proteins
- Haemoglobin
- Albumin
- Total serum proteins (fructosamine)

and compliance with dietary measures encouraged. Single random blood glucose estimations obtained at routine clinic visits are of limited value. The main disadvantage of day profiles obtained in hospital or in day-patients is that they are obtained in a highly artificial situation. The advantage of the capillary blood spot profile is that tests are performed in the real-life situation while at the same time the estimations are accurate. In this technique patients collect serial capillary blood samples by finger prick on to filter paper strips previously soaked in boric acid. When the series is complete the strips are posted to the laboratory for estimation. The disadvantage of this system is the delay in obtaining results.

Glycated haemoglobin

When haemoglobin from a normal adult is passed through a chromatographic column it separates into the major component haemoglobin A (HbA_0) comprising 92–94% of the total and several minor, fast-moving components collectively known as haemoglobin A_1 (HbA_1) comprising 6–8% of the total (Fig. 12.41, p. 744). The latter are structurally identical to HbA_0 except for the addition of a glucose group to the terminal amino acid of the B chain of the haemoglobin molecule (glycation). The rate of synthesis of HbA_1 is therefore a function of the exposure of the red blood cell to glucose. Since the glucose linkage to haemoglobin is relatively stable, HbA_1 accumulates throughout the life-span of the erythrocyte and its concentration reflects the integrated blood glucose concentration over a period approximating to the half-life of the red blood cell, i.e. 6–8 weeks. Measurement of HbA_1 can therefore be used as a supplement to blood glucose estimations to monitor the overall degree of diabetic control achieved. Figure 12.42 (p. 745) shows the close relationship between total HbA_1 and the mean blood glucose concentration in 40 patients with IDDM over 3 months. The very close correlation obtained between HbA_1 and mean blood glucose concentration supports the expectation that such measurements taken during a normal working day are more representative of the usual prevailing blood glucose levels than those obtained in hospital or in day-patients.

Glycation of haemoglobin is one example of the many glycosylation reactions which occur in the body. Glycated serum proteins ('fructosamine') can also be measured and, because of their shorter half-life, give an indication of glycaemic control over the preceding two weeks.

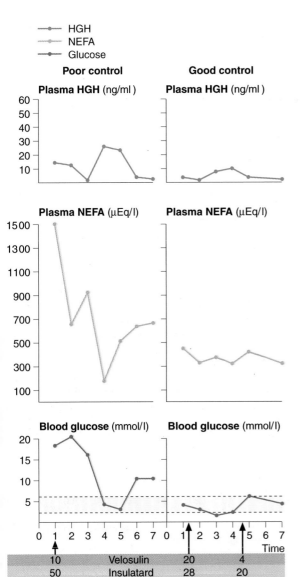

Legend:
- HGH
- NEFA
- Glucose

Poor control — **Good control**

Plasma HGH (ng/ml) — **Plasma HGH** (ng/ml)

Plasma NEFA (µEq/l) — **Plasma NEFA** (µEq/l)

Blood glucose (mmol/l) — **Blood glucose** (mmol/l)

10	Velosulin	20	4	
50	Insulatard	28	20	

Fig. 12.39 Blood glucose and plasma non-esterified fatty acids (1) fasting, (2) 1½ hours after breakfast, (3) and (4) before and 1½ hours after the midday meal, (5) and (6) before and 1½ hours after the evening meal, and (7) before going to bed, in a non-obese 14-year-old girl with IDDM, undertaking normal activity in the course of the day. Diabetes had been diagnosed 11 years previously and she was following a diet of 9.2 MJ distributed in 3 main meals and 3 snacks taken at mid-morning, mid-afternoon and bedtime. Her diabetes was poorly controlled by 60 units of insulin taken in a single daily dose before breakfast. Greatly improved control was achieved by a slight increase in the total daily amount of insulin given and by administering this in 2 doses. The broken lines in the upper panel indicate the physiological range for the blood glucose concentration.

Blood lipids

Concentration of serum lipids is another important index of overall metabolic control in diabetic patients and should be monitored regularly. Ideally the concentration of total cholesterol, triglyceride and HDL cholesterol should be measured in blood samples obtained from patients who have fasted overnight.

THERAPEUTIC GOALS

The ideal management for diabetes would allow the patient to lead a completely normal life, to remain not only symptom-free but in good health, to achieve a normal metabolic state and to escape the micro- and macroangiopathy associated with long-term diabetes. Nowadays diabetic patients rarely die in ketoacidosis but the major problem which has emerged is the excess mortality and serious morbidity and disability suffered by many of those whose duration of life has been extended by treatment. As indicated in the information box on page 745, the cost to the community and to the individual patient is enormous.

The factors which have been shown to be associated with increased mortality and morbidity in diabetic patients are listed in the second information box (p. 745).

Metabolic control and development of long-term complications of diabetes

Duration of diabetes and high HbA₁ are most closely associated with vascular complications. A graded relationship has been demonstrated between the duration and degree of sustained hyperglycaemia, *however caused and at whatever age it develops*, and the risk of vascular disease. *Note that there is nothing 'mild' about NIDDM as regards the development of complications.*

The possibility of reversing early vascular disease by improving metabolic control has been examined in several prospective, randomised, controlled clinical trials involving patients with early background retinopathy and minimal proteinuria. None of these independently conducted studies produced any evidence of reversal of either retinopathy or nephropathy, and indeed retinopathy worsened abruptly in some cases soon after control was improved. Despite this, in the long term the rate of progression of both retinopathy and nephropathy was reduced by continuing better control. These studies have had two effects. Firstly, they have stimulated a search for markers of early, reversible, retinal, renal and neural dysfunction, and microalbuminuria is now validated as a marker for the subsequent development not only of diabetic nephropathy and hypertension in patients with IDDM but also of increased mortality from large blood vessel disease in NIDDM. Secondly, the whole emphasis

Table 12.24 Blood glucose test strips and meters

Brand (manufacturer)	BG range (mmol/l)*	Visual reading	Meter	Test time
BM-Accutest (BM Diag)	1.1–33.3	—	✓	20 sec
BM-Test 1-44 (BM Diag)	1–44	✓	✓	2 min
Dextrostix (Bayer Diag)	1.4–14	✓	✓	1 min
Exactech (Medisense)	2.2–25	—	✓	30 sec
Glucostix (Bayer Diag)	1–44	✓	✓	2 min
Hypoguard (Hypoguard)	0–22	✓	✓	1–1.5 min
One Touch (Lifescan)	0–33.3	—	✓	45 sec

* Blood glucose

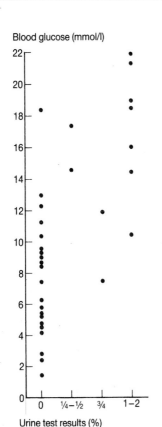

Fig. 12.40 Simultaneous urinary and blood glucose estimations performed over a 2-week period in a 14-year-old girl taking twice daily injections of insulin for 1 year. Note that when the urinary test records 0 the blood glucose concentration ranges from 1.5–18 mmol/l even when the bladder has been emptied 0.5–1 hour before passing the urine to be tested.

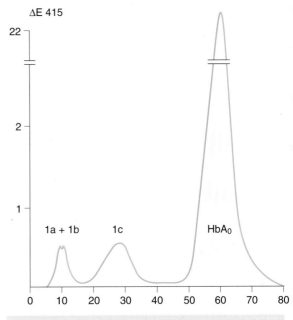

Fig. 12.41 Elution profile of human haemoglobin from chromatographic column.

in the management of diabetes has shifted to primary prevention of complications.

The Diabetes Control and Complications Trial (DCCT) was set up to answer the question: are diabetic complications preventable? Recent analysis of the data generated during the 9 years of this large and very carefully designed study (see further reading) shows a 60% overall reduction in the risk of developing diabetic complications in those with 'near-normal' glycaemia (mean total HbA_1 less than or equal to 9%), compared with those poorly controlled (mean HbA_1 less than or equal to 11%). In this study a comprehensive biochemical profile was performed regularly on all patients but no single factor other than total glycaemic control (as measured by HbA_1) had a significant effect on outcome.

The conclusions which can be drawn from this critically important study are clear and incontrovertible:

● *diabetic complications are preventable*

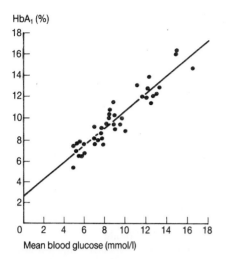

HbA$_1$ (%)

Mean blood glucose (mmol/l)

Fig. 12.42 The relationship between %HbA$_1$ and mean blood glucose levels in the previous 3 months. Each dot represents the mean blood glucose concentration for a single patient. Each patient collected capillary blood samples before and 2 hours after each main meal for 24 hours every 2 weeks for 3 months. Glycated haemoglobin is expressed here as HbA$_1$ (that is HbA$_{1a+1b+1c}$). HbA$_{1c}$ (the largest fraction) is sometimes reported alone, in which case the normal range is significantly lower than that for HbA$_1$.

THE CURRENT COST OF DIABETES IN THE UK

- 30% reduction in life expectancy
- Commonest cause of blindness in 20–65 age group
- 600 patients reach end-stage renal failure per annum
- Lower limb amputation rate increased 25-fold
- Use of hospital beds increased 6-fold
- 4.5% of total NHS budget

FACTORS ASSOCIATED WITH INCREASED MORTALITY AND MORBIDITY IN DIABETIC PATIENTS

- Duration of diabetes
- Early age at onset of disease
- High HbA$_1$
- Raised BP
- Proteinuria
- Obesity
- Hyperlipidaemia

- *the aim of treatment should be 'near-normal' glycaemia,* while at the same time avoiding serious hypoglycaemic episodes in insulin-treated patients.

In the DCCT serious hypoglycaemic episodes occurred 3 times more often in well- than in poorly-controlled patients. Although no deaths, major macro-vascular events or neurological/cognitive defects were associated with hypoglycaemia in this study (which did

---

DIABETES—AIMS OF MANAGEMENT

- **Near-normal glycaemia**
  HbA$_1$ $\leqslant 9.0\%$
  Mean blood glucose concentration (mmol/l)
  Fasting $\quad$ < 6.7
  2 hours postprandial $\quad$ < 11.1
- **No serious hypoglycaemic episodes**

---

not include patients with recurrent severe hypoglycaemia) an increased risk of hypoglycaemia may alter the risk–benefit ratio of good control in certain patients. Thus less intensive treatment may be indicated:

(1) in those with loss of awareness of hypoglycaemia for a variety of other reasons
(2) in those with severe macrovascular disease (particularly if they have a past history of myocardial infarction or cerebrovascular accident)
(3) for those who are very old and frail.

EDUCATING PATIENTS

It is essential that diabetic patients learn to manage all aspects of their management as quickly as possible and this can best be done on an outpatient basis while leading a relatively normal existence at home and work. However, patients requiring insulin have to be seen daily at first and, if this is not practicable, admission to hospital will be necessary. Hospital admission will also be required for patients presenting with ketoacidosis.

Every patient who is capable of learning must be taught how to perform capillary blood glucose estimations and tests of urinary ketones, to keep a record of the results and to understand their significance.

Those requiring insulin need to learn how to measure their dose of insulin accurately with an insulin syringe, to give their own injections and to adjust the dose themselves on the basis of blood glucose estimations and other factors such as illness, unusual exercise and hypoglycaemic episodes. They must be familiar with the symptoms associated with hypoglycaemia (information box p. 746). They must therefore have a working knowledge of diabetes and also ready access to medical advice when the need arises. Such education is time consuming but only in this way can patients safely undertake normal activities while maintaining good control.

It is a wise precaution for diabetic patients who are taking insulin or an oral hypoglycaemic drug to carry a card with them at all times stating their name and address, the fact that they are diabetic, the nature and dose of any insulin or other drugs they may be taking, and giving the name, address and telephone number of their family doctor and any specialist diabetic clinic they may be attending.

LONG-TERM SUPERVISION

Diabetic patients should be seen at regular intervals for the remainder of their lives either at a specialist diabetic clinic or by their general practitioner *if he or she has a particular interest and training in diabetes*. A check list for follow-up visits is detailed in the information box below. The frequency of visits is very variable, ranging from weekly during pregnancy to annually in the case of patients with well-controlled NIDDM.

CHECK LIST FOR FOLLOW-UP VISITS OF PATIENTS WITH DIABETES MELLITUS

- Body weight
- Urinalysis of fasting specimen for glucose, ketones, albumin (both macro and micro albuminuria)
- Glycaemic control
  HbA$_1$
  Inspection of home blood glucose monitoring record
- Hypoglycaemic episodes
  Number of serious (requiring assistance in treatment) and mild episodes
  Time when 'hypos' experienced
- BP (supine and erect)
- Visual acuity
  Ophthalmoscopy
- Lower limbs
  Peripheral pulses
  Tendon reflexes
  Perception of vibration sensation
  Feet: ulceration, callus skin indicating pressure areas, nails, need for chiropody

---

ACUTE COMPLICATIONS OF DIABETES

HYPOGLYCAEMIA

Hypoglycaemia, defined as a blood glucose concentration of less than 2.5 mmol/l, occurs commonly in diabetic patients treated with insulin and relatively infrequently in those taking a sulphonylurea drug. In most instances the patient has no difficulty in recognising the symptoms of hypoglycaemia and can take appropriate remedial action. However, in certain circumstances (e.g. during sleep) and particularly in certain types of patients (e.g. patients with long duration of IDDM) warning symptoms are not always perceived by the patient even when awake so that appropriate action is not taken and, if no assistance is available, eventually unconsciousness ensues.

Severe hypoglycaemia, defined as *hypoglycaemia requiring the assistance of another person for recovery*, can result in serious morbidity (see information box) and has a recognised mortality of 2–4% in insulin-treated patients. The unrecognised mortality is probably significantly higher than this. Sudden death during sleep in otherwise healthy young patients with IDDM has been described, and has been attributed to hypoglycaemia-induced cardiac arrhythmia. Recurrent severe hypoglycaemia is very disruptive and impinges on many aspects of the patient's life including employment, driving and sport. Risk of hypoglycaemia is the most important single factor limiting attainment of the therapeutic goal, namely normal/near-normal glycaemia in patients with IDDM.

Symptoms of hypoglycaemia

Common symptoms of hypoglycaemia are listed in the information box. They fall into two main groups: those related to acute activation of the autonomic nervous system and those secondary to glucose deprivation of the brain (neuroglycopenia). Symptoms of hypoglycaemia are idiosyncratic and ability to recognise their onset is an important aspect of the initial education of diabetic patients treated with insulin.

SYMPTOMS OF HYPOGLYCAEMIA

Autonomic	**Neuroglycopenic**	**Non-specific**
• sweating	• confusion	• nausea
• trembling	• drowsiness	• tiredness
• pounding heart	• speech difficulty	• headache
• hunger	• inability to	
• anxiety	concentrate	
	• incoordination	

MORBIDITY OF SEVERE HYPOGLYCAEMIA IN DIABETIC PATIENTS

• CNS	Coma
	Convulsions
	Brain damage
	Impaired cognitive function
	Intellectual decline
	Vascular events: transient ischaemic attack, stroke
• Heart	Cardiac arrhythmias
	Myocardial ischaemia
• Eye	Vitreous haemorrhage
	? worsening of retinopathy
• Other	Hypothermia
	Accidents

Awareness of symptoms

If unmodified insulin is administered to a normal person, symptoms of hypoglycaemia are usually experienced when the blood glucose is about 2.5 mmol/l and are fully developed at about 2.2 mmol/l. In diabetic patients who are chronically hyperglycaemic the same symptoms may develop at a higher blood glucose level; conversely patients who are frequently hypoglycaemic may not experience any symptoms even when the blood glucose concentration is well below 2.5 mmol/l. This therapy-induced loss of awareness of hypoglycaemia is usually reversible if the overall blood glucose level is allowed to rise and hypoglycaemic episodes avoided by appropriate adjustments to the insulin regime.

The incidence of impaired perception of symptoms of hypoglycaemia and an altered symptom profile increases steadily with duration of insulin treatment, and almost 50% of patients with IDDM are affected after 20 years of diabetes. This chronic form of hypoglycaemia unawareness is not reversible and intensive insulin therapy is inappropriate in such cases. The usual therapeutic goals need to be modified in such patients and daily self-monitoring of blood glucose is mandatory.

Causes and prevention

The main causes of hypoglycaemia in patients taking insulin or a sulphonylurea drug are listed in the information box.

CAUSES OF HYPOGLYCAEMIA

- Missed, delayed or inadequate meal
- Unexpected or unusual exercise
- Alcohol
- Poorly designed insulin regime, particularly that predisposing to nocturnal hypoglycaemia
- Defective glucose counter-regulation/unawareness of hypoglycaemia
- Gastroparesis due to autonomic neuropathy
- Other endocrine disorder, e.g. Addison's disease
- Malabsorption
- Factitious hypoglycaemia

The incidence of the most common causes, that is unpunctual or inadequate meals, unexpected or unusual exercise (Fig. 12.43), and ingestion of alcohol (p. 736) can all be reduced by adequate patient education. Exercise-induced hypoglycaemia occurs in treated, well-controlled, insulin-dependent diabetic patients because a key factor in the normal adaptation to exercise (p. 730, Fig. 12.33), namely decreased secretion of insulin, does not occur. Patients should be taught that if unusual exercise is anticipated the preceding dose of insulin should be reduced (the degree of reduction varying widely in individual patients but often being substantial) and extra

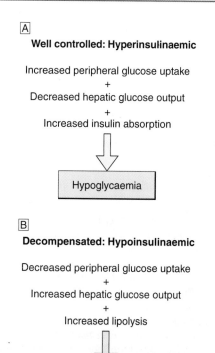

A

Well controlled: Hyperinsulinaemic

Increased peripheral glucose uptake

+

Decreased hepatic glucose output

+

Increased insulin absorption

↓

Hypoglycaemia

B

Decompensated: Hypoinsulinaemic

Decreased peripheral glucose uptake

+

Increased hepatic glucose output

+

Increased lipolysis

↓

Hyperglycaemia and ketonaemia

Fig. 12.43   The effect of exercise in diabetic patients being treated with insulin. [A] Well controlled: hyperinsulinaemic patients. [B] Decompensated: hypoinsulinaemic patients.

carbohydrate ingested. All patients taking insulin should carry with them glucose tablets (Dextrosol: 2.5 g glucose per tablet) at all times.

The incidence of nocturnal hypoglycaemia in patients with IDDM treated conventionally with a twice daily injection regime (Table 12.23, p. 742) is difficult to establish. It is certainly common and may occur in 50% of these patients. The basic cause is the physiological diurnal variation in the amount of insulin required to achieve homeostasis which is probably related to the diurnal rhythm in the secretion of counter-regulatory hormones such as glucocorticoids and growth hormone which are insulin antagonists (information box, p. 748). Thus if, as is common, an intermediate-acting depot insulin is taken before the main evening meal at 17.00–19.00 hours its peak action will coincide with the period of maximum sensitivity to insulin, namely 24.00–04.00 hours. This hypoglycaemia is usually not perceived by the patient and is therefore often undetected. However, on direct questioning patients may admit to poor sleep, morning headaches, 'hangover', chronic fatigue, vivid dreams or nightmares. Sometimes a relative may observe sweating (which may be profuse), restlessness, twitching or even

NOCTURNAL HYPOGLYCAEMIA IN IDDM

- **Incidence**   Uncertain, but common
- **Cause**   Variation in overnight requirement for insulin:
  24.00 – 04.00 h = 8 mU/kg/h
  04.00 – 08.00 h = 16 mU/kg/h

- **Diagnosis**   Accurate blood glucose estimations at 03.00 and 08.00 h

- **Treatment**   Split evening dose of insulin
  Take unmodified insulin only before the evening meal and depot insulin not before 23.00 h

convulsions. The only reliable way to make the diagnosis is to measure the blood glucose between 02.00 and 03.00 hours. The treatment is to split the evening dose of insulin. In most cases this solves the problem *provided that the depot insulin is not taken earlier than 23.00 hours*. Nevertheless it is a wise precaution for patients to measure the blood glucose concentration as they go to bed and to take additional carbohydrate if the reading is less than 6.0 mmol/l.

In response to a falling blood glucose there is normally increased secretion of a battery of hormones which counter the blood glucose lowering effect of insulin (Table 12.16, p. 729). Glucagon and adrenaline are the most important of these. Secretion of glucagon is impaired in most patients with long-standing IDDM and in some with NIDDM and as time goes on an increasing number of patients also develop a defective adrenaline response to hypoglycaemia so that glucose recovery fails to occur. Autonomic neuropathy may be involved in the deficient adrenaline response but there is some evidence that those who develop defective counter-regulatory responses also have dysfunction of hypothalamic or other central neuroendocrine mechanisms.

Management

Treatment of acute hypoglycaemia is described in the section on spontaneous hypoglycaemia (p. 773). It depends on the severity of the hypoglycaemia and whether the patient is conscious and able to swallow. Treatment may require oral carbohydrate if hypoglycaemia is recognised early, or parenteral glucose or glucagon. Glucagon, in addition to increasing hepatic breakdown of glycogen, stimulates the secretion of insulin and therefore should not be used to treat hypoglycaemia induced by an oral hypoglycaemic drug.

As soon as the patient is able to swallow, glucose should be given orally. Full recovery may not occur

immediately. Further, when hypoglycaemia has occurred in a diabetic using a long-acting depot insulin or a sulphonylurea, particularly chlorpropamide, the possibility of relapse within a day or more should be anticipated.

Repeated episodes of severe hypoglycaemia may lead to permanent intellectual deterioration. Following recovery it is important to try to identify a cause and make appropriate adjustments to the patient's therapy. Unless the reason for a hypoglycaemic episode is clear and will not recur the patient should reduce the next and subsequent dose of insulin by 20% and seek medical advice about further adjustments in dose. Patient education on the potential risks of inducing hypoglycaemia, regular blood glucose monitoring and treatment, including the need to have an accessible supply of glucose (and glucagon) are fundamental to prevention of this potentially dangerous side-effect of treatment. Relatives and friends also need to be aware of the symptoms and signs of hypoglycaemia and should be instructed as to how this should be managed (including how to give an intramuscular injection of glucagon).

DIABETIC KETOACIDOSIS

Prior to the discovery of insulin more than 50% of diabetic patients died in ketoacidosis. Today this complication should account for less than 2% of deaths among diabetics. However, both the incidence and the mortality rate are still regrettably high. Failure of the patient to understand the disease and to appreciate the significance of symptoms of poor control are the most common causes. Its prevention is largely a matter of education of both patients and doctors. A significant number of new patients still present in diabetic ketoacidosis and in established diabetics a common course of events is that patients develop an intercurrent infection, lose their appetite, and either stop or drastically reduce their dose of insulin (on either their own initiative or their doctor's advice) in the mistaken belief that under these circumstances less insulin is required. Any form of stress, particularly that produced by infection, may precipitate severe ketoacidosis in even the mildest case of diabetes.

A clear understanding of the biochemical basis and pathophysiology of this problem (p. 729) is essential for its efficient treatment. Hyperglycaemia and ketoacidosis are not always necessarily closely correlated. Even moderate hyperglycaemia may be associated with life-threatening acidosis, particularly in young patients with IDDM, while coma can occur, usually in elderly patients, with extreme hyperglycaemia and dehydration but no ketoacidosis. This metabolic state is known as **hyperosmolar diabetic coma**.

AVERAGE LOSS OF FLUID AND ELECTROLYTES IN AN ADULT WITH DIABETIC KETOACIDOSIS OF MODERATE SEVERITY

- Water   6 litres
- Sodium   500 mmol
- Chloride   400 mmol
- Potassium   350 mmol

The information box shows the average loss of fluid and electrolytes in moderately severe diabetic keto-acidosis in an adult. About half the deficit of total body water is derived from the intracellular compartment and occurs comparatively early in the development of acidosis with relatively few clinical features; the remainder represents loss of extracellular fluid sustained largely in the latter stages. It is at this time that marked contraction of the size of the extracellular space occurs, with haemo-concentration, a decreased blood volume, and finally a fall in blood pressure with associated renal ischaemia and oliguria.

Every patient in diabetic ketoacidosis is potassium depleted, but the plasma concentration of potassium gives very little indication of the total body deficit. Plasma potassium may even be raised initially due to disproportionate loss of water and catabolism of protein and glycogen. However, soon after treatment with insulin is started there is likely to be a precipitous fall in the plasma potassium due to dilution of extracellular potassium by administration of intravenous fluids, the movement of potassium into cells as a result of treatment with insulin, and the continuing renal loss of potassium.

The severity of ketoacidosis can be assessed rapidly by measuring the plasma bicarbonate; less than 12 mmol/l indicates severe acidosis. The hydrogen ion concentration in the blood gives an even more precise mea-sure but may not be so readily available. There is no simple and accurate quantitative method for determination of ketones in plasma although a test strip (keto-stix) can be used as a semiquantitative guide to the plasma concentration of acetoacetate and acetone.

Clinical features

The clinical features of coma due to ketoacidosis are listed in Table 12.25 where they are compared with those of hypoglycaemia. It should be remembered however that the state of consciousness is very variable in patients with diabetic ketoacidosis and a patient with dangerous ketoacidosis requiring urgent treatment may walk into the consulting room. For this reason the term diabetic ketoacidosis is to be preferred to 'diabetic coma' which suggests that there is no urgency until unconsciousness occurs. In fact it is imperative that energetic treatment is started at the earliest possible stage.

Management

Diabetic ketoacidosis is a medical emergency which should be treated in hospital. Intravenous fluid replacement is required since, even when the patient is able to swallow, fluids given by mouth may be poorly absorbed. Treatment must be checked against the plasma concentration of glucose, potassium and bicarbonate estimated at intervals of 1–2 hours initially. The components of treatment are:

- the administration of unmodified insulin by intra-muscular or intravenous injection
- fluid replacement
- potassium replacement
- the administration of antibiotics if infection is present.

Note that, although leucocytosis is invariably seen, this represents a stress response and does not necessarily indicate infection; note also that pyrexia may not be

Table 12.25 Differences in coma due to hypoglycaemia and ketoacidosis in IDDM

	Hypoglycaemic coma	Coma with ketosis
History	No food; too much insulin; unaccustomed exercise	Too little or no insulin; an infection; digestive disturbance
Onset	In good previous health; related to last insulin injection	Ill-health for several days
Symptoms	Hypoglycaemia; occasional vomiting from depot insulins	Of glycosuria and dehydration; abdominal pain and vomiting
Signs	Moist skin and tongue Full pulse Normal or raised systolic BP Shallow or normal breathing Brisk reflexes	Dry skin and tongue Weak pulse Low BP Air hunger Diminished reflexes
Urine	No ketonuria No glycosuria, if bladder recently emptied	Ketonuria Glycosuria
Blood	Hypoglycaemia Normal plasma bicarbonate	Hyperglycaemia Reduced plasma bicarbonate

Table 12.26 Guidelines for the management of diabetic ketoacidosis

TIME (h)	INSULIN (use only unmodified, clear insulin)	FLUID (i.v.)	POTASSIUM (i.v.)	OTHER
0	Start i.v. insulin infusion 5 U/h (Alternatively, 10–20 U i.m. followed by 5 U/h i.m. thereafter)	START i.v. 0.9% saline infusion, 1 litre in 30 min		Check capillary blood glucose. If ≥17 mmol/l obtain venous blood for urgent laboratory measurement of glucose, Na, K, Cl, Co_2, urea and pH or $[H^+]$. Test urine for ketones
0.5	Continue insulin 5 U/h i.v.	0.5 l of 0.9% saline in 30 min	If plasma K^+ >5.5 mmol/l give no KCl; 3.5–5.5 mmol/l give 20 mmol KCl/l of infused fluid; <3.5 mmol/l give 40 mmol KCl/l of infused fluid	If plasma Na^+ > 155 mmol/l give 0.45% rather than 0.9% saline until Na^+ falls to 140 mmol/l. If pH <7.0 ($[H^+]$ >100 nmol/l) give 300–500 ml 1.26% sodium bicarbonate over 30 min into large vein
1	Continue insulin 5 U/h i.v.	0.5 l of 0.9% saline in 1 h	As above	Recheck biochemistry
2	Continue insulin 5 U/h i.v. (higher rate if fall in blood glucose <3 mmol/h)	0.5 l of 0.9% saline in 2 h	As above	Recheck biochemistry
	When blood glucose <15 mmol/l Reduce rate of insulin infusion to 1–4 U/h	Change to 5% glucose infusion 0.5 l/2 h	Continue i.v. K^+ supplements	Continue to check biochemistry every 2–4 h

Continue with regimen until fluid deficit replaced, ketonuria abolished and adequate oral intake of carbohydrate feasible.

Average fluid deficit = 6 litres ⟨ 3.0 litres from EXTRA-cellular compartment: replaced by saline / 3.0 litres from INTRA-cellular compartment: replaced by glucose

A bedside capillary blood glucose measurement giving a reading ≥17 mmol/l using visually-read BM 1–44 strips can be very misleading since the actual blood glucose concentration is often considerably higher when measured accurately in the laboratory. Therefore an accurate measurement should be carried out at an early stage.

Additional procedures which may be required are:
Catheterisation: if after 3 hours no urine passed
Nasogastric tube to keep stomach empty (in unconscious or semi-conscious patients)
Central venous line if cardiovascular system compromised so that volume of fluid given can be adjusted accurately
Plasma expander if BP does not rise with i.v. saline.
Antibiotic if infection demonstrated or suspected.

Monitor Blood glucose and electrolytes hourly for 3 hours and every 2–4 hours thereafter; temperature, pulse, respiration, BP hourly; urinary output and ketones; ECG, osmolality, arterial pH in some cases.
†These guidelines for a typical 'average' case should be modified appropriately in the individual patient after considering the blood biochemistry and clinical features, e.g. see page 751 for section on treatment of hyperosmolar non-ketotic diabetic coma.

present initially because of vasodilatation secondary to acidosis. Guidelines for the management of ketoacidosis are shown in Table 12.26.

Insulin

If intravenous infusion of insulin (see Table 12.26) is not practical, a loading dose of 10–20 units unmodified (clear) insulin can be given by intramuscular injection immediately followed by 4–6 units hourly thereafter. The blood glucose concentration should fall by 3–6 mmol/l per hr. If there is no fall in the blood glucose concentration by 2 hours after treatment, then the dose of insulin should be doubled until a satisfactory response

is obtained. Ketosis, dehydration, acidaemia and stress combine to produce severe insulin resistance in some cases but most will respond to a low dose insulin regime. When the blood glucose concentration has fallen to 10–15 mmol/l the dose of insulin should be reduced to 1–4 units hourly.

Fluid replacement

The deficit of extracellular fluid should be made good by infusing isotonic saline (0.9% NaCl). Early rapid rehydration is essential otherwise the administered insulin will not reach the poorly perfused tissues. If the plasma sodium is greater than 155 mmol/l, 0.45% saline may be given initially instead of 0.9%. In patients who are severely acidotic (pH <7.0, $[H^+] > 100$ nmol/l), 300–500 ml of 1.26% sodium bicarbonate may be given over 30 min into a large vein, with caution, in place of the same volume of isotonic saline. *Correction of the total bicarbonate deficit should not be attempted* on any account since there is some evidence that rapid correction of acidosis may aggravate tissue hypoxia and also reduce the level of consciousness by causing a paradoxical acidosis of the cerebrospinal fluid. The combined administration of bicarbonate and insulin will also increase the risk of hypokalaemia, and potassium should be given along with bicarbonate.

The intracellular water deficit must be replaced by using 5 or 10% dextrose and not by more saline. It is best given when the blood glucose concentration approaches normal.

Potassium

As the plasma potassium is often high at presentation treatment with intravenous potassium chloride should be started cautiously (Table 12.26) and carefully monitored by frequent estimations. Sufficient should be given to maintain a normal plasma concentration and large amounts may be required (10–300 mmol in the first 24 hours).

Antibiotics

Infections must be carefully sought and vigorously treated since it may not be possible to abolish ketosis until they are controlled.

Non-ketotic hyperosmolar diabetic coma

The aetiology of this condition is discussed on page 730. Its treatment differs from that of ketoacidosis in two main respects. Firstly, these patients are usually relatively sensitive to insulin and approximately half the dose of insulin recommended for the treatment of ketoacidosis should usually be employed at least initially. Secondly, the plasma osmolality should be measured or, less accurately, calculated using the following formula based on plasma values in mmol/l:

$$2[Na^+] + 2([K^+] + [glucose] + [urea])$$

This value is normally 280–300 mOsm/l and if it is high (>360 mOsm/l), 0.45% saline should be given until the osmolality approaches normal, when 0.9% should be substituted. The rate of fluid replacement should be regulated on the basis of the central venous pressure, and plasma sodium concentration checked frequently. Too rapid a fall in osmolality may be associated with the development of cerebral oedema.

Lactic acidosis

In coma due to lactic acidosis the patient is likely to be: a diabetic taking a biguanide who is very ill and over-breathing but not so profoundly dehydrated as is usual in coma due to ketoacidosis; whose breath does not smell of acetone, with mild or even absent ketonuria yet whose plasma bicarbonate and pH are markedly reduced (pH < 7.2). The diagnosis is confirmed by a high (usually > 5.0 mmol/l) concentration of lactic acid in the blood. Treatment is with intravenous bicarbonate sufficient to raise the plasma pH to above 7.2, along with insulin and glucose. Despite energetic treatment the mortality in this condition is $> 50\%$.

Acute circulatory failure

Acute circulatory failure occurring in any of these types of acute metabolic decompensation should be treated as described on page 215.

LONG-TERM COMPLICATIONS OF DIABETES

The long-term results of treatment of diabetes are disappointing in many patients (p. 752). The information box shows that the excess mortality incurred by diabetic patients is mainly due to large blood-vessel disease, which is common in treated diabetic patients and accounts for about 70% of all deaths. The pathological changes associated with atherosclerosis in diabetic patients are similar to those seen in the non-diabetic population but they occur earlier in life and are more extensive and severe.

Disease of small blood vessels is specific to diabetes and is termed **diabetic microangiopathy**. It contributes to the mortality, particularly that incurred by younger people, by causing renal failure due to **diabetic nephropathy**.

Both types of vascular disease also cause substantial morbidity and disability: e.g. blindness due to diabetic retinopathy; difficulty in walking, chronic ulceration of the feet, bowel and bladder dysfunction due to diabetic neuropathy; angina, cardiac failure, intermittent claudication and gangrene due to atherosclerosis.

Pathophysiology

Some of the numerous pathological, biochemical and functional abnormalities found in long-standing poorly-controlled diabetic patients are listed in the information box on page 752.

The hallmark of diabetic microangiopathy at the level of ultrastructural pathology is thickening of the capillary basement membrane with associated increased vascular permeability throughout the body. The development of

MORTALITY IN DIABETICS

Mortality ratios for diabetics and matched controls

		Significance of increased ratio seen in diabetics
Overall	2.6	P < 0.001
• Coronary heart disease		
• Cerebrovascular disease	} 2.8	P < 0.001
• Peripheral vascular disease		
• All other causes including renal failure	2.7	P < 0.05

Approximate figures for causes of deaths in treated diabetic patients

• Atherosclerosis	70%
• Renal failure	10%
• Cancer	10%
• Infections	6%
• Diabetic ketoacidosis	1%
• Other	3%

FUNCTIONAL ABNORMALITIES WITH A POSSIBLE PATHOGENIC ROLE IN DIABETIC VASCULAR AND NEUROPATHIC DISEASE

Microangiopathy and neuropathy
- Protein glycosylation↑
- Capillary basement membrane↑
- Sorbitol synthesis↑
- *Myo*-inositol metabolism↓
- Capillary permeability↑
- Blood flow↑
- Red cell deformability↓
- Red cell aggregation↑
- Blood viscosity↑
- Platelet aggregation and adhesiveness↑
- Fibrinolysis↓
- Hypertension

Macroangiopathy
- Hyperlipidaemia
- Hyperinsulinaemia
- Hypertension
- Arterial endothelial permeability↑

the characteristic clinical syndromes of diabetic retinopathy, nephropathy, neuropathy and atherosclerosis are thought to result from the imposition of organ and tissue specific factors (anatomical, haemodynamic and metabolic) on the generalised vascular injury. For example, increased permeability of arterial endothelium, particularly when combined with hyperinsulinaemia (stimulating the uptake of lipid in large arteries) and hypertension, will increase the deposition of atherogenic lipoproteins in the wall of large vessels.

Although the precise mechanisms linking hyperglycaemia to the pathological changes underlying the clinical syndromes are not yet fully defined, it is thought that increased metabolism of glucose to sorbitol via the polyol pathway is of central importance in pathogenesis, since haemodynamic, vascular permeability and structural changes in capillaries are prevented in diabetic animals by treatment with a variety of structurally different aldose-reductase inhibitors. Glycation of structural proteins and the production of advanced glycation end products, with their deposition in various tissues, may underlie some of the structural and functional abnormalities of diabetic complications.

Whatever the mechanism of the noxious effect of long-standing hyperglycaemia it has been shown (both in long-term clinical and experimental animal studies involving animal models with spontaneous and chemically-induced diabetes) that the nearer the overall blood glucose concentration is to normal, the fewer and less severe are the abnormalities listed in the information box and the lower the incidence of the clinical syndromes arising from micro- and macroangiopathy.

DIABETIC RETINOPATHY

The fact that diabetic retinopathy is the most common cause of blindness in adults between 30 and 65 years of age in developed countries is all the more depressing when one realises that, although the precise mechanism underlying its development is still not completely defined, *retinal photocoagulation is an effective treatment provided it is given at an early stage when the patient is usually symptomless. This means that regular ophthalmoscopy, with the pupils fully dilated, is mandatory in all diabetic patients.*

Clinical features

The clinical features characteristic of diabetic retinopathy are listed in the information box below. These occur in varying combinations in different patients. Abnormalities of the capillary bed, which are not clinically visible, are the earliest lesions. They include capillary dilatation and closure.

CLINICAL FEATURES OF DIABETIC RETINOPATHY

- Microaneurysms
- Retinal haemorrhages
- Hard exudates
- Soft exudates
- Venous changes
- Neovascularisation
- Pre-retinal haemorrhage
- Vitreous haemorrhage
- Fibrosis

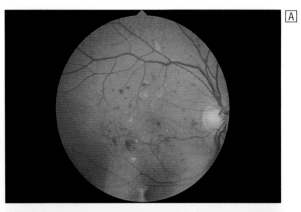

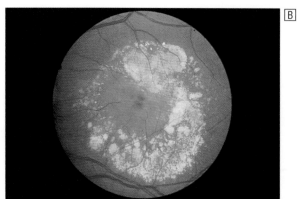

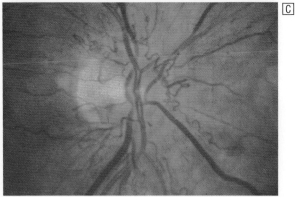

Fig. 12.44 [A] **Background diabetic retinopathy** showing dot and blot haemorrhages and a few hard exudates. [B] **Diabetic maculopathy** with ring of exudates surrounding macula. [C] **Proliferative diabetic retinopathy** showing new vessels at upper and lower edges of optic disc.

Microaneurysms

In most cases these are the earliest clinical abnormality detected. They appear as minute, discrete, circular, dark red spots near to but apparently separate from the retinal vessels (Fig. 12.44A). They look like tiny haemorrhages but photographs of injected preparations of retina show that they are in fact minute aneurysms arising mainly from the venous end of capillaries near areas of capillary closure.

Haemorrhages

These most characteristically occur in the deeper layers of the retina and hence are round and regular in shape and described as 'blot' haemorrhages (Fig. 12.44A). The smaller ones may be difficult to differentiate from micro-aneurysms and the two are often grouped together as 'dots and blots'. Superficial flame-shaped haemorrhages may also occur, particularly if the patient is hypertensive.

Hard exudates

These are characteristic of diabetic retinopathy. They vary in size from tiny specks to large confluent patches and tend to occur particularly in the perimacular area

(Fig. 12.44B). They result from leakage of plasma from abnormal retinal capillaries and overlie areas of neuronal degeneration.

Soft exudates

Sometimes referred to as 'cotton wool spots', these are similar to those seen in hypertension, and also occur particularly within five disc diameters of the optic disc. They represent arteriolar occlusions and are most often seen in rapidly advancing retinopathy or in association with uncontrolled hypertension.

Intra-retinal microvascular abnormalities

Intra-retinal microvascular abnormalities (IRMA) are dilated, tortuous capillaries which represent the remaining patent capillaries in an area where most have occluded.

Neovascularisation

This may arise from mature vessels on the optic disc or the retina in response to areas of ischaemic retina. The earliest appearance is that of fine tufts of delicate vessels forming arcades on the surface of the retina (Fig.

12.44C). As they grow they may extend forwards towards the vitreous. They are fragile and leaky and are liable to rupture causing haemorrhage which may be intraretinal, pre-retinal ('sub-hyaloid') or into the vitreous. Serous products leaking from these new vessel systems stimulate a connective tissue reaction, *retinitis proliferans*. This first appears as a white, cloudy haze among the network of new vessels. As it extends, the new vessels may be obliterated and the surrounding retina covered by a dense white sheet. At this stage bleeding is less common but retinal detachment can occur due to contraction of adhesions between the vitreous and the retina.

Venous changes

These include venous dilatation (an early feature probably representing increased blood flow), 'beading' (sausage-like changes in calibre) and increased tortuosity including 'oxbow lakes' or loops. These latter changes often indicate widespread capillary non-perfusion.

Classification

A classification of diabetic retinopathy based on prognosis for vision and indications for specialist referral, is shown in the information box.

Microaneurysms, abnormalities of the veins and small blot haemorrhages and hard exudates situated in the periphery will not interfere with vision unless they are associated with macular oedema in the perimacular or macular area. This is not easy to detect by ophthalmoscopy but should be suspected, particularly if there is marked impairment of visual acuity in association with mild peripheral background retinopathy and no other obvious pathology.

New vessels may be completely symptomless until sudden visual loss occurs from a haemorrhage into the vitreous. Although these frequently clear, the risk of recurrence is high and the more frequent the haemorrhage the slower and less complete the recovery. Fibrous tissue may seriously interfere with vision by obscuring the retina and/or causing retinal haemorrhage or detachment.

Prevention and management

Glycaemic control

Since it is clear that good metabolic control, particularly in the early years following the development of diabetes, reduces the risk of developing retinopathy, every effort should be made to achieve a metabolic state as near normal as is practicable in all diabetic patients from the time of presentation. Early diagnosis followed by effective treatment is particularly important for those with NIDDM, 15–20% of whom present with the com-

---

> **CLASSIFICATION OF DIABETIC RETINOPATHY BASED ON PROGNOSIS FOR VISION AND ACTION INDICATED**
>
> **'Background' retinopathy without maculopathy**
> - Venous dilatation
> - Peripheral: microaneurysms small blot haemorrhages small hard exudates
>
> **No immediate threat to vision**
> - Maximise control of blood glucose, lipids, and pressure; give advice to stop smoking and reduce intake of alcohol; observe carefully, i.e. fundoscopy *with dilated pupils* every 6–12 months
> - Refer for specialist opinion if rate of progression increases significantly
>
> **Pre-proliferative retinopathy and/or maculopathy**
> - Venous loops and beading
> - Clusters/sheets of micro-aneurysms and small blot haemorrhages and/or large retinal haemorrhages
> - Intra-retinal microvascular abnormalities
> - Multiple soft exudates
> - Macular oedema with reduced visual acuity
> - Perimacular exudates ± retinal haemorrhages of any size
>
> **Sight-threatening: refer for specialist opinion**
> - At this stage rapid lowering of the blood sugar may result in abrupt worsening of retinopathy with the appearance of soft exudates and an increased number of haemorrhages; it may be safer to lower the blood glucose gradually over a period of months
>
> **Proliferative retinopathy and/or exudative maculopathy**
> - Preretinal haemorrhage
> - Neovascularisation
> - Fibrosis
> - Exudative maculopathy
>
> **Urgent review and treatment by specialist mandatory**

---

plications already established. In some of these cases retinopathy is untreatable at diagnosis of diabetes while in others untreatable retinopathy is diagnosed only when the patient is referred for a specialist opinion after years of ineffective treatment of NIDDM. In other cases rapid reduction in blood glucose may result in initial deterioration (which is associated with failure of improved glycaemic control to reduce hyperperfusion) but despite this, long-term follow-up studies show that the rate of progression of retinopathy is significantly less in these intensively treated patients than in matched control subjects.

Screening

Regular screening for retinopathy is essential in all diabetic patients but is particularly important in those with risk factors. These include early onset, long duration of diabetes, hypertension, poor glycaemic control, pregnancy, use of the oral contraceptive pill, heavy smoking, abuse of alcohol, irregular attendance at specialist diabetes centres and evidence of microangiopathy elsewhere, particularly patients with neuropathy and persistent proteinuria.

Management

Pre-proliferative, proliferative and maculopathic retinopathy can be treated with retinal photocoagulation and has been shown to reduce severe visual loss by 50%. Photocoagulation is used:

- to destroy areas of retinal ischaemia (since it is thought that this plays a major role in the development of neovascularisation)
- to seal leaking microaneurysms and exudates
- to obliterate new vessels directly.

Two types of photocoagulation are available: xenon-arc (white light) and laser beam (monochromatic blue/green light). The latter is less uncomfortable for the patient and the smaller size of beam allows greater accuracy in delivering shots. This procedure can be done under local anaesthesia and in skilled hands is a simple procedure which carries little risk and can be very effective. New vessels can be eliminated and vision maintained in up to 90% of patients with new vessels on the retina and/or disc. Successfully treated patients must be reviewed regularly to check for further development of new vessels.

Vitrectomy may be used in selected cases with advanced diabetic eye disease causing permanent visual loss due to vitreous haemorrhage which has failed to clear or retinal detachment resulting from retinitis proliferans.

The more severe types of retinopathy may be accompanied by the development of new vessels on the anterior surface of the iris: 'rubeosis iridis'. These vessels may obstruct the anterior angle of the eye and the outflow of aqueous fluid, causing glaucoma. Various techniques for the treatment of rubeosis are now available

but the main method of management is the prevention of extension of the rubeosis by early retinal photocoagulation.

Cataract

Very rarely a type of cataract specific to diabetes occurs in young patients with poorly controlled diabetes. Senile cataract also occurs commonly in elderly diabetics but is probably no more common than in non-diabetic people in this age group. The indications for cataract extraction are similar to that operation in the non-diabetic population and depend on the degree of visual impairment caused by the cataract. An additional indication in the diabetic is when adequate assessment of the fundus is precluded or laser treatment to the retina is prevented. The extra-capsular method of extraction is preferable in diabetics and there is no contraindication to an intra-ocular lens.

DIABETIC NEUROPATHY

This is a relatively early and common complication in diabetic patients. Although it can cause severe disability in a few, it is symptomless in the majority. Like retinopathy it occurs secondary to the metabolic disturbance and the prevalence is related to the duration of diabetes and the degree of metabolic control. Although there is evidence that the central nervous system is affected in long-term diabetes the clinical impact of diabetes is mainly manifest on the peripheral nervous system.

Pathology

The main pathological features are listed in the information box below. They can occur in motor, sensory and autonomic nerves.

Classification

Various classifications of diabetic neuropathy have been proposed. One is shown in the information box (p. 756). None of the proposed classifications is entirely satisfactory since motor, sensory and autonomic nerves may be involved in varying combinations so that clinically mixed syndromes usually occur.

CLASSIFICATION OF DIABETIC NEUROPATHY

Somatic
- Polyneuropathy
  Symmetrical, mainly sensory and distal
  Asymmetrical, mainly motor and proximal
- Mononeuropathy (including mononeuritis multiplex)

Visceral (autonomic)
- Cardiovascular
- Gastrointestinal
- Genitourinary
- Sudomotor
- Vasomotor
- Pupillary

Clinical features

Symmetrical sensory polyneuropathy

This is frequently asymptomatic. The most common signs found on physical examination are loss of tendon reflexes in the lower limbs, diminished perception of vibration sensation distally, and 'glove-and-stocking' impairment of all other modalities of sensation. Symptoms include paraesthesiae in the feet and sometimes in the hands, pain in the lower limbs (dull, aching and/or lancinating, worse at night, and mainly felt on the anterior aspect of the legs), burning sensations in the soles of the feet, cutaneous hyperaesthesia and an abnormal gait (commonly wide-based) often associated with a sense of numbness in the feet. There may be perforating, relatively or completely painless, ulcers on the feet and painless distal arthropathy characterised by disorganisation of the joint (Charcot joints). There may also be some motor involvement causing muscle weakness and wasting. The toes may be 'clawed up' due to wasting of the interosseous muscles which results in increased pressure on the plantar aspects of the metatarsal heads with the development of callus skin at these sites. Callus skin may also develop at other pressure points. On investigation both motor and sensory conduction velocities are reduced and CSF protein may be raised.

Asymmetrical motor diabetic neuropathy

Sometimes called diabetic amyotrophy, this presents as severe and progressive weakness and wasting of the proximal muscles of the lower (and occasionally also the upper) limbs. It is commonly accompanied by severe pain mainly felt on the anterior aspect of the leg. Sometimes there may also be marked loss of weight ('neuropathic cachexia'). Hyperaesthesia and paraesthesiae are also common. The patient may look extremely ill and may be unable to get out of bed. Tendon reflexes may be absent on the affected side(s). Sometimes there are extensor plantar responses and again the CSF protein is commonly raised. This condition is now known to involve the lower motor neurones of the lumbosacral plexus. Other lesions involving this plexus, such as lower abdominal neoplasms and lumbar disc disease, must be excluded.

Mononeuropathy

Either motor or sensory function can be affected within a single peripheral or cranial nerve. The nerves most commonly affected are: the third and sixth cranial nerves resulting in diplopia due to impaired ocular movement; the ulnar and median nerves leading to the clinical picture of carpal tunnel compression syndrome; and the femoral, sciatic and lateral popliteal nerves leading to foot drop. Rarely, involvement of other single nerves results in bizarre paresis and paraesthesiae in the thorax and trunk.

Autonomic neuropathy

This is not necessarily associated with peripheral somatic neuropathy. Either parasympathetic or sympathetic nerves may be predominantly affected in any one or more system(s). Although autonomic neuropathy can affect virtually all bodily systems in any one patient, system involvement is patchy. The information box below lists the symptoms and signs arising from autonomic neuropathy affecting the various systems. The development of autonomic neuropathy is less clearly related to poor metabolic control than somatic neuropathy, and improved control rarely results in amelioration of symptoms. Five years after developing symptoms of autonomic neuropathy 50% of patients are dead—many from sudden cardiorespiratory arrest, the cause of which is unknown.

Management

Somatic neuropathy

Symptomatic relief and a degree of functional improvement can often be achieved in somatic neuropathy by maintaining a near normal blood glucose concentration ($HbA_1 < 9\%$) on a long-term basis. However, rapid improvement of glycaemic control in patients with symptomless somatic neuropathy may sometimes precipitate the development of severe symptomatic neuropathy in the short term. Continuing treatment of these cases also gives good results in the long term. This is true for proximal motor neuropathy as well as for the more common mainly sensory distal type. Intensive insulin treatment may be required not only to achieve

CLINICAL FEATURES OF AUTONOMIC NEUROPATHY

Cardiovascular
- Postural hypotension
- Resting tachycardia
- Fixed heart rate
- Sudden cardiorespiratory arrest

Gastrointestinal
- Dysphagia, due to oesophageal atony
- Abdominal fullness, nausea and vomiting, unstable diabetes, due to delayed gastric emptying ('gastroparesis')
- Nocturnal diarrhoea ± faecal incontinence
- Constipation, due to colonic atony

Genitourinary
- Difficulty in micturition, urinary incontinence, recurrent infection, due to atonic bladder
- Impotence and retrograde ejaculation

Sudomotor
- Gustatory sweating
- Nocturnal sweats without hypoglycaemia
- Anhidrosis—fissures in the feet

Vasomotor
- Feet feel constantly cold, due to loss of skin vasomotor responses
- Dependent oedema, due to loss of vasomotor tone and increased vascular permeability
- Bullous formation

Pupillary
- Decreased pupil size
- Resistance to mydriatics
- Delayed or absent response to light

Loss of awareness of hypoglycaemia
- Due to central hypothalamic dysfunction and altered glycaemic threshold for autonomic activation

an adequate degree of control but also to improve the general nutritional state. With intensive insulin treatment the prognosis is good for most patients with diabetic amyotrophy who recover over a period of months, up to 2 years.

The pain of diabetic neuropathy can be extremely distressing and unremitting particularly since it is commonly worse through the night, preventing sleep. It does not respond well to conventional analgesics but the tricyclic antidepressants, amitriptyline or imipramine, are often rapidly effective long before their anti-depressant effect is apparent. Side-effects include a dry mouth and postural hypotension, which may be particularly important if the patient also has autonomic neuropathy with associated postural hypotension.

Aldose reductase inhibitors are now available. These have been shown to reverse or prevent most of the acute changes seen in animal models of diabetic neuropathy but their place in the treatment of patients with neuropathy is still being assessed.

Postural hypotension

Postural hypotension may be improved by support stockings and fludrocortisone. When the latter is used patients require careful monitoring in relation to the possible development of hypertension or oedema.

Gastroparesis

The dopamine antagonists, metoclopramide and domperidone, are used in the treatment of gastroparesis but have several disadvantages including the fact that they tend to lose their effectiveness as time goes on, sometimes produce extrapyramidal reactions and may worsen impotence. Cisapride is a new pro-kinetic agent chemically related to metoclopramide which facilitates or restores motility throughout the gastrointestinal tract. It is thought to act mainly by indirectly enhancing acetylcholine release from the neurones of the myenteric plexus thereby increasing motor activity in gastrointestinal smooth muscle.

Diarrhoea

Diabetic diarrhoea is difficult to treat but a few patients respond to tetracycline.

Atonic bladder

Problems arising from a neurogenic bladder are also difficult to treat effectively. In a few cases stimulation of the detrusor muscle by a sympathomimetic drug such as carbachol, or bladder-neck resection, are effective but many end up with an indwelling catheter.

Impotence

Again there is no really satisfactory treatment for diabetic impotence which affects at least 25% of diabetic males. A variety of penile prostheses have been used; one of the simplest consists of a semi-rigid silicone rod implanted into the corpus cavernosa. Alternatively the patient may be taught how to inject the corpus cavernosa with papaverine or the prostaglandin E_1, alprostadil, before intercourse. However, priapism may be a troublesome side-effect which occasionally requires surgical decompression. It should be remembered that several antihypertensive drugs including beta-adrenoceptor antagonists and methyldopa can affect sexual function and that, although neuropathy is usually the cause of impotence in diabetic men, a few will have an endocrine cause and all should be screened for this.

Excessive sweating

Anticholinergic drugs such as propantheline may relieve gustatory sweating and nocturnal drenching sweats (which are not associated with hypoglycaemia) but have the disadvantage that gastric atony and urinary retention may worsen.

Prevention (see p. 752, 764)

THE DIABETIC FOOT

The foot is a frequent site for complications in patients with diabetes and for this reason foot care is particularly important. The clinical features which may be observed are listed in the information box.

CLINICAL FEATURES OF THE DIABETIC FOOT

- **Primarily neuropathic**
  Warm
  Bounding pulses
  Diminished sensation
  Pink skin
  Anhidrosis
  Callus formation
  Cracks and fissures
  Painless ulceration
  Digital gangrene
  Charcot joints
  Wasting of interosseous
    muscles
  Clawed toes
  Neuropathic oedema

- **Primarily ischaemic**
  Cold
  Absent pulses
  Sensation intact
  Skin blanches on elevation

  Painful ulceration
  Digital gangrene

  Oedema associated with
  cardiac decompensation

Tissue necrosis in the feet is a common reason for hospital admission in diabetic patients. Such admissions tend to be prolonged (weeks or months rather than days) and not unusually end with amputation at various levels.

Aetiology

Foot ulceration occurs as a result of trauma (which may be trivial) in the presence of neuropathy and/or peripheral vascular disease, with infection occurring as a secondary phenomenon following ulceration of the protective epidermis. In most cases all three components are involved but sometimes neuropathy or ischaemia may predominate. The clinical features of these two types of foot are shown in the information box above. Pure ischaemia accounts for a minority (probably about 10%) of foot ulcers in diabetic patients, neuropathy alone for 45% and the remainder are neuro-ischaemic.

The main factors involved in the development of ulceration in the primarily neuropathic foot are shown in Figure 12.45. The most common cause of ulceration is a plaque of callus skin beneath which tissue necrosis occurs. This eventually breaks through to the surface.

Management

The main components of medical management are listed in the information box. Removal of callus skin with a scalpel is usually best done by a chiropodist who has

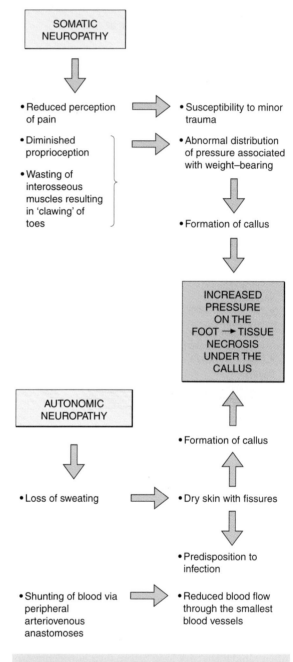

Fig. 12.45 Aetiology of ulceration in the neuropathic foot.

specialist training and experience in diabetic foot problems. Insulin may be required in patients with NIDDM who are either normally treated with dietary measures only or with diet and an oral hypoglycaemic drug, to improve glycaemic control and promote healing. Amputation may be necessary if there is extensive tissue and/or bony destruction or intractable ischaemic pain at rest in a limb in which vascular reconstruction has failed or is impossible due to extensive large blood vessel disease.

> **MEDICAL MANAGEMENT OF DIABETIC NEURO-ISCHAEMIC FOOT ULCERS**
>
> - Remove callus skin
> - Treat infection
> - Avoid weight bearing
> - Ensure good diabetic control
> - Control oedema
> - Take angiogram to assess feasibility of vascular reconstruction in some cases

> **DIABETIC FOOT—PRACTICE POINTS**
>
> - Prevention is the most effective and cost-effective way of dealing with the problem of tissue necrosis in the diabetic foot
> - A specialist chiropodist is an integral part of the diabetes team to ensure regular and effective chiropody and to educate patients in care of the feet

DIABETIC NEPHROPATHY

Diabetic nephropathy accounts for approximately 14% of all deaths in diabetic patients and some 25% of those developing diabetes under the age of 30 die from renal failure due to diabetic nephropathy.

Pathology

Figure 12.46 relates the renal histopathology to the development of diabetic nephropathy. The earliest functional renal change detected is glomerular hyperperfusion. This is followed by renal hypertrophy. At this stage renal morphology is normal although there may be microalbuminuria (albumin excretion > 30 μg/min) which is reversible by strict control of the blood glucose concentration and of hypertension, if present. Its importance is that it predicts the development of irreversible renal damage indicated by the development of proteinuria detectable by dipstix (> 150 mg/l).

Management

Once proteinuria is established, glomerular filtration declines steadily with time in a linear fashion. The rate of progression of the disease can be reduced by energetic treatment of hypertension and a low protein (40–60 g daily) diet. Since many patients are relatively young a diastolic blood pressure > 95 mmHg usually indicates the need for treatment of hypertension. Standard hypotensive drugs can be used but there are particular problems in their use in diabetic patients. For example, thiazide diuretics, by inhibiting the secretion of insulin, raise the blood glucose concentration in patients with NIDDM, while non-cardioselective beta-adrenoceptor antagonists, by inhibiting muscle glycogenolysis, may not only blunt the symptoms of hypoglycaemia in some patients taking a sulphonylurea or insulin but also aggravate impotence and peripheral vascular disease, both of which are common problems in these patients. Calcium antagonists and angiotensin-converting enzyme inhibitors are commonly used with a loop diuretic.

The management of patients with renal failure (serum creatinine > 200 μmol/l) is essentially the same as in other forms of chronic renal disease. Diabetes often becomes unstable and the dose of insulin required may have to be adjusted daily on the basis of capillary blood

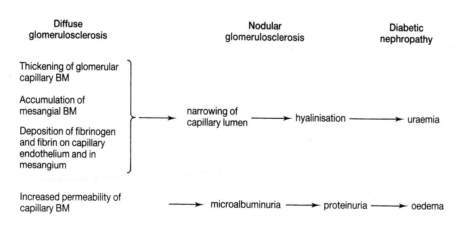

Fig. 12.46 **Renal histopathology and development of diabetic nephropathy** (BM: basement membrane).

glucose monitoring. Increased sensitivity to the action of exogenous insulin is often seen, resulting in an overall decrease in the dose of insulin required. Treatment with metformin should never be used since the risk of lactic acidosis increases with impaired renal function and long-acting sulphonylureas should be avoided and replaced by those which are metabolised rather than excreted (e.g. tolbutamide or glipizide).

When the serum creatinine level exceeds 450 μmol/l most patients are unwell and should be considered for renal support treatment. Unfortunately some will not qualify for active intervention because of another major disability arising from severe large blood-vessel disease, neuropathy or retinopathy. The results of haemodialysis are less good than in non-diabetics and most diabetic patients start treatment with continuous ambulatory peritoneal dialysis (CAPD). The results of renal transplantation in carefully selected cases can be almost as good as in non-diabetics and the use of cyclosporin has improved results in diabetic as in non-diabetic patients.

Large blood-vessel disease causing cardiac failure and ischaemic gangrene, and retinopathy and neuropathy show continued progression even after successful transplantation and need constant attention. Although characteristic glomerular and arterial changes develop in transplanted kidneys, recurrence of renal failure takes many years to develop.

SPECIAL PROBLEMS IN MANAGEMENT

DIABETES IN CHILDREN

Diabetes is relatively uncommon in children though its incidence is increasing. It always requires treatment with insulin. The therapeutic problem of matching the dose of insulin to the intake of food (which is often variable) raises practical difficulties but the principles of treating children with diabetes are the same as for adults who have IDDM. It is important to achieve as good control of the diabetes as is practicable to ensure normal growth and development and prevent the development of long-term complications of diabetes while at the same time avoiding serious hypoglycaemic episodes. This is particularly important in children since the brain may be more prone to damage than in adults. Thus children and their parents need to be educated in the management of diabetes to the limit of their ability. They need to have sufficient knowledge to make daily alterations in the dose of insulin on the basis of the results of preprandial capillary blood glucose measurements and consideration of factors such as exercise and illness. Families with a diabetic child require much support, and open access

to specialist advice by means of a 'hot line' telephone is an important component of this. The greater the integration of the medical paediatric and adult diabetes services, the less the trauma for diabetic children and their families as they grow up.

PREGNANCY AND DIABETES

Problems in diabetic pregnancy

Pregnancy in diabetic women is associated with an increased perinatal mortality rate (that is stillbirths and neonatal deaths within the first week of life). The main causes of this are intra-uterine death in the third trimester of pregnancy, prematurity (due to a high incidence of spontaneous premature labour and of elective premature delivery in an attempt to avoid late intra-uterine death), low birth weight and congenital malformation. Birth trauma is also more common due to a high incidence of excessively large, macrosomic babies.

Management of pregnancy in established diabetic women

All these problems are directly related to poor metabolic control and largely disappear if near normoglycaemia is maintained before and at conception and during pregnancy and delivery. The therapeutic goals and the components of a successful diabetic pregnancy are listed in the information box.

Gestational diabetes

Gestational diabetes, defined as diabetes diagnosed for the first time in pregnancy, is a common problem. It is associated not only with increased rates of perinatal mortality and neonatal morbidity but also with a high incidence (possibly as great as 80% at 25 years postpartum) of subsequent clinical diabetes (both insulin-dependent and non-insulin-dependent) in the mother. Normalisation of the metabolism, whether by treatment with dietary measures alone or, more commonly, with additional treatment usually in the form of insulin, undoubtedly reduces the fetal risk; its effect on diminishing the maternal risk of subsequent diabetes is less certain.

A screening procedure for gestational diabetes involving the measurement of true venous plasma glucose concentration 1 hour after a 50 g oral glucose load, followed by a formal 3-hour 100 g oral glucose tolerance test in suspicious cases, has been validated but is complicated. An accurate laboratory measurement of the basal (i.e. fasting or more than 3 hours after a meal) prevailing venous true plasma glucose concentration can be recommended for the following reasons:

- It is a simple test which avoids the need for special preparation and can be incorporated readily as part of routine antenatal care, thus encouraging assessment 2 or 3 times during pregnancy in all pregnant women.
- It is more physiological and relevant to the clinical problem, since the prevailing maternal blood glucose concentration is the important thing as far as the fetus is concerned.

Thus this measurement selects those in need of treatment. The information box gives the basal plasma glucose concentrations which indicate the need to consider instituting treatment.

HbA_1 is unreliable as a screening test for gestational diabetes and for assessing diabetic control during pregnancy because:

- it is too insensitive
- it changes too slowly
- it is affected by things other than changes in the blood glucose concentration, such as the influx of new young red cells into the circulation
- it reflects the overall integrated mean blood glucose concentration; it gives no information about fluctuations in the blood glucose level and may therefore be misleading.

Although measurements of glycated plasma albumin ('fructosamine') may be more useful than glycated hae-moglobin in pregnancy (since its rate of turnover is of the order of 2–4 weeks), it can only complement and not substitute for measurement of the blood glucose concentration which is the cornerstone of management in diabetic pregnancy.

Management of diabetes at delivery

Because of the risk of sudden intra-uterine death in the third trimester, diabetic women have traditionally been delivered at 36–38 weeks' gestation, either by caesarian section or by vaginal delivery following induction. Today improved metabolic control makes later delivery possible and most are now delivered between 38 and 39 weeks' gestation after induction of labour, or if necessary by caesarian section, while an increasing number are allowed to proceed to spontaneous vaginal delivery at term.

On the morning of delivery the usual breakfast and insulin should be replaced by an intravenous infusion of 10% dextrose with 10 units of unmodified insulin added to each 500 ml. This should be given at a rate of 100 ml hourly. The blood glucose concentration should be monitored at intervals of 1–2 hours and the concentration of insulin adjusted to keep the blood glucose concentration within the range 5–6 mmol/l. An alternative, easier and better method is to give the insulin separately from the glucose infusion by means of a constant rate infusion pump at a rate of 1–2 units hourly. Whatever method is used, administration of insulin should be stopped immediately on delivery and subcutaneous insulin resumed according to need, as determined by capillary blood glucose estimations. Little or no insulin may be required for 12 hours after delivery. Thereafter the pre-pregnancy dose of subcutaneously administered insulin can be gradually resumed.

SURGERY AND DIABETES

Surgery, whether performed electively or in an emergency, represents stress and invariably elicits secretion of the catabolic hormones cortisol, catecholamines, glucagon, and growth hormone in both normal and diabetic subjects. This results in increased glycogenolysis, gluconeogenesis, lipolysis, proteolysis and insulin resistance, while at the same time the release of insulin is suppressed. In the non-diabetic person these metabolic effects lead to a secondary increase in the secretion of insulin which exerts a restraining and controlling influence. In diabetic patients there is either absolute deficiency of insulin (IDDM) or insulin secretion is delayed and impaired (NIDDM) so that in untreated or poorly controlled diabetes the uptake of metabolic substrate is significantly reduced, catabolism is increased and ultimately metabolic decompensation in the form of diabetic ketoacidosis may develop in both types of diabetic patients. Starvation will exacerbate this process. In addition, hyperglycaemia impairs phagocytic function (leading to reduced resistance to infection) and wound healing. Thus surgery must be carefully planned and managed in the diabetic patient with particular emphasis on good metabolic control along with avoidance of hypoglycaemia which is obviously particularly dangerous in the unconscious or semiconscious patient.

Preoperative assessment

Careful preoperative assessment is mandatory and is summarised in the information box below. Much of this can be done on an outpatient basis but, if cardiovascular or renal function is impaired, there are signs of neuropathy (particular autonomic), diabetic control is poor, and alterations need to be made in the patient's usual treatment, then admission to hospital some days before operation will be required.

PREOPERATIVE ASSESSMENT IN DIABETIC PATIENTS

- Assess cardiovascular and renal function
- Check for signs of neuropathy, particularly autonomic
- Assess diabetic control
  Measure HbA$_1$
  Monitor preprandial blood glucose 4 times daily
- Review treatment of diabetes
  Replace long-acting with intermediate insulin
  Stop metformin and long-acting sulphonylureas: replace with insulin if necessary

---

Perioperative management

The management of diabetic patients undergoing surgery requiring general anaesthesia is summarised in Figure 12.47. Postoperatively the glucose/insulin/potassium infusion should be continued until the patient's intake of food is adequate, when the normal insulin or tablet regimen can be resumed. If the intravenous infusion has to be continued for more than 24 hours, plasma electrolytes and urea should be measured and urinary ketones checked daily. If the infusion is prolonged the concentration of potassium may require adjustment and if dilutional hyponatraemia occurs a parallel saline infusion may be necessary. If fluids need to be restricted, e.g. in patients with cardiovascular or renal disease, the volume of the glucose infusion can be halved by using a 20% dextrose solution and doubling the concentration of insulin and potassium. The infusion rate should then be 50 ml/hour. The insulin requirement is likely to be higher than that indicated in Figure 12.47 in patients with hepatic disease, obesity or sepsis and in

those being treated with corticosteroids or undergoing cardiopulmonary bypass surgery.

Surgical emergencies

If the patient is significantly hyperglycaemic and/or ketoacidotic this should be corrected first with an intravenous infusion of saline and/or glucose plus insulin 6 units per hour plus potassium as required on the basis of repeated plasma potassium levels. Subsequently treatment as described in Figure 12.47 can be used during and after the operation.

Emergency surgery in a patient with well-controlled insulin-dependent diabetes depends on when the last subcutaneous injection of insulin was given. If this was recent an infusion of glucose only may be sufficient but frequent monitoring is essential.

PROSPECTS IN DIABETES MELLITUS

Management

The scale of the clinical problem presented by diabetic patients with severe vascular disease, the knowledge that diabetic complications are preventable with good glycaemic control, the introduction of better methods of assessing diabetic control, the realisation that at present good control is achieved in only a minority of diabetic patients, and increased understanding of the deficiencies and limitations of conventional treatment with insulin, have led to a search for better methods of treating IDDM and these are listed in the information box above.

NEW SYSTEMS FOR DELIVERING INSULIN

- 'Open loop': pumps
- 'Closed loop': artificial pancreas
- Organ transplantation
  Whole pancreas
  Isolated islets

'Open-loop' systems are battery powered portable pumps providing continuous subcutaneous, intramuscular or intravenous infusion of insulin, delivered at fixed rates (a low basal rate and one or more higher rates before main meals) without reference to the blood glucose concentration. In practice the 'loop' is closed by the patient performing blood glucose estimations and the use of these devices requires a high degree of patient motivation; they have the particular disadvantage that if the pump fails the onset of ketosis tends to be more

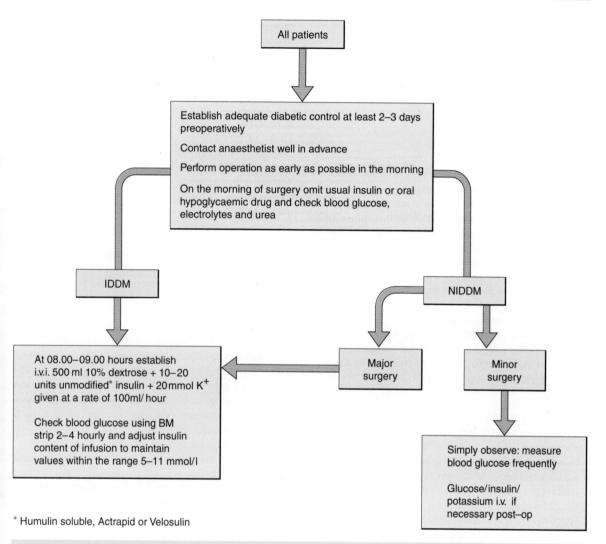

Fig. 12.47 Management of diabetic patients undergoing surgery and general anaesthesia. (IVI: intravenous infusion).

rapid than with conventional treatment because there is no subcutaneous depot of insulin. These systems will not be suitable for general therapeutic use until they are less expensive and incorporate an automatic failure alarm and a miniaturised glucose sensor. Unfortunately the latter is not yet available.

'Closed loop', sometimes referred to as 'artificial pancreas' systems, consist of three basic components: a glucose sensor, an insulin delivery pump and a computer control which regulates the administration of insulin on the basis of the blood glucose concentration. Ideally such a device should be small enough for implantation, deliver insulin intraportally and measure the blood glucose concentration rapidly without consuming blood. Existing systems deliver insulin peripherally, use blood

and are large, extracorporeal, relatively slow and unreliable, and very expensive.

Pancreatic transplantation is an alternative approach but there are particular problems relating to the exocrine pancreatic secretions and long-term immunosuppression is of course necessary. While results are steadily improving they remain significantly less good than for renal transplantation and it is questionable if it will ever be considered justifiable to transplant young diabetics before vascular disease is clinically apparent.

Transplantation of isolated pancreatic islets is an attractive concept theoretically: it is safe and the problem of the exocrine secretions is avoided. Progress is being made towards meeting the needs of supply and storage but the disadvantages of rejection and autoimmune destruction remain. Nevertheless, the development of methods of inducing tolerance to transplanted islets means that this may still prove the most promising approach in the long run.

Against this background thoughts have turned in recent years to the possibility of preventing diabetes itself.

Primary prevention of diabetes

From a public health standpoint the only cost-effective way of dealing with diabetes is to prevent it.

NIDDM is a disease of the prosperous and its development is associated with an affluent life-style. NIDDM is likely to arise in genetically predisposed individuals who eat too much and exercise too little. Effective health education could do much to reduce the incidence of clinically expressed disease, while screening for diabetes (particularly in high-risk groups such as the first-degree relatives of known cases) and more vigorous and early treatment of NIDDM would reduce the incidence of serious vascular disease in these patients.

The fact that the islet insulin-secreting cells are destroyed slowly over several years before clinical presentation of IDDM offers the hope that, in the future, it may be possible to prevent IDDM. This depends on:

- the availability of accurate, predictive markers for the development of clinical diabetes in genetically predisposed individual subjects (islet cell antibodies are being used for this purpose at present)
- an understanding of the precise sequence of events leading to pancreatic beta cell destruction
- the development of methods of intervention based on specifically targeted immunomodulation (p. 727, Fig. 12.31) which could be applied early in the prediabetic period before most of the insulin-secreting cells have been destroyed.

Rapid progress is being made in all these areas.

FURTHER READING

Alberti K G M M, Krall L P (eds) 1991 The Diabetes Annual, 6. Elsevier Science Publishers, Amsterdam. Contains review chapters on most aspects of diabetes
Caputo G M, Cavanagh P R, Ulbrecht J S, Gibbons G W, Karchmer A W 1994 Assessment and management of foot disease in patients with diabetes. New England Journal of Medicine 331: 854–860
The Diabetes Control and Complications Trial Research Group 1993 The effect of intensive treatment of diabetes on the development and progression of long-term complications in insulin-dependent diabetes mellitus. New England Journal of Medicine 329: 977–986
Frier B M 1993 Hypoglycaemia in the diabetic adult. Baillière's Clinical Endocrinology and Metabolism 7: 575–777

OTHER METABOLIC DISORDERS

Metabolism is as fundamental as life itself; in medicine the term 'metabolic' is usually restricted to disorders which can best be described in biochemical terms.

Many metabolic disorders are acquired. Others are congenital. The genetic aetiology of numerous inborn errors of metabolism has been identified with abnormalities of the structure or function of DNA and the pattern of their inheritance mapped by the study of a particular biochemical disorder. The vast majority of inborn errors of metabolism are rare and it would be inappropriate to describe them here. The reader will find much further information in specialised textbooks (p. 774).

Metabolic disorders may be classified in various ways, e.g. by the mode of inheritance or by the chemical factors involved. The specific enzyme deficiency responsible for the disorder or the body system principally affected may be named. Disorders of carbohydrate, protein or amino acid, lipid or mineral metabolism may be predominant features, and a few examples of these are given below.

Carbohydrate. Diabetes mellitus is by far the most frequent and important disorder of carbohydrate metabolism. Rare genetic errors lead to abnormalities in the metabolism of galactose (galactosaemia), fructose (fructosuria), and glycogen (glycogen storage diseases, such as von Gierke's disease, p. 885).

Amino acids. Inborn errors account for many relatively rare diseases such as cystinuria and the Fanconi syndrome. Phenylketonuria is also rare but leads to mental retardation if not detected in the neonatal period and treated with a special diet.

Purines. Gout is a classic example of a metabolic disorder and is described on page 883 along with other causes of arthritis.

LIPID DISORDERS

LIPOPROTEIN METABOLISM

The problem of transporting cholesterol and triglyceride through the aqueous environment of the plasma was solved by enveloping these hydrophobic neutral lipids in a coat of phospholipid and special proteins (called apolipoproteins) with the characteristic properties of detergents (Fig. 12.48). The phospholipid molecules are arranged on the surface of the lipoproteins with their polar head groups facing the surrounding aqueous environment and their fatty acid side chains penetrating the interior of the particles. The apolipoproteins are

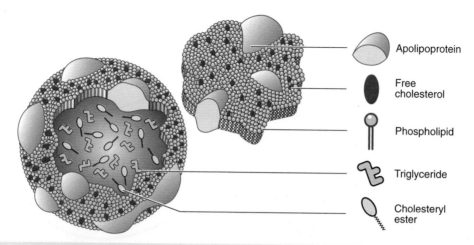

Fig. 12.48 Structural characteristics of a typical lipoprotein.

Apolipoprotein

Free cholesterol

Phospholipid

Triglyceride

Cholesteryl ester

interspersed in this surface matrix and act as recognition domains, permitting the specific interaction of the lipoproteins with the plasma enzymes and cell receptors which are responsible for their catabolism.

Lipoprotein metabolism can be thought of in terms of two interconnected transport pathways focusing on the liver (Fig. 12.49). One, the exogenous pathway, is responsible for the digestion, absorption and tissue dissemination of dietary fat. Through it each day flows about 100 g of triglyceride and 0.5 g of cholesterol. Digestive enzymes in the intestinal lumen hydrolyse these fats to free cholesterol, fatty acids and mono- and diglycerides which combine with bile salts to form the water soluble micelles responsible for carrying the lipids to absorptive sites in the small intestine. Under normal circumstances triglyceride absorption is virtually complete, while only about 50% of the cholesterol is taken up, the rest being lost in the faeces.

Following their absorption into the intestinal enterocytes, the component parts of the dietary fat are reconstituted to reform triglyceride and cholesteryl ester which are packaged in chylomicrons and secreted into the intestinal lymphatics, through which they reach the blood stream via the thoracic duct. In the circulation triglyceride is gradually removed by the action of the enzyme lipoprotein lipase, located on the endothelial surface of capillary beds in adipose tissue and cardiac and skeletal muscle. This process eviscerates the chylomicron, leaving a remnant which is taken up rapidly by the liver, depositing in the process dietary cholesterol in that organ. There the sterol may be incorporated into hepatocyte membranes, oxidised to bile acids or repackaged into the endogenous triglyceride-

rich counterpart of the chylomicron, the very low density lipoprotein (VLDL).

Among its many synthetic activities, the liver is responsible for the continuous production of VLDL which in the fasting state represents the body's primary source of circulating triglyceride energy. This particle is subject to the same lipase-mediated digestion process as the chylomicron except that in this case the resulting particle (intermediate density lipoprotein) is not cleared rapidly by the liver but instead undergoes additional remodelling to produce a cholesterol-enriched particle (low density lipoprotein) with a plasma half-life of about 3 days. LDL is ultimately removed from the circulation by the high affinity LDL receptor pathway or by other less well understood scavenger mechanisms which are thought to lead to the incorporation of LDL cholesterol into atheromatous plaques. Raised levels of LDL cholesterol therefore predispose to coronary heart disease.

In contrast to LDL with its associated risk of coronary heart disease, cholesterol-rich high density lipoprotein (HDL) particles protect against the condition. They are synthesised in both the liver and intestine and are able to remove cholesterol from peripheral tissues and transport it centripetally for hepatic excretion. This process is thought to be anti-atherogenic, consistent with the observation that raised values of circulating HDL reduce the risk of coronary heart disease.

Disorders of lipoprotein metabolism

Lipoprotein disorders or dyslipidaemias are among the commonest metabolic diseases seen in clinical practice. They are important because they may lead to a number of sequelae including coronary heart disease, dermato-

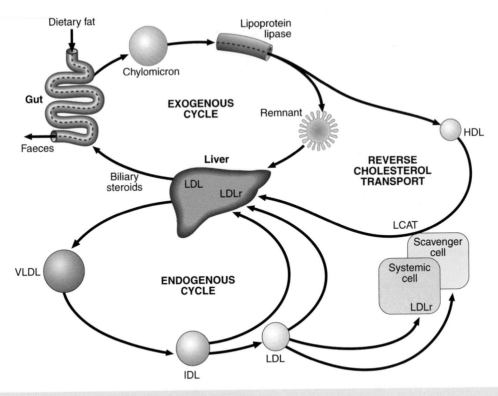

Fig. 12.49   The pathways of cholesterol transport through the plasma.

logical manifestations (xanthelasmata and xantho-mata), pancreatitis and (more rarely) neurological and ocular anomalies. Both hyper- and hypolipidaemias are recognised.

The hyperlipidaemias

Hyperlipidaemia is common and can be divided into **primary** anomalies which cannot be linked to an ident-ifiable underlying disease or **secondary** manifestations of some other condition (see information box). The lat-

ter usually disappear when the underlying condition is treated effectively.

PRIMARY HYPERLIPIDAEMIA

Classification

There is at present no satisfactory comprehensive classi-fication of lipoprotein disorders. Initially, attempts were made to define the abnormalities on the basis of their laboratory presentation. This classification, attributed to Fredrickson and his colleagues, is still clinically valuable (Table 12.27) but fails to identify the molecular or genetic defect(s) responsible for the condition. Conse-quently, patients with the same genetic defect may fall into two or more of the five Fredrickson categories; and progression of the condition or treatment may cause a patient to move from one category to another.

Recently, attempts have been made to introduce a genetic classification system (Table 12.27) but, as dif-ferent molecular defects are being discovered, this approach has become increasingly complex. So, until gene therapy or pharmacologic manipulation of molec-ular defects become real possibilities, genetic classi-fications are unlikely to prove widely useful in clinical

---

COMMON CAUSES OF SECONDARY HYPERLIPIDAEMIA	
Disease	**Dominant lipid and lipoprotein abnormality**
Diabetes mellitus	Raised triglyceride, VLDL, IDL
Alcohol excess	Raised triglyceride, VLDL
Chronic renal failure	Raised triglycerides, VLDL; low HDL
Drugs, e.g. thiazides, non-selective β-adreno-ceptor antagonists	Raised triglycerides, VLDL
	Raised triglycerides, VLDL
	Raised cholesterol, LDL
Hypothyroidism	Raised cholesterol, LDL
Nephrotic syndrome	Raised cholesterol, LDL

Table 12.27   Classification of the hyperlipoproteinaemias

Fredrickson type	Genetic classification	Defect	Risk
I	Lipoprotein lipase deficiency Apo CII deficiency	Mutated or absent lipoprotein lipase Mutated lipoprotein lipase cofactor	Pancreatitis
II	Familial hypercholesterolaemia Apo B_{3500} defect	Diminished or absent LDL-receptor interaction	CHD
III	Apo E_2 homozygosity	Mutated apolipoprotein E plus precipitating environmental factor	CHD and PVD
IV	Familial combined hyperlipidaemia Familial hypertriglyceridaemia	? ?	CHD Pancreatitis
V	Familial hypertriglyceridaemia	?	Pancreatitis

CHD = Coronary heart disease
PVD = Peripheral vascular disease

practice and most physicians will remain loyal to the older Fredrickson classification.

Clinical application of the Fredrickson classification

Type I hyperlipoproteinaemia

This autosomal recessive abnormality manifests itself in childhood as an intolerance of dietary fat and failure to thrive. It presents clinically as a widespread cutaneous papular rash, often accompanied by abdominal pain which may progress to full-blown pancreatitis. Metabolically, lipolysis of chylomicrons is defective, and these particles persist in the blood stream even in the fasting state and can be visualised directly as lipaemia in the retinal vessels. Plasma triglyceride values often exceed 50 mmol/l (i.e. 25 times the upper reference limit) and cholesterol may rise to 12–15 mmol/1 reflecting the increased amount of chylomicrons in the blood stream. In molecular terms, the disease results from faulty operation of the plasma enzyme lipoprotein lipase, either as a result of a mutation in the lipase gene itself or because of a sequence defect in its essential apolipoprotein cofactor, apo CII, which normally circulates in association with triglyceride-rich lipoproteins.

Management consists of limiting dietary fat intake to no more than about 30 g/day and, instead of natural breast or bottled milk, substituting short chain triglycerides, with fatty acid chain length of 12 carbon atoms on average. The latter do not contribute to chylomicron production but are transferred, albumin-bound directly to the liver via the portal venous system.

Type II hyperlipoproteinaemia

This rubric describes patients who present with elevated plasma LDL cholesterol levels. Most individuals in this category suffer from a polygenic inability to metabolise their normal dietary cholesterol load and generally it is possible to achieve a favourable clinical response by limiting their daily intake of sterol and substituting poly- or monounsaturated for saturated fat in their diet. One in 100 of these individuals, however, will harbour the monogenic autosomal condition known as familial hypercholesterolaemia. They usually develop tendon xanthomata and present with a personal and family history of premature coronary atherosclerosis (50% will have a myocardial infarction by the age of 50). It is rare for such individuals to show an adequate response to dietary restriction alone since heterozygotes will have twice normal LDL cholesterol values, and the rarer and more severely affected homozygotes, levels as high as 20 mmol/l. The disease results from defective or absent LDL receptors, and, as a consequence, retarded LDL clearance. The lipoprotein which accumulates in the blood stream is redirected into poorly controlled, potentially atherogenic catabolic routes. Treatment is aimed at maximising the efficiency of functional LDL receptors using bile acid sequestrant resins like cholestyramine (up to 24 g/day) or HMG CoA reductase inhibitors like pravastatin or simvastatin (10–40 mg/d). Recently, a new syndrome with all the features of familial hypercholesterolaemia has been described. It results from a sequence defect in apolipoprotein B, the recognition protein on LDL which causes it to bind to its receptor. This condition, known as the B_{3500} defect, responds well to sequestrant resin or statin therapy.

Type III hyperlipoproteinaemia (synonyms: familial dysbetalipoproteinaemia; remnant removal disease, floating beta disease)

Lipolysis of VLDL normally proceeds in the plasma via a transient particle intermediate in density and composition (called intermediate density lipoprotein or IDL) to LDL. However, roughly 1 in 5000 individuals accumulates this intermediate density particle in his or her plasma. The metabolic defect responsible for the condition is not yet clear, although two independent factors appear to combine together to produce it. First, the primary sequence of amino acids in apolipoprotein E, one of the VLDL proteins, is defective. This is clearly not the sole problem since 1 in 100 in the population harbours such a defect. Clinical expression of the condition must therefore be triggered by a second, probably environmental, aggravating factor. Interestingly, although the level of LDL in the plasma of type III hyperlipoproteinaemic subjects is reduced rather than elevated, they are predisposed to premature atherosclerosis. For this reason, it is likely that IDL is of particular significance in the pathogenesis of atherosclerosis.

Type III responds well to diet and drug therapy, particularly with the new generation of clofibrate analogues like fenofibrate, ciprofibrate, bezafibrate and gemfibrozil. These agents are very effective in reducing the high circulating IDL levels, but they do not, of course, correct the primary sequence defect in apolipoprotein E. Their actions must therefore be directed against those factors that operate synergistically with this defect to generate the characteristic clinical expression of the disease.

Type IV hyperlipoproteinaemia

Type IV hyperlipoproteinaemia is associated with accumulation in the plasma of VLDL of normal composition which, from metabolic studies, appears to be oversynthesised in some individuals and undercatabolised in others. In severe cases, where VLDL levels are very high, plasma LDL is commonly subnormal. However, it is not uncommon to see, in the families of affected individuals, some subjects with raised LDL and others with a combined increment in both VLDL and LDL. The origins of this condition, familial combined hyperlipidaemia, still await elucidation.

As is the case for the other hyperlipoproteinaemias, dietary modification always constitutes the first line of treatment of type IV hyperlipoproteinaemic subjects. Carbohydrate and alcohol restriction frequently achieves satisfactory control of their plasma triglyceride levels. Where the response is inadequate, however, it may be necessary to add nicotinic acid (3–4 g/day) or a clofibrate analogue to the regimen.

Type V hyperlipoproteinaemia

Although primary type V hyperlipoproteinaemia is rare, the phenotype is a not infrequent sequel to overindulgence in alcohol and to diabetes mellitus. It is, therefore, a disease of adult life and is characterised biochemically by the simultaneous accumulation of VLDL and chylomicra in the blood stream. It shares several clinical features with type I hyperlipoproteinaemia, such as eruptive xanthomata and pancreatitis, and, like the former, is not characterised by premature atherosclerosis.

Management again begins with diet, restricting carbohydrate and alcohol intake. Where this fails to resolve the problem, triglyceride-lowering agents like nicotinic acid or the fibrates are added to the regimen.

The hypolipoproteinaemias

The hypolipoproteinaemias are fortunately rare but, when they do occur, they often present with spectacular clinical features. Basically, they are of two main types. The first, abetalipoproteinaemia or hypobetalipoproteinaemia, results from defective secretion of apolipoprotein B containing lipoproteins (chylomicra, VLDL, IDL and LDL). This results in fat malabsorption, ataxic neuropathy, retinitis pigmentosa and acanthocytosis. There is no definitive treatment, though vitamin E administration may curb many of the morbid consequences of the condition.

The second deficiency state, Tangier disease, is associated with defective production of apolipoprotein A containing HDL particles. As a result cholesterol transport to the liver for excretion is obstructed and sterol esters accumulate in unusual peripheral sites within the reticuloendothelial system (e.g. tonsils, intestinal lymph nodes) and the cornea. Relapsing neuropathy is a feature of the condition which has no specific treatment.

SPONTANEOUS HYPOGLYCAEMIA

Multiple causes of hypoglycaemia are recognised in humans. By far the commonest is 'iatrogenic', which results from treatment with insulin or sulphonylurea drugs in patients with diabetes mellitus (see p. 746). Occasionally, hypoglycaemia is the presenting feature of an illness or occurs as an important epiphenomenon and is then considered to be 'spontaneous'. Hypoglycaemia is a biochemical abnormality (and not a clinical diagnostic entity per se), and is arbitrarily defined as a blood glucose concentration below 2.2 mmol/l. A blood glucose of this level is almost always pathological; it is accompanied by clinical manifestations and requires active investigation to establish the cause.

Because the human brain is vitally dependent on a continuous supply of glucose as its principal source of energy, disruption of glucose availability will rapidly cause malfunction from neuroglycopenia. Multiple counter-regulatory mechanisms therefore exist to prevent a dangerous decline in blood glucose, including the secretion of hormones such as glucagon and adrenaline, suppression of endogenous insulin secretion, and neurally activated release of neurotransmitters.

The main factors affecting glucose homeostasis are: the intake of nutrients, gastric emptying and intestinal absorption, hepatic production of glucose and the secretion of insulin and counter-regulatory hormones. Prevailing blood glucose concentration is a consequence of the rates of glucose influx into, and efflux from, the circulation. Homeostatic mechanisms normally maintain blood glucose in a narrow range of 3.5–6.5 mmol/l with very limited excursions associated with starvation and the ingestion of food.

Classification

The most useful classification of hypoglycaemia is based upon aetiology, and the main causes of spontaneous hypoglycaemia in adults are shown in the information box on page 771. Subdivision of hypoglycaemia into 'fasting' and 'reactive' types is now outdated.

The spectrum of causes of hypoglycaemia varies between hospital and community practice. In hospitalised patients, hypoglycaemia is associated with diabetic therapy, chronic renal failure, liver disease, infections, shock, pregnancy, neoplasia and burns. In the community, the majority of cases of hypoglycaemia are associated with the inadvertent misuse of insulin or excessive alcohol consumption. All other causes (see information box on page 771) are relatively rare in clinical practice.

Clinical features

Hypoglycaemia is usually episodic and recurs at irregular intervals. Symptomatic features which are common with acute insulin-induced hypoglycaemia (e.g. sweating, tremor, hunger and anxiety, see p. 746) are often absent in patients with spontaneous hypoglycaemia. A low blood glucose should be suspected in patients with altered consciousness, convulsions, abnormal neurological findings or odd behaviour. A high index of suspicion of hypoglycaemia should be maintained even when an obvious cause of cerebral abnormality is apparent, such as hemiplegic stroke, alcoholic intoxication or cerebral malaria. An accurate and reliable history may be difficult to obtain from the patient and an objective account from witnesses may be invaluable. Subacute or chronic neuroglycopenia often presents with deteriorating cognitive function over months or years, and psychiatric features may be prominent such as altered personality or even frank psychosis. In many instances, the only indication that hypoglycaemia is responsible is the finding of a low blood glucose on routine biochemical screening.

Investigations

A firm diagnosis of hypoglycaemia is usually based on 'Whipple's triad':

1. Symptoms are associated with fasting or exercise
2. Symptoms are relieved by glucose
3. A low blood glucose is demonstrated biochemically.

In addition, hypoglycaemia is often associated with inappropriately elevated plasma insulin concentrations.

Suspected hypoglycaemia (blood glucose <2.5 mmol/l) should be confirmed by laboratory analysis of venous blood or capillary glucose. Test strips for capillary blood glucose, which are used for monitoring diabetes, are not adequate to make a definitive diagnosis of hypoglycaemia. They are neither sufficiently sensitive nor accurate in the hypoglycaemic range and are often misread. Blood should be collected during the emergency presentation, both to confirm hypoglycaemia and for additional analyses, e.g. hormones, (insulin, C-peptide), alcohol and drugs which may identify a cause. This can prevent subsequent unnecessary and costly investigation, and has forensic and medico-legal importance in cases such as attempted suicide or deliberate poisoning with toxic substances.

The nature and timing of the blood samples for glucose measurement are of importance. Although arterial blood glucose concentration usually determines the presence of neuroglycopenia, normally venous or capillary blood samples are taken for glucose estimation. In the fasting state, no significant arteriovenous difference in blood glucose is present; but following administration of a glucose load (usually as oral liquid carbohydrate) the difference between venous and arterial blood glucose can be 1.0 mmol/l or greater, producing apparent but spurious hypoglycaemia in venous blood samples. The possible development of a large arteriovenous difference after glucose absorption precludes the use of oral glucose load tests in the evaluation of causes of hypoglycaemia.

INVESTIGATION OF SPONTANEOUS HYPOGLYCAEMIA

- **Provocation tests**
  Fasting: blood glucose and insulin measured following overnight (18 hours) fast ($\times 3$)
  Prolonged fast (72 hours) rarely needed
  Exercise: blood glucose measured following 30 minutes' vigorous exercise on treadmill or bicycle

- **Dynamic suppression tests**
  C-peptide suppression test: i.v. infusion of 0.125 U/kg soluble insulin for 60 minutes with measurement of plasma glucose, insulin and C-peptide at 30 minute intervals

Blood glucose

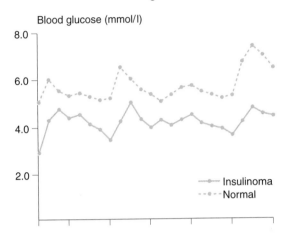

Plasma insulin

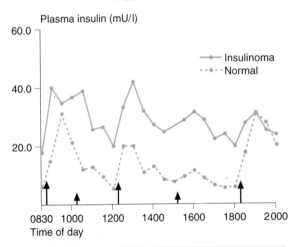

Fig. 12.50 Profiles of blood glucose and plasma insulin over a 12-hour period in six patients with insulinoma (●——●) and six normal subjects (●---●). Long arrows indicate main meals and small arrows indicate snacks. Mean plasma insulin was calculated from log transformed data.

It should also be noted that plasma glucose concentration is 15% higher than that estimated from whole venous blood.

Provocative tests for investigating suspected hypoglycaemia are summarised in the information box. Most patients with recurrent spontaneous hypoglycaemia will have a low blood glucose (<2.5 mmol/l) after an overnight fast (18 hours), but this should be confirmed on three separate occasions. In normal persons, blood glucose levels do not fall during exercise but in affected individuals hypoglycaemia may be precipitated by vigorous exercise for 30 minutes. A prolonged fast (72 hours) is rarely necessary, being a non-specific test which should be reserved for patients with demonstrated hyperinsulinism who have not developed symptomatic neuroglycopenia after overnight fasting, with or without exercise.

Plasma concentrations of insulin, C-peptide, pro-insulin and other hormones such as IGF-I and IGF-II may be estimated during confirmed hypoglycaemia. Characteristic patterns of plasma glucose and insulin are associated with different causes of hypoglycaemia.

A diagnosis of endogenous hyperinsulinism depends upon evidence of inappropriate insulin and/or C-peptide secretion in the presence of hypoglycaemia.

Other provocative tests, such as the measurement of plasma C-peptide during insulin-induced hypoglycaemia (C-peptide suppression test) may be of value in the investigation of insulin-secreting tumours. Most other forms of provocative test are seldom used or are obsolete.

TUMOUR-INDUCED HYPOGLYCAEMIA

Insulinomas are pancreatic islet-cell tumours that secrete insulin and usually cause recurrent fasting hypoglycaemia.

These are rare tumours (about 1–2 cases/million population per year) but are one of the commonest causes of fasting hypoglycaemia in non-diabetics (information box p. 771). Often the patient has had symptoms for many years prior to presentation. These may include drowsiness on waking or a variety of other symptoms which may result in referral to a neurologist or psychiatrist (fits, 'funny turns', faintness, abnormal behaviour, paraesthesiae). These characteristically occur before meals and are relieved by food or a sweet drink. The tumours are often relatively small (0.5–5 mm in diameter) and may be found in any part of the pancreas. About 10% of them are malignant. The key to diagnosis is the demonstration of fasting hyperinsulinaemia (i.e. a plasma insulin which is inappropriately high for the blood glucose—see the information box) and a failure of suppression of insulin secretion, as judged by C-peptide levels, during insulin-induced hypoglycaemia. The tumours can be difficult to localise by CT scanning or conventional ultrasound but endoscopic ultrasonography may help. If the tumour cannot be found in this way then multiple blood samples can be taken from the portal, superior mesenteric and splenic veins to measure insulin levels. A 'hot spot' may indicate the site of the tumour. For non-malignant tumours surgery is the

CAUSES OF HYPOGLYCAEMIA IN ADULTS

- **Pancreatic**
  Insulinoma*: benign, malignant, multiple and microadenomatosis
  Islet hyperplasia: nesidioblastosis or functional hyperinsulinism
  Pancreatitis
  Pluriglandular syndrome

- **Extrapancreatic neoplasms**
  Mesenchymal tumours*
  Haemangiopericytoma
  Primary hepatic carcinoma
  Various other tumours

- **Autoimmune hypoglycaemia**
  Autoimmune insulin syndrome
  Anti-insulin receptor antibodies

- **Toxic hypoglycaemia**
  Therapeutic hypoglycaemic agents: insulin, sulphonylureas*
  Alcohol*
  Drugs, e.g. quinine, salicylates, propranolol, pentamidine
  Poisons, e.g. certain types of mushroom

- **Essential reactive hypoglycaemia**
  Postgastrectomy: gastrointestinal motility disorders
  Early diabetes mellitus
  Alcohol-provoked
  'Idiopathic'; postprandial syndrome

- **Liver and kidney disease**
  Hepatocellular disease
  Advanced renal failure
  Congestive cardiac failure

- **Endocrine disease**
  Pituitary insufficiency
  Adrenocortical insufficiency
  Hypothyroidism
  Selective hypothalamic insufficiency

- **Inborn errors of metabolism**
  Adult glycogenolysis (liver glycogen disease)
  Hereditary fructose intolerance
  Defective gluconeogenesis

- **Miscellaneous**
  Sepsis
  Prolonged starvation: anorexia nervosa
  Dialysis
  Excessive exercise
  Diseases of the nervous system

*indicates common cause

treatment of choice but if the tumour cannot be found or is malignant then medical therapy may be appropriate (see below).

Hypoglycaemia may also occur as a preterminal feature of advanced malignancy, particularly in patients with extensive hepatic metastases, and also with some very large tumours such as fibrosarcoma. Some tumours secrete substances with insulin-like activity, but this is uncommon. An alternative mechanism for tumours affecting the liver is the loss of hepatic gluconeogenesis.

REACTIVE HYPOGLYCAEMIA AND POSTPRANDIAL SYNDROME

True reactive hypoglycaemia may occur in patients who have had previous gastric surgery or who have gastro-intestinal motility disorders and this may be a manifestation of the 'dumping' syndrome (Ch. 7). However, some individuals describe symptoms suggestive of, but not actually due to, hypoglycaemia occurring 1–2 hours after food. This is often investigated inappropriately with an extended oral glucose tolerance test. An oral liquid glucose load often provokes a fall in blood glucose to below 3.0 mmol/l in normal individuals, and in view of the potential arteriovenous glucose difference, mis-interpretation of these results may provoke an erroneous diagnosis of reactive hypoglycaemia. The suggested mechanisms for these symptoms include meal-induced hypotension, hyperventilation, altered glycaemic thresholds for neuroglycopenia, and neuroticism.

These patients should be evaluated with ambulatory blood glucose measurements or with a standard mixed meal with serial measurements of plasma glucose and insulin and recording of symptoms. Occasionally, asynchronous plasma concentrations of glucose and insulin may be demonstrated but the meal provocation test rarely provokes symptomatic or biochemical hypoglycaemia, in contrast to the extended oral glucose tolerance test which may yield false-positive results and has to be interpreted with caution.

Management

Emergency

The emergency treatment of severe hypoglycaemia should not be withheld to await the establishment of a

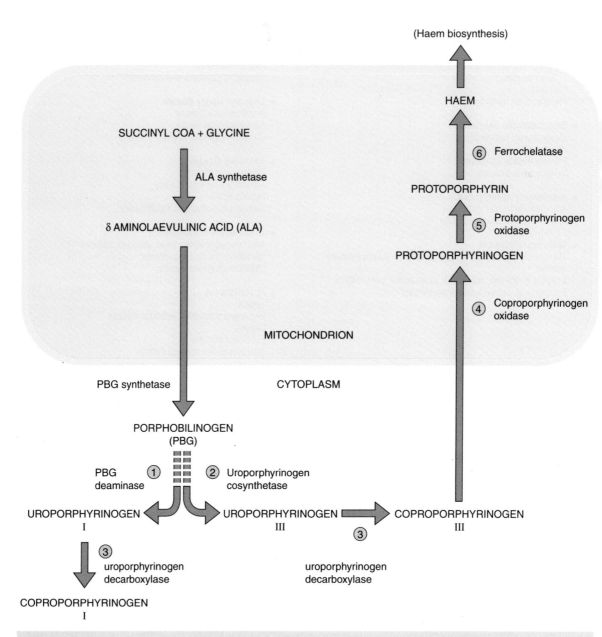

Fig. 12.51   Metabolic pathways for haem biosynthesis. Key: A block in porphyrin metabolism at the following sites results in a particular form of porphyria:

1 PBG deaminase	**Acute intermittent porphyria**
2 Uroporphyrinogen cosynthetase	**Congenital (erythropoietic) porphyria**
3 Uroporphyrinogen decarboxylase	**Porphyria cutanea tarda**
4 Coproporphyrinogen oxidase	**Hereditary coproporphyria**
5 Protoporphyrinogen oxidase	**Variegate porphyria**
6 Ferrochelatase	**Erythropoietic protoporphyria**

biochemical diagnosis. Reversal of hypoglycaemia is most effectively achieved with intravenous glucose given as 50 ml of 50% dextrose. Localised thrombophlebitis is a hazard. On regaining consciousness, the patient should be given oral carbohydrate and a continuous intravenous infusion of dextrose (5% or 10%) may be necessary to prevent recurrence of hypoglycaemia. Intramuscular glucagon (1 mg) may be of value but may be ineffective if hepatic glycogen stores are depleted, as in prolonged starvation, severe inanition or protracted hypoglycaemia.

The development of cerebral oedema should be considered in patients who fail to regain consciousness after blood glucose is restored to normal. Other causes of impaired consciousness, such as alcoholic intoxication, a post-ictal state or cerebral haemorrhage, should be excluded and computed tomography of the brain may be necessary. Cerebral oedema has a high mortality and morbidity and requires urgent treatment with mannitol and/or dexamethasone.

Long-term

Treatment of the underlying cause of hypoglycaemia will depend principally upon the specific diagnosis. Tumour-induced hypoglycaemia may require prolonged medical therapy if the tumour is not resectable surgically or cannot be located. Drugs such as diazoxide, combined with chlorothiazide, are beneficial and inhibit insulin secretion. Streptozotocin is used in treating malignant insulin-secreting tumours, particularly when metastatic disease is present. Octreotide (a long-acting synthetic analogue of somatostatin) may be useful in some cases. The doses of these drugs have to be determined on the basis of the response. Patients with true reactive hypoglycaemia usually respond to dietary measures with the exclusion of highly refined sugars (such as sucrose) and frequent, regular meals high in fibre content.

THE PORPHYRIAS

Haem is the ferrous iron complex of protoporphyrin IX which functions as a prosthetic group for the haemoproteins; its biosynthesis occurs in all aerobic cells (Fig. 12.51). The porphyrias are a heterogeneous group of rare disorders associated with inherited or acquired abnormalities of enzymes involved in the biosynthesis of haem, resulting in overproduction, accumulation and excretion of the intermediate compounds, the porphyrins. These are pigments formed of four pyrrole rings, each composed of delta-aminolaevulinic acid (ALA). The enzyme delta-ALA synthase is a rate-limiting step

Table 12.28 Classification and principal features of the porphyrias

Hepatic	Erythropoietic
Acute intermittent porphyria (AIP) Autosomal dominant Porphobilinogen synthase abnormality Precipitated by drugs and alcohol Abdominal pain, polyneuropathy, hypertension, neuropsychiatric disorders	**Congenital porphyria** Autosomal recessive Uroporphyrinogen synthase abnormality Extreme sensitivity to sunlight (severe scarring) Dystrophy of nails and teeth, blindness
Variegate porphyria Autosomal dominant Protoporphyrinogen oxidase abnormality Features of AIP and cutaneous porphyria Bullous eruption with sunlight	**Erythropoietic protoporphyria** Autosomal dominant Ferrochelatase abnormality Cutaneous photosensitivity, hepatic dysfunction
Hereditary coproporphyria Autosomal dominant Similar to variegate porphyria Very rare	
Porphyria cutanea tarda Autosomal dominant Hepatic uroporphyrinogen decarboxylase abnormality Association with alcohol; hepatic tumours	

in the rate of production of haem, and an increase in its activity results in overproduction of porphyrins. Porphyrins are categorised as uro-, copro- or protoporphyrins depending on their structure, and both uro- and coproporphyrins can be excreted in the urine. The urine may turn reddish-brown on standing, and excess porphobilinogen can be demonstrated with the use of Ehrlich's aldehyde reagent.

The excess production of porphyrins occurs either in the liver (hepatic porphyria) or in the bone marrow (erythropoietic porphyria). The classification of the porphyrias is shown in Table 12.28. The hepatic porphyrias present clinically as acute disorders, with the exception of porphyria cutanea tarda. The clinical manifestations take the form of neurological dysfunction and sensitivity of the skin to sunlight, and may be exacerbated by drugs, hormones or hepatic disease. The neurological syndrome includes acute abdominal pain and vomiting, peripheral neuropathy and mental disturbance including depression or frank psychosis. Skin photosensitivity and cutaneous eruptions are directly related to tissue accumulation of porphyrins. Acute intermittent porphyria may be precipitated by drugs (barbiturates and oestrogen-containing oral contraceptives) or alcohol. Management of acute episodes is mainly supportive, and affected patients must try to avoid possible precipitating factors.

FURTHER READING

Endo A 1992 The discovery and development of HMGCoA reductase inhibitors. Journal of Lipid Research 33: 1569–1582

Klag M J, Ford D E, Mead L A, He J, Whelton P K et al 1993 Serum cholesterol in young men and subsequent cardiovascular disease. New England Journal of Medicine 328: 313–318

Marks V, Teale J D 1993 Hypoglycaemia in the adult. Baillière's Clinical Endocrinology and Metabolism 7(3): 705–729

Pyorala K, de Backer G, Graham I, Poole-Wilson P, Wood D 1994 Prevention of coronary heart disease in clinical practice. European Heart Journal 15: 1300–1331

Shepherd J 1994 Lipoprotein metabolism. Drugs 47: 1–10

M.J. Mackie, C.A. Ludlam

13

Diseases of the blood

Blood diseases cover a wide spectrum of illnesses ranging from anaemias, one of the commonest disorders affecting mankind, to relatively rare conditions such as leukaemias and congenital coagulation disorders. Although the latter are uncommon, recent advances in their understanding at the cellular and molecular level are already beginning to impact on diagnosis and treatment.

Diseases affecting any system can, however, secondarily influence haematological parameters, making their study an integral part of the assessment of any medical disease. This assessment is facilitated by the ease of access to the blood and bone marrow.

BLOOD CELL FORMATION

STEM AND PROGENITOR CELLS

Major advances have been made in the understanding of blood cell formation from studies using in vitro culture techniques, purified growth factors and the application of this knowledge to clinical bone marrow transplantation. Up to 0.05% of bone marrow cells are stem cells. These are unique in the marrow because they are capable of self renewal and have the ability to divide and differentiate through a variety of stages to produce the mature cells found in the peripheral blood (Fig. 13.1). A small number of pluripotent stem cells give rise to progenitor cells which differentiate to produce lymphocytes and the multipotent precursor from which committed progenitors (colony forming cells—CFC) for the myeloid series are derived. This committed progenitor stage has been identified in tissue culture and the colony forming cells can be recognised for each of the mature cell types in the blood. Not only does this system result in the differentiation of all mature cells from the stem cells but it allows for significant amplification of the number of mature cells produced.

Growth factors

An increased understanding of cellular development has been matched by a dramatic expansion in knowledge about controlling factors. A large number of growth factors have been described (Fig. 13.2) and their action and interaction is proving to be complex. They are glycoproteins which can be produced by a variety of cells, in particular T lymphocytes, monocytes, endothelial cells and fibroblasts. Growth factors act not only on stem and progenitor cells but also affect the function of mature cells.

Growth factors responsible for stimulating the proliferation of myeloid cells are called colony stimulating

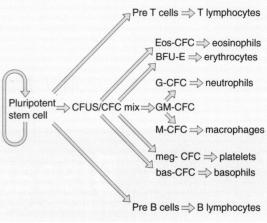

CFUS = Colony forming unit, spleen
CFC = Colony forming cells
BFU-E = Blast forming unit-erythrocytes
G-CFC = Granulocyte colony forming cells
GM-CFC = Granulocyte-macrophage colony forming cells
M-CFC = Macrophage colony forming cells
Meg-CFC = Megakaryocyte colony forming cells
Bas-CFC = Basophil colony forming cells

Fig. 13.1 Differentiation and maturation of haemopoietic cells.

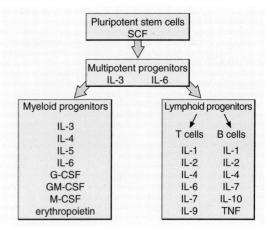

SCF = Stem cell factor
IL = Interleukin
G-CSF = Granulocyte colony stimulating factor
GM-CSF = Granulocyte/macrophage colony stimulating factor
M-CSF = Macrophage colony stimulating factor
TNF = Tumour necrosis factor

Fig. 13.2 Simplified action of growth factors.

factors (CSFs). Granulocyte CSF (G-CSF) acts to promote neutrophil production and granulocyte/macrophage CSF or GM-CSF promotes neutrophil and macrophage production. Both these CSFs are commercially available and are in clinical use. Various substances termed interleukins influence proliferation and differentiation of lymphoid precursors. However, it is recognised that certain interleukins interact with CSFs to modulate myeloid precursors and it has become increasingly apparent that interaction and synergy between growth factors is common.

It is difficult to detect many of the growth factors under basal conditions in the plasma. However, stimuli such as infection via activation of monocytes result in the production of tumour necrosis factor and interleukin-I. These lead to increased production of growth factors such as G-CSF and GM-CSF which stimulate the white cell count and help to combat infection.

ERYTHROCYTES

The earliest identifiable erythrocyte precursor in the marrow is the pro-erythroblast, a large cell with a nucleolated nucleus and deeply basophilic cytoplasm. This cell undergoes a rapid series of divisions so that the daughter cells do not have time to regrow between divisions and become progressively smaller. At the same time maturation proceeds with the formation of haemoglobin in the cytoplasm. Early, intermediate and late normoblasts can be identified.

Proliferation ceases at the intermediate normoblast stage and maturation is completed with condensation of the nuclear chromatin and eventual ejection of the nuclear remnant. At this stage the cell retains the capacity to synthesise haemoglobin due to the presence of ribosomes in the cytoplasm. This ribosomal material (RNA) gives the cell a faintly bluish colour with Romanowsky stains. This appearance seen on a conventionally stained blood film is termed increased polychromasia. Supravital staining with new methylene blue causes condensation of the ribosomes to form reticular material which makes the cells easy to identify. They are called reticulocytes and are easily counted. The reticulocyte matures into an adult red cell in about 3 days and is released to the circulation about half way through the period. Normally between 10 and 100×10^9/l reticulocytes are found in the circulating blood of healthy adults.

Under stress, reticulocytes can be released sooner from the marrow, raising the reticulocyte count without an increase in erythropoiesis. These 'marrow' reticulocytes can be recognised by their more dense central aggregate of reticulum when stained with supravital stains. However, an absolute increase in the number of reticulocytes usually reflects increased erythropoiesis.

After the first few days of life there are, in health, no nucleated red cells in the peripheral blood. The presence of normoblasts indicates excessive or abnormal blood formation or irritation of the bone marrow by invasion with foreign elements.

The mature erythrocyte is a circular biconcave disc with a mean diameter of 7.2 μm. There is an excess of membrane which is partly responsible for the biconcave shape but the maintenance of this shape requires energy supplied by glycolysis. This unusual morphology gives the erythrocyte considerable plasticity, enabling it to pass through capillaries and other structures of small diameter. In some disorders erythrocytes may lose membrane, becoming progressively more spherical and rigid. As a result they are more susceptible to destruction, particularly in the spleen which is uniquely adapted to filtering out such cells. The spleen also removes inclusion bodies such as Howell–Jolly bodies and Pappenheimer bodies (p. 783) from erythrocytes without destroying the cells. The red cell membrane has a lipid bilayer structure in which the membrane proteins are found. It is a complex dynamic structure, one function of which is to maintain high levels of potassium and low levels of sodium in the cell by means of ionic pumps. The surface of the membrane also carries antigenic determinants for the various blood groups.

Erythropoietin

Erythropoiesis is controlled by a hormone, erythropoietin, produced mainly in the kidneys by cells probably located in the tubules, which monitor the provision of oxygen to the tissues and respond to hypoxia by the production of erythropoietin (Fig. 13.3). Erythropoietin acts on the erythropoietic stem cells stimulating increased proliferation and reducing ineffective erythropoiesis. Recombinant erythropoietin has a defined role in the effective treatment of the anaemia associated with renal failure.

Haemoglobin

Haemoglobin in the erythrocyte provides the oxygen transport mechanism of the blood. Erythrocytes also carry carbon dioxide from the tissues to the lungs buffering the carbonic acid formed in the red cell (p. 588). Haemoglobin is a complex globular protein molecule, being a conjugate of a red pigment (haem) with protein (globin). Haem is formed under the control of the enzyme amino laevulinic acid synthetase by the condensation of glycine and succinyl coenzyme A to form amino laevulinic acid. There follows a series of synthetic steps which build the porphyrin ring culminating in the enzyme haem-synthetase (ferrochelatase) inserting iron

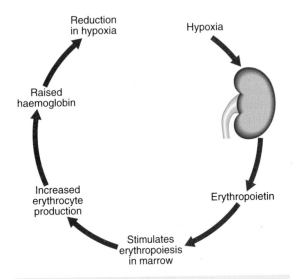

Fig. 13.3 Erythropoietin and erythropoiesis.

into the ring to form haem. Each step in this synthetic pathway requires its own enzyme; deficiencies of these enzymes give rise to the various forms of porphyria (p. 773).

The globin fraction of normal human haemoglobin comprises four polypeptide chains, two alpha chains of 141 amino acids and two other chains of 146 amino acids. The chains are the product of four structural genes, all on autosomal chromosomes. The genes and their polypeptide chains are designated alpha, gamma, beta and delta and are responsible for the production of the three main haemoglobins seen after birth, namely haemoglobins F, A and A2 (Table 13.1). The α genes are on chromosome 16 and the β, γ and δ genes on chromosome 11.

One molecule of oxygen is carried by each haem fraction of the haemoglobin molecule which is therefore capable of carrying four molecules of oxygen. Beta, gamma and delta chains are incapable of accepting oxygen until the alpha chains have taken up oxygen. When this occurs a configurational change in the haemoglobin

molecule prises open the haem pockets of the other chains, allowing them to accept oxygen. Thus the more oxygen the haemoglobin molecule has, the more easily it acquires further oxygen until it becomes saturated. In the tissues the reverse occurs, ready loss becoming more difficult as haemoglobin becomes desaturated.

This function can be influenced further by a product of glucose metabolism, 2-3 diphosphoglycerate (2-3-DPG). The concentration of 2-3-DPG in the erythrocyte affects the avidity of the haemoglobin molecule for oxygen by reversible combination with deoxygenated haemoglobin. Increased levels of 2-3-DPG decrease haemoglobin's oxygen affinity and improve release to the tissues. Under hypoxic conditions, 2-3-DPG levels in the erythrocytes increase as a compensatory mechanism. This is the first step in acclimatisation at high altitude and occurs within 24–48 hours, long before increased erythropoietin production stimulates an increase in erythrocyte numbers.

Iron metabolism

Iron is essential for the synthesis of the haem fraction of haemoglobin. It is also present in myoglobin and enzymes such as the cytochromes. Iron in food is absorbed from the upper small intestine, mainly in the ferrous form bound to amino acids and sugars, but also in haem from red meat. Iron readily takes the non-absorbable ferric form but the low pH in the stomach helps to preserve it in the ferrous form (Fig. 13.4).

Each cell obtains iron from the iron transport system (transferrin) in the blood by transfer across its membrane. The intestinal mucosal cell is no exception but it also receives iron by absorption from the gut lumen. When body stores of iron are adequate the intestinal mucosal cells are sloughed into the gut. Thus excessive iron absorption is prevented. The mucosal cell becomes iron depleted and therefore avid for iron when demand for iron increases, or the body stores are low. Absorption from the gut increases and the iron is passed rapidly to the iron transport system in the blood. Little is lost when the cell is sloughed.

Iron for erythropoiesis comes mainly from transferrin and almost all iron absorbed from the gut goes preferentially to the bone marrow to be used by the developing red cells. Increased erythropoiesis associated with a variety of disorders may promote iron absorption by using this iron even when iron stores are increased. Thus some forms of prolonged anaemia, not due to blood loss or iron deficiency, can be associated with excessive iron stores. Haem absorbed by the mucosal cell is split in the cell and iron liberated. The iron is then treated in the same way as that absorbed by other means. This is a very useful additional means of iron absorption provided mainly by red meat. Iron obtained from the catabolism

Table 13.1	Haemoglobin chain composition		
		Schematic	Written
	HbF	$\alpha\gamma$ $\gamma\alpha$	$\alpha_2\gamma_2$
	HbA	$\alpha\beta$ $\beta\alpha$	$\alpha_2\beta_2$
	HbA2	$\alpha\delta$ $\delta\alpha$	$\alpha_2\delta_2$

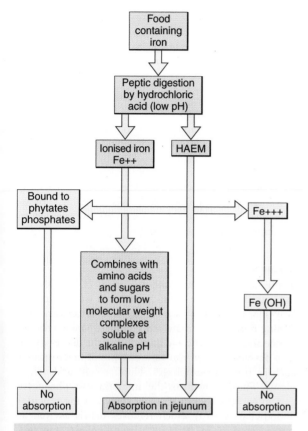

Fig. 13.4   Iron absorption.

of haemoglobin from destroyed red cells is recycled either to the bone marrow, or, if there is excess, to the iron stores. Iron is stored in cells in two forms—ferritin and haemosiderin.

Iron loss

The body conserves iron very effectively. A small amount is lost in sweat and urine. The total daily loss amounts to about 1 mg in males and 2 mg/day on average in menstruating females. Iron balance is thus precarious (Fig. 13.5).

Other factors which influence erythropoiesis include vitamin B_{12} (p. 787), folate (p. 788), thyroxine, vitamin C, vitamin E, androgens and trace elements such as copper and manganese.

Erythrocyte destruction

Destruction of all form elements of the blood occurs in the mononuclear-phagocyte system. The survival of mature erythrocytes in the peripheral blood is approximately 110–120 days as estimated by cross-transfusion experiments and represents the mean life span. A more

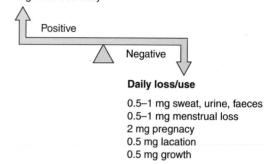

Dietary intake

1.5–2 mg absorbed daily

Daily loss/use

0.5–1 mg sweat, urine, faeces
0.5–1 mg menstrual loss
2 mg pregnacy
0.5 mg lacation
0.5 mg growth

Fig. 13.5   Normal iron balance.

practical technique for clinical use is to label the patient's erythrocytes with radioactive chromium and re-transfuse. The time taken for half of the radioactivity to disappear is estimated. The half-life of the radioactivity in normal erythrocytes is 25–35 days, which is shorter than the true half-life because of the elution of chromium from the cells.

LEUCOCYTES

Leucocytes are found in the blood as they migrate from bone marrow to the tissues. In any one individual the number is remarkably constant, showing only minor diurnal variation. The types of leucocytes are listed in the information box below.

MORPHOLOGICAL CHARACTERISTICS OF BLOOD LEUCOCYTES

Polymorphonuclear granulocytes
- Neutrophils   These cells are distinguished by the
- Eosinophils   granules in the cytoplasm which
- Basophils   stain either with neutral acid (eosin)
                       or alkaline (basic) reactions

Mononuclear cells
- Monocytes
- Lymphocytes

The neutrophil granulocyte

The production of neutrophil granulocytes takes place in the bone marrow, which holds a large reserve of neutrophils. Mature neutrophils leave the marrow and circulate in the blood, on average, for about 8 hours. They leave the circulation by adhering to the capillary endothelium (margination) and migration through the vessel wall into the tissues where they function. A considerable proportion of the neutrophils in blood is marginated. Certain stress factors such as exercise and emotion may return these cells to the circulation, raising the leucocyte count. The life span of neutrophils is about 3–4 days.

Immature granulocytes, such as myelocytes, are found in the blood when the production of leukocytes is being stimulated by severe pyogenic infection and an increase in the cytoplasmic granulation may also be seen (toxic granulation). In adults the appearance of significant numbers of more primitive forms in the blood, such as myeloblasts and promyelocytes, indicates a serious disturbance of marrow function, for example invasion by metastases or neoplastic change as in leukaemia.

Neutrophil granulocytes are phagocytic cells which ingest bacteria and fungi. Neutrophils are attracted to bacteria by chemotaxis, and phagocytosis is enhanced by opsonisation. Having engulfed a bacterium the neutrophils kill it by a number of processes:

1. production of hydrogen peroxide (oxygen dependent)
2. release of myeloperoxidase into the phagosome (oxygen dependent)
3. release of lysozyme, lactoferrin and pH reduction in the phagosome (oxygen independent).

The products of autodigestion of cells killed by organisms are potent stimulants of fresh neutrophil formation by the marrow. Pyrogens are also released. Neutrophils also ingest uric acid crystals and may disintegrate in the process, liberating tissue-damaging substances which cause local inflammation. Apart from responding to infection, neutrophils also produce a vitamin B_{12} binding protein, transcobalamin III, which explains the high levels of vitamin B_{12} in the serum in conditions in which there is a greatly increased number of neutrophils, e.g. chronic myeloid leukaemia.

The degree of segmentation of neutrophils varies from unsegmented to five segments. The number of segments appears to have no functional importance. A failure to segment with the formation of 'band' cells occurs in toxic conditions, and under such circumstances the degree of segmentation tends to diminish. This is commonly called a 'shift to the left'. A 'shift to the right' in which there is increased segmentation occurs in disorders such as a vitamin B_{12} and folate deficiency and iron deficiency.

Eosinophil granulocytes

These are also produced in the marrow. The absolute count in blood is normally less than $0.4 \times 10^9/l$. Factors influencing production are poorly understood but T lymphocytes appear to exert some control. Eosinophils are also phagocytic but less actively so than neutrophils. They are associated with allergic reactions, ingest antigen–antibody complexes and are concerned in processes involving foreign proteins, such as hypersensitivity reactions, and have a role in the containment of parasitic infections. Their numbers are severely reduced by corticosteroid therapy.

Basophil granulocytes

These are poorly phagocytic and possess the Fc portion of the IgE molecule on specific binding sites on the surface membrane. Activation of this by antigens results in degranulation of the cell with release of histamine. Thus basophils participate in hypersensitivity reactions in the same way as mast cells (tissue basophils). Basophils also contain heparin which may be released to participate in lipid metabolism.

Monocytes

These derive from the same precursors (CFC-GM) as the granulocyte. The monocyte is a cell with an irregularly shaped nucleus in a cloudy blue cytoplasm containing numerous minute red granules. Monocytes are motile and phagocytic and migrate into the tissues where they develop further into various types of macrophages such as tissue macrophages, Kupffer cells and osteoclasts. These constitute the mononuclear phagocyte system (previously but wrongly known as the reticuloendothelial system) which removes debris as well as microorganisms by phagocytosis and collects and presents antigenic material to lymphocytes. Lysis of tumour cells is another important function. Their production of platelet-derived growth factor is important in promoting healing and tissue remodelling. They also produce interleukin-I and tumour necrosis factor, mediators of the acute phase response. Production of tissue thromboplastin in response to bacterial endotoxin may activate the extrinsic coagulation mechanism and promote intravascular coagulation. Macrophages may survive for months.

Lymphocytes

These originate from committed stem cells in the bone marrow. Some migrate to the thymus where they become T (thymic) lymphocytes. Others become B (bursa) lymphocytes and a few become cytotoxic killer cells. About 75% of circulating lymphocytes are T cells. The rest are B cells and a few are 'null' cells showing neither T nor B characteristics. Both B cells and T cells respond to antigenic stimuli by transformation—in the case of B lymphocytes, to plasma cells producing immunoglobulin. T cells mediate cellular immunity. They are divided into 'helper' and 'suppressor' types. The life span of lymphocytes may vary from as short as a few

Table 13.2 Causes of spurious results from automatic full blood count analysers

Increased haemoglobin	Lipaemia, jaundice, very high white cell count
Reduced haemoglobin	Improper sample mixing, blood taken from a vein to which an infusion is flowing
Increased mean red cell volume	Cold agglutinins, non-ketotic hyper-osmolarity
Increased white cell count	Nucleated red cells
Reduced platelet count	Clots in the sample, platelet clumping or satellitism

Table 13.3 Reference range for haematological parameters

	Female	Male
Hb g/l	115–165	130–180
Hct	0.37–0.47	0.4–0.54
RBC × 10^9/l	3.8–5.8	4.5–6.5
ESR mm in 1 hour	0–7	0–5
MCV fl	76–98	
MCH pg	27–35	
MCHC g/dl	31–35	
RDW	11–16	
Platelets × 10^9/l	150–400	
WBC × 10^9/l	4.0–11.0	
Differential WBC		
Neutrophils	2.0–7.5 × 10^9/l (40–75%)	
Lymphocytes	1.5–4.0 × 10^9/l (20–45%)	
Monocytes	0.2–0.8 × 10^9/l (2–10%)	
Eosinophils	0.04–0.4 × 10^9/l (1–6%)	
Basophils	0.01–0.1 × 10^9/l (0–1%)	
Reticulocytes	10–100 × 10^9/l (0.2–2%)	
Serum ferritin	(female) 14–150 μg/l	(male) 17–300 μg/l
Serum vitamin B$_{12}$	140–725 ng/l	
Serum folate	1.9–9.0 μg/l	
Red cell folate	118–450 μg/l	
Red cell mass	(female) 20–30 ml/kg	(male) 25–35 ml/kg
Plasma volume	40–50 ml/kg	

days to many years. The latter may re-enter the circulation at intervals.

PLATELETS

These are discussed on page 826.

ASSESSMENT OF HAEMATOLOGICAL PARAMETERS

The full blood count

This is the haematology test which is requested most frequently by clinicians. Blood anticoagulated with EDTA is rapidly processed through an automatic analyser. A variety of technologies (particle sizing, radio frequency and laser instrumentation) are used to measure the haemoglobin, count the red cells, estimate the haematocrit and measure red cell parameters, e.g. mean cell volume (MCV), mean cell haemoglobin content and mean cell haemoglobin concentration. The absolute white count is measured and a differential count performed. The most modern version of analysers have the ability to provide a full five part differential. A platelet count is also measured. Thus a wealth of information is provided by what can be regarded as a simple test. It is important to appreciate that a number of conditions can lead to spurious results (Table 13.2). The reference values for a number of common haematological parameters in adults are given in Table 13.3.

Blood film examination

Although the technical advances of modern full blood count analysers have resulted in fewer blood films requiring examination, scrutiny of the blood film can often yield invaluable information (see Table 13.4). Analysers, in the main, are not able to recognise abnormal white cells such as blast cells or identify abnormalities of red cell shape and content (Howell–Jolly bodies, basophilic stippling, malarial parasites, etc.).

Bone marrow examination

Bone marrow examination is performed in adults either from the sternum or posterior iliac crest. Marrow may be simply aspirated or a bone marrow biopsy (trephine) performed. The latter cannot be obtained safely from the sternum and increasingly both aspirate and biopsy are performed from the posterior iliac crest. A biopsy is superior for assessing marrow cellularity and infiltration. Bone marrow examination is performed under local anaesthesia and can easily be undertaken as an outpatient procedure. Both aspiration and trephine biopsy can be carried out by the same needle but often separate needles are used (Fig. 13.6).

Marrow is examined not only for its morphological appearances but increasingly cell marker studies, karyotyping and molecular biology studies are undertaken as appropriate for the accurate diagnosis and assessment of malignant disease. Marrow can also be sent for culture in cases of suspected tuberculosis. The main indications for a bone marrow examination are shown in the information box.

FURTHER READING

Ogawa M 1993 Differentiation and proliferation of haemopoietic stem cells. Blood 81: 2844–2853

Steward W P 1993 Granulocyte and granulocyte-macrophage colony stimulating factors. Lancet 342: 153–157

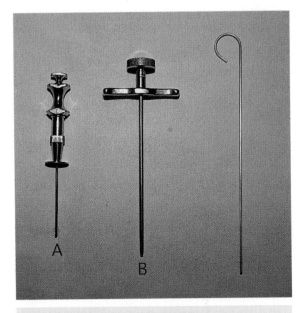

Fig. 13.6 A Bone marrow aspirate needle; B Bone marrow trephine needle (centre) with stylet (right).

MAIN INDICATIONS FOR BONE MARROW EXAMINATION

- **Marrow infiltration:**
  Leukaemia/lymphoma
  Secondary carcinoma
  Myelofibrosis
- **Cytopenia:**
  Neutropenia
  Thrombocytopenia
  Anaemia—complex cases or aplasia
- **Myeloproliferative disorders**

DISORDERS OF THE ERYTHROCYTES

ANAEMIA

Anaemia may be defined as a state in which the blood haemoglobin level is below the normal range for the patient's age and sex. At birth the haemoglobin level is high (200 g/l) because fetal haemoglobin has a higher oxygen affinity than adult haemoglobin. In the first 3 months of life lower affinity haemoglobin A replaces haemoglobin F. The haemoglobin level drops, due partly to removal of old and damaged red cells but also by reduced production, reaching about half the birth level when the baby is 3 months of age. Thereafter, the average level rises gradually until the child reaches

puberty when a further rise occurs which is more marked in males than in females. Adult males have haemoglobin levels on average of 20 g/l higher than adult females which reflects the stimulus of androgens on erythropoiesis. A haemoglobin level of 120 g/l is regarded as anaemic in an adult male but is normal in an adult female. Most adults who are otherwise in reasonably good health function satisfactorily if the haemoglobin is above 100 g/l, provided this lower level has not appeared quickly.

The presence of symptoms related to anaemia depends partly on its severity but also on how rapidly the anaemia develops. A patient who has had a reduction of haemoglobin from 130–80 g/l in 1 week may have severe symptoms while another patient who has anaemia which has developed slowly to a similar level over months may be asymptomatic.

CAUSES OF ANAEMIA

Decreased or ineffective marrow production
- Lack of iron, B_{12} or folate
- Hypoplasia
- Invasion by malignant cells

Peripheral causes
- Blood loss
- Haemolysis
- Hypersplenism

Classification

The classification of anaemias outlined in the information box above helps to guide the clinician in planning investigations as it reflects the underlying mechanisms. The commonest cause of anaemia is iron deficiency and the commonest reason for this is blood loss. However, anaemia is often multifactorial.

An alternative classification of anaemia is based on the size of the red cell which is most accurately indicated by the MCV. In the presence of anaemia:

- a normal MCV suggests either acute blood loss or the anaemia of chronic disease (ACD)
- a low MCV suggests iron deficiency or thalassaemia
- a high MCV suggests B_{12} or folate deficiency.

Flow charts can be developed indicating the pattern of investigation in an anaemic patient based on the MCV (Figs 13.7, 13.8).

Symptoms and signs of anaemia

Clinical features of anaemia reflect the diminished oxygen-carrying capacity of the blood. The severity depends

Table 13.4   Terms describing abnormal blood film appearances and their meaning

Microcytosis	The average size of the red cells is reduced. The mean cell volume will be reduced. It is commonly found in iron deficiency anaemia and other disorders of haemoglobin synthesis.
Macrocytosis	The average size of red cells is greater than normal. The mean cell volume will be increased. It is seen, for instance, in megaloblastic anaemias but its occurrence does not necessarily mean a megaloblastic change in the marrow. A common cause is excessive alcohol consumption.
Hypochromia	The red cells contain less than the normal amount of haemoglobin and they stain less deeply. They show greater than normal central pallor. Hypochromia is commonly associated with microcytosis and is a characteristic feature of disorders of haemoglobin synthesis, most commonly iron deficiency.
Anisocytosis	Inequality in the size of the red cells. It is found in many forms of anaemia but is very prominent in megaloblastic anaemia.
Poikilocytosis	Marked irregularity in the shape of the red cells. It is never present without anisocytosis and usually reflects dyserythropoiesis.
Elliptocytosis	Elliptical red cells; **ovalocytosis** refers to a less marked abnormality. Such cells are found in small numbers in a variety of disorders such as megaloblastic and hypochromic anaemias. The presence of a majority of cells being oval or elliptical indicates a hereditary disorder of dominant type which is usually of no clinical significance.
Target cells	Abnormally flat red cells with a central mass of haemoglobin surrounded by a ring of pallor and an outer ring of haemoglobin. They are commonly associated with liver disease, impaired or absent splenic function (hyposplenism) and haemoglobinopathies.
Polychromasia and reticulocytosis	Young red cells when stained by the Romanowsky method have a faint bluish colour (basophilia) due to residual ribosomal material. A blood film in which such cells are present in increased numbers along with those of normal orange colour is said to show polychromasia. This, like reticulocytosis (p. 777), indicates increased production of new red cells by the bone marrow.
Punctuate basophilia (Basophilic stippling)	Abnormally damaged young red cells may show scattered deep blue dots in the cytoplasm with Romanowsky staining. Such punctate basophilia may be found in any severe anaemia but the presence of many of these cells is most commonly seen in Beta thalassaemia and chronic lead poisoning where it may occur when the anaemia is slight.
Howell–Jolly bodies	Remnants of nuclear material left in the erythrocyte after the nucleus is extruded. They are normally removed by the spleen and their presence usually indicates a non-functioning or absent spleen. Their numbers are greatly increased in certain erythropoietic disorders, e.g. megaloblastic anaemia.
Pappenheimer bodies	Iron-protein complexes (sideroblastic granules) found in red cells in certain iron overload states and increased when the spleen is non-functioning or absent.
Nucleated red cells	Usually normoblasts, found in the blood when erythropoiesis is very vigorous or when there is irritation of the bone marrow, as in leukaemia or infiltration by secondary tumour.
Leucoerythroblastic	A blood picture in which primitive granulocytes and erythroblasts are simultaneously present in the peripheral blood. It is usually, but not necessarily, associated with anaemia and reflects bone marrow irritation, as in malignant infiltration of the marrow, or disordered haemopoiesis, as in myelofibrosis. It can occur as a reaction to severe haemolysis or bleeding.

on the degree of the anaemia and the rapidity of its development but is independent of its type. Symptoms and signs of anaemia are listed in Table 13.5.

IRON DEFICIENCY ANAEMIA

Iron deficiency anaemia is by far the commonest cause of anaemia in most parts of the world. The aetiology varies with the age, sex and country of residence of the patient.

Aetiology

Iron deficiency usually results from either loss of iron due to bleeding, an inadequate diet (p. 560) or malabsorption (p. 447). Occasionally iron may be lost in the urine in the form of haemosiderin. Loss due to bleeding in greater amounts than can be balanced in absorption is by far the most common cause.

There are periods in life when iron deficiency may be regarded as almost physiological. At birth the normal infant has a store in the form of a very high haemoglobin level and in addition some iron is available in the liver. This is adequate for erythropoietic requirements in the first few months of life. Thereafter a mild degree of deficiency appears because milk is a very poor source of iron. If weaning is delayed for 1 or 2 years, as is the custom in certain parts of the world, deficiency may become marked. The deficiency is fairly quickly corrected when the child is weaned to a good diet. Prematurity and haemorrhage from the cord at birth deprive the infant of the normal store of iron and deficiency may appear sooner and be more severe. Adolescents have a marked growth spurt and iron requirements may outstrip absorption. Food fads are not uncommon at this age, which may contribute to the problem.

Menstruation causes an average loss of 30 mg of iron per month, requiring increased absorption of approximately 1 mg daily. Although this loss disappears during pregnancy, the mother requires additional iron for the fetus, the placenta, her own increased red cell mass and blood loss at parturition. The daily requirements will be about 2.5 mg plus the basic requirement of 1 mg a day, a total of 3.5 mg. This increased demand for iron rises as pregnancy progresses, being greatest in the second half of pregnancy. Thus iron deficiency is more common in females than males during the reproductive years. In

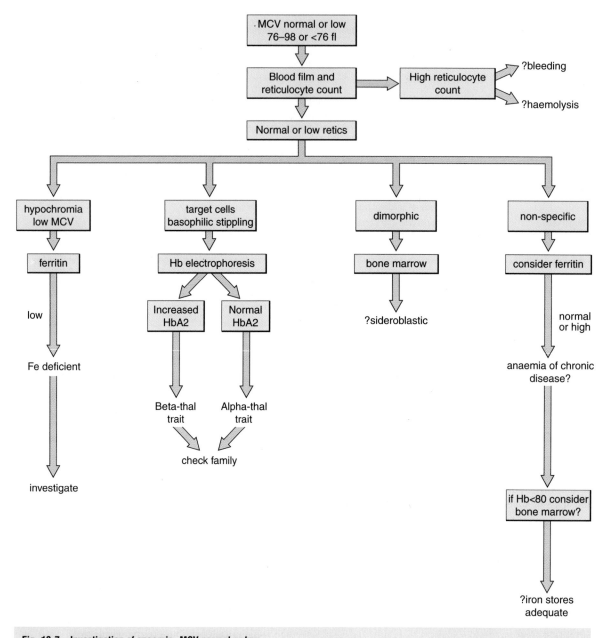

Fig. 13.7   Investigation of anaemia, MCV normal or low.

post-menopausal women and adult men the commonest cause of iron deficiency is gastrointestinal bleeding, for example, from erosions associated with anti-inflammatory drugs, neoplastic disease and peptic ulcers. In tropical and sub-tropical areas, infestation with hookworm and schistosomiasis is also very common and is the main cause of iron deficiency. A diet containing inadequate iron (p. 560) can cause or contribute to iron

deficiency anaemia at all ages. The elderly, particularly men living alone, are susceptible.

Clinical features

There are often no symptoms and the deficiency may be discovered incidentally. Vague symptoms of tiredness are insufficient to make some patients seek medical help. The symptoms and signs of iron deficiency are mainly

Table 13.5   Symptoms and signs of anaemia

Symptoms	Signs
Lassitude	Pallor of
Fatigue	skin
Breathlessness on exertion	mucous membranes
Palpitations	palms of hands
Throbbing in head and ears	conjunctivae
Dizziness	Tachycardia
Tinnitus	Cardiac dilatation
Headache	Systolic flow murmurs
Dimness of vision	Oedema
Insomnia	
Paraesthesia in fingers and toes	
Angina	

Table 13.6   Diagnostic features of iron deficiency

Haemoglobin	Variably reduced
Mean cell volume	Reduced
Erythrocyte count	Normal or reduced less than Hb level would suggest
Blood film	Hypochromia, microcytosis, oval and elliptical cells, poikilocytes in more severe cases
Leucocyte count differential	Normal
Platelet count	Normal or raised
Bone marrow iron stores	Empty
Plasma transferrin	Raised
Plasma iron	Reduced
Serum ferritin	Reduced

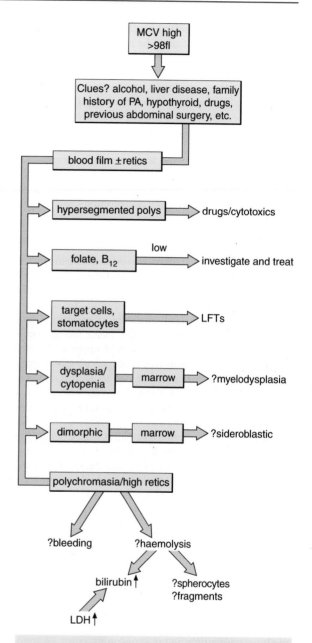

Fig. 13.8   Investigation of anaemia and high MCV.

those of anaemia (Table 13.5). However, there are some characteristic features. Angular stomatitis, glossitis and brittle finger nails are relatively frequent. Evidence of nail cracking is common but flattening or concavity of the nails (koilonychia) is rare. Dysphagia is very rare and when present should raise the possibility of a post-circoid web (Plummer–Vinson syndrome). Pica, the eating of strange items such as coal, earth, or foods in great excess such as tomatoes or greens, is more common than generally realised and may be uncovered only if the patient is specifically asked. Splenomegaly is uncommon unless the anaemia is severe and may then reflect other diseases such as portal hypertension in which the iron deficiency is also a feature.

Investigations (Table 13.6)

The first abnormality to appear is microcytosis, to be followed by hypochromia from the reduced amount of haemoglobin in the red cells. Elliptical cells may be found but often indicate other disorders (p. 791). The haematological findings are a reduced haemoglobin with normal or slightly reduced red cell count and a low mean cell volume (MCV) of less than 76 fl. The white cell and differential counts are usually normal, although hyper-segmentation of the neutrophils commonly occurs. The erythrocyte sedimentation rate (ESR) is usually lower than would be expected for the degree of anaemia or associated disease. A raised platelet count may suggest that bleeding is the cause of the deficiency. Bone marrow iron stores stained by the Prussian blue technique are found to be empty.

Iron deficiency suspected because of the finding of a low MCV is best confirmed by measuring the ferritin. However, inflammatory conditions such as rheumatoid arthritis and certain tumours raise the ferritin level and patients with these conditions who have iron deficiency may have a ferritin in the low/normal range. Unfortunately, the serum iron is subject to considerable diurnal variation and low levels are found in the presence of inflammation or infection. Iron absorption is increased in iron deficiency and the total iron binding capacity rises. Thus a low serum iron associated with a high total iron binding capacity is much more specific for iron deficiency. However, the total iron binding capacity may be reduced by poor nutrition.

Diagnosis of the cause of iron deficiency

The direction of the investigations will obviously be influenced by the age and sex of the patient, the history and the findings on examination. Excessive menstrual loss and repeated pregnancy are common causes. In the absence of any clear lead, evidence of gastrointestinal blood loss should first be sought using faecal occult blood tests, barium meal, enema and upper and lower gastrointestinal tract endoscopy. Negative barium studies or occult blood tests should not be accepted as evidence of the absence of lesions. Chromium labelled red cells may be used to measure blood loss into the gut. The level of radioactivity in the stool provides an accurate measurement of the amount of blood lost. Coeliac disease may present in adults as an isolated iron deficiency. The stools and urine should be examined in tropical countries for hookworm infestation and schistosomiasis. Patients in whom there is a known cause of intravascular red cell destruction, such as a prosthetic heart valve, should have urine tested for haemosiderin.

Management

Most patients can be treated orally and the cheapest preparation is dried ferrous sulphate given as a tablet containing 200 mg of the salt (60 mg elemental iron) 3 times daily. A small proportion of patients develop dyspepsia, constipation or diarrhoea. If this occurs more expensive proprietary preparations may be tried. Delayed-release preparations are to be avoided as they release little iron in the upper jejunum where absorption is best. Proprietary liquid preparations may be used. A response to oral medication usually appears in under 2 weeks. The haemoglobin should rise by 10 g/l every 7–10 days. If no response is seen, it may be that the patient is not taking the tablets. A check may be made by examining the stool, which will be grey or black if the patient is ingesting iron. Failure to respond to iron therapy may be due to poor compliance, continued blood loss, severe malabsorption or the wrong diagnosis.

Iron should be continued for 3–6 months after the haemoglobin level has returned to normal, to replenish iron stores. Continuous oral therapy may be required or the iron may be given parenterally to patients with malabsorption, or chronic loss as in haemosiderinuria.

Parenteral iron therapy

This is suitable for those very few patients who are genuinely unable to take iron by mouth because of pain, vomiting or diarrhoea, who are unable to absorb iron because of some disorder of the gastrointestinal tract or who are unreliable in taking oral preparations. Iron given by injection has also been used for the treatment of anaemia or rheumatoid arthritis, for the correction of severe anaemia in the late stages of pregnancy and following major operations. The recommended single dose of iron-sorbitol is 1.5 mg of iron per kg of body weight given daily. It is assumed that about 250 mg of iron are required to increase the haemoglobin level by 10 g/l but the total dose of iron should not exceed 2.5 g. Iron-sorbitol should be given by intramuscular injection, never intravenously.

MEGALOBLASTIC ANAEMIA

Haemopoietic tissue is one of a number of rapidly proliferating tissues in which DNA synthesis is intense. Both vitamin B_{12} and folate are essential for DNA synthesis, and deficiency of either or both causes a failure of DNA synthesis and disordered cell proliferation. Haemopoiesis is particularly susceptible and division of cells is delayed and eventually halted. Morphological changes appear in the marrow cells. In the erythrocyte series these changes are described as megaloblastic because the cells appear abnormally large. Changes also occur in the granulocyte precursors (giant metamyelocytes) and megakaryocytes, and disordered morphology can be seen in other rapidly dividing cells such as those of the gastrointestinal tract.

Cell division occurs rapidly in normal erythrocyte production. The cells do not have time to regrow to their full size between divisions and a progressive size reduction occurs. When DNA synthesis is impaired, the time between divisions increases, more cell growth occurs and the cells become larger. The cells also undergo fewer divisions, probably because the synthesis of haemoglobin is unimpaired. Haemoglobin production appears to be one of the factors limiting proliferation. Once a certain haemoglobin level has been reached, division stops. Thus in megaloblastic disorders not only do the erythrocyte precursors have time to grow to a larger size between divisions, they also undergo fewer divisions,

Table 13.7   Diagnostic features of a megaloblastic anaemia

Investigation	Result
Haemoglobin	Often reduced, may be very low
Mean cell volume	Usually raised, commonly > 120 fl
Erythrocyte count	Low for degree of anaemia
Reticulocyte count	Low for degree of anaemia
Leucocyte count	Low normal or reduced
Platelet count	Low normal or reduced
Blood film	Oval macrocytosis, poikilocytosis, red cell fragmentation, neutrophil hypersegmentation
Bone marrow	Increased cellularity, megaloblastic changes in erythroid series, giant metamyelocytes, dysplastic megakaryocytes, increased iron in stores, pathological non-ring sideroblasts
Serum iron	Elevated
Iron binding capacity	Increased saturation
Serum ferritin	Elevated
Plasma LDH	Elevated, often markedly

both factors contributing to the macrocytosis. The end products are abnormally large and misshapen red cells which are well haemoglobinised. As dysplasia becomes advanced erythrocyte fragments appear and the MCV may drop. Despite anaemia the reticulocyte count is low. There is usually leucopenia and thrombocytopenia.

The massive destruction of marrow cells from dyserythropoiesis liberates large quantities of enzymes including lactase dehydrogenase (LDH) which rises to very high levels in the blood. Eventually, in the absence of treatment, cell production fails. Excessive doses of antimetabolites such as those used in the treatment of cancer which interfere with DNA synthesis have similar effects and may induce severe dysplasia and morphological changes in the marrow and blood very similar to those produced by vitamin B_{12} and folate deficiency.

The findings on investigation of a megaloblastic anaemia whatever the cause are given in Table 13.7. Most patients with megaloblastic anaemia suffer from deficiency of either vitamin B_{12} or folate which is demonstrated by deficient blood levels of these vitamins.

Vitamin B_{12}

This is a cobalt-containing porphyrin, termed cobalamin. The absorption of vitamin B_{12} from the lower ileum is facilitated by gastric intrinsic factor, a glycoprotein synthesised by gastric parietal cells, which complexes with ingested vitamin B_{12} in the stomach. The complex is taken up at special binding sites in the ileum where the vitamin B_{12} is released to the ileal cells. Intrinsic factor is not absorbed. After absorption vitamin B_{12} is bound to a carrier protein in the plasma, transcobalamin II, transported to the tissues and taken up by cells as required. Vitamin B_{12} is stored in the liver where there may be up to 3 years' supply.

Deficiency of vitamin B_{12}

This vitamin is obtained mainly from animal foodstuffs. Vegetables alone are an inadequate source. Normal requirements of vitamin B_{12} are 1–2 μg daily. Deficiency takes at least 3 years to appear and occurs because of the factors listed in the information box below. A low serum B_{12} concentration may be secondary to a low serum folate level.

> **CAUSES OF VITAMIN B_{12} DEFICIENCY**
>
> - Inadequate diet (true vegans)
> - Intrinsic factor deficiency:
>   pernicious anaemia, gastrectomy
>   congenital deficiency without gastric atrophy (rare)
> - Disease of the terminal ileum
>   e.g. Crohn's disease
> - Vitamin B_{12} may be removed from the gut by:
>   bacterial proliferation in stagnant loops,
>   parasites such as the fish tapeworm

Prevalence

The majority of patients with vitamin B_{12} deficiency have Addisonian pernicious anaemia. This appears to be relatively uncommon in tropical countries.

ADDISONIAN PERNICIOUS ANAEMIA

The term Addisonian pernicious anaemia should be limited to megaloblastic anaemia due to a failure of secretion of intrinsic factor by the stomach other than from total gastrectomy. It is an autoimmune disease and in about 50% of patients antibodies to intrinsic factor can be demonstrated. The disease is rare before the age of 30, occurs mainly between 45 and 65 years and affects females more frequently than males.

Pathology

There is evidence of increased blood destruction, including unconjugated hyperbilirubinaemia and increased deposition of iron (haemosiderin) in the liver, spleen, kidneys and bone marrow. The gastric mucosa is thin and atrophic.

Clinical features

The onset is insidious and the degree of anaemia is often great before the patient consults the doctor. In addition to the general symptoms of anaemia (Table 13.5) there may be intermittent soreness of the tongue and periodic diarrhoea. The patient generally appears well nourished despite the fact that weight loss is a common feature. The skin and mucous membranes are pale and in severely anaemic patients the skin and conjunctivae may show a lemon yellow tint from a combination of anaemia and mild haemolysis; the surface of the tongue is usually smooth and atrophic, but sometimes it is red and inflamed. The spleen may be palpable. In many patients paraesthesiae occur in the fingers and toes and occasionally there are signs of sub-acute combined degeneration (p. 570), which can appear before the anaemia. Dementia may also occur. In young females there may be infertility.

Investigations

Helpful findings in the diagnosis of Addisonian pernicious anaemia are given in the information box below.

DIAGNOSTIC FEATURES OF ADDISONIAN PERNICIOUS ANAEMIA

Diagnostic findings
- Very low serum vitamin B_{12}, often less than 50 ng/l
- Anti-intrinsic factor antibodies in serum (present in 50%)

Corroborative findings
- Macrocytic dysplastic blood picture
- Megaloblastic marrow
- Abnormal vitamin B_{12} absorption test corrected by addition of intrinsic factor (Schilling Test)

OTHER CAUSES OF MEGALOBLASTIC ANAEMIA

Due to vitamin B_{12} deficiency

Dietary insufficiency

This is rare unless meat and other animal foodstuffs are not eaten. The deficiency is readily corrected by the parenteral administration of vitamin B_{12}. Thereafter the vitamin should be given by mouth.

Gastrectomy

Total resection of the stomach results in a complete loss of intrinsic factor production and failure to absorb vitamin B_{12}. The patient requires life-long vitamin B_{12} injections. Partial gastrectomy reduces vitamin B_{12} absorption, in some cases to the point that deficiency occurs. Gastritis may, in part, be responsible. The Schilling test often demonstrates reduced absorption. One annual injection of 1000 μg of hydroxocobalamin is adequate prophylaxis for a patient who has had a partial gastrectomy.

Disease of the terminal ileum

This should be suspected if the Schilling test is not corrected by the addition of adequate amounts of intrinsic factor.

Bacterial colonisation of the small intestine

This results in an abnormal Schilling test, both without and with intrinsic factor; this is corrected by the administration of tetracycline.

Folic acid and interaction with vitamin B_{12}

Folic acid (pteroylglutamic acid) and related compounds are known as folates. The body obtains folates by the breakdown of food polyglutamates to monoglutamates in the small intestine or mucosal cell. Folic acid as such is available only as a medicinal compound. In the plasma, folate appears as methyl tetrahydrofolate which is changed to tetrahydrofolate (THF) by a pathway for which vitamin B_{12} is essential (Fig. 13.9). Without this, active folate coenzymes are poorly formed. 5, 10 methylene THF is the form essential for the synthesis of DNA. Dihydrofolate from this step is reconverted to the THF by dihydrofolate reductase, an enzyme inhibited by the folate antagonist, methotrexate. Formyl THF (folinic acid) will bypass both the metabolic blocks created by vitamin B_{12} deficiency or methotrexate and acts as an antidote to this drug. Clinically folinic acid or folic acid must not be used to treat vitamin B_{12} deficiency or severe neurological damage may result although the anaemia may be corrected. Daily requirement of folate for a normal healthy adult is 100 μg.

Megaloblastic anaemia due to folate deficiency

Folate occurs mainly in the form of polyglutamates in both vegetable and animal foodstuffs. Much is destroyed by cooking. Body stores are relatively small, lasting only a few weeks. Folate is absorbed mainly in the jejunum. Its metabolism thereafter is shown in Figure 13.9. The causes of folate deficiency are shown in the information box below.

CAUSES OF FOLATE DEFICIENCY

- Diet—poor intake of vegetables
- Malabsorption—e.g. coeliac disease
- Increased demand—pregnancy
                —cell proliferation, e.g. haemolysis
- Drugs*—certain anticonvulsants (e.g. phenytoin) the contraceptive pill, certain cytotoxic drugs (e.g. methotrexate)

* usually only a problem in patients deficient in folate from another cause

---

Prevalence

Approximately 60% of all megaloblastic anaemias in Britain are due to folate deficiency. In tropical countries most megaloblastic disease is due to folate deficiency associated with malnutrition, infection and pregnancy.

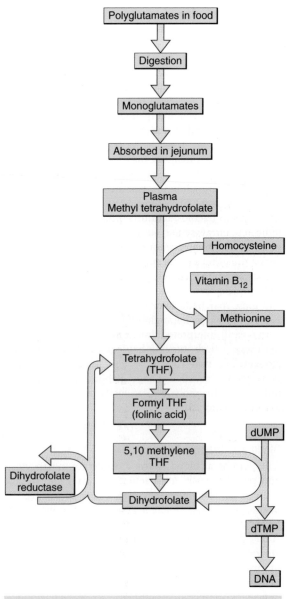

Fig. 13.9 Metabolic pathway showing interaction of vitamin B₁₂ and folate in the synthesis of DNA.

Clinical features

These are those of anaemia (Table 13.5) and of the underlying cause. Glossitis is less common than in vitamin B_{12} deficiency. Neurological problems are very rare.

Investigations

Diagnostic features of a folic acid deficiency anaemia are given in the information box below.

Management

The decision to give a blood transfusion in a patient with a megaloblastic anaemia is based on general principles concerning the clinical state of the patient. It should be seriously considered when the haemoglobin level is so low as to endanger life, for example under 40 g/l. In all types of chronic anaemia of sufficient severity to require transfusion the blood should be given very slowly, preferably as red cell concentrate, because of the danger of producing cardiac failure. A diuretic is given simultaneously (frusemide, 40–80 mg).

Vitamin B_{12} deficiency

Hydroxocobalamin is given parenterally in a dosage of 1000 μg twice during the first week, then 1000 μg weekly for a further 6 doses. Within 48 hours of the first injection the bone marrow shows a striking change from a megaloblastic to a normoblastic state. The serum iron drops precipitously and hypokalaemia may be a problem sufficient to require replacement therapy. Within 2 to 3 days the reticulocyte count begins to rise, reaching a maximum between the fifth and tenth days. The response may be delayed if there is coexisting inflammatory disease or if the patient has been transfused. There is a brief peak of erythrocyte output due to the maturation of the large number of cells held in maturation arrest by the vitamin B_{12} deficiency. Depending on the initial erythrocyte count the proportion of reticulocytes may rise above 50% but soon falls to below 10% as more normal production is resumed.

In some patients the rapid regeneration of the blood depletes the iron reserves of the body and recovery is halted. To prevent this, ferrous sulphate 200 mg daily should be given soon after the commencement of treatment. A combined deficiency of vitamin B_{12} and iron is recognised by the presence of macrocytosis and hypochromia—a dimorphic blood picture.

Maintenance treatment

The patient must have regular parenteral doses of hydroxocobalamin indefinitely (1000 μg i.m. every 3 months) for life. Blood counts should be performed annually and the assessment should never be made solely on clinical impression or on the haemoglobin level alone. The patient has a normal life expectancy with the maintenance of a normal blood count by adequate specific treatment. There is, however, a statistically significant increase in death from gastric carcinoma in patients with pernicious anaemia. Patients with subacute combined degeneration of the cord receive monthly hydroxocobalamin injections (p. 570).

If a patient with pernicious anaemia fails to respond to parenteral administration of adequate doses of hydroxocobalamin, it suggests that the diagnosis is wrong. The patient may be suffering from another type of megaloblastic anaemia which may be partially or completely refractory to hydroxocobalamin. Such patients respond to folic acid. An unsustained response may indicate depletion of iron stores and the need for oral iron therapy.

Folate deficiency

Treatment with a daily dose of 5 mg of folic acid by mouth is sufficient; 5 mg once a week is always adequate for maintenance therapy. Folic acid must never be given, other than with vitamin B_{12}, in Addisonian pernicious anaemia or other vitamin B_{12} deficiency anaemias, because of the risk of aggravating or precipitating neurological features of vitamin B_{12} depletion.

Megaloblastic change due to vitamin B_{12} deficiency is very rare in pregnancy. It is therefore reasonable to give folate supplements (350 μg daily) to all pregnant women. When a drug such as methotrexate inhibits dihydrofolate reductase, it is possible to employ folinic acid to overcome the metabolic block. Folinic acid may be given as tablets, 15 mg daily orally, or as an injection intravenously or intramuscularly at a dose of 3 mg/ml. Folinic acid mouthwashes are used to counteract the oral side-effects of folate antagonist drugs. Megaloblastic disorder caused by other cytotoxic drugs which inhibit DNA synthesis is not reversed by either vitamin B_{12} or folate administration.

HAEMOLYTIC ANAEMIA

Various abnormalities may shorten the normal red cell life span of 120 days, and anaemia develops when marrow output no longer compensates. The increased output of new erythrocytes is reflected in a raised reticulocyte count which gives an indication of the severity of the process. Normoblasts may be released under extreme stress. The catabolic pathways for haemoglobin degradation are overloaded and there is a modest increase in unconjugated bilirubin in the blood and increased re-absorption of urobilinogen from the gut,

which is excreted in the urine in increased amounts. Bilirubin does not appear in the urine. Jaundice is mild (p. 790).

Haemolysis may occur intravascularly or extravascularly. Haemoglobin liberated into the plasma is bound mainly by the alpha-2 globulin, haptoglobin, to form a complex too large to be lost in the urine. It is taken up by the liver and degraded. Some haemoglobin is partially degraded and bound to albumin to form methaemalbumin. If all the haptoglobin has been consumed, free haemoglobin may be lost in the urine. In small amounts this is re-absorbed by the renal tubules where the haemoglobin is degraded and the iron stored as haemosiderin. Sloughing of the renal tubular cells gives rise to haemosiderinuria which, if found, always indicates intravascular haemolysis. Haemoglobinuria occurs when greater amounts of haemoglobin are lost, giving the urine a black appearance (black water).

Extravascular haemolysis occurs in the phagocytic cells of the spleen, liver, bone marrow and other organs and there may be little or no depletion of haptoglobin. Estimation of the haptoglobin level in the blood is not always easily interpreted. Inflammatory disease and steroid therapy both increase haptoglobin levels. Ahaptoglobinaemia may occur as an inherited disorder. Nevertheless, absence of haptoglobin is usually a strong indicator of haemolytic disease. Its presence does not exclude haemolysis.

Blood and marrow findings

The peripheral blood shows a moderate macrocytosis and polychromasia from reticulocytosis while specific red cell abnormalities may give a clue to the type of haemolytic disease. There may be a polymorphonuclear leucocytosis. The marrow shows erythroid hyperplasia. A megaloblastic change usually reflects depletion of folate reserves. Increased erythropoietic turnover in the marrow is associated with increased serum lactic dehydrogenase levels which, in the absence of folate deficiency, closely follows the severity of the haemolytic disorder. Red cell survival can be measured crudely using radioactive chromium (^{51}Cr). Surface counting performed at the same time over liver and spleen may give an indication of the site of haemolysis. If transfusion has been given the patient's blood will contain a mixed cell population which is not suitable for ^{51}Cr studies. In these circumstances cross-matched donor cells should be used for labelling.

Aetiology

The causes of haemolytic anaemias are classified as congenital or acquired and are listed in Table 13.8.

Table 13.8   Causes of haemolytic anaemia

Congenital

Membrane abnormalities
   hereditary spherocytosis
   hereditary elliptocytosis
Haemoglobinopathies
   lack of haemoglobin chain synthesis
   thalassaemias
   Amino acid substitution on the haemoglobin chain
   haemoglobin S, C, D
Red cell enzyme defects
   glucose 6 phosphate dehydrogenase deficiency

Acquired

Immune
Isoimmune
Autoimmune
   warm antibody
   cold antibody
Alloimmune

Non-immune
Mechanical
   artificial cardiac valves
   burns
   microangiopathic
   march haemoglobinuria
Infections
Clostridium welchi, malaria
Drugs, chemicals
Dyserythropoietic
   paroxysmal nocturnal haemoglobinuria

CONGENITAL HAEMOLYTIC ANAEMIAS

The principal disorders are hereditary spherocytosis, glucose-6-phosphate dehydrogenase (G6PD) deficiency and the haemoglobinopathies (e.g. sickle-cell disease and thalassaemia). G6PD deficiency and haemoglobinopathies are most common in Black Africans; thalassaemia is most frequent in the Mediterranean area.

HEREDITARY SPHEROCYTOSIS

This is an autosomal dominant disorder in which the principal abnormality appears to be a deficiency of spectrin, a red cell membrane protein. Approximately 25% of patients have no family history. The erythrocyte envelope is abnormally permeable and the sodium pumps are overworked. The exact nature of the RBC defect may vary from family to family. The erythrocytes lose their biconcave shape, become spherical and are more susceptible to osmotic lysis. These spherocytes are destroyed almost exclusively by the spleen. The severity of the disorder is very variable even within an affected family. Haemolysis is mainly extravascular.

Clinical features

Symptoms vary from none to those of severe anaemia (Table 13.5). Episodic jaundice may be noted. The spleen is often but not always palpably enlarged. The severity of the disorder tends to vary in any one patient with episodes of increased haemolysis (haemolytic crises) at times. The transient hypoplasia of red cell production, which may normally occur in association with parvovirus infections, presents as aplastic crises in these patients because of the greatly increased red cell turnover. There is a liability to form pigment gallstones and occasionally cholecystitis may be the presenting event. Leg ulcers sometimes occur.

Investigations

The diagnosis is made by demonstrating a haemolytic state (p. 790) together with spherocytes in the blood film, increased osmotic fragility reflecting the spherocytes and the demonstration of the same disorder in other members of the family. The Coomb's test is negative. There is an increased loss of urobilinogen in the urine. Red cell survival studies with ^{51}Cr show destruction of red cells almost exclusively in the spleen. The differential diagnosis is from other causes of spherocytosis, particularly the various forms of immune haemolysis (p. 798).

Management

Splenectomy results in striking and usually permanent improvement both in the symptoms and in the anaemia and should be advised when:

- the anaemia causes persistent impairment of health
- severe haemolytic or aplastic crises have occurred
- other members of the family have died from the disease
- evidence of cholecystitis and cholelithiasis is present.

Opinion differs as to the desirability of operation for patients with no disability. The operation should be performed during a period of remission, and in young children should be deferred until they are as old as possible and should be preceded by vaccination against pneumococcal infection. Following splenectomy, resistance to some infections may be impaired and daily penicillin V, 250 mg 12-hourly, is prescribed for at least 5 years.

Severe haemolytic crises require treatment by blood transfusion. Blood must be matched very carefully and administered very slowly, as gross haemolytic transfusion reactions are common in this disease. Folic acid, 5 mg daily orally, is prescribed to support the increased erythropoiesis.

GLUCOSE-6-PHOSPHATE DEHYDROGENASE DEFICIENCY

Glucose-6-phosphate dehydrogenase (G6PD) is the first enzyme in the hexose monophosphate shunt of the Embden–Meyerhof glycolytic pathway from which red cells derive most of their metabolic energy. The function of this shunt is to service the enzymes glutathione reductase and glutathione peroxidase which protect the red cells against damage due to oxidation. This protective mechanism is crippled in the absence of G6PD and certain drugs in sufficient concentration can seriously injure the erythrocyte.

The deficiency is inherited as an X-linked disorder with a high frequency among Black Africans who possess an electrophoretic enzyme polymorphism with A and B type enzymes. The enzyme is A type (A-) in deficient Black Africans. In Caucasians only the normal B type enzyme is found and the deficient type is also B (B-). In West and East Africa about 20% of male (hemizygotes) and about 4% of females (homozygous for the abnormal gene) are affected and the enzyme activity is about 15% of normal. Heterozygous females have two populations of red cells, one deficient and the other normal. 100 million persons are affected by this disorder world-wide. The deficiency in Caucasian and Oriental populations is more severe, enzyme activity being less than 1% of normal. Favism (haemolytic anaemia from the ingestion of the broad bean, *Vicia faba*) is due to deficiency of G6PD of the severe variety (B-). Some cases of haemolytic disease of the newborn are caused by this deficiency. Other rare types of G6PD, biochemically different from the above, may be associated with congenital non-spherocytic haemolytic disease and occur sporadically in all races.

Many drugs in common clinical use, for example, some antimalarials and sulphonamides, are capable of precipitating haemolysis in individuals with G6PD deficiency. Infections may also potentiate the haemolytic action of drugs such as aspirin, chloramphenicol, and chloroquine.

Clinical features

Persons with G6PD deficiency normally enjoy good health but are liable to haemolysis if any of the incriminated drugs or foods are ingested. However, the haemolytic effect is dose related and will not be clinically detectable if the amount does not exceed a critical level. It is often possible to employ doses which are not toxic. The anaemia, when it occurs, may be rapid in onset, becoming obvious between 2 and 10 days after exposure to the precipitating agent, and may be sufficiently severe to cause haemoglobinuria as well as the other classical signs of haemolysis. In the relatively mild type of deficiency prevalent in Black people, only older cells which have lost enzyme activity are involved so that the haemolysis is to some extent self-limiting even when the offending agent is continued. Young red cells have high G6PD activity and remain viable until their enzyme complement decays. The enzyme deficiency is much more severe in the B- variety, and destruction tends to be greater. Anuria is an infrequent but serious complication.

Investigations

The diagnosis can be confirmed by estimating the G6PD activity of the red cell but this may not be entirely accurate if there is considerable reticulocytosis. A number of screening tests are also available. The characteristics of intravascular haemolysis are usually present: haemoglobinaemia, methaemalbuminaemia, haemoglobinuria, ahaptoglobinaemia and later haemosiderinuria.

Management

This is by removal of the toxic agent. Recovery is usually rapid but if the anaemia is severe, transfusion of red cells with a normal enzyme complement may be required. Thereafter, the patient should be advised to avoid drugs which may precipitate the disorder. Splenectomy is valueless.

HAEMOGLOBINOPATHIES

The haemoglobinopathies can be classified into two subgroups:

1. Where there is an alteration in the amino acid structure of the polypeptide chains of the globin fraction of haemoglobin, commonly called the abnormal haemoglobins; the best known example is haemoglobin S found in sickle-cell anaemia
2. Where the amino acid sequence is normal but polypeptide chain production is impaired or absent for a variety of reasons; these are the thalassaemias.

Abnormal haemoglobins are caused by amino acid substitutions in their polypeptide chains. These in turn reflect mutations in the structural genes controlling the production of these chains. There are several hundred haemoglobin variants known, some functionally normal, most not. Originally they were designated by letters of the alphabet, e.g. S, C, E and so on. Now this does not suffice and for some years new variants have been given names, often of the towns or districts in which they were discovered. Sickle-cell haemoglobin or haemoglobin S is the most important but haemoglobin C, D and E are also significant in some parts of the world, particularly when inherited along with haemoglobin S or with beta thalassaemia (p. 796).

Modern nomenclature includes a statement of the site of the amino acid substitution. Thus sickle haemoglobin may be defined as:

$$Hb\ S^{6GLU-VAL} \qquad Hb\ S^{A3GLU-VAL}$$

The second method is more accurate since it defines the helix or bend in which the substitution occurs.

Control of haemoglobin synthesis is inherited from both parents. Thus a normal adult can be depicted as having the haemoglobin genotype AA, sickle-cell trait by AS and sickle-cell anaemia or homozygous S disease by SS. The inheritance when both parents have sickle-cell trait can be shown thus:

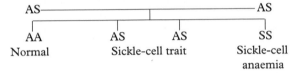

AS———————————————AS

AA   AS   AS   SS
Normal   Sickle-cell trait   Sickle-cell anaemia

There is a 1:4 chance with each pregnancy that the offspring will have sickle-cell anaemia.

SICKLE-CELL ANAEMIA

Epidemiology

The patient with sickle-cell trait is relatively resistant to the lethal effects of falciparum malaria in early childhood. The high incidence of this deleterious gene in equatorial Africa is thus explained by the selective advantage for survival it confers in an environment of endemic falciparum malaria. Patients with sickle-cell anaemia do not have correspondingly greater resistance to falciparum malaria. The geographical distribution of sickle-cell anaemia and other haemoglobinopathies is shown in Figure 13.10. The greatest prevalence of haemoglobinopathies occurs in tropical Africa where the heterozygote frequency is over 20%. In American Black populations sickle-cell trait has a frequency of 8%.

Pathogenesis

When haemoglobin S is deoxygenated, the molecules of haemoglobin polymerise to form pseudo-crystalline structures known as 'tactoids'. These distort the red cell membrane and produce characteristic sickle-shaped cells. The polymerisation is reversible when re-oxygenation occurs. The distortion of the red cell membrane, however, may become permanent and the red cell 'irreversibly sickled'. The greater the concentration of sickle-cell haemoglobin in the individual cell, the more easily are tactoids formed, but this process may be enhanced or retarded by the presence of other haemoglobins. Thus haemoglobin C participates in the polymerisation more readily than haemoglobin A, whereas haemoglobin F strongly inhibits polymerisation.

Most of the red cells in sickle-cell anaemia contain haemoglobin S and little else. They are very prone to sickle even in vivo under normal conditions. This happens particularly in those parts of the microvasculature which are sinusoidal and where the flow is sluggish. Sickled cells increase blood viscosity, traverse capillaries poorly and tend to obstruct flow, thereby increasing the sickling of other cells and eventually stopping the flow. Thrombosis follows and an area of tissue infarction results causing severe pain, swelling and tenderness (infarction crisis). In addition these cells are phagocytosed in large numbers by the mononuclear-phagocyte system, reducing their life span considerably and giving rise to haemolysis.

Clinical features

Patients with the sickle-cell trait (AS) have a normal full blood count and are clinically well. The patients with clinical problems have sickle-cell disease and are homozygous SS or inherit two abnormal haemoglobins, most commonly S&C (SC). The two major problems in sickle-cell disease are chronic anaemia due to reduced erythrocyte survival and episodes of tissue infarction (Fig. 13.11).

Anaemia

Problems do not arise until about the fourth month of life when haemoglobin F-containing cells give way to haemoglobin S-containing cells. The anaemia is haemolytic in type and severe, the haemoglobin seldom rising above 100 g/l and averaging approximately 80 g/l. Secondary folate deficiency is common and exacerbates the anaemia. When folate deficiency is chronic, growth may be retarded and puberty delayed. Episodes of increased sequestration and destruction of red cells (haemolytic crises) occur, sometimes for no apparent reason, and may lead to a swift fall in haemoglobin with rapidly enlarging spleen and liver. Aplastic crises occur in association with parvovirus infections as in hereditary spherocytosis (p. 791) but the effect of the temporary cessation of erythropoiesis may be more dramatic as the haemolysis is severe. The chronic anaemia is responsible for fatigue, reduced exercise tolerance, increased susceptibility to infection, cardiomegaly, leg ulcers and cholelithiasis. Hyperplasia of the marrow in the first year of life expands the marrow cavity producing bossing of the skull, prominent malar bones and protuberant teeth.

Infarction crises

These are characterised by episodes of severe pain which punctuate the patients' lives. They occur commonly in

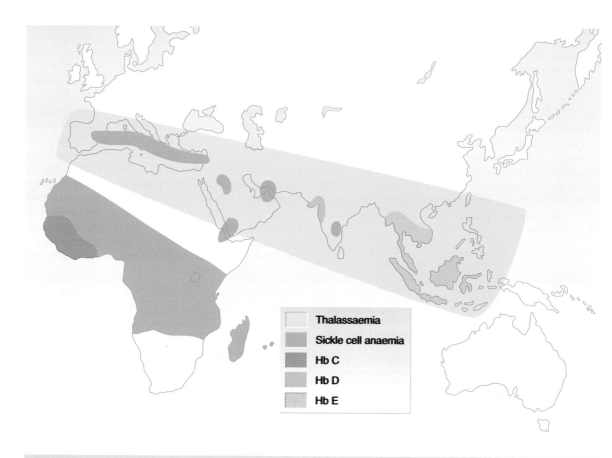

Fig. 13.10 The geographical distribution of the haemoglobinopathies.

bones and spleen but no tissue is exempt. In the infant they classically affect the fingers and toes, producing large fusiform swellings (dactylitis). Metacarpal and tarsal bones may be affected, and shortened digits due to epiphyseal involvement may occur. Mesenteric infarction may produce an acute abdominal emergency at any age. The renal papilla is another site of damage and infarction may give rise to painless haematuria. In adults aseptic necrosis of the head of the femur is a disabling complication. An acute chest syndrome occurs in 20–50% and resembles pneumonia but is probably due to pulmonary infarction. There is a significant risk of stroke (5–17%) which is associated with a high recurrence rate. Precipitating factors include dehydration, chilling and infection, but sometimes the attacks occur spontaneously. The onset is usually rapid and the pain excruciatingly severe (pain crisis) in the first 24 hours, thereafter abating over the next few days. Fever, increasing jaundice and malaise are frequent and, if persistent, may suggest the establishment of infection in the infarcted site. Salmonella osteomyelitis is common.

Pregnancy is hazardous unless careful ante-natal care is provided and as full term approaches, infarction crises in the bones may liberate large amounts of fat and bone marrow emboli. These cause diffuse micro-embolism of the lungs with pulmonary infarction, cor pulmonale and even death. A pseudo-toxaemia syndrome may develop. These complications may also be seen in the less severe haemoglobin SC disease. Sickle-cell anaemia should always be suspected in a patient who has had symptoms of anaemia and 'rheumatism' since infancy and who belongs to a race which is often affected. It should be considered in the differential diagnosis of many disorders in areas where sickle-cell anaemia is common. Patients must be adequately screened before major surgery and bloodless field surgery should never be employed because infarction of the entire limb below the tourniquet may occur.

Investigations

Diagnosis is based on the patient's race, history, clinical findings and investigations which demonstrate the pres-

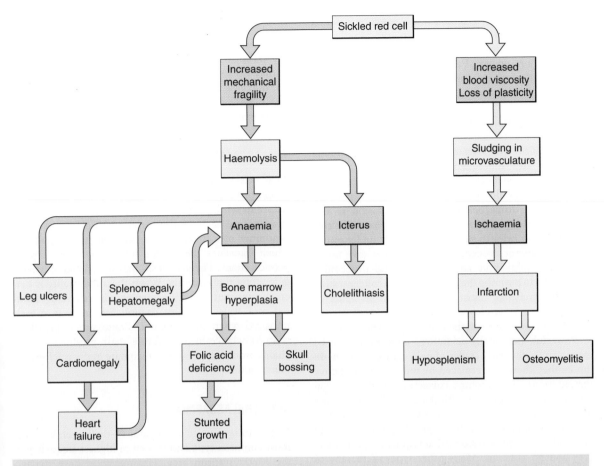

Fig. 13.11   Clinical effects of sickled red cells.

ence of Hb S and no other major abnormal haemoglobin in the blood. The haematological features in SS patients are anaemia with reticulocytosis, the blood film showing sickle cells, target cells and in patients over the age of 7, features of hyposplenism. Rapid screening tests are available to demonstrate the presence of sickle-cell haemoglobin but it is important to remember that these will be positive in both sickle-cell disease and trait. A family study should reveal that both parents carry the abnormal gene for Hb S. In this way true sickle-cell anaemia can be differentiated from other diseases in which haemoglobin S is combined with thalassaemia or some other abnormal haemoglobin such as C or D.

Ante-natal diagnosis is discussed on page 24.

Management

Preliminary experience with allogeneic transplantation has introduced the prospect of cure for the first time in the management of sickle-cell patients. However, its exact role remains to be defined and benefits must be balanced against the morbidity and mortality of the procedure. There are obvious economic implications especially as the disease is most prevalent in areas of the world where money for high technology medicine is limited.

General management is aimed at alleviation of the symptom and the promotion of lifestyle that will minimise the ill effects of the disorder. Regular folic acid supplements (5 mg daily) are prescribed to support the greatly increased erythropoietic activity. Exacerbation of the chronic haemolytic anaemia is commonly associated with infections which should be treated promptly and prevented, for example life-long antimalarials taken where appropriate. Young patients with hyposplenism should receive phenoxymethylpenicillin, one 250 mg tablet daily, and pneumococcal vaccine. Patients should avoid becoming chilled, dehydrated or exposed to hypoxia, for example high altitudes. An acute exacerbation of the anaemia may have no obvious precipitating cause. The spleen and liver may enlarge rapidly and the haemoglobin drops, sometimes with alarming speed (sequestration crisis). Parents should be taught to examine affected children for an enlarging spleen. Transfusion with red cell concentrate is urgently required.

The patient should be adequately hydrated in less severe illness and transfusion with red cell concentrate is used only if essential because of the risk of allo-antibody formation and subsequent reactions. Most patients become habituated to a haemoglobin level of about 80 g/l and should be transfused only when the haemoglobin drops below 50 g/l. Transfusion is also indicated for sequestration and aplastic crises. The role of transfusion prior to surgery is currently under evaluation. At present, it seems reasonable to reserve transfusion for ophthalmic and major surgical procedures with a view to lowering the haemoglobin S concentration to 30%. Exchange transfusion either on an acute or chronic basis is employed in the management of cerebrovascular disease and the acute chest syndrome.

Powerful, potentially addictive, analgesics may be necessary in the early stages of pain crises; after 24–48 hours they should be replaced by milder non-addictive preparations. The prompt correction of dehydration often helps to relieve pain. Antibiotics will be necessary if there are infective complications such as osteomyelitis. At the end of pregnancy these episodes may precipitate a pseudo-toxaemia syndrome that requires heparin therapy and no sedation. Many other types of therapy to prevent in vivo sickling have been tried but all have proved disappointing. The administration of hydroxyurea, which can elevate haemoglobin F, is under evaluation.

Prognosis

It is probable that in Africa few children with sickle-cell anaemia survive to adult life without medical attention. With standard medical care 15% will die by the age of 20 years and 50% by the age of 40.

HAEMOGLOBIN SC DISEASE

This disorder behaves like a mild variety of sickle-cell anaemia. Episodes of infarction are less frequent and anaemia is either absent or less severe. Aseptic necrosis of the femoral head, retinal vein thrombosis and painless haematuria are not uncommon complications. Pregnancy is the main hazard because the same complications occur as in sickle-cell anaemia, particularly fat and bone marrow embolisation of the lungs and pseudo-toxaemia.

HAEMOGLOBIN C DISEASE

This is a benign haemoglobinopathy which, in its homozygous form, is not associated with much morbidity. It may cause megaloblastic anaemia in pregnancy and considerable splenomegaly in adult life. No specific treatment is required other than folic acid supplements in pregnancy.

THALASSAEMIAS

Thalassaemia is an inherited impairment of haemoglobin production, in which there is partial or complete failure to synthesise a specific type of globin chain. The exact nature of the defect varies and it is probable that a number of different faults occur along the pathway which translates the genetic information into a polypeptide chain. The gene itself may be deleted; it usually is in alpha thalassaemia. When the abnormality is heterozygous, synthesis of haemoglobin is only mildly affected and little disability occurs. Synthesis is grossly impaired when the patient is homozygous and there is an imbalance in polypeptide chain production. The chains produced in excess precipitate in the cell forming Heinz bodies.

BETA-THALASSAEMIA

Failure to synthesise beta chains (β-thalassaemia) is the most common type and is seen in highest frequency in the Mediterranean area. Heterozygotes have thalassaemia minor, a condition in which there is usually mild anaemia and little or no clinical disability. Homozygotes (thalassaemia major) are either unable to synthesise haemoglobin A or at best produce very little and, after the first 4 months of life, develop a profound hypochromic anaemia. The diagnostic features are listed in the information box below.

Clinical Features

β-thalassaemia major
The anaemia is crippling and the probability of survival for more than a few years without transfusion is low. Bone marrow hyperplasia early in life may produce head bossing and prominent malar eminences. The skull radiograph shows a 'hair on end' appearance and general widening of the medullary spaces which may interfere with the development of the paranasal sinuses. Development and growth are retarded and folate deficiency may occur. Splenomegaly is an early and prominent feature. Hepatomegaly is slower to develop but may become massive especially if splenectomy is undertaken. Transfusion therapy inevitably gives rise to haemo-

DIAGNOSTIC FEATURES OF β-THALASSAEMIA

Major
- Profound hypochromic anaemia
- Evidence of severe red cell dysplasia
- Erythroblastosis
- Absence or gross reduction of the amount of haemoglobin A
- Raised levels of haemoglobin F
- Evidence that both parents have thalassaemia minor

Minor
- Mild anaemia
- Microcytic hypochromic erythrocytes (not iron deficient)
- Some target cells
- Punctate basophilia
- Raised resistance of erythrocytes to osmotic lysis
- Raised haemoglobin A2 fraction
- Evidence that one parent has thalassaemia minor

Table 13.9   Treatment of β-thalassaemia major

Problem	Management
Erythropoietic failure	Allogeneic bone marrow transplantation from HLA compatible sibling Hypertransfusion to maintain Hb > 100 g/l Folic acid 5 mg daily
Iron overload	Iron therapy forbidden Desferrioxamine therapy
Splenomegaly causing mechanical problems, excessive transfusion required	Splenectomy

siderosis. Cardiac enlargement is common and cardiac failure, in which haemosiderosis may play a part, is a frequent terminal event.

β-thalassaemia minor

β-thalassaemia minor is often detected only when iron therapy for a mild hypochromic anaemia fails. The diagnostic features are summarised in the information box. Symptoms are absent or minimal. Intermediate grades of clinical severity occur.

Management

The treatment of β-thalassaemia major is given in Table 13.9.

Prevention

It is possible to identify a fetus with homozygous β-thalassaemia by obtaining chorionic villus material for DNA analysis sufficiently early in pregnancy to allow termination of pregnancy. This examination is appro-priate if both parents are known to be carriers (β-thalassaemia minor) and will accept a termination.

ALPHA-THALASSAEMIA

The reduction or absence of alpha chain synthesis is common in South East Asia. There are two alpha gene loci on chromosome 16 and therefore four alpha genes. If one is deleted there is no clinical effect. If two are deleted there may be a mild hypochromic anaemia. If three are deleted the patient has haemoglobin H disease and if all four are deleted the baby is stillborn (hydrops fetalis). Haemoglobin H is a β-chain tetramer formed from the excess of chains. It is functionally useless. Treatment of haemoglobin H disease is similar to that of β-thalassaemia of intermediate severity. In some patients the disorder is due to a combination of alpha thalassaemia genes with genes which produce a functionally useless globin chain, Hb Constant Spring. The combinations are shown in the information box.

ALPHA-THALASSAEMIA

- **Cause**
  Failure of production of haemoglobin chain due to gene deletion
- **Age and sex**
  Both sexes from birth onward
- **Genetics**
  2 α chain genes from each parent
- **Presentation**
  Hydrops fetalis. All genes deleted
  Haemoglobin H. 3 genes deleted
  Mild hypochromic microcytic anaemia. 2 genes deleted
- **Treatment**
  Hydrops fetalis—none available
  Haemoglobin H—no specific therapy required; avoid iron therapy. Folic acid if necessary

ACQUIRED HAEMOLYTIC ANAEMIA

IMMUNE–AUTOIMMUNE

In this disorder antibodies are formed against red cell antigens and cause inappropriate destruction of cells. The two main types are categorised on the basis of the thermal characteristics of the antibody.

1. 'Warm' antibodies have a thermal optimum of 37°C and account for 80% of cases. The majority are IgG. A specificity, if it can be demonstrated, is usually to the Rhesus system.
2. 'Cold' antibodies have a thermal optimum of 4°C

but sometimes a thermal range of up to 37°C. These antibodies are IgM and bind complement. Cold antibodies are found in approximately 20% of autoimmune haemolytic anaemias.

WARM AUTOIMMUNE HAEMOLYTIC ANAEMIA

Many cases are idiopathic but some occur in association with chronic lymphatic leukaemia, lymphoma, systemic lupus erythematosus or certain drugs (e.g. methyldopa).

Clinical features

Patients of all ages are affected. Symptoms vary with the severity of the disease and its cause and are mainly those of anaemia (Table 13.5). In addition, in severe cases there may be fever, vomiting and prostration. Splenomegaly and sometimes hepatomegaly is present.

Investigations

The diagnosis is suggested by finding spherocytes and increased polychromasia on the blood film. It is established by demonstrating evidence of antibody on the red cells by the direct antiglobulin test (Coomb's test). This test detects the presence of antibodies on the surface of erythrocytes using an anti-human globulin antiserum (AHG). Antibodies being human globulin are recognised by the AHG which attacks them and causes agglutination of the erythrocytes. This is the 'direct' test. When antibodies are present in serum they must first be attached to red cells with the appropriate antigen before their presence can be detected as described above. This is known as the 'indirect' test. Elution of antibody from the red cells allows investigation of specificity against a panel of cells. The majority of these antibodies can be shown to have anti-Rhesus specificity. Of these, anti-e is the commonest. Identification of specificity, if possible, is useful as blood for transfusion which does not carry the specific antigen can be chosen.

Management

This is with prednisolone 40 mg daily for 3–4 weeks; thereafter the dose is slowly reduced. Response to treatment can be monitored with reticulocyte counts and haemoglobin estimations. The dose should be increased if relapse occurs and maintained for a further two to three weeks when reduction may be tried again. Blood transfusion is avoided unless an antibody specificity has clearly been identified and antigen-free blood is available. In life-threatening situations, the least incompatible blood available can be given, covered by high doses of prednisolone. Splenectomy should be considered if treatment fails from the beginning, or there is

a fall in the haemoglobin following reduction/cessation of steroids.

COLD AGGLUTININ DISEASE

Idiopathic cold agglutinin disease occurs mainly in the elderly. Symptoms reflect a tendency of the red cells to agglutinate and sludge in the microvasculature of the extremities where the blood is cooled. Raynaud's phenomenon (p. 273) is usually present and also acrocyanosis. A low-grade chronic haemolytic anaemia occurs. All these problems are worse in cold weather. Characteristic haematological features are a very high MCV and agglutination on the blood film; these features are reversed if the blood is warmed to 37°C. 'Cold' antibody is present in enormously high titres with anti I or i specificity. The antiglobulin test is almost always positive and demonstrates complement binding.

Treatment consists of keeping the extremities warm. Transfusion is possible but the specimen collected for transfusion must be kept warm during transport to the laboratory; the cross matched blood should be transfused via a blood warmer. Steroids and splenectomy are of little value but immunosuppressive therapy may decrease antibody levels in severe cases.

Cold antibody-type disease may also occur in association with Mycoplasma pneumonia infection and infectious mononucleosis when the haemolysis is usually self limiting. If found in lymphoma the haemolysis tends to be more chronic.

Paroxysmal cold haemoglobinuria is a rare cause of haemolysis in children. It can be associated with syphilis. It is characterised by the Donath Landsteiner IgG antibody which may be found and has anti-P specificity.

ISOIMMUNE HAEMOLYTIC DISEASE

The term isoimmune is used to indicate that the antigen and the antibody come from different persons. This distinguishes it from autoimmune disease in which the antigen and the antibody are from the same individual.

HAEMOLYTIC DISEASE OF THE NEWBORN (HDN)

This disorder, previously called erythroblastosis fetalis, occurs in either sex and is due to an attack on the fetal erythrocytes by maternal antibodies of IgG type which can pass the placental barrier. Causes are listed in the information box below.

The various degrees of severity of HDN are listed in the information box.

Rhesus HDN. In about 1 pregnancy in 10 the mother is Rh-negative and the fetus Rh-positive. However, haemolytic disease of the newborn is very rare in a first

CAUSES OF HAEMOLYTIC DISEASE OF THE NEWBORN

- **ABO incompatibility**
  This form is the commonest and is usually mild and can affect first pregnancies. It occurs in Group O mothers carrying A or B infants and is due to immune anti A or anti B
- **Rhesus incompatibility**
  This form occurs in Rhesus negative mothers carrying rhesus positive babies. The first pregnancy is seldom affected unless the mother has been previously sensitised
- **Other blood group system incompatibilities**
  e.g. anti-Kell. These are rare

TYPES OF HAEMOLYTIC DISEASE OF THE NEWBORN

- Haemolytic disease of the newborn is the mildest
- Icterus gravis neonatorum is more severe and carries the risk of severe brain damage unless treated urgently, but is compatible with survival
- Hydrops fetalis is the most severe and causes death in utero

pregnancy provided the mother has not previously been sensitised by transfusion (see below). Furthermore, sensitisation does not occur as often as might be anticipated and the risk of an Rh-negative woman having a baby with haemolytic disease of the newborn in any pregnancy other than the first is about 1 in 22. If a mother is Rh-negative and the father Rh-positive, the maternal serum must be tested for antibodies between the 32nd and 36th week of each pregnancy. Delivery should be undertaken in hospital. The infant will probably escape the disease if no antibodies are detected but nevertheless the cord blood should be tested for antibodies. If present, preventive treatment can be instituted.

Clinical features

These are of severe haemolytic anaemia with oedema and enlargement of the liver and spleen. Clinical jaundice may be absent for the first 24 hours after birth. Thereafter, deep unconjugated hyperbilirubinaemia leading to kernicterus may occur. The severity of the jaundice is largely due to the immaturity of the fetal liver which is unable to conjugate the large amounts of bilirubin. The haemoglobin level, which should normally be about 180 g/l at birth, falls rapidly. Enormous numbers of nucleated red cells and a reticulocytosis of 10–50% are seen in the blood film (erythroblastosis). The direct Coomb's test is positive.

Management

Exchange transfusion should be given to all severely affected infants (Hb <140 g/l, cord serum bilirubin >60 mmol/l, infant's serum bilirubin >300 mmol/l), as this is the only treatment which will overcome heart failure in a very anaemic infant and prevent deep jaundice and kernicterus. Early diagnosis is essential. Antenatal prediction from tests for antibodies in the maternal serum gives the infant the best chance. In mild cases simple transfusion and phototherapy will be sufficient and in some instances no treatment is required.

Prevention

The most common cause of primary Rh immunisation is transplacental haemorrhage during the third stage of labour. The likelihood of an Rh-negative woman developing anti-Rh antibodies is related to the number of Rh-positive red cells present in her circulation immediately after delivery. These can be stained and quantified. If found the mother should receive an injection of gammaglobulin containing a high titre of anti-D immunoglobulin within 72 hours of delivery. This will destroy the infant cells that have leaked into the mother's circulation and will prevent the development of antibodies in the mother and haemolytic disease in subsequent offspring.

NON-IMMUNE HAEMOLYTIC ANAEMIA

Mechanical

Shearing of red cells may occur as a result of incompetent heart valves and when cells are forced through fibrin deposited in the vasculature. The latter may be deposited by a number of processes resulting in microangiopathic haemolysis. This may occur in disseminated malignancy, toxaemia of pregnancy, the accelerated phase of hypertension and in the haemolytic uraemic syndrome. Direct mechanical trauma has been associated with vigorous contact activities such as karate or prolonged marching (March haemoglobinuria). Thermal injury in severe burns may result in haemolysis in which characteristic small spherocytes can be seen in the film. An important laboratory finding in the majority of mechanically induced haemolytic anaemias is the demonstration of red cell fragmentation on the blood film. As the haemolysis is mainly intravascular haemosiderin may be found in the urine.

Infections

Malarial infection usually with *Plasmodium falciparum* often results in a mild degree of haemolysis. Less frequently there is severe intravascular haemolysis, blackwater fever. The parasites should be seen in the red blood cells on the blood film and the management is discussed on page 152. Clostridium perfringens septicaemia may cause devastating intravascular haemolysis characterised by spherocytosis. The mechanism is thought to be the production of lecithinase activity. The organism is sensitive to penicillin.

Drugs and chemicals

Dapsone and salazopyrin may result in haemolysis in patients who are not G6PD deficient. The mechanism is oxidant and individual variation in drug metabolism is an important factor. Dapsone is acetylated and slow acetylators are much more prone to haemolysis. The demonstration of Heinz bodies is a strong pointer to the diagnosis. Haemolysis has been described following exposure to arsenic gas, copper, chlorate, nitrites and nitrobenzene derivatives. Anaemia is a feature of lead poisoning but this is not predominantly haemolytic. Several enzymes of haem synthesis are inhibited and basophilic stippling is a characteristic finding on the blood film due to pyrimidine-5'-nucleotidase inhibition.

APLASTIC ANAEMIA

PRIMARY IDIOPATHIC ACQUIRED

The annual prevalence in the United States and United Kingdom is approximately 3–6 cases per million; the disease is much more common in certain parts of the world, for example China. The basic problem is failure of the stem cells to a varying degree producing hypoplasia of the marrow elements. An autoimmune mechanism may be responsible in a proportion of cases.

Clinical features

The disorder may occur at any age, the peak incidence being around 30 years. The onset is insidious and the clinical problems are due to the reduction or virtual absence of production of erythrocytes, granulocytes and platelets. Infections and haemorrhage are the most troublesome complications and may be lethal. Bleeding occurs in the skin and mucous membranes. Haematuria and epistaxis are common. Intracranial bleeding is always a risk. Necrotic mouth and throat ulcers and monilial infections reflect the neutropenia.

Investigations

Known causes of hypoplastic and aplastic anaemia must first be excluded. A careful inquiry into exposure to drugs, chemicals and radiation should be made. A history of viral illness, particularly hepatitis, may be important. A full blood count demonstrates a pancytopenia.

Neutropenia is the most marked aspect of the leucopenia, although leucopenia may not be the first abnormality. The anaemia is normocytic, normochromic and often marked. Platelet production is often the most severely affected and the last to recover. The bone marrow should be examined by aspiration and trephine. The latter provides a better assessment of cellularity and an aspirate may be difficult to obtain (dry tap).

Management

All patients will require blood product support and aggressive management of infection. The curative treatment for young (<20 years) patients with severe idiopathic aplastic anaemia is allogeneic bone marrow transplantation if there is an available donor. Those with a compatible sibling donor should proceed to transplantation as soon as possible. Successful pre-transplant conditioning can be achieved with cyclophosphamide alone. In older patients, immunosuppressive therapy gives equivalent results.

A number of drugs have been investigated, for older patients and those without a donor including androgens, steroids, cyclosporin and anti-lymphocyte/anti-thymocyte globulin. These approaches, in the main, reflect the likelihood that an immunological mechanism is involved in a significant proportion of cases. Antilymphocyte globulin has been the most successful agent although haematological responses are often incomplete and long term follow up has revealed a proportion of cases developing myelodysplasia. Short term toxicity is in the form of serum sickness. More recently there has been an interest in the combination therapy; females with severe aplastic anaemia appear to benefit particularly from a combination of antilymphocyte globulin, androgens and steroids.

Prognosis

The prognosis of severe aplastic anaemia managed with supportive therapy only is poor and more than 50% of patients die, usually in the first year. However, the survival of over 60% has been reported after bone marrow transplantation in young patients and similar results can be achieved with immunosuppressive regimens involving antithymocyte globulin.

SECONDARY APLASIA

Causes of this condition are listed in the information box on page 801. It is not practical to list all the drugs which have been suspected of causing aplasia but it is important to investigate the reported side-effects of all drugs taken over the preceding months. In some instances the cytopenia is more selective and affects only one cell line, most often the neutrophils. Frequently this is an incidental finding unassociated with ill health. It probably has an immune basis but this is difficult to prove.

The clinical features and methods of diagnosis are the same as for primary idiopathic aplastic anaemia. An underlying cause should be treated or removed but otherwise the management is as for the idiopathic form. Bone marrow transplantation may have to be considered in young patients who have HLA matched sibling donors.

CAUSES OF ACQUIRED APLASTIC ANAEMIA

- **Drugs**—cytotoxic drugs, idiosyncratic[1]
- **Chemicals**[2]
- **Radiation**
- **Viral hepatitis**
- **Pregnancy**
- **Paroxysmal nocturnal haemoglobinuria**

Key
1. antibiotics—chloramphenicol, sulphonamides
   anti rheumatic agents—penicillamine, gold, phenylbutazone, indomethacin
   antithyroid drugs
   anticonvulsants
2. Benzene toluene solvent abuse—glue sniffing
   Insecticides—chlorinated hydrocarbons (DDT), organo-phosphates and carbonates

---

ANAEMIA OF CHRONIC DISEASE (ACD)

This is a common type of anaemia particularly in hospital populations. Characteristic features are as follows:

1. The anaemia occurs in the setting of chronic infections, chronic inflammation, or neoplasia.
2. The anaemia is not related to bleeding, haemolysis or marrow infiltration.
3. The anaemia is generally mild in the range 85–115 g/l and is usually associated with a normal MCV (normocytic normochromic) but up to 25% may have a reduced MCV.
4. The serum iron is low but iron stores are normal or increased as indicated by the ferritin or stainable marrow iron.

Pathogenesis

The pathogenesis of this type of anaemia is thought to involve abnormalities of iron metabolism and erythropoiesis. Recent interest is centred on the role of erythropoietin and the inhibitory effect of various cytokines (interleukin I and tumour necrosis factor alpha) on erythropoiesis. Erythropoietin levels appear to be lower than would be expected for the degree of anaemia. Administration of erythropoietin to patients with rheumatoid arthritis has a beneficial effect on the anaemia.

Management

A particular problem is to distinguish the ACD associated with a low MCV from iron deficiency. The ferritin level is elevated in inflammatory conditions and the serum iron is low in both the ACD and iron deficiency. A ferritin in the low/normal range (up to 100 mcg/1) in the setting of disorders associated with the ACD may indicate iron deficiency. Examination of the marrow is useful to assess iron stores. A trial of oral iron could be given in difficult situations. A positive response occurs in true iron deficiency but not in ACD. Measures which reduce the severity of the underlying disorder generally help to improve the ACD.

ERYTHROCYTOSIS AND POLYCYTHAEMIA

A raised haemoglobin usually but not always indicates an absolute increase in the number of circulating red cells. In some patients, however, the apparently high haemoglobin level may be due to reduction in plasma volume. This may occur because of dehydration or because of unknown mechanisms associated with stress (Fig. 13.12). A genuine increase in red cell numbers occurs as a secondary phenomenon or is due to a primary myeloproliferative disorder, primary proliferative polycythaemia. The causes of secondary erythrocytosis are given in the information box.

CAUSES OF SECONDARY ERYTHROCYTOSIS

- **Increased production of erythropoietin secondary to hypoxia**
  High altitude
  Lung disease
  Cyanotic congenital heart disease
  Smoking
  High affinity haemoglobins
- **Inappropriate erythropoietin production**
  Renal, liver, lung, uterine and cerebellar tumours

STRESS, SPURIOUS, OR LOW PLASMA VOLUME POLYCYTHAEMIA

Some patients with a high haemoglobin have a red cell mass which is normal or even low. The main abnormality is a reduced plasma volume. A number of terms have been used but this condition is now termed 'low plasma volume polycythaemia'. It often occurs in individuals who are stressed and is associated with hypertension and other risk factors for occlusive vascular disease. The management involves the removal as far as possible of any risk factors for vascular disease. The role of venesection is controversial but should be considered in patients with a haematocrit above 0.55.

PRIMARY PROLIFERATIVE POLYCYTHAEMIA (PPP)

PPP is one of a group of disorders of the pluripotential stem cells called 'myeloproliferative disorders' (p. 803) which have features in common and may progress from one form to another.

Clinical features

PPP occurs mainly in patients over the age of 40 years and is more common in males than females. There may be no symptoms and the disorder is diagnosed incidentally. Common complaints are lassitude, loss of concentration, headaches, dizziness, blackouts, pruritus, epistaxis and 'indigestion'. Some patients present with manifestations of peripheral vascular disease or a cerebrovascular accident. The patients often have a high colour with suffused conjunctivae; retinal vein engorgement may be found. The spleen is palpable in 75% of patients at diagnosis. Thrombotic complications may occur and peptic ulceration is common, sometimes complicated by bleeding.

Investigations

Diagnosis is established along the lines indicated in the information box below. In some patients the results listed in the information box may be only marginally abnormal and the diagnosis is uncertain. The finding of a raised red cell mass together with splenomegaly is virtually diagnostic. Measurement of the erythropoietin level and if available determination of the in vitro culture characteristics of the marrow may be helpful in difficult cases. Marrow from patients with PPP grows in culture without the addition of erythropoietin.

Management

Venesection is the simplest therapeutic measure and the best to use if the diagnosis is in doubt; 500 ml of blood (less if the patient is elderly) is removed and the venesection repeated within a day or two if necessary until the haematocrit reading is reduced to < 45%. Clinical improvement occurs rapidly with the reduction of blood viscosity. Iron deficiency will eventually appear but iron therapy is withheld until the disease has been controlled by other methods of treatment. Radioactive phosphorus (5 mCi of ^{32}P i.v.) is an effective form of treatment for

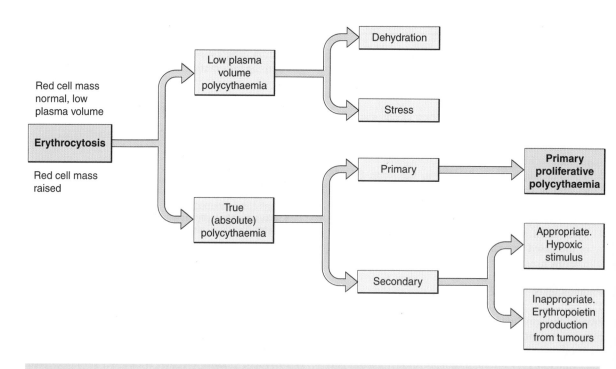

Fig. 13.12 Erythrocytosis and polycythaemia.

THE DIAGNOSIS OF PRIMARY PROLIFERATIVE POLYCYTHAEMIA

Positive features
- Elevated red cell mass
- Splenomegaly
- An associated elevation of white cell and platelet counts
- Hypercellular marrow with hyperplasia of erythropoiesis/granulopoiesis and megakaryocytes
- Absent iron stores
- Elevated neutrophil alkaline phosphatase score
- Elevated serum B_{12} levels
- Absence of secondary causes of erythrocytosis

FURTHER READING

Hoffbrand A V, Pettit J E 1993 Essential haematology, 3rd edn. Genetic defects of haemoglobin. Blackwell Scientific, Oxford. See ch 6, p 94–120

Means R T, Krantz S B 1992 Progress in understanding the pathogenesis of the anaemia of chronic disease. Blood 80: 1639–1645

older patients when the diagnosis is certain. The full effect on the haemoglobin will not appear for three months but the white cell count and platelet count respond more quickly. Further doses may be required but often there is good disease control for periods up to 18 months. The major problem with radioactive phosphorus is that it has a leukaemogenic potential. Chemotherapy with hydroxyurea until the disease is brought under control is equally effective but requires more supervision and more frequent blood counts than radioactive phosphorus. However, hydroxyurea may be less leukaemogenic and is preferred for patients under 50 years. Other treatments used in the past are busulphan which can use irreversible bone marrow depression in case of accidental overdose and chlorambucil which is associated with an increased incidence of secondary acute leukaemia.

Prognosis

The median life span after diagnosis in treated patients exceeds 10 years. Some patients survive more than 20 years. The disease may convert to another myeloproliferative disorder, for example essential thrombocythaemia, and about 15% develop myelofibrosis. Acute leukaemia develops principally in those patients who have been treated with radioactive phosphorus. Despite more efficient treatment, deaths still occur because of thrombotic events.

OTHER MYELOPROLIFERATIVE DISORDERS

There are a number of other myeloproliferative conditions in addition to primary proliferative polycythaemia which are closely related and are either malignant or pre-malignant. These include myelofibrosis (p. 812), chronic myeloid leukaemia (p. 810) and essential thrombocythaemia (p. 831).

DISORDERS OF THE WHITE CELLS

Reactive changes

Tables 13.10–13.14 indicate a variety of causes of neutrophilia (10), lymphocytosis (11), monocytosis (12), eosinophilia (13) and basophilia (14). Tables 13.15, 13.16 list causes of neutropenia and lymphocytopenia and Table 13.17 drug induced neutropenia. Such lists cannot be exhaustive but give a guide to the commoner associations.

LEUKAEMIAS AND MYELOPROLIFERATIVE DISORDERS

Leukaemias are a group of malignant disorders of the haemopoietic tissues characteristically associated with

Table 13.10 Causes of neutrophilia

Infection	Bacterial
Inflammation	Gout, rheumatoid arthritis
Trauma	
Drugs	Steroids, lithium
Malignant disease	Gastric, bronchogenic, breast
Metabolic/endocrine	Renal failure, gout, acidosis
Haematological	Myeloproliferative disorders
Haemorrhage	
Myocardial infarction	

Table 13.11 Causes of lymphocytosis

Malignancy	Acute and chronic lymphatic leukaemia, Non-Hodgkin's lymphoma
Infections	Mononucleosis syndromes
	Epstein–Barr virus
	Cytomegalovirus
	Toxoplasmosis
	HIV
	Herpes simplex
	Other viruses—measles, mumps, chickenpox, infectious hepatitis, acute infectious lymphocytosis
	Other infections—pertussis, brucellosis
Miscellaneous	Serum sickness
	Thyrotoxicosis

Table 13.12   Causes of monocytosis

Haematological disorders	Acute monocytic leukaemia
	Acute myelomonocytic leukaemia
	Chronic myelomonocytic leukaemia
	Hodgkin's disease
	Chronic neutropenias
Gastrointestinal disease	Ulcerative colitis
	Crohn's disease
Collagen vascular diseases	Systemic lupus erythematosus
	Polyarteritis nodosa
	Rheumatoid arthritis
Infections	Tuberculosis
	Subacute bacterial endocarditis
	Syphilis
Sarcoidosis	

Table 13.13   Causes of eosinophilia

Parasite infection	many including strongyloidiasis, hookworm disease, schistosomiasis, scabies
Allergic disorders	hay fever, asthma
Skin disorders	eczema, psoriasis, dermatitis herpetiformis
Tumours	myeloproliferative disorders, lymphoma, carcinomatosis
Hypereosinophilic syndromes	Loeffler's syndrome
Sarcoidosis	
Polyarteritis nodosa	

Table 13.14   Causes of basophilia

Myeloproliferative disease	Ulcerative colitis
Carcinoma	Infections—Influenza
Mastocytosis	Chickenpox
Hypothyroidism	Tuberculosis

Table 13.15   Causes of neutropenia

Congenital	
Acquired	
Drugs	See table 13.17
Infection	Viral—hepatitis
	Bacterial—miliary TB, typhoid, brucellosis
Malignancy	Usually secondary to marrow invasion
Hypersplenism	
Systemic lupus erythematosus	
Megaloblastic anaemia	

Table 13.16   Causes of lymphocytopenia

Immunoglobulin disorders leading to decreased production	Ataxia telangiectasia, thymic dysplasia
Increased destruction	Cytotoxic drugs
	Corticosteroids
	Radiotherapy
	Anti-thymocyte globulin
Increased intestinal lymph loss	Severe right sided heart failure
	Whipple's disease
	Intestinal lymphectasia
Miscellaneous	Advanced carcinoma, advanced Hodgkin's, AIDS, sarcoidosis, miliary TB, renal failure

Table 13.17   Drugs associated with neutropenia

Group	Examples
Analgesics/anti-inflammatory agents	Phenylbutazone, oxyphenylbutazone, gold, diflunisal
	Penicillamine, naproxen
Anti-thyroid	Carbimazole, methimazole, propylthiouracil
Anti-arrhythmias	Quinidine, procainamide, tocainide
Anti-hypertensives	Captopril, enalapril, nifedipine
Anti-depressants/ psychotropics	Amitriptyline, dothiepin, mianserin
Anti-malarials	Maloprim, fansidar, chloroquine
Anti-convulsants	Phenytoin, sodium valproate, carbamazepine
Antibiotics	Sulphonamides, penicillins, cephalosporins
Miscellaneous	Cimetidine, ranitidine, chlorpropamide, zidovudine

increased numbers of primitive white cells (blasts) in the bone marrow. The course of the disease may vary from a few days or weeks to many years depending on the type of leukaemia.

Epidemiology

The incidence of leukaemia of all types in the population is approximately 10 per 100 000 per annum of which just under half are acute leukaemia. Males are affected more frequently than females, the ratio being about 3:2 in acute leukaemia, in chronic lymphocytic leukaemia 2:1 and in chronic myeloid leukaemia 1.3:1. Geographic variation in incidence does occur, the most striking being the rarity of chronic lymphocytic leukaemia in the Chinese and related races. Acute leukaemia occurs at all ages. Acute lymphoblastic leukaemia shows a peak of incidence in the 1–5 age group. All forms of acute leukaemia have their lowest incidence in young adult life and there is a striking rise over the age of 50. Chronic leukaemias occur mainly in middle and old age.

Aetiology

The cause of the leukaemia is unknown in the majority of patients. Several factors, however, are associated with the development of leukaemia and these are listed in the information box below.

Terminology and classification

The terms 'acute' and 'chronic', when applied to leukaemia, refer to the clinical behaviour of the disease. In acute leukaemia the history is usually brief and life expectancy, without treatment, short. In chronic leu-kaemias the patients may have been unwell for months and survival is measured in years. A significant number of chronic leukaemias are discovered incidentally.

Not all leukaemias are associated with an increased leucocyte count or even the appearance of abnormal cells in the blood. The diagnosis is made from an examination of the bone marrow.

FACTORS ASSOCIATED WITH THE DEVELOPMENT OF LEUKAEMIA

- **Ionising radiation**
  A significant increase in myeloid leukaemia followed the atomic bombing of Japanese cities. An increase in leukaemia was observed after the use of radiotherapy for ankylosing spondylitis and diagnostic radiographs of the fetus in pregnancy
- **Cytotoxic drugs**
  These, particularly alkylating agents, may induce myeloid leukaemia, usually after a latent period of several years
- **Exposure to benzene in industry**
- **Retroviruses**
  One rare form of T cell leukaemia/lymphoma appears to be associated with a retrovirus similar to the viruses causing leukaemia in cats and cattle
- **Genetic**
  There is a greatly increased incidence of leukaemia in the identical twin of patients with leukaemia. Increased incidence occurs in Down syndrome and other genetic disorders
- **Immunological**
  Immune deficiency states are associated with an increase in haematological malignancy
  Occasionally, acute leukaemia presents as an aplastic anaemia

---

The classification of leukaemia is given in Tables 13.18 and 13.19.

Although leukaemias are divided into lymphoid or myeloid varieties, recent advances have shown that this division may be artificial because in acute leukaemias the two types may coexist in the same patient. Nevertheless there is a value in maintaining the distinction as the drug therapy of the two main types is substantially different.

The sub-classification of the lymphoblastic varieties is possibly of greater value for the subtype dictates greater variation in treatment. The 'common' type which constitutes 70% of all patients responds well to treatment

Table 13.18 A classification of leukaemia

Acute	Chronic
Lymphoblastic	Lymphatic
Myeloid	Myeloid

Table 13.19 Subclassifications of leukaemia

Acute lymphoblastic	Acute myeloid
Common type (pre B)	FAB* classification
T cell	M1, undifferentiated
B cell	M2, differentiated
Undifferentiated	M3, promyelocytic
	M4, myelomonocytic
	M5, monocytic
	M6, erythrocytic
	M7, megakaryocytic
Chronic lymphatic	**Chronic myeloid**
Common B cell	Ph.^{x} positive
Rare T cell	Ph.^{x} negative, BCR^{xx} positive
	Ph.^{x} negative, BCR^{xx} negative
	Eosinophilic leukaemia

FAB* = French, American, British
Ph.^{x} = Philadelphia chromosome
BCR^{xx} = Breakpoint Cluster Region

and carries the best chance of long-term remission. The classification of acute myeloblastic leukaemia into seven varieties reflects the variable degree of maturation of the granulocyte series, the common involvement of the monocyte series with the granulocyte series and also the involvement of erythrocytic and megakaryocytic elements.

ACUTE LEUKAEMIA

There is a failure of cell maturation in acute leukaemia. Proliferation of cells which do not mature leads to an increasing accumulation of useless cells which take up more and more marrow space at the expense of the normal haemopoietic elements. Eventually this proliferation spills into the blood. The evolution of acute leukaemia is illustrated schematically in Figure 13.13. Acute myeloblastic leukaemia is about four times more common than acute lymphoblastic leukaemia in adults. In children the lymphoblastic variety is more common.

Clinical features

The patient usually presents with non-specific 'flu-like' symptoms or vague malaise and tiredness. A bleeding tendency manifests, such as purpura, epistaxis and gum bleeding. Mouth ulcers, herpes labialis and sore throats are common. Often the diagnosis is not obvious from the symptomatology and is uncovered by laboratory investigation. On examination the spleen and liver may be enlarged, particularly when the disease is advanced. There may be cervical lymphadenopathy secondary to pharyngeal sepsis but enlarged lymph nodes due to the disease are a common feature particularly of the lymphoblastic form.

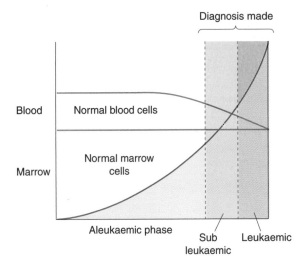

Fig. 13.13 Development of leukaemia.

OTHER INVESTIGATIONS FOR ACUTE LEUKAEMIA

- **Haemostatic function**
  Coagulation screen
  Fibrinogen
  D-dimers
- **Renal function**
  Plasma urea
  Plasma creatinine

- **Hepatic function**
  Total protein
  Albumin
  Bilirubin
  Alkaline phosphatase
  AST/ALT
- **Cellular proliferation**
  Plasma LDH
  Plasma urate

Investigations

Blood examination usually shows anaemia with a normal or raised MCV. The leucocyte count may vary from as low as $1 \times 10^9/1$ to as high as $500 \times 10^9/1$ or more. In the majority of patients the count is below $100 \times 10^9/1$. The blood film appearance of blast cells and other primitive cells are usually diagnostic. Sometimes the blast cell count may be very low in the peripheral blood and a bone marrow examination is necessary to establish the diagnosis. Severe thrombocytopenia is usual but not invariable.

The bone marrow is the most valuable diagnostic investigation and will provide material for cytology, cytogenetics and immunological phenotyping. A trephine biopsy should be taken if no marrow is obtained (dry tap). The marrow is usually hypercellular with replacement of normal elements by leukaemic blast cells in varying degrees (but more than 30% of the cells). The presence of Auer rods in the cytoplasm of blast cells indicates a myeloblastic type of leukaemia.

Other basic investigations required at diagnosis are given in the information box below.

Management

The general strategy for acute leukaemia is given in Figure 13.14. The first decision must be whether or not to give specific treatment. However, specific treatment is generally aggressive and has a number of side-effects; it may not be appropriate for the following groups of patients:

1. the very elderly (over 80 years of age).
2. patients with other serious disorders.

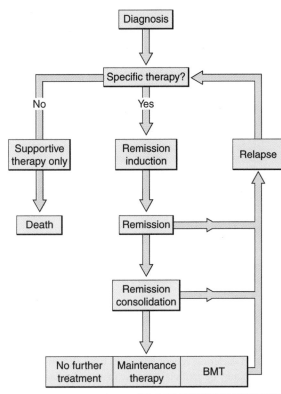

Fig. 13.14 Treatment strategy in acute leukaemia.

3. patients who decline specific therapy.
4. patients with types of leukaemia known to be very unresponsive to specific treatment (secondary leukaemias).

In these patients supportive treatment only should be offered which can effect considerable improvement in well-being. These decisions must, if possible, be made with the understanding and co-operation of the patient and his or her relatives.

Specific therapy

If a decision to embark on specific therapy has been taken, the patient should be prepared in the ways listed in the information box below. It is unwise to attempt aggressive management of acute leukaemia unless adequate services are available for the provision of the various forms of supportive therapy outlined later. Such treatment should only be directed by physicians experienced in the management of leukaemic patients.

The aim of treatment is to destroy the leukaemic clone of cells without destroying the residual normal stem cell compartment from which repopulation of the haemopoietic tissues will occur. There are three phases, remission induction, consolidation and maintenance.

PREPARATIONS FOR SPECIFIC THERAPY IN ACUTE LEUKAEMIA

- Existing infections should be identified and treated (e.g. urinary tract infection, oral candidiasis, dental, gingival and skin infections)
- Anaemia corrected with red cell concentrate infusion
- Thrombocytopenic bleeding controlled with platelet transfusion
- If possible, insertion of a central venous catheter (e.g. Hickman line) to facilitate access to the circulation for delivery of chemotherapy
- Careful explanation of the therapeutic regimen to the patient

---

1. **Remission induction**: In this phase the bulk of the tumour is destroyed by combination chemotherapy. The patient often goes through repeated periods of severe bone marrow failure requiring intensive support and in-patient care from specially trained medical and nursing staff.
2. **Remission consolidation**: If remission has been achieved by induction therapy, residual disease is attacked by therapy during the consolidation phase. This includes intrathecal drug therapy to deal with disease which may have survived in the sanctuary of the nervous tissues where it is not easily reached by systemic chemotherapy. Cranial irradiation is also given for the same purpose, particularly in acute lymphoblastic leukaemia.
3. **Remission maintenance**: If the patient is still in remission after the consolidation phase for acute lymphoblastic leukaemia a period of maintenance therapy is given consisting of a repeating cycle of drug administration. This may extend for up to 2 years if relapse does not occur and is usually given on an outpatient basis. Thereafter, specific therapy is discontinued and the patient observed. This phase is not thought to be of benefit in patients with acute

Table 13.20 Drugs commonly used in the treatment of acute leukaemia

Lymphoblastic	Myeloid
Induction	
Vincristine (i.v.)	Daunorubicin (i.v.)
Prednisolone (oral)	Cytosine arabinoside (i.v.)
L-asparaginase (i.v.)	Etoposide (i.v. and oral)
Daunorubicin (i.v.)	Thioguanine (oral)
Methotrexate (intrathecal)	
Consolidation	
Daunorubicin (i.v.)	Cytosine arabinoside (i.v.)
Cytosine (i.v.)	Amsacrine (i.v.)
Etoposide (i.v.)	Mitozantrone (i.v.)
Maintenance	
Prednisolone (oral)	
Vincristine (i.v.)	
Mercaptopurine (oral)	
Methotrexate (oral)	

myeloblastic leukaemia who have been brought into complete remission by induction and consolidation therapy.

The detail of the treatment schedules for these treatments will be found in specialist texts. The drugs most commonly employed for the two main varieties of acute leukaemia are given in Table 13.20. If a patient fails to go into remission with induction treatment, alternative drug combinations may be tried but generally the outlook is poor. Alternatively, a decision may be taken not to give any further specific therapy and to provide supportive treatment only. Disease which relapses during treatment or soon after the end of treatment carries a poor prognosis and is difficult to treat. The longer after the end of treatment relapse occurs, the more likely it is that further treatment will be effective.

Supportive therapy

Aggressive and potentially curative therapy which involves periods of severe bone marrow failure would not be possible without adequate and skilled supportive care. The following problems commonly arise.

Anaemia: Anaemia is treated with red cell concentrate infusion to maintain a haemoglobin above 100 g/l.

Bleeding: Thrombocytopenic bleeding requires platelet transfusions unless the bleeding is trivial. Freshly harvested platelets from five donors are pooled and provided as a pack. One or two packs daily may be required if bleeding is severe. Coagulation abnormalities occur and need accurate diagnosis and treatment as appropriate, usually with fresh frozen plasma. The role of prophylactic platelet transfusion is controversial. However, many units give platelets in an attempt to keep the count above 10×10^9/l.

Infection: Fever (greater than 38°C) lasting over 1 hour in a neutropenic patient (absolute neutrophil count $< 1.0 \times 10^9$/l) indicates possible septicaemia. Parenteral antibiotic therapy is essential. Empirical therapy with a combination of an aminoglycoside (e.g. gentamicin) is given with acylureido penicillin (e.g. azlocillin). This combination is synergistic and bacteriocidal and should be continued for at least 5 days after the fever has resolved. The organisms most commonly associated with severe neutropenia are Gram-positive bacteria such as *Staphylococcus aureus* and *Staphylococcus epidermidis*. The Gram-negative infections with organisms such as *Escherichia coli*, Pseudomonas and Klebsiella are more likely to cause rapid clinical deterioration and these organisms must be covered with the initial empiric therapy. Gram-positive infection, particularly when the patient has an indwelling i.v. catheter, may require vancomycin. Patients with lymphoblastic leukaemia are susceptible to infection with the protozoan sp. *Pneumocystis carinii* which causes a severe pneumonia. Diagnosis may be difficult and is obtained either from bronchial washings or open lung biopsy. Treatment is with high dose co-trimoxazole, initially intravenously with change to oral treatment as soon as possible.

Oral and pharyngeal monilial infection is common. Prophylaxis with oral nystatin is standard practice: 1 ml of suspension (100 000 units) held in the mouth for as long as possible 4 times per day. Lozenges are less effective. For established infection nystatin suspension or amphotericin suspension, 1 ml (100 mg per ml) 4 times per day or amphotericin lozenges, 10 mg dissolved slowly in the mouth 4 times per day, should be given. Therapy with fluconazole is often effective in severe cases.

For systemic fungal infection with candida or pulmonary aspergillosis, intravenous amphotericin is required: 0.5–1 mg/kg per day for at least three weeks. The addition of flucytosine, 100–200 mg/kg daily given intravenously or orally in 4 divided doses may enhance the therapeutic effect of amphotericin. However, flucytosine is myelotoxic and may delay recovery from bone marrow failure. Amphotericin is nephrotoxic and hepatotoxic. Renal and hepatic function should be monitored closely, particularly if the patient is receiving antibiotics which are also nephrotoxic. Potassium supplementation is usually required.

Herpes simplex infection occurs frequently round the lips and nose during ablative therapy for acute leukaemia. Acyclovir (200 mg 5 times per day) may be prescribed prophylactically to patients with a history of cold sores or elevated titres to herpes simplex. The intravenous dose is 5 mg/kg over 1 hour repeated every 8 hours. Herpes zoster can also be treated in the early stage with acyclovir at a dose of 10 mg/kg, 8-hourly intravenously for 5 days. Cytomegalovirus infection has become a problem in some leukaemia units. Treatment is difficult but a combination of ganciclovir and immunoglobulin can be tried.

The value of isolation facilities, such as laminar flow rooms, is debatable but may contribute to the awareness of staff for careful barrier nursing practice. The isolation is often psychologically stressful for the patient.

Metabolic problems: Continuous monitoring of renal, hepatic and haemostatic function is necessary, together with fluid balance measurements. Patients are often severely anorexic and may find drinking difficult. The necessary fluids and electrolytes often must be given intravenously for as long as necessary. Renal toxicity occurs with some antibiotics (e.g. aminoglycosides) and anti-fungal agents (amphotericin).

Psychological support: Psychological support of the patient is very important. The patient should be continuously kept informed, questions answered and fears allayed as far as possible. An optimistic attitude from the staff is vital. Delusions, hallucinations and paranoia are not uncommon during periods of severe bone marrow failure and septicaemic episodes, and should be met with patience and understanding.

Alternative chemotherapy: Gentle chemotherapy not designed to achieve remission may be used to curb excessive leucocyte proliferation. Drugs used for this purpose include hydroxyurea up to 4 g daily and mercaptopurine up to 150 mg daily. The effect is to reduce the leucocyte count without inducing bone marrow failure.

Prognosis

Without treatment the median survival of patients with acute leukaemia is about 5 weeks. This may be extended to a number of months with supportive treatment. Patients who achieve remission with specific therapy have a better outlook. Around 80% of adult patients less than sixty years of age with acute lymphoblastic leukaemia and acute myeloblastic leukaemia achieve remission. Remission rates are lower for older patients. However, the relapse rate continues to be high. Median survival for acute lymphoblastic leukaemia patients is about 30 months and for acute myeloblastic leukaemia patients about 13 months if remission is achieved. Bad prognostic factors for survival are given in the information box below.

Allogeneic bone marrow transplantation (BMT)

This is the only therapeutic measure which holds out the hope of 'cure' for persons with a variety of haematological disorders, particularly those listed in the information box below.

Healthy marrow from a donor is injected intravenously into a recipient who has been suitably 'conditioned'. The conditioning therapy used most frequently is high dose cyclophosphamide and total body irradiation. Conditioning ablates the recipient's haemopoietic and immunological tissues. The injected cells 'home' to the marrow and produce enough erythrocytes, granulocytes and platelets for the patient's needs in about 3–4 weeks. It takes up to 3 or more years to regain good lymphocyte function and immunological stability. During this period, particularly in the first year, the patient is at great risk from opportunistic infections.

The preferred donors are histocompatible siblings and the best results are obtained in patients aged under 20. Older patients can be transplanted, but results become progressively worse with age. The patient must be sufficiently stable psychologically to contend with the period of illness during the transplantation process. The patient should be free of other disorders which might seriously limit life span. Bone marrow transplantation requires specialised supervision and supportive facilities with fully trained staff. It is best performed in units established for the care of acute leukaemias under the primary care of haematologists, with the cooperation of immunologists, microbiologists, radiotherapists and full laboratory services.

Bone marrow transplantation may be syngeneic (identical twin donor) or allogeneic (non-identical donor). Disorders for which allogeneic transplantation

is currently offered are shown in the information box below.

Transplantation is also a possibility for resistant acute leukaemia and selected patients with lymphoma. The role of allogeneic BMT in patients with haemoglobinopathies such as sickle-cell disease is controversial.

The main complications of allogeneic bone marrow transplantation are outlined in the information box.

Graft-versus-host disease (GVHD)

Problems of GVHD and interstitial pneumonitis may cause serious morbidity and death if the graft is successful. Even low-grade GVHD, which is probably advantageous in terms of survival, can reduce the quality of life. GVHD is due to the cytotoxic activity of donor T lymphocytes which become sensitised to their new host which they regard as foreign. This may cause either an acute or chronic form of GVHD.

Acute GVHD: The acute GVHD usually appears 14–21 days after the graft, although it may appear earlier or up to 70 days later. It can affect the skin, liver and gut. It may vary from being mild to lethal. It appears to be associated with infection, although the relationship is not fully understood. Methotrexate, cyclosporin, antithymocyte globulin, high dose corticosteroids and T cell depletion of the donor marrow have all been used to try and prevent the disorder. The more severe forms prove very difficult to control; high dose steroids may be helpful.

Table 13.21   Infection during recovery from bone marrow transplant

Infection	Period after BMT	Treatment
Herpes simplex	0–4 weeks	Acyclovir
Bacterial, fungal	0–4 weeks	As for acute leukaemia (see p. 806)
Cytomegalovirus	7–21 weeks	If patient CMV negative, use CMV negative blood products. Hyperimmune immunoglobulin and granulovir for documented infections
Varicella zoster	After 13 weeks	Acyclovir, 10 mg/kg per day for 1–2 weeks i.v.
Pneumocystis carinii	8–26 weeks	Co-trimoxazole
Interstitial pneumonitis (non-infective)	6–18 weeks	No specific therapy Prednisolone, 60 mg daily orally may be tried

Chronic GVHD: This may follow acute GVHD or arise independently; it occurs later than acute GVHD. It often resembles a connective tissue disorder, although in mild cases a rash may be the only manifestation. Chronic GVHD is usually treated with steroids/Cyclosporin which can be used in cases associated with thrombocytopenia. Associated with chronic GVHD is a graft versus leukaemia effect which results in a lower relapse rate.

Infection is the other major problem during recovery from BMT. Details are given in Table 13.21. The long term survival for patients undergoing allogeneic bone marrow transplantation in acute leukaemia is around 50%. 30% succumb to procedure-related morbidity (GVHD, pneumonitis) and in 20% the disease relapses.

Autologous bone marrow transplantation

In this procedure the patient's own marrow is harvested to be given back again after intensive therapy. It may be used for disorders which do not primarily involve the haemopoietic tissues or in patients in whom very good remissions have been achieved in conditions such as acute leukaemias and high-grade lymphomas. In acute leukaemias the procedure carries a lower procedure-related mortality rate than with allogeneic bone marrow transplantation but there is a high relapse rate (50%). The issue of whether the bone marrow should be treated (purged) in an attempt to remove any residual leukaemia cells is controversial. The results of randomised trials are awaited to determine the role of autografting in acute leukaemia.

CHRONIC LEUKAEMIA

CHRONIC MYELOID LEUKAEMIA

Chronic myeloid leukaemia is a disorder of proliferation which is unrestrained and excessive. Maturation proceeds fairly normally. The disease occurs chiefly between the ages of 30 and 80 years with a peak at 55 years. The ratio of males to females is 1.3:1. It is rare, with an annual incidence in the UK of 1/100 000. The disease is found in all races. The aetiology is unknown.

Cytogenetic and molecular aspects

90% of patients with chronic myeloid leukaemia have a chromosome abnormality known as the Philadelphia (Ph) chromosome. This is a shortened chromosome 22 and is the result of a reciprocal translocation of material with chromosome 9. The break on chromosome 22 occurs in the BCR (breakpoint cluster region). The fragment from chromosome 9 that joins the BCR carries the Abelson (ABL) oncogene which forms a chimeric gene with the remains of the BCR. This chimeric gene codes for 210 kDa protein with tyrosine kinase activity which may play a causative role in the disease. Some Ph negative patients also have evidence of the same molecular abnormality.

Natural history

The disease has three phases: a chronic phase in which the disease is responsive to treatment, is easily controlled and is essentially a benign neoplasm; an accelerated phase (not always seen) in which disease control becomes more difficult; and a blast crisis phase in which the disease transforms into an acute leukaemia, either myeloid (70%) or lymphoblastic (30%) which is relatively refractory to treatment. Blast crisis occurs randomly and is the cause of death in the majority of patients. Patient survival is therefore dictated by the timing of the blast crisis, which cannot be predicted.

Clinical features

The frequency of the more common symptoms at presentation is given in Table 13.22. About 11% of patients are asymptomatic at diagnosis. On examination the principal clinical finding is splenomegaly, which is present in 90% of patients. In about 10% the enlargement is massive, extending to over 15 cm below the costal margin. The spleen is usually firm, smooth and painless but occasionally infarction may occur, giving rise to

Table 13.22 Symptoms at presentation of chronic myeloid leukaemia

Symptoms	Percentages
Tiredness	37
Weight loss	26
Breathlessness	21
Abdominal pain and discomfort	21
Lethargy	13
Anorexia	12
Sweating	11
Abdominal fullness	10
Bruising	7
Vague ill health	7

Table 13.23 Causes of splenomegaly

Congestive
Intrahepatic portal hypertension
  cirrhosis
  hepatic vein occlusion
Extrahepatic portal hypertension
  thrombosis, stenosis or malformation of the portal or splenic vein
Cardiac
  chronic congestive cardiac failure

Infective

Bacterial	endocarditis
	septicaemia
	tuberculosis
	brucellosis
	salmonella
Viral	hepatitis
	Epstein-Barr
	cytomegalovirus
Protozoal	malaria, leishmaniasis
	trypanosomiasis
Fungal	histoplasmosis

Inflammatory/granulomatous disorders
  Felty's syndrome, SLE
  sarcoidosis

Haematological
Red cell disorders
  megaloblastic anaemia
  haemoglobinopathies
Autoimmune haemolytic anaemias
Myeloproliferative disorders
  chronic myeloid leukaemia
  myelofibrosis, primary polycythaemia, essential thrombocythaemia
Neoplastic
  leukaemias, lymphomas

Other malignancies
Secondary—rare

Storage disease
Gaucher's disease
Nieman–Pick disease

Miscellaneous
Cysts, amyloid, hyperthyroidism

exquisite tenderness. A friction rub may be heard in cases of splenic infarction. Other causes of massive splenomegaly apart from chronic myeloid leukaemia are myelofibrosis, lymphoma and malaria. Hepatomegaly occurs in about 50% of patients.

Lymphadenopathy is unusual. A list of causes of splenomegaly is shown in Table 13.23.

Investigations

Examination of the blood usually shows a normocytic normochromic anaemia. The mean haemoglobin is 105 g/l with a range 70–150 g/l. The mean leucocyte count is 220×10^9/l with a range of 9.5–600. The mean platelet count is 445×10^9/l with a range of 162–2000. In the blood film the full range of granulocyte precursors from myeloblasts to mature neutrophils is seen with peaks at the myelocyte and mature granulocyte stage of maturation. Myeloblasts are usually less than 10%. There is often an absolute increase in eosinophils and basophils and nucleated red cells are common. If the disease progresses through an accelerated phase the percentage of the more primitive cells increases. There is a dramatic increase in the number of circulating myeloblasts as the disease enters blast transformation. In about a third of patients very high platelet counts are seen during treatment, both in chronic and accelerated phase, but usually drop dramatically at blast transformation. Basophilia tends to increase as the disease progresses.

The peripheral blood is the most useful diagnostically but bone marrow material should be obtained for chromosome analysis to demonstrate the presence of the Philadelphia chromosome. Increasingly DNA analysis is being undertaken to demonstrate the presence of the chimeric Abelson-BCR gene. Other characteristic findings on investigation include a very low neutrophil alkaline phosphatase score and very high vitamin B_{12} levels in the plasma. Lactate dehydrogenase levels are also substantially elevated.

Management

No specific therapy is required if the patient is asymptomatic and the leucocyte count not greatly elevated. In the majority of patients, however, treatment is necessary.

Chemotherapy

The two most widely used drugs, both given orally, are busulphan and hydroxyurea. Although control of the leucocyte count is smoother with busulphan than hydroxyurea it carries greater risk of serious marrow suppression and, rarely, of serious interstitial pulmonary fibrosis (busulphan lung). Hydroxyurea is currently the most widely used oral agent to provide initial control of the disease. A daily dose of around 2–4 g is used initially and the dose tailored to maintain the white count in the normal range. After some months of satisfactory maintenance treatment the drug can be stopped, sometimes for as long as a year or more, and reintroduced when the leucocyte count rises above $20 \times 10^9/l$. It is seldom possible to stop hydroxyurea for long periods as the leucocyte count tends to rise quickly. None of these treatments diminishes the Philadelphia chromosome or affects the onset of blast cell transformation. They therefore do little to prolong life but they do substantially improve the quality of life. Two types of treatment given in chronic phase affect survival.

Alpha interferon: this is given intramuscularly or subcutaneously at 3–9 mega units daily. It can induce and maintain control of this disease in chronic phase in about 70% of patients. In addition, however, reduction in the percentage of Ph positive cells is seen in about 20% and apparent elimination of the Ph chromosome in about 5%. There is evidence that interferon prolongs survival in those who achieve a significant reduction in Philadelphia positive cells. Only prolonged follow-up will determine whether such patients are cured. Interferon therapy causes 'flu-like' symptoms initially, tiredness, somnolence, weight loss, dizziness, nausea, vomiting, loss of taste, diarrhoea and headache. Some of these side-effects may be controlled with paracetamol; others such as severe bone pain and severe weight loss are reasons for discontinuation. The majority of patients tolerate the therapy well, particularly if the dose can be reduced to 3 mega units 3 times per week. It is probably unwise to use interferon therapy in patients over 75 years of age because of neurotoxicity. During treatment the aim should be to maintain the leucocyte count at low levels between 2 and $5 \times 10^9/l$.

Allogeneic or syngeneic bone marrow transplant from a matched sibling donor provides the only means of obtaining long-term remission in this disease. It is available to those under the age of 40 years who have a suitable donor. The best results are obtained in patients in early chronic phase when about 60% can expect prolongation of survival and possible cure. The results of transplantation in accelerated and blast transformation phases are poor. As only few patients have available matched family donors there is increasing interest in transplantation using matched unrelated volunteer donors. Such a transplant carries higher morbidity and mortality but may offer up to 40% the prospect of long-term survival. Various autografting approaches are also under evaluation.

Treatment of the accelerated phase and blast crisis of the disease is more difficult. In accelerated phase hydroxyurea can be an effective single agent; low dose cytosine arabinoside can also be tried. When blast transformation occurs, the type of blast cells should be ascertained by cytochemical and immunological techniques. If lymphoblastic, the response to appropriate treatment (p. 807) is better than if myeloblastic. Response to treatment for the latter is very poor. There is a strong case for supportive therapy only, particularly in older patients.

Prognosis
Patients treated conventionally have a 15% risk of death in the first 12 months and thereafter an annual risk of 20–25%. Median survival is about 3 years but a few patients survive over 10 years.

Philadelphia chromosome negative chronic myeloid leukaemia
About half of these patients have the classical molecular abnormality (BCR positive) without a demonstrable Ph chromosome. They behave as Ph chromosome positive patients and they should be managed in the same way. The remainder (BCR negative) tend to be older, mostly males, with lower platelet counts and higher absolute monocyte counts, and respond poorly to treatment. Median survival is less than 1 year.

MYELOID METAPLASIA AND MYELOFIBROSIS

Myeloid metaplasia is the appearance of precursors of red cells, granulocytes and platelets in abnormal sites such as the liver and spleen and is usually associated with a leucoerythroblastic blood picture (p.783). This is not a phenomenon compensating for loss of marrow activity but is evidence of disordered behaviour by the precursor cell lines.

MYELOFIBROSIS

Myeloid metaplasia is seen in myelofibrosis. Early in myelofibrosis the marrow may have little fibrous tissue and be hypercellular with an excess of all cell lines, particularly megakaryocytes. As the disease progresses fibrous tissue increases and may eventually fill most of the marrow space. The fibrosis is a reactive response to the disease process, not part of the neoplastic disorder.

Clinical features
These are very variable. Most patients with myelofibrosis suffer lassitude, weight loss, night sweats and some intolerance of heat. The spleen may be greatly enlarged and splenic infarcts may occur. Rarely splenomegaly is absent.

Investigations
Anaemia, sometimes macrocytic, is common. The leucocyte count varies with an increase in granulocytes and usually a leucoerythroblastic blood picture. The erythrocytes show very characteristic tear drop poikilocytes. The platelet count may be very high, normal or low and giant forms are seen in the blood film. The

neutrophil alkaline phosphatase score is frequently raised, as are urate levels. The marrow is often difficult to aspirate and a trephine biopsy shows an excess of megakaryocytes and increased reticulin and fibrous tissue replacement. Folate deficiency is very common.

Management

Treatment is largely supportive with blood transfusion. Folic acid (5 mg daily) may be helpful. Androgen therapy (oxymetholone 50 mg daily if tolerated) and corticosteroids (prednisolone 40 mg daily), however, have also been tried, albeit with very little success. Cytotoxic therapy with drugs such as hydroxyurea up to 2 g daily should be used very cautiously to try to reduce the spleen size or a very high white count. Splenectomy may be required if the grossly enlarged spleen is causing distress or because transfusion requirements are excessive, but the outcome is unpredictable. Prognosis is variable and survival may exceed 10 years. The disease is progressive with steady deterioration. Bone marrow transplantation should be considered for young patients.

CHRONIC LYMPHOCYTIC LEUKAEMIA

This is the commonest variety of leukaemia. The ratio male:female is 2:1 and the majority of patients are over the age of 45 with a peak at 65. The disease is very rare in the Chinese and related races. In this disease B lymphocytes, which would normally respond to antigens by transformation and antibody formation, fail to do so. An ever-increasing mass of immuno-incompetent cells accumulate to the detriment of immune function and normal bone marrow haemopoiesis. The receptor profile of the lymphocytes almost always demonstrates a B cell type of disease. T cell disease occurs rarely (5%). The light chains of immunoglobulins produced by these B cells tend to be either kappa or lambda in type indicating in the majority of cases a monoclonal expansion of cells. The B cells of chronic lymphatic leukaemia characteristically express a T cell antigen, CD5.

Clinical features

The onset is very insidious. Tiredness and vague ill-health are common although about 25% of patients are symptom free and the disorder is found incidentally. The development of anaemia tends to be slower than in chronic myeloid leukaemia and the presenting feature is usually the finding of firm, rubbery, discrete and painless lymph nodes in the cervical, axillary and inguinal regions. A list of the causes of lymphadenopathy is given in Table 13.24. The spleen is usually palpable but smaller than in chronic myeloid leukaemia. The liver

Table 13.24 Causes of lymphadenopathy

Infective	
Bacterial	streptococcal, TB
Viral	Epstein–Barr, HIV
Protozoal	toxoplasmosis, brucellosis
Fungal	histoplasmosis, coccidioidomycosis
Neoplastic	
Primary	leukaemias, lymphomas
Secondary	e.g. lung, breast, thyroid, stomach
Connective tissue disorders	rheumatoid arthritis, SLE
Sarcoidosis	
Amyloidosis	
Drugs	phenytoin

may also be enlarged. As a result of immunosuppression there is an increasing tendency to recurrent infections.

Investigations

Peripheral blood examination usually shows a mild but gradually increasing anaemia. Haemolytic anaemia may occur and is usually warm auto-immune in type. In the majority of patients the leucocyte count is between 50 and $200 \times 10^9/1$ although it may occasionally be greatly increased up to $1000 \times 10^9/1$. About 95% or more of these cells are lymphocytes which are predominantly of the small variety. Lymphoblasts are rare but undifferentiated lymphocytes may increase in number in the terminal stages. The platelet count is either low normal or only mildly reduced. Examination both by aspiration and trephine is required to assess the degree of marrow involvement. Folate deficiency may occur. Estimations of total proteins and immunoglobulin levels should be undertaken to establish the degree of immunosuppression which is common and progressive. In some patients immunoglobulin levels may be raised and there may be a monoclonal band. Urate levels are seldom raised because cell turnover is low.

Staging

The disease may be staged according to the criteria of the widely accepted international classification which is given in the information box below.

Management

The treatment depends upon the stage of the disease.

Clinical Stage A. No specific treatment required. Life expectancy is normal in older patients. The patient should be reassured.

Clinical Stage B. No treatment may be required if asymptomatic. Chemotherapy with chlorambucil may be initiated in symptomatic patients. Local radiotherapy to lymph nodes which cause discomfort may be given.

Clinical Stage C. Anaemia may require transfusion with red cell concentrate. Bone marrow failure, if present, is treated initially with prednisolone, 40 mg daily for 2–4 weeks. A degree of bone marrow recovery is usually achieved.

Cytotoxic therapy

Chlorambucil, 5 mg orally daily, over long periods with dose adjustment according to blood counts, will reduce the abnormal lymphocyte mass and produce symptomatic improvement in most patients. Alternatively, chlorambucil may be given as intermittent high dose therapy, 0.4 mg/kg every 2 weeks incrementing by 0.1 mg/kg until the maximum tolerated dose is reached. This is continued until the desired therapeutic effect is obtained. In Stage C disease there is some evidence that more aggressive combination chemotherapy might be beneficial but this is controversial. Fludarabine, a synthetic nucleoside, appears to be the most active drug and is undergoing intensive evaluation.

Radiotherapy

Total body irradiation employing very small doses spread over 5 weeks in 10 fractions is also effective and well tolerated, especially by the elderly. Local radiotherapy may be used to reduce spleen size or treat local problems due to the disease.

Infections

These must be vigorously treated with antibiotics as appropriate. Recurrent viral or non-specific infections (often respiratory) sometimes respond to immunoglobulin replacement therapy. Acyclovir is indicated for herpetic infections.

Splenectomy

This may be required to treat auto-immune haemolytic anaemia or gross splenic enlargement.

Prognosis

The overall median survival is about 6 years. Clinical Stage A patients have a median survival over 12 years and Stage C patients between 2 and 3 years. 50% of patients die of infection and 30% of causes unrelated to chronic lymphocytic leukaemia. Unlike chronic myeloid leukaemia, chronic lymphocytic leukaemia rarely transforms to an acute phase.

HAIRY CELL LEUKAEMIA

This is a lymphoproliferative chronic B cell disorder.

Clinical features

The male:female ratio is 6:1 and the median age is 50. Presenting symptoms are generally those of ill health and recurrent infections. Splenomegaly occurs in 90% but lymph node enlargement is unusual.

Investigations

Severe neutropenia, monocytopenia and the characteristic hairy cells in blood and bone marrow are typical. These cells usually type as B lymphocytes but characteristically express CD25 and FMC7. A characteristic test is the demonstration that the acid phosphatase staining reaction in the cells is resistant to the action of tartrate. The neutrophil alkaline phosphatase score is almost always very high.

Management

Splenectomy was the mainstay of treatment until the introduction of alpha interferon. This drug when commenced at 3 mega units daily, reducing eventually to 3 times a week, subcutaneously is very effective at controlling the disease although complete remissions are seldom obtained. Agents such as deoxycoformycin and 2-chlorodeoxyadenosine are under evaluation as they may induce a complete remission.

PROLYMPHOCYTIC LEUKAEMIA

This is another variant of chronic lymphatic leukaemia found mainly in males over the age of 60; 25% are of the T cell variety. There is massive splenomegaly with little lymphadenopathy and a very high leucocyte count, often in excess of $400 \times 10^9/l$. The characteristic cell is a large lymphocyte with a prominent nucleolus. Treatment is generally unsuccessful and the prognosis very poor. Leucophoresis for very high white counts, splenectomy and chemotherapy may be tried.

THE MYELODYSPLASTIC SYNDROME (MDS)

This syndrome consists of a clonal group of disorders which represent steps in the progression to the development of leukaemia. It is characterised by variable cytopenia, hypo-granular neutrophils with nuclear hyper or hypo-segmentation and hypercellular marrow with dysplastic changes in all three cell lines. The syndrome is being recognised more frequently; its exact incidence is uncertain but is thought to be more common than acute leukaemia. Usually the disease presents as a primary problem in elderly patients although it may occur as a secondary complication of treatment for malignant disease in younger patients.

The syndrome comprises the following conditions:

1. refractory anaemia
2. refractory anaemia with ring sideroblasts
3. chronic myelomonocytic leukaemia
4. refractory anaemia with excess of blasts (RAEB)
5. refractory anaemia with excess of blasts in transformation (RAEB-t).

Diagnosis

The diagnosis should be considered in a patient with a cytopenia with the dysplastic features indicated above. A marrow aspiration should be performed, which is usually hypercellular with evidence of dysplasia. Blast cells may be increased but do not reach the 30% level which indicates acute leukaemia. Chromosome analysis frequently reveals abnormalities, particularly of chromosomes 5 or 7.

Prognosis

The first two conditions are relatively chronic disorders while the latter three presentations show a more aggressive course with a tendency to terminate as acute myeloid leukaemia. Thus patients with refractory and sideroblastic anaemia may survive for years but prognosis in the other three conditions is measured usually in months.

Management

Treatment is unsatisfactory. Support in the form of transfusion of blood and platelets and treatment of infection is required for all. Aggressive antileukaemic therapy is not generally successful. Differentiating agents such as retinoic acid have not fulfilled their promise. Low dose cytosine arabinoside (20 mg subcutaneously, twice daily), produces occasional remission but this is short lived. Allogeneic transplantation should be considered in younger patients who have a donor but results indicate only a 30% success rate.

THE LYMPHOMAS

This group of malignant neoplasms is divided into two main types: Hodgkin's disease and non-Hodgkin's lymphoma (NHL). The latter accounts for approximately 70% of lymphomas and has an annual incidence of 11/100 000. Its incidence is increasing. In the younger age group this is related to NHL occurring secondary to HIV infection.

HODGKIN'S DISEASE

This disease is characterised by progressive, painless enlargement of lymphoid tissues throughout the body. It occurs in both sexes but more commonly in men, with two peaks of incidence, one in adolescence and early adult life and a second in the 45–75 age group. The pathogenesis is unknown, although the Epstein–Barr virus has been implicated.

The pathological hallmark of HD is the Reed–Sternberg cell (Fig. 13.15). There is still debate about its exact origin, although it is felt to be the malignant cell. The disease can be defined pathologically into four types, which are listed in the information box.

> **PATHOLOGICAL CLARIFICATION OF HODGKIN'S LYMPHOMA**
> - lymphocyte predominant
> - nodular sclerosing
> - mixed cellularity
> - lymphocyte depleted

The nodular sclerosing variety is the most commonly encountered, particularly in young women: the mixed cellularity type, commoner in older men, is second and the, lymphocyte predominant is third. Lymphocyte depleted is the least often seen and is sometimes difficult to distinguish from a high grade non-Hodgkin's lymphoma. Lymphocyte predominant HD is now thought to represent a low grade NHL.

Clinical features

The onset is insidious, usually with enlargement of one group of superficial nodes which may fluctuate in size. While the cervical nodes are often the first to be involved, the disease may also appear to start in the mediastinal and axillary nodes and more rarely in abdominal, pelvic and inguinal areas. Involved lymph nodes are usually painless, discrete and rubbery, though tenderness does occur in some patients, particularly when the nodes have enlarged rapidly. The overlying skin is freely mobile. Extension of the disease from the lymph nodes to adjac-

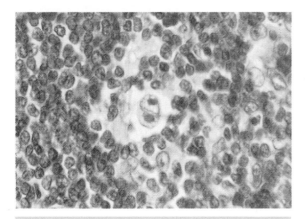

Fig. 13.15 Hodgkin's disease: Reed–Sternberg cell.

Table 13.25 Clinical stages of Hodgkin's disease (Ann Arbor Classification)	
Stage	**Definition**
I	Involvement of a single lymph node region (I) or extra-lymphatic site (IE)
II	Involvement of two or more lymph node regions (II) or an extra-lymphatic site and lymph node regions on the same side (above or below) the diaphragm (IIE)
III	Involvement of lymph node regions on both sides of the diaphragm with (IIE) or without (III) localised extra-lymphatic involvement or involvement of the spleen (IIIS) or both (IIISE)
IV	Diffuse involvement of one or more extra-lymphatic tissues, e.g. liver or bone marrow. The lymphatic structures are defined as the lymph nodes, spleen, thymus, Waldeyer's ring, appendix and Peyer's patches

ent tissues may occur and is found particularly in the mediastinum. Pressure by node masses on neighbouring structures may cause a variety of problems, such as dysphagia, breathlessness, venous obstruction, jaundice and paraplegia. Splenomegaly is uncommon at the onset of the disease and even when present does not always signify organ involvement; but absence of splenomegaly does not exclude involvement by disease.

Extranodal disease is very uncommon, particularly in contrast to NHL. General features may include progressive weakness, loss of weight and drenching night sweats. Fever may be present. Some patients have a low-grade pyrexia and others experience swinging fevers. The classical Pel–Ebstein intermittent fever is seldom encountered because the disease has been modified by treatment. Pruritus is troublesome in about 10% of patients. Some patients experience discomfort at the site of disease infiltration shortly after an alcoholic drink.

Staging

Hodgkin's disease is thought to arise in one area and spread to others. It is important to establish the extent of the disease at the time of diagnosis because staging largely determines the therapeutic approach. Clinical staging investigations required include chest radiographs, computed tomography, and marrow trephine and aspirate. Magnetic resonance imaging is not more sensitive than computed tomography for detecting enlarged nodes. A laparotomy is rarely performed to establish the extent of intra-abdominal disease but when undertaken does enable pathological staging to be made. There are four clinical stages based primarily on the extent of the disease (Table 13.25).

Each stage is sub-divided into A or B categories according to whether or not they have systemic symptoms. The symptoms that place a patient in the category are: unexplained weight loss of more than 10% of the body weight in the previous 6 months; unexplained fever above 38°C; and heavy night sweats.

The disadvantage of this classification is that it does not take account of the bulk of disease which is prognostically important.

The full blood count may be numerically normal. A normochromic and normocytic anaemia may be found and occasionally there is an immune haemolytic component. There is no diagnostic change in the white cells although a modest eosinophilia occurs in about 10–15% of patients. The total white cell count may be normal but is sometimes considerably raised with a neutrophil leucocytosis. Lymphopenia, when it occurs, has a bad prognosis and is an indicator of lymphocyte depletion. In the terminal phase there may be leucopenia and thrombocytopenia which may be as much a reflection of treatment as of the disease. Bone marrow involvement is uncommon (15%) at the onset of the disease but may be found later. The diagnosis can be established with certainty only by tissue biopsy, usually of a lymph node. Liver biopsy may provide the diagnosis in patients with hepatic enlargement.

Management

There are two main modalities of treatment, radiotherapy and chemotherapy (p. 817). Megavoltage radiotherapy can eliminate the disease in a high proportion of patients provided the disease is localised. Chemotherapy alone or combined with radiotherapy is employed when there is any suspicion that the disease is more widespread. The indications for radiotherapy and chemotherapy are given in the information box below.

Radiotherapy

Megavoltage radiotherapy to a dose of 3500–4000 cGy is given over a period of 4 weeks, 5 days each week, to involved areas and a slightly lower dose to adjacent areas.

Table 13.26   The ChlVPP regimen

Drug	Dose		
Chlorambucil	6 mg/m²	(up to 10 mg total)	Days 1–14 orally
Vinblastine	6 mg/m²	(up to 10 mg total)	Days 1 and 8 i.v.
Procarbazine	100 mg/m²		Days 1–14 orally
Prednisolone	40 mg/m²		Days 1–14 orally

Extensive radiotherapy prejudices future chemotherapy by destroying too much of the bone marrow reserves. The tendency is, therefore, to opt for chemotherapy if the disease is extensive, to be followed by radiotherapy if necessary.

Chemotherapy

Combination chemotherapy is highly effective in obtaining lasting remissions. A widely used regimen in the United Kingdom is given in Table 13.26 and is a variation of the MOPP and MVPP regimens which employ mustine hydrochloride as the alkylating agent. In the ChlVPP regimen chlorambucil replaces mustine. The drugs are given on a 28-day cycle for a minimum of 6 pulses and up to 9 if necessary. The chlorambucil-based regimen is better tolerated, causing less vomiting and depilation than that based on mustine hydrochloride. The regimen using vinblastine (MVPP) is less neurotoxic than that employing vincristine (MOPP). Chlorambucil can be given orally. All regimens are myelotoxic and bone marrow tolerance is monitored with repeated blood counts. Dose modification or delay may be required if leucocyte and platelet counts do not recover adequately by the time the next pulse of chemotherapy is due. There is a small (5%) risk that patients treated with chemotherapy, particularly if combined with radiotherapy, will develop acute leukaemia, usually 7–10 years later. Attempts have been made to compile regimens that do not carry this risk, and one employs doxorubicin (Adriamycin), bleomycin, vinblastine and decarbazine (ABVD) although the last drug is now often replaced by VP16. This may be used as an alternating regimen with ChlVPP or as salvage therapy.

Combined modality treatment

This is employed usually where there is bulk disease. The chemotherapy is given first and radiotherapy subsequently to the original sites of bulk disease which have been shrunk by the chemotherapy.

Relapse

Patients who relapse while on therapy have a poor prognosis. The same drugs may be used again if relapse occurs more than one year after the cessation of chemotherapy; otherwise salvage chemotherapy or radiotherapy is required. Autologous bone marrow transplantation may be employed for patients whose marrow is not involved and who have relapsed, or for the type of disease that carries poor prognosis.

Chemotherapy has an appreciable risk of inducing sterility in males which may be permanent. It is less of a risk in females, in whom evidence of premature menopause may also appear. Because many of these patients are young, males in particular may require counselling about the effect of chemotherapy and should be offered the possibility of sperm storage. In women replacement hormone therapy may be required to preserve the skeleton if premature menopause occurs.

Prognosis

The disease is fatal if untreated. The 5 year survival rate in patients with stage IA disease treated with radiotherapy exceeds 90% and in stage IIA disease it is greater than 70%. In more advanced disease the results of chemotherapy are very satisfactory and more than 50% of patients remain disease free after 10 years. Just how effective combination chemotherapy is, remains to be determined because many patients who have been treated in this way are still alive. The prognosis with regard to histological type matters less when chemotherapy is used. Chronic relapsing disease occurs in some patients who may survive with repeated treatment for over 20 years.

NON-HODGKIN'S LYMPHOMA (NHL)

In this group of disorders there is a malignant monoclonal proliferation of lymphoid cells, the majority of cases identifiable as B cell and a minority as T cell (15%). Non-Hodgkin's lymphomas merge with lymphoblastic and lymphocytic leukaemias with which they have many features in common.

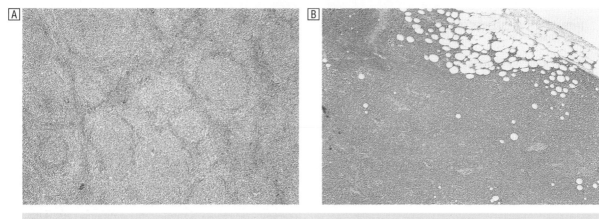

Fig. 13.16   Non-Hodgkin's lymphoma: Ⓐ (low-grade), follicular or nodular pattern and Ⓑ (high-grade), diffuse pattern of histology.

Pathology and classification

In the past the most widely used classification was that of Rappaport, which had the merit of simplicity. It drew attention to the division between lymphomas which retained a nodular structure (nodular or follicular) and those in which the architecture was lost (diffuse) (Fig. 13.16). Another classification, the Kiel, has also been widely adopted. More recently an 'International Working Formulation' has been developed in an attempt to produce a single standard classification. Patients are allotted to one of three grades: low, intermediate, and high. The criteria by which patients are allotted are complex but this grading provides a practical guide for the clinician and can be easily understood. For treatment purposes intermediate and high grade lymphomas are often taken as one group. The size of the lymphoid cells is also a guide to prognosis. Small cell disease (mature lymphocytes) is associated with low grade and large cell disease (immature lymphoid cells) with high grade disease. Most nodular lymphomas are low grade disease and most diffuse lymphomas high grade. Low grade lymphomas carry the best prognosis and high grade the worst. However, high grade lymphomas may respond better to treatment and patients can achieve long term remission if treated properly. 80% of low grade NHL and 20% of high grades have a chromosome abnormality which is a translocation involving chromosomes 14 and 18. The bc12 oncogene is on chromosome 18 and the bc12 product inhibits programmed cell death (apoptosis). This is thought to be an important step in the pathogenesis of the lymphoma.

Staging

The Ann Arbor classification outlined in the section on Hodgkin's disease is used (p. 816). Unlike Hodgkin's lymphoma the disease in NHL is frequently widespread at the time of diagnosis (Stage III or IV), often involving not only lymph nodes but also extra nodal sites such as the gastrointestinal tract. Early involvement of bone marrow is typical of nodular lymphoma. Extra lymphatic tissue involvement at the time of presentation is more common and almost every organ or tissue in the body may be the site of initial disease. In gastrointestinal lymphomas the stomach is most frequently and the rectum least frequently involved. Thyroid lymphomas tend to be associated with gastrointestinal involvement. Some skin lymphomas are T cell in type, for example mycosis fungoides. Most lymphomas originating in extra-lymphatic tissues are of the diffuse variety and have a rather poor prognosis unless they are well localised.

Epidemiology

These lymphomas occur at all ages, are rare under 2 years and become more frequent with increasing age. Males are more frequently affected than females. Nodular lymphomas occur mainly in adults between the ages of 30 and 60. NHL may be associated with HIV infection. In the USA 3% of AIDS cases present with NHL and about 15% of NHLs might be HIV related. These lymphomas are usually high grade and commonly involve extranodal sites.

Clinical features

Lymph node enlargement is the most common presenting finding and is usually painless unless it has developed rapidly. The nodes are discrete and firm. The patient usually complains of tiredness, lassitude, loss of weight and occasionally fever and sweating. However, the patient may be symptom free. When the presentation is extra lymphatic the symptoms will reflect the tissues involved. Frequently the diagnosis of lymphoma is an unexpected finding at laparotomy or during some other investigative procedure. Because of the association between HIV infection and NHL a history of high risk activity should be sought. Weakness of the legs progressing to paraplegia may be due to an extradural lymphoma compressing the cord. Pressure effects in other areas may cause dysphagia, breathlessness, vomiting, intestinal obstruction or ascites and limb oedema. Pain is the main symptom of bone involvement which may present with a pathological fracture.

One variety of low grade NHL, the lymphoplasmacytoid variety (frequently called Waldenstrom's macroglobulinaemia) is associated with IgM paraprotein production. Symptoms of hyperviscosity may result such as tiredness, mental confusion, headaches and nose bleeds. These symptoms may require plasmapheresis for rapid relief.

Physical examination often reveals more widespread node involvement than noticed by the patient. Unexplained lymphadenopathy which fails to resolve spontaneously within a few weeks should always be suspect. Lymphomatous nodes may wax and wane in size and the shrinkage of nodes does not exclude a diagnosis of lymphoma. Splenomegaly usually indicates that the spleen is involved.

Investigations

The diagnosis is made by lymph node biopsy. Often the node is superficial and easily accessible but more invasive techniques may be required if nodes are situated, for example, deep in the abdomen. Such nodes can be biopsied under CT scan guidance (Fig. 13.17) or via the laparoscope. Laparotomy may be required for diagnostic purposes if inadequate samples are obtained. Bone marrow aspiration and trephine biopsy should be performed early in the investigation because marrow involvement is common and indicates stage IV disease. Blood counts usually show normal values unless there is splenomegaly with hypersplenism or a complicating autoimmune haemolytic anaemia when a reduced haemoglobin level, reticulocytosis and positive direct antiglobulin test (Coomb's test) will be found (p. 798). In some patients there may be an overspill of lymphoma cells into the peripheral blood. Thrombocytopenia is uncommon. Moderate degrees of anaemia may be present if there is considerable bone marrow involvement. HIV testing should certainly be carried out in patients in high risk groups.

Immunophenotyping of blood, lymph node and marrow lymphoid cells provides invaluable information on cell lineage (B or T or other), the degree of cell differentiation and cell clonality. It may also identify patients who are non-lymphomatous and may demonstrate lymphoma in patients thought not to be. An assessment of immune competence is also important and immunoglobulin levels should be measured. A monoclonal band may be found in some patients.

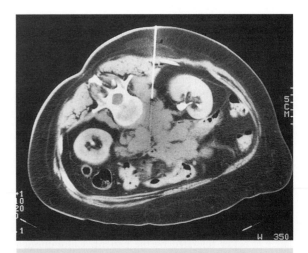

Fig. 13.17 CT guided percutaneous needle biopsy of retroperitoneal nodes involved by lymphoma.

FACTORS DETERMINING MANAGEMENT STRATEGY IN NON-HODGKIN'S LYMPHOMA

- Age of the patient
- Degree of ill health (concomitant disease)
- Histological grade
- Staging of the disease
- HIV status
- Patient's wishes

Management

Treatment strategy in lymphoma is determined by factors listed in the information box. There are two principal modalities of treatment, radiotherapy and chemotherapy.

Radiotherapy

Radiotherapy, if used, is usually given as 'involved field' treatment. No benefit is gained in survival terms from more extensive treatment.

Chemotherapy

This may be given as simple single agent treatment or as combination therapy with multiple drug regimens designed to optimise tumour toxicity and minimise damage to the normal tissues, particularly the haemopoietic tissues.

Disease relapsing during chemotherapy generally carries a poor prognosis unless alternative therapy is available. If relapse occurs years after cessation of therapy, response to the same chemotherapy as was originally used may be effective.

Management of low grade lymphoma

No specific therapy may be required if the disease is not advanced. Some patients can be observed for years before active measures are indicated. Where treatment is required, either radiotherapy or chemotherapy may be used. The indications are:

Stage I and IIA	Involved field radiotherapy
Stage IIB, III and IV	Chemotherapy, single agent or combination
	Whole body irradiation.

Treatment with radiotherapy is used for very localised disease as there is the possibility of cure. No combination chemotherapy regimen has been shown to induce longer survival than single agent chlorambucil therapy and the latter is better tolerated by the patient. Chlorambucil can be as a daily dose or be given for 3 days at 20 mg/m^2 every month. Dose reduction will be necessary if the leucocyte and platelet count fall significantly below the normal range. Once response has been achieved, therapy can be discontinued sometimes for a number of years, and the same treatment used again on relapse. Eventually the disease becomes more aggressive with the appearance of more primitive lymphocytes. At this stage combination chemotherapy is very often required and the palliative use of radiotherapy for local problems can be useful.

Interferon has an effect in low grade NHL but whether it is superior to conventional therapy is undetermined. One possible role is as an agent for maintenance therapy. Autologous bone marrow transplant usually with marrow purging is being investigated and results are awaited.

Prognosis

At present all but local low grade NHL should be considered incurable. However, the median survival is of the order of eight years.

Management of high grade lymphoma

The indications for radiotherapy and chemotherapy in high grade lymphoma are:

Stage I disease (adequately staged): involved field radiotherapy

Stage II, III and IV disease: intensive combination chemotherapy to the limit of patient tolerance.

Over 90% of these patients require chemotherapy. Stage I disease is uncommon and difficult to prove. Intensive combination chemotherapy (e.g. using cyclophosphamide, adriamycin, vincristine, and prednisolone—CHOP.) will induce long-term remission in over 40% of patients with the most malignant varieties of high grade lymphoma. Younger patients with good performance status and without bulky disease will achieve superior results. The treatment should extend to the limits of tolerance and may require the services of highly specialised units capable of supporting patients with severe bone marrow failure, as for the treatment of acute leukaemia (p. 807).

Two particular subtypes of high grade NHL deserve particular mention.

LYMPHOBLASTIC LYMPHOMA

This is a highly malignant lymphoma usually of T cell phenotype found in young persons. Over 70% are males, adolescent or young adults. Presentation is with bulky mediastinal disease in about 50%, and 30% have marrow involvement at diagnosis. There is a tendency to develop CNS disease. Aggressive chemotherapy similar to poor prognosis acute lymphoblastic leukaemia is given together with CNS prophylaxis.

BURKITT'S LYMPHOMA

This form of lymphoblastic B cell non-Hodgkin's lymphoma occurs predominantly in tropical Africa and New Guinea, although it also occurs less frequently in other parts of the world. There is strong evidence that the Epstein-Barr (EB) virus plays an important aetiological role. The majority of patients are children with a peak incidence between the ages of 4 and 8 years, although cases found outside the tropics show an older age distribution and a lower incidence of EB viral infection.

Clinical features

The disorder affects predominantly extranodal tissues with a marked predilection for the mandible and the maxillary bones. This may cause marked bone deformity, loosening of the teeth and, if the orbit is involved, extrusion of the eye with loss of sight. In the abdomen, involvement of the kidneys, adrenals, ovaries or lymph nodes, often bilaterally, may give rise to abdominal tumours. Extradural lesions of the spinal cord may cause sudden onset of paraplegia. Other sites which may be involved include the long bones, the salivary glands, the thyroid, testes and the heart. Bilateral tumours of the breast may be seen in young adult women. Abdominal tumours are the most common finding in patients outside the tropics and lymph nodes and marrow are more frequently involved.

Investigations

The cytological appearance of Burkitt's lymphoma is characteristic with lymphoblast-type cells showing vacuolation in the cytoplasm and nucleus. Histologically the 'starry sky' appearance created by histiocytes scattered amongst sheets of primitive lymphoid cells is typical. Chromosome analysis shows an 8/14 translocation in a high proportion of cases and less often 2/8 or 8/22 translocation. Antibody to EB viral capsid antigen is found in most patients with the African variety.

Management
Response to chemotherapy is very good, particularly in the African variety if the disease is localised. Cyclophosphamide is given intramuscularly, 40–60 mg/kg every 2 weeks for up to 6 doses. Prophylactic intrathecal methotrexate may also be used because meningeal involvement often occurs later in the disease. The response to treatment is often dramatic with resolution of the disease following the first dose of cyclophosphamide. Disease found randomly throughout the world in an older age group is much more difficult to treat and requires aggressive chemotherapy often combined with autologous transplantation.

Bone marrow transplantation in lymphoma
Although patients with relapsed lymphoma can be treated, long term response is unusual. Thus younger patients with relapsed disease, particularly if it is still responsive to chemotherapy, are treated with further intensive chemotherapy supported either with autologous marrow or peripheral blood stem cells collected from the patient. Complete disease control has been achieved in around 50% of patients although longer follow-up is required to determine whether any cures have been achieved. A similar therapeutic approach has also been evaluated in first remission in patients with poor prognostic features or with difficult categories of lymphoma such as lymphoblastic or Burkitt's.

MULTIPLE MYELOMA

This is a malignant disorder of plasma cells. The disease is very uncommon under the age of 30. Thereafter, it becomes increasingly frequent, with a peak incidence between 60 and 70 years; the incidence is 4/100 000. Males are affected rather more frequently than females and Black people of Central African origin two to three times more often than Caucasians.

Immunopathology
Normal plasma cells are derived from B lymphocytes by transformation after exposure to antigenic stimuli; individual plasma cells manufacture immunoglobulins with only one type of light chain. In myeloma, and in other related malignant disorders of B lymphocytes, all the malignant cells produce the same immunoglobulin which indicates that the tumour is derived originally from one cell by cloning; the disease is, therefore, mono-

Table 13.27 Classification of multiple myeloma

Type of paraprotein	Relative frequency %
IgG	55
IgA	21
Light chain only	22
Others (D, E, non-secretory)	2

clonal. The immunoglobulin is called a paraprotein and appears on electrophoretic strips as a clear-cut band. Each of the five normal types of immunoglobulin has light chains of either lambda or kappa variety. In myeloma the paraprotein produced belongs to one of these immunoglobulin types and has one or other of the two light chains. In some patients only part of the immunoglobulin molecule is produced by the tumour cells, most commonly the light chains. These appear in the urine as Bence–Jones proteinuria and if myeloma is associated only with light chains it is known as Bence–Jones myeloma. The classification of myeloma by type of paraprotein, and their relative frequency, are given in Table 13.27. Patients with a myeloma which produces complete immunoglobulin molecules may also excrete increased amounts of light chain in their urine (Bence–Jones proteinuria). In some this appears as a new phenomenon later in the disease and usually indicates an acceleration of the disease.

Pathology
In the majority of patients the bone marrow is heavily infiltrated with atypical plasma cells which are usually larger and paler staining than normal plasma cells and contain nucleoli. Some cells may be multinucleated. Progressive replacement of the marrow occurs with eventual reduction of the normal cell lines, inducing variable cytopenia. Osteoclasts are stimulated and absorption of bone occurs producing diffuse osteoporosis. Local tumour formation by the myeloma causes punched out translucencies in the bone radiograph (Fig. 13.18). Rarely the disease may present as a solitary plasmacytoma either in bone or soft tissue. Excessive production of the myeloma paraprotein is associated with progressive reduction in normal immunoglobulin levels and impairment of immune function.

Clinical features
There is a long pre-clinical phase, in some instances up to 25 years, and the disorder may be discovered incidentally by laboratory tests during this phase. The patient may be observed for years before symptoms appear. The symptoms and their mechanism are given in Table 13.28.

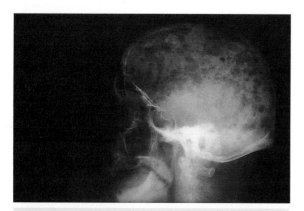

Fig. 13.18 Translucencies in skull radiograph—multiple myeloma.

Table 13.29 Rationale for investigations in multiple myeloma

Problem	Investigations
Renal function	Urea and electrolytes, creatinine, urate
Presence of hypercalcaemia	Blood calcium Albumin
Presence of bone fractures	Radiographs Blood alkaline phosphatase Isotope bone scan
Degree of immune paresis	Plasma immunoglobulin
Degree of bone marrow failure	Blood counts Reticulocyte count
Degree of haemostasis	Bleeding time Coagulation screen
Blood viscosity	Plasma viscosity
Disease activity	Serum β_2 microglobulin

Investigations

A diagnosis of myeloma requires the detection of at least two of the following abnormalities: monoclonal immunoglobulin or light chains in blood or urine, infiltration of the marrow with malignant plasma cells, or osteolytic bone lesions. (Fig. 13.18).

Once a diagnosis has been established further investigations should be undertaken to clarify the questions listed in Table 13.29. The points listed in the information box should be noted.

Management

Myeloma may sometimes be diagnosed when the disease is at an early stage and not causing symptoms. At this stage, it is reasonable to observe the patient as no specific treatment may be required for several years. Treatment should be started if the patient is symptomatic or if there is other evidence of disorder due to the myeloma.

Supportive treatment

All patients must drink at least 3 litres of fluid daily indefinitely to preserve normal renal function unless there is no evidence of renal impairment, a serum

POINTS TO NOTE IN DIAGNOSIS OF MYELOMA

- In the absence of fractures or bone repair the plasma alkaline phosphatase and the bone scan are normal
- Serum β_2-microglobulin estimations may provide a useful assessment of prognosis
- The absence of immune paresis (reduction of normal immunoglobulins below normal levels) should cast doubt on the diagnosis
- Only about 5% of patients with ESRs persistently above 100 mm in the first hour have myeloma

β_2-microglobulin level of less than 4 mg/l and less than 0.1 unit of free light chains per gram creatinine in the urine. The high fluid intake is particularly important in patients with compromised renal function. Although vigorous hydration may completely reverse renal impairment some individuals will have to be considered for dialysis. A high fluid intake also helps to manage a raised calcium. The availability of diphosphonates has greatly helped the management of acute hypercalcaemia and

Table 13.28 Multiple myeloma: the relationship between pathology, the effect of the disease process, and symptoms

Pathology	Effect	Symptoms
Marrow involvement with malignant plasma cells	Bone erosion due to stimulation of osteoclasts Pathological fracture Hypercalcaemia Bone marrow failure: anaemia	Pain Severe local pain Lethargy, thirst Tiredness
Excess production of paraprotein and light chains	Renal damage Increased blood viscosity Amyloidosis—renal damage	None until uraemic None until severe, then blurred vision, headache, vertigo, stupor, coma Azotaemia
Reduction in number of normal plasma cells	Impaired immune function	Susceptibility to infection, particularly respiratory

15 mg or 30 mg of pamidronate by slow intravenous infusion will usually result in a sustained fall in calcium. Allopurinol 300 mg orally daily is required in the early stages of treatment to prevent excessive formation of uric acid.

Chemotherapy

A regimen which includes adriamycin, BCNU, cyclophosphamide and melphalan in 6 weekly pulses achieves the best results if the patient can tolerate aggressive therapy. It is unsuitable for patients over 75. A more gentle regimen consists of melphalan 7 mg/m^2 daily for 4 days every 4–6 weeks with or without prednisolone 40 mg/m^2 for 4 days. Cytopenic patients can be given cyclophosphamide i.v. 300 mg/m^2 weekly. Treatment is continued until 'plateau phase' after which further treatment is of no benefit. Plateau phase is that stage at which the patient's paraprotein level, haemoglobin and β-microglobulin level have become stable and the patient remains well or only minimally symptomatic over a period of at least 3 months. Interferon is currently being investigated to determine if it has a role in prolonging the maintenance phase. Further chemotherapy with the same or other regimens may be offered if the patient relapses and further response may be obtained. Eventually the disease becomes increasingly refractory to treatment. In an effort to achieve better disease control in younger patients intensive therapy with the marrow rescue has been employed. Most patients with myeloma are not young enough to undergo allogeneic transplantation, but promising results have been obtained in a few. Autologous bone marrow transplantation is also being evaluated.

Radiotherapy

Radiotherapy is uniquely useful in the treatment of local problems such as severe bone pain, pathological fractures and tumorous lesions. Hemi-body irradiation in which the lower half of the body and then 6–8 weeks later the upper half is irradiated, may be employed for disseminated skeletal pain but is moderately toxic to bone marrow and lungs.

Prognosis

Without treatment the disease progresses relentlessly to death. The outlook for the majority of patients is considerably improved with treatment and a few may survive for many years. The median survival is still of around 2–3 years with treatment. Poor prognostic signs at the time of diagnosis are shown in the information box. Prognosis should be guarded in any individual until

the response to treatment has been assessed; this may take 6 months or more.

POOR PROGNOSTIC FEATURES AT DIAGNOSIS IN MULTIPLE MYELOMA

- A haemoglobin concentration less than 70 g/l
- Severe hypoalbuminaemia
- Intractable renal failure
- Thrombocytopenia
- High β_2-microglobulin levels
- Plasma cell leukaemia

FURTHER READING

Armitage J O 1993 Treatment of non-Hodgkin's lymphoma. New England Journal of Medicine 328: 1023–1029
Foon K A, Gale R P 1992 Therapy of acute myelogenous leukaemia. Blood Reviews 6: 15–25
Hirst W J R, Mufti G J 1993 Management of myelodysplastic syndromes. British Journal of Haematology 84: 191–196
Kantarjian H M, Deisseroth A, Kurzrock R, Estrov W, Talpaz M 1993 Chronic myelogenous leukaemia: a concise update. Blood 82: 691–703
Montserrat E, Rozman C 1993 Chronic lymphatic leukaemia. Blood Reviews 7: 164–174
Vrba W J, Longo D 1992 Hodgkin's disease. New England Journal of Medicine 326: 678–687

BLOOD TRANSFUSION

The modern transfusion service is able to prepare a number of components from each donated unit of blood; very little whole blood is used in adult practice. This enables each product to be stored under ideal conditions, prolonging its life and making available the appropriate product for a particular clinical situation. Red cell concentrates are prepared by removing the plasma, which is further processed, and substituting additive electrolyte solutions to maintain the functions of the red cells and ensure that the viscosity of the product allows rapid transfusion where necessary. The decision to transfuse red cells is made on clinical grounds. Patients with chronic anaemias may be relatively asymptomatic. The loss of approximately 20% of the whole blood volume can be corrected by crystalloid solutions. The transfusion of one unit of red cells generally raises the haemoglobin by 10 g/l.

The use of products for haemostatic disorders will be discussed later in this chapter.

THE ABO BLOOD GROUP SYSTEM

A large number of blood group antigens have been identified. The ABO system is particularly important as naturally occurring antibodies are found in the plasma of patients who lack the appropriate antigen. The antibodies to the other blood group antigens (Rhesus, Duffy, Kell, Kidd, etc.) only develop in individuals who lack the particular antigen and who are exposed to the antigen, either by transfusion or during pregnancy. The frequency of the ABO blood groups in the United Kingdom is given in Table 13.30. If blood taken from a group A individual is given to a Group B patient a severe, possibly fatal, haemolytic reaction will result.

THE RHESUS (Rh) SYSTEM

This system consists of three sets of antigen, Ee, Ce and Dd (d denotes absence of D). A particular set (e.g. CDe) is inherited from each parent. Antibodies to the Rh system rarely occur naturally and arise because of exposure during pregnancy or transfusion. In routine clinical transfusion practice individuals are typed as Rh D positive (85% of the UK population) or negative. The D antigen is the most immunogenic and anti D is responsible for most of the clinical problems which arise with the Rh system.

PRINCIPLES OF THE CROSS MATCH

In order to ensure that no antibody/antigen reaction leads to haemolysis blood is firstly selected for a patient on the basis of his ABO and Rh D group. However, it is possible that the patient could have an antibody to any of the other groups. The cross match procedure basically is a check to see that there is compatibility between the patient's serum and the red cells from the potential donor units. Donor cells and patient's serum are reacted together under conditions which would result in agglutination of cells which have reacted with an antibody. If such a reaction occurs blood cannot be issued. The nature of the antibody has to be determined and donor units selected which lack the antigen to which the particular antibody is directed. The grouping and cross matching of blood on a routine basis when no incompatibility is found should be accomplished in under 40 minutes. Blood should not be issued if an incom-

patibility is found until a full explanation for the incompatibility has been determined and compatible blood identified. Most hospitals have available Group O negative blood for use in extreme emergency situations, in which there is judged, on clinical grounds, to be no time for formal grouping and matching.

HAZARDS OF TRANSFUSION

The transfusion of blood products is not without its complications and about 5% of patients receiving a transfusion will have a reaction. Most of the reactions are relatively mild but they can be severe, even fatal. The symptoms related to transfusion reactions are nonspecific (Table 13.31).

It is often very difficult to distinguish on clinical grounds between a transfusion reaction from other complications which may occur during a patient's hospitalisation. The appreciation of these symptoms may obviously be extremely difficult in the anaesthetised

Table 13.31 Symptoms associated with transfusion reactions

Symptoms	Frequency (%)	Symptoms	Frequency (%)
Chills	55	Nausea, vomiting	7
Fever	47	Lumbar pain	5
Urticaria	35	Haemoglobinuria	5
Tachycardia	28	Hypotension	2
Chest tightness	7	Jaundice	1
Breathlessness	7		

Table 13.32 Classification of transfusion reactions

Acute (during or within 72 hours)	Delayed (after 72 hours)
Immunological	**Immunological**
Haemolytic: haemolytic transfusion reactions	Haemolytic: delayed haemolytic transfusion reactions
	Post-transfusion purpura
Nonhaemolytic:	Graft-versus-host disease
febrile nonhaemolytic reactions	Allo-immunisation (particularly HLA)
allergic reactions—urticarial —anaphylactoid	
noncardiac pulmonary oedema	
Non-immunological	**Non-immunological**
Circulatory overload	Iron overload
Physical damage:	Viral hepatitis (A, B, C)
overheating	HIV/AIDS
freezing	Other transmissible diseases:
incompatible solutions	syphilis
Bacterial contamination	malaria
Metabolic effects of stored blood:	CMV, etc.
hypothermia	
increased O_2 affinity	
potassium changes	
micro-aggregates	
Dilutional coagulation defects	

Table 13.30 The ABO system

Phenotype	Antigens	Naturally occurring antibodies	Frequency (%)
O	O	anti A, anti B	46
A	A	anti B	42
B	B	anti A	9
AB	AB	nil	3

patient. The safest approach is to assume that the event is transfusion related, stop the transfusion and begin the appropriate investigations (see below). Transfusion reactions can be classified as acute, if they occur within 72 hours, or delayed (Table 13.32).

A detailed discussion of all the complications listed should be sought in specialist texts. Certain conditions, such as the various types of viral hepatitis, HIV infection and iron overload are discussed elsewhere. The signs and symptoms, causation and management of acute haemolytic reactions, febrile non-haemolytic reactions and haemolysis are considered in the information boxes.

ACUTE HAEMOLYSIS

- **Aetiology**
  Haemolysis due to antibody destruction of incompatible red cells, usually involving the ABO system
- **Clinical features**
  Usually commence within minutes of the infusion of the incompatible unit
  Chills/rigors and fever
  Lumbar pain and/or chest tightness
  Burning sensation at infusion site
  Development of shock and/or bleeding
  In anaesthetised patients—hypotension, bleeding and pyrexia
- **Management**
  Stop the transfusion
  Check the identity of the patient and the blood unit
  Monitor patient's pulse, blood pressure and urine output
  Send unit(s) of blood back to the laboratory
  Check full blood count, bilirubin and coagulation screen
  Re-group and cross match patient's samples and units of blood
  Support patient's circulatory volume and haemostatic status

N.B. Rarely blood may be bacterially contaminated producing a similar shock-like picture
Take blood cultures

SAFE TRANSFUSION PRACTICE

The clinician expects to be supplied with high quality blood products. In many parts of the world the responsibility for selecting and testing donors, the preparation, quality control and storage of blood products is the responsibility of a specially organised Blood Transfusion Service. Transfusion laboratories based in local hospitals will match the product with the patient and the clinician exerts little control over these areas. However, the cause of the majority of fatal haemolytic transfusion reactions is a clerical error due to faulty labelling of the specimen and/or a failure to correctly identify the recipient. This type of error can be minimised by following the procedures outlined in principle below. Individual hospitals will frequently have their

---

FEBRILE NON-HAEMOLYTIC TRANSFUSION REACTIONS

- **Aetiology**
  Anti white cell or anti HLA antibodies reacting with white cells in the unit. Occurs in 1% of transfusions but especially in multi-transfused or multiparous individuals
- **Clinical features**
  Usually occurs after more than one Unit has been transfused
  Fever/chills
  Urticaria
- **Management**
  Stop the transfusion
  Exclude a haemolytic reaction
  Symptomatic treatment for pyrexia
  Consider pre-medication with antihistamines and/or steroids if further blood required
  Use of leuco-depleted blood in patients who have more than two consecutive febrile, non-haemolytic transfusion reactions

---

DELAYED HAEMOLYTIC TRANSFUSION REACTION

- **Aetiology**
  This occurs 5–7 days after transfusion. The transfusion has stimulated the production of an antibody which was not detected at the initial cross match
- **Clinical features**
  Anaemia
  Jaundice
- **Management**
  A diagnosis suggested by the finding of polychromasia and spherocytes on the blood film
  Serological investigation to demonstrate a blood group antibody which previously had not been detected
  Compatible blood made available using serological findings

---

own policies for drawing blood for transfusion and the administration of blood products which should be followed. A clinician drawing blood for cross matching should: positively identify the patient at the bedside, label the tubes and request form after identifying the patient, and ensure that all the information requested by the Transfusion Laboratory is given both on the tube and request form. This information must match!

The person administering blood should: positively identify the patient at the bedside, ensure that the patient identification and the identification of the units match, check that the ABO and Rh D group of the patient and units is identical, inspect the units for evidence of damage, ensure that the checking procedures are validated by another member of the nursing or medical staff, and complete the necessary documentation indicating the detailed identification of the units transfused.

FURTHER READING

Hoffbrand A V, Pettit J E 1993 Essential Haematology, 3rd edn. Blackwell Scientific, Oxford

HAEMOSTASIS

The prevention of bleeding depends upon maintaining the integrity of the blood vessel walls by mechanisms which ensure that any breaches are rapidly sealed by deposition of platelets and fibrin. This process can be arbitrarily divided into two stages. Firstly during primary haemostasis the vessel constricts, activated platelets adhere to the damaged wall and subsequently aggregate to form a platelet plug which arrests haemorrhage. In the ensuing secondary haemostasis the platelet plug is stabilised by deposition of a network of fibrin. The initial platelet plug formation takes place over a few minutes whilst its stabilisation by fibrin, within the mass of aggregated platelets, takes longer. Although haemostasis is arbitrarily divided into these two stages they are closely interrelated. There are receptors on the activated platelet surface for components of the coagulation cascade, ensuring that each of these is brought into close proximity resulting in a greatly enhanced rate of fibrin generation compared to the reactions that occur in plasma without platelets.

The dissolution by fibrinolysis of both haemostatic plugs and thrombus is initiated by tissue plasminogen activator released from local endothelial cells. This converts fibrin bound plasminogen to plasmin which hydrolyses fibrin into many degradation products. One of these is the crosslinked D fragments of fibrin and it is quantitated in the D-dimer assay.

PLATELETS

Each megakaryocyte liberates several thousand individual platelets into the circulation where each has a lifespan of approximately 10 days. They are complex highly specialised cells capable of responding quickly and specifically to a variety of activators, e.g. ADP, thrombin and collagen, by contracting into spheres and sending out long pseudopodia which adhere to subendothelial vessel wall components, e.g. collagen and neighbouring platelets. Von Willebrand factor is a plasma protein which is an essential bridge between the platelets and collagen fibrils of the damaged vessel wall; its deficiency in von Willebrand's disease leads to an haemorrhagic diathesis which resembles a platelet disorder rather than that of a coagulation factor deficiency.

Table 13.33 Screening tests for assessing a patient for a bleeding disorder

Investigation	Normal Range	Situations in which the test is abnormal
Platelet count	$150–350 \times 10^9/l$	Thrombocytopenia Congenital Acquired
Bleeding time	Less than 8 minutes	Thrombocytopenia Thrombopathy Congenital Acquired, e.g. aspirin, von Willebrand's disease
Prothrombin time	12–14 seconds	Deficiency of factors II, V, VII, X Liver disease Warfarin therapy *DIC
Activated partial thromboplastin time	30–40 seconds	Deficiency of factors II, V, VIII, IX, X, XI, XII Haemophilia A and B von Willebrand's disease *DIC
Fibrinogen	1.5–3.0 g/dl	Congenital hypofibrinogenaemia

* Disseminated intravascular coagulation

Within the platelet cytoplasm are three types of storage organelles; alpha granules containing a variety of coagulation factors, for example fibrinogen and von Willebrand factor; dense granules which store low molecular weight substances, for example ADP and serotonin, and lysosomes containing acid hydrolases. When platelets are activated the contents of these granules are discharged and promote further platelet aggregation and fibrin deposition on the platelet surface. This possesses many well characterised glycoproteins which act as receptors for external activators and transmit external stimuli into the cytoplasm. During activation arachidonic acid is liberated from membrane lipids and converted by the platelet enzyme cyclo-oxygenase and thromboxane synthetase to thromboxane B_2 which is a very potent stimulator of platelet aggregation. Aspirin, and other non-steroidal anti-inflammatory drugs, being potent inhibitors of cyclo-oxygenase, reduce platelet function resulting in a predisposition to haemorrhage.

Platelet function can be assessed by performing a standardised template bleeding time test. In this investigation a small incision is made on the forearm below a sphygmomanometer cuff inflated up to 40 mmHg. The bleeding time is prolonged in those with platelet functional defects, thrombocytopenia and von Willebrand's disease (Table 13.33).

Thrombocytopenia causes characteristic bleeding with purpura, bruising and mucosal haemorrhage from

Table 13.34   Components of the coagulation system

Factor	Synonym	Half-life	Treatment of single deficiency
I	Fibrinogen	4 days	Cryoprecipitate
II	Prothrombin	3 days	Concentrate II, IX, X
V	Proaccelerin	12–15 h	Fresh frozen plasma
VII	Proconvertin	4–6 h	Concentrate VII
VIII	Antihaemophilic factor	12–15 h	Concentrate VIII
IX	Christmas factor	20 h	Concentrate IX
X	Stuart–Prower factor	10–15 h	Concentrate II, IX, X
XI	Plasma thromboplastin antecedent (PTA)	3 days	Concentrate XI
XII	Hageman factor		—
XIII	Fibrin stabilising factor	12–15 days	Concentrate XIII
	Platelets	3–4 days	Platelet concentrate

the nose, mouth, gastrointestinal and genito-urinary tracts. A severe reduction in platelet numbers may result in optic fundal haemorrhage and life-threatening intracranial bleeding.

COAGULATION SYSTEM

The coagulation cascade consists of a series of soluble inactive zymogens. When activated each is capable of activating one or more subsequent components of the cascade by proteolysis. The individual components are given Roman numerals, for example factor VIII, and are listed in Table 13.34. Each factor can be assayed by its coagulant activity in vitro and this is indicated by the suffix 'C', e.g. factor VIIIC. When an inactive zymogen is activated this is denoted by 'a', e.g. factor IIa (thrombin). Historically the cascade has been considered to be composed of two parts; the extrinsic system which starts with the activation of factor VII by tissue factor, and the intrinsic system which is initiated by collagen and negatively charged surfaces which activate factor XII (Fig. 13.19). The principal physiological haemostatic mechanism is believed to be via the extrinsic system which is initiated by the expression of tissue factor by, for example, endothelial cells at the site of haemorrhage. The rate of successive reactions is greatly enhanced when the plasma coagulation factor components are attached to specific receptors on the platelet surface. The rate of reaction is also greatly increased by the initial traces of thrombin formed; this activates components of the haemostatic system in a positive feedback loop, for example, platelets and factors V, VIII and XI. Thus from a relatively simple trigger very quickly there is an explosive activation of platelets and the coagulation factors which lead to the formation of a fibrin stabilised platelet plug.

The extrinsic system is assessed with the prothrombin time (PT) in which test plasma is incubated with tissue factor and calcium. The reaction proceeds preferentially with the activation by factor VIIa of factor X (rather than factor IX). Thus the prothrombin time is particularly sensitive to a deficiency of factors VII, X and V. The activated partial thromboplastin time (APTT) is determined by adding an activator to plasma, for instance a suspension of kaolin, along with an extract of phospholipid (to mimic the platelet membrane). The APTT is prolonged with a deficiency of factor II, V, VIII, IX, X, XI or XII. Neither the PT nor the APTT is sensitive to minor deficiencies of fibrinogen or a lack of factor XIII, an enzyme which cross-links molecules of fibrin to enhance the strength of the polymerising fibrin; both these factors therefore need to be measured by specific assays.

Deficiencies, either congenital or acquired, of single or multiple components of the coagulation system, result in a bleeding diathesis, for example haemophilia. This is characterised by joint and muscle haemorrhage and prolonged bleeding after surgery or trauma. Occasionally autoantibodies may arise, sometimes in association with autoimmune disorders, which specifically inhibit one of the components, such as factor VIII, resulting in a severe bleeding disorder, for example acquired haemophilia. It may be very difficult to treat patients with these autoantibodies because when the factor which is deficient is transfused it is quickly neutralised by the antibody.

The plasma contains several proteins which inhibit

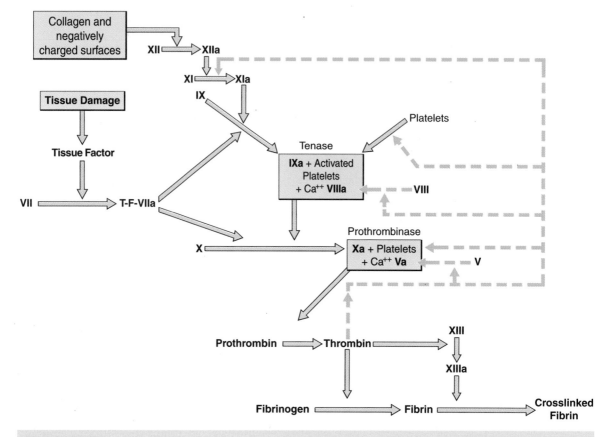

Fig. 13.19 Coagulation cascade. The diagram illustrates the interrelationship between coagulation factors and platelets. Tissue factor is the most important initiator of the cascade. Note the central role of thrombin, particularly its importance in the positive feedback loops causing further activation of the haemostatic system.

activated clotting factors to prevent too extensive activation of the haemostatic system, which might lead to excessive aggregation of platelets and deposition of fibrin within the circulation (Table 13.36). A deficiency of these may lead to an increased level of circulating activated clotting factors predisposing to thrombosis.

ASSESSMENT OF PATIENTS WITH A POSSIBLE BLEEDING DISORDER

History

Prior to laboratory investigation, a careful history of all bleeding episodes is essential as well as a full clinical examination. A history of bleeding is often remarkably reproducible particularly after dental extraction; if a socket oozes for 2 days after removal of a tooth on one occasion this is likely to occur again following each subsequent extraction.

It is important to consider the following points when taking a history.

1. *Site of bleeds:* Muscle and joint bleeds indicate a coagulation defect, whereas purpura, prolonged bleeding from superficial cuts, epistaxis, gastrointestinal haemorrhage or menorrhagia indicate a failure of primary haemostasis due to a platelet disorder, thrombocytopenia or von Willebrand's disease. Recurrent bleeds at a single site suggest a local structural abnormality.
2. *Duration of history:* It may be possible to assess whether the patient has a congenital or acquired disorder by whether the propensity to bleeding is lifelong or a short history suggestive of an acquired cause.
3. *Precipitating causes:* Bleeding arising spontaneously indicates a more severe defect than if haemorrhage only arises after trauma.
4. *Surgery:* Enquiry about all operations is useful but

particularly dental extractions, tonsillectomy and circumcision as these are all stressful tests of the haemostatic system. Bleeding that starts immediately after surgery indicates defective platelet plug formation whereas that which comes on after several hours is more indicative of failure of platelet plug stabilisation by fibrin due to a coagulation defect.

5. *Family history:* Absence of relatives with clinically significant bleeding does not exclude a hereditary bleeding diathesis; about one third of cases of haemophilia, for example, arise in individuals without a family history.

6. *Systemic illnesses:* Many diseases, or their treatment, may occasionally be associated with bleeding but it is particularly important to consider the possibility of hepatic or renal failure, paraproteinaemia or a collagenosis.

7. *Drugs:* Almost any medicine can potentially produce bleeding either by depressing marrow function with consequent thrombocytopenia or by interacting with warfarin. Non-steroidal anti-inflammatory drugs inhibit platelet function; the effect of aspirin may last for up to 10 days after a single tablet.

Examination

Superficial examination may reveal bruises and purpura or scars due to poor healing following prolonged superficial bleeding. Telangiectasia of lips and tongue are diagnostic of hereditary haemorrhagic telangiectasia. Joints should be carefully scrutinised for evidence of haemarthroses. A full general medical examination is important because it may give clues of systemic illness, for example stigmata of liver disease; splenomegaly may cause thrombocytopenia due to hypersplenism.

Investigations

Screening investigations and their interpretation are given in Table 13.33. If the patient has a history strongly suggestive of a bleeding disorder and all the preliminary tests give normal results, it may be appropriate to perform further investigations. The clinical history may be a useful guide as to whether attention should be directed to platelet function (or von Willebrand's disease) or coagulation disturbance, for example haemophilia.

DISORDERS OF PRIMARY HAEMOSTASIS

Platelet functional disorders, thrombocytopenia, von Willebrand's disease, along with diseases affecting the vessel wall, may all result in failure of the initial platelet plug formation in primary haemostasis. In this section

disorders due to an increased platelet count, thrombocytosis, will also be considered.

VESSEL WALL ABNORMALITIES

Abnormalities of the vessel walls both congenital and acquired, for example vasculitis, may result in a propensity to purpuric lesions. Causes of non-thrombocytopenic purpura are set out in the information box.

CAUSES OF NON-THROMBOCYTOPENIC PURPURA

- Senile purpura
- Factitious purpura
- Henoch–Schönlein purpura
- Vasculitis
- Paraproteinaemias
- Purpura fulminans
- Embolic purpura

HEREDITARY HAEMORRHAGIC TELANGIECTASIA

Hereditary haemorrhagic telangiectasia is a dominantly inherited condition in which telangiectasia and small aneurysms are found on the fingertips, face, nasal passages, tongue and gastrointestinal tract. A small group of these patients also develop pulmonary arteriovenous malformation. Patients present either with recurrent bleeds, particularly epistaxis, or iron deficiency due to occult gastrointestinal bleeding. Treatment can be difficult because of the multiple bleeding points but regular iron therapy often allows the marrow to compensate for blood loss. Local cautery or laser therapy may prevent single lesions from bleeding. A variety of medical therapies have been tried, for example oestrogens, but none has been found to be universally effective.

EHLERS–DANLOS DISEASE

Ehlers–Danlos is a congenital disorder of collagen synthesis in which the capillaries are poorly supported by subcutaneous collagen and echymoses are commonly observed.

QUALITATIVE DISORDERS OF PLATELETS

Even in the presence of a normal platelet count an individual may bleed if the function of the platelets is reduced. Congenital abnormalities include rare disorders of the membrane glycoproteins, for example thrombasthenia and Bernard–Soulier syndrome, or the presence of defective platelet granules, for example a deficiency of dense granules giving rise to storage pool disorders. Such patients exhibit bleeding of platelet type which varies between patients, some presenting with severe recurrent bleeds whilst others are only diagnosed because of excessive post-operative haemorrhage. Mild functional disorders, which only cause excessive bleeding after trauma or surgery, are often not diagnosed and are probably relatively common.

Many drugs inhibit platelets. Aspirin and other non-steroidal drugs inhibit platelet cyclo-oxygenase preventing the conversion of arachidonic acid to the potent platelet aggregator thromboxane B_2. Other drugs which inhibit platelets are listed in the information box.

DRUGS INHIBITING PLATELET FUNCTION

- **Non-steroidal anti-inflammatory drugs**
  Aspirin
  Indomethacin
  Phenylbutazone
  Sulphinpyrazone
- **Antibiotics**
  Penicillins
  Cephalosporins
- **Dextran**
- **Heparin**
- **Beta-blockers**

QUANTITATIVE DISORDERS OF PLATELETS

THROMBOCYTOPENIA

A reduced platelet count may arise by one of three mechanisms; failure of megakaryocyte maturation, excessive platelet consumption after their release into the circulation or their sequestration in an enlarged spleen. The common causes of thrombocytopenia are listed in Table 13.35.

Spontaneous bleeding does not usually occur until the platelet count falls below about $30 \times 10^9/1$ unless their function is also compromised, for example following aspirin ingestion. Purpura and spontaneous bruising are characteristic but there may also be oral, nasal, gastrointestinal or genito-urinary bleeding. Severe thrombocytopenia results in optic fundal haemorrhage (Fig. 13.20) which may be a prelude to a rapidly fatal intracranial bleed.

Investigations to ascertain the possible cause of thrombocytopenia should be directed towards the conditions listed in Table 13.35. A blood film may give diagnostic information, for example acute leukaemia. Examination of the bone marrow will reveal whether there is an infiltrate such as carcinoma, a reduced

Table 13.35   Causes of thrombocytopenia

Marrow disorders
Hypoplasia:
  Idiopathic
  Drug-induced—cytotoxic, antimetabolites, thiazides
Infiltration:
  Leukaemia
  Myeloma
  Carcinoma
  Myelofibrosis
  Osteopetrosis
B_{12}/folate deficiency

Increased consumption of platelets
Disseminated intravascular coagulation (DIC)
Idiopathic thrombocytopenic purpura (ITP)
Viral infections—e.g. Epstein-Barr virus, HIV
Bacterial infections—e.g. Gram-negative septicaemia

Hypersplenism
Lymphomas
Liver disease

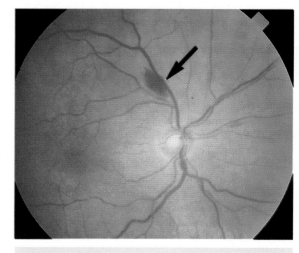

Fig. 13.20   Superficial fundal haemorrhage in patient with a platelet count of $5 \times 10^9/l$.

number of megakaryocytes, for example hypoplastic anaemia, or an increased number of megakaryocytes indicating excessive peripheral destruction, for example idiopathic thrombocytopenic purpura.

Thrombocytopenia causing clinically significant bleeding constitutes an haematological emergency which should be promptly investigated and appropriately treated. Treatment should be directed to the underlying condition as well as specific treatment to raise the platelet count when appropriate. For thrombocytopenia in general platelet transfusions should be given only if the platelet count is less than $10 \times 10^9/1$, or to treat troublesome bleeding such as persistent epistaxis, or potentially life threatening bleeding, for example gastrointestinal haemorrhage. Such transfusions provide only temporary relief because the survival of the platelets in the circulation is only a few days at most and in many instances may be only a matter of minutes or hours if the thrombocytopenia is due to increased platelet consumption as in idiopathic thrombocytopenic purpura or disseminated intravascular coagulation.

IDIOPATHIC THROMBOCYTOPENIC PURPURA (ITP)

The presence of auto-antibodies, often directed against platelet membrane glycoprotein IIb-IIIa, causes the premature removal of platelets by the monocyte-macrophage system. Occasionally antigen-antibody immune complexes adhere to platelets at their Fc receptor resulting in their premature removal from the circulation.

Clinical features

In children, ITP often presents 2–3 weeks after a viral illness with the sudden onset of purpura and sometimes oral and nasal bleeding. The peripheral blood film is normal apart from a greatly reduced platelet number whilst the bone marrow reveals an obvious increase in megakaryocytes. It is important to ascertain that the child does not have any other systemic illness and in particular disseminated intravascular coagulation.

In adults, ITP more commonly affects females and has a more gradual insidious onset. It is unusual for there to be a history of a preceding viral infection. At presentation some cases may be associated with symptoms or signs of a collagenosis or rheumatoid arthritis, whilst in others these disorders may become apparent several years later. The condition is likely to become chronic, with remissions and relapses.

Management

Children

If the child has only mild bleeding symptoms it is usual to withhold any specific treatment as the condition in the majority of instances is self limiting within a few weeks. The presence of moderate to severe purpura, bruising or epistaxis and a platelet count less than $10 \times 10^9/1$ is an indication for prednisolone 2 mg/kg daily. The platelet count usually rises promptly within 1–3 days. Persistent epistaxis, gastrointestinal bleeding, retinal haemorrhages or any suggestion of intracranial bleeding should be treated immediately by a platelet transfusion. If fresh bleeding persists for more than a few days following the introduction of steroids, intravenous immunoglobulin should be given.

Adults

Treatment with prednisolone 1 mg/kg daily is less rewarding than in children; often the platelet count rises

in response to therapy but falls again when the dose is reduced or stopped. As with children persistent or potentially life threatening bleeding should be treated with platelet transfusion. Intravenous immunoglobulin (IVIgG) (1 g/kg) should be given if the patient is very haemorrhagic or the bleeding is immediately life threatening. The mechanism by which IVIgG raises the platelet count remains uncertain although increasing evidence indicates that it may be due to blocking of monocyte-macrophage Fc receptors.

Relapses should be treated by increasing the dose of prednisolone. If a patient has two relapses it is customary to consider splenectomy. This should be preceded by pneumococcal, meningococcal and *Haemophilus influenzae* vaccination. Because so many adults with ITP eventually require splenectomy it is prudent to vaccinate all patients at presentation (subcutaneously; if given by the customary intramuscular route it may result in an haematoma) before they become immuno-suppressed with a prolonged course of steroids. Splenectomy is curative in about 70% of patients and in the remainder the aim should be to keep the patient free of symptoms rather than treat the platelet count alone. Often such patients have counts of 20–$30 \times 10^9/1$ without symptoms; some require long term maintenance with prednisolone at 5 mg/day. If significant bleeding persists despite splenectomy and a small dose of steroids, vincristine, immunosuppressive therapy, for example cyclophosphamide, or repeated infusions of intravenous immunoglobulin should be considered.

THROMBOCYTOSIS

An increase in platelet count may occur either as a direct result of malignant proliferation of megakaryocytes or as nonspecific reactive response to chronic bleeding or inflammation. Secondary thrombocytosis is much more common than the primary malignant disorder. Malignant increase of megakaryocytes may occur alone resulting in essential thrombocythaemia or may be accompanied by a more fundamental defect of the bone marrow stem cell as in chronic myeloid leukaemia, polycythaemia rubra vera or myelofibrosis. Causes of a raised platelet count are set out in the information box.

ESSENTIAL THROMBOCYTHAEMIA

The malignant proliferation of megakaryocytes results in a raised level of circulating platelets which may, in addition, have aberrant function.

Clinical features

Patients may present with excessive bruising and bleeding or with venous or arterial thrombosis. Splenomegaly

CAUSES OF A RAISED PLATELET COUNT

Reactive thrombocytosis	Malignant thrombocytosis
• Chronic inflammatory disorders	• Essential thrombocythaemia
• Malignant disease	• Polycythaemia rubra vera
• Tissue damage	• Myelofibrosis
• Haemolytic anaemias	• Chronic myeloid leukaemia
• Post-splenectomy	
• Post-haemorrhage	

Table 13.36   Inhibitors of the coagulation system

Inhibitor	Action	Reduced concentration

Antithrombin III	Inhibits factors IIa, IXa, Xa, XIa	Congenital
		Acquired
		    Heparin therapy
		    *DIC

Protein C	Inactivates factors Va and VIIIa	Congenital
		Acquired
		    Warfarin
		    *DIC

Protein S	Co-factor for protein C	Congenital
		Acquired
		    Warfarin
		    Pregnancy

* Disseminated intravascular coagulation

may be present but in some patients the blood film reveals changes due to splenic atrophy, for example Howell–Jolly bodies, as a result of asymptomatic splenic infarction. In most individuals the condition is chronic with the platelet count only gradually increasing.

Management

Treatment is by intravenous radioactive phosphorus (^{32}P), hydroxyurea or alkylating agent, for example busulphan. On rare occasions the platelets rise rapidly, sometimes accompanied by blast cells in the peripheral blood, and this condition is megakaryocytic leukaemia and should be treated like acute myeloid leukaemia.

DISORDERS OF SECONDARY HAEMOSTASIS

Coagulation factor disorders (Table 13.36) can either arise from single factor, usually congenital, deficiency, for example factor VIII, resulting in haemophilia A, or from multiple factor deficiencies which are often acquired, for example secondary to liver disease or warfarin therapy. Of the single congenital deficiencies haemophilia A and B are the commonest although, rarely, any of the coagulation factors may be reduced. The congenital disorders almost exclusively arise as a result of an abnormality in the structural gene coding for the coagulation factor. (Table 13.34.)

CONGENITAL BLEEDING DISORDERS

HAEMOPHILIA A

Of the various congenital disorders of coagulation factors the commonest is that causing a reduction of factor VIII resulting in haemophilia A, which affects 1/10 000 individuals. Factor VIII is primarily synthesised by the liver but other organs such as the spleen, kidney and placenta may also contribute to the plasma level. Plasma factor VIII has a half life of about 12 hours and is carried non-covalently bound to the von Willebrand factor. The very large 286 kilobase factor VIII gene is located on the X chromosome and consists of 26 exons. Many different defects in the gene have been identified, for example single base changes resulting in amino acid substitutions or nonsense codons (causing premature chain termination), deletions or inversions. The normal factor VIII gene has been cloned and small amounts of synthetic factor VIII have been manufactured to treat patients. It is anticipated that within the next few years this supply will greatly increase, potentially providing an almost unlimited amount of factor VIII for treating patients.

Genetics

The factor VIII gene is localised on the X chromosome making haemophilia A a sex-linked disorder. Thus on pedigree grounds all daughters of haemophiliacs are obligate carriers and sisters have a 50% chance of being a carrier. If a carrier has a son, he has a 50% chance of having haemophilia, and a daughter has a 50% chance of being a carrier. Haemophilia 'breeds true' within a family. All members will have the same abnormality of the factor VIII gene; thus if one individual has severe haemophilia all others affected will also have a severe form of the disorder. Female carriers of haemophilia tend to have reduced factor VIII levels because of random inactivation of the X chromosome in the developing fetus (lyonisation). An indication of carriership can be ascertained by measurement of factor VIII/vWF ratio which is reduced in carriers compared to normal individuals.

The use of molecular genetic techniques has revolutionised the identification of carriers and the antenatal diagnosis of haemophilia. Tracing of the haemophilia gene within families can now be accomplished using gene probes which detect restriction fragment length polymorphisms (RFLPs). The most useful probes are those that detect an endonuclease restriction site within the gene and these are known as 'genomic' probes. Other probes detect endonuclease sites close to the gene and these 'linked' probes are less reliable because recombination between the factor VIII gene and the endonuclease site may occur during meiosis. Antenatal diagnosis can be undertaken in a female who has a high probability of being a carrier. This is accomplished by chorion villus sampling (CVS) at about 10–11 weeks' gestation, sexing the fetus and using informative factor VIII probes. Alternatively the fetus can be sexed at 16 weeks' gestation by amniocentesis and, if male, a fetal blood sample obtained at about 19–20 weeks. The CVS technique is preferable because it allows for the possibility of therapeutic termination at about 10–12 weeks compared to 20 weeks following fetal blood sampling.

Clinical features

Although haemophilia A is a congenital disorder it is unusual for excessive bleeding to be noticed until babies are about 6 months old when superficial bruising or a haemarthrosis may occur. This apparent delay in presentation is due to the relative inactivity of babies in the first few months of life and it is only when they begin to move about that more trauma results in bleeding. It is not uncommon for children to be initially classified as having non-accidental injury unless all such children are appropriately investigated for the presence of a bleeding disorder (Table 13.33).

The normal factor VIII level is 50–150% and is usually measured by a clotting assay. In haemophilia the propensity to bleeding is related to the plasma factor VIII level. The severity of haemophilia is set out in the information box.

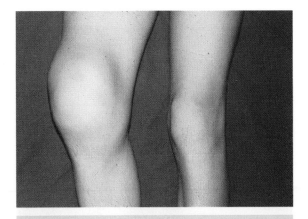

Fig. 13.21 Large haemarthrosis in right knee of boy with haemophilia A.

SEVERITY OF HAEMOPHILIA		
	Factor VIII or IX level	
		Clinical presentation
• Severe	<2%	Spontaneous haemarthroses and muscle haematomas
• Moderate	2–10%	Mild trauma or surgery cause haematomas
• Mild	10–50%	Major injury or surgery result in excess bleeding

Individuals with severe haemophilia (factor VIII < 2%) experience recurrent haemarthroses in large joints (Fig. 13.21). These usually begin spontaneously without apparent trauma and the joints most commonly affected are knees, elbows, ankles and hips. A typical severe haemophiliac may have one or two bleeds each week. The patient is aware that bleeding has started because he experiences an abnormal sensation in the joint. If treatment is not given at this stage bleeding continues, resulting in a hot, swollen, very painful joint. Without treatment severe pain and swelling may last for many days before gradually subsiding. Recurrent bleeds into joints lead to synovial hypertrophy, destruction of the cartilage and secondary osteoarthrosis (Fig. 13.22).

The resultant limitation of movement may greatly reduce the function of joints, making walking difficult.

Muscle haematomas are also characteristic of haemophilia. These occur most commonly in the calf and psoas muscles but they can arise in almost any muscle. Although relatively less common than haemarthroses a single episode can leave severe lasting damage if not effectively treated. A large psoas bleed, for example, may extend to press on the femoral nerve with consequent parasthaesia in the thigh and weakness of the quadriceps; although some of this injury may be reversible the patient is often left with some weakness in the leg. Furthermore if the bleed does not resolve completely recurrences at the same site may occur, leading to progressive muscle and nerve damage. Calf haematomas are also serious because of the inflexible fascial sheath surrounding the soleus and gastrocnemius muscles. Untreated haemorrhage causes a rise in pressure with eventual ischaemia, necrosis, fibrosis and subsequent contraction and shortening of the Achilles tendon (Fig. 13.23).

Although joint and muscle bleeds are the commonest sites for haemorrhage, bleeding can occur at almost any site. It is particularly serious if it takes place in a confined anatomical space associated with vital structures. The

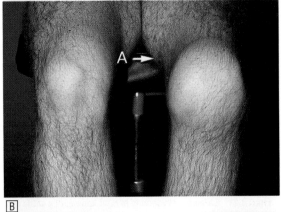

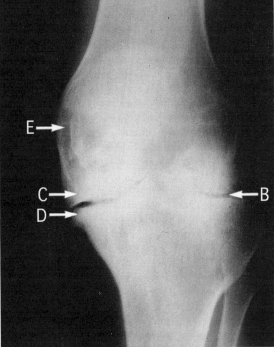

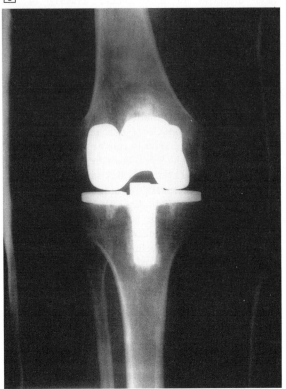

Fig. 13.22 Chronic haemophilic arthropathy of left knee.
Ⓐ Repeated bleeds have led to broadening of the femoral epicondyles. Unilateral atrophy of the quadriceps (A) is easily seen. Ⓑ Radiograph confirms broadening of femoral epicondyles. There is no cartilage present as evidenced by the close proximity of the femur and fibia (B); sclerosis (C), osteophyte (D) and bony cysts (E) are present. Ⓒ A haemophiliac's stiff joint with minimal flexion has been replaced by a prosthesis. This enabled the joint to have a greatly extended range of motion which very markedly improved the patient's mobility.

intracranial area is one such site and unless it is treated very promptly, haemorrhage here is often fatal (Fig. 13.24).

Individuals with moderate haemophilia usually only experience haemorrhage after minor trauma and those with the mild form of the disorder following more major trauma or surgery. Whereas severe haemophilia is usually diagnosed within the first 2 years of life individuals with moderate and mild forms may escape diagnosis until adulthood.

Management
Bleeding episodes should be treated early by raising the factor VIII level. This is most commonly accomplished by intravenous infusion of factor VIII concentrate prepared from blood donor plasma. Such concentrates are freeze-dried and stable at 4°C and can therefore be stored in domestic refrigerators. This facility, which allows many patients to treat themselves at home, revolutionised haemophilia care in the 1970s; prior to this, patients had to travel to hospital to receive treatment for

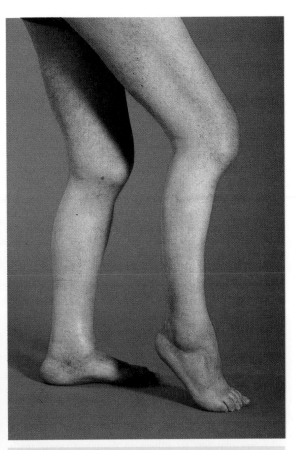

Fig. 13.23   Atrophy in an adult of the calf followed an inadequately treated gastrocnemius haematoma as a child. The increased pressure of the haematoma caused ischaemia of the muscle, this being followed by necrosis, fibrosis and subsequent contraction to give the equinus deformity.

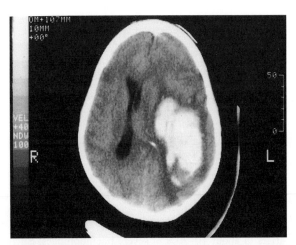

Fig. 13.24   The CT scan reveals a major intracerebral haematoma which arose apparently spontaneously in a severe haemophiliac.

each bleed with fresh frozen plasma or cryoprecipitate. All factor VIII concentrates are now prepared from donors who are not perceived as having an increased risk of viral carriage, for example HIV. The plasma is screened for the presence of antibodies to hepatitis B and C viruses and HIV and the final product is treated either by heat or chemicals to inactivate any residual viruses. Concentrates prepared with these precautions have an extremely good safety record and viral transmission is now very rare.

In addition to factor VIII concentrate therapy, resting either in bed or with a splint of the bleeding site helps reduce continuing haemorrhage. Once bleeding has settled the patient should be mobilised and given physiotherapy to restore strength to the surrounding muscles.

Although factor VIII concentrates have transformed the lives of haemophiliacs by allowing many to lead near-normal lives this freedom has been bought at the cost of side-effects from repeated injections of concentrate (Table 13.37). Many patients treated before 1985, when concentrates were first treated with heat or chemicals to destroy viruses, became infected by the hepatitis and human immunodeficiency viruses. As a result most severe haemophiliacs have been exposed to hepatitis B virus and have developed immunity as evidenced by the development of anti-HBs. A small number become chronic HBsAg carriers and may infect sexual partners, who should therefore be offered hepatitis B immunisation. They are also at risk of delta virus infection (p. 493). All potential recipients of pooled blood products should be offered hepatitis A and B immunisation because it will protect against hepatitis A, B and D infection. Hepatitis C virus was ubiquitously transmitted by concentrates prior to 1985, resulting in virtually all recipients becoming infected. It is clear that many of these patients have hepatitis and a significant proportion are progressing to cirrhosis. Treatment with interferon therapy is likely to benefit a proportion of patients.

Prior to 1985, HIV was transmitted to haemophiliacs by concentrates, resulting in approximately 60% of severe haemophiliacs becoming infected. The clinical consequences are very similar to other individuals who have become infected with HIV (p. 89) although their clinical course is perhaps more like those who become infected intravenously, for example the drug abusers, than those who become infected sexually. Kaposi's sarcoma, for example, is rare in haemophiliacs compared to homosexuals.

The other serious consequence of factor VIII infusion is the development of anti factor VIII antibodies which

Table 13.37   Long term sequelae of haemophilia

Complications due to repeated haemorrhages
Arthropathy of large joints, e.g. knees, elbows
Atrophy of muscles secondary to haematomas
Mononeuropathy resulting from pressure by haematomas

Complications due to therapy
Antifactor VIII antibody development
Virus transmission
  Hepatitis A virus—acute self-limiting illness
  Hepatitis B virus—5–10% become chronic HBsAg carriers
  Hepatitis C virus—chronic progressive liver disease
  Hepatitis D virus—only arises in those with HBsAg
  Human Immunodeficiency virus—AIDS
  Parvovirus—Acute systemic self-limiting illness

arises in about 10–20% of severe haemophiliacs. Such antibodies rapidly neutralise therapeutic infusions, making treatment relatively ineffective. Individuals may be treated with porcine factor VIII because the antibody has less activity against the animal factor VIII than against human. Alternatively, infusions of activated clotting factors, e.g. VIIa or Feiba (Factor Eight Inhibitor Bypassing Activity—an activated concentrate of factors II, IX and X) may stop bleeding.

In individuals with a basal factor VIII level of 0.07% or greater it may be possible to raise the level approximately three- to five-fold with intravenous desmopressin (0.3 μg/kg). This is often sufficient to treat a mild bleed or cover minor surgery such as dental extraction. Injections can be repeated 6–8-hourly although the response to second and subsequent infusions is not as good due to the development of tachyphylaxis. Desmopressin is an important form of therapy because it may avoid patients' being exposed to blood products.

Surgery in haemophiliacs can be safely performed provided the patient does not have an inhibitor to factor VIII and receives appropriate doses of concentrate. A single infusion of factor VIII is usually adequate for simple dental extractions, in an individual with severe haemophilia, along with a 10-day course of tranexamic acid (a fibrinolytic inhibitor) and antibiotic. Major surgery, for example orthopaedic surgery, requires twice-daily therapy for 14 days or longer.

HAEMOPHILIA B (CHRISTMAS DISEASE)

Aberrations of the factor IX gene, which is also present on the X chromosome, results in a reduction of the plasma factor IX level giving rise to haemophilia B. This disorder is clinically indistinguishable from haemophilia A and is less common. The frequency of bleeding episodes is related to the severity of the deficiency of the plasma factor IX level. Treatment is with a factor IX concentrate; it is used in much the same way as factor

VIII for haemophilia A. Carrier identification and antenatal diagnosis can be accomplished with gene probes, although different ones from that for the factor VIII gene.

VON WILLEBRAND's DISEASE

Genetics
The gene for von Willebrand Factor (vWF) is located on chromosome 12 and therefore the disorder is inherited in an autosomal fashion. In most families it has the appearance of being inherited in a dominant manner; rarely it appears in a clinically severe form with almost undetectable levels of vWF. In these circumstances the patient usually inherits a different abnormal vWF gene from each parent and is thus a compound heterozygote. Probes are available to trace the gene in a family although in most instances antenatal diagnosis is not indicated because of the relatively mild nature of the disorder.

The vWF is a protein, synthesised by endothelial cells and megakaryocytes, that performs two principal functions. It acts as carrier protein for factor VIII to which it is non-covalently bound. A deficiency of vWF therefore results in a secondary reduction in the factor VIII level. Its other function is to form bridges between platelets and subendothelial components, for example collagen, allowing platelets to adhere to damaged vessel walls. A deficiency of vWF therefore also leads to prolonged primary haemorrhage after trauma.

Clinical features
As vWF participates, along with platelets, in primary haemostasis, patients present with haemorrhagic manifestations which are similar to individuals with reduced platelet function. Superficial bruising, epistaxis, menorrhagia and gastrointestinal haemorrhage are common. Bleeding episodes are usually much less common than in severe haemophilia and excessive haemorrhage may only be observed after trauma or surgery. Within a single family the disease is of very variable expression so that some members may have quite severe and frequent bleeds whereas others are relatively little troubled.

Investigations
The disorder is characterised by finding a reduced level of vWF which is often accompanied by a secondary reduction in factor VIII and a prolongation of the bleeding time.

Management

Many episodes of mild haemorrhage can be successfully treated with desmopressin which raises the vWF level resulting in a secondary increase in factor VIII. For more serious or persistent bleeds haemostasis can be achieved with some factor VIII concentrates which contain considerable quantities of vWF in addition to factor VIII.

ACQUIRED BLEEDING DISORDERS

DISSEMINATED INTRAVASCULAR COAGULATION

Clinical features

Disseminated intravascular coagulation (DIC) can be initiated by a variety of different mechanisms in a number of diverse but distinct clinical situations, as set out in the information box below. Endothelial damage, due to many causes, for example endotoxin produced during Gram-negative septicaemia, may activate platelets, leucocytes and factor XII leading to initiation and promotion of the coagulation cascade. The presence of thromboplastin from damaged tissues, placenta, fat embolus or following brain injury, may also activate coagulation. Intravascular coagulation takes place with consumption of platelets, factors V and VIII and fibrinogen. This results in a potential haemorrhagic state, due to the depletion of haemostatic components, which may be exacerbated by activation of the fibrinolytic systems secondary to the deposition of fibrin.

CAUSES OF DISSEMINATED INTRAVASCULAR COAGULATION

- **Infections**   *E. coli*
                     Neisseria meningococcus
                     Streptococcus pneumoniae
                     Malaria
- **Obstetric**   Abruptio placentae
                     Retained dead fetus
                     Pre-eclampsia
                     Amniotic fluid embolism
- **Cancers**   Lung
                     Pancreas
                     Prostate

Investigations

DIC should be suspected when any of the conditions in the above information box are encountered. Definitive diagnosis depends on the finding of thrombocytopenia, prolongation of the prothrombin time (due to factor V and fibrinogen deficiency) and activated partial thromboplastin time (due to factors V, VIII and fibrinogen deficiency), a low fibrinogen concentration and increased levels of D-dimer (evidence of fibrin lysis).

Management

Therapy should be aimed at treating the underlying condition causing the DIC, for example intravenous antibiotics for suspected septicaemia. Exacerbating factors such as acidosis, dehydration, renal failure and hypoxia should be corrected. If the patient is bleeding, blood products to correct identified abnormalities such as platelets and/or cryoprecipitate (which is enriched in factor VIII and fibrinogen) should be given. It may also be reasonable to treat severe coagulation abnormalities in the absence of frank bleeding to prevent sudden catastrophic haemorrhage, for example intracranial bleed or massive gastrointestinal haemorrhage.

LIVER DISEASE

In severe parenchymal liver disease bleeding may arise from many different causes. Local anatomical abnormalities are often the site of major bleeding, for example oesophageal varices or peptic ulcer, and this may be difficult to arrest because of deficiencies in components of the haemostatic system. These may arise because of reduced hepatic synthesis, for example factors II, VII, IX, X and fibrinogen; DIC, reduced clearance of plasminogen activator, or thrombocytopenia secondary to hypersplenism. Treatment should be reserved for acute bleeds or to cover interventional procedures, for example liver biopsy.

Cholestatic jaundice reduces vitamin K absorption and leads to a deficiency of function of factors II, VII, IX and X due to reduced gamma carboxylation. This deficiency can be readily and effectively treated with vitamin K_1 10 mg daily parenterally for several days.

RENAL FAILURE

The severity of the haemorrhagic state in renal failure is proportional to the plasma urea concentration. Bleeding manifestations are of platelet type, with gastrointestinal haemorrhage being particularly common. The causes are multifactorial including anaemia, mild thrombocytopenia and the accumulation of low molecular waste products, normally excreted by the kidney, that inhibit platelet function. Treatment is by dialysis to reduce the urea concentration, and platelet concentrate infusions; red cell transfusions may raise the haemoglobin and decrease the propensity to bleed. Increasing the concentration of vWF, either by cryoprecipitate or desmopressin, may promote haemostasis.

FURTHER READING

British Committee for Standards in Haematology, Haemostasis and Thrombosis Task Force 1990 Guidelines on oral anticoagulation, 2nd edn. Journal of Clinical Pathology 43: 177–183

Hoyer L W 1994 Haemophilia A. New England Journal of Medicine 330: 38–47

VENOUS THROMBOSIS

Both arterial and venous thrombosis may arise either because of damage to vessels, for instance atheroma or varicose veins, or as a result of changes in the plasma or cellular elements. Predisposing conditions for venous thromboembolism are listed in Table 13.38.

DEEP VENOUS THROMBOSIS see p. 275.

PULMONARY EMBOLISM see p. 277.

HAEMATOLOGICAL DISORDERS PREDISPOSING TO VENOUS THROMBOEMBOLISM

When a thrombotic event arises in an individual under the age of 40 years, particularly in the absence of a predisposing factor, or if there is a family history of thrombosis, investigations should be undertaken to assess whether there is a predisposing plasma abnormality. A deficiency of a circulating anticoagulant or the presence of an antiphospholipid antibody will increase the propensity to thrombosis. A reduced level of plasminogen-activated inhibitor is also associated with both arterial and venous thrombosis. The mechanisms controlling this inhibitor of tissue plasminogen activator are ill understood but in most instances these are not apparently familial unlike a deficiency of a circulating anticoagulant, for example antithrombin III, which is usually inherited in an autosomal dominant fashion. In a few individuals thrombosis may result from a deficiency of tissue plasminogen activator synthesis and release from endothelial cells. Investigations for an haematological condition predisposing to thrombosis are given in the information box.

ANTITHROMBIN III DEFICIENCY

Antithrombin III is a protease inhibitor which inactivates factors IIa, IXa, Xa and XIa especially in the presence

Table 13.38 Factors predisposing to venous thrombosis

Age greater than 40 years
Obesity
Varicose veins
Previous DVT
Oral contraceptive
Pregnancy/puerperium
Dehydration
Immobility
Surgery especially if > 30-minute duration
                      abdominal or pelvic
                      orthopaedic to lower limb

Medical conditions
Myocardial infarction/heart failure
Inflammatory bowel disease
Malignancy
Nephrotic syndrome
Behçet's syndrome
Homocystinuria

Haematological disorders
Polycythaemia rubra vera
Essential thrombocythaemia
Myelofibrosis
Paroxysmal nocturnal haemoglobinuria

Deficiency of anticoagulants
Antithrombin III
Protein C
Protein S

Antiphospholipid antibody—lupus anticoagulant
                              —anticardiolipin antibody

INVESTIGATIONS OF AN INDIVIDUAL WHO MAY HAVE AN HAEMATOLOGICAL CONDITION PREDISPOSING TO THROMBOSIS

- Haemoglobin
- White cell count
- Platelet count
- Antithrombin III
- Protein C
- Protein S
- Lupus anticoagulant ⎱ Antiphospholipid antibody
- Anticardiolipin antibody ⎰
- Activated protein C resistance
- Plasminogen activator inhibitor

of heparin (which greatly potentiates its activity). Congenital deficiency of antithrombin III is associated with a predisposition to venous thromboembolism. Such patients may be relatively resistant to anticoagulation with heparin because of the low level of antithrombin III which is necessary for heparin to produce its anticoagulant effect.

PROTEIN C AND S DEFICIENCIES

Protein C is a vitamin K-dependent protein which, when activated by traces of thrombin in the presence of protein

S, inactivates factors Va and VIIIa. Thus a deficiency of either protein C or S results in a prothrombotic state due to reduced inhibition of activated factor V and VIII. A deficiency of either factor is usually inherited in an autosomal fashion.

ACTIVATED PROTEIN C RESISTANCE

A further disorder associated with recurrent venous thrombosis has recently been described, and it appears to be the commonest genetic abnormality resulting in thrombophilia. It was originally characterised as an inability of the patient's plasma clotting time to lengthen in the presence of activated protein C (APC). Further investigation revealed that the abnormality resided in the substrate for APC, namely factor Va; a substitution of argenine by glutamine at position 506 prevents its cleavage and hence inactivation. Factor Va will therefore tend to persist, resulting in a tendency to venous thrombosis.

The mutation has been identified in about 3–5% of healthy individuals and about 20–40% of those with a history of venous thrombosis at a young age. The risk of venous thrombosis, in individuals with this mutation, is substantially increased if the patient has a second plasma abnormality, e.g. a lupus anticoagulant.

ANTIPHOSPHOLIPID ANTIBODY SYNDROME

In the recently recognised antiphospholipid antibody syndrome an antibody in the patient's plasma has activity against enzymic reactions in the coagulation cascade that are enhanced by platelet membranes (or in vitro by phospholipid). The antibody, in vitro, has the effect of prolonging the APTT because it interacts with the phospholipid in the reaction tube and inhibits the binding or enzymic interactions of the coagulation components. It also prolongs the Russell Viper Venom Time of plasma, an effect that can be neutralised by adding platelet membranes. When the antibody inhibits coagulation in these ways it is known as the lupus anticoagulant. In some individuals the antibody can be detected because it binds to cardiolipin when it is known as an anticardiolipin antibody. The term antiphospholipid antibody encompasses both a lupus anticoagulant and anticardiolipin antibody; some individuals are only positive for one of these activities whereas in others both activities are present.

Clinical features

The antiphospholipid antibody is associated with a constellation of clinical conditions (Table 13.39). As the term lupus anticoagulant implies, the antibody was first detected in individuals with systemic lupus ery-

Table 13.39 Antiphospholipid syndrome

The clinical features are mainly related to arterial or venous occlusion which may affect one or several organs.

Haematologic
Thrombocytopenia
Autoimmune haemolytic anaemia

Cardiac
Myocardial infarction
Pulmonary hypertension
Valvular disease, e.g. mitral

Neurological
Cerebral ischaemia
  single lesions
  multi-infarct dementia
Migraine
Epilepsy
Chorea
Transverse myelopathy

Renal
Renal vein thrombosis
Glomerular thrombosis

Endocrine
Adrenal thrombosis—Addison's disease

GI tract
Bowel ischaemia
Budd–Chiari syndrome

Skin
Livedo reticularis
Recurrent skin ulcers

Obstetric
Recurrent spontaneous abortions
Intrauterine growth retardation

thematosus when it was found to be associated with a history of thromboembolism. The antibody has now been found in some individuals with a history of arterial or venous thromboembolism, often at a young age. The antibody is also associated with recurrent spontaneous abortions as well as intrauterine fetal growth retardation. The mechanism by which the antibody predisposes to thrombosis is unclear but it may be related to either maintaining platelets in an activated state within the circulation or possibly inhibiting the fibrinolytic activity of endothelial cells.

MANAGEMENT OF THROMBOEMBOLISM

The use of fibrinolytic drugs, such as tissue plasminogen activator or streptokinase, or anticoagulants, for example heparin or warfarin, depends upon the site, extent and age of the thrombus and whether it is arterial or venous. Prior to any antithrombotic therapy it is essential to consider whether the patient has a significant contraindication to anticoagulant therapy. On occasions antithrombotic therapy may have to be given to a patient who has a contraindication and in this instance the potential benefits have to be weighed against the risk of serious haemorrhage. Indications and contraindications to anticoagulation are given in the information boxes.

INDICATIONS FOR ANTICOAGULATION

Indications for heparin anticoagulation

- Treatment and prevention of deep venous thrombosis
- Pulmonary embolism
- Myocardial infarction—to prevent
  1. coronary reocclusion after thrombolysis
  2. mural thrombosis
- Unstable angina pectoris
- Acute peripheral arterial occlusion

Indications for warfarin anticoagulation	Therapeutic corrected prothrombin ratio (INR)
- Prophylaxis against deep venous thrombosis	2.0
- Treatment of deep venous thrombosis and pulmonary embolism - Arterial embolism - Mitral stenosis with atrial fibrillation - Transient ischaemic attacks	2.0–3.0
- Recurrent deep venous thrombosis - Mechanical prosthetic cardiac valves	3.0–4.5

CONTRAINDICATIONS TO ANTICOAGULATION

- Recent surgery especially to eye or CNS
- Preexisting haemorrhagic state
  e.g. liver disease
  renal failure
  haemophilia
  thrombocytopenia
- Preexisting structural lesions
  e.g. peptic ulcer
- Recent cerebral haemorrhage
- Uncontrolled hypertension

ANTICOAGULANT THERAPY

Heparin

Heparin produces its anticoagulant effect by potentiating the activity of antithrombin III which inhibits the procoagulant enzymic activity of factors IIa, IXa, Xa and XIa. The therapeutic indications for heparin use are listed in the information box below. For the treatment of established venous thrombosis a loading dose of 5000 Units should be given intravenously followed by a continuous infusion of 20 U/kg hourly initially. The level of anticoagulation should be assessed after 6 hours and if satisfactory then daily by use of a coagulation test which is appropriately sensitive to heparin, for example APTT. It is usual to aim for a patient time which is 1.5–2.5 times the control time of the test. Treatment should continue for 3–10 days depending upon the extent of the thrombus. In most patients it is appropriate to start warfarin therapy at the same time as heparin as it takes several days to decrease the concentration of the vitamin K-dependent clotting factors.

Warfarin

Warfarin inhibits the vitamin K-dependent carboxylation of factors II, VII, IX and X in the liver. Carboxylation of glutamyl residues of these coagulation factors increases their negative charge and allows them to bind, via calcium bridges, to negatively charged phospholipid surfaces particularly on the platelet. The recognised indications for warfarin therapy are listed in the information box (left).

Therapy with warfarin must be initiated with a loading dose, for example 10 mg orally, on the first day, and subsequent daily doses depending on the prothrombin time ratio. This should be in the range 2.0 to 4.5; the degree of anticoagulation depends on the clinical circumstances and the appropriate prothrombin ratio is given in the information box above. Following a single episode of venous thromboembolism it is usual to continue oral anticoagulation for 3 to 6 months, but if the patient has a prothrombotic condition warfarin may need to be continued on a long term basis. It is important to remember that nearly all drugs can potentially modify the degree of warfarin therapy, such as non-steroidal anti-inflammatory drugs, and therefore the prothrombin ratio should be checked 2 or 3 days after stopping or starting any other medicine.

If the patient bleeds, the anticoagulant effect of warfarin may be reversed by vitamin K_1, 5 mg slowly intravenously; the effect becomes apparent within about 6 hours although it may not fully reverse anticoagulation for one or two days. If the patient has a serious haemorrhage, reversal can be effected quickly by giving coagulation concentrate containing factors II, IX and X (50 U/kg) or if unavailable, fresh frozen plasma.

During the next few years it is likely that there will major developments in anticoagulant therapies. LMWH seems to be as effective as standard heparin, and as the dose does not require to be monitored and adjusted its use is likely to increase. The leech anticoagulant, hirudin, which is now synthesised by recombinant DNA technology, is a potent specific thrombin antagonist.

This enzyme has a pivotal role in the haemostatic system and its inhibition may make hirudin good therapy both for prevention and treatment of thromboembolism.

THROMBOLYTIC THERAPY

Therapeutic fibrinolytic therapy now has an established place in the management of occlusive thromboembolism. It should be considered for all patients with myocardial infarction (see p. 256) and it is being increasingly used to good clinical effect in peripheral arterial thromboembolism, extensive deep venous thrombosis and massive life-threatening pulmonary embolism.

The most commonly used agents are streptokinase and alteplase (recombinant tissue plasminogen activator). Following infusion streptokinase combines with plasminogen to become an activator of plasminogen resulting in the formation of plasmin. Alteplase directly converts plasminogen to plasmin. As streptokinase is a non-human protein it elicits a brisk anti-streptokinase antibody response and it can therefore only be used for 3–5 days and further therapy can only be given after two years. Alteplase is human tissue plasminogen activator and therefore does not elicit a specific antibody response.

Streptokinase and alteplase hasten dissolution of thrombus by several different mechanisms:

(i) They diffuse into the thrombus to convert plasminogen, bound to fibrin, to plasmin.
(ii) Alteplase, and to a lesser extent the streptokinase-plasminogen complex, have an affinity for fibrin which further increases their local concentration in the thrombus. Although alteplase might appear on a theoretical basis to be a safer drug, clinical experience has demonstrated that for an equivalent lytic dose it is associated with a greater degree of intracranial haemorrhage leading to stroke compared to streptokinase.
(iii) All the activators lead to enhanced proteolytic activity which reduces the level of coagulant proteins, e.g. fibrinogen.
(iv) The resultant fibrin degradation products have anti-thrombin and antiplatelet activity which will help reduce the formation of further thrombus.

In general, prolonged infusions, e.g. over 12 hours, tend to result in a greater haemorrhagic tendency due to the longer duration of enhanced fibrinolysis and also because there is greater depletion of circulating coagulation factors.

All patients in whom a definitive diagnosis of myocardial infarction has been made should be considered for treatment as quickly as possible with fibrinolytic therapy and aspirin, bearing in mind that there are contraindications to such therapy (see information box, p. 262). Streptokinase is the preferred therapy because it is associated with a lower incidence of intracranial haemorrhage than alteplase; it is also considerably less expensive.

Alteplase (along with intravenous heparin) should be used in those individuals who have had streptokinase within the previous two years or who have had severe allergic reactions to streptokinase.

Thrombolytic therapy, particularly with alteplase, is being used increasingly to good effect in patients with acute peripheral arterial thromboembolism. All such patients require angiograms and the lytic agent is infused via the arterial catheter into the thrombus.

The treatment of extensive deep venous thrombosis and pulmonary embolism by fibrinolytic therapy is under very active investigation by clinical trials at present. In carefully selected individuals, particularly those with massive pulmonary embolism leading to hypotension and hypoxia, thrombolytic therapy may be indicated particularly if the patient has not responded to full heparinisation which is the initial immediate treatment of choice.

The use of either streptokinase or alteplase results in a propensity to bleed. Invasive procedures, including both arterial and venous punctures, should be kept to a minimum and drugs should not be given by the intramuscular route. All patients should be carefully monitored for evidence of bleeding. For short infusions, e.g. up to 3 hours, it is not necessary to monitor changes in the coagulation screen. As the tendency to bleed increases with prolonged infusions it is prudent to monitor such therapy with an APTT, fibrinogen and full blood count, including platelets, to assess whether there has been a large decrease in components of the haemostatic system. This may be useful in the continuing management of individuals with serious venous thromboembolism.

For minor haemorrhage, e.g. at venepuncture site, sustained local pressure should be applied. For more serious bleeding, consideration should be given to stopping the infusion of lytic agent. Should life-threatening haemorrhage be suspected, e.g. an intracranial bleed, the infusion should be stopped and aprotinin or cyclokapron given immediately along with fresh frozen plasma or cryoprecipitate (depending upon the result of a coagulation screen). Patients suspected of having internal haemorrhage should be immediately investigated by appropriate techniques, e.g. cranial CT scan for suspected intracranial haemorrhage or abdominal ultrasound for retroperitoneal haematoma, after the fibrinolytic therapy has been reversed.

PREVENTION OF VENOUS THROMBOSIS

Heparin can be used to prevent DVT formation both following surgery and in immobilised medical patients.

The usual dose is 5000 U 12-hourly subcutaneously and should be started pre-operatively and continued until the patient is fully mobile. Patients particularly at risk of post-operative thrombosis are those over the age of 40 years who have abdominal surgery which lasts more than half an hour. Any individual who has any of the additional risk factors in Table 13.38 is also at increased likelihood of thrombosis and every care should be taken to ensure that, so far as possible, the risk can be lessened prior to surgery, for instance the haemoglobin reduced in polycythaemia.

Standard heparin contains molecules which range in molecular weight from approximately 5000 to 35 000 Daltons. Recently low molecular weight derivations of standard heparin (LMWH) have been prepared and are now licensed for use in the prevention of post-operative venous thromboembolism after hip and knee ortho-paedic surgery because this is associated with a high risk of thrombosis which cannot be adequately prevented by subcutaneous standard heparin. LMWH has greater anti-Xa than antithrombin activity, has a longer half life and is less tissue-bound than standard heparin. It is not necessary to monitor the level of anticoagulation; it does not readily prolong the APTT and can only effectively be measured using an anti-Xa assay. It is given either as a standard dose or a dose related to the patient's weight. In future it may allow for effective and safe treatment of DVTs at home because blood levels do not need to be monitored.

FURTHER READING

Bick R L 1994 Common bleeding and clotting disorders. Medical Clinics of North America 78(3): 511–772
British Committee for Standards in Haematology, Haemostasis and Thrombosis Task Force 1992 Guidelines on the use and monitoring of heparin. Journal of Clinical Pathology 46: 97–103
Hirsh J 1991 Heparin. New England Journal of Medicine 324: 1565–1574
Meade T W 1994 Haemostatic function, arterial disease and the prevention of arterial thrombosis. Baillière's Clinical Haematology 7: 1–760
Thromboembolic Risk Factors (THRIFT) Consensus Group 1992 Risk of and prophylaxis for venous thromboembolism in hospital patients. British Medical Journal 305: 567

J. F. Smyth

Oncology

Oncology is the study of tumours. Neoplasia means abnormal new growth, which may be benign or malignant. Cancer is a term that is used to describe a wide variety of malignant diseases, the management of which requires several medical disciplines. Traditionally physicians have played a lesser role than surgeons or radiotherapists in the treatment of these diseases but the development of cytotoxic drugs and major advances in palliative care have resulted in the greater involvement of physicians in the overall management of malignancy. The use of cytotoxic drugs, and medicines to control the symptoms of advanced malignancy, require specialised knowledge and experience but since cancer impinges on every medical discipline, it is necessary for all doctors to be aware of the basic principles of investigating and managing malignant diseases. This chapter reviews these basic principles and outlines some aspects of the aetiology and pathology of tumours, the assessment of tumour burden, the use of radiotherapy, chemotherapy and hormone therapy, and possible approaches to the prevention of these diseases, many of which may be associated with avoidable causes.

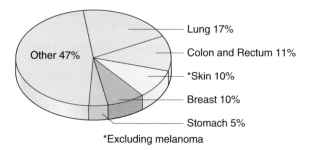

Fig. 14.1   Cancer mortality—UK 1988.

CLINICAL PRESENTATION

INCIDENCE

Cancer is second only to coronary artery disease as being the commonest cause of death in the Western world. For example, in Scotland during 1990 (the most recent year for which complete figures are available), 31 480 new cancer patients were registered, and there were 15 030 deaths. This gives an incidence of 5555 per million of population for males and 6746 for females. Based on current incidence rates it is estimated that 1 in 3 people will develop cancer at some time during their life.

Throughout the Western world the commonest sites of malignant disease are the lung, large bowel and breast (Fig. 14.1). Over the past 25 years the incidence of lung cancer in men has increased by 125%, and even more significantly in women concomitant with their increased consumption of cigarettes. The incidence of colonic, prostatic and bladder cancer has also shown an increase but during the past decade there has been a decrease in the incidence of carcinomas arising in the stomach, uterus, rectum and oesophagus.

Progress in diagnosis and treatment has had a significant effect on survival for some cancers, but ironically the best results have been achieved in relatively rare cancers such as testicular tumours and Hodgkin's lym-

phoma. The commonest cancers such as lung and large bowel remain the most refractory. Figure 14.2 illustrates 5-year survival data for patients first diagnosed in 1983.

Age

Age has a bearing on the incidence of specific cancers, and more than 70% of all new cases occur in patients over 60 years old. In children, cancer is the leading cause of death between the ages of 3 and 13 years, about half of these being due to acute lymphoblastic leukaemia. For the age group in the third and fourth decades, cancer is three times as common in women as in men but men are at greater risk than women between the ages of 60 and 80.

AETIOLOGY

In a recent survey of the trend in mortality from cancer in the USA it has been estimated that up to 90% of all such deaths could be attributed to potentially avoidable factors, namely tobacco, alcohol, diet, reproductive and sexual behaviour, occupation, pollution and geographical features.

Cigarette smoking

Tobacco is the most clearly identified cause of cancer; this causes more than 50 000 deaths per year in the UK—one third of all cancer deaths. The public health campaigns emphasising the indisputable association between cigarette tobacco and lung cancer are beginning to prove successful, and there are indications that cigarette consumption is at last starting to decline. There is, however, still a continuing need for such education, aimed particularly at the young to warn them of the dangers of cigarette smoking.

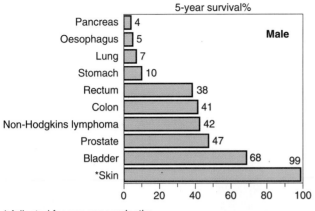

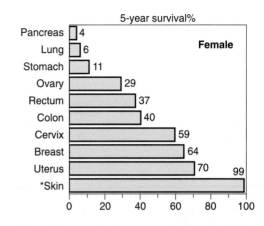

* Adjusted for non-cancer deaths

Fig. 14.2   Five-year survival rates in Scotland, 1983–87.

CANCERS ASSOCIATED WITH TOBACCO

- Lung
- Mouth
- Larynx
- Oesophagus
- Bladder

Diet

It appears easier to influence dietary habits but research is needed to identify the specific agents responsible for the development of tumours where diet appears to play a role, such as gastrointestinal carcinomas. Epidemiological aspects of diet are very difficult but foodstuffs may cause cancers in some of the following ways:

1. By being direct carcinogens.
2. Carcinogens may be produced by cooking.
3. Micro-organisms may produce carcinogens in stored foods.
4. Foodstuffs may act as substrates for the formation of carcinogens in the body.
5. Foodstuffs may alter the bacterial flora of the bowel, thereby producing carcinogens.

Geographical distribution

Studies of the geographical distribution of the incidence of different cancers give some leads as to the possible influence of particular environmental or social factors in causation.

The incidence of carcinoma of the *oesophagus* varies greatly from country to country (over a 200-fold range) with a particularly high incidence in the geographical band covering eastern and southern Africa, Iran, Afghanistan, Soviet and central Asia, Mongolia and northern China. Suggestions that diet or cooking practices are involved are as yet unconfirmed.

The incidence of carcinoma of the *pancreas* is increasing in most of the developed countries but is relatively rare in Japan, whereas the reverse is true for stomach cancer, which is particularly prevalent in Japan.

It has been known for a long time that the incidence of *breast* cancer varies appreciably in different parts of the world, being high in the USA and low in the Orient but increasing over two generations of orientals who emigrate to the USA. Population migration represents a natural experiment where the assumption of incidence levels of the host country strongly suggests an environmental rather than a genetic aetiology. Breast cancer incidence rates increase with age, but the rate of increase is greater up to age 50 than afterwards. If the currently observed increases in incidence rates in younger women in previously low-risk parts of the world, such as Asia and South America, continue throughout their life-span, then it is estimated that by the year 2000 the annual world-wide incidence of breast cancer will be in excess of 1 million. Several aetiological factors are known to be associated with breast cancer, such as an increased risk for women having an early menarche and late menopause. The older the age at which a woman has her first full-term pregnancy the higher is the risk of developing breast cancer, but lactation has a protective influence.

The incidence of carcinoma of the *uterine cervix* has increased in recent years particularly amongst younger women. This has coincided with changing social patterns of greater sexual freedom and the use of oral contraception, suggesting that a sexually transmissible agent may be the aetiological factor responsible. The screening of women who have started sexual activity at an early age or have had multiple partners should be

Table 14.1 Proportions of cancer deaths attributed to various aetiological factors*

Factors or class of factors	Percent of all cancer deaths	
	Best estimate	Range of acceptable estimates
Tobacco	30	25–40
Alcohol	3	2–4
Diet	35	10–70
Food additives	<1	−5–2
Reproductive and sexual behaviour	7	1–13
Occupation	4	2–8
Pollution	2	<1–5
Industrial products	<1	<1–2
Medicines and medical procedures	1	0.5–3
Geophysical factors	3	2–4
Infection	10?	1–?
Unknown	?	?

* Reproduced with permission from Doll R, Peto R 1981 The Causes of Cancer. Oxford Medical Publications, Oxford

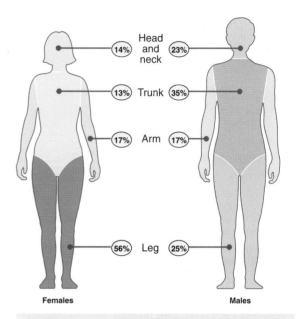

Fig. 14.3 Percentage distribution of malignant melanoma on parts of the body.

encouraged because early detection can result in cure. As further aetiological factors are identified, it is reasonable to predict that other screening procedures will become useful for certain groups although at present there is no indication for screening the entire population.

There is evidence that both environmental and genetic factors are important in the pathogenesis of malignant *melanoma*. Of great concern is the fact that the incidence of malignant melanoma is rising rapidly. The rate per 100 000 population per year in Scotland has increased from 3.4 in 1979 to 7.1 in 1989 for men, and 6.6 to 10.4 for women. This represents an 82% overall increase over 11 years.

Melanoma is rare in black and oriental people, suggesting that skin-pigment plays a role in protecting against its development. Although not proven, there is support for sunlight being involved in the aetiology of this disease. Although in most parts of the world the incidence between the sexes is equal, women tend to develop melanoma in the legs and exposed parts of the limbs more frequently than men, who have a higher incidence of lesions on the trunk (Fig. 14.3). Furthermore, studies from Norway, Canada, the USA and Australia show that the incidence of melanoma increases as one approaches the equator, consistent with greater exposure to ultraviolet light.

Table 14.1 illustrates the best estimate for the effect of various factors on cancer deaths.

Viruses

It has been suspected that viruses may be involved in the pathogenesis of human neoplasms. Indirect evidence suggests that viruses may act as cofactors in the devel-

opment of some malignant diseases; viral particles can be demonstrated in the cells of certain malignancies, the enzyme reverse transcriptase (of oncornavirus-type) has been demonstrated in human cancer cells, and the nuclei of some malignant cells have been shown to contain DNA base sequences complementary to the base sequences of known tumour viruses. If viruses do produce cancer there are many possible ways in which a virus may interact with the host tissue. One mechanism is illustrated by the Epstein–Barr virus, which is responsible for producing glandular fever (infectious mononucleosis, p. 109). Under certain conditions—particularly in tropical Africa and southern China—the virus gets inserted into the DNA of a reticuloendothelial cell, or of an epithelial cell in the nasopharynx, and gives rise to a Burkitt's lymphoma or a nasopharyngeal carcinoma—the cells of which contain a mixture of viral DNA in combination with their own.

Oncogenes

The fact that viral information can be integrated into the genome of a human cell, and thereby transform that cell into a malignant one, has led to major advances in our understanding of the molecular genetics of cancer. It is now recognised that there exist regulatory genes known as tumour suppressor genes whose normal function is to prevent malignant transformation. The latter might be triggered by exposure to a carcinogen (e.g. tobacco) or by a spontaneous mutation. Conversely normal cells contain growth promoting genes known as

Table 14.2 Association of proto-oncogenes with various cancers

Disease	Proto-oncogene	Mechanism
Small cell lung carcinoma	c-myc I-myc n-myc	Amplification
Breast carcinoma	c-myc c-erb-B2	Amplification
Cervical carcinoma	c-myc	Amplification
Burkitt's lymphoma	c-myc	Translocation
Chronic myelogenous leukaemia	c-myc	Translocation
Colon carcinoma	c-ras	Point mutation

Table 14.3 Classification of cancers

Type	Tissue or cell of origin	Examples
Carcinoma	Endoderm or ectoderm	Epithelial lining of gut (e.g. adenocarcinoma of colon) or bronchus (e.g. squamous cell or small cell carcinoma of bronchus).
Sarcoma	Mesoderm	Osteosarcoma Fibrosarcoma
Leukaemia	White blood cell	Acute lymphoblastic leukaemia
Lymphoma	Monocyte, macrophage	Hodgkin's disease

proto-oncogenes where inappropriate activation (by a carcinogen or mutation) to produce oncogenes could similarly result in malignant transformation. Examples of tumour suppressor genes and oncogenes are given in Chapter 1, pages 22–23.

Amplification of proto-oncogenes may occur as an occasional event in many types of tumour or consistently as an abnormality of a specific proto-oncogene in a particular tumour type. Some examples of the association of proto-oncogenes with specific cancers are illustrated in Table 14.2. The proteins encoded by the large number of oncogenes that have been identified are mostly unknown, and hence the effects of gene amplifications are unclear. In the case of C-erb-B2 the protein appears to be a transmembrane growth factor regulator. Recent evidence in patients with various cancers suggests that the greater the amplification of the oncogene, the poorer the prognosis. For an explanation of the translocation mechanism, see page 18.

PATHOLOGY

A fundamental principle of oncology is to establish, usually by biopsy, the pathological nature of any lesion suspected of being neoplastic before making decisions about management.

The first distinction to be made is between benign and malignant lesions. Benign tumours represent the accumulation of cells which have been transformed to reproduce in abnormal numbers but under circumstances where they remain within the tissue of origin. Malignant tumours are composed of cells which are capable of invading adjacent tissues and leaving the tissue of origin to disseminate and form metastases. The histological distinction between benign and malignant lesions will depend, amongst other factors, on the pleomorphism of the cells, the presence of aberrations in the nucleus, increased numbers of mitoses and whether or not there is evidence of invasion into surrounding tissues.

Biologically there is a continuum between the benign and malignant state that can cause great difficulties in diagnosis. The concept of 'pre-cancerous' conditions has led to terms such as 'carcinoma in situ', which can be confusing. To be preferred is the term 'intraepithelial neoplasia', which recognises the continuum between dysplasia or atypical hyperplasia and 'carcinoma in situ'. A grading system is frequently used with intraepithelial neoplasia to indicate increasing degrees of severity, e.g. for cervical cancer CIN-1, CIN-2, CIN-3, where CIN-1 represents minimal morphological change and CIN-3 the carcinoma in situ state where the entire epithelium from basement membrane to the surface is composed of malignant cells.

Cancers are classified into four major groups (Table 14.3). Within a given tissue there may be major differences in the cell type from which the tumour has arisen. Thus for example bronchogenic carcinomas are classified histologically into four major groups: squamous carcinomas, adenocarcinomas, small cell and large cell undifferentiated carcinomas.

Such distinctions are essential to clinical management since the choice between surgery, radiotherapy and chemotherapy will depend on whether the lesion is benign or malignant, and whether or not the particular histological subtype is sensitive to radiotherapy or chemotherapy. As regards the latter, there is a great variation in the sensitivity of different tumours to different cytotoxic drugs, and therefore appropriate therapy can be prescribed only when the tumour tissue has been accurately classified.

Although there is evidence to support the concept that many human tumours arise from the transformation of a single cell, i.e. are clonal in origin, it is not unusual to find a mixed histological picture; for example in the testis, teratomas and seminomatous tissue may occur together, and in the lung, squamous and small-cell undifferentiated tumours may present in the same biopsy specimen.

In addition to defining whether the tumour is benign or malignant and from which cell type it arises, it is useful to define the degree of differentiation or anaplasia of the cancer cell since for many tumour types this has been shown to correlate with prognosis and response to treatment.

Cytology

Whilst most histology is performed on tissue that is obtained by surgical biopsy, in certain circumstances it is possible to achieve excellent classification from cytology alone. Thus, for example, sputum may be examined for malignant bronchogenic cells, pleural or peritoneal effusions may provide suitable cells for diagnostic purposes and smears can be prepared from the uterine cervix. Increasing use is being made of needle aspiration for cytological diagnosis. A fine-gauge needle can be inserted into breast lumps, subcutaneous deposits, intra-thoracic or hepatic lesions, and a smear for cytological evaluation can be made from the aspirated material. In experienced hands, this technique has many advantages over the more conventional surgical biopsy technique, mainly because of speed and simplicity.

Immunohistochemistry

The production of polyclonal and, more recently, monoclonal antibodies has made a very significant contribution to the further identification and classification of histological and cytological preparations of tumour tissues. Highly specific antibodies raised against tumour antigens can be labelled with fluorescein or used in immunohistochemical techniques to detect tumour cell products such as enzymes, hormones or receptors. This technique can be used for the more confident distinction between benign and malignant tissues, and to differentiate between histological subtypes of similar tumours; for example, in a histologically undifferentiated bronchogenic tumour a monoclonal antibody that stains positively for mucin, used in conjunction with one that detects keratin, may help distinguish an adenocarcinoma from a squamous carcinoma. Similarly, immunophenotyping (as it is called) of lymphomas and leukaemias can greatly enhance the distinction between morphologically related subtypes. Such categorisation is important in predicting the natural history of an individual patient's illness and in selecting the most appropriate therapy.

Tumour markers

Malignant cells appear different histologically and vary biochemically from their normal counterparts but attempts to identify biochemical abnormalities unique to the cancer cell have proved unrewarding. Nevertheless it is now appreciated that the presence of viable tumour tissue in the body may be detectable by the presence in the blood of biochemical products known as 'tumour markers'. These are normal metabolic constituents that are found either in abnormal amounts or at an inappropriate time of life, for example fetal proteins being re-expressed in adult life.

Tumour markers of this type can be useful in a number of different clinical situations. In theory tumour markers might be useful for screening whole populations for undetected cancers but in practice this has not proved useful, for the following reasons. The predictive value of a screening test depends on the sensitivity of the test, its specificity and the prevalence of the particular disease. Sensitivity refers to the number of times a test is positive for patients known to have the disease, i.e. true positives, and specificity refers to the incidence of true negatives, i.e. that the test should prove negative in people known to be free of the disease. Unfortunately sensitivity is inversely related to specificity. For example it is known that some gastrointestinal tumours contain carcino-embryonic antigen (CEA), a substance that is present in the gut during fetal life but which is not found in normal adult gastrointestinal tissues. Radio-immuno-assays of CEA in blood have shown an overall 67% positivity in patients with colorectal carcinoma but the test is also positive in alcoholic cirrhosis (70%), emphysema (57%) and diabetes mellitus (38%), amongst many other diseases. Screening the population at large for subclinical carcinomas of the colon with this method would therefore fail because of lack of specificity.

However, the presence of a tumour marker can be of clinical value in monitoring the progress of individual patients known to have a given malignancy. For example testicular teratomas not infrequently secrete another oncofetal protein—alpha-fetoprotein (AFP). Figure 14.4 illustrates a typical case where during the months following surgical resection of the primary tumour, a rising level of AFP was associated with (and preceded) the clinical appearance of metastases. The successful use of chemotherapy was associated with a disappearance of the abnormal tumour marker.

Human chorionic gonadotrophin (normally produced only by placental tissue) is another tumour marker seen in testicular teratoma while the production of placental alkaline phosphatase is associated with approximately 40% of testicular seminomas.

Table 14.4 illustrates some of the tumour markers currently in use to aid in prognosis and/or follow the effects of treatment.

Human chorionic gonadotrophin is only one of a variety of hormones which can be produced ectopically by tumours (Table 14.5). The levels of these hormones, or

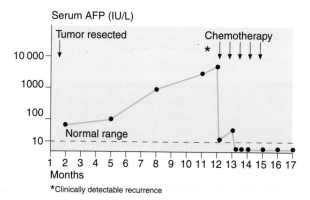

*Clinically detectable recurrence

Fig. 14.4 Serum alpha-fetoprotein (AFP) levels in a young man with testicular teratoma. The levels of AFP fluctuate with disease state and can be used to monitor the effects of the treatment.

Table 14.4 Serum tumour markers

Cancer	Marker
Testicular (germ cell)	Alpha-fetoprotein (AFP) β-human chorionic gonadotrophin (β-HCG)
Choriocarcinoma	β-HCG
Ovary	Ca-125
Prostate	Prostate Specific Antigen (PSA)
Hepatocellular carcinoma	Alpha-fetoprotein
Colorectal	CEA

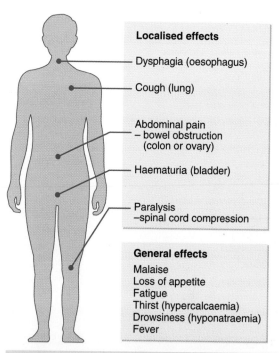

Fig. 14.5 General and localised effects of malignant disease.

the biochemical consequences of their production, can be useful markers of the viability of residual tumour following treatment, therefore indicating whether or not further therapy is required.

CLINICAL FEATURES

Malignant diseases manifest themselves in a variety of ways resulting from general or localised effects. Some of these are illustrated in Figure 14.5. The presence of an abnormal accumulation of cells may, by virtue of its physical bulk alone, produce clinical symptoms and signs. Thus for example painless swellings in the breast or in muscle may indicate an underlying carcinoma or sarcoma respectively. Lymphomas usually present as painless enlargements of lymph nodes or spleen. Intracranial space-occupying lesions may cause focal manifestations, fits, headaches, vomiting and papilloedema. Tumours in the distal colon may partially obstruct the lumen of the bowel with a resulting change in bowel habit. Bronchogenic tumours may cause cough or short-

ness of breath resulting from partial or complete occlusion of an airway.

Haemorrhage

Malignant tumours not infrequently present as haemorrhage from an eroded epithelial surface. For example, bronchogenic carcinomas may present with haemoptysis, gastric carcinomas with iron deficiency anaemia or, occasionally, haematemesis, colonic carcinoma with bleeding per rectum, and renal and bladder carcinomas with haematuria.

Pain

This is often thought to be an inevitable accompaniment of malignant disease but in fact it is not a common symptom especially at presentation of most cancers. When pain does occur, it usually reflects either nerve compression or distension of an organ. The most common peripheral nerve compressions are due to involvement of the brachial plexus (carcinomas of the lung or breast), the sacral plexus (carcinomas of the rectum or cervix) or the paraspinal nerves (carcinomas of the pancreas). Metastatic tumours in the liver may cause pain as a result of distension and stretching of its capsule. Bone pain resulting from primary, or more commonly, secondary deposits usually occurs in the weight-bearing

Table 14.5 Hormones produced by tumours

Ectopically-produced hormones	Clinical hormone syndromes	Associated neoplasms
ACTH	Cushing's syndrome	Small cell bronchogenic ca
HCG (human chorionic gonadotrophin)	Gynaecomastia, precocious puberty	Small cell bronchogenic ca, hepatoblastoma
AVP (arginine vasopressin)	Inappropriate ADH (AVP) syndrome	Small cell bronchogenic ca, ca pancreas (rare)
PTHrP (parathyroid hormone related protein)	Hypercalcaemia	Squamous cell bronchogenic ca, kidney ca, ovarian ca
OAF (osteoclast activating factor)	Hypercalcaemia	Myeloma
Erythropoietin	Erythrocytosis	Uterine fibromyoma, cerebellar haemangioblastoma
Chorionic somato-mammotrophin or HPL (human placental lactogen)	None	Small cell bronchogenic ca
GH (growth hormone)	? Hypertrophic pulmonary osteoarthropathy	Small cell bronchogenic ca
GH releasing factor	Acromegaly	Bronchial carcinoid, pancreatic islet carcinoid
HCG (TSH-like)	Hyperthyroidism	Choriocarcinoma
Prolactin	Galactorrhoea	Hypernephroma
Enteroglucagon	Gastrointestinal abnormalities and symptoms	Renal tumour
CRF (corticotrophin-releasing factor)	Cushing's syndrome	Bronchial carcinoid, prostatic ca
Calcitonin	None	Small cell bronchogenic ca, medullary ca, thyroid and breast ca
VIP (vasoactive intestinal polypeptide)	Watery diarrhoea	Small cell bronchogenic ca

bones, and results from compression secondary to weakening of the structural component of the bone. Pathological fractures may arise as a consequence. Patients may present with referred pain, most frequently in the shoulder, hip or knee, as when a nerve root is involved directly or by metastases.

Cachexia

This is a profound state of general ill health—malnutrition, wasting, anaemia and muscle weakness. It is a clinical feature of many malignant diseases presenting at an advanced stage, especially carcinomas of the gastrointestinal tract, lung, ovary and testis. It is, however, not a universal phenomenon and is rare in breast cancer and in tumours of the central nervous system, and uncommon in leukaemia and lymphomas.

Cachexia may arise as a direct result of malnutrition from a tumour in the gastrointestinal tract. Malabsorption may arise rarely as a consequence of tumour replacing the absorptive epithelia but more commonly from reduced exocrine function (from carcinomas of the pancreas), or loss of bile from carcinomas of the upper gastrointestinal tract that obstruct biliary outflow. Loss of taste and the malaise that accompanies many malignant diseases may contribute to poor food intake but all of these factors in promoting malnutrition do not of themselves fully explain the cachexia of malignancy.

Although many patients will have a negative nitrogen balance, others who are in positive balance may show caloric deficit. It has been shown that in the cachexia accompanying malignant disease, caloric expenditure remains high with an elevated basal metabolic rate despite reduced dietary intake (the reverse of the situation that follows starvation) which indicates that this phenomenon results from a profound systemic derangement of host metabolism, the pathogenesis of which remains unclear.

Paraneoplastic features

In addition to generalised clinical features that are commonly associated with the presentation of a malignant disease, there are a variety of syndromes for which the term 'paraneoplastic' has been used. These syndromes include many that arise as a result of the secretion into the blood of tumour products (usually polypeptide hormones) which produce clinical symptoms and signs as a consequence of their action on target organs remote from the primary tumour (see Table 14.5).

A number of neurological paraneoplastic syndromes have been described for which the tumour product remains unknown. These include peripheral neuropathies, a myasthenia-like syndrome and subacute cerebellar degeneration. Whilst all of these syndromes may improve with successful treatment of the primary tumour, complete resolution is rare.

Dermatomyositis and polymyositis present as gradually progressive muscle weakness predominantly affecting the proximal musculature, coming on over a period of months. Whilst these disorders are not universally associated with malignancy, patients suffering from them have a greatly increased risk of an underlying neoplasm compared with the general public, and malignancies of the breast, lung and gastrointestinal and genito-urinary tract should be considered.

Acanthosis nigricans is a rare condition characterised by the appearance of black velvety verrucose lesions in the flexures around the neck, axillae and groin. It is particularly seen in patients with carcinomas of the stomach.

FURTHER READING

Bishop J M 1986 From proto-oncogene to oncogene: the molecular genetics of cancer. Advances in Oncology No. 4: 3–8
Doll R, Peto R 1981 The causes of cancer. Oxford Medical Publications, Oxford. A short resumé of the known epidemiological factors
Franks L M, Teich N M 1991 Introduction to the Cellular and Molecular Biology of Cancer. Oxford University Press, Oxford
Glover D M, Hames B D 1989 Oncogenes. Oxford University Press, Oxford

PRINCIPLES OF MANAGEMENT

As a general rule, patients should be informed that they have a malignant disease prior to starting treatment but not necessarily of the exact prognosis.

The first interview with a patient suspected of having a malignant disease should be performed in a quiet and unhurried manner. In addition to a routine history of symptoms and previous illnesses, it is important to ascertain whether patients already know that they have a malignant disease and what this means to them. The patient will be helped very considerably by positive assurance that symptoms can almost always be improved even if the underlying disease cannot be eradicated.

Cure or palliation

In order to plan the optimal management for an individual patient, it is necessary to consider two questions:

1. Is the tumour still localised to its site of origin?
2. Is it a realistic aim to 'cure' the patient, or should treatment be focused on palliation of symptoms?

Tumours that have not metastasised are amenable to local forms of treatment (e.g. surgery or radiotherapy)

whilst tumours that have already disseminated require systemic treatment with chemotherapy or hormonal therapy. It is frequently necessary to use a combination of these measures, particularly if aiming for complete eradication of the tumour. Radiotherapy and chemotherapy both act by causing damage to DNA. This will occur not only in tumour cells but in any normal host cells that are exposed to treatment. Hence the doses of either form of treatment are limited by the tolerance of normal tissues, rather than by the 'sensitivity' of the cancer cells. Some host toxicity is inevitable and for this reason it is important to decide whether or not cure is feasible in order to minimise treatment-related toxicity in circumstances where an aggressive therapeutic approach would be inappropriate.

Staging

It is usually necessary to perform specialised investigations to determine the extent of dissemination of the tumour prior to selecting treatment—the process of 'staging' the tumour. Staging investigations take time and the delay causes anxiety for the patient.

Staging is important both for the selection of appropriate treatment, and to provide information about prognosis. Usually advancing stage indicates a worse prognosis, even if the tumour has not yet metastasised. Inadequate or inaccurate staging may lead to under- or over-treatment, resulting in failure to cure or unnecessary toxicity respectively.

The internationally recognised staging system is known as the TNM classification. This is shown in Table 14.6. An example for lung cancer is shown in Table 14.7.

The TNM system is a clinical staging system but if

Table 14.6	TNM classification
T*	Extent of primary tumour
N*	Extent of regional lymph node involvement
M	Presence or absence of metastases
Extent of disease	
T0	Excised tumour
T1	
T2	Increases in primary tumour size
T3	
Increased involvement of nodes	
N1	
N2	Increasing involvement
N3	
Presence of metastases	
M0	Not present
M1	Present

* Exact criteria of size and region of nodal involvement have been defined for each anatomical site.

Table 14.7 TNM for lung cancer

TX	Positive cytology only	
T1	<3 cm	
T2	>3 cm/extends to hilar region/invades visceral pleura/partial atelectasis	Primary tumour
T3	Chest wall, diaphragm, pericardium, mediastinum, pleura, etc., total atelectasis	
T4	mediastinum, heart, great vessels, trachea, oesophagus, etc., malignant effusion	
N1	Peribronchial, ipsilateral hilar	
N2	Ipsilateral mediastinal	Lymph node
N3	Contralateral mediastinal, scalene or supraclavicular	

Table 14.8 Stage grouping for lung cancer

Stage	T	N	M
Occult carcinoma	TX	N0	M0
0	Tis	N0	M0
I	T1	N0	M0
	T2	N0	M0
II	T1	N1	M0
	T2	N1	M0
IIIA	T1	N2	M0
	T2	N2	M0
	T3	N0, N1, N2	M0
IIIB	Any T	N3	M0
	T4	Any N	M0
IV	Any T	Any N	M1

Table 14.9 Eastern Cooperative Oncology Group performance status scale

0	Fully active, able to carry on all usual activities without restriction and without the aid of analgesics
1	Restricted in strenuous activity but ambulatory and able to carry out light work or pursue a sedentary occupation. This group also contains patients who are fully active, as in grade 0, but only with the aid of analgesics
2	Ambulatory and capable of all self-care but unable to work. Up and about more than 50% of waking hours
3	Capable of only limited self-care, confined to bed or chair more than 50% of waking hours
4	Completely disabled, unable to carry out any self-care and confined totally to bed or chair

to assess the overall degree of functional impairment that the disease is causing the patient at the time of diagnosis. A variety of 'performance status' scales have been devised such as the Eastern Cooperative Oncology Group (ECOG) scale shown in Table 14.9. These have been found useful in assessing prognosis and also the efficacy and toxicity of treatment.

INVESTIGATIONS TO DEFINE TNM STATUS

- **Tumour**
  Palpation
  Inspection including endoscopy (e.g. bronchoscopy, cystoscopy)
  Radiology (conventional, CT, Magnetic Resonance Imaging)
  Cytology/aspiration/biopsy

- **Nodes**
  Palpation
  Aspiration
  Biopsy
  Radiology (lymphangiogram/CT scanning)

- **Metastases**
  Biochemical screening (e.g. liver function tests)
  Radionuclide scans (e.g. liver, brain, bone)
  Ultrasound of liver
  Radiology (e.g. chest radiograph, CT scan of liver, brain, thorax)
  Laparoscopy
  Laparotomy

supplemented by the pathological examination of biopsied or resected specimens the suffix p is added.

Having defined the T, N and M status of the tumour, it is then possible to group patients into different stages. For example in lung cancers the stage groupings are as shown in Table 14.8.

The TNM system is increasingly being used for the majority of malignant diseases, particularly to facilitate comparisons of the results of treatments in different international centres. For certain diseases it has proved useful to define staging systems which differ from the TNM classification, as for example the Ann Arbor staging for Hodgkin's lymphoma and Duke's classification for carcinomas of the rectum.

The investigations required to define the T, N or M status of a tumour vary for different diseases. Examples are shown in the information box below.

Performance status

In addition to the anatomical assessment of tumour extent evaluated by staging procedures, it is important

Evaluation of response

With presently available therapies most methods of cancer treatment are associated with significant morbidity. It is thus essential to evaluate the response to therapy as accurately as possible and use properly defined criteria for evaluating response so as to make valid comparisons between different treatments. The concept of 'survival time', especially the traditional use of 'five year survival', places too much emphasis on cure. Since palliation is a much commoner objective in management planning, more subtle criteria are required than crude survival figures.

The terms universally accepted for evaluating treatment are defined as shown in the information box.

The term 'complete response' may or may not indicate true eradication of the tumour and for any given disease these terms can only reflect the ability to detect viable tumour.

TERMS FOR EVALUATING TREATMENT

- **Objective response**
  Any response that fulfils the criteria of complete or partial response

- **Complete response**
  Complete disappearance of all known disease in the absence of any new lesions appearing

- **Partial response**
  A reduction in size by at least 50% of the tumour in the absence of any new lesions appearing

- **No response**
  No change, or an increase or decrease of 25% in the size of the tumour in the absence of new lesions

- **Progressive disease**
  Increase in the size of the tumour by 25% or the development of any new lesions

---

PRINCIPLES OF RADIOTHERAPY

It is important that physicians should be familiar with an outline of the procedures involved when their patients are referred for this form of treatment.

Radiotherapy involves the exposure of a defined area of the body to a source of ionising radiation under carefully controlled conditions. Treatment planning involves accurate localisation of the tumour and prescription of multiple daily fractions of irradiation for a specified period of time. The biological effect of radiation depends on the amount of energy absorbed per unit mass. The unit of absorbed dose is the gray and is equivalent to 1 joule per kilogram.

Ionising radiation damages cells by interaction with nuclear DNA thus preventing the normal reproduction of that cell. As with cytotoxic drugs there is only a relative selectivity in this process, and normal (non-malignant) cells are readily damaged by radiation. For this reason radiotherapy planning must take into account the exact anatomical distribution of the tumour in order to minimise the exposure of normal tissues whilst at the same time ensuring that all of the diseased tissues are included in the treated area. Great care is taken to ensure that the patient can be accurately and reproducibly repositioned whilst radiotherapy is being undertaken.

Patients are usually treated in the supine position although the prone position may be more suitable for some abdominal and pelvic tumours. In order to immobilise the area to be treated, moulds, casts and shells are constructed for the individual patient.

With the patient comfortably positioned and the treatment area immobilised, the tumour is localised by a variety of techniques such as the placement of radio-opaque seeds in the tumour or the use of contrast media as in conventional radiography. Increasingly computed tomography is being used to assist in planning radiotherapeutic treatment, especially since CT can provide information about tumour margins in the transverse plane in which most radiotherapy is administered.

Radiotherapy localisation is usually carried out on specialised equipment known as a simulator which is designed to allow isocentric rotation and thus to simulate the exact axis distance of the treatment machine. Computers are now used to integrate the information obtained from simulators in order to select the optimum configuration, energy and variable loading of different treatment beams. This ensures that the least possible dose of radiation will be given to critical normal tissues and that a homogeneous high level of dose will be given to the tumour.

To maximise the absorbed dose within the tumour area and minimise the dose to normal tissues, treatment is given through multiple portals, for example as a four-field box technique for the pelvis, or through fields at right angles to each other with wedge filters to even the dose distribution where the beams overlap. Compensating filters are used to overcome variations in thickness of the areas to be treated through multiple ports. Since the human body is not a symmetrical cube, the routine use of these filters allows for the lack of consistent tissue thickness and ensures a more homogeneous dose distribution throughout the target.

Teletherapy

Most radiotherapy is performed with 'teletherapy' techniques, i.e. where a beam of photons is used to irradiate the tumour from outside the patient. Alternatively for specific sites, 'brachytherapy' is used whereby a source of radiation is implanted in a body cavity or within the tumour itself. Teletherapy techniques include the use of low energy ortho- or kilovoltage sources and the more widely used megavoltage sources. Low energy radiation (50–100 kVp range) is useful for treating carcinomas of the skin and lip, and orthovoltage (250–300 kVp) machines are sometimes used for the palliative treatment of bone metastases and lesions of the chest wall. However, orthovoltage machines are unsuitable for the treatment of more deep-seated tumours.

^{60}Cobalt machines and linear accelerators are the most widely used teletherapy equipment. Both of these types can be used isocentrically, i.e. the radiation source can be mounted in a gantry which can be rotated around the axis of the patient thus allowing direction of multiple beams to the centre of the target volume with great accuracy. ^{60}Cobalt machines provide a less well-defined beam of radiation than a linear accelerator. In general, ^{60}cobalt or 4MV linear accelerators are used for treating carcinomas of the head and neck and breast, 6MV linear accelerators for lymphomas and lung cancers, and high energy accelerators for some deep-seated abdominal and pelvic tumours. In addition to producing X-rays, the high energy linear accelerators can be used to produce accelerated electrons. The latter are charged particles which are absorbed within a finite range of tissue and can be useful in the treatment of superficial lesions where it is desirable to spare underlying tissues. Thus, for example, electrons may be employed (with advantage) for the treatment of some lesions of the head and neck, lymph nodes near the spinal cord, and lesions of the chest wall such as occur in breast carcinoma.

Brachytherapy

Brachytherapy is performed with sealed sources of radioactivity introduced for a few days into a body cavity or tumour, for example the insertion of ^{137}caesium into the uterus for treating carcinoma of the cervix. The advantages of brachytherapy are that a relatively high dose of radiation can be administered to a very limited volume of tissue thereby sparing any adverse effects on normal adjacent tissues. Such treatments are often supplemented by teletherapy to treat the larger volume where microscopic disease may be present.

Fractionation of dose

Radiotherapy is most frequently prescribed in daily fractions of 200 centigray (cGy) for 5 days a week where, depending on the tumour type and management plan, treatment may continue for 3–6 weeks. This fractionation of dose is used in order to increase the tumouricidal effect without increasing normal tissue damage. Many patients, particularly those treated with target volumes greater than 500 cm^3, will experience some malaise and fatigue. Nausea and anorexia are common and vomiting is a frequent problem if it is necessary to irradiate very large volumes, particularly in the upper abdomen. Acute skin reaction usually consists of mild erythema best treated by keeping the skin dry. Oral and pharyngeal mucosal reactions are common if the area receives high

radiation doses. Particular attention to oral hygiene is required and close inspection for candidiasis essential.

Radiation effects on the bone marrow may occur. Minor decreases in lymphocyte count are common and a frequent check on the peripheral blood must be made throughout treatment. Maintenance of haemoglobin is important since hypoxia may render the tumour less sensitive to radiation damage. Irradiation of the gastrointestinal tract may result in temporary dysphagia, diarrhoea, tenesmus or production of mucus per rectum.

PRINCIPLES OF CHEMOTHERAPY

During the 1940s research into the action of mustard gas showed that sulphur and nitrogen mustard could destroy dividing cells in lymph nodes and the bone marrow. The potential therapeutic benefit was explored in treating some lymphomas with nitrogen mustard, which was then developed as the first clinically useful cytotoxic drug. Study of the effects of altering folic acid metabolism in leukaemic cells resulted in the second cytotoxic drug of therapeutic value—the antifolate, methotrexate. Thereafter many naturally occurring substances were tested, resulting in some 35 effective antineoplastic drugs.

Classification of anticancer drugs

Anticancer drugs are divided into 6 main groups (Table 14.10). The site of action of each group is shown in Figure 14.6.

Antimetabolites

Methotrexate acts to inhibit folate metabolism by preventing the cell from replenishing its source of reduced folates necessary for purine and pyrimidine synthesis (p. 787). The term 'antimetabolite' is used for this group of drugs.

Alkylating agents

Nitrogen mustard is thought to destroy cells by the process of alkylation—the addition of an alkyl group to constituents of DNA, thus interfering with replication and transcription of further nucleic acid.

Plant alkaloids

These inhibit cell division by binding to tubulin and disrupting the mitotic spindle.

Antibiotics

The compounds grouped together as antibiotics include doxorubicin and actinomycin which act by intercalating

Table 14.10   Classification of anticancer drugs

Group	Examples
1. **Antimetabolites** (metabolism of substance in parenthesis is interrupted)	Methotrexate (folic acid) 6-Mercaptopurine (hypoxanthine) 6-Thioguanine (guanine) 5-Fluorouracil (uracil) Cytosine arabinoside (cytidine)
2. **Alkylating agents**	Nitrogen mustard Cyclophosphamide Chlorambucil Busulphan Melphalan Iphosphamide
3. **Plant alkaloids**	Vinblastine Vincristine Vindesine VP-16-213 VM 26
4. **Antibiotics**	Doxorubicin Daunorubicin Actinomycin D Bleomycin Mitomycin C
5. **Nitrosoureas**	BCNU CCNU Streptozotocin
6. **Miscellaneous synthetic compounds**	DTIC Cisplatin Procarbazine Hexamethylmelamine Hydroxyurea Mitozantrone

between base pairs and DNA, and bleomycin which causes breaks in both single and double-stranded DNA.

Nitrosoureas
The mechanism of action of this group probably involves alkylation.

Miscellaneous synthetic compounds
Alkylation and other metabolic lesions may be involved.

Therapeutic index
Unfortunately none of these biochemical events is confined to the metabolism of malignant cells. Systemic exposure to these cellular poisons therefore must inevitably result in some damage to normal host tissues, particularly to those which rely on rapid cell division such as the bone marrow and gastrointestinal tract. In addition to their relative lack of selectivity, anticancer drugs are very potent because they act at low concentrations. Together with a tendency towards steep dose-response curves, these factors all account for the narrow 'therapeutic index' of cytotoxic drugs (see Fig. 14.7).

The narrow therapeutic index of antineoplastic drugs means that the greatest care is required in their administration. Whenever anticancer drugs are used, it is necessary to monitor the peripheral blood count and be aware of any functional disturbances such as dysphagia or diarrhoea. Since the maximum dose of any cytotoxic drug that can be prescribed on any one occasion is governed by its toxicity to normal cells, only partial tumour shrinkage results from any single treatment. It is therefore necessary to administer these drugs repeatedly, the total duration of treatment varying from a few months to several years. To prevent damage to host tissues,

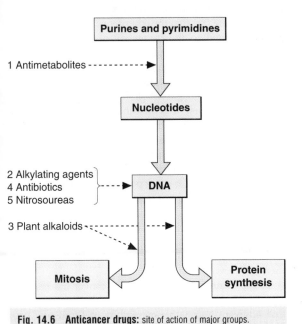

Fig. 14.6   Anticancer drugs: site of action of major groups.

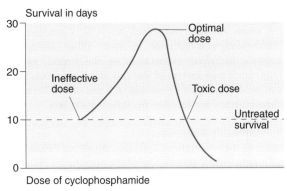

Fig. 14.7   Dose-response curve for cyclophosphamide in mice bearing the L1210 leukaemia. Too low a dose is ineffective but beyond a narrow therapeutic range too high a dose kills the animals from haematological toxicity.

Table 14.11   Choice of drug—three phases of clinical trials

Phase	Aims	Type of malignant disease
I	Determine acute toxicology Discover pharmacokinetics and pharmacodynamics	Advanced disease refractory to known chemotherapy
II	Determine range of activity	Wide variety of malignant diseases
III	Determine efficacy in particular tumour types by large-scale randomised trials	Specific malignant diseases

intermittent administration is necessary to allow host tissue to recover between treatments. Damage to bone marrow results in depression of the blood counts 10–14 days later. Thus many cytotoxic drug regimens are given on 21-day cycles to preserve bone marrow integrity.

Choice of drug

To select the most appropriate drug it is necessary to know the range of activity against disease for the various drugs, and to use those which have the minimum toxicities in relation to the particular patient. This information is obtained through a sequence of three phases of clinical trials which are shown in Table 14.11.

Combination chemotherapy

The theory behind combination chemotherapy is that simultaneous disruption of the metabolism of a tumour cell at more than one site may have far more profound effects on the cell than a single metabolic lesion. Thus for example in Hodgkin's disease, a treatment with the four-drug combination of nitrogen mustard, vincristine, procarbazine and prednisolone yields complete remissions in more than 80% of patients whereas when these same drugs were used singly they produced remissions in only 15–20% of cases. Similarly, combination chemotherapy for acute leukaemia has increased the remission rate from 20% to 90%. Combination chemotherapy is valuable in many other malignant diseases including carcinomas of the breast, ovary, lung, testis and several of the childhood tumours. The five general principles governing the use of combination chemotherapy are listed in the information box.

Multimodality treatment

Since in many situations cytotoxic drugs are capable of shrinking only a proportion of the tumour, increasing attention has been paid to the use of chemotherapy in conjunction with surgery or radiotherapy. Thus chemotherapy can be used to reduce tumour bulk prior to local therapy with surgery or radiotherapy, as for example in treating head and neck tumours, or drug treatment can be introduced after primary resection or irradiation to

GENERAL PRINCIPLES OF COMBINATION CHEMOTHERAPY

- Each drug in the combination should have been demonstrated to have some activity on its own against the tumour type for which the combination is being used
- Drugs with a similar mechanism of action should not be combined
- As far as is possible the major dose-limiting toxicity of each drug should differ from that of the other components of the combination
- Since it is rarely possible to avoid some overlap in toxicity to host tissues, it is usually necessary to reduce the dose of each of the component drugs compared with the optimal dose which would be used if the drugs were prescribed individually
- There should be no known adverse interaction between the drugs

prevent the growth of subclinical micrometastases. The latter use of chemotherapy is frequently referred to as 'adjuvant' chemotherapy, and is now widely used for treating breast carcinomas, lymphomas, and several tumours in children.

Caution must be exercised to prevent additive damage to host tissues, particularly to bone marrow if the radiotherapy and chemotherapy are used together, but the principle of combining local and systemic therapy has many potential advantages since as a general principle small tumours are much more susceptible to chemotherapy than large ones. This is explained in part by the fact that drugs penetrate small tumours more effectively but also by the fact that the emergence of drug resistance may be related to the frequency of mutations in the tumour, and the potential number of such events increases with the growth of a tumour.

One major difficulty with adjuvant chemotherapy is to decide for how long it should be continued. In obvious advanced tumours, it is possible to measure tumour shrinkage and continue treatment for as long as benefit lasts. Conversely drug resistance is detectable and thus further inappropriate chemotherapy can be avoided. However, in the 'adjuvant' setting where there is no measurable tumour, it is not possible to be certain in the short term whether or not treatment is proving effective. Clinical trials have demonstrated that, for curable tumours in children, it is necessary to continue chemotherapy for 1–2 years. For lymphomas and carcinomas in adults, the optimum duration of adjuvant chemotherapy is less certain.

Of the common tumours, breast cancer has been researched in the greatest detail and it is now accepted that adjuvant chemotherapy results in significant prolongation both of disease-free and overall survival, especially for premenopausal women where tumours do not contain oestrogen receptors (see below). The most widely used adjuvant treatment is a combination of cyclophosphamide, methotrexate and 5-fluorouracil (CMF) administered for 6 months after primary surgery.

The problem of drug resistance continues to be the subject of major attention for cancer research workers. Distinction is made between 'intrinsic' and 'acquired' drug resistance. The former is typified by malignant melanoma or renal cell cancer, where currently available drugs have little or no effect on cancer growth. Conversely, 'acquired' resistance is exemplified by small cell lung cancer—a disease that is initially highly sensitive to a range of cytotoxic drugs, but where drug resistant clones of cells eventually emerge and the disease recurs. Many biological factors contribute to the development of acquired drug resistance but one major process that has been revealed involves the enhanced production of a glycoprotein termed p180. This normally occurring transmembrane protein can be produced in greatly enhanced quantity by genetic amplification as a cancer cell reacts to the presence of a perceived poison (a cytotoxic drug). p180 acts as a transport pump which extrudes drug from within the cell, thereby rescuing itself from cytotoxic damage. This form of drug resistance is seen in response to several classes of anticancer drug, e.g. doxorubicin, the vinca alkaloids and the epipodophylotoxins. Research is now focused on finding ways to block the amplification of p180 and thereby prevent the emergence of this type of drug resistance.

It is possible to rank many malignant diseases into groups comprising those for which chemotherapy contributes to cure, those for which effective control prolongs useful life and those for which benefit is less certain or unproven. These are listed in the information box.

Side-effects of chemotherapy

Due to the relatively poor selectivity of presently available anticancer drugs, it is impossible to avoid some damage to normal host tissues, resulting in a variety of side-effects. Table 14.12 illustrates one representative study of side-effects. Nevertheless, when properly administered and monitored, many cytotoxic drugs can be given without producing symptomatic side-effects. For example, the effect on the bone marrow should not cause significant symptoms provided adequate time is allowed between cycles of treatment and the blood count is monitored prior to subsequent treatment.

Mouth ulceration and diarrhoea result from necrosis of the rapidly dividing epithelial cells lining the gut. Appropriate timing of chemotherapy can prevent this but sometimes it is necessary to adjust the dose of the drug if an individual is particularly sensitive. For many

---

CONTRIBUTION OF CHEMOTHERAPY TO MANAGEMENT OF VARIOUS MALIGNANT DISEASES

Tumours for which chemotherapy can be curative
- Acute lymphoblastic leukaemia in children
- Burkitt's lymphoma
- Hodgkin's lymphoma
- Wilms' tumour
- Rhabdomyosarcoma
- Testicular teratoma
- Choriocarcinoma
- Diffuse histiocytic lymphoma
- Ewing's sarcoma

Tumours highly sensitive to chemotherapy— remissions prolong life
- Breast carcinoma
- Ovarian carcinoma
- Small cell anaplastic lung carcinoma
- Non-Hodgkin's lymphoma
- Chronic lymphocytic leukaemia
- Acute myeloid leukaemia
- Medulloblastoma

Tumours sensitive to chemotherapy—life sometimes prolonged
- Gastric carcinoma
- Pancreatic carcinoma
- Myeloma
- Soft tissue sarcoma
- Bladder carcinoma
- Anaplastic thyroid carcinoma

Tumours refractory to available chemotherapy
- Squamous cell lung carcinoma
- Colorectal carcinoma
- Carcinoma of the oesophagus
- Melanoma

Table 14.12   Rank order of the distressing side-effects of chemotherapy*

Symptom	Rank
Being sick (vomiting)	1
Feeling sick (nausea)	2
Loss of hair	3
Thought of coming for treatment	4
Length of time treatment takes at clinic	5
Having to have a needle	6
Shortness of breath	7
Constantly tired	8
Difficulty sleeping	9
Affects family or partner	10
Affects work/home duties	11
Trouble finding somewhere to park	12
Feeling anxious or tense	13
Feeling low, miserable (depression)	14
Loss of weight	14

(* from Coates et al 1983—see Further Reading)

patients the worst side-effect of chemotherapy (and sometimes radiotherapy) is emesis—nausea and/or vomiting. The events leading to nausea and vomiting almost certainly include a direct central nervous system response to many cytotoxic drugs. Recent research has identified the importance of receptors for 5-hydroxy-tryptamine (5HT) in the small bowel and in the brain, which are triggered by the presence of some chemo-therapeutic drugs, e.g. cisplatinum. Stimulation of these receptors results in a release of 5HT in the brain which in turn triggers the vomiting centre and causes emesis. Development of highly selective $5HT_3$ receptor antagonists has resulted in a new generation of effective antiemetics. For the cytotoxic drugs which are known to cause nausea and vomiting, it is necessary to prescribe antiemetics prior to and following administration of the cytotoxic drug.

Nausea and vomiting

Not all cytotoxic drugs cause emesis, and individuals vary considerably in the degree to which they experience the problem. As illustrated in Table 14.13 cisplatinum and other platinum–containing compounds are the most emetogenic of all cytotoxic drugs and hence prophylaxis is necessary. Nausea may persist for 5–7 days after starting therapy, and therefore antiemetic treatment must be continued for this period. For most patients given platinum the combination of ondansetron or granisetron and dexamethasone affords the best antiemetic treatment (Table 14.14).

Cytotoxic drugs such as the alkylating agents cyclo-phosphamide, iphosphamide and nitrogen mustard cause emesis of less severity and shorter duration. Antiemetic therapy should however be administered, and as with platinum therapy it is important to administer the antiemetic prior to the cytotoxic treatment, since prevention is very much more successful than trying to stop nausea and/or vomiting once they have started. For these alkylating agents and for the widely used anthracycline doxorubicin, dexamethasone, metoclopramide, lorazepam, prochlorperazine or domperidone are usually successful in abolishing emesis. Recommended doses of these antiemetics are given in Table 14.14. There is increasing use of antiemetics in combinations of two or more drugs.

Alopecia

Alopecia is associated with the administration of some cytotoxic drugs, particularly doxorubicin and cyclo-phosphamide. If such drugs are prescribed, it is important to warn the patient in advance and, if appropriate, to arrange for a wig to be fitted. Alopecia is almost always reversible on cessation of therapy.

Psychological effects

The psychological effect of chemotherapy over a period of many months is one which the physician must be aware of. If properly counselled, many patients tolerate being informed of their diagnosis and also their early treatment remarkably well, only to become anxious and depressed as treatment continues even though their tumour may be obviously responding. Awareness of this is essential and constant reassurance and support are necessary.

Growth

The chronic toxicity of cancer chemotherapy is important now that increasing numbers of patients are surviving for longer periods. Data from the follow-up of children cured of malignant disease have shown that physical growth can be stunted by the use of combinations of cytotoxic drugs with radiation but there is conflicting evidence as to whether or not these agents cause significant intellectual impairment.

Fertility

This is preserved for the majority of prepubertal children treated with cytotoxic drugs but for adults fertility may be lost. This is particularly the case for men. For women the problem is more variable depending on their premorbid menstrual pattern and the length of time prior to the expected menopause. Many patients suffering from malignant diseases may be subfertile at the time of diagnosis and amenorrhoea is common for the months during which women are receiving treatment. Nevertheless, this is not a universal finding and since cytotoxic drugs are potentially teratogenic, patients of both sexes should be advised to use contraceptive measures whilst they are receiving chemotherapy.

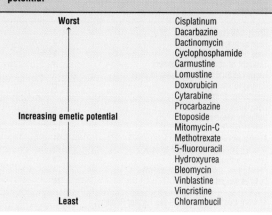

Table 14.13 Common cytotoxic drugs in rank order of emetic potential

Worst	Cisplatinum
	Dacarbazine
	Dactinomycin
	Cyclophosphamide
	Carmustine
	Lomustine
	Doxorubicin
	Cytarabine
	Procarbazine
Increasing emetic potential	Etoposide
	Mitomycin-C
	Methotrexate
	5-fluorouracil
	Hydroxyurea
	Bleomycin
	Vinblastine
	Vincristine
Least	Chlorambucil

Table 14.14 Commonly used antiemetic regimes

Cytotoxic drug	Antiemetic	Dose-regime
Cisplatinum	Ondansetron Dexamethasone	8 mg i.v. 12-hourly or 8-hourly 16 mg in 20 ml normal saline given i.v. over 10–15 minutes at time of cisplatinum administration
Cyclophosphamide, Iphosphamide	Dexamethasone	As above
Nitrogen Mustard, DTIC	Lorazepam	2–4 mg i.v. every four hours
Doxorubicin	Domperidone	10–20 mg orally or by suppository every 4–8 hours

It is now established that children who receive curative treatment for cancer may successfully produce children of their own in adult life. The number of successful pregnancies in this situation is only approximately half that of the normal population, but the frequency of congenital malformations amongst second generation children is no greater than that expected.

Second malignancy

Cytotoxic drugs may be associated with the eventual development of a second malignancy in a small proportion of patients. The cases have usually been of acute myelomonocytic leukaemia developing 5–10 years following the use of alkylating agents. In a study of over 5000 cases of ovarian cancer treated with alkylating agents, it was shown that the risk of developing acute leukaemia was 36 times that of the normal population. However, only certain classes of anticancer drug are associated with this rare phenomenon, which has arisen only as a result of developing therapies which may cure the primary tumour.

PRINCIPLES OF ENDOCRINE THERAPY

Tumours which develop in organs that are known to be under hormonal control sometimes retain hormonal dependency. This can be used therapeutically either by withdrawing the source of the hormone, by prescribing an anti-hormone or by the administration of another hormone. Carcinomas of the breast, prostate, endometrium and thyroid are the diseases currently amenable to endocrine therapy. The therapeutic use of adrenal corticosteroids is exceptional in that these compounds influence non-endocrine-related tumours, e.g. the lymphomas and leukaemias.

The biological effect of hormones such as oestrogen and progesterone is dependent on the hormone binding to a cytoplasmic receptor protein that transports the hormone to the nucleus where it interacts with DNA to modulate gene expression. Oestrogen receptors can be assayed in biopsies of breast tumours or lymph nodes containing metastases. It has been found that for about 65% of patients whose tumours possess a significant amount of this receptor protein, removal of the source of oestrogen will be therapeutically useful whilst for those in whom this protein is absent, hormonal therapy is usually of no benefit. The presence of progesterone-receptor further increases the likelihood of hormone sensitivity. The development of techniques to predict hormone sensitivity has had a major influence on the management of patients with breast carcinomas. If oestrogen receptor activity is present, then premenopausal patients may benefit from oophorectomy and both pre- and postmenopausal patients may respond to the administration of tamoxifen, a compound that blocks oestrogen binding.

The use of ablative procedures such as adrenalectomy has now been superseded by the availability of aminoglutethimide, which achieves the same result by 'medical' rather than surgical means. In order to prevent excess secretion of ACTH (as a result of the failure to produce the 11-hydroxycorticosteroids), it is necessary to prescribe glucocorticoid together with aminoglutethimide. Tumour response to tamoxifen and aminoglutethamide may not be manifest for 6–12 weeks from the start of therapy and it is therefore necessary to wait for this period before making decisions about further management.

Oestrogens are useful in the palliation of prostate cancer, but have significant risks and have a similar response rate (c.80%) to that of orchidectomy which removes the major source of testosterone.

A class of endocrine compounds has recently been introduced into clinical practice which are long-acting agonists of luteinising hormone releasing hormone (LHRH). By down-regulating receptors on pituitary gonadotrophs these substances have the potential to suppress gonadal activity on a temporary basis and by a potentially reversible mechanism. This is not associated with the side-effects of direct suppression achieved with the use of oestrogens or androgens. The two malignant conditions in which LHRH agonists have been evaluated most thoroughly are the treatment of breast and prostatic cancer. For premenopausal women with hormonally sensitive breast cancer (oestrogen receptor positive) LHRH antagonists offer a medical alternative to the surgical removal of the ovaries or a permanent menopause induced by radiation. Clinical trials of the agonist leuprolide given as a subcutaneous injection of 1 mg show that it provides sustained suppression of plasma oestradiol. An alternative is administration of nasal spray preparations such as buserelin which has to be given 6 times daily. Although medical oophorectomy is achieved by this means the relatively low morbidity and cost of ovariectomy considered together with the fact that breast cancer, even in pre-menopausal women, frequently occurs beyond the time at which women will wish to have further children, suggests that surgery may be preferable for some patients.

For the management of prostate cancer it has been shown that daily subcutaneous injections of leuprolide produce marked suppression of testosterone. This provides a potential medical alternative to surgical castration.

Progestogens are compounds related to the progesterone produced by the corpus luteum and placenta. Some women with metastatic endometrial carcinoma may benefit from these drugs, particularly patients with well differentiated tumours.

Papillary carcinomas of the thyroid remain under the influence of thyroid-stimulating hormone (TSH) and the administration of thyroid hormone may be useful as a result of its inhibiting pituitary secretion of TSH. Initial treatment of these tumours is surgical, with total thyroidectomy followed by ablation dose of radioactive iodine to remove any residual normal thyroid. The patient is then established on thyroid hormone replacement therapy and serum thyroglobulin levels used to monitor progress.

The major advantage of hormonal therapy over chemotherapy is that the side-effects of endocrine treatment are usually less severe than those associated with cytotoxic drugs. Tamoxifen rarely causes acute toxicity but aminoglutethimide can cause drowsiness, depression and transient rashes in some patients. The use of oestrogen in elderly men with prostate cancer warrants special caution in view of its known propensity to exacerbate the fluid retention that may be associated with cardiovascular disease and the increased incidence of thromboembolic disease.

MANAGEMENT OF PAIN

Pain is relatively rare as a presenting symptom of early or localised malignant disease, but patients often associate the diagnosis of cancer as leading inevitably to severe and intractable pain, and many need reassurance that such a situation is both rare and preventable. However, advanced cancer is frequently associated with some degree of pain and its management forms an essential part of palliative medicine.

Accurate definition of the site and cause of pain

This is essential before deciding on therapy; for example, bone pain as caused by myeloma or metastases from tumours such as breast cancer often has two components—a background of diffuse aching pain unrelated to activity, and localised intensive pain triggered by touch or weight bearing. Abdominal colic is typically of sudden, intermittent type, whereas headache arising from raised intracranial pressure tends to be more constant. Musculo-skeletal and joint pains are usually localised, as are the consequences of nerve entrapment such as can result from tumour infiltration (for example of the brachial plexus), or collapsed vertebrae secondary to bone metastases.

Assessment of the severity of pain

This should be recorded in the patients' notes so that the results of analgesic therapy can be *regularly reviewed*. Several grading systems are used, such as the one shown in the information box below.

SCALE FOR GRADING PAIN

- Grade 1: Pain relieved by occasional mild analgesics
- Grade 2: Pain requiring regular mild analgesics
- Grade 3: Pain requiring regular medium strength analgesics
- Grade 4: Pain requiring regular strong analgesics
- Grade 5: Pain not controlled by regular strong analgesics

Only 10–15% of patients with cancer fall into the category of grade 4 or 5. It cannot be over-emphasised that successful pain control requires not only the selection of the analgesic most appropriate to the particular cause of painful stimulus, but the *regular* administration of therapy to constantly suppress pain and prevent its re-emergence. As indicated in the above grading of pain, analgesics can be classified as mild, medium or strong in terms of their effect.

Relief of pain

Mild analgesics

Widely used mild analgesics include paracetamol, aspirin, dextropropoxyphene, and flurbiprofen. Nonsteroidal anti-inflammatory drugs (NSAIDs) such as

Table 14.15   Mild and medium strength analgesics

Mild	Dose	Side-effects
Paracetamol	1 g 4-hourly	Hepatotoxic (rare)
Aspirin (with codeine)	300–600 mg (with 8–16 mg codeine) 4-hourly	Gastritis
Dextropropoxyphene	65–130 mg 6-hourly See BNF for details	Constipation, sedation
NSAIDs		Gastritis
Medium	**Dose**	**Side-effects**
Dihydrocodeine	30–60 mg 4-hourly	Constipation, sedation
Dipipanone (with cyclizine)	10 mg ⎱ 6-hourly 30 mg ⎰	Sedation

flurbiprofen are particularly useful for pain arising in bone—a frequent site of metastases.

Medium strength analgesics

Dihydrocodeine and dipipanone are useful as medium strength analgesics. Dihydrocodeine is the most commonly used of these and is well tolerated apart from causing constipation. Co-proxamol (dextropropoxyphene and paracetamol) is equally effective and may be preferred since constipation is less of a problem. Dipipanone is stronger than dihydrocodeine and provides useful analgesia for grade 3 symptoms. Examples of doses of mild and medium strength analgesics are given in Table 14.15.

Strong analgesics

Dextromoramide, morphine and diamorphine are the most widely used potent analgesics. Dextromoramide is limited by short duration of action (approximately 2 hours) but for the same reason is valuable for 'breakthrough' pain that may occur occasionally when a patient is on long-term opiates. Morphine and diamorphine play an essential role in the management of severe chronic pain, but these substances are all too often prescribed in sub-optimal ways. Two common mistakes are the overcautious prescription for fear of inducing addiction, and prescribing 'cocktails' containing substances such as cocaine and chlorpromazine (e.g. Brompton's mixture). Addiction is irrelevant in the management of severe pain in advanced malignancy, and the stimulant or sedative effects of cocaine or chlorpromazine can induce confusion, anxiety and emotional distress. There is little to choose between morphine and diamorphine, but the availability of slow release oral morphine is useful for ambulant patients, and the greater solubility of diamorphine can be useful in reducing the volume of parenteral injection. MST Continus tablets contain morphine in different strengths (10, 30, 60 and

100 mg), and are formulated to provide slow release for up to 12 hours. For these and standard formulations of morphine and diamorphine the dose must be titrated to the needs of the individual patient. For oral administration of standard preparations the dose must be repeated every 4 hours and dosage will vary from 20–100 mg or more. Intravenous administration of high dose may be appropriate for hospitalised patients, but the introduction of highly accurate slow-release pumps has enabled opiates to be given by continuous subcutaneous administration. The two major advantages of this are that these portable devices allow patients to remain ambulant, and that even very large doses can be given without causing significant central nervous system depression resulting in lethargy and confusion. Constipation is an inevitable consequence of prolonged administration of opiates and patients requiring these should always be given regular laxatives at the same time. Stool softeners such as dioctyl sodium sulphosuccinate and compounds that stimulate peristalsis such as bisacodyl are appropriate to ease constipation.

Localised techniques for pain relief

In addition to systemic analgesics, there are a number of localised techniques that may prove useful for the management of severe, intractable pain. These include the injection of anaesthetics, neurosurgical ablation and transcutaneous electrical nerve stimulation (TENS). The principal advantage of such techniques is to spare the systemic effects of strong analgesics (drowsiness, constipation, etc.) but this has to be balanced with the morbidity of the procedure. The use of anaesthetics includes a wide range of procedures where techniques now exist to target most major divisions of the nervous system. A relatively widely used technique is that of spinal opioid administration including epidural, intrathecal or subarachnoid administration of opioids. Spinal opioids are particularly appropriate for patients with deep constant somatic pain, but intermittent somatic pain (for example that caused by a pathological fracture) may also respond.

Neurosurgical procedures have become less widely used with improvements in analgesic medication, and ablative procedures should only be used when pharmacological pain therapies have failed. Ablative procedures include peripheral neurectomy, sympathectomy, cordotomy and hypophysectomy.

Electrical nerve stimulation (TENS) is used in several forms—for example, continuous, pulsed or acupuncture-like. The types of pain for which TENS may have particular use include predominantly nociceptive pain—for example, pain from metastatic bone disease or abdominal pain from hepatomegaly — and neuropathic pain due to compression of a nerve, for example a lumbar nerve compressed by a retroperitoneal tumour.

TERMINAL CARE

An essential component of oncological medicine is the management of patients in the terminal phase of their illness. Psychological support is the most important aspect but this can be provided only if positive measures are taken to relieve pain, to ensure adequate and appropriate nutrition and treat specific symptoms such as cough, pruritus and nausea. Successful symptomatic treatment allows patients to prepare themselves mentally for death, and the relief of physical distress will also help the patient's family to cope with impending bereavement.

An individual patient's reaction to the inevitability of death from a malignant disease depends on a host of interrelated variables including his or her cultural and religious background, age, education, the duration of the illness and the reactions of dependants. Nevertheless certain common patterns of behaviour are recognisable. A period of initial disbelief and denial is often replaced by a period of depression which is almost universal but many patients, with or without medical intervention, enter a final phase of peacefully accepting the inevitability of death.

When to tell patients that they have a terminal illness is a matter of experience. Death does not necessarily represent a failure of treatment and it is essential that those caring for the terminally ill do not avoid discussion of the processes of terminal illness. Such avoidance can only enhance the patient's sense of loneliness and isolation.

It is not always appropriate to present all of the facts to a patient, most especially on a single occasion, and time must be spent to determine patients' awareness of their situation, and their expectations. Non-committal, even ambiguous statements about the future may be appropriate but the patient should never be told what is known to be untrue.

Preparation for death is not the sole responsibility of the medical profession and, especially for patients dying in hospital, it is important to make provision for the adequate access of relatives, friends and other professionals such as the clergy when patients request their support. Religious belief does not necessarily make death any easier and even for patients who hold such beliefs it should not be forgotten that fear of the unknown is something shared by patients and all those who are caring for them.

The most important principle of managing terminal illness is to provide adequate time for talking with the patient. In a busy world this is difficult and it is sometimes easier to use the lack of time as an excuse for avoiding demanding consultations that drain the doctor's emotional resources. Nevertheless, to develop the ability to listen to patients and to learn from them how best to provide psychological support during terminal illness can be one of the most rewarding experiences in medicine.

FURTHER READING

Chabner B 1982 Pharmacologic Principles of Cancer Treatment. Saunders, Philadelphia. A detailed account both preclinical and clinical

Coates A, Abraham S, Kaye S B et al 1983 On the receiving end: patient perception of the side-effects of cancer chemotherapy. European Journal of Cancer and Clinical Oncology 19/2: 203–208

De Vita V T, Hellman S, Rosenburg S A 1993 Cancer, Principles and Practice of Oncology, 4th edn. J P Lippincott Co., Philadelphia

Doyle D, Hanks G, Macdonald N 1993 Oxford Textbook of Palliative Medicine. Oxford University Press, Oxford

Tobias J S 1992 Clinical practice of radiotherapy. Lancet 339: 159–163

Withers H R 1992 Biological basis of radiation therapy. Lancet 339: 156–159

Diseases of the connective tissues, joints and bones

The Rheumatic Diseases comprise a heterogeneous group of disorders of connective tissue, joints and bones in which musculoskeletal pain and stiffness are prominent.

PREVALENCE

Rheumatic diseases affect people of all ages and ethnic groups. Their frequency increases with age and as many as 40% of persons over the age of 65 years in the UK have had some kind of rheumatic disorder. In Britain 20 million people experience a rheumatic complaint each year. Five million suffer from osteoarthritis, 500 000 have rheumatoid arthritis and there are 12 000 children with juvenile chronic arthritis. Rheumatic complaints account for 20–25% of all consultations in general practice and 15% of all those on a GP's list in the UK consult their doctor each year with a musculoskeletal problem (Fig. 15.1). In Europe rheumatic diseases are the commonest cause of physical impairment in the community and about a third of all people with physical disabilities have a rheumatic disease as the primary cause of their disability. In the UK about a quarter of a million people are severely disabled by a rheumatic disease. No other group of disorders is responsible for greater loss of earnings, and the cost to the United States economy attributed to the musculoskeletal disorders is more than 20 billion dollars per annum.

CLASSIFICATION

The World Health Organization (WHO) classifies common rheumatic complaints under four headings:

- Back pain
- Regional periarticular or 'soft tissue' disorders
- Osteoarthritis and related disorders
- Inflammatory arthropathies.

A more detailed classification of diseases of joints, connective tissue and bones is given in the information box.

BACK DISORDERS

LOW BACK PAIN

Non-specific low back pain of mechanical origin is second only to the common cold as a cause of self-limiting symptoms and disability in the community.

CLASSIFICATION OF RHEUMATIC DISEASES

- **Inflammatory joint diseases**
  Rheumatoid arthritis
  Ankylosing spondylitis
  Reiter's disease
  Psoriatic arthritis
  Enteropathic arthropathy
  Juvenile chronic arthritis
  Behçet's syndrome
  Whipple's disease
- **Infectious arthritis**
  Bacterial
  Viral
  Fungal
- **Connective tissue diseases**
  Systemic lupus erythematosus
  Mixed connective tissue disease
  Progressive systemic sclerosis
  Polymyositis
  Polyarteritis nodosa
  Churg–Strauss vasculitis
  Wegener's granulomatosis
  Giant cell arteritis
  Takayasu's disease
- **Crystal deposition diseases**
  Gout
  Chondrocalcinosis
- **Osteoarthrosis**
- **Soft tissue rheumatism**
- **Miscellaneous**
- **Disorders of bone**

Epidemiology

It has been calculated that more than three-quarters of the world's population experience back pain at some time in their lives and in developed Western countries low back pain is the commonest cause of sickness-related absence from work. In the United Kingdom approximately 10% of people who suffer episodes of low back pain consult their general practitioner annually. This results in more than 2 million consultations and more than 50 million days lost from work each year. In the USA the annual cost of low back pain, including direct medical costs, work-related sickness payments, time lost from work and related litigation approaches 30 billion dollars.

More than 90% of episodes of low back pain are of mechanical origin and most resolve spontaneously within 1–2 weeks. In about 30% of patients episodes can last as long as a month but chronic low back pain of more than 3 months' duration accounts for less than 3% of all cases.

Mechanical low back pain is particularly associated with occupations that involve heavy lifting, bending or twisting such as manual labouring or nursing but people whose jobs involve awkward static posture or prolonged driving are also at increased risk. Episodes of occupationally related low back pain are twice as common in adults over the age of 40 years. The overall prevalence is similar in both sexes but recurrences are commoner in men (20% in one year). Job dissatisfaction, depression,

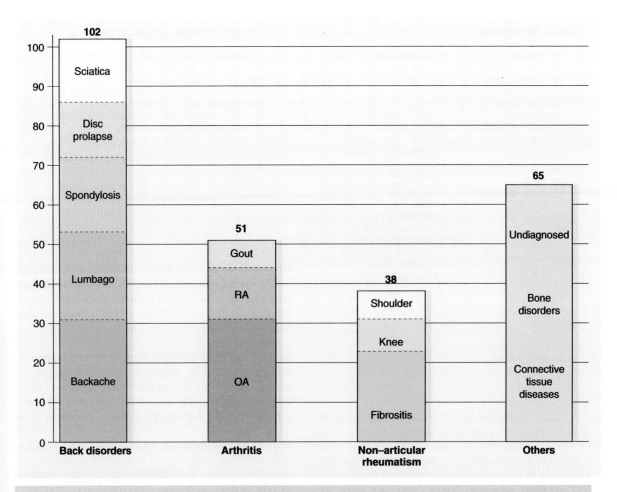

Fig. 15.1   Rheumatic complaints in an Edinburgh general practice. Annual number of patient consultations/2500 population. Total 256 = 10% of all patients registered.

obesity, smoking, alcohol and socio-economic deprivation have also been implicated as risk factors.

Aetiology
The common type of short-lived mechanical low back pain is not associated with a definable aetiology or spinal pathology. The causes of rarer but more serious chronic back pain are listed in the information box (p. 866).

Clinical features
Mechanical low back pain is characteristically acute in onset and frequently associated with a definite history of lifting or bending. Radiation of pain to the thighs can be associated with sprains of muscles, ligaments and apophyseal joints as well as with nerve root irritation. However, pain which radiates down the back of the leg beyond the knee and pain which is aggravated by coughing, sneezing and straining at stool is usually associated with disc protrusion or other causes of nerve root compression. Radicular pain is frequently sharp and lancinating in quality and associated with signs of lumbar nerve root compression (Table 18.62, p. 1105). Other medical and systemic causes of low back pain are usually more insidious in onset, more prolonged in duration and not so obviously influenced by posture and movement. Back pain due to sacroiliitis or spondylitis is uniquely ameliorated by physical activity and exercise as well as being associated with prolonged early morning and inactivity stiffness (see p. 905).

Systematic enquiry may give important clues to rarer causes of back pain. Anorexia, weight loss or dyspepsia may point to a penetrating peptic ulcer, gastric or pancreatic tumour, while changes in bowel habit, prostatism or gynaecological symptoms can be clues to colon cancer, prostatic metastases, endometriosis or uterine/ovarian malignancies.

CAUSES OF BACK PAIN

- **Mechanical**
  Prolapsed intervertebral disc
  Lumbar spondylosis
  Spondylolysis/
  spondylolisthesis
  Spinal stenosis
  Congenital abnormalities
  Non-specific

- **Inflammatory**
  Infections
  Sacroiliitis
  Ankylosing spondylitis
  Arachnoiditis

- **Metabolic**
  Osteoporosis
  Osteomalacia
  Hyperparathyroidism
  Renal osteodystrophy
  Paget's Disease

- **Neoplastic**
  Metastases
  Myeloma
  Reticuloses
  Osteoid osteoma
  Intrathecal tumours

- **Referred pain**
  Peptic ulcer
  Pancreas
  Bowel
  Kidney
  Aortic aneurysm
  Endometriosis
  Ovary
  Retroperitoneal fibrosis
  Herpes zoster
  Hip disease
  Polymyalgia rheumatica

- **Other**
  Scheuermann's
    osteochondritis
  Diffuse idiopathic
    skeletal hyperostosis
    (DISH)
  Fibromyalgia

TESTS FOR FUNCTIONAL LOW BACK PAIN*

- Tenderness to superficial touch
- Simulation tests, e.g. pain on axial loading or spinal rotation in one plane
- Distraction tests, e.g. limited straight leg raising but able to sit with legs flexed to 90°
- Regional inconsistencies, e.g. symptoms and sensory loss that fail to follow neuroanatomy
- Overreaction to examination with illness behaviour.

3/5 positive tests strongly suggest a non-organic cause for symptoms.

* After Waddell G 1982 An approach to backache. British Journal of Hospital Medicine 28: 187–219

A history of intermittent claudication may be an indication of severe peripheral vascular disease, spinal stenosis or lateral canal stenosis.

Social and psychiatric assessment are also important as primary and secondary illness behaviour are relatively frequent in patients with chronic low back pain, particularly when litigation or insurance claims are pending.

Local tenderness over the spine, loss of lumbar lordosis and postural changes associated with muscle spasm and an uncompensated non-structural scoliosis are common physical signs associated with all causes of mechanical low back pain. Disc prolapse and other causes of nerve root compression can frequently be established by careful neurological assessment and the diagnosis of early sacroiliitis and spondylitis may be entirely dependent on physical assessment (p. 905) in the early stages.

Clinical tests that help to identify individuals with functional, non-organic back pain are shown in the information box.

Investigations

Blood tests are rarely helpful in patients with acute low back pain. A low haemoglobin and raised CRP or ESR may augment a clinical suspicion of inflammation or malignancy. A raised acid phosphatase or prostate specific antigen (PSA) is associated with metastatic carcinoma of the prostate and raised alkaline phosphatase with other bone metastases and Paget's disease. Myelomatosis is associated with a monoclonal band on immunoelectrophoresis and the presence of urine light chains (Bence–Jones proteinuria).

Plain radiographs are indicated in all patients whose pain has not resolved spontaneously within one month, but are only of clear diagnostic value in a minority of patients with sacroiliitis, ankylosing spondylitis, Paget's disease, lytic or sclerotic metastases, myelomatosis, osteoporotic crush fractures or spinal infections. Disc degeneration can be associated with loss of disc height and gas formation in the nucleus pulposus as well as with vertebral sclerosis and osteophyte formation but radiological signs of lumbar spondylosis are common in middle-aged and elderly people in the absence of symptoms. Minor congenital abnormalities such as spina bifida occulta and transitional vertebrae are not associated with low back pain. Bone scintigraphy with ^{99m}Tc bisphosphonate is the imaging technique of choice for detecting the presence and extent of metastases and Paget's disease, and can also be useful for the identification of fractures and bone infection when plain radiographs are negative. Magnetic resonance imaging is rapidly becoming the imaging modality of choice for defining most difficult spinal pathology where surgery is being considered (Fig. 15.2). Computed tomography is however superior for detection of subtle abnormalities of the bony architecture of the spine and sacroiliac joints in patients with back pain and normal plain radiographs. Myelography (Fig. 15.3) and CT myelography are particularly useful for the pre-operative assessment of the site of tumours, disc herniation and nerve root entrapment and are also employed when MRI is contraindicated because of the presence of a cardiac pacemaker or ferromagnetic clips. EMG and nerve conduction studies with or without measurement of

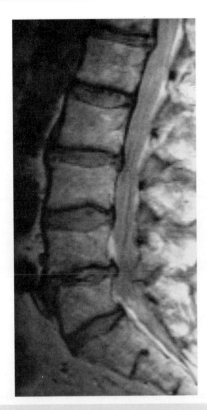

Fig. 15.2 Prolapsed L4/5 lumbar intervertebral disc.
Sagittal MRI shows loss of disc height with anterior and posterior disc protrusion.

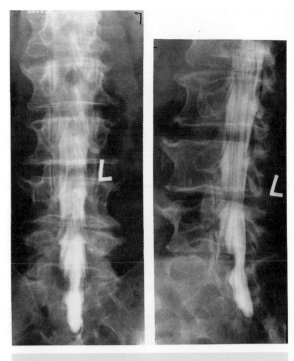

Fig. 15.3 Prolapsed L5/S1 lumbar intervertebral disc.
Myelogram showing nerve root obliteration and cord compression.

somatosensory evoked responses are occasionally required to confirm the localisation of nerve root lesions.

Even the most sophisticated investigation techniques seldom reveal treatable new pathology in patients with chronic low back pain of more than a year's duration.

Management

Most episodes of mechanical low back pain settle spontaneously in 1–2 weeks with nothing more than 1–2 days' bed rest on a firm mattress, explanation, reassurance and simple analgesics. Short-term home help or nursing services may be required and mobilisation can be facilitated by provision of a temporary lumbar corset and/or exercise physiotherapy. The McKenzie technique of passive extension and postural correction can speed up return to work, as can manipulation in some cases.

Chiropractic manipulation has also been shown to be superior to hydrotherapy and traction in patients with chronic low back pain but controlled clinical trials have failed to show that treatment with short wave diathermy, ultrasound, acupuncture or transcutaneous nerve stimulation (TENS) have anything more than a placebo effect.

Epidural corticosteroid injections are occasionally used in patients with nerve root compression that has failed to respond to more conservative treatment and facet joint injections of steroid and/or local anaesthetic are sometimes used under fluoroscopic control in patients with apophyseal joint pathology simulating nerve root irritation, but the efficacy of such injections remains uncertain.

Intractable low back pain may be helped by the judicious use of tricyclic antidepressants to augment analgesia or relieve depression while psychological counselling and social support are indicated in selected cases. Surgery is required in less than 1% of patients with low back pain.

LUMBAR SPONDYLOSIS

Degenerative changes in the discs and lumbar spine are almost universal in the elderly.

Aetiology

Disc degeneration is age-related and starts in the third decade. Reduction in the molecular size of the proteoglycans of the nucleus pulposus is associated with loss of viscoelastic properties. Increased load bearing by the annulus is followed by focal damage and disc herniation in some cases (Fig. 15.4). Simultaneously

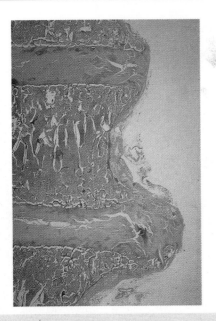

Fig. 15.4 Lumbar spondylosis. Low-power cross-section of vertebral column showing disc degeneration and osteophytosis.

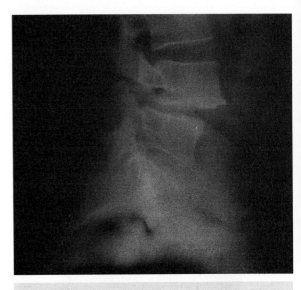

Fig. 15.5 Spondylolytic spondylolisthesis. Lateral radiograph showing L4/5 spondylolisthesis with defect in posterior element (spondylolysis).

the development of osteoarthritic changes in the spinal apophyseal joints leads to increases in sheer stress and disc damage with cleft formation and osteophyte formation around the vertebral margins. The combination of disc prolapse and osteophytosis can result in direct nerve root compression and indirect ischaemic neuronal damage.

Clinical features

Advanced lumbar spondylosis is frequently associated with low back pain but the clinical features are very variable and there is a poor correlation between symptoms and radiographic changes. Postural low back pain is often provoked by prolonged sitting, standing, bending or lifting. Acute episodes with symptoms and signs of nerve root compression are similar to those following acute disc prolapse (p. 1102), and investigation and management follow the same lines.

SPONDYLOLYSIS AND SPONDYLOLISTHESIS

Spondylolysis describes a simple defect in the pars interarticularis. In spondylolisthesis one vertebra slips forward on the one below and this is usually associated with spondylolysis (Fig. 15.5).

Aetiology and classification

The types and causes of spondylolisthesis are shown in the information box.

Clinical features

Uncomplicated spondylolysis is not associated with symptoms but spondylolisthesis is variably associated with low back pain aggravated by standing and walking. More severe cases can result in nerve root compression or a lumbar stenosis syndrome and the vertebral slip is occasionally palpable.

Investigations

Spondylolysis and spondylolisthesis can be easily diagnosed with lateral or oblique radiographs of the lumbar spine (Fig. 15.5). MRI may be required if there is nerve root involvement.

Management

Postural advice and muscle strengthening exercises are all that are required in milder cases. Surgical fusion is indicated in patients with severe and recurrent low back pain and surgical decompression is mandatory prior to fusion in patients with significant lumbar stenosis or symptoms of cauda equina compression.

CAUSES OF SPONDYLOLISTHESIS

- Congenital
- Isthmic: stress failure or fracture of pars interarticularis
- Degenerative
- Post traumatic
- Pathological: metastatic destruction of posterior elements
- Post-surgical

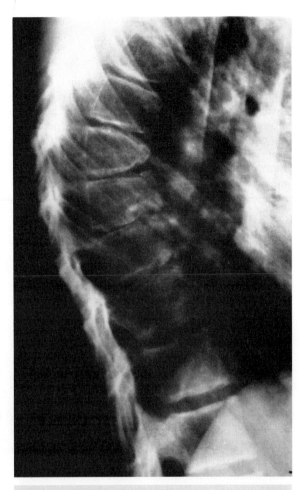

Fig. 15.6   Scheuermann's disease.

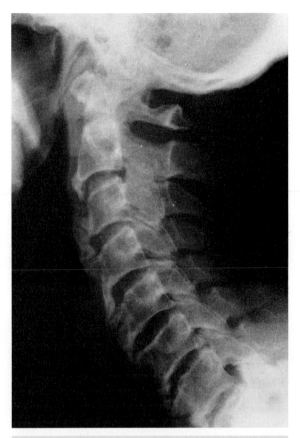

Fig. 15.7   Diffuse idiopathic skeletal hyperostosis (DISH).

ARACHNOIDITIS

Severe low back pain with or without nerve root symptoms can be associated with chronic inflammation of the nerve root sheaths in the spinal canal. Chronic arachnoiditis may be a complication of meningitis or spinal surgery but is seen most frequently as a late complication of myelography with oil-based contrast agents. The diagnosis can be confirmed by MRI or radiculography but no satisfactory treatment is available.

SCHEUERMANN'S OSTEOCHONDRITIS

This is a disorder of unknown aetiology which is seen predominantly in male adolescents who develop a painless dorsal kyphosis in association with irregular ossification of the vertebral end plates (Fig. 15.6). Back pain, aggravated by exercise and relieved by rest, occurs if the vertebrae of the upper lumbar spine are affected

and secondary spondylosis can follow in middle age. Excessive exercise and heavy manual labour before epiphyseal fusion has occurred may aggravate the problem. Treatment is with rest and protective postural exercises. The deformity is seldom severe enough to warrant corrective surgery.

DIFFUSE IDIOPATHIC SKELETAL HYPEROSTOSIS (DISH)

DISH, also known as *Forrestier's disease* and *ankylosing hyperostosis*, is a chronic age-related disorder characterised by exuberant new bone formation. The condition is defined radiologically by the presence of flowing ossification along the antero-lateral aspect of at least four contiguous vertebral bodies (Fig. 15.7). It is distinguished from lumbar spondylosis by the preservation of disc height and the absence of the vacuum phenomenon or marginal sclerosis of the vertebral bodies, and distinguished from ankylosing spondylitis by the absence of sacroiliitis or apophyseal joint fusion.

Epidemiology

DISH is a common disorder in the elderly with a prevalence of 10% in males and 8% in females over the age of 65 years. It is seldom seen below the age of 45. The prevalence in male Pima Indians is greater than 50% and this may reflect their high prevalence of obesity and diabetes mellitus.

Aetiology and pathogenesis

DISH appears to be the result of a systemic disturbance which results in excessive proteoglycan production at entheses prior to ossification and hyperostosis. It occurs more frequently in association with gout, obesity, hypertension, Type II diabetes mellitus and hyperinsulinaemia but growth hormone and somatomedin levels are not increased. Hyperostosis occurs predominantly on the right hand side of the thoracolumbar spine, except in patients with situs inversus, suggesting that the presence of the aorta influences the development of ossification in some way.

Clinical features

The development of DISH is associated with restriction of movements of the neck and spine but seldom with pain in the axial skeleton. Heel pain can occur in association with calcaneal spur formation and DISH may be associated occasionally with a form of hypertrophic hip osteoarthrosis. Extraspinal ossification at other sites such as the olecranon and patella is seldom associated with symptoms. Dysphagia, cervical myelopathy and lumbar stenosis are rare complications.

Investigations

The diagnosis is established with simple radiographs. MRI, CT or myelography are only required if lumbar stenosis is suspected.

Management

In the absence of any specific therapy, management involves general advice with regard to weight loss and the maintenance of musculoskeletal fitness. Heel pads and suitable footwear are generally more effective than steroid injections for patients with heel pain and calcaneal spurs. Insulin, oral hypoglycaemic drugs and thiazide diuretics which can increase plasma insulin levels should be avoided if possible.

FURTHER READING

Deyo R A, Bigos S J, Maravilla K R 1989 Diagnostic imaging procedures for the lumbar spine. Annals of Internal Medicine III; 856–867
Waddell G 1982 An approach to backache. British Journal of Hospital Medicine 28: 187–219

REGIONAL PERIARTICULAR OR 'SOFT TISSUE' DISORDERS

Musculoskeletal aches and pains are extremely common and become more frequent with increasing age. More than one-third of all 'rheumatic complaints' cannot be attributed to defined diseases of the spine, peripheral joints or connective tissues. Many are trivial, self limiting and cause little disability. Others can be more troublesome. The neck, shoulder girdle, back and gluteal muscles are the commonest sites for many of these complaints. Muscular spasm of reflex origin is a prominent feature and must be differentiated from limitation of movement due to structural damage. Absence of signs of systemic illness and a normal ESR will help to distinguish these **regional rheumatic disorders** from the inflammatory connective tissue diseases.

Certain factors may be of importance in precipitating attacks in susceptible individuals. Exposure to cold and damp has always been suspected as a cause of nonarticular 'rheumatic' complaints. Unaccustomed physical effort, undue fatigue, minor injuries and poor posture have also been incriminated. Any reduction in muscular efficiency will render an individual more prone to sprains of tendons, ligaments and extra-articular soft tissue structures.

Diffuse muscular pain and stiffness is common in certain infections, particularly of viral origin, such as influenza, rubella and measles. Localised pain occurs in epidemic myalgia (Bornholm disease), while myalgic 'encephalomyelitis' (chronic fatigue syndrome or post-viral syndrome) is characterised by relapsing episodes of prolonged fatigue following physical or mental effort. Many anxious and depressed people complain of aches and pains, particularly in the region of the neck, shoulders or lower back.

NECK PAIN

Neck pain, stiffness and restriction of movements are a frequent consequence of trauma and degenerative disorders of the cervical spine.

Epidemiology

Transient episodes of acute neck pain and stiffness occur in 40–50% of all adults with an increasing incidence in those over the age of 45 years. Many attacks appear to be precipitated by awkward sleeping posture and most resolve spontaneously within 1–4 days.

Neck pain of mechanical origin is less common than low back pain as a cause of industrial disability but assembly line workers and heavy manual labourers are at particular risk. Violinists and other performing artists are prone to recurrent neck pain of postural origin.

More prolonged neck pain and stiffness lasting up to 2–3 months is a frequent sequel of 'whiplash' flexion/hyperextension injuries in up to 50% of all serious car collisions even in the absence of fracture or nerve root injury. More protracted disability in such patients is often associated with compensation claims and secondary psychological problems.

Aetiology

The common types of transient acute neck pain and stiffness are not associated with definable aetiology or spinal pathology. Other causes of neck pain are listed in the information box.

CAUSES OF NECK PAIN

- **Mechanical**
  Acute stiff neck
  Postural
  Whiplash injury
  Disc prolapse
  Cervical spondylosis
  Thoracic outlet/
    neurovascular
    syndromes

- **Inflammatory**
  Infections
  Ankylosing spondylitis
  Juvenile chronic
    arthritis
  Rheumatoid arthritis
  Polymyalgia rheumatica

- **Metabolic**
  Osteoporosis
  Osteomalacia
  Paget's disease
  Crystal arthropathies

- **Neoplastic**
  Metastases
  Myeloma
  Reticulosis
  Intrathecal tumours

- **Other**
  Torticollis
  Fibromyalgia

- **Referred pain**
  Angina pectoris
  Aortic aneurysm
  Pancoast tumour
  Diaphragm
  Pharynx
  Cervical lymph nodes
  Teeth
  Acromio-clavicular
    joints
  Shoulder

Clinical features

Mechanical neck pain is characteristically acute in onset and associated with restriction of neck movements and a history of awkward posture or trauma. The pain is frequently referred to the occiput or shoulders as well as the nuchal muscles, and neck pain associated with acute disc prolapse may be aggravated by coughing and sneezing. Occipital, retro-orbital and temporal referral of pain suggests pathology in the atlas, axis or third cervical vertebra while interscapular pain and anterior chest wall pain masquerading as angina may be associated with lesions of the lower cervical spine (C6 and C7). Neck pain associated with disc protrusions or cervical spondylosis is frequently complicated by cervical

radiculopathy with characteristic radiation of pain, paraesthesiae, sensory loss, muscle weakness, wasting and reflex changes in the arm (see p. 1028).

Inflammatory, metabolic and neoplastic diseases are associated with neck pain that is more insidious in onset, more prolonged in duration and usually not so obviously influenced by posture and movement.

Investigations

Blood tests are rarely helpful in patients with acute neck pain. A low haemoglobin and raised CRP or ESR may augment a clinical suspicion of infection, inflammation or malignancy. A raised acid phosphatase or PSA is associated with metastatic carcinoma of the prostate and raised alkaline phosphatase with other bone metastases or Paget's disease. A monoclonal paraprotein band on serum immuno-electrophoresis and/or the presence of urine light chains may point to multiple myelomatosis.

AP and lateral radiographs are indicated in all patients with prolonged neck pain and can be helpful in detecting sepsis, spondylitis, myelomatosis, lytic or sclerotic metastases and Paget's disease. Cervical spondylosis is associated with loss of disc height, vertebral sclerosis and osteophyte formation and oblique radiographs are sometimes helpful in demonstrating foraminal encroachment by osteophytes in patients with radicular symptoms (Fig. 15.8). Bone scintigraphy with ^{99m}Tc bisphosphonate can be useful in detecting the presence and extent of metastases and Paget's disease as well as bone infection and fracture when pain radiographs are negative. Magnetic resonance imaging and computed tomography are equally effective in delineating large disc prolapses and extramedullary tumours. Enhanced CT with simultaneous radiculography is more reliable in the pre-operative assessment of patients with radicular pain but MRI has become the imaging modality of choice for detecting minor disc prolapse as well as spinal cord pathology (Fig. 15.9). EMG and nerve conduction studies with or without measurement of somatosensory evoked responses are occasionally needed to confirm the localisation of nerve root lesions. Lumbar puncture and CSF examination are essential in patients with suspected meningitis or subarachnoid haemorrhage.

Management

Most episodes of mechanical and postural acute neck pain will resolve in less than a week with nothing more than simple analgesics, a soft collar and strong reassurance. Bed rest and traction can sometimes be effective in patients with more severe and more prolonged acute neck pain associated with disc prolapse and radiculopathy but as traction can rarely be associated with vertebral artery damage or neurological complications it should never be used in patients with radiographic

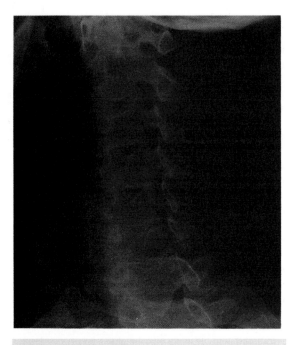

Fig. 15.8 Cervical spondylosis. Oblique radiograph of cervical spine showing foraminal encroachment by osteophyte.

evidence of advanced cervical spondylosis or other pathology. Chronic cervical pain syndromes are best treated conservatively with postural advice, muscle strengthening exercises and the occasional judicious use of analgesics and a cervical collar during acute exacerbations. Surgery is only rarely required in patients with symptoms and neurological signs of radiculopathy or progressive cervical myelopathy.

TORTICOLLIS

● *Congenital torticollis* results from painless flexion and rotation of the head and neck secondary to unilateral contracture of the sternomastoid muscle.
● *Acute torticollis* is associated with severe neck pain and muscle spasm secondary to a variety of causes (see information box).
● *Spasmodic torticollis* is a form of severe and painful

CAUSES OF ACUTE TORTICOLLIS

● Disc prolapse
● Apophyseal joint subluxation
● Pharyngitis
● Cervical adenitis
● Juvenile chronic arthritis

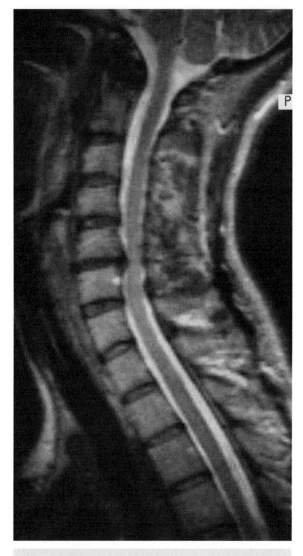

Fig. 15.9 Cervical disc prolapse. MRI of cervical spine showing disc prolapse at C5/6.

muscle dystonia which is usually unassociated with any other evidence of an extra-pyramidal neurological disorder.

Rarely it can be a late complication of encephalitis. Local injection of paralysing doses of Botulinum toxin can give symptomatic relief.

CERVICAL SPONDYLOSIS

Disc degeneration with associated osteophyte formation and osteoarthritis of the spinal apophyseal joints, collectively termed cervical spondylosis, is almost universal in elderly people.

Aetiology and pathogenesis

See lumbar spondylosis, page 867.

Clinical features

Two thirds of patients over the age of 65 years experience neck pain in association with cervical spondylosis but there is a poor correlation between symptoms and radiographic signs. Cervical radiculopathy is associated with characteristic radiation of pain, paraesthesiae, sensory loss, muscle weakness, wasting and reflex changes in the arm (see p. 1028). Drop attacks and vertigo precipitated by neck extension are common consequences of vertebro-basilar ischaemia while visual disturbance, unsteadiness, nausea, dyspnoea and cardiac arrhythmias are rarely the result of sympathetic nerve stimulation. Dysphagia is occasionally caused by massive osteophyte formation.

FIBROMYALGIA (FIBROSITIS, MYOFASCIAL PAIN SYNDROME)

This is a poorly defined syndrome of chronic musculoskeletal pain that affects about 2% of all patients seen in general practice and as many as 20% of patients referred to rheumatologists in the USA.

Clinical features

The syndrome is characterised by diffuse muscle pain, stiffness and fatigue in association with focal point tenderness (see information box). Additional features frequently include tension headaches, dysmenorrhoea and symptoms of an irritable bowel syndrome suggesting a strong psychosomatic component. A proportion of patients have some features of anxiety and depression.

Investigations

Radiographs and laboratory investigations (FBC, ESR, CPK and serological tests for RF and ANF) are only helpful in excluding other more serious pathology. EMG and nerve conduction studies are normal but most patients have a disturbance of stage IV non-rapid eye movement sleep on EEG.

Management

Strong medical reassurance coupled with advice from a physiotherapist about posture and improving physical fitness can sometimes be helpful. A small evening dose of a tricyclic antidepressant may improve sleep but the condition tends to have a chronic and protracted course in most patients.

FIBROMYALGIA: TENDER POINTS

● Occiput	Bilateral at suboccipital muscle insertion
● Low cervical	Bilateral at intertransverse spaces C5–7
● Trapezius	Bilateral at mid point of the upper border
● Supraspinatus	Bilateral at the origins above the scapula near the medial border
● Second rib	Bilateral at the 2nd costochondral junction
● Lateral epicondyle	Bilateral, 2 cm distal to the epicondyle
● Gluteal	Bilateral in upper outer quadrants of buttocks in anterior fold of muscle
● Greater trochanter	Bilateral posterior to the trochanteric prominence
● Knees	Bilateral at the medial fat pad proximal to the joint line

Diagnosis requires the presence of pain on digital palpation in at least 11/18 tender point sites.

SHOULDER PAIN

Shoulder pain is a feature of disorders affecting the acromio-clavicular joint as well as the glenohumeral joint and periarticular structures. The shoulder is also a common site for referred pain in patients with ischaemic heart disease, cervical radiculopathy or abdominal pathology involving the diaphragm. Most frequently shoulder pain is the result of extra-articular traumatic, degenerative or inflammatory lesions of the capsule or 'rotator cuff' of tendons.

Most painful shoulders can be diagnosed and managed without the need for imaging. Radiographs are required however if shoulder pain persists and ultrasound or MRI is occasionally required to localise rotator cuff tears and distinguish tears from tendonitis.

Supraspinatus tendonitis

This results from impingement of the tendon on the acromion. It is characterised by a 'painful arc' on abduction of the arm which can be abolished by external rotation. There is localised tenderness over the greater tuberosity of the humerus and a radiograph may show calcification in the supraspinatus tendon (Fig. 15.10). Rupture of calcific material into the subacromial bursa occasionally results in acutely painful gout-like attacks of inflammatory subacromial bursitis. Fluid aspirated

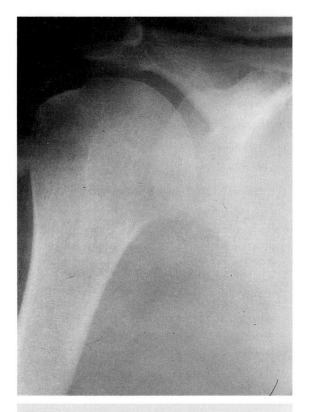

Fig. 15.10 Supraspinatus tendonitis. Radiograph showing soft tissue calcification.

restriction of movements alone. A frozen shoulder may be a late consequence of a rotator cuff lesion and sometimes follows myocardial infarction, hemiplegia, herpes zoster, breast or thoracic surgery.

Treatment is with analgesics and local corticosteroid injection in the early phase and mobilising exercises after the pain has resolved.

The natural history is for slow but complete recovery, the complete cycle sometimes taking as long as 2 years.

Shoulder-hand syndrome

This syndrome is characterised by burning pain, vasomotor changes and severe limitation of movement of the hand in association with restriction of shoulder movements. A radiograph of the hand shows patchy osteoporosis after some weeks or months. It is a manifestation of reflex sympathetic dystrophy and may be a sequel to the same disorders that precede a frozen shoulder. Epilepsy, barbiturates and anti-tuberculous drugs can also be predisposing factors. Exaggerated illness behaviour is a feature in some patients.

Treatment is aimed at mobilising the affected limb. Analgesics, a short course of systemic corticosteroids, sympathetic nerve block and physiotherapy each have their advocates in this difficult situation. The prognosis for recovery is less certain than in frozen shoulder.

from the bursa beneath the acromion contains crystals of calcium hydroxyapatite.

Treatment is with local injection of steroid.

Degenerative changes in the rotator cuff may extend to involve the long head of biceps and the infraspinatus tendon.

Bicipital tendonitis

This condition can be recognised by pain and tenderness in the bicipital groove aggravated by resisted flexion of the elbow.

Infraspinatus tendonitis

This form of tendonitis is associated with pain on resisted external rotation with **subscapularis** lesions causing pain on resisted internal rotation of the arm.

Capsulitis

In this common and disabling condition (frozen shoulder) there is severe spontaneous shoulder pain initially associated with capsular tenderness and painful restriction of all shoulder movements and later with painless

ELBOW PAIN

Elbow pain may be referred from the shoulder, cervical spine or brachial plexus but periarticular soft tissue lesions are common.

Lateral epicondylitis

Commonly referred to as 'tennis elbow', this condition is associated with partial tears of the origin of the extensor muscles at the lateral epicondyle. Local tenderness and pain on active wrist extension are characteristic and treatment is with local corticosteroid injection, ultrasound and/or advice concerning inappropriate use.

Medial epicondylitis

'Golfer's elbow' results from similar lesions in the origin of the common flexor tendon at the medial epicondyle and treatment is also with local corticosteroid injections, ultrasound and general advice concerning musculoskeletal protection.

Olecranon bursitis

This can follow local trauma but infection, gout and rheumatoid arthritis are also important causes that need to be considered.

HAND AND WRIST PAIN

Extra-articular causes of hand pain include tenosynovitis, median nerve compression in the carpal tunnel, lower brachial plexus lesions, C8/T1 radiculopathy and a thoracic outlet syndrome as well as algodystrophy, angina pectoris and Raynaud's phenomenon.

Trigger finger

This results from stenosing tenosynovitis in the flexor tendon sheath with intermittent locking of the finger in flexion. A local corticosteroid injection usually relieves the problem and surgical decompression is only occasionally required.

De Quervain's tenosynovitis

Results from traumatic or work-related tenosynovitis of the tendon sheaths of abductor pollicis longus and extensor pollicis brevis. Pain on moving the thumb and wrist is associated with tenderness in the 'anatomical snuffbox' between the tendons and pain on forced ulnar deviation of the wrist with the thumb apposed to the palm (Finkelstein's sign). Treatment is primarily with rest and splinting but local corticosteroid injection is occasionally required. Surgical decompression is very rarely necessary.

Dupuytren's contracture

A relatively painless disorder in which flexion of the fingers results from fibrosis and contracture of the superficial palmar fascia. Inability to extend the fingers is associated with puckering of the skin and the presence of palpable nodules. The fourth finger is usually the earliest to be affected and the condition is age-related and occurs four times more frequently in men. Undetermined genetic factors are clearly involved with a dominant pattern of inheritance. An association with knuckle pads, plantar fibromatosis and Peyronie's disease in some patients suggests the possibility of a generalised susceptibility to fibrosis in connective tissues. Dupuytren's contracture can also occur in association with alcohol misuse, epilepsy and chronic pulmonary disorders but must be distinguished from cheirarthropathy in patients with diabetes mellitus and flexor tendon tenosynovitis in patients with rheumatoid arthritis and other types of inflammatory polyarthritis. Local protection, stretching exercises and strong reassurance are all that are required in most patients but progressive deformities with functional impairment necessitate fasciectomy in a few.

HIP PAIN

Pain in the region of the hip is frequently associated with periarticular tendonitis or bursitis as well as with bone disorders and arthritis of the hips and sacroiliac joints. Common causes of referred pain are shown in the information box.

REFERRED PAIN IN THE HIP REGION	
• **Sacroiliac joints**	Buttock
• **Thoraco-lumbar spine**	
T12–L1	Greater trochanter
L2–L4	Inguinal region + anterior thigh
• **Abdominal pathology**	
Psoas abscess	Groin+anterior thigh
Pelvic inflammation	aggravated by resisted
Retroperitoneal	hip flexion
haemorrhage	
Femoral/inguinal	Groin+anterior thigh
hernias	
• **Vascular disease**	
Aortic aneurysm	Claudication
Iliac artery thrombosis	buttock or thigh

Trochanteric bursitis

This condition is associated with aching or burning pain over the lateral aspect of the hip and thigh which is aggravated by walking, squatting and resisted abduction of the hip. There may be local tenderness and swelling over the greater trochanter.

Radiographs may show periosteal irregularity and some calcification around the trochanter. Treatment is with rest, analgesics and local corticosteroid injection.

Iliopsoas bursitis

Iliopsoas bursitis occurs in association with inflammatory or degenerative arthritis of the hip. Patients may present with a painless or painful inguinal swelling, a swollen leg or symptoms and signs of femoral nerve compression. The diagnosis can be confirmed by ultrasound, CT, MRI or arthrography. If treatment with local corticosteroid is ineffective, surgical excision is required.

Iliogluteal bursitis

Alternatively called 'Weaver's bottom', this condition is associated with pain and tenderness over the ischial tuberosities aggravated by sitting and lying. Treatment is with local corticosteroid injection and the avoidance of local pressure.

Adductor tendonitis

Associated with groin pain which is aggravated by abduction and resisted adduction of the hip, this is usually a sports related problem in gymnasts or horseback riders. Treatment is with rest and analgesics, and corticosteroid injections are seldom required.

KNEE PAIN

Periarticular causes of knee pain in adults include ligament injuries, tendonitis, enthesitis and bursitis.

Prepatellar bursitis

'Housemaid's knee' most frequently follows the trauma of prolonged or unaccustomed kneeling but infection and gout need to be considered and the bursa aspirated for microscopy and culture if there is any doubt. Most cases settle with rest and the avoidance of kneeling alone.

Infrapatellar bursitis

Characterised by the finding of swelling and tenderness adjacent to the insertion of the patellar tendon into the tibial tubercle when the knee is extended.

Anserine bursitis

Presents as pain and tenderness on the medial side of the lower femur. Women with valgus deformities of the knees are particularly susceptible but it may be hard to distinguish from **pes anserinus tendonitis** and **medial ligament sprains** in runners. Treatment is with rest and analgesics and local corticosteroid injection.

Impingement of a medial patellar **plica** can be associated with pain over the medial femoral condyle and a sensation of snapping. The diagnosis is confirmed by detecting an inflamed plica on arthroscopy and the problem is relieved by arthroscopic resection.

Pellegrini–Steida disease

This is further cause of pain and tenderness over the medial side of the lower femur. It follows injuries to the medial collateral ligament and is characteristically associated with calcification at the ligament insertion on radiograph. Symptoms usually settle with rest and analgesics alone.

Anterior knee pain

Characteristically the pain is worse at night and aggravated by sporting activities. It is a common problem in adolescent girls. In a small proportion of these patients there is evidence of non-progressive fibrillation of the articular cartilage of the patella on arthroscopy—chondromalacia patellae. The condition is self-limiting and treatment should be conservative with quadriceps strengthening exercises, stretching of the hamstrings and the avoidance of high heels.

Osgood–Schlatter's disease

This condition is due to apophysitis of the tibial tubercle. Adolescents present with pain, swelling and tenderness at the patella tendon insertion aggravated by resisted extension of the knee. Lateral radiographs show fragmentation of the tibial tubercle. In most patients symptoms settle with rest and disappear altogether following fusion of the tibial tubercle.

Anterior tibial compartment syndrome

Characterised by severe pain in the front of the lower leg aggravated by exercise and relieved by rest. Symptoms result from fascial compression of the muscles in the anterior tibial compartment and may be associated with a foot drop. Treatment is by surgical decompression.

FOOT AND ANKLE PAIN

Pes planus

Pes planus, or 'flat foot' results from loss of the longitudinal arch of the foot. Pain is only experienced following ligament sprains, excessive walking or weight gain, or if there is associated spasm of the peroneal muscles. Acquired causes of pes planus include trauma, constitutional hypermobility, rheumatoid arthritis and neuropathic arthropathies. Medial arch supports in well-fitting shoes and/or intrinsic muscle strengthening exercises will relieve symptoms in most cases but individually moulded rigid orthotics are required for patients with hyperpronated feet provided the foot is not rigid as a result of fusion of the tarsal bones (tarsal coalition).

Pes cavus

'Claw foot' is characterised by the presence of a high medial arch and secondary metatarsal callosities with clawing of the toes. Rarely it is associated with neurological disorders such as Friedreich's ataxia, spina bifida or poliomyelitis. Foot pain can be ameliorated with medial arch supports and metatarsal insoles in most patients and surgical intervention with fasciectomy or osteotomy are only very rarely indicated.

Hallux valgus

This deformity with secondary bursitis (bunions) and osteoarthritis of the first MTP joints is commonly associated with local forefoot pain and flattening of the transverse metatarsal arch. The problem is more common in women as a consequence of wearing narrow high-heeled shoes. Surgical correction is required in patients with intractable pain and severe deformity but most patients respond to adjustment of footwear alone.

Hallux rigidus

Associated with severe intermittent aching pain and restriction of movements of the first metatarsophalangeal joint, this is usually secondary to osteoarthritis in the elderly but occasionally occurs as a primary problem without obvious cause in young adults. Treatment is with wide-fitting shoes with rigid soles and metatarsal bars. Arthrodesis is only rarely required.

Morton's neuroma

The name given to an entrapment neuropathy of the interdigital nerves which occurs most frequently between the third and fourth metatarsal heads in middle aged women who wear ill-fitting shoes. Neuralgic, lancinating pain which is characteristically aggravated by wearing shoes may be associated with local sensory loss and a palpable tender mass between the metatarsal heads. Many patients respond to adjustment of footwear with or without a local corticosteroid injection but surgical excision is occasionally required.

Non-articular causes of **hind foot** pain in adults include **Achilles tendon tears, Achilles tendonitis** and **retrocalcaneal bursitis**. Pain and local tenderness at the Achilles tendon insertion in boys can be associated with **retrocalcaneal apophysitis** (Sever's disease). Achilles tendon ruptures require surgical repair but other causes of pain behind the heel are managed conservatively with rest, local protective padding and a raised heel; corticosteroid injections are contraindicated.

Plantar fasciitis

Associated with pain and tenderness under the heel on standing or walking, in some cases this results from an inflammatory enthesitis as part of a seronegative spondarthritis (see p. 905) and may or may not be associated with the presence of a calcaneal spur on radiograph. Treatment is with silicone heel pads, ultrasound or occasionally local corticosteroid injection.

FURTHER READING

Borenstein D G, Wiesel S W 1989 Low Back Pain: Medical Diagnosis and Comprehensive Management. Saunders, Philadelphia
Hadler N M 1993 Occupational Musculoskeletal Disorders. Raven Press, New York

OSTEOARTHRITIS AND RELATED DISORDERS

OSTEOARTHRITIS

Osteoarthritis (OA, osteoarthrosis, arthrosis or degenerative joint disease) is not a single disease. Rather it is the end result of a variety of patterns of joint failure. To a greater or lesser extent it is always characterised by both degeneration of articular cartilage and simultaneous proliferation of new bone, cartilage and connective tissue. The proliferative response results in some degree of remodelling of the joint contour. Inflammatory changes in the synovium are usually minor and secondary.

Epidemiology

Radiological and autopsy surveys show a steady rise in degenerative changes in joints from the age of 30. By the age of 65, 80% of people have some radiographic evidence of osteoarthritis although only 25% may have symptoms. Males and females are both affected but OA is more generalised and more severe in older women. Geographical surveys show differences in both the prevalence of OA and the pattern of joint involvement. OA of the hips is much more frequent in Caucasians than in Blacks or Chinese. Twin and family studies show the importance of genetic factors, particularly in the nodal form of primary generalised osteoarthritis, and associations have been reported with the $HLA-A_1B_8$ and alpha-1-antitrypsin MZ phenotypes. Obesity and body mass index are particularly associated with knee OA while osteoporosis and smoking appear to have a modest protective effect. Cold, damp climates are associated with more symptoms but not with greater radiological prevalence.

Aetiology and pathogenesis

OA is classified as primary if the aetiology is unknown and secondary when degenerative joint changes occur in response to a recognisable local or systemic factor. The causes of secondary osteoarthritis are listed in the information box on page 879. Developmental abnormalities are believed to be of major importance in the aetiology of OA of the hip in the vast majority, and type II collagen gene defects have been identified in a few families in whom familial, premature, polyarticular OA is associated with an epiphyseal or spondyloepiphyseal dysplasia. Epidemiological surveys suggest that physical factors involved in occupations such as farming are also important determinants in hip OA. Abnormal surface contacts and weight-bearing alignments lead to increased local mechanical stress and wear. Post-traumatic malalignment and incongruity of joints are well established as important predisposing causes of premature OA.

Metabolic diseases lead to degeneration of cartilage by very different mechanisms. In **alkaptonuria** (ochronosis) the genetically determined defect of homogentisic acid oxidase results in the accumulation of a pigmented polymer that binds to collagen, rendering it brittle and prone to mechanical degradation. There may be other inborn errors of metabolism where unknown colourless metabolites induce changes in the biochemical composition of cartilagenous matrix in a similar way and so predispose to OA. **Crystal deposition** of calcium pyrophosphate dihydrate or hydroxyapatite may alter the properties of cartilage matrix directly and low grade crystal inflammation may play a part in pathogenesis, but recent studies suggest that cartilage matrix changes precede crystal formation.

It is uncertain whether the degenerative joint disease seen in **acromegaly** is a consequence of joint incongruity following cartilage overgrowth or whether the endocrine disturbance results in a mechanically defective matrix. **Paget's disease**, Gaucher's disease and various diseases associated with **aseptic necrosis** result in pathological changes in subchondral bone with consequent altered stresses on the overlying articular cartilage. Thus OA can be the end result of disorders in which defective cartilage matrix disintegrates under the influence of normal mechanical stresses, and disorders in which normal cartilage matrix fails secondary to the application of abnormal mechanical loads (Fig. 15.11).

Current concepts of the pathogenesis of OA are based on the assumption that whatever the provoking cause, the final pathway of changes in articular cartilage will be identical. Two mechanical hypotheses merit consideration. The first suggests that the initiating event is fatigue fracture of the collagen fibre network which is followed by increased hydration of the articular cartilage with

unravelling of the proteoglycans and loss of proteoglycans into the synovial fluid. There is some evidence of augmented neutral protease and collagenolytic activity but collagen may also be lost simply as a result of mechanical attrition.

The alternative hypothesis suggests that the initial lesions are microfractures of the subchondral bone following repetitive loading. Healing of these microfractures leads to significant loss of resilience of the subchondral bone, which in turn creates a sheer stress gradient in the adjacent articular cartilage. As the process evolves the cartilage surface becomes fibrillated and deep clefts appear with reduplication and proliferation of chondrocytes within them. Simultaneous proliferative changes commence at the joint margins with formation of osteophytes. Eventually articular cartilage is lost altogether in areas of maximum mechanical stress and the underlying bone becomes hardened and eburnated. Cysts may form but bony ankylosis does not occur (Fig. 15.12). The associated biochemical changes in articular cartilage are summarised in the information box.

BIOCHEMICAL CHANGES IN OA CARTILAGE

- ↑H_2O
- ↓Collagen, proteoglycan, monomer size, hyaluronate, keratan sulphate and chondroitin sulphate
- ↑Chondroitin 4:6 ratio
  Expression of foetal chondroitin sulphate epitopes
- ↑Collagen and proteoglycan synthesis
- ↑Collagenase and proteoglycanase

Clinical features

The joints most frequently involved are those of the spine, hips, knees and hands. The disease is confined to one or only a few joints in the majority of patients. Common patterns of joint involvement include the nodal and non-nodal types of primary generalised OA with prominent involvement of the knees and hands (distal interphalangeal joints, proximal interphalangeal joints, carpometacarpal joints of thumbs), as well as OA confined to the knees or hips. The symptoms are gradual in onset. Pain is at first intermittent and aching and is provoked by the use of the joint and relieved by rest. As the disease progresses, movement in the affected joint becomes increasingly limited, initially as a result of pain and muscular spasm, but later because of capsular fibrosis, osteophyte formation and remodelling of bone. There may be repeated effusions into joints, especially after minor twists or injuries. Crepitus may be felt or even heard. Associated muscle wasting is an important factor in the progress of the disease, as in the absence of normal muscular control the joint becomes more prone

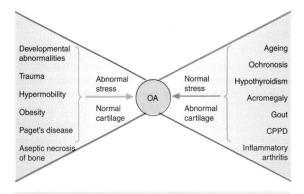

Fig. 15.11 Secondary osteoarthritis. Crude classification of mechanisms of cartilage failure.

CAUSES OF SECONDARY OSTEOARTHROSIS

- **Developmental**
  Perthes' disease
  Slipped capital femoral
    epiphysis
  Epiphysiolysis
  Hip dysplasia
  Epiphysial dysplasias
  Intra-articular acetabular
    labrum
- **Traumatic**
  Intra-articular fracture
  Menisectomy
  Occupational, e.g. elbows of
    pneumatic drill operators
  Hypermobility, e.g.
    Ehlers–Danlos
    syndrome
  Long leg arthropathy
- **Metabolic**
  Alkaptonuria
    (ochronosis)
  Haemochromatosis
  Wilson's disease
  Chrondrocalcinosis

- **Endocrine**
  Acromegaly
- **Inflammatory**
  Rheumatoid arthritis
  Gout
  Septic arthritis
  Haemophilia
- **Aseptic necrosis**
  Corticosteroids
  Sickle-cell disease
  Caisson sickness
  SLE and other
    collagenoses
- **Neuropathic**
  Tabes dorsalis
  Syringomyelia
  Diabetes mellitus
  Peripheral nerve
    lesions
- **Miscellaneous**
  Paget's disease
  Gaucher's disease

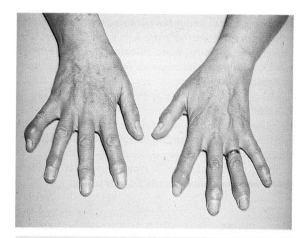

Fig. 15.13 Nodal osteoarthritis. Hands of patient with primary generalised OA showing prominent involvement of the distal interphalangeal (DIP) joints with Heberden's nodes.

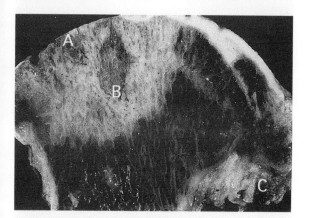

Fig. 15.12 The pathology of osteoarthritis. Cross-section of head of femur in patient with advanced OA. Note (A) loss of articular cartilage, (B) cyst formation and (C) bone sclerosis as well as osteophyte formation and remodelling of the femoral head.

to injury. Pain arises from trabecular microfractures, traumatic lesions in the capsule and periarticular tissues and a low grade synovitis. Nocturnal aching may be attributable to hyperaemia of the subchondral bone.

Nodal osteoarthritis

This is a clinically distinct form of primary generalised OA which occurs predominantly in middle-aged women. Characteristically it affects the terminal inter-

phalangeal (IP) joints of the fingers with the development of gelatinous cysts or bony outgrowths on the dorsal aspect of these joints (Heberden's nodes, Fig. 15.13). The onset is sometimes acute with considerable pain, swelling and inflammation. Although these lesions may be associated with a good deal of deformity, they seldom cause serious disability. Similar lesions may affect the proximal IP joints (Bouchard's nodes) and the disorder also frequently involves the carpometacarpal joints of the thumbs, the spinal apophyseal joints, the hips and the knees. A strong family history of Heberden's nodes is usual in such patients and though the existence of multi-generation families with the disorder appears to suggest a single autosomal dominant gene, careful family studies reveal polygenic inheritance in both nodal and non-nodal primary generalised osteoarthritis (PGOA). Patients with nodal PGOA are also more susceptible to secondary OA, again emphasising the multifactorial aetiology of this disorder.

Erosive OA

A more severe form of nodal PGOA characterised by episodic symptoms and signs of local joint inflammation with the development of destructive subchondral erosions and instability in the proximal and distal interphalangeal joints.

Non-nodal PGOA

Characterised by a more equal sex incidence and less prominent distal interphalangeal joint disease.

Osteoarthritis of the knees

Often associated with obesity and hand OA in women. The medial and patello-femoral compartments are usually first involved and more advanced disease is associated with varus knee deformities. Isolated knee OA may however be a consequence of varus knee deformities associated with medial meniscectomy and dysplasias such as Blount's disease.

Isolated hip OA

Frequently secondary to definable predisposing causes such as inequality of leg lengths, preceding hip disease, acetabular dysplasia or occupational trauma. The superior pole of the hip is typically affected in such cases, whereas hip disease in PGOA is usually medial or concentric.

Investigations

The blood count and ESR are characteristically normal. Synovial fluid is viscous and has a low cell count; apatite crystals can rarely be detected (Table 15.4, p. 896). Cartilage degradation products such as keratan sulphate and pyridinoline cross links derived from collagen are increased in the synovial fluid and urine but these are too non-specific and variable to be useful for diagnosis or following progress.

Radiographs show loss of joint space and formation of marginal osteophytes. Subchondral bone sclerosis, bone remodelling and cyst formation are seen in more advanced cases (Figs 15.14 and 15.15). Isotope scintigraphy with ^{99m}Tc bisphosphonate shows increased uptake of isotope in OA joints that are destined to develop progressive damage.

Management

Treatment is directed towards relieving symptoms, maintaining and improving joint function and minimising handicap. Patient education and the encouragement of a positive approach are particularly important in osteoarthritis. While the pathological changes of OA are irreversible, the overall prognosis for maintaining function is generally good and a great deal can be done to alleviate symptoms. Improving muscle strength and maintaining mobility are just as important as the avoidance of undue trauma and physical stress to affected joints. Simple joint protection techniques include such measures as the fitting of rubber heels to reduce jarring and minimise the risk of slipping, the provision of built-up shoes to equalise leg lengths, weight loss in obese patients with OA of the knee or hip and the provision of a suitable walking stick. Occasionally patients are advised to change their occupation, transfer to lighter work or give up unduly strenuous hobbies; more often modification of existing activities to avoid prolonged standing or walking is all that is required.

Simple non-narcotic analgesics such as paracetamol or coproxamol are the drugs of first choice for relieving

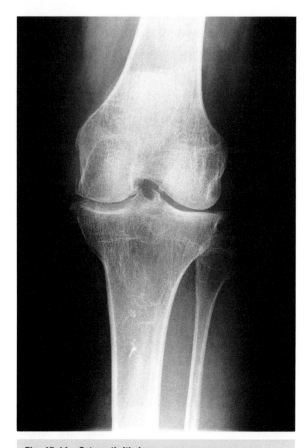

Fig. 15.14 Osteoarthritis knee. Weightbearing radiograph showing joint space narrowing with osteophyte formation, and early subchondral bone sclerosis.

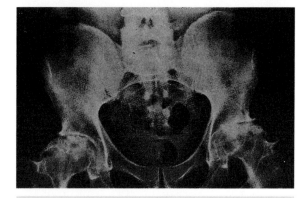

Fig. 15.15 Osteoarthritis of the hips showing loss of articular cartilage, sclerosis, cyst formation and bone remodelling with early protrusio acetabulae. Note previous acetabular osteotomy on right hip.

pain in OA. Some patients obtain better symptom control with small, analgesic doses of non-steroidal anti-inflammatory drugs (NSAIDs). Larger, anti-inflammatory doses are usually no more effective and carry an increased risk of causing gastric erosion or haemorrhage, particularly in elderly debilitated women. Prostaglandin synthetase inhibitors are also liable to cause impairment of renal function and fluid retention in patients with renal insufficiency and/or cardiac disease. On the other hand concerns that some NSAIDs may be associated with cartilage damage, due to inhibition of proteoglycan metabolism or the excessive use of damaged joints, are probably exaggerated.

Although there is evidence that some NSAIDs such as diclofenac, piroxicam and tiaprofenic acid, and other agents such as glycosaminoglycan peptide complex, pentosan polyphosphate and hyaluronan may have a chondroprotective effect in in-vitro and animal experiments there is no clear clinical evidence that these or any other drugs are of value as disease modifying agents for human OA.

Occasionally intra-articular or periarticular corticosteroid injections can be helpful, especially in the knee. Hydrotherapy may be useful for patients with OA of the hip associated with pain and muscle spasm.

Surgery needs to be considered in patients with more advanced hip and knee disease (see Table 15.10, p. 903). Precision osteotomy can prolong the life of malaligned joints as well as relieving pain by reducing intraosseous pressure. Hip and knee arthroplasties can transform the quality of life of patients with intractable pain and disability.

FURTHER READING

Docherty M, Watt I, Dieppe P 1983 Influence of primary generalised osteoarthritis on the development of secondary osteoarthritis. Lancet ii: 8–11

Felson D T 1988 Epidemiology of hip and knee osteoarthritis. Epidemiological Reviews 10: 1–28

Knettner E K, Schleyerbach R, Peyron J G et al (eds) 1988 Articular Cartilage and Osteoarthritis. Raven Press, New York

Moskowitz R W (ed.) 1993 Osteoarthritis. Rheumatic Disease Clinics of North America 19: 523–763

CRYSTAL DEPOSITION DISEASES

A variety of crystals are associated with acute and chronic arthritis, periarthritis, tendonitis and deposition in connective tissues (Table 15.1)

CALCIUM PYROPHOSPHATE DIHYDRATE (CPPD) DEPOSITION
(Chondrocalcinosis, pyrophosphate arthropathy)

CPPD crystals are deposited in fibrous and articular cartilage, where they are associated with degenerative

Table 15.1 Crystal associated arthropathies and deposition in connective tissue

Crystal	Associations
Calcium pyrophosphate dihydrate (CPPD)	Acute pseudogout Variety of patterns of chronic inflammatory/degenerative arthritis Chondrocalcinosis

Basic calcium phosphate
  Hydroxyapatite
  Octacalcium phosphate
  Tricalcium phosphate
  Dicalcium phosphate dihydrate
	Calcific periarthritis/tendonitis
	Acute/chronic inflammatory arthritis
	Destructive arthropathy
	Soft tissue calcinosis

Calcium oxalate Aluminium phosphate	Acute arthritis in patients on renal dialysis
Monosodium urate (MSU)	Acute/chronic gouty arthritis Renal calculous disease Tophi
Xanthine	Acute arthritis (rare) Renal calculous disease Asymptomatic deposition in muscles
Cholesterol	Chronic synovial effusions RA/OA
Cysteine Cystine	Acute arthritis
Charcot–Leyden (lysophospholipase)	Synovial fluid and tissues with eosinophilia

changes. Shedding of crystals into the joint space provokes an attack of synovitis—**pseudogout.** Autopsy and radiological surveys indicate that chondrocalcinosis is a common age-related finding often unassociated with symptoms of articular disease. The menisci and articular cartilage of the knee are the commonest sites.

Aetiology

Chondrocalcinosis and pseudogout are clearly not a single disease. The majority of cases are sporadic and no underlying cause can be found. Genetic factors are important in some families with increases in intracellular pyrophosphate concentrations in some kindreds and a collagen gene defect in others. A variety of metabolic disorders clearly predispose to chondrocalcinosis and these are listed in the information box.

No common determinant comparable to the hyperuricaemia of gout has been identified, but pyrophosphate concentrations are increased in synovial fluids. This, coupled with the association with hypophosphatasia, has suggested that the disease may be a consequence of defective pyrophosphatase activity.

Clinical features

Pyrophosphate arthropathy can mimic many other conditions. Six clinical patterns of disease are described in the information box overleaf.

CHONDROCALCINOSIS (PYROPHOSPHATE ARTHROPATHY)

- **Familial**
- **Sporadic**
- **Metabolic**
  Hyperparathyroidism
  Haemochromatosis
  Hypothyroidism
  Hypomagnesaemia
  Hypophosphatasia
  Gout
  Ochronosis
  Wilson's disease

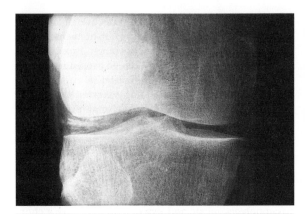

Fig. 15.16 Chondrocalcinosis. Radiograph of knee showing calcification of meniscus in patient with calcium pyrophosphate deposition disease.

CHONDROCALCINOSIS—PATTERNS OF CLINICAL DISEASE

- **Type A: Pseudogout**
  As with gout the affected joint becomes suddenly painful, warm, swollen and tender. The knee is the site of more than half of all attacks, the duration of which can vary from a few days to four weeks. Subacute or 'petite' attacks are not uncommon and there may be polyarticular clustering of acute attacks. Men are affected more frequently than women

- **Type B: Pseudo-rheumatoid arthritis**
  In a few patients there is a subacute inflammatory polyarthritis which may last for several months

- **Type C: Pseudo-osteoarthritis with superimposed acute attacks**

- **Type D: Pseudo-osteoarthritis without acute attacks**
  Types C and D account for nearly half the patients. Women are more frequently affected. Prominent involvement of the wrists and MCP joints clearly distinguishes pseudo-osteoarthritic chondrocalcinosis from primary generalised osteoarthrosis

- **Type E: Asymptomatic**
  This is the most common

- **Type F: Pseudo-neuropathic**
  Severe destructive changes resembling those of Charcot joints can occur in the knee and shoulder in the absence of any neurological defect (Fig. 15.17)

Investigations

Radiographs show CPPD in articular cartilage, the menisci of the knees (Fig. 15.16), the labrum of the acetabulum and glenoid cavity, the triangular cartilage of the wrist and the symphysis pubis. Examination of synovial fluid under polarising light microscopy allows CPPD crystals to be distinguished from monosodium urate crystals. X-ray diffraction techniques differentiate CPPD from calcium phosphate and calcium hydroxy-apatite crystals found in synovial fluid in osteoarthritis and other forms of degenerative joint disease.

Management

Joint aspiration and intra-articular injection of corticosteroids are the most effective means of treating acute attack of pseudogout. NSAIDs and colchicine are less effective than they are in classical gout.

BASIC CALCIUM PHOSPHATE (BCP) CRYSTAL DEPOSITION

Controlled deposition of the BCP crystal hydroxyapatite (HA) is essential for the formation of normal bone, dentine and enamel. Deposition of HA and other BCP crystals in connective tissues occurs in a variety of disorders associated with damage to collagen (see information box).

DISORDERS ASSOCIATED WITH CONNECTIVE TISSUE DAMAGE AND DEPOSITION OF BCP

- Rotator cuff injuries
- Hip arthroplasty
- Paraplegia
- Myositis ossificans
- Prolapsed intervertebral discs
- Calcific aortic valves
- Scleroderma
- CREST syndrome
- Dermatomyositis
- Paget's disease
- Chronic dialysis
- Vitamin D intoxication

Calcific periarthritis

Acute calcific periarthritis is characterised by periarticular inflammation in association with juxta-articular deposition of HA crystals. The shoulder region is most frequently affected in middle-aged men or women, but monoarticular/polyarticular attacks can also occur at the hip, knee, ankle, elbow and wrist. The cause of calcific periarthritis of the shoulder is usually unknown but the problem may be familial or secondary in patients with chronic renal failure undergoing dialysis.

Acute inflammation results from peritendonitis or bursitis following sudden release of HA crystals from a primary deposit in the tendon.

Radiographs usually show evidence of a calcinotic deposit in the supraspinatus tendon (Fig. 15.10, p. 874), the rotator cuff or subacromial bursa and these occasionally disappear following an acute attack. Identification of the crystals from the bursal fluid requires x-ray diffraction, infrared spectroscopy or electron microscopy and is not required in clinical practice.

Acute attacks usually respond to treatment with non-steroidal anti-inflammatory drugs (NSAIDs) or colchicine, and aspiration, corticosteroid injection or surgical excision are very rarely indicated.

APATITE-ASSOCIATED DESTRUCTIVE ARTHROPATHY
('Milwaukee' shoulder/knee syndrome, cuff-tear arthropathy)

This is an unusual but distinctive type of destructive arthropathy seen in the elderly. Women are affected more than men. The shoulders and knees are the main joints affected but the wrists, hips and midtarsal joints are also rarely involved. Sudden onset of pain and swelling in the dominant shoulder is associated with the presence of a large cool effusion, variable pain on moving the joint and the rapid development of joint subluxation and destruction. Radiographs show evidence of rotator cuff defects with upward migration and destruction of the humeral head but little in the way of bone remodelling or osteophyte formation. Some cases are associated with calcific periarthritis. Synovial fluid analysis shows large volumes of relatively non-inflammatory fluid with numerous crystals of CPPD and HA as well as elevated levels of collagenase and neutral protease activity.

Treatment is with simple analgesics, NSAIDs and supportive physiotherapy as well as with joint aspiration and intra-articular injection of corticosteroid. Rarely surgical intervention with a shoulder joint spacer or replacement arthroplasty are required.

GOUT

Gout is not a single disease. The term is used to describe a number of disorders in which crystals of monosodium urate monohydrate derived from hyperuricaemic body fluids give rise to inflammatory arthritis, tenosynovitis, bursitis or cellulitis, tophaceous deposits, urolithiasis

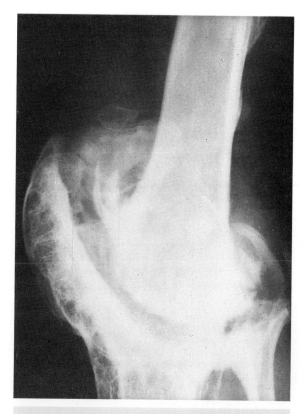

Fig. 15.17 Pseudoneuropathic CPPD disease. Radiograph of knee showing severe destructive and proliferative changes.

and renal disease. Hyperuricaemia is a necessary but not a sufficient prerequisite for clinical manifestations of gout.

Epidemiology
Gouty arthritis is predominantly a problem of post-pubertal males and is seldom seen in women before the menopause. Asymptomatic hyperuricaemia is 10 times more common. Serum uric acid concentrations are distributed in the community as a continuous variable and are determined by a number of demographic factors of which age, sex, body bulk and genetic constitution are the most important. Serum uric acid levels are higher in urban than in rural communities and are positively correlated with intelligence, social class, weight, haemoglobin, serum proteins and a high protein diet.

Hyperuricaemia is arbitrarily defined as a serum uric acid level greater than two standard deviations from the mean, i.e. above 0.42 mmol/1 in adult males and 0.36 mmol/1 in adult females.

Aetiology
The concentration of uric acid in body fluids depends on a balance between purine synthesis plus ingestion

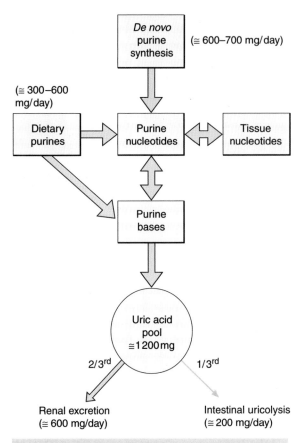

Fig. 15.18 The uric acid pool. Origins and disposal of uric acid in normal man.

and uric acid elimination through the kidneys and intestine (Fig. 15.18). Purine nucleotide synthesis and degradation are regulated by a network of enzyme pathways (Fig. 15.19).

Various genetic and environmental factors lead to hyperuricaemia and gout by decreasing the excretion of uric acid and/or increasing its production, as shown in the information box.

Diminished renal excretion of uric acid

In more than 75% of patients with gout there appears to be a genetically-determined defect in fractional urate excretion which results in an inability to increase uric acid excretion in response to a purine load.

Increased production of uric acid

This is at least partly responsible for hyperuricaemia in 20–25% of gout patients. In the absence of significant renal impairment such patients are hyperexcretors of uric acid. Specific enzyme defects resulting in an increase in *de novo* purine synthesis should be suspected:

- in the absence of disorders resulting in increased turnover of purines
- if gout develops at an unusually early age
- if there is a family history of gout commencing at an early age
- if uric acid lithiasis is the first presenting feature.

Idiopathic

The enzyme defect(s) responsible for most cases of gout with increased synthesis of purine de novo remain to be discovered.

Deficiency of hypoxanthine-guanine-phosphoribosyl transferase (HGPRT)

The Lesch–Nyhan syndrome is a rare X-linked recessive inborn error of metabolism in which gout and severe overproduction of uric acid are associated with choreoathetosis, spasticity, a variable degree of mental deficiency and compulsive self-mutilation. The enzyme

---

FACTORS PREDISPOSING TO HYPERURICAEMIA AND GOUT

Diminished renal excretion of uric acid

- Renal failure
- Drugs
  - Diuretics
  - Pyrazinamide
  - Low doses aspirin
- Lead poisoning
- Hyperparathyroidism
- Myxoedema
- Down syndrome

- Lactic acidosis
  - Alcohol
  - Exercise
  - Starvation
  - Vomiting
  - Toxaemia of pregnancy
  - Type I glycogen storage disease
- Unidentified inherited defect

Increased production of uric acid

- **Increased turnover of purines**
  Myeloproliferative disorder, e.g. polycythaemia vera
  Lymphoproliferative disorders, e.g. chronic lymphatic leukaemia
  Psoriasis—severe, exfoliative
- **Increased purine synthesis de novo**
  HGPRT deficiency
  PRPP synthetase overactivity
  Glucose-6-phosphatase deficiency
  Idiopathic

HGPRT—Hypoxanthine-guanine phosphoribosyl transferase
PRPP—Phosphoribosyl pyrophosphate

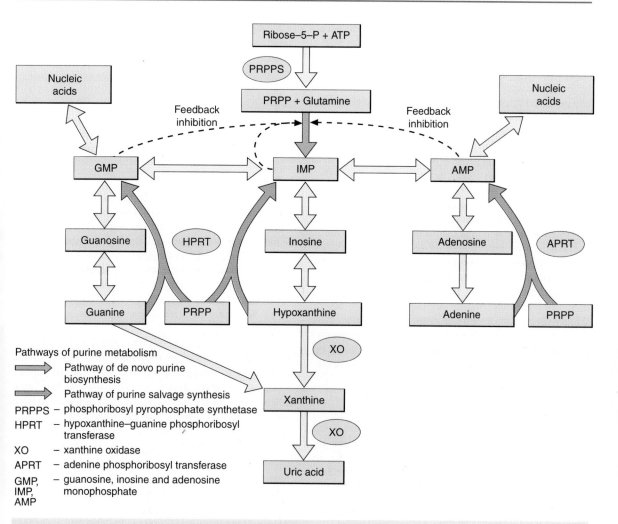

Fig. 15.19 Pathways of purine metabolism in mammalian cells.

defect can be detected in red cell lysates; female carriers can be identified from skin fibroblast cultures or hair root analysis, and pre-natal detection can be undertaken using amniotic fluid cells. The elucidation of the mechanism whereby this deficit in the activity of a purine salvage enzyme leads to primary purine overproduction has been a key to the understanding of purine metabolism and the development of allopurinol for the treatment and prevention of gout.

Phosphoribosyl pyrophosphate (PRPP) synthetase overactivity

Severe gouty arthritis and uric acid lithiasis is seen from an early age in families with inborn errors of metabolism resulting in increased activity in this enzyme. The defect can be detected in red cell lysates.

Glucose-6-phosphatase deficiency

Children with glycogen storage disease Type I (von Gierke's disease) who survive to adult life develop severe gout and hyperuricaemia as a consequence of impaired uric acid excretion secondary to lactic acidosis and also of increased purine synthesis de novo. The enzyme defect can be detected only in the liver, kidney or intestine.

Clinical features

Acute gout

The metatarso-phalangeal joint of a great toe is the site of the first attack of acute gouty arthritis in 70% of patients; the ankle, the knee, the small joints of the feet and hands, the wrist and elbow follow in decreasing order of frequency. The onset may be insidious or explosively sudden, often waking the patient from sleep. The affected joint is hot, red and swollen with shiny overlying skin and dilated veins; it is excruciatingly painful and tender. Very acute attacks may be accompanied by fever, leucocytosis and a raised ESR and are occasionally preceded by prodromal symptoms such as anorexia, nausea or a change in mood. If untreated, the attack lasts for days or weeks but it eventually subsides spontaneously. Resolution of the acute attack may be accompanied by local pruritus and desquamation.

Some patients have only a single attack, or suffer another only after an interval of many months or years. More often there is a tendency to have recurrent attacks. These increase in frequency and duration so that eventually one attack may merge into another and the patient remains in a prolonged state of subacute gout. Acute attacks are occasionally polyarticular, and tenosynovitis, bursitis or cellulitis may be the presenting feature.

Acute attacks may be precipitated by sudden rises in serum urate following dietary excess, alcohol, severe dietary restriction or diuretic drugs, or by sudden falls following initiation of therapy with allopurinol or uricosuric drugs. Acute attacks may also be provoked by trauma, unusual physical exercise, surgery or severe systemic illness.

Chronic gout

First attacks of gouty arthritis are seldom associated with residual disability but recurrent acute attacks are followed by progressive cartilage and bone erosion in association with deposition of tophi and secondary degenerative changes. Severe functional impairment and gross joint deformities may occur in chronic tophaceous gout. Tophi are frequently found in the cartilage of the ear, bursae and tendon sheaths.

Urate urolithiasis

This occurs in about 10% of patients with gout attending British hospital clinics. The incidence is much higher in hot climates. The formation of urate calculi is also favoured by:

- hyperuricosuria
- purine overproduction
- excessive purine ingestion
- uricosuric drugs and defects in tubular resorption of uric acid
- low urine pH, e.g. in chronic diarrhoeal diseases or following ileostomy.

Chronic urate nephropathy

This results from a combination of renal tubular obstruction, uric acid calculi, hypertension, glomerulo-sclerosis and secondary pyelonephritis. It is rare in the absence of well-established chronic gouty arthritis.

Other manifestations

Gout and hyperuricaemia are frequently associated with obesity, type IV hyperlipoproteinaemia, diabetes mellitus, hypertension and ischaemic heart disease. Hyperuricaemia itself does not, however, appear to be a risk factor for vascular disease or diabetes mellitus.

Investigations

The serum urate level is usually raised but it is important to appreciate that this does not prove the diagnosis because asymptomatic hyperuricaemia is very common. Whenever possible synovial fluid should be aspirated and examined under polarising light (Fig. 15.20). Acute attacks of gout can occur when the serum urate level is normal. This is usually seen in patients who have received treatment with allopurinol, a uricosuric agent or an NSAID with uricosuric side-effects such as azapropazone.

Joint radiographs are seldom useful in establishing the diagnosis. Although they may show characteristic punched-out erosions associated with the soft tissue swelling of urate tophi, occasionally flecked with calcium, the diagnosis will be clinically apparent in such patients and in others the erosions may be indistinguishable from those seen in various forms of inflammatory arthritis.

Management

NSAIDs are the agents of choice. It is important to start treatment as early as possible, to use adequate doses and to avoid salicylates and diuretics. Patients known to have gout should keep a supply of a NSAID with which they are familiar so that an acute attack can be aborted as soon as the first symptoms are noticed. Indomethacin (50 mg 6-hourly orally), or naproxen (500 mg 8-hourly orally) are given until the acute attack subsides. Treatment is then continued with lower doses for 7–10 days. Colchicine is highly effective but causes vomiting and diarrhoea in many patients in the doses that need to be used (1 mg at once followed by 0.5 mg 2-hourly orally).

Prevention

Prolonged administration of drugs which lower the serum urate level should be considered following the resolution of the acute attack in patients with:

- recurrent attacks of gouty arthritis
- tophi or evidence of chronic gouty arthritis
- associated renal disease
- gout and markedly raised serum urate.

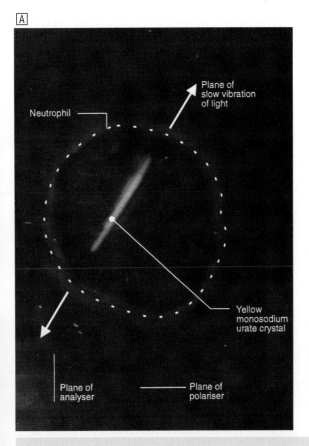

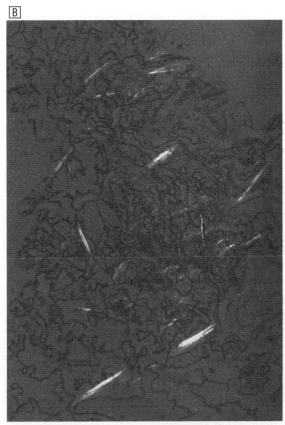

Fig. 15.20 [A] **Photograph and overlying diagram of needle-shaped crystal of monosodium urate in polymorphonuclear leucocyte** from joint fluid of patient with acute gouty arthritis. [B] **Typical birefringence of monosodium urate crystals present in synovial tissue.**

Allopurinol

This is the drug of choice for long-term prophylaxis because of its convenience and low incidence of side-effects. It lowers the serum urate by inhibiting xanthine oxidase which is responsible for the conversion of xanthine and hypoxanthine to uric acid. Oral treatment is commenced with 300 mg once daily together with colchicine 0.5 mg 12-hourly to avert the acute attacks of gouty arthritis which frequently follow initiation of hypouricaemic drug therapy. It is important not to commence treatment with allopurinol until several weeks have elapsed after the last acute attack and to continue concurrent administration of colchicine for several months. The dose of allopurinol may have to be adjusted in the range of 300–900 mg daily to bring the serum urate within the normal range. If renal function is impaired lower doses (100 mg daily) should be used.

Uricosuric agents

These can also be very effective in lowering the serum urate level, reducing the frequency of acute attacks of gout and decreasing the size of the tophi. Probencid 0.5–1 g 12-hourly orally or sulphinpyrazone 100 mg 8-hourly are given with colchicine 0.5 mg 12-hourly orally. Salicylates must be avoided as they antagonise the uricosuric effects of these drugs. Uricosuric drug therapy is contraindicated:

- in gout with overproduction of uric acid and gross uricosuria
- in patients with renal failure (ineffective)
- in patients with urate urolithiasis.

Benzbromarone 100 mg daily can be used in patients with moderate renal impairment when other uricosuric agents are ineffective.

Diet

There is no need for severe dietary restrictions but excessive purine intake and overindulgence in alcohol should be avoided. Gradual weight loss is encouraged in obese patients and is associated with a fall in serum urate. Severe calorie restriction must be avoided as it causes lactic acidosis and a rise in serum urate.

Surgery

This is occasionally required to deal with a large or ulcerating tophus.

Asymptomatic hyperuricaemia

This does not require prophylactic treatment in the absence of a history, family history or clinical evidence of gout. A search should be made for causes of secondary hyperuricaemia (p. 882). Obese subjects should lose weight gradually and have their blood pressure and renal function monitored annually.

FURTHER READING

Emmerson B T 1991 Identification of the causes of persistent hyperuricaemia. Lancet 337: 461–463
Fam A G 1992 Calcium pyrophosphate crystal deposition disease and other crystal deposition diseases. Current Opinion in Rheumatology 4: 574–582
Terkeltaub R A, Ginsberg M H 1991 The inflammatory reaction to crystals. Rheumatic Disease Clinics of North America 14: 353–364

INFLAMMATORY JOINT DISEASE

RHEUMATOID ARTHRITIS

Rheumatoid arthritis (RA) is the commonest form of chronic inflammatory joint disease. In its typical form RA is a symmetrical, destructive and deforming polyarthritis affecting small and large synovial joints with associated systemic disturbance, a variety of extra-articular features and the presence of circulating anti-globulin antibodies (rheumatoid factors). Characteristically the course of the disease is prolonged with exacerbations and remissions but atypical, asymmetrical and incomplete forms are not uncommon.

Epidemiology

Rheumatoid arthritis occurs throughout the world and in all ethnic groups. Climate, altitude and geography do not appear to influence its prevalence but a higher proportion of patients in Western and urban communities have more severe and disabling disease. The overall prevalence of RA in Caucasian populations is about 1% with a female to male ratio of 3:1. The disease starts most commonly between the third and fifth decades but the age of onset follows a normal distribution curve and no age group is exempted. With an annual incidence of new cases of about 0.02%, 5% of women and 2% of men over the age of 55 years are affected.

A diagnosis of rheumatoid arthritis can be established in patients with clinical features of inflammatory arthritis of 6 weeks' duration. The revised criteria for the diagnosis of RA used for epidemiological purposes are shown in the information box below.

CRITERIA FOR THE DIAGNOSIS OF RHEUMATOID ARTHRITIS

(American Rheumatism Association 1988 Revision)

- Morning stiffness (>1 hour)*
- Arthritis of 3 or more joint areas*
- Arthritis of hand joints*
- Symmetrical arthritis*
- Rheumatoid nodules
- Rheumatoid factor
- Radiological changes

* Duration of six weeks or more

Diagnosis of RA made with 4 or more criteria.

Aetiology

Although the cause of rheumatoid arthritis remains tantalisingly obscure, there is increasing evidence that the disease is triggered by T-lymphocyte activation in genetically predisposed individuals with defined HLA class II haplotypes. HLA-DR4 is the major susceptibility haplotype in most ethnic groups but DR1 is more important in Indians and Israelis and DW15 in Japanese; alleles of DW10, DW13 and DW14 have also been implicated.

The molecular basis for disease susceptibility resides in a shared epitope found in the third allelic hypervariable region of HLA-DR beta 1 between amino acid residues 67 and 74 which flank the T-cell recognition site (Figs 15.21, 15.22). Whether or not one or more exogenous or auto-antigenic peptides can bind this disease susceptibility epitope to initiate or perpetuate disease is still unclear, but it is of interest that an Epstein–Barr virus glycoprotein (GP110) contains the identical amino acid sequence. The search for other potential mechanisms for persistent antigenic stimulation and altered immune reactivity include a search for the presence of retroviral or parvoviral gene products, partially degraded bacterial cell wall peptidoglycans, cross reaction between bacterial or viral antigens and articular components, viral induction of immune complexes or viral immunosuppression. The possibility that RA is a superantigen-driven disorder has also been raised. Alternatively it has been suggested that sensitisation to self antigens could be a consequence of enzymatic or free radical damage to proteins such as immunoglobulin (IgG) or Type II collagen, the development of anti-idiotypic antibodies or a defect in glycosation of IgG.

Clinical evidence for the importance of genetic factors

		66	67		70				74	75
	DR1	D	L	L	E	Q	R	R	A	A	A
Haplotypes associated with RA	DR4, DW4	D	L	L	E	Q	K	R	A	A	A
	DR4, DW14	D	L	L	E	Q	R	R	A	A	A
	DR4, DW15	D	L	L	E	Q	R	R	A	A	A
	DRW10	D	L	L	E	R	R	R	A	A	A
	DR4, DW10	D	I	L	E	R	E	R	A	A	A
Haplotypes not associated with RA	DR4, DW53	D	L	L	E	D	R	R	A	E	A
	DR7	D	I	L	E	D	A	R	G	Q	A

One letter amino acid code

A=Ala, D=Asp, E=Glu, G=Gly, I=Ile, K=Lys, L=Leu, Q=Gln, R=Arg

Fig. 15.21   The RA susceptibility determinant: a common epitope on the third hypervariable region of HLA-DR beta 1 which is shared by 85% of patients with rheumatoid arthritis.

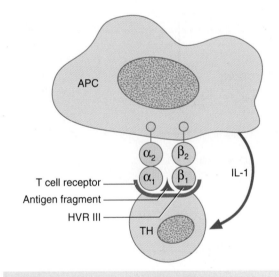

Fig. 15.22   Antigen presentation by class 2 molecules: schematic diagram. APC—antigen presenting cell. TH—T helper lymphocyte (CD4). HVR III—3rd hypervariable region of DR β_1.

Table 15.2   Evidence for cellular activation, autoimmunity and immune complex pathology in RA

Cellular activation	Autoantibodies	Immune complex pathology
DR expression (dendritic and synovial lining cells)	Rheumatoid factors (IgM, IgA, IgG)	IgG-IgG IgG-IgM complexes in synovial fluid
Endothelial cell expression of adhesion molecules	Antinuclear factor Anticollagen antibodies	Complement activation with ↓ C3, C4, CH50
Leucocyte emigration CD4 lymphocytes B lymphocytes Plasma cells Monocytes Cytokine production (IL-1, TNF$_\alpha$, IL-6, IL-2) Prostaglandins Leucotrienes Metalloproteinases Acute phase proteins Heat shock proteins O$_2$ free radicals		

T-cell receptors, immunoglobulin genes and cytokine gene polymorphisms may also be involved in genetic susceptibility to RA.

Whatever the initiating stimulus, RA is characterised by persistent cellular activation, autoimmunity and the presence of immune complexes at sites of articular and extra-articular lesions (Table 15.2). The development of amyloidosis in some patients provides further clinical evidence for chronic immune stimulation while the striking remissions of activity that can follow lymphocyte depletion by thoracic duct drainage, lymphocytophoresis or cytotoxic drug therapy attest to the importance of lymphocytes and cellular immunity. Thus rheumatoid arthritis is both an extra-vascular immune complex disease and a disorder of cell-mediated immunity in which the events depicted in Figure 15.23 lead to chronic inflammation, granuloma formation and joint destruction. The severity of tissue damage is related to joint movement and physical stress as well as the activity of the inflammatory disease, indicating that mechanical factors are also important in pathogenesis.

Pathology (Fig. 15.24)

The earliest change is swelling and congestion of the synovial membrane and the underlying connective tissues, which become infiltrated with lymphocytes (especially CD4 T cells), plasma cells and macrophages. Effusion of synovial fluid into the joint space takes place during active phases of the disease. Hypertrophy of the synovial membrane occurs with the formation of lymphoid follicles resembling an immunologically active lymph

comes from an increase in the frequency of disease in first degree relatives of patients with RA and a higher concordance rate of disease in identical twins (30%) compared with that in non-identical twins (5%). 50–75% of Caucasian patients with RA are HLA-DR4 positive compared with 20–25% of the population at large. Tissue typing studies, however, in families with multiple cases of RA suggest that HLA genes may only account for 30% of the genetic determinants involved. Current research is exploring the possibility that specific

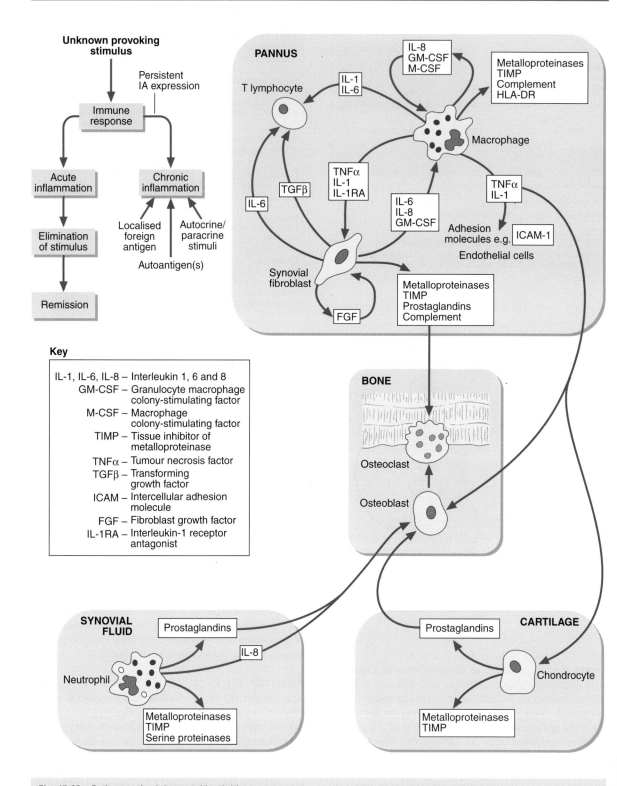

Key

IL-1, IL-6, IL-8 – Interleukin 1, 6 and 8

GM-CSF – Granulocyte macrophage colony-stimulating factor

M-CSF – Macrophage colony-stimulating factor

TIMP – Tissue inhibitor of metalloproteinase

TNFα – Tumour necrosis factor

TGFβ – Transforming growth factor

ICAM – Intercellular adhesion molecule

FGF – Fibroblast growth factor

IL-1RA – Interleukin-1 receptor antagonist

Fig. 15.23   Pathogenesis of rheumatoid arthritis: possible sequence of events and network of cytokines and mediators.

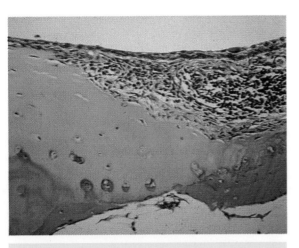

Fig. 15.24   Pathology of rheumatoid arthritis: synovial pannus eroding articular cartilage.

PATTERNS OF ONSET IN RHEUMATOID ARTHRITIS

• Insidious	70%		• Oligoarticular	44%
• Acute	15%		• Polyarticular	35%
• Systemic	10%		• Monoarticular	21%
• Palindromic	5%			

node. Inflammatory granulation tissue (pannus) is formed, spreading over and under the articular cartilage which is progressively eroded and destroyed. Later, fibrous adhesions may form between the layers of pannus across the joint space and fibrous or bony ankylosis may occur. Muscles adjacent to inflamed joints atrophy and there may be focal infiltration with lymphocytes.

Subcutaneous nodules have a characteristic histological appearance. There is a central area of fibrinoid material consisting of swollen and fragmented collagen fibres, fibrinous exudate and cellular debris, surrounded by a palisade of radially arranged proliferating mononuclear cells. The nodules have a loose capsule of fibrous tissue. Similar granulomatous lesions may occur in the pleura, lung, pericardium and sclera. Lymph nodes are often hyperplastic, showing many lymphoid follicles with large germinal centres and numerous plasma cells in the sinuses and medullary cords. Immunofluorescence shows that the plasma cells in the synovium and lymph nodes synthesise rheumatoid factors.

Clinical features

In the majority of patients the onset is *insidious*, with joint pain, stiffness and symmetrical swelling of a number of peripheral joints but other disease patterns can occur (see information box). Initially, pain may be experienced only on movement of joints, but rest pain and especially early morning stiffness are characteristic features of all kinds of inflammatory arthritis.

In the typical case the small joints of the fingers and toes are the first to be affected. Swelling of the proximal, but not the distal, interphalangeal joints gives the fingers a 'spindled' appearance (Fig. 15.25) and swelling of the metatarsophalangeal joints results in 'broadening' of the

forefoot. As the disease progresses with or without intervening remissions, there is a tendency for it to spread to involve the wrists, elbows, shoulders, knees, ankles, subtalar and midtarsal joints. The hip joints become involved only in the more severely affected, but neck pain and stiffness from cervical spine disease is common. The temporomandibular, acromioclavicular, sternoclavicular and crico-arytenoid joints are sometimes affected, as indeed are all synovial joints.

In 10–15% of patients the disease starts as an acute *polyarthritis* with severe systemic symptoms. A more insidious *systemic onset* with fever, weight loss, profound fatigue and malaise without joint symptoms occurs less often, particularly in middle-aged men, and this can cause diagnostic confusion with malignant disease or chronic infections. The onset is *palindromic* in some patients with recurrent acute episodes of joint pain and stiffness in individual joints lasting only a few hours or days. In about a third of such cases the disease sooner or later evolves into a more typical arthritis. The onset of RA in the elderly can be indistinguishable from polymyalgia rheumatica with pain and stiffness in the region of the hip and shoulder girdles without apparent synovitis. The presence of rheumatoid factor in such patients may be a clue to the true diagnosis before typical joint changes have developed.

Progression

As the disease advances, muscle atrophy, tendon sheath and joint destruction result in limitation of joint motion, joint instability, subluxation and deformities. At first deformities are correctable, but later permanent contractures develop and the joints may become completely disorganised.

Characteristic deformities include flexion contractures of the small joints of the hands and feet, the knees, hips and elbows. Anterior subluxation of the metacarpophalangeal joints is common with ulnar deviation of the fingers. Other finger deformities lead to greater loss of hand function. These include the 'swan neck' deformity (hyperextension of the proximal interphalangeal joint with fixed flexion at the distal interphalangeal joints—Fig. 15.25B), the *boutonnière* or 'button-hole' deformity (fixed flexion of the proximal interphalangeal joint and extension of the terminal inter-

A

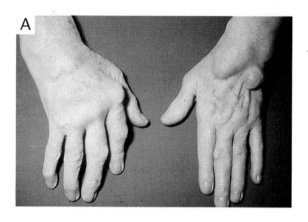

B

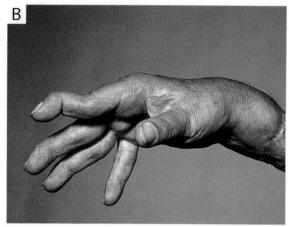

Fig. 15.25   The hand in rheumatoid arthritis. [A] Ulnar deviation of the fingers with wasting of the small muscles of the hands and synovial swelling at the wrists, the extensor tendon sheaths, the MCP and PIP joints. [B] Swan neck deformity of the fingers.

phalangeal joint) and a Z deformity of the thumb. Dorsal subluxation of the ulnar styloid of the wrist is common and may contribute to rupture of the 4th and 5th extensor tendons when these are already the site of tenosynovitis.

In the forefoot, subluxation of the metatarsophalangeal joints is followed by clawing of the toes, callosities over the exposed metatarsal heads and a painful sensation of 'walking on pebbles'. In the hindfoot, calcaneal erosions may develop at the insertion of the Achilles tendon, and valgus deformities at the subtalar joint are common.

Tenosynovitis and bursitis are integral features of RA as tendon sheaths and bursae are also lined with synovium. 'Triggering' of the fingers may be associated with nodules in the flexor tendon sheaths which can progress to permanent flexion contractures or tendon rupture if left untreated.

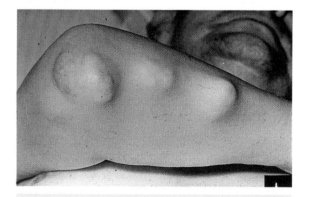

Fig. 15.26   Rheumatoid nodules.

Popliteal cysts (Baker's cysts) communicate with the knee but fluid is prevented from returning to the joint by a valve-like mechanism. The high pressure generated by flexion of the knee, especially when effusions are present, can cause gradual extension or rupture of the cyst into the calf. Rupture is accompanied by calf pain, swelling, tenderness and pitting oedema. Diagnostic confusion with deep vein thrombosis can usually be avoided by careful consideration of the history but ultrasound examination, venogram or arthrogram are occasionally required to establish the correct diagnosis (Fig. 15.27).

Extra-articular features

Rheumatoid arthritis is a systemic disease. Anorexia, weight loss, lethargy and myalgia occur commonly throughout its course and may precede the onset of articular symptoms by weeks or months. The many extra-articular features of the disease are listed in Table 15.3.

Lymphadenopathy is usually found in nodes draining actively inflamed joints but more generalised lymphadenopathy can give rise to diagnostic confusion when arthritis is minimal or quiescent. The nodes are discrete and non-tender. Histology shows a reactive hyperplasia which can be mistaken for lymphoma.

Periarticular osteoporosis, muscle weakness and wasting are prominent adjacent to inflamed and functionally impaired joints. **Generalised osteoporosis, muscle wasting and skin atrophy** occur as global secondary complications of systemic inflammation and circulating catalytic cytokines (IL-1, IL-6, TNFα). Although often seen early in the course of the disease they progress to become major features in very active or advanced cases.

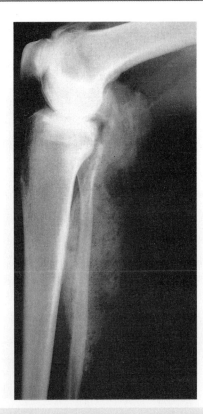

Fig. 15.27 Rupture of knee joint in rheumatoid arthritis.
Arthrogram showing radio-opaque contrast medium in popliteal cyst and tissues of the calf.

Table 15.3 Extra-articular manifestations of rheumatoid disease	
Systemic Fever Weight loss Fatigue Susceptibility to infection	**Vasculitis** Digital arteritis Ulcers Pyoderma gangrenosum Mononeuritis multiplex Visceral arteritis
Musculoskeletal Muscle wasting Tenosynovitis Bursitis Osteoporosis	**Cardiac** Pericarditis Myocarditis Endocarditis Conduction defects Coronary vasculitis Granulomatous aortitis
Haematological Anaemia Thrombocytosis Eosinophilia	**Pulmonary** Nodules Pleural effusions Fibrosing alveolitis Bronchiolitis Caplan's syndrome
Lymphatic Splenomegaly Felty's syndrome	
Nodules Sinuses Fistulae	**Neurological** Cervical cord compression Compression neuropathies Peripheral neuropathy Mononeuritis multiplex
Ocular Episcleritis Scleritis Scleromalacia Keratoconjunctivitis sicca	**Amyloidosis**

Subcutaneous nodules occur in about 20% of patients. They are usually seen at sites of pressure or friction such as the extensor surfaces of the forearms below the elbow (Fig. 15.26), the scalp, sacrum, scapula and Achilles tendon, as well as the fingers and toes. Ulceration and secondary infection are common. Nodules are almost invariably associated with positive tests for rheumatoid factor.

Ocular manifestations

Episcleritis is a frequent and benign feature in patients with nodular seropositive disease. The intermittent inflammation of the superficial sclera is usually painless. It is not associated with visual disturbance and requires no specific therapy. **Scleritis** is a rarer but more serious condition. The eye is red and painful with inflammatory changes throughout the sclera and uveal tract. The pupil may be irregular from adhesions (synechiae) which can cause secondary glaucoma and visual impairment. **Scleromalacia** may follow episodes of scleritis and is seen as a blue discoloration of the white of the eye. **Scleromalacia perforans** follows necrosis of the sclera and may require grafting or enucleation of the eye. **Ker-** atoconjunctivitis sicca (secondary Sjögren's syndrome) occurs in 10% of RA patients. Lack of lacrimal secretions results in grittiness, burning or itching associated with sticky mucous threads. Diagnosis can be confirmed by finding a reduction in the rate of tear secretion (Schirmer test).

Cardiovascular manifestations

Asymptomatic **pericarditis** occurs in about a third of patients with seropositive RA. **Pericardial effusions** and **constrictive pericarditis** are rarer complications. Very rarely granulomatous lesions lead to **heart block, cardiomyopathy, coronary artery occlusion or aortic regurgitation**.

Vasculitis

Raynaud's phenomenon (see p. 273, Ch. 5) can occur throughout the course of the disease as well as in the prodromal period. Diffuse **necrotising vasculitis** is seen particularly in patients with nodules and positive tests for rheumatoid factor. Clinical manifestations vary with the size and site of the vessel involved. Small vessel disease of the terminal arterioles or capillaries is often associated with no more than nail fold infarcts, leg ulcers or purpura. Large areas of skin necrosis or digital gangrene have more serious clinical significance and may herald the onset of **malignant rheumatoid disease**.

Such patients are often febrile with severe systemic disturbance and multiple extra-articular manifestations. A larger vessel arteritis, histologically resembling polyarteritis nodosa, may result in catastrophic mesenteric, renal, cerebrovascular or coronary artery occlusion. Such patients frequently have evidence of circulating immune complexes, hypergammaglobulinaemia, cryoglobulins and hypocomplementaemia.

Pulmonary manifestations See page 389.

Neurological manifestations

Entrapment neuropathies result from compression of peripheral nerves by hypertrophied synovium. Median nerve compression in the carpal tunnel is the most common and may be an early clinical manifestation of the disease. Others include ulnar nerve compression at the elbow, peroneal nerve palsy at the knee and posterior tibial nerve entrapment in the flexor retinaculum at the ankle (tarsal tunnel syndrome). A more diffuse symmetrical **peripheral neuropathy** can occur and is usually limited to symptoms and signs of mild 'glove and stocking' sensory loss. **Mononeuritis multiplex** follows occlusion of vasa nervorum in patients with arteritis. **Cervical cord compression** can result from subluxation of the cervical spine at the atlanto-axial joint or at a subaxial level. Atlanto-axial subluxation is a common finding in long-standing rheumatoid arthritis and can be diagnosed from lateral radiographs of the cervical spine taken in full flexion (Fig. 15.28). Although usually associated with no more than neck pain radiating to the occiput, it can result in cord compression and sudden death if the neck is manipulated inadvertently under an anaesthetic. Progressive cervical myelopathy may develop more insidiously with limb weakness, difficulty in holding up the head and tetraparesis. These problems occur more often following subluxation at a subaxial level and may require operative decompression and fixation.

Haematological manifestations

A normochromic normocytic anaemia of chronic disease which does not respond to oral iron is very common in active rheumatoid disease. The picture is frequently complicated by true iron deficiency secondary to gastrointestinal blood loss from treatment with nonsteroidal anti-inflammatory drugs. Thrombocytosis is a feature of active systemic inflammation. Much less frequently there may be a macrocytic anaemia associated with folate deficiency. **Felty's syndrome** is the association of splenomegaly and neutropenia with rheumatoid arthritis. The features are listed in the information box below.

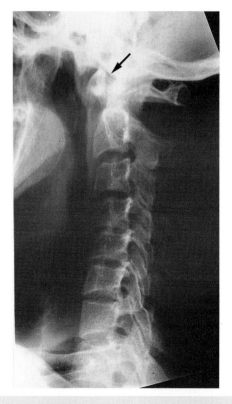

Fig. 15.28 Subluxation of cervical spine in rheumatoid arthritis. Lateral radiograph in flexion shows atlanto-axial subluxation (>4 mm gap between odontoid peg and arch of atlas, arrowed).

FELTY'S SYNDROME

- Age onset 50–70
- F > M
- Caucasian > Blacks
- Incidence <1% RA patients
- Longstanding RA
- Deforming but inactive disease
- Seropositive
- **Common clinical features**
  Splenomegaly
  Lymphadenopathy
  Weight loss
  Skin pigmentation
  Keratoconjunctivitis sicca
  Nodules
  Vasculitis
  Leg ulcers
  Recurrent infections
- **Laboratory findings**
  Anaemia
  Neutropenia
  Thrombocytopenia
  Impaired T and B cell immunity
  Abnormal liver function

Complications

Septic arthritis may complicate rheumatoid arthritis, particularly in patients with long-standing nodular seropositive disease. In debilitated patients, fever and leucocytosis may be absent and the signs of infection limited to malaise and slight exacerbation of inflammation in one or more joints. *Staphylococcus aureus* is commonly implicated secondary to invasion from an ulcerated nodule or infected skin lesion. **Amyloidosis** is a complication of prolonged active disease and is found in 25–30% of patients at autopsy, making rheumatoid arthritis a leading cause of secondary amyloidosis.

Investigations

These are listed in the information box.

INVESTIGATIONS IN RHEUMATOID ARTHRITIS

To establish diagnosis
- Clinical criteria
- Markers of inflammation
- Serological tests
- Radiographs
- Synovial analysis

To document extent of pathological changes
- Radiographs
  Occasionally:
- Arthrography
- Scintigraphy
- Ultrasound
- CT scanning
- MRI

To monitor disease activity in response to therapy
- Clinical measures
- ESR, plasma viscosity or acute phase proteins (e.g. CRP)
- Haemoglobin

To assess progression of disease
- Radiographs
- Functional index
- Outcome assessment

To monitor for safety of drug therapy
- Haematology
- Urinalysis
- Biochemistry
- Other tests

Serological tests

Rheumatoid factors (RF) are immunoglobulins of the IgG or IgM class which react with the Fc portion of IgG. In clinical immunological practice RF of the IgM class can be detected and measured semiquantitatively by testing the ability of the patient's serum to agglutinate carrier particles coated with IgG. Polystyrene particles coated with human IgG are used in the latex slide test. Sheep or human erythrocytes coated with rabbit anti-erythrocyte antibodies are used in the Rose Waaler sheep-cell agglutination test (SCAT), the human erythrocyte agglutination test (HEAT) and the differential agglutination test (DAT). The latex fixation test is simple and sensitive but less specific so that it is frequently used as a screening test. The erythrocyte tests are less sensitive but more specific. Significant titres which exclude 95% of the normal population are: SCAT 1:32; DAT 1:16; latex 1:20; but positive tests are more frequently found in the normal elderly population. Sensitive nephelometric tests have recently been developed.

The Rose Waaler test is positive in 70% of patients with RA but may not become so for 1–2 years. Positive tests are also found in other autoimmune diseases and chronic infections and these are listed in the information box below.

DISEASES WHICH MAY BE ASSOCIATED WITH POSITIVE RHEUMATOID FACTOR TESTS

Autoimmune and connective tissue diseases
- Rheumatoid arthritis
- Sjögren's syndrome
- Systemic lupus erythematosus
- Progressive systemic sclerosis
- Polymyositis/dermatomyositis
- Fibrosing alveolitis
- Chronic active hepatitis
- Liver cirrhosis
- Sarcoidosis
- Waldenström's macroglobulinaemia

Chronic infections
- Infectious mononucleosis
- Infectious hepatitis
- Bacterial endocarditis
- Tuberculosis
- Syphilis
- Yaws
- Leprosy
- Kala-azar
- Schistosomiasis
- Filariasis

Up to 30% of patients with rheumatoid arthritis have positive tests for antinuclear factor.

Synovial analysis

Analysis of synovial fluid is an important diagnostic procedure in patients presenting with a joint effusion and essential for the immediate diagnosis of joint infections and crystal arthropathies. Synovial fluid analysis can however also be useful in the differential diagnosis of inflammatory and degenerative arthropathies (Table 15.4).

Low levels of synovial fluid complement (CH_{50}, C_3, C_4) reflecting activation of the classical pathway of complement by immune complexes are only found in patients with classical rheumatoid arthritis. Blood contamination can follow a traumatic tap but evenly blood-stained haemarthroses are characteristically associated with haemophilia and von Willebrand's disease, villonodular synovitis, neuropathic joints, pyrophosphate arthropathy and resolving infections, as well as traumatic arthropathies.

Table 15.4   Synovial fluid analysis

	Colour	Viscosity	Clarity	Cell count/mm^3	Other tests
Normal	Colourless	Very high	Clear	0–200	—
OA	Colourless	High	Clear	200–4000	—
RA	Yellow	Low	Cloudy	2000–40 000	Low complement
Seronegative inflammatory arthritis	Yellow	Low	Cloudy	2000–40 000	Normal complement
Gout/Pseudogout	Variable	Low	Variable	2000–40 000	Crystals MSU/CPPD on polarising microscopy
Septic arthritis	Yellow	Low	Very turbid	>50 000	Gram stain culture and GLC

Synovial biopsy

This is seldom useful in distinguishing different types of inflammatory arthritis but it can be undertaken by blind needle biopsy, arthroscopy or open surgery if tuberculosis or a tumour are suspected.

Arthroscopy

This is particularly useful for excluding meniscal tears in the knee and it can also be used to establish the extent of erosive cartilage damage.

Imaging techniques

Radiographs are most frequently used to follow the progression of erosive inflammatory disease. The stages are listed in the information box below. Other imaging techniques such as arthrography, scintigraphy, ultrasound, CT scanning and MRI are occasionally used to establish the extent of local pathology in joints.

STAGES OF RADIOLOGICAL PROGRESSION IN RHEUMATOID ARTHRITIS

I	Periarticular osteoporosis
II	Loss of articular cartilage ('joint space')
III	Erosions
IV	Subluxation and ankylosis

Management

Because the aetiology of rheumatoid arthritis is unknown, treatment is empirically directed towards:

- relief of symptoms
- suppression of active and progressive disease
- conservation and restoration of function in affected joints.

To a greater or lesser extent these are achieved by combining:

- treatment of the patient—drugs, rest, physiotherapy, surgery with
- modification of the environment—aids, appliances, housing, occupation, statutory social benefits.

In a chronic and frequently progressive disease characterised by exacerbations and remissions over many years, as well as by systemic, psychiatric and social complications, periodic assessment of radiological progression, disease activity and disability are required (see information boxes). General practitioners and hospital physicians have a special responsibility to coordinate a team of medical specialists, orthopaedic surgeons, occupational therapists, physiotherapists, nurses, social workers and other health professionals in an integrated programme of multidisciplinary care and rehabilitation.

Patient education, counselling and continuing medical support are usually required for successful management while physical rehabilitation, reconstructive surgery and environmental adaptation assume increasing importance when advancing joint damage and deformity are associated with functional impairment.

Repeated medical, functional and social assessment are required if patients are to maintain their maximum physical, psychological, social and vocational potential, and outcome should be assessed using a comprehensive health status questionnaire (Table 15.5) as well as simple process measures.

ASSESSMENT OF DISEASE ACTIVITY IN RHEUMATOID ARTHRITIS

Clinical
- Pain (visual analogue scale)
- Early morning stiffness (minutes)
- Joint tenderness (number of inflamed joints, articular index)

Laboratory
- Acute phase proteins
- Erythrocyte sedimentation rate
- Plasma viscosity

General treatment in the active phase

Physical rest, anti-inflammatory drug therapy and maintenance exercises are the cornerstones of treatment for exacerbations of rheumatoid arthritis. Admission to hospital is necessary in a minority of patients when wide-

GRADING OF FUNCTION IN RHEUMATOID ARTHRITIS

- I   Fit for all activities—no handicap
- II   Moderate restriction—independent despite some limitation of joint movement
- III Marked restriction—limited self-care. Some assistance required
- IV   Confined to chair or bedbound—largely incapacitated and dependent

Table 15.5   Outcome measures in rheumatoid arthritis

Functional
Grip strength
Activities of daily living
Functional index

Health status questionnaire

Dimensions	Subdimensions	Components (e.g.)
Death		
Disability	Upper	Grip, feed,
	Lower	walk, climb
Discomfort	Physical	Pain, fatigue
	Psychological	Depression, anxiety
Iatrogenic	Medical	Dyspepsia, haemorrhage
	Surgical	Prosthesis, infection and loosening
Economic	Direct	Drugs, consultations
	Indirect	Loss of work, social

spread active polyarthritis is associated with signs of constitutional disturbance and there has been no response to rest at home and optimal doses of non-steroidal anti-inflammatory drugs (NSAIDs).

The rest from physical and emotional stress provided by 2–3 weeks in hospital is usually sufficient to induce a marked remission of symptoms without recourse to strict bed-rest. The time in hospital allows for detailed assessment by all members of the arthritis team. It ensures that the programme of medical and physical rehabilitation best suited to the individual's needs can be started under supervision and it provides an opportunity to plan the solution of outstanding functional and social problems with appropriate aids and social services.

In a few patients a period of complete bed-rest may be required to induce a remission. In these circumstances it is essential to prevent the development of 'bed deformities'. The mattress should be firm or fracture boards inserted beneath it. A back rest with the minimum number of pillows should be in position during the day and only one firm pillow used at night. Pillows behind the knees must be avoided and a bed cage with padded

footrest provided. Foot and quadriceps exercises should be performed daily, along with maintenance exercises for muscle groups in unaffected limbs.

Anaemia of chronic disease responds best to induction of disease remission, and oral iron is only indicated in those patients with super added true iron deficiency. Folic acid is occasionally required to treat an associated macrocytic anaemia.

Local measures in the active phase

Rest splints. These can be useful to support a particularly painful joint, such as the knee or wrist, and splints are used to prevent or correct flexion deformities.

Intra-articular corticosteroid injections. These are particularly useful for settling inflammation in isolated joints that remain painful and inflamed despite general measures. Local injection of a long-acting microcrystalline corticosteroid such as methyl-prednisolone acetate (20–80 mg large joints; 4–10 mg small joints) or triamcinolone hexacetonide (10–30 mg large joints; 2–6 mg small joints) can bring symptomatic relief lasting weeks or months. Repeated injections at short intervals, particularly in weight-bearing joints, should be avoided. Local injection of a corticosteroid is also the treatment of choice for bursitis, tenosynovitis and carpal tunnel syndrome when rest, splints, and other general measures have not been effective.

Non-steroidal anti-inflammatory drugs

These are the mainstay of therapy for active inflammatory arthritis in optimal anti-inflammatory doses (Table 15.6). They can be very effective in relieving pain and stiffness but they do not alter the course of the disease and the margin between effective and toxic doses is often small.

Inhibition of prostaglandin synthetase is a major pharmacological action common to all these agents but simultaneous inhibition of the cytoprotective effect of prostanoids on gastric mucosa makes them all liable to cause gastrointestinal side-effects such as dyspepsia, ulceration and haemorrhage. NSAID-associated upper gastrointestinal haemorrhage is the most frequent serious adverse drug-related event to be reported to the Committee on Safety of Medicines. Elderly women are particularly susceptible and case control studies suggest that a fifth of all admissions to hospital in patients over the age of 60 with bleeding gastric or duodenal ulcers are directly attributable to taking NSAIDs. About 1% of RA patients receiving NSAID drugs are admitted to hospital each year with a major GI bleed although the overall risk of an individual developing a life-threatening gastrointestinal side-effect following treatment with an NSAID is approximately 1/10 000. Treatment with these agents should be avoided in patients with peptic

Table 15.6 Non-steroidal anti-inflammatory drugs (NSAIDs)	
Drug	**Usual oral dose**
CARBOXYLIC ACIDS	
Salicylic acids	
Aspirin	600–900 mg 4-hourly
Aloxiprin	1200 mg 6-hourly
Benorylate	10 ml 12-hourly
Diflusinal	500 mg 12-hourly
Salsalate	1–1.5 g 12-hourly
Trilisate	1–1.5 g 12-hourly
Anthranilic acids	
Mefenamic acid	500 mg 6-hourly
Propionic acids	
Fenbufen	300 mg morning
	600 mg evening
Fenoprofen	600 mg 6-hourly
Flurbiprofen	100 mg 8-hourly
Ibuprofen	400–800 mg 6-hourly
Ketoprofen	100 mg 8-hourly
Naproxen	500 mg 12-hourly
Tiaprofenic acid	200 mg 8-hourly
Acetic acids	
Diclofenac	50 mg 8-hourly
Naphthylalkanones	
Nabumetone	1 g daily
Heterocyclic acetic acids	
Tolmetin	400 mg 6-hourly
Indole acetic acids	
Indomethacin	25–50 mg 8-hourly
Sulindac	200 mg 12-hourly
Pyranocarboxylic acids	
Etodolac	200 mg 12-hourly
ENOLIC ACIDS	
Pyrazolones	
Azapropazone	600 mg 12-hourly
Phenylbutazone	100 mg 8-hourly
(severe, active ankylosing	
spondylitis only)	
Oxicams	
Piroxicam	20 mg daily
Tenoxicam	20 mg daily

ulceration but it is important to realise that endoscopic evidence of ulcers is found in 20% of NSAID-treated patients even in the absence of symptoms. When NSAID treatment cannot be avoided, peptic ulcers can be made to heal by concomitant administration of H2 antagonists (cimetidine, ranitidine) or prostaglandin E analogues (misoprostol). The risk of NSAID-induced gastric ulceration can be reduced by the simultaneous administration of misoprostol 100–200 μg 6-hourly to high-risk patients. These include physically disabled debilitated patients, the elderly and patients with a previous history of peptic ulceration.

Other side-effects of NSAIDs include fluid retention, rashes, interstitial nephritis, occasional hepatotoxicity and rarely asthma and anaphylaxis.

It is advisable to start with one of the established, less expensive NSAIDs, with a low incidence of side-effects, for a trial period of about 2–3 weeks. Another NSAID with which the clinician is familiar can be tried if the response is not satisfactory but simultaneous administration of more than one NSAID generally results in an increase in the risk of adverse events without significant therapeutic benefit.

Simple analgesics

Drugs without appreciable anti-inflammatory action include peripherally acting agents such as paracetamol and centrally acting narcotic analgesics such as dextropropoxyphene, dihydrocodeine and nefopam. Although centrally acting narcotic analgesics should generally be avoided in the management of rheumatic diseases, simple analgesics are frequently used as additions to therapy when pain relief is inadequate and combination drugs such as co-proxamol (paracetamol and dextropropoxyphene) can be safe and effective when used in moderate doses.

Slow acting antirheumatic drugs

The addition of a 'second-line' or 'disease-modifying' (DMARD) suppressive antirheumatic drug should be considered in all patients where symptoms and signs of active inflammatory arthritis have persisted for 3–4 months despite adequate general measures and optimal doses of a NSAID. Drugs of this type do not possess immediate anti-inflammatory effects but will improve joint pain, stiffness and swelling and reduce systemic symptoms, acute phase proteins, sedimentation rate and rheumatoid factor titre over a period of months. If started early they may have a marginal effect in reducing the rate of radiological progression of disease but their main benefit is in inducing a symptomatic remission for 1–2 years in 40–60% of patients. They are usually introduced in a pyramidal fashion starting with the safest agent (Fig. 15.29) because they are all potentially associated with serious adverse reactions.

Antimalarials. Chloroquine phosphate (250 mg/daily, orally) or hydroxychloroquine sulphate (200 mg 12-hourly, orally) can be used as an adjunct to basic therapy. Clinical benefit is noted in about half the patients in 4–12 weeks and the drug should be discontinued if there is no effect within 6 months. Occasional side-effects include nausea, diarrhoea, rashes, haemolytic anaemia, ototoxicity and neuromyopathy and there is a small risk of ocular toxicity after more than a year of therapy. Deposits of the drug in the cornea may produce disturbances of vision which tend to disappear when the drug is withdrawn. More rarely retinopathy can result in permanent visual impairment. If the drug is effective it is advisable to check visual acuity, macular function with an Amsler grid and the ophthalmoscopic appear-

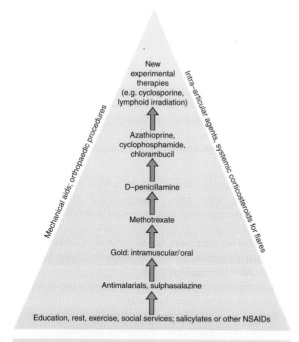

Fig. 15.29 The pyramidal approach to therapy in rheumatoid arthritis.

muscular gold but the full blood count including platelets and routine urinalysis do need to be monitored regularly.

Methotrexate, penicillamine and parenteral gold are slow acting suppressive antirheumatic drugs which have been shown to decrease the progression of erosive changes as well as reduce the activity of the disease in 50–60% of patients. Because of a high incidence of toxic effects, treatment with these agents should only be considered as an addition to basic therapy when there are clear indications for the use of a disease-modifying drug and the patient has failed to respond to antimalarials or sulphasalazine. Indications for use are listed in the information box below.

INDICATIONS FOR DISEASE-MODIFYING DRUGS

- Persistent symptoms and signs of inflammatory arthritis despite optimum therapy with NSAIDs
- Evidence of progressive radiological damage
- Troublesome extra-articular manifestations
- Palindromic rheumatoid arthritis

Methotrexate is now the drug of choice in patients with active or aggressive disease who have failed to respond to sulphasalazine. It works more quickly than other second line agents with significant improvement in symptoms in 4–6 weeks. It is administered as an oral pulse of 5–15 mg weekly with a 5 mg dose of folic acid on the day following methotrexate to reduce the incidence of adverse reactions. Methotrexate is only rarely associated with bone marrow suppression or acute disturbances of liver function but full blood counts and liver function tests must be monitored regularly and care must be taken to avoid drug interaction with sulphonamides. Increased susceptibility to infection is an important consideration and acute pulmonary toxicity is a rare but unpredictable problem in 5–10% of patients. The silent development of progressive hepatic fibrosis has been recorded and the drug should not be given to patients who are taking alcohol regularly.

Penicillamine. This treatment is commenced with a single evening dose of 125 or 250 mg orally and dosage is increased by no more than 250 mg monthly to a maximum of 1 g daily. Clinical benefit is noted several weeks after an effective dose has been achieved and reaches a maximum only after 4–6 months.

Rashes, loss of taste, nausea, vomiting and serious febrile reactions can occur early after starting treatment. Later side-effects include mouth ulcers, proteinuria and the nephrotic syndrome. Very rarely diseases resembling systemic lupus erythematosus, myasthenia gravis, pemphigus and Goodpasture's syndrome can occur. Throm-

ance of the maculae after one year and at 6-monthly intervals thereafter. In order to reduce the risks of ocular toxicity antimalarials are often given for only 10 months in each year. In some patients the dose can be halved without exacerbation of symptoms. Although antimalarials are generally less effective than other DMARDs, their use is associated with fewer patient drop-outs for toxicity.

Sulphasalazine has a good benefit-to-risk profile and is frequently used as the first choice of DMARDs. Approximately 50% of patients respond in 3–6 months. Nausea and vomiting can be troublesome but these symptoms can usually be avoided if treatment is started with 500 mg of the enteric coated preparation daily, increasing to 1 g 12-hourly over a period of 4 weeks. Depression, rashes, megaloblastic anaemia and hepatitis are rarer side-effects and the full blood count and liver function tests should be monitored monthly.

Auranofin. This oral gold compound is less toxic than parenteral preparations but short- and medium-term efficacy are also less. The usual dose is 6 mg daily but this can be increased to 9 mg daily if there has been no response after 3–4 months. Diarrhoea is a common side-effect during the early phases of treatment. Mouth ulcers, dermatitis, proteinuria and bone marrow suppression are significantly less likely than with intra-

bocytopenia and pancytopenia may occur at any time and are potentially the most serious toxic effects.

Patients should be monitored, initially at weekly intervals, by urinalysis and full blood counts, including platelets. Proteinuria and mild thrombocytopenia are indications for cessation of therapy followed by re-introduction of the drug at a lower dose if the abnormalities disappear. It is advisable to withdraw penicillamine altogether if the side-effects recur. Febrile reactions and pancytopenia are absolute indications for drug withdrawal. The likelihood of side-effects with penicillamine is increased in slow sulphoxidisers.

Parenteral gold. After a test dose of 10 mg, weekly intramuscular injections of 50 mg sodium aurothiomalate are given until a response is obtained, usually by 2–3 months. The intervals between injections are progressively increased provided the remission is maintained and the drug is continued indefinitely. Gold injections should be stopped if there has been no clinical benefit after 6 months.

Adverse effects include pruritic rashes, exfoliative dermatitis, mouth ulcers, enterocolitis, proteinuria and the nephrotic syndrome, thrombocytopenia, agranulocytosis and aplastic anaemia. All are potentially serious and preclude further therapy. Patients who are HLA-DR3 positive are particularly at risk of developing a gold-induced immune complex glomerulonephritis. Monitoring should include a routine urinalysis and full blood counts with platelets, initially prior to each injection.

Pruritus may respond to antihistamines, and exfoliative dermatitis, thrombocytopenia, agranulocytosis and nephropathy to corticosteroids. Patients with agranulocytosis almost invariably recover if they can be protected from serious infection; those with aplastic anaemia have a more serious prognosis. Dimercaprol (BAL) combines with heavy metals to form a stable compound which is rapidly excreted in the urine; 3 mg/kg body weight should be administered intramuscularly 6-hourly for 3–4 days in patients with aplastic anaemia who have not responded to withdrawal of gold injections after 4–5 days.

Other disease-modifying antirheumatic drugs

Dapsone is associated with slow clinical improvement and reduction of acute phase proteins but haemolytic anaemia can be a troublesome side-effect, particularly in slow acetylators. Other compounds which have been shown to have slow acting antirheumatic activity include the antibacterial agent rifampicin, the antihypertensive agent captopril, the penicillamine analogues 5-thiopyridoxine, pyrithioxine and thyopronine, the pentapeptide thymosin and the cytokine gamma interferon.

Corticosteroids have a very potent anti-inflammatory activity but doses required to maintain adequate

symptomatic relief on a long-term basis are accompanied by an unacceptable level of side-effects and it remains uncertain to what extent they possess the disease-modifying properties of the slow acting antirheumatic agents. Indications for their use are therefore restricted and a slow acting antirheumatic agent is usually commenced simultaneously with a view to gradual withdrawal of corticosteroid therapy when remission has been obtained.

The main indications for the use of systemic corticosteroids are:

- in exceptionally severe exacerbations which are not remitting with rest, intra-articular injections of corticosteroids and non-steroidal anti-inflammatory drugs
- when other measures fail to control persistently disabling symptoms in breadwinners or young mothers who have to return to work
- in some elderly patients when acute disease is threatening to render them bedbound
- in life- or sight-threatening visceral disease such as severe pericarditis, polyarteritis or scleritis.

Prednisolone is the corticosteroid of choice. It should ideally be administered as a single morning oral dose of no more than 7.5 mg daily to minimise suppression of the hypothalamo-pituitary-adrenal axis. An evening dose of 5 mg is sometimes more useful in overcoming intractable early morning stiffness. Enteric coated tablets may be preferred in patients with a previous history of peptic ulceration. The potential side-effects of steroids are numerous (Table 15.7). Infection and osteoporosis are particularly troublesome in patients with RA and patients commencing systemic steroid therapy should be given oral calcium supplements.

Immunomodulation

Because rheumatoid arthritis is associated with evidence of both immune hyperreactivity and suppression of some cell-mediated immune responses, both immunosuppressive and immunostimulant drugs have been considered for the management of the disease. Increased understanding of the complexity of regulation of the immune system and the immunopharmacology of cytotoxic and immunostimulant drugs makes it clear that these agents may have variable and even paradoxical effects on the expression of immune responses depending on the dose, the timing of administration and the subpopulation of cells predominantly affected. Net immune stimulation may result from treatment with a drug which predominantly inhibits a suppressor cell subpopulation of lymphocytes while functional immunosuppression can follow use of an immunostimulant which selectively activates these cells. Many immuno-

Table 15.7 Side-effects of systemic corticosteroid therapy

Endocrine	**Immunological**
Moon face	Suppresion delayed
Truncal obesity	hypersensitivity
Hirsutism	Reactivation of tuberculosis
Impotence	Susceptibility to infection
Menstrual irregularity	
Suppression of hypophyseal	**Gastrointestinal**
pituitary adrenal axis	Peptic ulceration
Growth suppression	Pancreatitis
Metabolic	**Cardiovascular**
Negative Ca^{2+}, K^+, and N balance	Hypertension
Sodium and fluid retention	Congestive cardiac failure
Hyperglycaemia	
Hyperlipoproteinaemia	**Ocular**
	Glaucoma
Musculoskeletal	Posterior subcapsular cataracts
Myopathy	
Osteoporosis	**Neurological**
Avascular necrosis	Changes in mood and personality
	Psychosis
Dermatological	Benign intracranial hypertension
Striae, acne	
Skin atrophy	
Bruising	
Impaired wound healing	

Table 15.8 Mechanism of action of immunomodulating drugs

Drug	Class	Effects
Azathioprine	Purine analogue	Inhibits purine synthesis DNA and RNA
Cyclophosphamide	Alkylating agent	Direct binding DNA, RNA and proteins
Methotrexate	Folic acid antagonist	Binds dihydrofolate reductase. Blocks de novo purine and thymidylate synthesis
Cyclosporin A	Fungal polypeptide	Inhibits IL-2 transcription: CD4 and cytotoxic lymphocytes

regulatory drugs are cell cycle specific so their action depends on the relationship of the cell cycle to target function. Receptors for growth factors and cytokines as well as the processing and release of these peptides are important targets for potential immunomodulation but nearly all the drugs currently in use were originally developed for the chemotherapy of malignant diseases. They tend therefore to be rather nonspecific cytotoxic and cytostatic agents which predominantly interfere with events involved in the cellular proliferation of all cells without specificity for receptors involved in the processes of cellular differentiation.

In practice a number of cytotoxic and immunostimulant agents have been found empirically to have both symptomatic and slow acting disease-modifying activity in rheumatoid arthritis. The effects are mediated as much by anti-inflammatory as by immunoregulatory activity and their usefulness is very strictly limited by immediate and potential long-term toxicity.

The indications for use of these agents at present are limited to:

- life-threatening extra-articular manifestations which have failed to respond to corticosteroids or second-line agents
- severe active symptomatic and progressive joint disease that has failed to respond to all other forms of therapy
- patients receiving unacceptably high doses of corticosteroids in whom dose reduction has not been possible.

Mechanisms of action of commonly used agents are summarised in Table 15.8 and toxic effects in Table 15.9.

Azathioprine has been shown to be effective in both high (2.5 mg/kg) and low (1.25 mg/kg) oral doses. Adverse effects include vomiting, stomatitis, diarrhoea, hepatitis and particularly bone marrow suppression and susceptibility to infection. Monitoring is with fortnightly or monthly full blood counts.

Cyclophosphamide has a narrow therapeutic range but is effective in a daily oral dose of 1–2 mg/kg. Adverse effects include alopecia, azoospermia, anovulation, cystitis, nausea and vomiting, susceptibility to infection, bone marrow suppression and teratogenesis. Monitoring is by fortnightly or monthly full blood counts and routine urinalysis. Toxicity may be reduced by intermittent intravenous infusion or oral boluses (0.5–1.5 g/m^2) every 1–3 months.

Cyclosporin is effective in doses of 2.5–4 mg/kg daily given in divided oral doses 12-hourly. Adverse effects include anorexia, nausea, hepatotoxicity, hypertension and dose related impairment of glomerular filtration. The full blood count, urinalysis and plasma creatinine should be monitored weekly at first and later every 2–4 weeks.

Novel approaches to immunotherapy

Targeted immunotherapy with a variety of mouse, chimeric and humanised monoclonal antibodies is superseding non-specific immunosuppression in the hope that the risks of infection can be reduced, but all such approaches remain experimental. Targets include CD4, CD5, CD7 and CD25 (IL-2 receptor) on lymphocytes, CDW52 on monocytes and lymphocytes (campath-1H), adhesion molecules (ICAM-1) and other cytokines and cytokine receptors such as TNFα and the IL-1 receptor. Recent placebo-controlled trials of anti-TNFα monoclonal antibody therapy have demonstrated good short-term efficacy and safety.

Levimasole This is an antihelminthic which has been shown to augment T lymphocyte responses as well as polymorph and macrophage chemotaxis and phago-

Table 15.9 Toxic effects of immunosuppressive drugs

	Azathioprine	Methotrexate	Cyclophosphamide	Chlorambucil	Cyclosporin A
GI Tract	+	++	+	+	+
Bone marrow	++	++	++	+++	+
Bladder	0	0	+++	0	0
Kidneys	0	+	0	0	+++
Liver	+	+++	0	0	++
Lungs	+	+++	+	+	0
Gonads	0	0	+++	+++	0
Fetus	±	+++	±	±	±
Neoplasia	+++	0	++	++	+

0 = no toxicity
+++ = severe toxicity

cytosis. It can be effective in patients with rheumatoid arthritis as a single weekly dose of 150 mg. Adverse effects include febrile reactions, vomiting, urticarial and vasculitic rashes. A high risk of agranulocytosis even with weekly monitoring of blood counts precludes its use routinely.

Medical synovectomy
Synovial obliteration can be achieved with osmic acid or a variety of radiocolloids if pain, effusion and synovitis persist despite local corticosteroid injections, systemic drug therapy and physical measures. Yttrium-90 silicate is used for large joints such as the knee and erbium-159 acetate for the small joints of the hands. Joints are immobilised for 72 hours to reduce spread to regional lymph nodes. Patients under the age of 45 should not be treated in this manner.

Surgical treatment and rehabilitation
There are many circumstances in the overall management of patients with severe and progressive rheumatoid arthritis when orthopaedic surgical procedures are required to relieve pain and conserve or restore locomotor function (Table 15.10).

Surgical decompression and synovectomy of the wrist and tendon sheaths of the hands are often needed when non-steroidal anti-inflammatory drugs, local injections of corticosteroids and simple physical measures have failed to relieve a carpal tunnel syndrome or flexion contractures of the fingers resulting from fibrosis and nodule formation. Flexor and extensor tendon synovectomy, the latter often accompanied by resection of a subluxated ulnar styloid, can be important measures in preventing tendon ruptures. Synovectomy of joints will not prevent disease progression but may be indicated for pain relief when drug therapy, local rest, intra-articular injections and radiocolloids have failed to provide symptomatic relief.

At a later stage, when tendons, cartilage and bone have been eroded and the mechanics of joints disturbed, reconstructive tendon surgery, osteotomy, arthrodesis and a variety of arthroplasties with or without prostheses play a major part in the rehabilitation of the patient.

If surgical treatment is to be successful the aims and consequences of each operation should be carefully considered as part of an integrated programme of management and rehabilitation. This is often best achieved where physicians and surgeons with special experience work together in a combined rheumatology/orthopaedic clinic with other allied health professionals. Assessment of motivation, social support and environment are no less important than careful consideration of the patient's general health and detailed assessment of the extent of disease in other joints, the integrity of the cervical spine, the presence or absence of infection, arteritis or osteoporosis. In particular it must be appreciated that whereas many patients with slowly progressive disease can be maintained mobile and functionally independent by a series of major joint replacements carried out over a number of years, it is seldom possible to mobilise a patient who has been chair- or bedbound for a long period by multiple joint replacement during a single lengthy hospital admission. In these and other circumstances pain relief and functional independence are better served by provision of a suitable wheelchair, home adjustments, physical aids and social services.

When a patient cannot return to a former occupation it may be necessary to suggest a change of employment

Table 15.10   Some useful surgical procedures in rheumatoid arthritis and osteoarthrosis

Procedure	Joint(s)	Indication
Soft tissue release (decompression)	Carpal tunnel	Median nerve compression
	Tarsal tunnel	Posterior tibial nerve entrapment
	Flexor tendon sheaths, hand	Relief of 'trigger fingers'
	Rerouting ulnar nerve at elbow	Ulnar nerve entrapment
Tendon repairs and transfers	Extensor tendons, hands	Rupture extensor tendons
	Flexor tendons, thumb and fingers	Rupture flexor tendons
Synovectomy	Wrist and extensor tendon sheaths (+ excision ulnar)	Pain relief and prevent extensor tendon rupture
Osteotomy	Keller's operation	Correct hallux valgus
	Femoral osteotomy	Pain relief. Correct deformity early OA hip
	Tibial osteotomy	Pain relief. Correct deformity unicompartmental OA knee
Excision arthroplasty	Radial head	Pain subluxation radio-ulnar joint
	Lateral end clavicle	Pain acromio-clavicular joint
	Fowler's operation metatarsal head resection	Forefoot pain MTP joint subluxation
Joint replacement	Hip, knee, elbow, shoulder, ankle, MCP joints hands	Pain relief. Maintain, restore and improve function
Arthrodesis	Interphalangeal joint thumb or fingers	Improve hand function
	MCP joint thumb	Improve pinch grip
	Wrist	Pain relief. Improve grip
	Ankle and subtalar joints	Pain relief. Stabilise hind foot

where less strain will be thrown on the damaged joints. Although disablement resettlement officers, industrial rehabilitation units and Government retraining centres are sometimes helpful in such circumstances it should be emphasised that patients have the best chance of returning to active work with their former employers. It cannot be stressed too strongly that adequate treatment in the early stages and throughout the course of the disease enables most patients to return to some form of wage-earning activity. Disabilities of all kinds can be reduced even in the 25% of patients running a severe progressive course.

Prognosis

The course and prognosis in rheumatoid arthritis is very variable. In those patients with disease of such severity as to require admission to hospital, review after ten years shows that: 25% will have a complete remission of symp-

toms and remain fit for all normal activities; 40% will have only moderate impairment of function despite exacerbations and remissions of disease; 25% will be more severely disabled; 10% will be severely crippled (this rises to 20% after 20 years). The overall prognosis is much better if the many patients in the community are considered whose symptoms are never of such severity as to require admission to hospital. A poor prognosis may be associated with:

- high titres of rheumatoid factor
- insidious onset of disease
- more than a year of active disease without remission
- early development of nodules and erosions
- extra-articular manifestations and
- severe functional impairment.

Mortality is greatly increased in RA patients with functional impairment. The 5-year survival for severely disabled RA patients is reduced by 50% and the prognosis in such patients is similar to that for patients with 3-vessel coronary artery disease or Stage IV Hodgkin's disease.

Patients with Sjögren's syndrome require scrupulous oral and ocular hygiene and the instillation of artificial tears (hypromellose eye drops). Drug hypersensitivity is sometimes a problem. Corticosteroids are used in Felty's syndrome but the outcome is unsatisfactory. Splenectomy is reserved for patients with serious or life-threatening infections and is followed by remission in 60% of patients.

PSORIATIC ARTHRITIS

This is a seronegative inflammatory arthritis found in patients with psoriasis, a past or family history of psoriasis or with characteristic changes in the nails.

Epidemiology

Psoriatic arthritis occurs in about 1/1000 of the general population and in 7% of patients with psoriasis. 20% of all patients with seronegative polyarthritis have psoriasis while the prevalence of psoriasis in seropositive rheumatoid arthritis is no higher than that in the general population, suggesting that the association of the skin disease with seronegative arthritis does not arise by chance alone. The onset is usually between the ages of 25 and 40 years.

Clinical features

Five distinct clinical patterns of psoriatic arthritis are recognised and are listed in the information box below. An inflammatory arthritis affecting the distal interphalangeal joints which are not typically involved in RA is the most characteristic form of psoriatic arthropathy

CLINICAL PATTERNS OF PSORIATIC ARTHROPATHY

- Asymmetrical oligoarthritis   70%
- Sacroiliitis/spondylitis   40%
- Symmetrical seronegative arthritis   15%
- Distal interphalangeal joint arthritis 15%
- Arthritis mutilans   5%

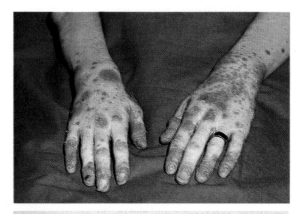

Fig. 15.30 Psoriatic arthritis. Arthritis in DIP joints with associated nail changes (hyperkeratosis).

and is almost invariably associated with nail changes (Fig. 15.30). However, an asymmetrical or symmetrical seronegative arthritis resembling RA is more common.

Sacroiliitis and spondylitis indistinguishable from classical ankylosing spondylitis can occur alone or in association with any of the clinical patterns of peripheral arthritis.

Extra-articular features are limited to:

1. skin lesions which may be widespread scaling lesions, typically over extensor surfaces, or insignificant and confined to such areas as the scalp, natal cleft and umbilicus where they are easily overlooked
2. nail changes including pitting, onycholysis, subungual hyperkeratosis and horizontal ridging
3. iritis.

Investigations
The ESR is usually only moderately raised and there may be a mild normochromic normocytic anaemia in active cases. Tests for rheumatoid factor and antinuclear factor are negative. Radiographs showing asymmetrical disease, terminal IP joint involvement and relatively little periarticular osteoporosis may help to distinguish psoriatic arthritis from rheumatoid arthritis. The changes in the axial skeleton resemble those in ankylosing spondylitis.

Management
NSAIDs are usually all that are required to control symptoms. Sulphasalazine and gold can be used in persistently symptomatic progressive cases without exacerbation of the psoriasis but the antimalarials chloroquine and hydroxychloroquine may give rise to exfoliative reactions. Methotrexate and other immunosuppressive drugs are given occasionally in an attempt to control progressive arthritis mutilans or extensive incapacitating skin disease. The retinoid etretinate (30 mg daily) has been shown to be effective in treating the arthritis as well as the skin lesions but it must be avoided in young women because of potential teratogenicity and its use can be complicated by mucocutaneous side-effects, hyperlipidaemia, myalgias and extra-spinal calcification. Photochemotherapy with methoxypsoralen and long-wave ultra violet light (PUVA) is primarily used for patients with severe skin lesions but it can also help some patients with synchronous exacerbations of inflammatory arthritis. Splints and prolonged rest are avoided because of the increased tendency to fibrous and bony ankylosis but intra-articular steroid injections can be used with good effect in persistently active and symptomatic joints.

Prognosis
This is better than for rheumatoid arthritis with the exception of those rare patients with arthritis mutilans.

SPONDARTHRITIDES

This is a group of diseases in which an inflammatory arthritis, characterised by persistently negative tests for IgM rheumatoid factor, is variably associated with a number of other common articular, extra-articular and genetic features. These are listed in the information box. The features held in common by the spondarthritides are shown in the second information box.

THE SPONDARTHRITIDES

- Ankylosing spondylitis
- Reiter's disease
- Reactive arthritis
- Behçet's syndrome
- Juvenile chronic arthritis
- Enteropathic arthritis
  Ulcerative colitis
  Crohn's disease

Current concepts of the aetiology of these disorders are that they may arise as an abnormal response to infection in genetically predisposed persons carrying the HLA-B27 antigen. In some an inciting organism has been identified, as in Reiter's disease which can follow bacterial dysentery or chlamydial urethritis, or in the reactive arthritis following infection with *Yersina enterocolitica*. In the others the infectious agent remains obscure. It is uncertain whether possession of HLA-B27 predisposes towards disease because:

- it is merely a marker for an immune response gene
- susceptibility to infection is increased as a result of cross-reactivity between an HLA-B27 determined host gene product and an antigen carried by the invading organism
- the inciting organism modifies HLA-B27 positive cellular receptors in such a way as to initiate an autoimmune reaction or render the cells more susceptible to cytotoxic lymphocytes.

ANKYLOSING SPONDYLITIS

In its typical form this is a chronic inflammatory arthritis with a predilection for the sacroiliac joints and spine and characterised by progressive stiffening and fusion of the axial skeleton.

Epidemiology

Typically, ankylosing spondylitis is a disease with a peak onset in the second and third decades and a male to female ratio of about 4:1. More than 90% of affected persons carry the histocompatibility antigen HLA-B27. The overall prevalence varies from 0.5–1% in most communities but is much greater in the Pima and Haida Indians who have a high prevalence of HLA-B27. First degree relatives of patients with ankylosing spondylitis have a greatly increased incidence of psoriatic arthritis, inflammatory bowel disease and Reiter's syndrome. Chronic prostatitis is more common than would be anticipated but it is not possible to isolate organisms from prostatic fluid. Faecal carriage of some *Klebsiella* species is increased in ankylosing spondylitis and this may be related to exacerbation of the disease.

Pathology

Biopsy material from peripheral joints shows changes similar to those found in rheumatoid arthritis. Bony ankylosis, however, occurs more frequently. The charac-teristic **enthesopathy** comprises multiple foci of inflammation with lymphocytes and plasma cells at ligamentous attachments with adjacent erosion of bone. Healing of similar lesions at the junction of the vertebral bodies and annulus fibrosus of the intervertebral discs leads to the new bone formation (syndesmophytes) which is the hallmark of the disease.

Clinical features

The onset is usually insidious with recurring episodes of low back pain and stiffness sometimes radiating to the buttocks or thighs. Characteristically the symptoms are worse in the early morning and after inactivity. Occasionally the onset may be acute, resembling a lumbar disc protrusion. A few patients present with symptoms referable to the dorsal or cervical spine but such cases usually reveal evidence of previous sacroiliitis and lumbar spine involvement.

Chest pain aggravated by breathing results from involvement of the costovertebral joints. Plantar fasciitis, Achilles tendonitis and tenderness over bony prominences such as the iliac crest, ischial tuberosity and greater trochanter are typical. 25% of patients have an attack of acute anterior uveitis during the course of the disease and this may occasionally be the presenting feature. A peripheral joint is first affected in 10% and in a further 10% symptoms begin in childhood as one variety of pauciarticular juvenile chronic arthritis.

Early signs include failure to obliterate the lumbar lordosis on forward flexion, pain on sacroiliac compression, and restriction of movements of the lumbar spine in all directions. As the disease progresses, stiffness increases throughout the spine, and chest expansion frequently becomes restricted. Severe spinal fusion and rigidity occurs in only a minority and in most of these is not associated with much deformity. A few develop kyphosis of the dorsal and cervical spine, which can be incapacitating especially when associated with hip involvement.

Iritis occurs in up to 25% of patients but other extra-articular features are rare. These manifestations are listed in the information box.

Investigations

The erythrocyte sedimentation rate (ESR) is usually raised but may be normal. Tests for rheumatoid factor are negative and synovial fluid complement levels are not depressed.

Radiological signs of sacroiliitis begin in the lower part of the joints with irregularity and marginal sclerosis eventually progressing to fusion. In the lumbar spine there may be 'squaring' of the vertebrae owing to ossification of the anterior longitudinal ligament, syndesmophyte formation, erosion and sclerosis at the anterior corners of the vertebrae and facetal joint changes. Progressive ossification results in the typical 'bamboo' spine (Fig. 15.31). Erosive changes may be seen in the symphysis pubis, the ischial tuberosities and peripheral joints. Osteoporosis and atlanto-axial dislocation can occur.

Radionuclide bone scanning may reveal evidence of sacroiliitis or spinal involvement when radiographs are negative but the increased uptake of the bone-seeking isotope is non-specific and reflects bone blood flow and turnover.

Management

The principles are to relieve pain and stiffness, maintain a maximal range of skeletal mobility and avoid the development of deformities. Early in the disease patients should be trained to perform regular exercises at home and encouraged to take up active non-contact sports like swimming. Poor bed and chair posture must be avoided.

NSAIDs are used to relieve symptoms but do not themselves alter the course of the disease. A few patients with spondylitis find phenylbutazone the most effective drug; it can usually be given safely even over prolonged periods provided a daily oral dose of 300 mg is not exceeded.

The addition of EC sulphasalazine 500 mg 6-hourly orally can be helpful in patients with persistent peripheral arthritis and has been shown to be of marginal benefit in suppressing the axial disease.

Radiotherapy is occasionally indicated if the response to drug therapy is unsatisfactory. It does not affect the course of the disease and earlier regimens of treatment, when excessive radiation was employed, were associated with a tenfold increase in the risk of developing leukaemia.

Local corticosteroid injections can be used for plantar fasciitis and the management of other manifestations of enthesopathy. Systemic steroids are sometimes required for treatment of acute iritis.

Hip disease may require surgery, and total hip arthroplasty has largely obviated the need for difficult spinal surgery in those with advanced deformity.

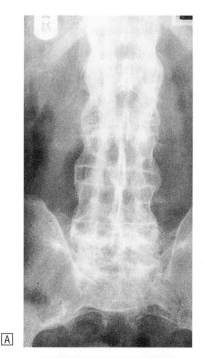

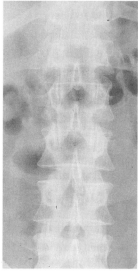

Fig. 15.31 Advanced ankylosing spondylitis. [A] Radiograph of spine showing obliteration of sacro-iliac joints and 'bamboo' appearance due to ligamentous ossification. [B] Corresponding radiograph of normal spine.

Prognosis

75% or more of patients with ankylosing spondylitis are able to remain in employment without significant loss of time from work. Restriction of chest movements does not predispose to pulmonary infection but systemic complications and especially hip involvement carry a worse prognosis.

REITER'S DISEASE

Classically this is the triad of non-specific urethritis, conjunctivitis and arthritis that follows bacterial dysentery or exposure to sexually transmitted infection. Incomplete forms are frequent and include the commonest variety of inflammatory arthritis seen in young men. When arthritis alone follows sexual exposure or enteric infection the term **reactive arthritis** is frequently used. The bacteria implicated in reactive arthritis are listed in the information box below.

ARTHRITOGENIC BACTERIA IMPLICATED IN REACTIVE ARTHRITIS

- Salmonella
- Shigella
- Campylobacter
- Yersinia
- Chlamydia

Epidemiology

1–2% of patients with non-specific urethritis seen at clinics for sexually transmitted diseases have Reiter's disease and there is a similar incidence following outbreaks of shigellosis. A male with HLA-B27 runs a 20% risk of getting the disease following an attack of shigella dysentery. Although predominantly a disease of young men, the apparent 50:1 male to female ratio is spuriously high as urethritis is frequently ignored in women and children.

Clinical features

The onset is typically acute with the simultaneous development of urethritis, conjunctivitis (in about 50%) and an inflammatory oligoarthritis affecting the large or small joints of the lower limbs, 1–3 weeks following sexual exposure or an attack of dysentery. There may be considerable systemic disturbance with fever, weight loss and vasomotor changes in the feet.

Often the onset is more insidious and many patients present with no more than monoarthritis of a knee or an asymmetrical inflammatory arthritis of some interphalangeal joints. Symptoms and signs of urethritis or conjunctivitis may have been minimal or forgotten. In such patients heel pain, Achilles tendonitis or plantar fasciitis are valuable clues while the presence of circinate balanitis or the rash of keratoderma blenorrhagica can establish the diagnosis even in the absence of the classical triad and without an overt history of sexual promiscuity or dysentery. The skin lesions can vary from faint

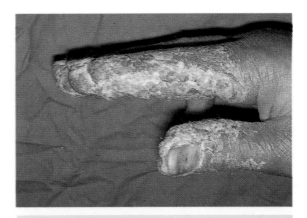

Fig. 15.32 Reiter's syndrome. Subungual hyperkeratosis and keratoderma blenorrhagica.

macules, vesicles and pustules on the hands and feet to marked hyperkeratosis with plaque-like lesions spreading to the scalp and trunk. These may be associated with severe nail dystrophy and massive subungual hyperkeratosis (Fig. 15.32).

Ocular involvement is normally limited to mild bilateral conjunctivitis which subsides spontaneously within a month. Acute iritis occurs at the outset in 10% of patients. It is distinguished from simple conjunctivitis by injection of the ciliary vessels around the cornea, by a constricted, irregular or unreactive pupil and by cells in the anterior chamber on slit lamp examination. Unlike the conjunctivitis it requires urgent treatment. Chronic iritis may lead to glaucoma and blindness.

The urethritis is usually associated with minor dysuria and a clear sterile discharge. Sometimes it is asymptomatic and detected only by finding mucoid threads in the first voided specimen of early morning urine. Occasionally there may be severe dysuria, haematuria and suprapubic discomfort from an associated acute haemorrhagic cystitis and prostatitis.

The arthritis is usually self-limiting, with spontaneous remission of symptoms within 2–3 months of onset. There is, however, a recurrence rate of about 15% per annum not necessarily related to further overt exposure to infection. Low back pain and stiffness from sacroiliitis are common and 15–20% of patients develop spondylitis. Iritis occurs in 30% of patients with recurring arthritis. Other extra-articular features are less common and are listed in the information box below.

Investigations

The ESR is often greatly raised during the acute phase and may remain so long after joint symptoms have settled. Polymorphonuclear leucocytosis and an anaemia of chronic disease are further indications of

REITER'S SYNDROME: EXTRA-ARTICULAR FEATURES

- Conjunctivitis
- Iritis
- Urethritis
- Pericarditis/pleurisy
- Aortic incompetence
- Cardiac conduction defects
- Meningoencephalitis
- Peripheral neuropathy

active systemic disturbance. The synovial fluid has the characteristics of a low viscosity inflammatory effusion with leucocyte counts as high as 50 000/cu.mm but it is sterile on culture. Giant synovial macrophages can be seen but synovial fluid complement levels are not depressed as they are in seropositive rheumatoid arthritis. Serum tests for rheumatoid factor and antinuclear factor are negative. Tissue typing reveals HLA-B27 in more than 70% of cases.

Radiological examination reveals periarticular osteoporosis, reduction of joint space and erosive changes especially when there has been prolonged or recurrent inflammatory arthritis. The changes are often accompanied by marked periostitis especially in the metatarsals, phalanges and pelvis; there may be large and 'fluffy' calcaneal spurs. Sacroiliitis is indistinguishable from that seen in ankylosing spondylitis but the spinal changes include early isolated bony spurs and paravertebral ossification. These are also seen in psoriasis but not in ankylosing spondylitis.

Management

This is mainly symptomatic and supportive. Rest and NSAIDs are required during the acute phases together with judicious aspiration of joints and intra-articular or other local steroid injections. Systemic corticosteroids are rarely required. Iritis is a medical emergency requiring topical, subconjunctival or systemic corticosteroids. Severe progressive arthritis and intractable keratoderma blenorrhagica occasionally warrant cytotoxic drug therapy. The non-specific urethritis is usually treated with a short course of tetracycline and there is now some evidence that it reduces the frequency of arthritis in sexually acquired cases.

10% of patients have evidence of active disease 20 years after the onset. Spondylitis, chronic erosive arthritis, recurrent acute arthritis and uveitis are the major causes of long-term morbidity.

ARTHRITIS AND INFLAMMATORY BOWEL DISEASE

Two patterns of seronegative inflammatory arthritis are associated with ulcerative colitis and Crohn's disease.

Enteropathic synovitis

An acute, often migratory, non-erosive oligoarthritis occurs in the course of the disorder in 12% of patients with ulcerative colitis and 20% of those with Crohn's disease. The knees, ankles and other weight-bearing joints are most commonly affected but the wrists and small joints of the fingers and toes can also be involved. The arthritis tends to follow exacerbations of the underlying bowel disease sometimes in association with aphthous mouth ulcers, iritis and erythema nodosum. It ceases to be a problem following total colectomy for ulcerative colitis. The higher prevalence in Crohn's disease may reflect the greater difficulty in eradicating the bowel problem.

Sacroiliitis (16%) and ankylosing spondylitis (6%)

These are also seen in the course of these disorders, but they pursue an independent course and often precede the bowel disease.

BEHÇET'S SYNDROME

This disease is rare in Western Europe but more common in Japan and Eastern Mediterranean countries where it has an association with HLA-B5.

Clinical features

Major criteria are recurrent aphthous stomatitis, skin lesions, iritis and genital ulceration. Minor criteria are inflammatory arthritis of large joints, intestinal ulcerations, meningoencephalitis, epididymitis and thrombophlebitis. In the presence of all four major criteria the syndrome is said to be 'complete'; in the presence of three, 'incomplete'. The arthritis is mono-articular or oligo-articular and non-erosive. It most frequently involves the knees, ankles, wrists and elbows. Occasionally the sacroiliac joints are affected.

Management

Treatment is symptomatic with NSAIDs; corticosteroids and immunosuppressive therapy are reserved for the more serious systemic manifestations.

WHIPPLE'S DISEASE (see p. 455).

JUVENILE CHRONIC ARTHRITIS

The five main patterns of chronic arthritis that commence in childhood are listed in the information box below.

SYSTEMIC ONSET JUVENILE CHRONIC ARTHRITIS (STILL'S DISEASE)

This pattern of disease is most common between the ages of 1 and 5 years.

Clinical features

Lymphadenopathy, hepatosplenomegaly, pleurisy, pericarditis and a high intermittent fever are associated with myalgias, arthralgias and eventually polyarthritis. Weight loss and retardation of growth may be striking and there is often a characteristic evanescent macular rash which tends to appear when the temperature is raised. Remission of symptoms usually occurs within 6 months but half the children have recurrent attacks and one quarter develop a severe chronic polyarthritis.

POLYARTICULAR JUVENILE CHRONIC ARTHRITIS

Seronegative polyarticular disease

This can occur at any age. Four or more large joints are commonly first affected acutely or insidiously. Inflammatory arthritis in the proximity of growing epiphyses may result in growth acceleration or arrest. Early fusion in the cervical spine and mandible gives rise to the short stiff neck and receding chin very characteristic of adults who have had juvenile chronic arthritis. The overall prognosis is good and only 10–15% have severe destructive arthritis.

Seropositive polyarticular disease

The onset is usually after the age of 8 years. The disease resembles severe adult onset rheumatoid arthritis with progressive erosive joint changes in more than half of those affected. Extra-articular features include nodules and vasculitis. Antinuclear factor tests are positive in 75%.

PAUCIARTICULAR JUVENILE CHRONIC ARTHRITIS

This involves four or fewer joints. At least two distinct subsets can be identified.

Young girls with mono- or pauciarticular arthritis but seldom any constitutional symptoms. HLA-DR5 and positive tests for antinuclear factor appear to be markers for chronic iritis which can occur in up to half of this group. Three-monthly slit lamp examinations are required if this complication is to be detected and treated early enough to preserve normal vision.

Older boys with mono- or pauciarticular arthritis affecting hips, knees or ankles. Sacroiliitis is common and there is frequently a family history of iritis, ankylosing spondylitis or another spondarthritis. 75% of these boys are HLA-B27 positive and in some the disease gradually evolves into ankylosing spondylitis in early adult life.

The differential diagnosis of acute arthritis in childhood includes bacterial, viral and reactive arthritis as it does in adults and also rheumatic fever, leukaemia and osteomyelitis.

Management

The principles of management in juvenile chronic arthritis do not differ from those in adult rheumatoid arthritis but special consideration is given to maintaining the child's education and helping parents to develop a sensible, vigilant but not overprotective approach to the child's disease. Bed-rest may be essential during acute phases but care must be taken to avoid development of flexion deformities of the hips and knees, by regular prone lying and appropriate lightweight splints. Whenever possible the child should be kept mobile and ambulant and daily physiotherapy is given throughout to maintain a good range of joint movements and muscle strength. Hydrotherapy in a warm pool is particularly useful.

Until recently aspirin was the drug of choice and its use in JCA is an exception to the recommendation that aspirin should not be given to children aged under 12 years because of the risk of Reye's syndrome. Naproxen (5 mg/kg) is safe and effective in children and experience is accumulating with other NSAIDs. Disease-modifying antirheumatic drugs can be used with the same precautions as in adults.

Corticosteroids are reserved for children with severe systemic disease, those with chronic iritis not responding to local therapy and where very active joint disease does not respond to other measures. The use of corticotrophin or alternate day corticosteroids should always be considered because daily doses of prednisolone as low as 3 mg can inhibit growth in children under the age of 5 years. Older children can be taught to give their own injections of corticotrophin if this has to be continued for any length of time. Corticosteroids do not arrest the progression of disease. Immunosuppressive drugs are used only in persistently active disease associated with amyloidosis.

Surgery is usually limited to the rehabilitation of children with deformities. Soft tissue release operations may be helpful in eliminating difficult flexion contractures, and osteotomies may be required when joints have been allowed to fuse in poor positions. Total hip arthroplasty can be considered for severely damaged joints as soon as growth has ceased.

HENOCH–SCHÖNLEIN (ANAPHYLACTOID) PURPURA

This is a small vessel vasculitis which is associated with abdominal pain and an acute arthritis affecting one or more joints for a few days at a time. The disease frequently follows an upper respiratory infection and usually lasts for less than 3 months. Boys are affected twice as frequently as girls. Non-thrombocytopenic purpura is found characteristically over the buttocks and lower legs, and up to half the children affected have angio-oedema. Intussusception, rectal bleeding and renal involvement are features of more severe cases.

INFECTIVE ARTHRITIS

SEPTIC ARTHRITIS

This can accompany septicaemia at any age. *H. influenzae* is the commonest causative organism in infancy, whereas staphylococcal and streptococcal infections are usually responsible in older children and adults. Other organisms which may be implicated are gonococci, pneumococci, meningococci, *Escherichia coli, Pseudomonas* and *Proteus*. Important predisposing factors include debilitating illnesses, diabetes mellitus, immunodeficiency disorders and immunosuppression. Joint trauma, surgery, penetrating injury and intra-articular injections may lead to bacterial joint infections and septic arthritis may complicate rheumatoid arthritis and other established arthritides.

Clinical features

Characteristically, septic arthritis has an abrupt onset with severe pain and swelling of a single joint associated with a swinging fever, severe malaise and a polymorphonuclear leucocytosis. Large joints are most frequently affected and the joint is hot, tender and swollen with an effusion and marked limitation of movement. The diagnosis may be missed when more than one joint is involved, in patients with rheumatoid arthritis or when the presentation is less acute in patients receiving corticosteroids or immunosuppressive drugs.

Investigations

It is essential to establish the diagnosis early by joint aspiration and blood culture. The synovial fluid is typically turbid with a high polymorphonuclear cell count ($>50\ 000$ cells/mm³ with $>80\%$ neutrophils, see Table 15.4). Organisms may be easily and immediately identified on Gram stain but special culture techniques are required especially for gonococci and anaerobic organisms. Elevated levels of lactic and succinic acid detectable by gas liquid chromatography suggest bacterial infection.

Radiographs show no more than soft tissue swelling initially. Later there may be periarticular osteoporosis, joint space narrowing, periostitis and articular erosions. In more long-standing infections the joint margins have a peculiar 'rubbed-out' appearance. Radionuclide imaging with gallium shows changes earlier than on plain radiographs and is especially useful in detecting infection in the axial and other deeper inaccessible joints.

Management

In all patients where bacterial infection is suspected treatment should be commenced with high parenteral doses of a broad spectrum antibiotic as soon as joint aspiration and blood cultures have been completed; it is continued until the responsible organism and its sensitivity have been established. Appropriate antibiotics must then be administered for several weeks. Antibiotics readily cross the inflamed synovial membrane and there is no need to inject them intra-articularly.

The joint should be rested and immobilised with a splint and daily joint aspiration undertaken until no more fluid reaccumulates. If the fluid becomes loculated or too thick for aspiration, surgical drainage is required.

Prognosis

The prognosis for recovery without joint damage is directly related to the speed with which antibiotic therapy is instituted.

ARTHRITIS ASSOCIATED WITH OTHER SPECIFIC INFECTIONS

Gonococcal arthritis

This is more common in females than males and not infrequently commences at the time of a menstrual period within 2–3 weeks of genital infection. Joint involvement is usually asymmetrical and polyarticular with an acute, or subacute, migratory polyarthralgia or polyarthritis. Tenosynovitis, an 'additive' as opposed to a 'flitting' pattern of joint involvement and a macular, vesicular or pustular rash are important diagnostic clues even in the absence of overt genital gonorrhoea.

The diagnosis can be established by cultures of synovial fluid, blood or skin lesions or from the genital tract. However, the organism is only identified in joint fluid in 20% of patients. Most patients respond to penicillin, 1 mega unit daily for 2 weeks, with dramatic improvement in 3–4 days.

Meningococcal infection

This can be associated with:

- an acute transient polyarthritis that is seen simultaneously with the characteristic petechial rash
- a purulent monoarthritis which usually occurs after 5 days, or
- a flitting polyarthralgia in patients with chronic meningococcaemia.

Penicillin is the treatment of choice.

Brucellosis

This is associated with polyarthralgia or transient polyarthritis. Much more rarely there may be a septic arthritis or spondylitis. Destructive lesions in one or more contiguous vertebrae lead to severe pain, disc narrowing and marginal proliferation of osteophytes with early bony fusion of vertebrae. Chronic bursitis and osteomyelitis may also occur. Diagnosis is established by blood and synovial fluid cultures coupled with rising antibody titres. Management is given on page 126.

Tuberculosis of joints

This is usually secondary to an established focus in the lungs or kidneys. Articular infection is rarely seen except in malnourished or socially deprived elderly or immigrant groups, following the eradication of bovine tuberculosis in Britain. A single large joint is affected in more than three-quarters of all patients. Clinical features include joint pain, stiffness, swelling and restriction of movements associated with anorexia, weight loss and night sweats. In the early stages of the disease, radiographs show only periarticular osteoporosis and soft tissue swelling. Later there is narrowing of the joint space, bony erosion and collapse of subchondral bone with little associated periosteal reaction. The tuberculin skin test is strongly positive and diagnosis can sometimes be made by direct bacteriological examination and culture of synovial fluid. In other patients synovial biopsy is required. After antibiotic control has been established (see pp. 360–361), synovectomy may be required in those with extensive disease.

Leprosy

This can have a number of osteoarticular manifestations. Joint deformities of the hands and feet are common as a sequel to peripheral nerve involvement and these may be complicated by neuropathic (Charcot) joints. Osteomyelitis may complicate digital ulceration and hypersensitivity reactions may resemble rheumatoid arthritis.

Syphilitic arthritis

Congenital syphilis may be associated with painful paraarticular swelling due to epiphyseal involvement soon after birth or painless effusions of the knees (Clutton's joints) in adolescents. Acquired secondary syphilis may be associated with a migrating polyarthralgia resembling rheumatic fever and Charcot (neuropathic) joints are a feature of tabes dorsalis.

Lyme arthritis (see p. 137).

Fungal infections

These are rare. Blastomycosis, histoplasmosis and sporotrichosis can be associated with destructive lesions of bones and joints. Histoplasmosis and coccidiomycosis may also be associated with erythema nodosum and a benign polyarthritis.

Viral infections

A number of viral infections are commonly associated with arthralgia and transient polyarthritis. These include hepatitis B, mumps, chickenpox, infectious mononucleosis, adenoviral, enteroviral, parvoviral and arboviral infections. Hepatitis-associated arthritis occurs in up to 30% of patients with hepatitis B. Typically it is associated with fever and rash and precedes the onset of jaundice. Rubella arthritis follows 1–7 days after the rash or 2–6 weeks after vaccination in 30–40% of adults. A symmetrical inflammatory polyarthritis may be associated with symptoms of carpal tunnel compression or tenosynovitis. Joint pain, stiffness and swelling, which may be severe, usually settle in 1–4 weeks but the condition may persist with intermittent arthralgia for some months. Posterior cervical lymphadenopathy and a high lymphocyte count in the synovial fluid may be helpful in diagnosis.

MISCELLANEOUS DISORDERS OF SYNOVIAL JOINTS

Acromegaly

This is associated with a symmetrical arthropathy in 50% of patients. The small joints of the hands, wrists and knees are particularly affected, as is the spine. Hypertrophy of synovium and articular cartilage are characteristically associated with periosteal new bone formation, osteophytosis, 'tufting' of the terminal phalanges and premature osteoarthrosis and hypertrophic spondylosis.

Amyloidosis

Amyloidosis, a multisystem disease, may be generalised or localised. It may be primary, or secondary to conditions such as rheumatoid arthritis, chronic suppuration, lepromatous leprosy and myelomatosis, and associated with carpal tunnel compression and a polyarthritis superficially resembling rheumatoid arthritis. The synovium is infiltrated with amyloid protein and the diagnosis can be made by finding fragments of amyloid tissue in the synovial fluid.

Hyperlipidaemia

Type II hyperlipidaemia can be associated with a migratory polyarthritis, and widespread xanthomas with tendon deposits. Type IV hyperlipidaemia can be associated with arthralgia and morning stiffness and also hyperuricaemia and gout.

Sarcoidosis

Erythema nodosum and hilar lymphadenopathy are frequently associated with a symmetrical non-destructive inflammatory arthritis especially affecting the knees, ankles and wrists. A more specific asymmetrical destructive arthritis affects similar joints especially in black people and biopsy of the synovium in these shows evidence of noncaseating granulomas. Radiologically there may be 'punched out' cystic bone lesions and also 'cortical erosions' and joint destruction.

FURTHER READING

Ansell B M 1986 Juvenile chronic arthritis. Current Orthopaedics 1: 81–89

Brooks P M 1993 Clinical management of rheumatoid arthritis. Lancet 341: 286–290

Gladman D D, Schuckett R, Russell M L et al 1987 Psoriatic arthritis (PsA)—an analysis of 220 patients. Quarterly Journal of Medicine 238: 127–141

Goldenberg D L, Reed J L 1985 Bacterial arthritis. New England Journal of Medicine 312: 764–771

Keat A E 1983 Reiter's syndrome and reactive arthritis in perspective. New England Journal of Medicine 309: 1606–1615

Scott D L, Huskisson E C 1992 The course of rheumatoid arthritis. Baillière's Clinical Rheumatology 6: 1–21

Sewell K L, Trentham D E 1993 Pathogenesis of rheumatoid arthritis. Lancet 341: 283–286

Tugwell P 1992 Cyclosporine in RA: efficacy and safety. Seminars in Arthritis and Rheumatism 21(6), Suppl 3: 30–38

Winchester R 1994 The molecular basis of susceptibility to rheumatoid arthritis. Advances in Immunology 56: 389–466

CONNECTIVE TISSUE DISEASES

SYSTEMIC LUPUS ERYTHEMATOSUS (SLE)

This is a multisystem connective tissue disease characterised by the presence of numerous autoantibodies,

Table 15.11 Immunological abnormalities detectable in the blood of patients with SLE

Antinuclear antibodies
  Anti-DNA-histone (and LE cells)
  Anti-DNA (single strand)
  Anti-DNA (double strand)
  Anti-RNA
  Anti-Sm
  Anti-U$_1$ RNP
  Anti-Ro/SS-A
  Anti-La/SS-B
  Anti-MA
  Anti-PCNA
	Antineuronal antibodies

	Biological false positive tests for syphilis
	Circulating anticoagulants (anti-cardiolipin antibodies)
Depression of CH$_{50}$ and C3 and C4	Anti-thyroid (and other organ specific autoantibodies)
Antibodies against erythrocytes, leucocytes and platelets	Rheumatoid factors
	Cryoglobulins
	Circulating immune complexes

DNA – deoxyribonucleic acid
RNA – ribonucleic acid
Sm, Ro, La, MA – antibodies identified by initials of patients in whom they were discovered
CH$_{50}$ – Total haemolytic complement activity
C3, C4 – complement components

circulating immune complexes and widespread immunologically determined tissue damage.

Epidemiology

SLE affects individuals throughout the world but occurs more frequently in the United States and the Far East. Americans of African origin are particularly susceptible, with a prevalence as high as 1/250 among females. The increasing use of sensitive tests for antinuclear antibodies suggests that mild and incomplete cases frequently occur. The onset is most commonly in the 2nd and 3rd decades, with a female/male ratio of 9:1. The sex incidence is more equal in children and the elderly.

Aetiology and pathogenesis

Although the cause of SLE remains obscure, current concepts suggest that this is a multifactorial disorder in which there is profound disturbance of immune regulation. A defect of suppressor T lymphocytes is associated with polyclonal B lymphocyte activation and the uncontrolled production of autoantibodies and immune complexes (Tables 15.11 and 15.12).

Evidence for genetic factors in the aetiology of the disease includes:

- its occurrence in monozygotic twin pairs
- a higher than expected prevalence of SLE, other connective tissue diseases, antinuclear antibodies and immune complexes in related family members
- inherited deficiency of isolated complement components, notably C2 in some patients

Table 15.12   Frequency (%) diagnostically useful autoantibodies in connective tissue diseases

.	dsDNA	Sm	RNP	Jo-1	PM-Scl	Scl–70	Centromere	XR	Ro	La
Systemic lupus erythematosus	60	20	25	—	—	—	—	—	25	10
Mixed connective tissue disease	—	Occ	100	Occ	—	—	—	—	20	Occ
Primary Sjögren's (sicca syndrome)	Occ	—	Occ	—	—	—	—	—	75	40
Progressive systemic sclerosis	—	—	Occ	—	—	20	Occ	—	Occ	—
CREST	—	—	—	—	—	—	30	—	—	—
Myositis	—	—	15	25	10	—	—	—	10	—
Primary biliary cirrhosis	Occ	—	—	—	—	—	10	10	5	—
Chronic active hepatitis	Occ	—	—	—	—	—	—	25	—	—

Occ   Occasionally
CREST   Calcinosis, Raynaud's syndrome, oesophageal involvement, sclerodactyly, telangiectasia

- increased prevalence of the histocompatibility antigens HLA-B8 and DR3.

Evidence for the influence of environmental factors includes:

- the provocative effect of sunlight
- the induction of lupus erythematosus by drugs
- the importance of oestrogens as determinants of disease expression. Exacerbations commonly occur in pregnancy and the puerperium and prevalence is increased in fertile women, those using oral contraceptives and men with Klinefelter's syndrome.

There is evidence of viral infection in animal models of SLE but not in humans.

Immunologically-mediated tissue damage results from at least two different mechanisms in SLE:

- Direct Type II antibody-mediated cytotoxicity. Brain damage and abortion may be a consequence of cytotoxicity by cold reactive antibodies which cross-react with neural and trophoblast tissues
- Immune complex (and complement) mediated Type III hypersensitivity. The renal and vascular lesions of SLE appear to be a consequence of deposition of circulating DNA-Anti-DNA and other complexes in tissues.

Clinical features

Arthritis, arthralgia and fever

These are the commonest presenting features. Unlike other types of inflammatory arthritis, symptoms may begin during pregnancy and there may be a past history of spontaneous abortions. The arthritis can be transient and migratory or a more persistent seronegative polyarthritis. Chronic inflammatory arthritis and tenosynovitis may lead to deformities and contractures but erosive changes are very uncommon.

Skin lesions

These are seen in more than two-thirds of patients. In addition to the classical, photosensitive erythematous 'butterfly' rash (Fig. 15.33) across the face, there may be lesions of discoid lupus or a vasculitic rash. The latter may present as purpura or periungual erythema with 'chilblain-like' lesions or digital infarcts. Livedo reticularis and Raynaud's phenomenon (see p. 273) are common while bullous eruptions and panniculitis ('lupus profundus') occur more rarely. Alopecia can be a useful diagnostic pointer and is seen in more than 50% of patients. Painful oral or nasopharyngeal ulcers are less common.

Cardiopulmonary features

These include pericarditis, myocarditis and endocarditis, pleurisy, fibrosing alveolitis and acute lupus pneumonitis as well as a 'shrinking lung syndrome' with progressive elevation of the diaphragms and linear scars from recurrent pulmonary infarction (see p. 390, Ch. 6). Lung function tests reveal impairment of ventilation and diffusion in these and many patients without overt clinical or radiological evidence of pulmonary involvement. Verrucous (Libman–Sacks) endocarditis may be demonstrated by echocardiography.

Renal involvement

This carries the worst prognosis. It may result in the nephrotic syndrome and renal failure or it may be limited to insignificant proteinuria or the presence of red cells or casts (see p. 646).

Central nervous system involvement

This occurs in up to half the patients. In the majority it is limited to mild psychiatric disturbance or epilepsy but in a few there may be severe depression, dementia, organic psychosis, cranial nerve lesions, hemiplegia, normochromic anaemia of chronic disease, a Coombs' positive haemolytic anaemia, leucopenia, thrombocytopenia and immunological abnormalities.

Immunological findings

The immunological abnormalities found in SLE are given in Tables 15.11 and 15.12 on pages 912 and 913.

Antinuclear antibodies (ANF). These can be detected by indirect immunofluorescence in the serum of more than 90% of patients but positive tests are found in many other conditions and these are listed in the information box below. Positive tests in low titre have no clinical significance and are frequently found in normal elderly people. The LE cell test is less sensitive, very time-consuming and hardly more specific.

ANTINUCLEAR ANTIBODIES: DISEASE ASSOCIATIONS

- SLE
- Mixed connective tissue disease
- Polymyositis
- Scleroderma
- Polyarteritis
- Sjögren's syndrome
- Rheumatoid arthritis

- Juvenile chronic arthritis
- Fibrosing alveolitis
- Chronic liver disease
- Thyroiditis
- Myasthenia gravis
- Leukaemia

Anti-DNA antibodies and immune complexes. Radioimmunoassays for antibodies to undenatured double stranded DNA have much greater specificity but anti-DNA antibodies are present in the serum in significant amounts in only about half the patients at any one time. High levels of anti-DNA antibodies coupled with depressed total haemolytic complement (CH_{50}) activity and low C3 and C4 complement components suggest that there is activation of the classical complement pathway by active immune complex disease. Further evidence for circulating immune complexes may be obtained by finding a cryoprecipitate or by using one of a number of tests for CIq binding. Tissue evidence for immune complex deposition comes from detection of complement components and immunoglobulins by immunofluorescence at the dermoepidermal junction of normal skin (lupus 'band' test) or in organ biopsies.

The lupus anticoagulant. This is an anticardiolipin antibody which may also give rise to false positive biological tests for syphilis. Lupus anticoagulant activity is detected by a prolongation of the partial thromboplastin time (PTTK, APTT) which is not correctable by the addition of normal plasma or by a prolongation of the dilute prothrombin time. Anticardiolipin antibodies are detected by ELISA. High titres are associated with thrombocytopenia, thrombotic manifestations, pulmonary hypertension and neurological problems such

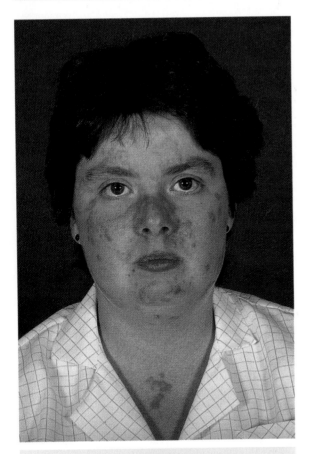

Fig. 15.33 Systemic lupus erythematosus. 'Butterfly' distribution facial rash.

transverse myelitis, chorea, cerebellar ataxia or peripheral neuropathy. The more severe manifestations are associated with a poor prognosis.

Other manifestations

Gastrointestinal symptoms are frequent but non-specific. Abdominal pain can be due to peritonitis, perisplenitis, pancreatitis or vasculitis. Gastric or duodenal perforation may be complications of corticosteroid therapy; colonic or gallbladder perforations are more likely to be a consequence of necrotising arteritis. Lymphadenopathy is found in half the patients and a moderately enlarged spleen in 20–30%. Ocular findings include keratoconjunctivitis sicca, episcleritis, retinal vasculitis and soft exudates.

Investigations

The ESR is usually raised in active disease but the C-reactive protein rarely so in the absence of infection. Haematological findings may include a normocytic

as chorea, strokes or TIAs and in some cases recurrent abortion (the **anti-phospholipid antibody syndrome**).

Management

Acute and life-threatening manifestations of SLE require systemic corticosteroid therapy, often initially in oral doses of 40–80 mg prednisolone or equivalent daily. 'Pulse' therapy with methylprednisolone (1 g intravenously on 3 successive days) is occasionally required in patients with proliferative glomerulonephritis and rapidly deteriorating renal function. With remission of disease careful attempts are made to withdraw steroids or maintain patients on very low doses or alternate day regimes of steroid therapy. Articular symptoms and less severe inflammatory manifestations should be managed without corticosteroids whenever possible, but NSAIDs must be used with care in patients with renal disease. Antimalarials are particularly useful in the management of patients with troublesome skin and joint lesions and they can reduce the frequency of severe exacerbations of disease.

Immunosuppressive drugs are reserved for patients with severe diffuse proliferative glomerulonephritis who are not responding adequately to corticosteroids and for those requiring maintenance steroid doses so high as to cause severe side-effects.

The combination of plasma exchange and immunosuppressive drug therapy may be useful in some patients with serious steroid-resistant exacerbations.

Patients with thrombotic problems associated with the antiphospholipid antibody syndrome are managed with small doses of aspirin and anticoagulants.

Prognosis

Prognosis for life has improved dramatically over the last 30 years and the 5-year survival should now be better than 90%. Much of this apparent improvement results, however, from the detection of milder cases using highly sensitive immunological tests for diagnostic purposes. Patients with severe renal, neurological or pulmonary involvement have the worst prognosis. Renal biopsy can provide a guide to prognosis. Infection is an important cause of morbidity, particularly in patients receiving high doses of corticosteroids and immunosuppressives. Pregnancy is not contraindicated provided the disease is in reasonable remission and renal, cardiac and cerebral functions are intact.

Drug-induced SLE

Positive tests for antinuclear factor are frequently encountered in patients receiving procainamide, hydralazine, anti-convulsants, oral contraceptives and pheno-

thiazines. Much more rarely a syndrome resembling SLE develops. Fever, polyarthritis, skin lesions, lymphadenopathy, serositis and pulmonary infiltrates are frequent, but renal disease and neurological manifestations are rare. Complement levels are usually normal and antibodies to double stranded DNA absent. Slow acetylators of hydralazine and those with the HLAL-DR4 histocompatibility antigen appear to be particularly at risk. Remission usually follows drug withdrawal. Occasionally a short course of corticosteroids is required.

Chronic discoid lupus erythematosus

This is more common than SLE. The skin lesions are characterised by photosensitivity, erythema, scaling, follicular plugging and telangiectasia. In most patients the disease is limited to the skin. ANF tests are positive but anti-DNA antibodies are not usually found and complement levels are normal. SLE may occasionally supervene.

MIXED CONNECTIVE TISSUE DISEASE (MCTD)

This is characterised by overlapping clinical features suggesting systemic lupus erythematosus, progressive systemic sclerosis (see below) and polymyositis in association with very high titres of a circulating antinuclear antibody with specificity for a ribonuclease sensitive extractable nuclear antigen (ENA) identified as a nuclear ribonucleoprotein (nRNP).

Clinical features

Women are affected four times more commonly than men. The onset is usually in the 3rd or 4th decade but may be at any age. Raynaud's phenomenon with 'sausage' swelling of the fingers, skin changes resembling dermatomyositis or scleroderma and a mild inflammatory polyarthritis are typically associated with proximal muscle weakness and tenderness and abnormal oesophageal motility. Diffuse interstitial pulmonary fibrosis is not uncommon but cardiac, renal and central nervous system involvement are very rare. The ESR and muscle enzymes are usually moderately raised. The condition is further characterised by a good response to low dosage steroid therapy.

SYSTEMIC SCLEROSIS AND RELATED SCLERODERMA SYNDROMES

This is a heterogeneous group of disorders of connective tissue characterised by fibrosis and degenerative changes in the skin and many internal organs (see information box).

SYSTEMIC SCLEROSIS AND SCLERODERMA SYNDROMES

- Systemic sclerosis
  - Diffuse cutaneous scleroderma
  - Limited cutaneous (CREST syndrome)
- Localised scleroderma
  - Morphoea
  - Linear scleroderma
- Overlap syndromes
- Undifferentiated connective tissue diseases
- Chemically induced
  - Occupational
  - Drugs
- Pseudo-scleroderma syndromes

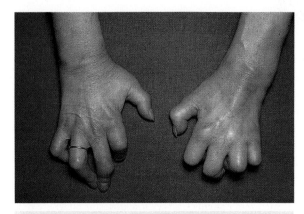

Fig. 15.34 Scleroderma. Hands showing tight shiny skin, sclerodactyly, flexion contractures of the fingers and thickening of an extensor tendon sheath.

Epidemiology

The prevalence of systemic sclerosis is about 10–20/100 000 population with an annual incidence of 1–2/100 000 and a 4:1 female to male ratio. HLA associations include the DR1, DR2, DR3, DR5 and DRW52 Class II alleles. Environmental risk factors include exposure to silica dusts, vinyl chloride, epoxy-resins and trichlorethylene.

Pathogenesis

Immunologically-mediated inflammation in genetically predisposed individuals is followed by intimal thickening in small blood vessels and excessive production and cross-linking of type I collagen. There is evidence of T lymphocyte and complement activation as well as autoimmunity with the presence of autoantibodies to nuclear antigens (Table 15.11, p. 912). Endothelial injury results in the release of the powerful vaso-constrictor endothelin as well as in secondary platelet activation with a release of other vasoconstrictor mediators (5-hydroxytryptamine, thromboxane A$_2$ and ADP).

Clinical features

The onset is most frequently in the 30–50 age group. Severe **Raynaud's phenomenon** (p. 273) is usually the presenting complaint and may precede other features by months or years. Critical digital ischaemia leads to ulceration, infarction, pulp atrophy and gangrene.

Skin changes (Fig. 15.34)

Initially there is often well-demarcated non-pitting oed-ema and induration associated with 'sausage' swelling and restriction of movement of the fingers. Later the skin becomes shiny, with atrophy and ulceration of the fingertips with or without associated calcinosis. The skin of the face, limbs and trunk is variably affected and there may be striking pigmentation and telangiectasia. As

scleroderma advances, the face may become taut and mask-like with 'beaking' of the nose and difficulty in opening the mouth. Tightening of skin over bony pro-minences results in flexion contractures and liability to trauma.

Musculoskeletal manifestations

These include arthralgia and a mild non-erosive inflammatory arthritis often characterised by 'leathery' crepitus in affected tendon sheaths or joints. Muscle weakness and wasting results from both disuse atrophy and low-grade myositis.

Gastrointestinal tract

This is involved in the majority of patients. Reflux oeso-phagitis associated with a sliding hiatus hernia is a com-mon problem and loss of oesophageal peristalsis is often detected on recumbent barium swallow examination even in the absence of dysphagia. Dilatation of segments of large and small bowel occur less frequently, causing intermittent abdominal pain, constipation, distension and obstruction; there may be diarrhoea and mal-absorption secondary to bacterial overgrowth. Systemic sclerosis may be associated with primary biliary cirrhosis and with Sjögren's syndrome.

Pulmonary fibrosis

This occurs in the majority of patients and is covered in detail on page 389.

Other manifestations

Cardiac involvement is usually secondary to systemic rather than pulmonary hypertension but pericarditis, cardiomyopathy, heart block and aortic valve lesions can also occur. Renal involvement may develop at any stage of the disease and is an important cause of morbidity and mortality. Cranial or peripheral nerve lesions occur rarely.

Investigations

The ANF is positive in about 50% of patients with a nucleolar or speckled staining pattern. Antibodies to single stranded RNA and to an extractable nuclear antigen anti-Scl-70 (anti-topoisomerase I) occur in 20% and may be a marker for pulmonary involvement. Anti-DNA antibodies are not detected and complement levels are normal.

Nailfold capillaroscopy shows evidence of dilated, tortuous and 'dropped out' capillary loops in a high proportion of patients with Raynaud's phenomenon destined to develop a connective tissue disease.

Management

No form of drug therapy has been proved to be effective in arresting the course of systemic sclerosis. Corticosteroids may produce some symptomatic benefit in early disease where inflammatory oedema or associated myositis and/or arthritis are prominent features and penicillamine can interfere with collagen cross linking. Nifedipine and prostacyclin infusions may occasionally be helpful in patients with severe Raynaud's phenomenon. Captopril or other ACE inhibitors can be dramatically effective in patients with renal crises and accelerated hypertension.

Attention should be paid to protecting the limbs from cold, the urgent treatment of chest infections and therapy for cardiac, respiratory and renal failure. Articular symptoms should be managed with NSAIDs. Episodes of steatorrhoea often respond to a short course of a broad spectrum antibiotic.

Prognosis

The outlook appears to be worse in those with late onset disease, widespread skin involvement of the trunk, and renal, cardiac or respiratory disease. The overall 5-year survival is about 70%.

Limited scleroderma (CREST syndrome)

This comprises a subset of patients whose skin disease is limited to sites distal to the elbow and knee with only occasional involvement of the face and neck. Calcinosis (Fig. 15.35), Raynaud's phenomenon, oEsophageal involvement, Sclerodactyly and Telangiectasia are the features of the CREST syndrome. An anticentromere antinuclear antibody with specificity for a protein of the

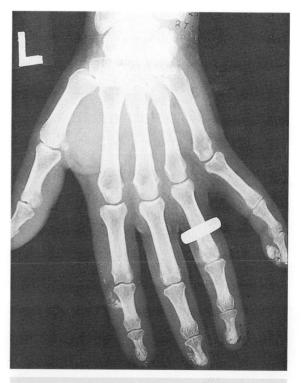

Fig. 15.35 Scleroderma. Radiograph of hand showing soft tissue calcinosis.

chromosomal kinetochore is present in the serum (Table 15.12, p. 913).

Morphoea and linear scleroderma

These are localised forms of disease limited to characteristic, well-demarcated lesions of the skin and subcutaneous connective tissues. Serological findings are similar to those of systemic sclerosis and very occasionally systemic features develop.

Eosinophilic fasciitis

This is a scleroderma-like condition characterised by pain, swelling and tenderness of the hands, forearms and feet where induration of the skin and subcutaneous tissues is not associated with Raynaud's phenomenon or systemic sclerosis. Carpal tunnel compression may be an early feature and the onset frequently follows abnormal exercise. Eosinophilia and hyperglobulinaemia are characteristic and the diagnosis is confirmed by finding an inflammatory cell infiltrate with prominent eosinophils in association with marked fibrosis of the subcutaneous fascia. Eosinophilic fasciitis responds to corticosteroids but is usually self-limiting.

Pseudo-scleroderma

Other conditions which may give rise to induration or brawny oedema of the skin that must be considered in the differential diagnosis of scleroderma include scleredema, scleromyxoedema, amyloidosis and acromegaly.

POLYMYOSITIS AND DERMATOMYOSITIS

These are diffuse connective tissue disorders in which muscle weakness and inflammatory changes in muscle and skin are the predominant features.

Epidemiology

They are rare disorders with an incidence of 2–10/million population per annum but occur throughout the world in all races and at all ages. The aetiology is obscure but persons with HLA-B8/DR3 appear to be genetically predisposed.

Clinical features

It is possible to define five clinical subsets which are listed in the information box below.

MYOSITIS SUBSETS

- Adult polymyositis
- Adult dermatomyositis
- Adult polymyositis with malignancies
- Childhood dermatomyositis
- Polymyositis in other connective tissue diseases

Adult polymyositis

Adult polymyositis occurs three times more frequently in women than in men. The onset is usually insidious in the 3rd to 5th decade. The patients may experience difficulty in climbing stairs or rising from a low chair and on examination there is weakness of the pelvic and shoulder girdle muscles. Sometimes the onset is more abrupt with rapid progression of muscular weakness. Involvement of pharyngeal, laryngeal and respiratory muscles can lead to dysphagia, dysphonia and respiratory failure within a few days. In the majority of cases progression is less rapid and profound. Spontaneous remissions are followed by some return of muscle strength but there may be atrophy, calcinosis and fibrosis in damaged muscles causing flexion contractures. Muscle pain and tenderness are unusual except in very acute illness. Mild arthralgia or inflammatory arthritis, Raynaud's phenomenon and erythematous rashes on the elbows and knuckles are frequent associated features.

Adult dermatomyositis

This is also more common in women. Acute or subacute muscle weakness is accompanied by periorbital oedema and a characteristic purple 'heliotrope' rash on the upper eyelids. In addition there may be a photosensitive, erythematous, scaling rash on the face, shoulders, upper arms and chest with red patches over knuckles, elbows and knees. Muscle pain, tenderness and weight loss are common, as are arthralgia and mild inflammatory polyarthritis.

Inflammatory myositis associated with malignancy

Less common than was previously thought, this is seen only after the age of 40 years, particularly in association with ovarian, gastric and nasopharyngeal carcinoma. The onset of symptoms is usually insidious and the clinical picture does not differ from that of typical polymyositis or dermatomyositis. The associated carcinoma may not become apparent for 2–3 years. Its resection is sometimes associated with remission of the myositis.

Childhood dermatomyositis

This most commonly affects children between the ages of 4 and 10 years. Muscle weakness is usually accompanied by the typical rash of dermatomyositis. Muscle atrophy, contractures and subcutaneous calcification may be widespread and severe. Recurrent abdominal pain due to vasculitis is also a feature.

Investigations

Serum aminotransferases, aldolase and creatinine phosphokinase are usually raised and are useful guides to the activity of the disease. Tests for rheumatoid factor and ANF are often positive and there may be antibodies to an extractable nuclear antigen (PM-Scl, Jo-1, Mi). Electromyography may show characteristic changes which can be very helpful in distinguishing polymyositis from peripheral neuropathy. Muscle biopsy shows fibre necrosis and regeneration in association with an inflammatory cell infiltrate. MRI can be used to detect active myositis non-invasively. Screening for malignancy is usually limited to relatively non-invasive investigations such as chest radiograph, mammography, pelvic/abdominal ultrasound, urinalysis and a search for tumour markers in the serum.

Management

Prednisolone, 40–60 mg daily, is used initially to induce a remission. Muscle enzyme levels may fall before clinical improvement is noted. The dose is then gradually reduced whilst continuing to monitor muscle strength and serum enzyme levels. Doses of 10–15 mg prednisolone daily are often needed to maintain remission. Immunosuppressive therapy is occasionally used when there is no response to corticosteroids. The use of splints and physiotherapy to prevent contractures should not be neglected. Prognosis is closely related to the presence or absence of associated malignancy and to the age of onset, being poorer in older patients.

SJÖGREN'S SYNDROME

This is an autoimmune disorder of unknown aetiology characterised by lymphocytic infiltration of the salivary and lacrimal glands leading to xerostomia and kerato-conjunctivitis sicca. In some patients sicca symptoms predominate—**Primary Sjögrens (sicca syndrome)**, while in others it is associated with another connective tissue disease such as RA, SLE, PSS or MCTD—**Secondary Sjögren's syndrome**. The main features of primary and secondary Sjögren's syndrome are contrasted in the information box.

Investigations

The salivary flow rate is reduced and reduction in lacrimal secretion can be demonstrated by use of the Shir-mer tear test. If necessary the diagnosis can be confirmed by demonstrating focal lymphocytic infiltration in the minor salivary glands in a lip biopsy. Biopsy of a major salivary gland is only necessary if there is concern that the patient may have developed a lymphoma. Patients with Sjögren's syndrome are characterised by having a wide range of autoantibodies (see information box above).

Management

Lacrimal substitution with hypromellose or other 'artificial tear drops' can relieve symptoms of kerato-conjunctivitis sicca in mild cases. Soft contact lenses can be useful for corneal protection in patients with filamentary keratitis, and occlusion of the lacrimal ducts is occasionally needed. Treatment of xerostomia is more difficult and none of the available saliva substitutes is very effective. Vaginal dryness is treated with lubricants such as KY jelly. Systemic corticosteroids and immuno-suppressive drugs are only occasionally indicated to control severe extra-glandular manifestations of Sjögren's syndrome.

PRIMARY AND SECONDARY SJÖGREN'S SYNDROME

PRIMARY SJÖGREN'S (SICCA) SYNDROME	**SECONDARY SJÖGREN'S SYNDROME**
• Age onset 40–60	• Age onset 40–60
• F > M	• F > M
• HLA-B8 DR3	• HLA-B8 DR3
	• Incidence 10% RA patients
• **Common clinical features**	• **Common clinical features**
Kerato conjunctivitis sicca	Mild keratoconjunctivitis sicca
Xerostomia	Dry mouth
Salivary gland enlargement	
• **Rarer clinical features**	• **Other associated autoimmune disorders**
Anaemia, leucopenia	Systemic lupus erythematosus
Thrombocytopenia	Progressive systemic sclerosis
Lymphadenopathy	Primary biliary cirrhosis
Hepatomegaly	Chronic active hepatitis
Hyperglobulinaemic purpura	Myasthenia gravis
Vasculitis	Polymyositis
Neuropathy	Thyroiditis
Myositis	
Fibrosing alveolitis	
Glomerulonephritis	
Renal tubular acidosis	
Lymphoreticular malignancy	
• **Autoantibodies frequently detected**	• **Autoantibodies frequently detected**
Rheumatoid factor	Rheumatoid factor
ANF	ANF
SS-A (Anti-Ro)	Salivary duct
SS-B (Anti-La)	Gastric parietal cell
Salivary duct	Thyroid
Gastric parietal cell	
Thyroid	

RELAPSING POLYCHONDRITIS

This is an acute, systemic, episodic disorder characterised by inflammation and destruction of cartilage.

Epidemiology

Relapsing polychondritis is extremely rare with an estimated annual incidence of only 3.5/million. It presents most frequently in the 40's and 50's but cases have been reported at all ages. In 30% of patients there is an associated autoimmune or connective tissue disease but unlike other autoimmune disorders it appears to occur with equal frequency in both sexes and there is no known association with HLA antigens.

Clinical features

The principal clinical features are summarised in the information box.

RELAPSING POLYCHONDRITIS: CLINICAL FEATURES

- **Ears**
  Auricular chondritis
  Conductive deafness
  Nerve deafness
  Vestibular damage
- **Nose**
  Nasal tenderness
  Saddle nose deformity
- **Throat**
  Hoarseness
  Stridor
  Laryngeal/tracheal
  stricture

- **Eyes**
  Episcleritis/scleritis
  Uveitis/keratitis
- **Joints**
  Sero-negative arthritis
- **CVS**
  Conduction defects
  Valvular disease
  Small/large vessel
  vasculitis
- **Kidneys**
  Proliferative
  glomerulonephritis

Most patients present with pain and swelling of the pinna of the ear or nose with or without an associated seronegative arthritis.

Investigations

Laboratory abnormalities during acute phases include non-specific indices of systemic inflammation (anaemia of chronic disease, leucocytosis, thrombocytosis, elevated ESR and acute phase proteins) and raised levels of serum antibodies to type II collagen and a 148 kDa cartilage specific protein. Positive tests for other autoantibodies usually reflect an associated autoimmune or connective tissue disease. Pulmonary function tests and CT scanning are often required to define the extent of laryngo-tracheal involvement and audiometry, ECG and echocardiography are required when there is deafness or cardiovascular disease. The tissue diagnosis can be confirmed by biopsy in patients with auricular chondritis, and renal biopsy may show a proliferative glomerulonephritis in patients with proteinuria or active urinary sediments.

Management

Mild episodes of auricular and nasal chondritis and seronegative arthritis usually respond to nonsteroidal anti-inflammatory drugs with or without low dosage corticosteroids. Other more serious manifestations require treatment with high dosage prednisolone (1 mg/kg) and sometimes cytotoxic drugs.

FAMILIAL MEDITERRANEAN FEVER

This is a rare genetic disorder which is largely restricted to Armenians, Sephardic Jews and other ethnic groups originating from the Middle East and Eastern Mediterranean. Inheritance is usually autosomal and recessive but families with dominant inheritance have been described.

Clinical features

The disease is characterised by repetitive episodes of high fever, peritonitis, pleurisy and inflammatory arthritis with the independent development of renal amyloidosis and renal failure. Typical acute attacks resolve spontaneously without residua in 12–72 hours but joint effusions and synovitis, especially in the knees and hips, may persist between febrile episodes with progressive damage to articular cartilage. The onset of symptoms is usually in childhood or early adolescence but the frequency of attacks varies greatly from regular weekly bouts of fever to occasional, irregular episodes with months or years of intervening spontaneous remission. Myalgia, erysipelas-like skin lesions and cutaneous vasculitis can occur in some patients but the presence of haematuria or persistent proteinuria usually signals the development of renal amyloidosis.

Investigations

Acute attacks are associated with a raised ESR and non-specific rises in acute phase proteins such as C reactive protein and fibrinogen as well as the serum amyloid A protein. Peritoneal, pleural and synovial aspirates are characteristically sterile exudates with a predominance of polymorphonuclear leucocytes. Chest radiographs may demonstrate small pleural effusions, and straight radiographs of the abdomen may show multiple small bowel fluid levels. Patients with protracted hip pain may show loss of articular cartilage and/or radiological evidence of osteonecrosis. Histological evidence of renal amyloidosis is established by renal biopsy.

Management

Prophylactic oral colchicine (1–2 mg/day) prevents the development of renal amyloidosis and suppresses acute attacks in two-thirds of patients. Renal transplantation and hip arthroplasty are necessary in a small minority.

SYSTEMIC VASCULITIS

The vasculitides are a group of disorders in which inflammation in blood vessel walls leads to impairment of blood flow, ischaemia, variable organ damage and associated systemic disturbance.

Vasculitis can be divided into three main categories depending on the size of vessel affected:

- Large arteries
  Giant cell arteritis
  Takayasu's disease
- Medium size arteries
  Systemic necrotising vasculitides
- Small vessel disease of arterioles
  capillaries and venules.

A more detailed classification is given in the information box below. It is important to recognise however that a systemic necrotising vasculitis can occur in the course of connective tissue diseases such as rheumatoid arthritis, systemic lupus erythematosus, progressive systemic sclerosis and childhood dermatomyositis or as the predominant clinical manifestation in four different systemic disorders.

CLASSIFICATION OF SYSTEMIC VASCULITIS

- **Systemic necrotising vasculitis**
  Polyarteritis nodosa
  Churg–Strauss vasculitis
  Microscopic polyarteritis
  Wegener's granulomatosis
- **Lymphomatoid granulomatosis**
- **Hypersensitivity vasculitis**
  Serum sickness, drug reactions
  Henoch–Schönlein purpura
  Infections
  Neoplasms
- **Vasculitis associated with connective tissue disease**
  Rheumatoid arthritis
  Systemic lupus erythematosus
  Progressive systemic sclerosis
  Polymyositis
- **Large vessel arteritis**
  Giant cell arteritis
  Takayasu's disease
- **Kawasaki's disease**

POLYARTERITIS NODOSA (PAN)

Classical PAN is a necrotising vasculitis affecting medium sized arteries.

Epidemiology

PAN is a rare disorder with an annual incidence of only 5–10/million in most populations.

All age groups can be affected, with a peak incidence in the 4th and 5th decades and a male to female ratio of 2:1. The incidence is ten times higher in the Inuit population of Alaska where hepatitis B infection is endemic.

Aetiology and pathogenesis

In most cases the aetiology of PAN is unknown. In 5–50%, however, depending on the population studied, PAN is associated with circulating immune complexes containing the hepatitis B surface antigen. Other viruses implicated include hepatitis A, cytomegalovirus, parvovirus and HIV. Immune complex deposition is associated with endothelial cell damage, intimal proliferation, panarteritis, fibrosis, organ infarction and aneurysm formation.

Clinical features

Clinical presentation is very variable. The major features are listed in Table 15.13. Some patients present with non-specific features of systemic illness such as fever, weight loss and profound fatigue. Myalgia, arthralgia and a non-erosive polyarthritis are common. In others there is evidence of obvious vasculitic damage with skin lesions such as ulcers, palpable purpura, cutaneous infarcts or gangrene. Mononeuritis multiplex results from arteritic involvement of the vasa nervorum. In some patients the presentation is with severe hypertension and/or renal impairment and a significant number present as an acute surgical emergency with abdominal pain, peritonitis, pancreatitis, major gastrointestinal haemorrhage, gut or gall bladder infarction. Testicular pain, leg and jaw claudication can occur as a result of vascular occlusion and about a third of patients have some lung involvement with chest pain, consolidation or variable pulmonary infiltrates. The frequency of organ involvement is shown in Figure 15.36.

MICROSCOPIC POLYARTERITIS

In this variety of polyarteritis necrotising glomerulonephritis is the major feature but progressive renal insufficiency may be preceded by non-specific symptoms of systemic illness and/or a variety of features of systemic vasculitis (Fig. 15.36).

Table 15.13   Clinical manifestations of polyarteritis nodosa

Systemic inflammation Fever Weight loss Myalgia/Muscle wasting	70%	**GI tract** Abdominal pain Peritonitis Organ infarction	20%
Renal disease Renal impairment (30%) Hypertension (40%)	70%	**Cardiovascular** Myocardial infarction Congestive cardiac failure	15%
Joint disease Arthralgia (50%) Arthritis (20%)	70%	**Pulmonary**	10%
		Eye Scleritis Retinitis	10%
Skin lesions Palpable purpura Infarction Ulcers Livedo reticularis	50%	**ENT**	10%
		CNS Epilepsy Stroke	5%
Neuropathy Mononeuritis multiplex Symmetrical sensori-motor	50%	**Other** Testicular pain Leg and jaw claudication	10%

CHURG–STRAUSS VASCULITIS

Asthma, allergic rhinitis, pulmonary infiltrates and eosinophilia are the major features in this syndrome which is also associated with multisystem necrotising vasculitis (Fig. 15.36).

WEGENER'S GRANULOMATOSIS

This form of systemic vasculitis characteristically presents with upper and lower respiratory tract lesions in association with a focal glomerulonephritis. Systemic features of a major multisystem disorder (Fig. 15.36) may be preceded by months or years of recurrent rhinitis, epistaxis, sinusitis, serous otitis media or a shorter history of pulmonary symptoms such as cough, haemoptysis, chest pain or dyspnoea. In some patients with **limited Wegener's granulomatosis** there is little in the way of systemic necrotising vasculitis, and local granuloma formation predominates with chronic sinusitis, nasal and orbital destruction or cavitating lung lesions.

Investigations

A normochromic, normocytic anaemia of chronic disease with a polymorphonuclear leucocytosis, thrombocytosis, raised ESR and elevated acute phase proteins are non-specific features of systemic inflammation in all types of systemic necrotising vasculitis. Eosinophilia is characteristic in patients with Churg–Strauss vasculitis and Wegener's granulomatosis with pulmonary lesions. Complement activation with reduced circulating levels of C_3, C_4 and CH_{50} are sometimes found in patients with active glomerulonephritis, and tests for antibodies to hepatitis B surface antigen are positive in some pat-

ients with PAN. Raised levels of antibodies to factor VIII related antigen are an indication of endothelial cell damage in all forms of vasculitis. Tests for rheumatoid factor are sometimes positive in patients with PAN and Wegener's granulomatosis.

Anti-neutrophil cytoplasmic antibodies (ANCAs) can be useful for diagnosis. Granular staining of the neutrophil cytoplasm, the classical or C-ANCA, is found in about 80% of patients with Wegener's granulomatosis while perinuclear staining (P-ANCA) is characteristically found in patients with microscopic polyarteritis.

Biopsy of clinically involved organs or tissue such as skin, muscle, kidney, nerve or nasal mucosa should be undertaken to obtain histological confirmation of diagnosis.

Renal or coeliac-axis angiography is indicated when there is no clear evidence of specific organ pathology. It may reveal evidence of segmental artery narrowing and aneurysm formation in PAN and other types of systemic necrotising vasculitis.

Management

PAN, microscopic polyarteritis and Wegener's granulomatosis are usually treated with high dosage oral prednisolone (1 mg/kg/daily) and cyclophosphamide (2 mg/kg/daily) or fortnightly intravenous boluses of prednisolone (10 mg/kg) and cyclophosphamide (15 mg/kg) from the outset. Churg–Strauss vasculitis frequently responds to high dosage steroids alone. Doses of prednisolone and cyclophosphamide are reduced gradually following induction of remission, and full blood counts must be carefully monitored. The dose of cyclophosphamide is reduced in patients with renal

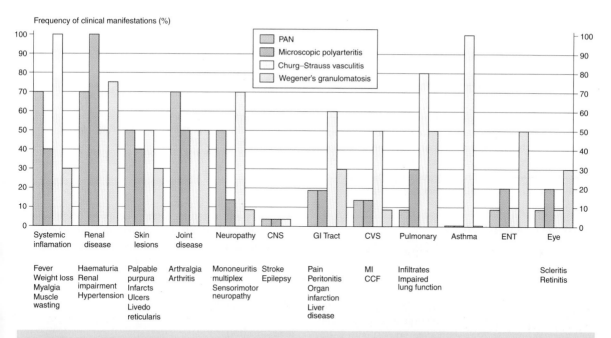

Fig. 15.36 Necrotising vasculitis. Frequency of clinical manifestations in polyarteritis nodosa, microscopic polyarteritis, Churg–Strauss vasculitis and Wegener's granulomatosis.

insufficiency and Mesna is given concurrently to reduce the risk of haemorrhagic cystitis. Other potential side effects are shown in Table 15.9 (p. 902). Plasma exchange is rarely undertaken in patients with severe or resistant disease and azathioprine plus alternate day steroids are sometimes preferred for maintenance of remission. Trimethoprim/sulphamethoxazole (co-trimoxazole) can be used for treating patients with limited Wegener's.

Prognosis

The use of cytotoxic drugs has transformed the prognosis for patients with Wegener's granulomatosis. What was once a disease with a 100% mortality in 2 years now has a better than 80% 5-year survival. The prognosis in PAN and Churg–Strauss vasculitis is similarly good but life expectancy is less in patients with microscopic polyarteritis.

LYMPHOMATOID GRANULOMATOSIS

This is a multisystem disorder with prominent pulmonary involvement that resembles Wegener's granulomatosis and the Churg–Strauss syndrome. Pathologically it is characterised by a focal angiocentric and angiodestructive T lymphocyte proliferation with lymphocyte, histiocyte and plasma cell infiltrates in arteries and veins.

Clinical features

These are usually cough and breathlessness but skin, renal and CNS lesions are common.

Investigations

There are non-specific rises in acute phase proteins and the ESR with evidence of a pleural effusion, pulmonary infiltrate or cavitating nodule on chest radiography. CT scans or MRI can be used to identify space-occupying lesions in the brain and the CSF has a high protein and cell count with atypical lymphocytes in patients with CNS involvement. Diagnosis is confirmed by biopsy.

Management

Treatment with prednisolone and cyclophosphamide will induce remission of disease in about 50% of patients.

HYPERSENSITIVITY VASCULITIS

Cutaneous leucocytoclastic vasculitis affecting small and medium sized vessels in the skin can be associated with hyperglobulinaemia, serum sickness, drug reactions, infections and malignant tumours.

Clinical features

There is palpable purpura and/or urticaria. Associated arthralgia, arthritis, abdominal pain and glomerulonephritis are characteristic of anaphylactic or **Henoch–Schönlein purpura** (see p. 910). Hypersensitivity vasculitis is an immune complex disorder and investigations sometimes reveal evidence of circulating IgG, IgM or IgA immune complexes as well as leucocytoclasis and immune complex deposition in skin biopsies.

Management
Treatment with antihistamines to control symptoms associated with urticaria is all that is required in mild cases but corticosteroids and pulses of cyclophosphamide are occasionally required in patients with severe systemic disease and glomerulonephritis.

GIANT CELL ARTERITIS (GCA)

CRANIAL ARTERITIS, POLYMYALGIA RHEUMATICA

Giant cell arteritis is a relatively common form of large vessel vasculitis occurring predominantly in elderly people. The annual incidence is approximately 10/100 000 in the general population in Europe. The mean age at onset is 70 years (range 50–90) with a 2:1 female to male ratio.

Pathology
Giant cell arteritis is characterised by an inflammatory infiltrate of lymphocytes, plasma cells, 'giant' macrophages and eosinophils throughout the arterial wall with predominant necrosis of the media and fragmentation of the internal elastic lamina.

Affected vessels may become occluded. The pathological process is of unknown cause, but may have an autoimmune basis because it occurs more frequently in patients with other autoimmune disorders such as thyroid disease or rheumatoid arthritis. The external carotid artery and its branches are particularly susceptible, and the ophthalmic, vertebral and subclavian vessels are often involved. Less commonly, the internal carotid, coronary and mesenteric arteries are affected.

CRANIAL ARTERITIS

Clinical Features
Three-quarters of patients present with severe headaches which may be associated with scalp tenderness. The onset can be acute or insidious and is often associated with constitutional symptoms of anorexia, fatigue, weight loss, fever, depression and general malaise. Visual problems such as diplopia, scintillating scotomata, transient blindness and ptosis are common. More permanent visual loss can result from ischaemic optic atrophy secondary to vasculitis in the posterior ciliary

---

CLINICAL FEATURES OF GIANT CELL ARTERITIS

- Headache, scalp tenderness
- Malaise, anorexia, weight loss
- Fever
- Arthralgia
- Muscle tenderness and stiffness (not weakness)
- Visual impairment
- Arm and jaw claudication
- Brain-stem ischaemia/infarction (ataxia, diplopia, dysarthria, syncope)
- Cerebral hemisphere infarction

---

arteries. Central retinal artery occlusion occurs much more rarely. Giant cell arteritis may also cause transient ischaemic attacks, brain stem infarcts and jaw claudication. Examination may reveal thickened and tender temporal arteries. The diagnosis should be suspected in any elderly patient with visual impairment, especially if headache and malaise are present.

Investigations
The erythrocyte sedimentation rate (ESR) is usually elevated above 50 mm/hour and may be more than twice this level. Temporal artery biopsy may prove the diagnosis but is not always positive, and treatment should be started immediately if clinical suspicion is strong, because the risk of further visual loss is high.

Management
Treatment is with high dose steroids (prednisolone 60–100 mg daily) initially, reducing the dose gradually over the first few weeks to a maintenance level of 10–20 mg daily as guided by the ESR response. The symptoms improve dramatically within a day or two of starting steroids but visual failure is usually permanent. If clinical suspicion is high, and the ESR elevated, steroids should be started immediately; temporal artery biopsy may be delayed for 48 hours before histological resolution is likely to take place. Maintenance therapy is required for at least a year, and sometimes for the rest of the patient's life.

POLYMYALGIA RHEUMATICA

Presentation with severe pain and stiffness in the neck, back, shoulders, upper arms and thighs, often associated with profound and prolonged early morning stiffness, is more common. Physical signs are usually limited to slight tenderness of the acromio-clavicular or sterno-clavicular joints but occasionally there may be evidence of mild inflammatory arthritis in a more peripheral joint. There is no associated primary myositis or muscle tenderness. Whereas in patients with cranial arteritis there may be arterial tenderness or absence of pulsation, the peripheral arteries are usually clinically normal in patients presenting with polymyalgia rheumatica although approximately one-third of patients do develop features of cranial arteritis at some point in the course of their disease. The risk of serious ocular complications is low, however.

Investigations

The ESR is markedly raised in the majority of patients and there may be a normochromic, normocytic anaemia of chronic disease. Temporal artery biopsy shows evidence of giant cell arteritis in 15–40% of patients with polymyalgia rheumatica but it is safe to assume that the true frequency of vasculitis is 100%.

Management

The response to corticosteroid therapy is dramatic. Treatment should be commenced with oral prednisolone (15 mg daily). The diagnosis should be reviewed if there is no striking remission of symptoms within a week. It is usually possible to begin tapering the dose of prednisolone 4–8 weeks after starting treatment and most patients can be maintained in clinical remission with 5–7 mg prednisolone daily.

Prognosis

Nearly all patients require corticosteroid therapy for 2 years but most can be weaned from steroids by 5 years. A few patients have a more prolonged chronic illness. The need for maintenance prednisolone should be reviewed by an attempt at gradual steroid withdrawal in all patients after 2 years, and the risks of relapse need to be balanced against the risks of steroid side-effects. Prophylactic calcium supplements should be given from the onset of therapy to all patients and the addition of a small dose of azathioprine needs to be considered as a steroid sparing manoeuvre in patients whose disease cannot be maintained in clinical remission with less than 10 mg of prednisolone daily.

TAKAYASU'S DISEASE

Takayasu's disease, also called pulseless disease or the aortic arch syndrome, is a chronic inflammatory granulomatous panarteritis which affects the aorta, its major branches and occasionally the pulmonary arteries.

Epidemiology

It has a low incidence of 1–3/million population per year in Europe and the United States but occurs much more frequently in Mexico and the Far East. The occurrence of this rare disorder in twins suggests that genetic factors

are important but little else is known about its aetiology or pathogenesis There may be an association with HLA-B5. The condition occurs most often in young women under the age of 40 years and there is a female:male ratio of approximately 8:1.

Clinical features

The clinical features are summarised in the information box.

TAKAYASU'S DISEASE: CLINICAL FEATURES

- **Systemic inflammation**
  Fever/sweats
  Fatigue
  Weight loss
  Arthralgia/myalgia
  Anaemia
- **Vascular insufficiency**
  Headaches
  Syncope
  Arm claudication
  Angina
- **Cardiovascular**
  Hypertension
  Myocardial infarction
  Aortic reflux
- **Other problems**
  Panniculitis
  Pleurisy
  Glomerulonephritis

In some patients there is a long phase of non-specific systemic illness prior to the development of vascular complications when examination typically reveals the presence of vascular bruits and diminished or absent pulses. The upper limbs are typically affected more than the lower limbs.

Investigations

A normocytic, normochromic anaemia of chronic disease, mild leucocytosis and raised ESR are non-specific features of systemic inflammation. Chest radiographs may show widening of the aorta as well as cardiomegaly. Arch aortography or intravenous digital subtraction angiography is usually required to reveal stenoses in the aortic arch or its branches (Type I), atypical coarctation with involvement of the descending aorta (Type II) or a mixed picture (Type III).

Management

Most patients respond to high dose oral prednisolone (1–2 mg/kg daily) but additional pulses of cyclophosphamide, and vascular surgery, are needed in a few. The 5-year survival in treated patients is 90%.

KAWASAKI'S DISEASE (MUCOCUTANEOUS LYMPH NODE SYNDROME)

This is an acute systemic disorder occurring predominantly in children under the age of 5 in which mucocutaneous lesions are associated with a vasculitis that characteristically involves the coronary arteries.

The annual incidence in Japan is 70–80/100 000 children under the age of 5 but it is much less common elsewhere in the world. Boys are affected three times as often as girls. The clinical picture and epidemic occurrence in Japan suggest an infective aetiology but no definite aetiological virus or bacterium has been identified. The principal clinical features are listed in the information box. Cardiovascular complications include coronary aneurysms, transient coronary artery dilatation, myocardial infarction, pericarditis and effusions and cardiac failure.

KAWASAKI'S DISEASE

- Fever persisting for more than 5 days
- Bilateral conjunctival congestion
- Erythema lips, tongue and buccal mucosa
- Acute non-purulent cervical lymphadenopathy
- Polymorphous exanthema
- Erythema of palms and soles (oedema followed by desquamation)

Diagnosis with 5/6 features, or 4/6 plus evidence of coronary aneurysm

---

In addition to a polymorphonuclear leucocytosis, thrombocytosis and raised acute phase proteins, positive tests for anti-neutrophil cytoplasmic antibodies (ANCA) and anti-endothelial cell antibodies are found. Coronary vessel abnormalities can be visualised by two-dimensional echocardiography or coronary angiography. Treatment is usually with aspirin (5 mg/kg daily) and high dosage intravenous gammaglobulin (400 mg/kg daily for 4 days). Most children recover and the overall mortality is less than 2%.

FURTHER READING

Churg A, Churg J (eds) 1991 Systemic Vasculitides. Ikagu-Shoin, New York
Lahita R G (ed.) 1992 Systemic lupus erythematosus, 2nd edn. Churchill Livingstone, New York
Tan E M 1989 Antinuclear antibodies: diagnostic markers for autoimmune diseases and probes for cell biology. Advances in Immunology 44: 93–151

DISEASES OF BONE

PHYSIOLOGY

Bone is a specialised form of metabolically active, mineralised connective tissue. It consists of cells of monocyte-macrophage origin (bone-forming osteoblasts, bone-resorbing osteoclasts, resting osteocytes) and an organic matrix of type I collagen, proteoglycan and some bone-specific glycoproteins. The skeleton contains more than 99% of the body calcium in the form of a crystalline calcium phosphate complex (hydroxyapatite). The tubular mid-sections of long bones (diaphyses), which make up 80% of the skeletal mass, are composed of circumferential lamellae of compact, cortical bone consisting of longitudinally orientated osteons surrounding central Haversian canals which carry the capillaries. Extracellular fluid reaches the bone osteocytes by a radial system of canaliculi and there are lateral vascular communications with the periosteal vessels through Volkmann's canals. The distal ends of the long bones (metaphyses), the vertebrae and the flat bones are composed of more loosely packed cancellous bone. Although it accounts for only 20% of the skeletal mass, the trabecular surface area of this cancellous bone is as large as that of compact bone, rendering it relatively more susceptible to metabolic diseases. It is important to realise that bone is bounded by a number of distinct cellular surfaces—the endosteal, periosteal, Haversian and trabecular envelopes.

The size and shape of bones change rapidly in the growing phase of infancy as part of the modelling process. The marrow cavity and outer cortex expand due to endosteal resorption and periosteal accretion of bone, and bone turnover may be as high as 200% per annum. Following skeletal maturity this is reduced to less than 5% but the rate of endosteal resorption is reduced less than that of periosteal accretion. Thus while the outer diameter of normal older bones is greater than that of younger, the cortex is progressively thinned with advancing years. Deformities and short stature may be a consequence of diseases interfering with the modelling process during the growing period. Examples include metabolic diseases such as rickets, inflammatory diseases such as polyarticular juvenile chronic arthritis, and bone dysplasias such as osteopetrosis.

Modern methods of bone histomorphometry, in which iliac biopsies are obtained following double tetracycline labelling, have revealed a second form of bone turnover or remodelling. This occurs throughout life and accounts for more than 95% of turnover in the mature skeleton. Remodelling occurs in 'programmed packages'; the sequence of cellular events is invariably one of activation of osteoclasts followed by a period of osteoblastic formation along the freshly resorbed trabecular surface. The whole sequence is completed in 4–6 months in healthy adults. Trauma and hyperthyroidism are two of the numerous factors that can activate the remodelling process, while oestrogens suppress it. Fluoride uncouples the remodelling sequence and stimulates osteoblastic activity.

Increased turnover of bone, whatever the cause, is associated with a rise in the plasma alkaline phosphatase and the bone-specific glycoprotein osteocalcin, and an increase in the urinary excretion of hydroxyproline and pyridinoline cross links.

A classification of bone disease is given in the information box.

CLASSIFICATION OF DISEASES OF BONE

- **Infections**
- **Metabolic and endocrine diseases**
  Rickets and osteomalacia
  Nutritional deficiency, e.g. calcium
  Osteoporosis
      Post menopausal
      Association with endocrine disease, e.g. in
      hypogonadism, Cushing's syndrome and
      hypopituitarism
  Iatrogenic, e.g. corticosteroid therapy
  Chronic wasting diseases, e.g. rheumatoid arthritis
      or malignancy
  Hereditary diseases, e.g. osteogenesis imperfecta
  Idiopathic juvenile osteoporosis
  Hyperparathyroidism
- **Paget's disease**
- **Disorders of collagen**
  e.g. Marfan's syndrome
- **Mucopolysaccharidoses**
  e.g. Hurler's syndrome and Hunter's syndrome
- **Skeletal dysplasias**
- **Neoplastic disease**
  Primary, benign or malignant
  Secondary malignant

INFECTIONS

OSTEOMYELITIS

This is most commonly encountered in children under the age of 12.

Clinical features

The onset is abrupt with fever, malaise and severe pain at the site of bone infection. When this is close to a joint there may be a 'sympathetic' effusion which can cause diagnostic confusion with septic arthritis. Isotope scanning and careful delineation of the site of bone tenderness can be helpful in establishing the correct diagnosis but radiographic changes do not occur for some days or weeks.

Staphylococci are the most frequent organisms responsible and in about half the cases haematogenous spread has occurred from a boil or superficial infection. Hypogammaglobulinaemia, malnutrition or debilitating illness may all be predisposing factors. Salmonella can also cause osteomyelitis and this infection is a common complication of sickle-cell anaemia.

Management

After taking blood for culture as soon as the diagnosis is suspected, an antibiotic, for example sodium fusidate, must be commenced and continued in adequate doses for long enough to eliminate the infection. Delay in starting treatment or inadequate therapy may result in chronic indolent bone infection (Brodie's abscess) with sequestrum formation. Surgical exploration and decompression are required if there is not an immediate response to antibiotics.

Tuberculous osteomyelitis

This has become much less common in Britain since the elimination of bovine tuberculosis but there is evidence of a recent increase among the elderly population and immigrant communities. The spine is affected in 50% of patients.

Typically the infection starts at the margins of vertebral bodies, with subsequent invasion of the disc space. Destruction of bone leads to angular kyphosis (Fig. 15.37). A paravertebral 'cold' abscess may form and track to the thigh, chest wall or neck (Fig. 15.38). The hip, knee, ankle or wrist joint may be affected by spread from adjacent bone. Tuberculous dactylitis and sacroiliitis are unusual but characteristic lesions.

The treatment of tuberculosis is described on pages 360–362.

RICKETS AND OSTEOMALACIA

Rickets and osteomalacia are metabolic bone diseases characterised by increased amounts of unmineralised osteoid and a decrease in the rate of bone formation. Vitamin D metabolism is depicted in Figure 15.39. The causes of rickets and osteomalacia are shown in the information box.

RICKETS

Rickets is the characteristic result of deficiency of vitamin D in children. When the epiphyses have fused the corresponding deficiency disease is osteomalacia. Both mainly affect the bones but they differ in details.

Infants in their first year are susceptible to rickets

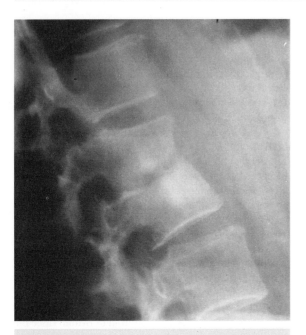

Fig. 15.37 Tuberculous osteomyelitis of lumbar spine. Lateral radiograph showing bone and disc destruction with angular kyphosis.

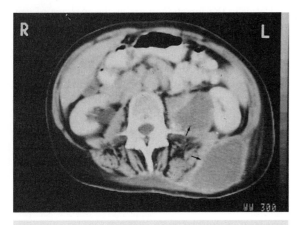

Fig. 15.38 Spinal tuberculosis. Abdominal CT scan showing large paravertebral 'cold' abscess.

CAUSES OF RICKETS AND OSTEOMALACIA

Vitamin D deficiency
- Dietary deficiency
- Lack of synthesis in skin
- Decreased absorption
  Coeliac disease
  Hepatobiliary disorders
  Pancreatic disease
  Gastric and intestinal surgery
- Defective metabolism
  Drugs (anticonvulsants, sedatives, rifampicin)
  Chronic renal failure
    Renal osteodystrophy
    Dialysis bone disease
  Vitamin D dependent rickets

Hypophosphataemia with normal vitamin D
- Familial hypophosphataemic rickets
- Inherited and acquired renal tubular defects (e.g. Fanconi syndrome, cadmium poisoning, multiple myelomatosis)

Osteomalacia with normal calcium phosphate and vitamin D
- Hypophosphatasia
- Fibrogenesis imperfecta
- Aluminium bone disease

skin to sunlight and very low dietary intakes of vitamin D. High phytate intake in chapatti flour may contribute by inhibiting calcium absorption. The disease is also liable to occur in premature babies.

Clinical features

The infant with rickets has often received sufficient calories and may appear well nourished, but is restless, fretful and pale, with flabby muscles, and is prone to respiratory and gastrointestinal infections. Development is delayed; the teeth often erupt late and there is failure to sit, crawl, stand and walk at the normal ages.

The bony changes are the most characteristic signs of rickets. The earliest lesion is often craniotabes—small round unossified areas in the membranous bones of the skull, yielding to the pressure of the finger, with a crackling feeling. This sign suggests the possibility of rickets in an infant under one year of age but it is not pathognomonic. It is not found over this age.

Two other early signs are enlargement of the epiphyses at the lower end of the radius and swelling of the costochondral junctions of the ribs ('rickety rosary,' Fig. 15.40). Later there may be 'bossing' of the frontal and parietal bones and delayed closure of the anterior fontanelle. Later still, there may be deformities of the chest. In the second or third year of life, deformities such as kyphosis develop as a result of the new gravitational and muscular strains caused by sitting up and standing. At

because of the inadequate vitamin D in cows' milk. If they are always kept indoors or completely covered whenever they are taken outside they are never exposed to sunlight. By the second year the infant is able to crawl about in the sunshine and spontaneous healing usually occurs.

The disease is now uncommon in countries where vitamin D is freely available. In Britain clinical rickets occurs in Asian immigrant children, often of school-going age, from a combination of little exposure of the

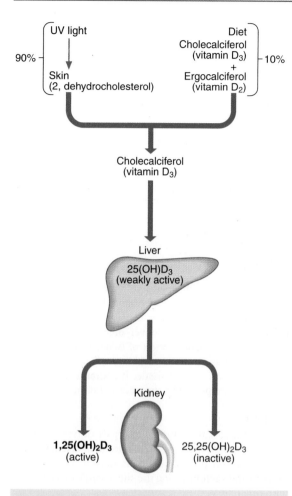

Fig. 15.39 Vitamin D metabolism in man.

In the diagram:

UV light → Skin (2, dehydrocholesterol) — 90%

Diet: Cholecalciferol (vitamin D_3) + Ergocalciferol (vitamin D_2) — 10%

↓

Cholecalciferol (vitamin D_3)

↓

Liver: $25(OH)D_3$ (weakly active)

↓

Kidney

$1,25(OH)_2D_3$ (active) $25,25(OH)_2D_3$ (inactive)

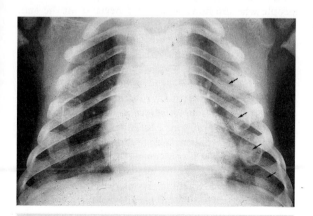

Fig. 15.40 Radiograph showing 'rickety rosary' in young child.

the same time there may be enlargement of the epiphyses at the lower ends of the femur, tibia and fibula. When the rachitic child begins to walk, deformities of the shafts of the leg bones develop, so that 'knock knees' or 'bow legs' are seen. Pelvic deformities can follow severe rickets in later childhood and lead to serious difficulties at childbirth.

When there is a reduction in ionised plasma calcium, infantile tetany may result, with spasm of the hands and feet and of the vocal cords. The latter causes a high-pitched distressing cry and difficulty in breathing. Epileptic fits may also occur.

Investigations

Radiological examination of the wrist will show characteristic changes in the epiphyses at the lower ends of the radius. The zones of epiphyseal cartilages are thickened and the distal ends of the shafts are widened. When fully developed this shows as a typical 'saucer' deformity.

Biochemical findings vary according to aetiology and are summarised in Table 15.14. Where rickets occurs as a result of dietary deficiency of vitamin D, the plasma calcium tends to fall from its normal level (p. 1148). More commonly the serum phosphate falls due to the parathyroid glands' responding to a slight reduction in calcium by increasing the excretion of phosphate in the urine.

Clinical rickets may occur when the levels of calcium and phosphorus in the plasma are still within normal limits but an increase in alkaline phosphatase is of diagnostic value. This enzyme is formed by the osteoblasts which, unable to make bone without a sufficient supply of calcium, liberate into the circulation the excess of this enzyme which they cannot use. Plasma 25-hydroxy-cholecalciferol, the main circulating form of vitamin D, is absent or very low.

Management

The two essentials of treatment are the provision of a supplement of vitamin D and an ample intake of calcium, the best source of which is milk.

A therapeutic dose of vitamin D varies from 25 to 125 μg (1000–5000 i.u.) daily, depending on the severity of the disease and age of the child. For comparison the prophylactic dose is 10 μg (400 i.u.) or less daily, depending on the sunlight.

Treatment of tetany is described on page 706.

Monitoring

The earliest evidence of healing in rickets is provided by radiological examination of the growing ends of the bones. Serum calcium and phosphorus provide an unreliable guide. The raised serum alkaline phosphatase does not usually fall for several weeks after treatment is

Table 15.14 Biochemical findings in rickets and osteomalacia

	Dietary deficiency	Vitamin D resistant rickets	Renal phosphate depletion	Renal osteodystrophy
Plasma calcium	↓	Normal	Normal	↓
Plasma phosphate	↓	↓	↓	↑
Alkaline phosphatase	↑	↑	↑	↑
1,25(OH)$_2$D3	↓	Normal	↑	↓

initiated. The therapeutic dose of vitamin D should be continued so long as this enzyme remains elevated; thereafter it can be reduced to the prophylactic dose of 10 μg daily.

Rickets is not a fatal disease per se, but the untreated rachitic child is always at risk of infections, notably bronchopneumonia. The skeletal changes, if mild in degree, usually tend to heal spontaneously as the child gets older, but in severe cases pigeon chest, spinal curvature, knock knees, bow legs or contracted pelvis persist.

Secondary and vitamin D resistant rickets

In malabsorption, e.g. in coeliac disease, rickets is common. Children on long-term anti-epileptic drugs are liable to develop rickets; these drugs induce changes in liver microsomal enzymes which convert vitamin D to inactive metabolites.

Occasional cases of rickets are resistant to ordinary therapeutic doses of vitamin D. The commonest type of vitamin D resistant rickets is **familial hypophosphataemic rickets,** an X-linked dominant condition in which there is renal tubular loss of phosphate. There are also two types of 'vitamin D dependent rickets', in one of which 1α hydroxylation of 25 OH vitamin D is impaired; in the other form there appears to be end-organ resistance to the active metabolite. Alfacalcidol is useful in these conditions.

Prevention

The natural means of prevention is regular exposure to the sun's UV light. There is no need for oral intake of vitamin D in tropical and subtropical countries except in the elderly housebound and chronic sick (see below). In high latitude northern countries very little UV light gets through the atmosphere in winter. Modern infant milk-based formulae include adequate vitamin D and there appears to be enough in breast milk for full-term infants for the first few months of life. After infancy North American children and adults are protected by added vitamin D in liquid milk. In Britain, however, none of the common foods is a good source of vitamin D. Growing children may benefit from a daily sup-

plement of 10 μg daily during the winter months. There are many suitable and inexpensive preparations. Cod liver oil is still effective but unpopular because of its taste.

OSTEOMALACIA

Osteomalacia, which means softening of bone, is primarily due to a deficiency of vitamin D (see information box on page 928 for other causes). This results in a failure to replace the turnover of calcium and phosphorus in the organic matrix of bone. Hence the bone content is demineralised and bony substance becomes replaced by soft osteoid tissue. It contains less calcium and phosphate per 100 g than normal bone.

Aetiology

Osteomalacia is the adult counterpart of rickets. It was formerly common in women in purdah in oriental countries, living on poor cereal diets devoid of milk, kept indoors and seldom seeing the sun. Symptoms occurred with pregnancy.

The disease may be due to malabsorption from any cause, including operations like partial gastrectomy, and in countries like the UK which do not have the insurance of fortification of milk with vitamin D it can occur in people who are housebound and never sit in the sun. Chronic renal disorders are a less important cause. Adults who have to take anti-epileptic drugs for years are likely to develop osteomalacia.

Clinical features

Skeletal discomfort is usually present and persistent, and ranges from backache to severe pain. Bone tenderness on pressure is common. Muscular weakness is often present and the patient may find difficulty in climbing stairs or getting out of a chair. A waddling gait is not unusual. Tetany may be manifested by carpopedal spasm and facial twitching. Spontaneous fractures may occur, independent of the pseudo-fractures described below. The biochemical changes in the blood are the same as in rickets.

Radiological examination shows rarefaction of bone

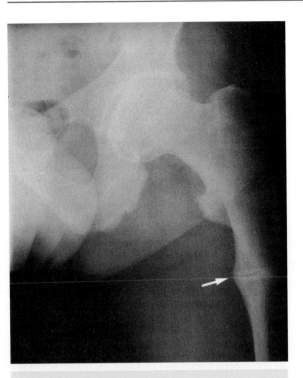

Fig. 15.41 Osteomalacia. Radiograph of femur showing pseudofracture (Looser's zone).

and commonly translucent bands (pseudo-fractures or Looser's zones, Fig. 15.41), often symmetrical, at points submitted to stress. Common sites are the ribs, the axillary border of the scapula, the pubic rami and the medial cortex of the upper femur. Pseudo-fractures are pathognomonic when well developed.

Histological examination of stained undecalcified sections of bone obtained by biopsy shows the presence of excess osteoid tissue.

Management

When osteomalacia is primarily due to defective intake, treatment is essentially the same as for rickets, namely 25–125 μg vitamin D daily. The response is usually dramatic. If there is evidence of malabsorption the dose should be increased or given intramuscularly at weekly intervals. If the disease is secondary to renal disorders alfacalcidol (p. 573) should be used.

Maintenance treatment with vitamin D will be required for all cases of osteomalacia in which the cause cannot be removed. In addition a good diet should be given which includes milk, cheese or yoghurt.

Prevention

Free access to sunshine and an adequate intake of dairy produce, supplemented when necessary with prophy-

lactic vitamin D (10 μg daily), will prevent nutritional osteomalacia. Particular attention in these prophylactic measures should be given to people in geriatric and mental hospitals and to old people living alone whose exposure to sunshine is limited and also to those who have had gastric surgery. Patients on long-term antiepileptic therapy should be given prophylactic doses of vitamin D.

OSTEOPOROSIS

Osteoporosis is defined as a decrease in the absolute amount of bone, leading to fractures following minimal trauma. In other words, osteoporosis is too little bone of normal mineral content and hence in contrast to osteomalacia the calcium phosphate per 100 g bone is normal. Osteoporosis is by far the commonest form of metabolic bone disease in developed countries, and is a major public health problem.

Epidemiology

Bone mass is determined by genetic and environmental factors and reaches a peak before the age of 40 years.

Age-related bone loss is greatly accelerated in women after the menopause and women lose approximately 30% of their cortical bone and 50% of their trabecular bone during their lifetime. Colles' fractures, femoral neck fractures and vertebral fractures are all related to osteoporosis. 25% of women over the age of 60 suffer vertebral fractures and 30% hip fractures. It has been calculated that four-fifths of the 37,500 femoral neck fractures occurring annually in England and Wales are at least in part attributable to osteoporosis. With a mean hospital stay of 40 days and mortality of 16% the annual cost of these fractures has been estimated at £165 million. There are about a quarter of a million femoral neck fractures in the United States each year, and the annual cost of treating osteoporosis-related problems is 6 billion dollars. Lifetime oestrogen exposure is an important determinant of bone mass but a number of risk factors for osteoporosis have been identified (see information box).

RISK FACTORS FOR OSTEOPOROSIS

Endogenous	Exogenous
● Female	● Low calcium intake
● Asian/Caucasian	● Reduced physical activity
● Small stature	● Cigarette smoking
● Thin physique	● Alcohol abuse
● Family history	● Aluminium antacids
● Nulliparity	● Surgical menopause
● Early menopause	● Steroid therapy
● Advanced age	

Table 15.15   Involutional osteoporosis

	Type I Menopause related	Type II Age related
Age (years)	50–70	>70
Sex ratio (F:M)	6:1	2:1
Type bone lost	Trabecular	Trabecular/cortical
Fractures	Colles' Crush vertebrae	Hip Wedge vertebrae
Parathyroid hormone Calcium absorption Vitamin D metabolism (25(OH)D$_3$ 1,25(OH)$_2$D$_3$)	Secondary decrease	Primary decrease

Table 15.16   Disorders associated with secondary osteoporosis

Disorder	Bone formation	Bone resorption
Cushing's syndrome	Decreased	Increased
Hyperthyroidism	Increased	Increased
Hypervitaminosis A	Increased	Increased
Heparin therapy	Increased	Increased
Immobilisation	Decreased	Increased
Anticonvulsant drug therapy	Increased	Increased

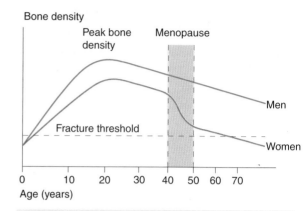

Fig. 15.42   Changes in bone mass with age in men and women. Postmenopausal osteoporosis with increased risk of fractures follows reduction of bone mass below fracture threshold in postmenopausal women with low initial peak bone mass.

Clinical features

Two types of involutional osteoporosis can be distinguished (Table 15.15). Type I is associated with forearm fractures, back pain and crush vertebral fractures in the post-menopausal period, while Type II, which is age related, occurs later and is associated with progressive loss of height, thoracic kyphosis and wedge fractures ('Dowager's hump') and hip fractures. Factors which predispose to falls in the elderly are obviously also important but fractures become much more likely when bone mass has fallen below a notional fracture threshold (Fig. 15.42). Other diseases predispose to osteoporosis by inhibiting bone formation or accelerating the rate of bone loss (Table 15.16).

Investigations

Plasma biochemical measurements are usually normal but the alkaline phosphatase and osteocalcin may be raised following a recent fracture and the calcium and hydroxyproline:creatinine ratio in the urine is increased after the menopause due to accelerated bone resorption. Radiographs show decreases in bone density and a more prominent trabecular pattern as well as the characteristic wedge and crush fractures in the spine but it has been calculated that at least 40% of bone mineral must be lost before changes are detectable on plain radiographs. The recent development of single and dual photon absorptiometry and dual X-ray absorptiometry allows measurement of bone mineral at forearm, hip or vertebral sites with an in vivo precision of about 1%. Skeletal scintigraphy with bone-seeking isotopes can help to reveal recent fractures and exclude other pathology. Quantitative histomorphometry on trans-iliac bone biopsies following tetracycline labelling is only required in difficult cases where osteomalacia and other pathology needs to be excluded.

Management

Effective treatment for established osteoporosis is difficult once bone mass has fallen below the fracture threshold so emphasis is placed on preventing osteoporosis in high-risk subjects (information box p. 931). Physical exercise, ensuring an adequate calcium intake (1500 mg daily) and avoiding cigarette smoking and alcohol abuse are encouraged. Hormone replacement therapy (HRT) should be considered in women with low bone mass following the menopause. Progestogens are added to oestrogen (0.625 mg conjugated equine oestrogen) to prevent the development of endometrial carcinoma, and transdermal oestrogen patches can be used to reduce risk of venous thrombosis and pulmonary embolism. A history of hypertension, stroke, ischaemic heart or thromboembolic disease are no longer regarded as absolute contraindications to HRT as oestrogen therapy is associated with decreased cardiovascular mortality. If bone loss is not too severe, treatment of established symptomatic osteoporosis can be undertaken with antiresorptive drug therapy (calcium supplements, HRT, bisphosphonate or calcitonin) and in selected very severe cases with recurrent symptomatic spinal fractures, bone-stimulating drug therapy with anabolic steroids and/or fluoride can be attempted.

PAGET'S DISEASE (OSTEITIS DEFORMANS)

Paget's disease, which is characterised by softening, enlargement and bowing of bones, is uncommon before the age of 40 years but increasingly frequent thereafter. There is increased blood flow through affected bones with resorption followed by excessive osteoblastic bone formation resulting in a high rate of bone turnover, raised levels of plasma alkaline phosphatase and increased urinary excretion of hydroxyproline and pyridinoline cross links. This activity is reflected in abnormal isotope bone scans and radiological evidence of localised bone enlargement, altered trabecular pattern and alternating areas of rarefaction and increased density. Recent evidence suggests that Paget's disease may be associated with a paramyxovirus infection of osteoclasts.

Clinical features

Men are more commonly affected and there may be a family history of the disease. Often the condition is symptomless and detected only when radiological examination is made for some other reason. In others there is pain of a deep aching character often aggravated by weight bearing. The pelvis, femur, tibia, lumbar spine and skull are common sites of bone involvement. The increased vascularity may cause warmth of the affected part on palpation; rarely widespread arteriovenous shunting causes high output cardiac failure. Enlargement and deformity of bones develop when the condition is advanced. Bowing of the femur and tibia is characteristic and Paget's disease may predispose to secondary osteoarthrosis of the hip or knee (Fig. 15.43). Fractures may occur spontaneously or after minor trauma but they usually heal normally. Skull involvement may result in headache, progressive enlargement of the cranium and deafness from compression of the auditory nerves. Paraplegia can follow vertebral involvement. Osteogenic sarcoma is an uncommon late complication.

Investigations

The serum calcium and phosphate are usually normal with high levels of alkaline phosphatase and increased hydroxyproline and pyridinoline excretion during phases of active disease.

Management

Calcitonin is used for severe bone pain not controlled by analgesics. Subcutaneous injection of 100 units of synthetic salmon calcitonin (Salcatonin) 3 times weekly can be continued for 6 months and is recommended if pain recurs. Mithramycin and the bisphosphonate etidronate, which reduce bone turnover, are less

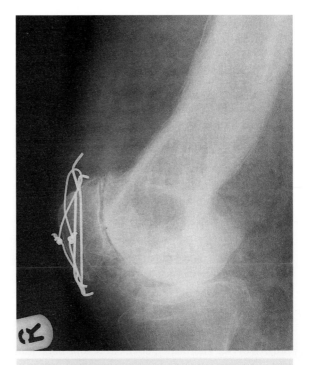

Fig. 15.43 Paget's disease of bone. Radiograph showing thickening and bowing of tibia with secondary osteoarthritis. The patella has been wired following a pathological fracture.

satisfactory alternatives, but the second generation bisphosphonate pamidronate (APD) has become the drug of choice for patients with bone pain. Confinement to bed may be followed by rapid mobilisation of calcium with hypercalcaemia, hypercalciuria and formation of renal calculi. Such patients should be given a high fluid intake and measures must be taken to lower the serum calcium if it becomes dangerously high. Pain due to secondary degenerative joint disease is treated with NSAIDs. Hip arthroplasty is occasionally required. Osteogenic sarcoma is treated with early surgery but has a poor prognosis.

AVASCULAR NECROSIS (OSTEONECROSIS)

Osteonecrosis is associated with a wide range of disorders that lead to ischaemic necrosis of cortical and trabecular bone (see information box p. 934). Fractures interfering with the blood supply to certain bone sites are numerically the most important cause and avascular necrosis of the femoral and humeral heads, scaphoid and talus are most frequently encountered. One-fifth of all subcapital fractures of the femoral neck are complicated by avascular necrosis of the femoral head but there is also evidence of osteonecrosis in about 20% of femoral heads removed from patients who have had total hip arthroplasties for OA or inflammatory joint disease. Other well defined pathogenic mechanisms include vasculitis affecting the extraosseous arteries and obliteration of intraosseous sinusoids by thrombi, sickled erythrocytes, fat and nitrogen amboli. The intraosseous circulation can also be impaired by pressure from metastases or lipid laden cells in storage disorders such as Gaucher's disease.

Osteonecrosis also occurs without obvious associated disease at a number of well-defined regional bone sites (see information box).

Clinical features

Bone pain present at rest and worse at night is typical but non-specific, and osteonecrosis can develop in the absence of symptoms.

Investigations

Plain radiographs may be normal at first but there is a typical sequence of radiographic changes as the disorder progresses (see information box). An isotope bone scan with ^{99}Tc diphosphonate will show increased uptake of the bone-seeking isotope and CT scans can show early sclerotic changes when plain radiographs are normal. MRI is however the imaging modality of choice and a high/low signal 'double line', which is pathognomonic of osteonecrosis, can be detected in about two-thirds of cases.

Management

Patients are usually advised to avoid weight bearing with the use of crutches in the early stages and pain relief with analgesics and non-steroidal analgesic anti-inflammatory drugs is frequently required. Nitrates and other peripheral dilators have been used widely for patients with sickle-cell crisis and the use of externally applied pulsed electromagnetic fields is currently being evaluated. Surgical approaches include bone decompression in the early stages and osteotomy to reduce mechanical stresses on affected bone segments but joint replacement is often required in patients with more advanced disease and secondary OA.

FURTHER READING

Coe F L, Favus M J 1992 Disorders of Bone and Mineral Metabolism. Raven Press, New York
Dempster D W, Lindsay R 1993 Pathogenesis of osteoporosis. Lancet 341: 797–801
Mundy G R, Martin T J (eds) 1993 Physiology and Pharmacology of Bone. Springer, Berlin
Riggs B. L, Melton G J 1992 The prevention and treatment of osteoporosis. New England Journal of Medicine 327: 620–627

DISORDERS ASSOCIATED WITH AVASCULAR NECROSIS OF BONE

- Fractures and trauma
- Radiotherapy
- Caisson disease
- Sickle-cell anaemia
- Gaucher's disease
- Chronic liver disease
- Alcoholism
- Pancreatitis
- Cushing's syndrome
- Corticosteroid therapy
- Organ transplantation
- Chronic renal dialysis
- Systemic lupus erythematosus
- Rheumatoid arthritis
- Other connective tissue disorders
- Diabetes mellitus
- Metastatic malignancies
- Pregnancy

REGIONAL TYPES OF OSTEONECROSIS

Disorder	Bone site	Age	Sex
Legg–Perthes' disease	Femoral head	5–12	M and F
Freiberg's disease	Metatarsal head	10–16	F
Kohler's disease	Tarsal navicular	5–10	M
Kienböck's disease	Lunate	Young adults	M and F
Osteonecrosis femoral condyle	Medial femoral condyle	Elderly	F > M

STAGES OF RADIOGRAPHIC PROGRESSION IN AVASCULAR NECROSIS OF THE HIP

I	Diffuse osteoporosis of femoral head
II	Cysts with sclerotic margin
III	Subchondral area of lucency ('crescent sign')
IV	Triangular area of bone sclerosis
V	Bone collapse, remodelling of femoral head and secondary OA

DISORDERS OF COLLAGEN AND PROTEOGLYCAN

OSTEOGENESIS IMPERFECTA

This is a collective name for a heterogeneous group of rare inherited disorders of Type I collagen characterised by brittle bones and abnormalities of the skin, tendons, teeth and sclerae. The current classification (Table 15.17) is based on clinical features and patterns of inheritance but research is revealing a wide range of molecular defects with mutations in the genes coding for the pro alpha 1 (1) and pro alpha 2 (1) collagen chains which do not allow easy prediction of the clinical phenotype.

Table 15.17 Osteogenesis imperfecta

| Type | Bone fragility | Clinical features | | | Inheritance |
		Blue sclerae	Dental defects	Deafness	
I	Mild, late fractures	Yes	Some	Some	Autosomal dominant
II	Extreme (lethal), perinatal fractures	Yes	Some	–	Sporadic new mutations
III	Severe fractures, deformity	Blue at birth Not adults	Some	Some	Autosomal recessive Sporadic new mutations
IV	Short stature, brittle bones	No	Some	Some	Autosomal dominant

MARFAN SYNDROME

This is another phenotypically heterogeneous dominantly inherited condition in which abnormalities of alpha 2 (1) collagen have been described. Skeletal disproportion (span greater than height) is associated with arachnodactyly, sternal depression, lens dislocation and a high arched palate. Cardiac complications can include mitral valve prolapse, aortic incompetence and dissection of the aorta.

EHLERS-DANLOS SYNDROME

This is the name given to a group of conditions in which genetically determined abnormalities of collagen are associated with skin laxity, hypermobility of joints and a range of more serious features including scoliosis, short stature, ocular fragility, skin bruising and visceral vascular catastrophes (Table 15.18). Biochemical defects include a deficiency of Type II collagen (ED Type III), lysyl oxidase deficiency (ED Type V), a defect in procollagen cleavage (ED Type VII), abnormal copper metabolism (ED Type IX) and a defect in fibronectin (ED Type X).

HOMOCYSTINURIA

This is an inborn error of methionine metabolism in which deficiency of the enzyme cystathionine synthetase is associated with mental retardation, venous thromboses, osteoporosis and skeletal features resembling the Marfan syndrome. The diagnosis is made by finding homocystine in the urine, and patients respond to treatment with pyridoxine (20–300 mg daily).

MUCOPOLYSACCHARIDOSES

These form a group of inborn errors of glycosaminoglycan metabolism in which lysosomal enzyme defects lead to abnormal substrate accumulation and a wide variety of clinical features (Table 15.19). All are associated with stiff joints and short stature except for the Morquio syndrome which is associated with hypermobility and atlantoaxial subluxation. The diagnoses are confirmed by identification of the urinary metabolites and detection of the enzyme defects in fibroblast cultures. Treatment by enzyme replacement therapy has had limited success in slowing progression in selected cases.

SKELETAL DYSPLASIAS (Table 15.20)

The skeletal dysplasias form a large and heterogeneous group of conditions which cause bone and joint deformity. Those with predominant epiphyseal involvement such as multiple epiphyseal dysplasia may be associated with premature osteoarthrosis. Those with predominant metaphyseal involvement such as achondroplasia are associated with short-limbed dwarfism. There are disorders such as osteogenesis imperfecta, idiopathic juvenile osteoporosis and hereditary osteolyses in which decreased bone density, fractures and bone loss are prominent features and others, such as osteopetrosis and sclerosteosis where increased bone density occurs.

Osteogenesis imperfecta is associated with a variety of mutations of the type I collagen gene which lead to defective collagen formation by osteoblasts. By contrast osteopetrosis is associated with excessive bone formation secondary to defective resorption of bone by osteoclasts, and some types can be successfully treated by marrow transplantation of normal osteoclasts in infancy. One type of osteopetrosis in man is associated with renal tubular acidosis and deficiency of carbonic anhydrase II while one type in mice results from a defect in the gene for macrophage colony-stimulating factor.

Skeletal abnormalities are prominent in a number of hereditary disorders of connective tissue such as the Marfan syndrome or neurofibromatosis as well as inborn errors of metabolism such as the mucolipidoses and

Table 15.18   Ehlers–Danlos syndromes

Type	Skeletal	Skin extensibility	Bruising	Other	Inheritance
		Clinical features			
I	Hypermobility Deformities	Gross	Marked	Pseudotumours	Autosomal dominant
II	Minimal	Mild	Mild	—	Autosomal dominant
III	Hypermobility	Mild	Mild	Dislocations, OA	Autosomal dominant
IV	Digital hypermobility	Thin skin	Gross	Vascular catastrophes	Autosomal dominant Autosomal recessive
V	Minimal	Mild	Mild	—	X-linked
VI	Hypermobility	Moderate	Moderate	Scoliosis, ocular fragility	Autosomal recessive
VII	Hypermobility	Moderate	Moderate	Short stature	Autosomal dominant Autosomal recessive
VIII	Hypermobility	Mild	Mild	Periodontitis	Autosomal dominant
IX	Hypermobility	Moderate	Moderate	Bowing long bones	X-linked
X	Hypermobility	Mild	Mild	—	X-linked Autosomal dominant

Table 15.19   The mucopolysaccharidoses

Type	Name	Clinical features	Inheritance	Urine MPS	Enzyme deficiency
MPS-I H	Hurler	Cloudy cornea Mental deficiency	Autosomal recessive	Dermatan/heparan sulphate	Alpha-L-iduronidase
MPS-I S	Schele	Cloudy cornea Stiff joints	Autosomal recessive	Dermatan/heparan sulphate	Alpha-L-iduronidase
MPS-I H/S	Hurler–Schele	Intermediate phenotype	Autosomal recessive	Dermatan/heparan sulphate	Alpha-L-iduronidase
MPS-II	Hunter	Stiff joints Mild general mental deficiency	X-linked	Dermatan/heparan sulphate	Iduronate sulphatase
MPS-III (a–d)	San Filippo (a–d)	Stiff joints CNS defects	Autosomal recessive	Heparan sulphate	a) Heparan N-sulphatase b) N-acetyl alpha D-glucosaminidase c) Acetyl-CoA alpha glucosaminidase N-acetyltransferase d) N-acetylglucosamine-6-sulphate sulphatase
MPS-IV	Morquio (a and b)	Cloudy cornea Aortic incompetence Hypermobile joints	Autosomal recessive	Keratan sulphate	a) Galactosamine-6-sulphate sulphatase b) Beta galactosidase
MPS-VI	Maroteaux–Lamy	Stiff joints Mild severe bone, cornea, heart valve changes	Autosomal recessive	Dermatan sulphate	Arylsulphatase Beta
MPS-VII	Sly	Mental retardation Dysostosis Hepatosplenomegaly	Autosomal recessive	Dermatan/heparan sulphate	Beta glucuronidase
MPS-VIII	DiFerrante	Short stature Dysostosis	Autosomal recessive	Keratan/heparan sulphate	Glucosamine-6-sulphate sulphatase

Table 15.20 Skeletal dysplasias

Epiphyseal	**Miscellaneous**
Multiple epiphyseal dysplasias	Neurofibromatosis
Chondrodysplasia punctata	Marfan syndrome
Dysplasia epiphysealis hemimelica	Cleido-cranio dysplasias
Hereditary arthro-ophthalmopathy	Nail-patella syndrome
Metaphyseal	**Increased bone density**
Achondroplasia	Osteopetrosis
Hypochondroplasia	Dysosteosclerosis
Lethal forms short limbed dwarfism	Pycnodysostosis
Chondroectodermal dysplasia	Sclerosteosis
Metaphyseal chondrodysplasias	Diaphyseal dysplasias
Hypophosphatasias	Pachydermperiostitis
Vertebral	**Anarchic bone**
Brachyolmia	Diaphyseal aclasis
	Ollier's disease
Vertebral and Epiphyseal	Maffucci's disease
Spondyloepiphyseal dysplasias	Melorheostosis
Vertebral and Metaphyseal	
Spondylometaphyseal dysplasia	
Vertebral, epiphyseal and metaphyseal	
Pseudochondroplasia	
Metatrophic dwarfism	
Kniest disease	
Diastrophic dwarfism	
Parastremmatic dwarfism	
Dygve–Melchior–Clauson disease	

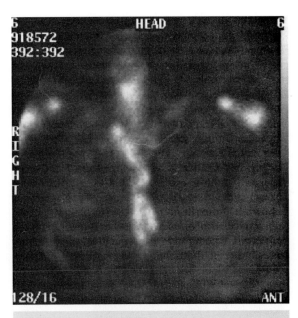

Fig. 15.44 Isotope bone scan showing increased local uptake at sites of bony metastases.

homocystinuria. The reader is referred to McKusick's book for details of all these groups of conditions.

FURTHER READING

Beighton P 1988 Inherited Disorders of the Skeleton, 2nd edn. Churchill Livingstone, Edinburgh
McKusick V A 1994 Mendelian Inheritance in Man, 10th edn. Johns Hopkins University Press, Baltimore

NEOPLASTIC DISEASES OF BONE

Malignant tumours of bone can cause diffuse skeletal aches and pains that are not infrequently dismissed as being 'rheumatic'.

Metastases

Most commonly these result from carcinoma of the bronchus, breast or prostate. Secondary deposits from most primary tumours appear typically as osteolytic on radiological examination and are frequently associated with a rise in serum alkaline phosphatase. Only prostatic metastases are commonly osteosclerotic and associated with a rise in serum acid phosphatase. Metastatic deposits can often be localised by skeletal isotope scans before radiological changes are apparent (Fig. 15.44) and widespread bone metastases can occur even in the absence of symptoms. A number of malignancies are hormone dependent, and useful remission can sometimes be obtained following hypophysectomy or administration of androgens to patients with metastatic breast cancer, or dienoestrol to those with prostatic metastases. Local radiotherapy and cytotoxic chemotherapy can occasionally be helpful in symptomatic management.

Multiple myeloma (pp. 821–822)

This disorder may also present with skeletal aches and pains associated with 'punched-out' osteolytic lesions on radiological examination. Unlike metastatic carcinoma these deposits usually fail to take up bone-seeking isotopes and the serum alkaline phosphatase is normal.

PRIMARY BONE TUMOURS

These are less common than secondary bone tumours. Ivory *osteomas* are benign tumours which occur most frequently in the vault of the skull and are not usually associated with symptoms. Cancellous osteomas (osteochondromas or exostoses) are slender out-growths of bone which arise from the metaphyses of long bones or from flat bones of the pelvis and scapulae. They may give rise to pressure symptoms and most frequently present during adolescence. Diaphyseal aclasis (multiple exostosis) is a rarer disorder inherited as an autosomal dominant and seen in younger children.

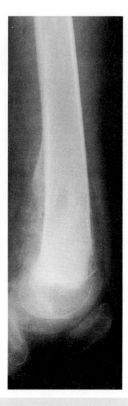

Fig. 15.45   Osteosarcoma of lower end of femur. Radiograph showing triangular area of new bone formation at periosteal margin.

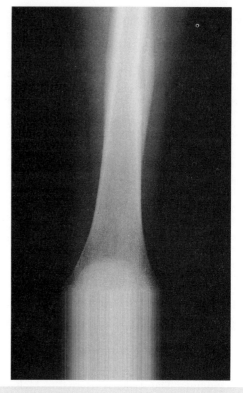

Fig. 15.46   Ewing's tumour of femur. Radiograph showing typical appearance with periosteal new bone formation.

PRIMARY OSTEOSARCOMAS

Occurring most frequently in the lower end of the femur, the upper end of the tibia and the upper end of the humerus, these are tumours of young people rarely seen after the age of 20. Swelling with or without vague aching is the presenting symptom and the bone may be tender and warm. Radiographs show a characteristic increase in radiolucency associated with bone expansion, triangular areas of new bone formation at the periosteal margin and a 'sun-ray' appearance due to new bone formation (Fig. 15.45). Early blood-borne metastases to the lungs are common and the 5-year survival is less than 10% despite treatment with radiotherapy and amputation.

FIBROSARCOMAS

Fibrosarcomas are of two types. Endosteal fibro-sarcomas arise within bones and give rise to destructive lesions as they grow out. They metastasise to both the local lymph nodes and the lungs and are associated with a poor prognosis despite treatment with radiotherapy or amputation. In contrast periosteal fibrosarcomas seldom

invade bone or metastasise to distant sites. Treatment is by local excision, repeated in the event of recurrence.

BENIGN OSTEOCHONDROMAS

These arise from cartilage within the long bones or small bones of the fingers. Multiple enchondromatosis is an unusual disorder of childhood in which multiple chondromas give rise to unsightly swellings attached to bones. Malignant change is very rare in chondromas.

CHONDROSARCOMAS

These occur in the long bones, pelvis or scapulae of adults. Pain and swelling are the presenting features and bone radiographs show only loss of bone density associated with some speckled calcification. Amputation is the treatment of choice and the 5-year survival is better than 50%.

EWING'S TUMOUR

A highly malignant bone neoplasm which affects children between the ages of 5 and 15, Ewing's tumour probably arises from the marrow endothelium and has characteristic radiographic features. Areas of osteolytic bone destruction are surrounded by layers of periosteal new bone formation giving lesions an 'onion skin' appearance (Fig. 15.46). Pain, swelling and tenderness may be associated with fever and leucocytosis so that these tumours can easily be mistaken for osteomyelitis. The 5-year survival is virtually nil despite radiotherapy and amputation.

GIANT CELL TUMOURS OF BONE

These may be benign or malignant. They usually occur in young adults and present with pain and swelling of a long bone in the neighbourhood of a joint. Radiographs show a typically eccentric tumour with a 'soap bubble' appearance. With local excision the prognosis is relatively good even for malignant tumours.

OSTEOID OSTEOMA

A rare cause of severe bone pain which is characteristically worse at night and relieved by NSAIDs, osteoid osteoma occurs between the ages of 10 and 30 in any bone except the skull. There may be warmth, swelling and tenderness on palpation and radiographs show some increase in sclerosis with a characteristic area of translucency surrounding a central nidus. Excision of the nidus cures the symptoms and these lesions do not recur.

Diseases of the skin

Large community studies in the UK and USA have revealed that between 20 and 30% of the population has a skin disease requiring attention, but only one in five of these will seek medical help. In spite of this some 10% of those who go to their family doctors do so with skin problems; self medication is much more common than treatment prescribed by doctors.

Skin diseases can harm affected individuals in a number of ways as shown in the information box below.

THE FOUR Ds

- **Discomfort**
  Most often itching or pain (e.g. eczema, post-herpetic neuralgia)
- **Disfigurement**
  Leading to embarrassment and withdrawal from society (e.g. birth marks, acne vulgaris and psoriasis)
- **Disability**
  Leading to loss of work and wages (e.g. dermatitis of the hands and feet)
- **Death**
  Rare but still seen (e.g. angioedema, metastatic skin cancer and widespread blistering)

Although there are reputed to be over 2000 skin conditions, this chapter covers only those which are commonly seen in general practice and the general medical clinic, some which are unusual but have distinctive clinical features, and those which are skin markers of systemic disease. Infections and infestations of the skin are dealt with in Chapter 4 and connective tissue disorders, which often involve the skin, are described in Chapter 15.

Every clinician has ample opportunity to look at the skin, when listening to or examining a patient. This chapter will explain the significance of what he or she sees; there is no branch of medicine more dependent on clinical acumen and experience and less dependent on the laboratory.

NORMAL STRUCTURE AND FUNCTION OF THE SKIN

The skin of an adult weighs an average of 4 kg and covers an area of 2 m^2. It has three layers: the outer **epidermis**, an avascular epithelium, which is firmly attached to, and supported by, connective tissue in the underlying **dermis**; beneath the dermis a layer of loose connective tissue, the **hypodermis**, which often contains abundant fat (Fig. 16.1).

Keratinocytes make up about 90% of the epidermal cells, their main function being to synthesise insoluble proteins, keratins. Keratinocytes are generated by division of cells in the basal layers of the epidermis and move outwards, die in the granular layer and become the flattened dead cells in the most superficial horny layer, finally being shed at the surface. In normal skin this process takes about 4 weeks but in some conditions (e.g. psoriasis) it is greatly accelerated.

Two types of dendritic cell make up the remaining 10% of the epidermal cells.

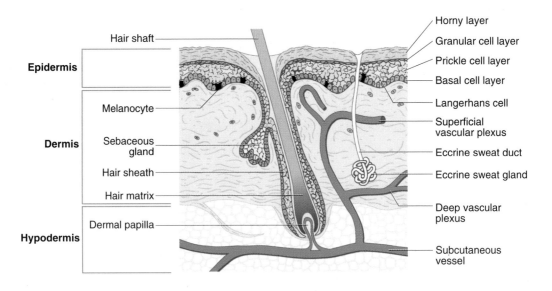

Epidermis
- Hair shaft
- Horny layer
- Granular cell layer
- Prickle cell layer
- Basal cell layer
- Langerhans cell

Dermis
- Melanocyte
- Sebaceous gland
- Hair sheath
- Hair matrix
- Superficial vascular plexus
- Eccrine sweat duct
- Eccrine sweat gland

Hypodermis
- Dermal papilla
- Deep vascular plexus
- Subcutaneous vessel

Fig. 16.1 Structure of normal hairy skin.

Table 16.1 Functions of the skin

Function	Structure/cell involved
Protection against	
Chemicals, particles	Horny layer
Ultraviolet radiation	Melanocytes
Antigens, haptens	Langerhans cells, lymphocytes, mononuclear phagocytes, mast cells
Microbes	Horny layer, Langerhans cells, mononuclear phagocytes, mast cells
Preservation of a balanced internal environment	Horny layer
Prevents loss of water, electrolytes and macromolecules	
Shock absorber	Dermis and subcutaneous fat
Strong, yet elastic and compliant covering	
Sensation	Specialist nerve endings
Calorie reserve	Subcutaneous fat
Vitamin D synthesis	Keratinocytes
Temperature regulation	Blood vessels, eccrine sweat glands
Lubrication and waterproofing	Sebaceous glands
Protection and prising	Nails
Body odour (more important in animals)	Apocrine sweat glands
Psycho-social	Hair, nails

- **Langerhans cells** are modified macrophages that circulate between the epidermis and the local lymph nodes. Their prime function is presentation of antigen to T lymphocytes in, for example, an allergic contact dermatitis reaction. The Langerhans cell may also play a part in immunosurveillance of viral and tumour antigens.
- **Melanocytes** are found mainly in the basal layer; they are the only epidermal cells capable of synthesising melanin, which they transfer to surrounding keratinocytes.

The dermis is vascular and supports the epidermis structurally and nutritionally. It is separated from the epidermis by a basement membrane zone and has three components: cells (many fibroblasts and a few mononuclear phagocytes, lymphocytes, Langerhans cells and mast cells), fibres (collagen, reticulin and elastin) and an amorphous ground substance (mostly the glycosaminoglycans, hyaluronic acid and dermatan sulphate). The dermis also supports hair, sweat and sebaceous glands, cutaneous muscles and nerves, and blood and lymphatic vessels.

The functions of the skin are summarised in Table 16.1.

DIAGNOSIS OF SKIN DISORDERS

The key to successful treatment is accurate diagnosis. This requires a careful history, thorough examination of the skin, hair and nails and the judicious use of the laboratory. Often it is best to have a quick look at the skin before obtaining a full history as this should prompt the right questions.

History

The principles of a general medical history should be followed with emphasis on the events surrounding the onset of the skin lesions and on the progression of the disease. A careful inquiry into drugs, a past or family history of skin disorders and details of the occupation and any hobbies are important. The more difficult the diagnosis—the more important the history.

Examination

To examine the skin properly the lighting must be uniform and bright, the patient undressed (if necessary) and make-up and dressings removed. The signs to note are shown in the information box.

SIGNS OF RASH TO NOTE

- **Distribution**. Is it symmetrical or asymmetrical? Is it dermatomal? Are any areas spared?
- **Morphology of individual lesions**. Appreciation of the definitions in Table 16.2 will save much time in describing lesions. The colour, surface contour, geometric shape, texture, temperature and even smell of lesions often warrant further description
- **Configuration of lesions**. Are the lesions discrete, confluent, grouped, circinate or linear?

A **magnifying lens** is essential; rashes and lesions cannot often be diagnosed at arm's length. A lens or

Table 16.2 Terms used to describe skin lesions

PRIMARY LESIONS		SECONDARY LESIONS (which evolve from primary lesions)	
Macule	Small flat area of altered colour or texture	Scale	A flake arising from the horny layer
Papule	Small solid elevation of skin, less than 0.5 cm in diameter	Crust	Looks like a scale, but is composed of dried blood or tissue fluid
Nodule	A solid mass in the skin, usually greater than 0.5 cm in diameter	Ulcer	An area of skin from which the whole of the epidermis and at least the upper part of the dermis has been lost
Plaque	Elevated area of skin greater than 2 cm in diameter but without substantial depth	Excoriation	An ulcer or erosion produced by scratching
Vesicle	Circumscribed elevation of skin, less than 0.5 cm in diameter, and containing fluid	Erosion	An area of skin denuded by a complete or partial loss of the epidermis
Bulla	Circumscribed elevation of skin over 0.5 cm in diameter and containing fluid	Fissure	A slit in the skin
Pustule	A visible accumulation of pus in the skin	Sinus	A cavity or channel that permits the escape of pus or fluid
Abscess	A localised collection of pus in a cavity, more than 1 cm in diameter	Scar	The result of healing, in which normal structures are permanently replaced by fibrous tissue
Wheal	An elevated white compressible, evanescent area produced by dermal oedema	Atrophy	Thinning of skin due to diminution of the epidermis, dermis, subcutaneous fat
Papilloma	A nipple-like mass projecting from the skin	Stria	A streak-like, linear, atrophic, pink, purple or white lesion of the skin due to changes in the connective tissue
Petechiae	Pinhead-sized macules of blood in the skin		
Purpura	A larger macule or papule of blood in the skin		
Ecchymosis	A larger extravasation of blood into the skin		
Haematoma	A swelling from gross bleeding		
Burrow	A linear or curvilinear papule, caused by a burrowing scabies mite		
Comedo	A plug of keratin and sebum wedged in a dilated pilosebaceous orifice		
Telangiectasia	The visible dilation of small cutaneous blood vessels		

glass slide can also be pressed on lesions to determine if they are vascular and to unmask their true colour.

The terminology commonly used in skin diseases is given in Table 16.2.

Investigation

Biopsy

This is performed, either with a special 'punch' biopsy instrument or a scalpel. Select an early and typical lesion, if possible one on a non-exposed site and where minimal scarring may be anticipated (avoid the upper back, shoulder tips and presternal area, where keloids commonly develop, and the lower legs of obese women). Use 1% xylocaine for local anaesthesia. Remove the specimen, avoiding crushing, and place in formol-saline. The wound is sutured; firm compression for a few minutes stops oozing. Fine sutures are used on the face. Stitches on the head are usually removed in 4–5 days, from the anterior trunk and arms in 7 days and from the back and legs in 10 days.

THE ECZEMAS

The terms eczema and dermatitis are now used synonymously. They refer to a distinctive reaction pattern of the skin showing a combination of signs which depends on the duration of the rash and the type of eczema.

Clinical features common to all eczemas

The reaction is similar in all types but varies according to the duration of the rash. The signs of acute eczema and chronic eczema are listed in the information box below.

Pathology

In the acute stage oedema of the epidermis (spongiosis) progresses to the formation of intra-epidermal vesicles, which may enlarge and rupture. In the chronic stage there is less oedema and vesication but more thickening

ACUTE ECZEMA

- Redness and swelling, usually with ill-defined margin
- Papules, vesicles and more rarely large blisters
- Exudation and cracking
- Scaling

CHRONIC ECZEMA

- May show all of the above features, though it is usually less vesicular and exudative
- Thickening. Lichenification, a dry leathery thickening with increased skin markings, is secondary to rubbing and scratching and is most often seen in atopic eczema
- Fissures and scratch marks
- Pigmentation

Table 16.3 Some common allergens

Allergen	Present in
Nickel	Jewellery, jean studs, bra clips
Dichromate	Cement, leather, matches
Rubber chemicals	Clothing, shoes, tyres
Colophony	Sticking plaster, collodion
Paraphenylenediamine	Hair dye, clothing
Balsam of Peru	Perfumes, citrus fruits
Neomycin benzocaine	Topical applications
Parabens	Preservative in cosmetics and creams
Wool alcohols	Lanolin, cosmetics, creams
Epoxy resin	Resin adhesives

of the epidermis (acanthosis); this is accompanied by a variable degree of vasodilation and T helper lymphocytic infiltration in the upper dermis.

Classification

There are two groups of eczema: exogenous (or contact) and endogenous (or constitutional). While overlap between the two groups is common, distinction between them is critical for treatment because avoidance of incriminating contactants takes precedence over other measures in the management of contact eczema. The information box following shows the basic classification.

CLASSIFICATION OF THE ECZEMAS

- **Exogenous**
  Irritant
  Allergic
- **Endogenous**
  Atopic
  Seborrhoeic
  Discoid
  Asteatotic
  Gravitational
  Neurodermatitis
  Pompholyx

EXOGENOUS ECZEMAS

IRRITANT CONTACT ECZEMA

Detergents, alkalis, acids, solvents and abrasive dusts are common causes. There is a wide range of susceptibility to weak irritants. Irritant contact eczema accounts for the majority of industrial cases and work

loss. The elderly, those with fair and dry skin and those with an atopic background (personal or family history of asthma, hay fever or eczema) are especially vulnerable. Napkin eczema in babies is common and due to irritant ammoniacal urine and faeces.

Strong irritants elicit an acute reaction at the site of contact whereas weak irritants most often cause chronic eczema, especially of the hands, after prolonged exposure.

ALLERGIC CONTACT ECZEMA

This is due to a delayed hypersensitivity reaction (p. 44) following contact with antigens or haptens. Previous exposure to the allergen is required for sensitisation and the reaction is specific to the allergen or closely related chemicals. Common allergens and their origin are listed in Table 16.3.

The eczema reaction occurs wherever the allergen contacts the skin and sensitisation persists indefinitely. It is important to determine the original site of the rash before secondary spread obscures the picture, as this often provides the best clue to the contactant. There are many easily recognisable patterns, e.g. eczema of the earlobes, wrists and back due to contact with nickel in costume jewellery, watches and bra clips; eczema of the hands and wrists due to rubber gloves. Oedema of the lax skin of the eyelids and genitalia is a frequent concomitant of allergic contact eczema (Fig. 16.2).

ENDOGENOUS ECZEMAS

ATOPIC ECZEMA

Atopy is a genetic predisposition to form excessive IgE antibodies to inhaled, injected and ingested antigens and

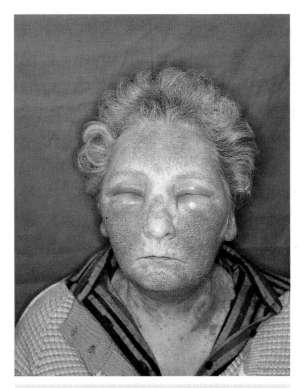

Fig. 16.2 Allergic contact eczema. This was caused by the application of an antihistamine cream. The acute eczematous reaction and bilateral periorbital oedema are typical.

ATOPIC ECZEMA: DISTRIBUTION AND CHARACTER OF RASH

- **Infancy**—the eczema is often acute and involves the face and trunk. The napkin area is frequently spared
- **Childhood**—the rash settles on the backs of the knees, fronts of the elbows, wrists and ankles (Fig. 16.3)
- **Adults**—the face and trunk are once more involved, lichenification is common

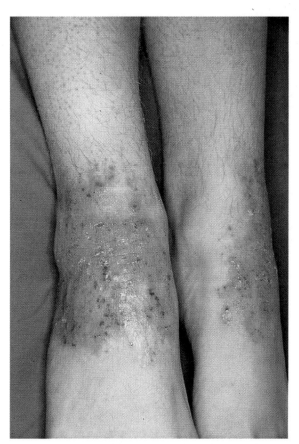

Fig. 16.3 Subacute eczema on the fronts of the ankles of a teenager: sites of predilection, along with the cubital and popliteal fossae, in atopic eczema.

to develop one or more of a group of diseases which include asthma, hay fever, urticaria, food and other allergies and this distinctive form of eczema. About 15% of the population have at least one atopic manifestation.

The inheritance of atopic eczema is controversial. The disorder is concordant in 86% of monozygotic twins but only in 21% of dizygotic ones. Atopic diseases are inherited more often from the mother than from the father and eczema, asthma and hay fever tend to run true to type within each family. Autosomal dominant, recessive and polygenic modes of inheritance have been suggested by different workers. Recently it has been proposed that a gene on chromosome 11q 13 is important in atopy. Interestingly, this site coincides with the β subunit gene of the high affinity IgE receptor found on mast cells and Langerhans cells.

The cardinal feature of atopic eczema is itch, and scratching may account for most of the signs. Atopic eczema usually begins before the age of 6 months but, paradoxically, seldom presents during the neonatal period. The rash remits spontaneously in at least two-thirds of children before the age of 10. The distribution and character of the rash vary with age as shown in the information box and in Fig. 16.3.

SEBORRHOEIC ECZEMA

The name is a poor one because the condition is unrelated to seborrhoea but it is used so often that it cannot be discarded. Its cause remains unknown though the yeast-like fungus, *Pityrosporum orbiculare*, appears to be a perpetuating factor. The condition often runs in families but the precise mode of inheritance is unclear.

The three common patterns involving seborrhoeic

eczema are shown in the information box below. This type of eczema is associated with a tendency to dandruff.

PATTERNS OF SEBORRHOEIC ECZEMA

- Scalp, ears, face and eyebrows
- Presternal and interscapular skin
- Flexures of axillae, umbilicus, breasts and groin

ASTEATOTIC ECZEMA

This is frequently seen in the hospitalised elderly, especially when the skin is dry; low humidity caused by central heating, overwashing and diuretics are contributory factors. It occurs most often on the lower legs as a rippled or 'crazy paving' pattern of fine fissuring on an erythematous background.

GRAVITATIONAL (STASIS) ECZEMA

This occurs on the lower legs and is often associated with signs of venous insufficiency (oedema, red or bluish discolouration, loss of hair, induration, haemosiderin pigmentation and ulceration).

POMPHOLYX (DYSHIDROTIC ECZEMA)

Pompholyx, sometimes provoked by heat or emotional upset, may occur in nickel-sensitive patients after they ingest small amounts of nickel in food. Bouts of recurrent vesicles or bullae affect the palms, fingers and soles.

DISCOID ECZEMA

This common form of eczema is seen most often on the limbs of elderly males. The lesions are more discrete than those of other types of eczema and are usually multiple, coin-shaped, vesicular and crusted.

Complications of eczema

These are listed in the information box below.

Investigation of eczema

Patch testing to allergens

This is used in suspected cases of allergic contact eczema. Patch testing to irritants (which cause reactions in everybody) is not advised.

Standard dilutions of the test substance are applied to the back under aluminium discs and the patches secured in place for 48 hours. The sites are inspected for eczema-

---

COMPLICATIONS OF ECZEMA

- **Superinfection**—most often with bacteria (*Staph. aureus*) but also with yeasts (*Candida albicans*) and viruses (atopic eczema patients are especially prone to papilloma virus, herpes simplex and molluscum contagiosum infections). Superinfection is encouraged by the use of local steroids
- **Reaction to local medicaments**
- **Psychological factors**—anxiety states are common and compensation neuroses may dominate the picture in cases of industrial dermatitis

---

tous reactions 1 hour after removal and after a further 48 hours.

Prick testing

This is used for a few patients with stubborn atopic eczema if food or inhalant allergens are suspected as exacerbating factors. It detects immediate (IgE-mediated) hypersensitivity. Commercially prepared dilute antigens and a control are placed as single drops on the volar aspect of the forearm. The skin is pricked through the drop (using a fresh sterile needle for each test and without drawing blood) and the drop removed with a tissue. After 10 minutes the sites are inspected for wheal and flare reactions and positive responses measured. The radio allergosorbent test (RAST) is a blood test which measures IgE antibodies against specific ingestant and inhalant antigens; although more expensive than prick testing it has largely replaced this technique because of safety and convenience.

Both patch and prick testing should be carried out only by trained personnel.

Culture

This is for bacterial yeast and fungal pathogens where superinfection is suspected.

General management of eczema

The main points are listed in the information box below.

GENERAL MANAGEMENT FOR ALL TYPES OF ECZEMA

- Explanation, reassurance and encouragement
- Avoidance of contact with irritants
- Careful use of topical steroids

Lotions and creams are preferable in acute eczema and ointments in chronic cases; they are usually applied twice daily. Only 1% hydrocortisone should be used on the face and in infancy. Even in adults it is seldom necessary to prescribe more than 200 g of a low potency steroid (e.g. 1% hydrocortisone), 50 g of a moderately potent steroid (e.g. 0.05% clobetasone butyrate) or 30 g of a potent steroid (e.g. 0.1% betamethasone valerate) per week. Very potent topical steroids (e.g. 0.05% clobetasol proprionate) should not be used long-term. The side-effects of strong or extensive local steroid therapy should always be borne in mind when patients are applying these preparations for years on end. They include skin thinning (with striae, fragility and purpura), enhanced or disguised infections and systemic absorption (causing suppression of the pituitary-adrenal axis and even Cushingoid features).

Bland emollients (e.g. emulsifying ointment) are used regularly either directly on the skin or in the bath. They not only prevent excessive water loss from an already dry skin, but also help to reduce the amount of local steroid used. Emollient soap substitutes (e.g. aqueous cream) are also helpful. Sedative antihistamines (e.g. trimeprazine tartrate) are of value if sleep is interrupted.

Specific measures (for certain types of eczema) additional to general treatment

Irritant contact eczema

This is treated by using protective clothing, especially gloves, and barrier creams which allow the skin to be cleaned easily.

Allergic contact eczema

As for irritant contact eczema but a change of job is often unavoidable.

Atopic eczema

Some advise that cow's milk and eggs should be avoided for the first 6 months of life by children with atopic parents. After this the role of diet is debatable. Similarly, the place for gamma-linolenic acid as a dietary supplement remains controversial. Routine inoculations are allowed during quiescent phases of eczema though children who are allergic to eggs should not be inoculated against measles, influenza and yellow fever. Systemic antibiotic treatment (e.g. erythromycin or flucloxacillin) is indicated for treating bacterial superinfection which is usually due to *Staphylococcus aureus*.

Seborrhoeic eczema

Local antiseptic, steroid and antifungal steroid (e.g. vioform-hydrocortisone and miconazole nitrate-hydrocortisone) are often helpful.

Gravitational eczema

Local steroids (see above) should be applied only to eczematous areas and not to ulcers. Neomycin should be avoided as sensitisation is common in this setting.

Treatment of this type of eczema should also include the elimination of oedema by leg elevation and graded compression bandages.

FURTHER READING

Bos J D, Kapsenberg M L, Sillevis Smitt J H 1994 Pathogenesis of atopic eczema. Lancet 343: 1338–1341
Cronin E 1992 Final diagnoses in patients referred for patch testing. Contact Dermatitis 27: 77–83
Hunter J A A, Herd R M 1994 Recent advances in atopic dermatitis. Quarterly Journal of Medicine 87: 323–327

ERYTHEMATOUS SCALY ERUPTIONS

PSORIASIS

Psoriasis is a non-infectious, inflammatory disease of the skin, characterised by well-defined erythematous plaques with large, adherent, silvery scales.

The main abnormality in psoriasis is increased epidermal proliferation due to excessive division of cells in the basal layers and a shorter cell cycle time. The transit time of keratinocytes through the epidermis is shortened and the epidermal turnover time falls from 28 to 5 or 6 days.

1–3% of most populations has psoriasis. It is commonest in Europe and North America. It may start at any age but is rare under 10 years and often seen between 15 and 40 years. The course of disease is unpredictable but is usually chronic with exacerbations and remissions.

Aetiology

Basic defect

This remains unknown but the following factors are involved:

- **Genetic.** There is frequently a genetic predisposition. A child with one affected parent has a 15% chance of developing the disease and this rises to 50% if both parents are affected. If non-psoriatic parents have a child with psoriasis the risk for subsequent children is about 10%. Psoriasis is probably heterogeneous but some have considered inheritance to be polygenic and others autosomal dominant with incomplete penetrance. Recently family studies in the USA have identified a susceptibility gene at the distal end of chromosome 17q, though this marker appears to be independent of HLA CW6 and those antigens of the major histocompatibility complex linked with CW6 with which psoriasis is strongly associated.
- **Biochemical.** It is not known if biochemical abnormalities are the cause or result of increased epidermal

proliferation. There are increased levels of prosta-glandins, leukotrienes and hydroxyeicosatetraenoic (HETE) acids in the epidermis. These may cause both the increased cellular proliferation seen in psoriasis and the inflammatory changes. Increased activity of phospholipase A$_2$ appears to be primarily responsible for these changes.

Decreased cAMP and increased cGMP are found in lesions, and beta-adrenoceptor antagonist drugs may exacerbate psoriasis by inhibiting cAMP formation. Polyamines are elevated in lesional skin, due to increased activity of ornithine decarboxylase, and may be intimately associated with cellular proliferation. Plasminogen activator is greatly increased in the lesions of psoriasis and its level parallels the epidermal mitotic rate.

Finally, the level of calmodulin, a calcium binding protein, is greatly raised in lesions and falls with successful treatment. The calcium–calmodulin complex may regulate epidermal cell proliferation by influencing phospholipase A$_2$ and cAMP phosphodiesterase (catalyses cAMP conversion to AMP) activity.

- **Immunopathological.** The inflammatory reaction may be part of an immunological response to as yet unknown antigens. Immune complexes to epidermal antigens have been detected in damaged skin and may activate complement, thereby attracting neutrophils to the area. Certain interleukins (IL-1, IL-2, IL-6 and IL-8) and growth factors (TNFα and TGFα) are elevated, and adhesion molecules are expressed or upregulated in lesions of psoriasis. The dermal mononuclear infiltrate is mainly of T lymphocytes, most of which are of the helper type. The beneficial effect of cyclosporin A in psoriasis may be due to its anti-T helper cell effect.
- **Dermal.** There is substantial evidence to suggest that the increased epidermal cell proliferation of psoriasis is related to the increased replication and metabolism of dermal fibroblasts. Both dermal and epidermal abnormalities appear to be necessary for the sustenance of psoriasis.

Given the basic defect, an individual may not inevitably develop psoriasis but certain precipitating factors make this more likely.

Precipitating factors
Although there appears to be no obvious precipitating factor in about 70% of exacerbations of psoriasis the factors shown in the information box (right) are responsible for the minority of flare-ups.

FACTORS CAUSING FLARE-UPS OF PSORIASIS

- **Trauma**
When the condition is erupting lesions appear in areas of skin damage such as scratches or surgical wounds (Köbner phenomenon)
- **Infection**
Beta-haemolytic streptococcal throat infections often precede guttate psoriasis
- **Sunlight**
Rarely, ultraviolet radiation may worsen psoriasis.
- **Drugs**
Antimalarials, beta-adrenoceptor antagonists and lithium may worsen psoriasis and the rash may 'rebound' after stopping systemic corticosteroids or potent local corticosteroids
- **Emotion**
Anxiety precipitates some exacerbations

Pathology
The histology of psoriasis is depicted in Figure 16.4.

Clinical features

Stable plaque psoriasis
This is the most common type. Individual lesions are well demarcated and range from a few millimetres to several centimetres in diameter (Fig. 16.5). The lesions are red with dry, silvery-white scaling, which may be obvious only after scraping the surface. The elbows, knees and lower back are commonly involved.

Other sites of predilection include:

- **Scalp.** This site is often involved, presumably due to repeated trauma from brushing and combing. Areas of marked scaling are interspersed with normal skin producing a lumpiness which is more easily felt than seen. Significant hair loss occurs only if there is gross involvement.
- **Nails.** Involvement of the nails is common with 'thimble pitting', onycholysis (separation of the nail from the nail bed) (Fig. 16.6) and subungual hyperkeratosis. It often reflects the severity of the psoriasis elsewhere.
- **Flexures.** Psoriasis involving the natal cleft, submammary and axillary folds is not scaly but red, glistening and symmetrical (Fig. 16.7).
- **Palms.** Psoriasis here is often difficult to recognise, as individual plaques may be poorly demarcated and barely erythematous.
- **Napkin area.** This may give the first hint of a psoriatic tendency in an infant.

Guttate psoriasis
This is usually seen in children and adolescents and may be the first sign of psoriasis. The rash often appears

Normal　　　　　**Psoriasis**

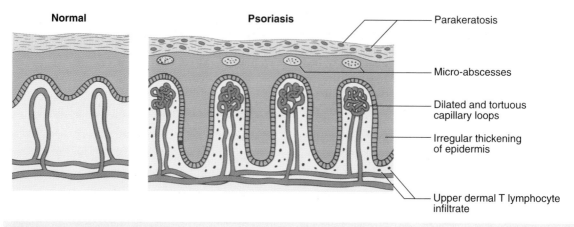

- Parakeratosis
- Micro-abscesses
- Dilated and tortuous capillary loops
- Irregular thickening of epidermis
- Upper dermal T lymphocyte infiltrate

Fig. 16.4　The histology of psoriasis.

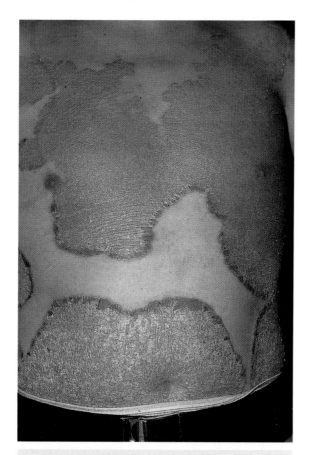

rapidly and individual lesions are droplet-shaped, small (seldom greater than 1 cm in diameter) and scaly. Bouts of guttate psoriasis usually clear in a few months, but patients may develop the plaque pattern later.

Erythrodermic psoriasis

The skin becomes universally red and scaly. Shivering compensates for the considerable heat loss. This unpleasant variant may be initiated by the irritant effect

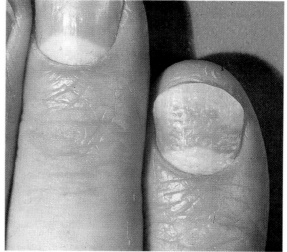

Fig. 16.5　Large sharply circumscribed plaques of psoriasis. The silvery scaling of the lower (untreated) plaque is typical.

Fig. 16.6　Coarse pitting of the nail and separation of the nail from the nail bed (onycholysis). These are both classic features of psoriasis.

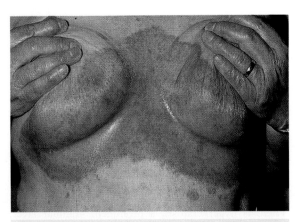

Fig. 16.7   Flexural psoriasis showing the glistening but not scaly rash.

of tar or dithranol or the withdrawal of systemic or potent topical corticosteroids.

Pustular psoriasis

The generalised form is a rare but serious type of psoriasis. The onset is sudden with myriads of small sterile pustules erupting on an erythematous base. The patient is ill with a swinging pyrexia, coinciding with the appearance of new pustules, and requires hospital admission. The localised form is more common. It most often involves the palms and soles. The eruption consists of numerous small sterile pustules lying on an erythematous base which leave brown macules or scaling in their wake. Some regard this as a separate disease entity.

Complications

Psoriatic arthropathy is a possible complication (see p. 903, Ch. 15), occurring in about 5% of psoriatics. Distal arthritis involves the terminal interphalangeal joints of the toes and fingers, especially those with marked nail changes. Other patterns include: involvement of a single large joint, a variety which mimics rheumatoid arthritis and which may be destructive; and one involving the sacro-iliac joints and lumbar spine (associated with HLA-B27). Tests for rheumatoid factor are usually negative in true psoriatic arthropathy and nodules are absent.

Investigations

Few are indicated. Biopsy is seldom necessary because the clinical picture is usually characteristic. Throat swabbing for beta-haemolytic streptococci should be performed in guttate psoriasis and an ASO titre may be helpful. Skin scrapings and nail clippings may have to

be examined to exclude tinea. Radiology and tests for rheumatoid factor are important in assessing arthritis.

Management

General measures

Explanation, reassurance and instruction are vital and must relate to the patient's or parent's intelligence. Both doctor and patient must keep the disease in perspective, so that treatment does not become more troublesome than the disease itself.

Physical and mental rest help to support the specific management of acute flare-ups of psoriasis. Concomitant depression and anxiety should be treated.

Local measures

- **Coal tar preparations.** Crude coal tar and its distillation products have been used to treat psoriasis for many years. Their main mode of action is probably by inhibiting DNA synthesis.

  Many products are available; in general the messier, less refined preparations (e.g. 10% strong coal tar solution and 4% tar paste) are more effective than the more refined and cleaner proprietary ointments. They are applied to the patches of psoriasis once or twice daily. Surprisingly, no increase in skin cancer has been found in patients treated for years with tar preparations. Salicylic acid (1–2%), sometimes added to tar preparations to remove scaling, is useful in the management of scalp psoriasis.

- **Dithranol.** This also inhibits DNA synthesis. Although it is irritant and more tricky to use than coal tar, its use has become widespread. The most popular regimen is short contact therapy in which the cream is applied to lesions for no longer than 30 minutes and then washed off. Initially 0.1% dithranol cream is used but, depending on the response, the strength may be increased stepwise to 2% over a few weeks. Dithranol stains normal skin purple-brown but the discolouration peels off after a few days.

  Eruptive and unstable patches of psoriasis are unsuitable for treatment with coal tar or dithranol and those with limited experience of their use should select test patches of psoriasis for initial treatment. Coal tar preparations and dithranol are best avoided on the face, genitalia and body folds because they are irritating.

- **Calcipotriol.** This recently introduced vitamin D analogue reduces epidermal proliferation and restores a normal horny layer. It is applied twice daily and, providing no more than 100 g is used each week, it does not cause hypercalcaemia and hypercalciuria. Patients like calcipotriol as it is odourless, colourless and does not stain. Irritation, which is usually transient, is the main side-effect.

- **Topical corticosteroids.** These are liked by patients and some doctors because they are clean and effective initially. However, there are few indications for their long-term use as, on their withdrawal, psoriasis may relapse rapidly or even change to an unstable phase which is more difficult to manage than previously. Their use should be limited as shown in the information box below.

LIMITATIONS ON USE OF TOPICAL CORTICOSTEROIDS FOR PSORIASIS

- The face, ears, genitalia and flexures where tar and dithranol are seldom tolerated
- Patients who cannot use tar or dithranol because of allergic or irritant reactions
- Unresponsive psoriasis of the scalp, palms and soles

Only mild steroids should be used on the face but moderately potent ones are suitable for elsewhere. Tar–steroid combinations are a useful stepping stone to pure tar preparations, while steroid–antifungal combinations are helpful for flexural psoriasis.

- **Ultraviolet radiation.** Most patients improve with natural sunlight and many clear their psoriasis by sunbathing during holiday periods. During the winter 6–8-week courses of medium-wave ultraviolet radiation (UVB) given in specialist centres 2–3 times weekly are often helpful. In the majority of patients sunbeds (emitting long-wave ultraviolet waves—UVA) are not beneficial. Combination therapies with UVB, coal tar preparations and dithranol are used to clear psoriasis more quickly than can be achieved by monotherapies.
- **Systemic treatment.** This will be considered by a dermatologist if extensive psoriasis fails to respond to the local measures outlined above. The most commonly used systemic treatments are photochemotherapy with PUVA (psoralen + UVA), retinoids (acitretin), methotrexate and cyclosporin A. All of these treatments have potential side-effects and patients receiving them require regular, specialist supervision.

LICHEN PLANUS

Lichen planus is a condition characterised by intensely itchy papules involving the flexor surfaces, genitalia and mucous membranes.

Aetiology

The cause is unknown but an immune pathogenesis is suspected as there is an association with some autoimmune diseases such as myasthenia gravis with thymoma and graft-versus-host disease. Rashes with clinical and histological features of lichen planus can occur in patients taking drugs, the most common culprits being gold and other heavy metals, sulphonamides, penicillamine, antimalarials, antituberculous drugs and thiazide diuretics. It also occurs in those handling colour developers.

Pathology

There is hyperkeratosis, a prominent granular layer, basal cell degeneration and a heavy T lymphocyte infiltration in the upper dermis. Degenerating basal cells may form 'colloid bodies'. The T cell–basal cell interaction leaves a 'sawtooth' dermoepidermal junction. The picture suggests an immune reaction to an unknown epidermal antigen.

Clinical features

Lichen planus tends to start on the distal limbs, most commonly the volar aspects of the wrists (Fig. 16.8), and the lower back. Intensely itchy flat-topped, pink-purplish papules appear and some develop a characteristic fine white network on their surface (Wickham's striae). New lesions may appear at the site of trauma (Köbner's phenomenon) and the rash may spread rapidly to become generalised. Individual lesions may last for many months and the eruption as a whole tends to last about one year, often leaving marked post-inflammatory pigmentation. Mucous membrane involvement, comprising an asymptomatic fine white lacy network or

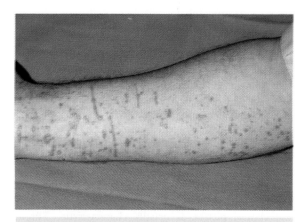

Fig. 16.8 Lichen planus. Glistening discrete papules involving the volar aspects of the forearm and wrist. Note the lesions along scratch marks (Köbner phenomenon).

pin-head sized white papules, occurs in about two-thirds of patients. The nails are usually normal but in 10% they may be affected with changes ranging from longitudinal grooving to destruction of the nail fold and bed. Variants of the classic picture are rare and often challenging diagnostically. They include annular, atrophic, bullous, follicular, hypertrophic and ulcerative types.

Diagnosis

This is usually clearcut clinically but a biopsy may be required. Other erythematous scaly conditions should be considered in the differential diagnosis, including: guttate psoriasis, pityriasis rosea, pityriasis lichenoides and drug eruptions.

Management

The condition is self-limiting. Moderately potent or potent local corticosteroids may be required for the intense itch. Systemic corticosteroid courses of up to three months may be required for acute widespread disease, ulcerative oral lesions and nail destruction. Acitretin, an oral retinoid, may help some patients with stubborn lichen planus.

PITYRIASIS ROSEA

This is a self-limiting condition of unknown cause. An infectious agent has been suspected but not proven; the disorder is not contagious.

Clinical features

Most patients develop a large, 2–5 cm in diameter plaque (the herald plaque) before the others. After several days many smaller, pink, oval and scaly plaques appear, mainly on the trunk but also on the neck and thighs. A delicate peripheral (collarette) scale appears as the lesions evolve. The lesions on the back are distributed parallel to the ribs giving a 'Christmas-tree' distribution. Purpuric lesions are rare. The eruption fades spontaneously in 4–10 weeks.

Diagnosis

This is made on clinical grounds. Disorders most likely to be confused include guttate psoriasis, pityriasis versicolor, tinea corporis and secondary syphilis. A drug eruption should also be excluded.

Management

Active treatment is seldom needed. A moderately potent topical corticosteroid may help the itching.

FURTHER READING

Barker J N W N 1991 The pathophysiology of psoriasis. Lancet 338: 227–230
Black M M, Newton J A 1986 Lichen planus. In: Thiers B G H, Dobson R C (eds) The Pathogenesis of Skin Disease. Churchill Livingstone, New York
Menter A, Barker J N W N 1991 Psoriasis in practice. Lancet 338: 231–234

DISORDERS OF THE PILOSEBACEOUS UNIT

ACNE VULGARIS

This disorder affects many teenagers. Its prevalence is similar in both sexes but the peak age of severity in females is 16–17 years and in males 17–19 years. Acne clears by the age of 23–25 years in 90% of patients but some 5% of women and 1% of men still need treatment in their thirties or even forties.

Aetiology

Many factors, rather than a single one, combine to cause chronic inflammation of blocked pilosebaceous follicles (Fig. 16.9).

Sebum secretion is increased, but this alone need not cause acne: for example, patients with acromegaly or Parkinson's disease have high sebum secretion rates but no acne. The sebum secretion rate may remain high after acne has healed.

Hormones are another factor and androgens from the testes, ovaries and adrenals are the main hormones which stimulate sebum secretion. In acne the sebaceous glands appear to be unduly sensitive to normal levels of these hormones.

Increased and abnormal keratinisation at the exit of the pilosebaceous follicle obstructs the flow of sebum. Bacteria play a pathogenic role. *Proprionobacterium acnes* is a normal skin commensal. It colonises the pilosebaceous ducts, breaks down triglycerides releasing free fatty acids, produces substances chemotactic for inflammatory cells and induces the ductal epithelium to secrete pro-inflammatory cytokines.

Acne is often familial. The inheritance pattern is probably polygenic.

Clinical features

Lesions are limited to the face, shoulders, upper chest and back. Seborrhoea (greasy skin) is often present. Open comedones (blackheads) due to plugging by keratin and sebum of the pilosebaceous orifice, or closed comedones (whiteheads) due to accretions of sebum and keratin deeper in the pilosebaceous ducts, are always

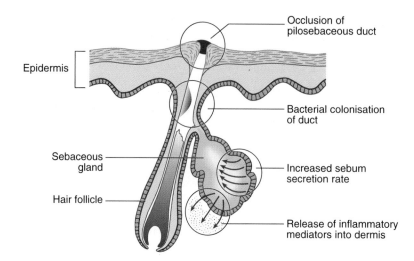

Occlusion of
pilosebaceous duct

Epidermis

Bacterial colonisation
of duct

Sebaceous
gland

Increased sebum
secretion rate

Hair follicle

Release of inflammatory
mediators into dermis

Fig. 16.9   The pathogenesis of acne.

evident. Inflammatory papules, nodules and cysts occur (Fig. 16.10A), with one or two types of lesion predominating. Scarring may follow.

There are less common variants of acne:

- Conglobate acne is severe with many abscesses and cysts, often connected by intercommunicating sinuses; scarring is severe.
- Acne fulminans is a type of conglobate acne accompanied by fever, joint pains and a high erythrocyte sedimentation rate.
- Excoriated acne manifests as discrete denuded areas caused by picking and is seen most often in early teenage girls.
- Infantile acne is rare and is due to transplacental stimulation of the infant's adrenals. It may last up to 3 years and may be the forerunner of severe acne in adolescence.
- Exogenous acne may be caused by tars, chlorinated hydrocarbons, oils and oily cosmetics; comedones dominate the clinical picture.
- Drug-induced acne may result from treatment with corticosteroids, androgenic steroids, lithium, oral contraceptives and anti-convulsant therapy.
- Acne associated with virilisation may be due to an androgen-secreting tumour of the adrenals, ovaries or testes.
- Non-classical late-onset congenital adrenal hyperplasia due to 21-hydroxylase deficiency may also present with severe cystic acne refractory to therapy with antibiotics or retinoic acid. The gene frequency for this condition is very high in Ashkenazi Jews (19%), inhabitants of former Yugoslavia (12%) and Italians (6%).

Investigations

None are usually necessary though swabs may be needed to exclude a pyogenic infection, anaerobic infection or

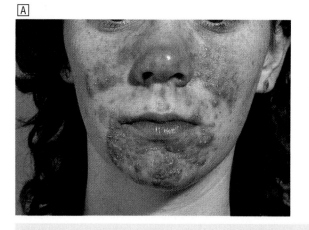

A

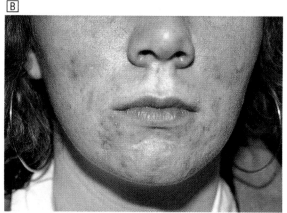

B

Fig. 16.10   Unpleasant cystic acne in a teenager, A before and B after prolonged systemic antibiotic treatment with minocycline.

Gram-negative folliculitis. Full endocrinological assessment is required for the investigation of acne associated with virilisation to exclude an androgen-secreting tumour or non-classical 21-hydroxylase deficiency (see p. 717, Ch. 12).

Management

Comedo-papular acne is managed by local treatment alone; pustular-cystic and scarring acne require local and systemic treatment.

Local measures

Regular washing with soap and water is essential. Antibacterial skin cleansers containing chlorhexidine such as Hibiscrub are also useful. Preparations containing benzoyl peroxide and retinoic acid are the cornerstone of local treatment and many proprietary products are available. They are irritant and drying and although some care is required to gauge an appropriate and regular regimen of application, most are applied once daily at night. Local clindamycin and erythromycin are helpful. The beneficial effect of ultraviolet B is usually short-lived.

Systemic measures

Antibiotics are used initially. They should not be used for less than 3 months and may even be necessary for 2 or 3 years. Oxytetracycline (up to 250 mg 6-hourly), minocycline (100 mg daily) and erythromycin (up to 250 mg 6-hourly) are suitable doses for adults with moderate acne, but larger doses may be required. Patients taking long-term antibiotics should be reviewed regularly for side-effects which fortunately are rare, though they include potentially dangerous benign intracranial hypertension (with tetracyclines).

Isotretinoin (13-cis-retinoic acid) is a very valuable addition to the list of drugs used for treating severe acne. It reduces sebum secretion dramatically and is given in a 4-month course. Although sebum secretion eventually rebounds to its former level after the drug is stopped, the acne does not usually recur. Minor side-effects, especially drying of the skin and mucous membranes, are common but well tolerated. Rarely, abnormalities of liver function occur and limit treatment. The main problem is that the drug is highly teratogenic and females requiring it must have a negative pregnancy test before treatment and take an oral contraceptive for at least a month before the course of isotretinoin, during the course and for 3 months after. Pregnancy tests at monthly reviews are also advisable.

Hormonal treatment in the form of a combined anti-androgen (cyproterone acetate)/oestrogen pill, taken in courses as an oral contraceptive, is available in many countries and may help women with persistent acne resistant to treatment with antibiotics. Monitoring is as for any female on an oral contraceptive.

Physical measures

Cysts can be incised and drained under local anaesthetic. Intralesional injections of triamcinolone acetonide (0.1–0.2 ml of a 10 mg/ml solution) hastens the resolution of stubborn cysts.

ROSACEA

Rosacea is a persistent facial eruption of unknown cause characterised by erythema and pustules. Sebum secretion is normal though sebaceous gland hyperplasia and associated inflammation is seen histologically.

Clinical features

The disorder is commonest in middle age. The cheeks, chin and central forehead are affected (Fig. 16.11). Intermittent blushing is followed by fixed erythema and telangiectasia. Dome-shaped papules and pustules but no comedones occur. Rhinophyma, with erythema, sebaceous gland hyperplasia and overgrowth of the soft tissues of the nose, is sometimes associated. Blepharitis and conjunctivitis are complications.

Diagnosis

This is often obvious on clinical grounds but acne, seborrhoeic eczema, photosensitivity and systemic lupus erythematosus must be distinguished.

Management

Mild cases may respond to local metronidazole gel. Usually an 8–10 week course of a tetracycline or erythromycin is required (dose as for acne) and repeat courses are often necessary. Plastic surgery may be required for rhinophyma.

FURTHER READING

Bork K 1993 Drug induced acne. Current Opinion in Dermatology 85–90

Cunliffe W 1989 Acne. Dunitz, London

Marks R 1992 Rosacea, flushing and perioral dermatitis. In: Champion R H, Burton J L, Ebling F J G (eds) Textbook of Dermatology, 5th edn., 1851–1863. Blackwell Scientific Publications, Oxford

---

SKIN ULCERATION DUE TO VASCULAR DISEASE

LEG ULCERS

Leg ulcers affect 1% of adults and are twice as common in women as in men. Approximately 50% are due to

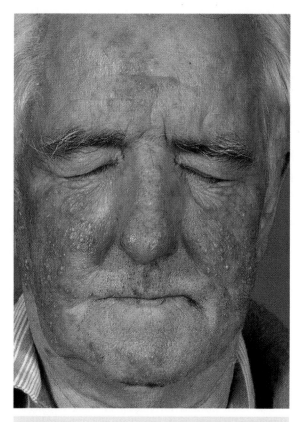

Fig. 16.11 Rosacea. The colour is distinctive and the papulo-pustular rash involves the cheeks, centre of forehead and chin.

Table 16.4 Main causes of leg ulceration	
Venous hypertension	(see text)
Arterial disease	Atherosclerosis
	Vasculitis
	Buerger's disease
Small vessel disease	Diabetes mellitus
	Vasculitis
Abnormalities of blood	Sickle cell disease
	Spherocytosis
	Cryoglobulinaemia
	Immune complex disease
Neuropathy	Diabetes mellitus
	Leprosy
	Syphilis
Tumour	Squamous cell carcinoma
	Basal cell carcinoma
	Malignant melanoma
	Kaposi's sarcoma
Trauma	Injury
	Artefact

venous disease, 10% arterial disease, 25% mixed venous/arterial disease and the remainder due to rare causes (Table 16.4).

LEG ULCERATION DUE TO VENOUS DISEASE

Damage to the venous system of the leg results in oedema, haemosiderin deposition, eczema, fibrosis and ulceration.

Aetiology

In the normal leg there is a superficial low-pressure venous system connected to the deep, high-pressure veins by perforating veins. Muscular activity, aided by valves in the veins, pumps blood from the superficial to the deep system and towards the heart. Incompetent valves in the deep and perforating veins result in the retrograde flow of blood to the superficial system ('venous hypertension') causing a rise in capillary hydrostatic pressure. Fibrinogen is forced out through the capillary walls and fibrin is deposited as a pericapillary cuff blocking the diffusion of oxygen and nutrients to

the skin. The skin ulcerates when a critical degree of hypoxia is reached.

Incompetent veins leading to venous hypertension may be due to deep vein thrombosis (p. 275), congenital or familial valve incompetence, infection or deep venous obstruction (e.g. from a pelvic tumour).

Clinical features

The problem usually starts in middle age. Leg ulcers are more likely to occur and to persist in obese people. Varicose veins, although often present, are not inevitable. The first symptom is frequently heaviness of the legs followed by the development of oedema. Haemosiderin pigmentation and ivory-coloured scarring may then be seen, sometimes associated with venous eczema (p. 947). The signs progress to lipodermatosclerosis, the firm induration, due to fibrosis of the dermis and subcutis, which may produce the well-known 'inverted champagne bottle' appearance. Ulceration, often precipitated by minor trauma or infection, soon occurs. Ulcers are seen typically around the medial malleolus but may encircle the ankle (Fig. 16.12). If conditions are favourable the ulcers will heal by granulation and small epithelial islands at the base and with epithelial growth from the edges. Healing is often slow and may never be complete. Recurrent ulceration is common even after good healing.

Complications

Chronic venous ulcers are invariably colonised by bacteria. Only if infection becomes overt, as suggested by an increase in the purulent discharge, increased pain, surrounding cellulitis or lymphangitis, is systemic antibiotic treatment required. Contact dermatitis to an oint-

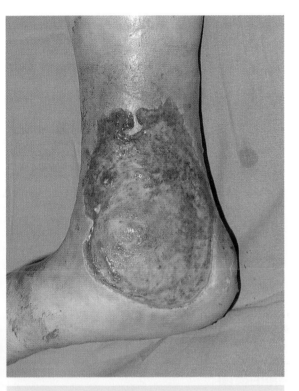

Fig. 16.12   A large venous ulcer overlying the medial malleolus.

ment, dressing or bandage is not uncommon. The usual culprits are preservatives, lanolin and neomycin. Lipo-dermatosclerosis may cause lymphoedema leading to hyperkeratosis and the so-called 'mossy foot'. A squamous cell carcinoma developing in a venous ulcer (Marjolin's ulcer) is rarely responsible for its failure to heal.

Diagnosis

Other causes of leg ulceration (Table 16.4) should be sought if the signs are atypical. All patients with chronic leg ulceration deserve a urine test to exclude diabetes, a full blood count to exclude anaemia and a Doppler ultrasound examination to assess the arterial circulation if the peripheral arterial pulses cannot easily be felt. Venography will help to detect surgically remediable causes of venous incompetence. Swabbing for bacterial pathogens is indicated in a long-standing ulcer especially if it is extending rapidly, painful, very purulent or complicated by the development of cellulitis, lymphangitis or septicaemia.

Management

- General management includes dietary advice for the obese and the encouragement of gentle exercise.

- Oedema should be reduced by the regular use of compression bandages, keeping the legs elevated when sitting and the judicious use of diuretics.
- The exudate and slough should be removed with normal saline solution or 0.5% aqueous silver nitrate or 5% aqueous hydrogen peroxide. If the ulcer is very purulent, soaking the leg for 15 minutes in 1:10 000 dilution of aqueous potassium permanganate may be helpful.
- Dressings commonly used for venous ulceration include antibiotic-impregnated tulle dressings, non-adhesive absorbent dressings (alginates, charcoals, hydrogels or hydrocolloids) and dry non-adherent dressings.
- The frequency of dressings depends on the state of the ulcer. Very purulent and exudative ulcers may need daily dressings whilst the dressing on a clean, healing ulcer may only require changing every week.
- Paste bandages, impregnated with zinc oxide or ich-thammol, help to keep dressings in place and provide protection.
- Surrounding venous eczema is treated by a mild or moderately potent topical corticosteroid. The corticosteroid should not be applied to the ulcer itself.
- Oral antibiotic therapy, given in short course, is only necessary for the treatment of overt infection (see above). An anabolic steroid, stanozolol, may help lipodermatosclerosis, but side-effects (fluid retention, hepatotoxicity) may limit its use.
- Surgery. Vein surgery may help some younger patients with persistent venous ulcers. Pinch grafts may hasten the healing of clean ulcers but do not influence their rate of recurrence.

LEG ULCERATION DUE TO ARTERIAL DISEASE

Deep, painful and punched-out ulcers on the lower leg, especially if they occur on the shin and foot and are preceded by a history of intermittent claudication, are likely to be due to arterial disease (Table 16.4). The foot is cyanotic and cold and the skin surrounding the ulcer is atrophic and hairless. The peripheral arterial pulses are absent or reduced. Doppler studies are required and, if arterial insufficiency is confirmed, then compression bandaging should be prohibited and advice from a vascular surgeon sought.

PRESSURE SORES

Pressure sores are caused by ischaemia due to sustained or repeated pressure on skin overlying bony prominences. Up to a third of patients over 70 years old in hospital develop pressure sores, especially those with a fractured neck of femur. The morbidity and mortality of those with deep ulcers is high.

Aetiology

The main factors responsible for pressure sores are:

- Prolonged immobility and recumbency, e.g. paraplegia, arthritis and apathy.
- Diminished sensation, e.g. neurological disease.
- Vascular disease, e.g. atherosclerosis.
- Malnutrition, general debility and severe systemic illness, e.g. alcoholism and malignant cachexia.

Clinical features

The sore starts as a localised area of erythema and progresses to a superficial blister or erosion. If the cause is not corrected, deeper damage occurs with the development of a black eschar which, when removed or shed, leaves a deep and penetrating ulcer, often colonised by *Pseudomonas aeruginosa*. The skin overlying the sacrum, greater trochanter, ischial tuberosity, tuberosity of calcaneus and lateral malleolus is especially susceptible.

Management

This is not easy but the following are important:

- Prevention by regular turning of recumbent patients and the use of antipressure mattresses in susceptible patients.
- Treatment of malnutrition and the general condition.
- Debridement: regular cleansing with normal saline or 0.5% aqueous silver nitrate; appropriate systemic antibiotic if spreading infection; antibacterial preparations locally; absorbent dressings (see leg ulcers, above); semipermeable dressings such as Opsite.
- Plastic surgical reconstruction may be indicated in the young when the ulcer is clean.

FURTHER READING

Lowthian P 1983 Nursing aspects of pressure sore prevention. In: Barbenel J C, Forbes C D, Low G D O (eds) Pressure Sores. Macmillan, London

Margolis D J 1993 The healing of recalcitrant leg ulcers. Current Opinion in Dermatology 31–6

BULLOUS DISEASES

Blisters, resulting from cleavage at various levels in the skin (Fig. 16.13), are the primary lesions in some rare but important disorders. Epidermolysis bullosa are a group of largely genetically determined conditions whereas pemphigus, bullous pemphigoid and dermatitis

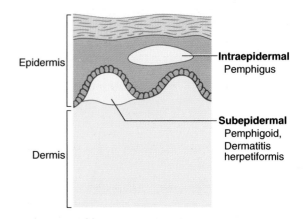

Fig. 16.13 The level of cleavage in acquired primary bullous diseases.

herpetiformis are acquired disorders with an immune pathogenesis.

INHERITED

EPIDERMOLYSIS BULLOSA

There are several types of epidermolysis bullosa; the main ones are listed in Table 16.5. They are all characterised by an inherited tendency to develop blisters after minimal trauma.

Simple epidermolysis bullosa

Defective keratin genes have recently been shown to cause this subgroup. The condition may be so mild that it is manifest by just occasional blisters on the palms and soles but blisters may be more widespread in some variants. Blisters heal without scarring. The nails and oral mucosa are unaffected.

Table 16.5 Classification and level of blister in epidermolysis bullosa (EB)

Type of epidermolysis bullosa	Mode of inheritance	Level of blister
Simple	Autosomal dominant	Epidermal basal cell
Junctional	Autosomal recessive	Lamina lucida
Dystrophic	Autosomal dominant	Dermis below lamina densa
Dystrophic	Autosomal recessive	Dermis below lamina densa

Junctional epidermolysis bullosa

This is due to an abnormality in the basal lamina involving defective anchoring filaments. The condition is present at birth and is often lethal. The newborn child shows large raw areas and flaccid blisters which heal slowly. The nails and oral mucosa are involved.

Dystrophic epidermolysis bullosa

This is due to defective type VII collagen, the main structural component of the anchoring fibrils found just below the basal lamina.

Blisters in the autosomal dominant type appear in late infancy. They are most common on sites subjected to friction, e.g. knees, elbows and fingers. They heal with scarring and leave milia. The nails may be involved but the mouth is seldom affected.

Blisters may be present at birth or appear soon after delivery in the autosomal recessive type. They are seen most often on the hands, feet, knees and elbows. They heal with scarring which may be so severe that the hands and feet become useless balls which have lost all the digits. The teeth, mouth and upper oesophagus are all affected; oesophageal strictures may require operative intervention.

Management of epidermolysis bullosa

There is no specific treatment for any form. Large blisters should be pricked and the blister fluid released. Dressings, to minimise friction, may be helpful. Superinfection should be treated with an appropriate local or systemic antibiotic. Systemic corticosteroids and phenytoin are disappointing in the treatment of the junctional and dystrophic types.

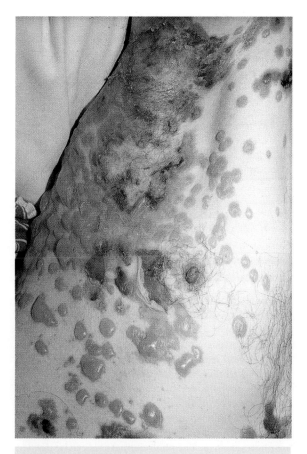

Fig. 16.14 Pemphigoid: large tense and unilocular blisters clustered in and around the axilla.

ACQUIRED

PEMPHIGUS, PEMPHIGOID AND DERMATITIS HERPETIFORMIS

Some distinguishing features of these primary bullous diseases are given in Table 16.6. and Fig. 16.13. A typical example of pemphigoid is shown in Figure 16.14.

The diagnosis is often clear on clinical grounds but biopsy of an early blister and 'normal' perilesional skin (dermatitis herpetiformis) is usually performed. Direct immunofluorescence on the biopsy specimen to detect fixed antibodies and indirect immunofluorescence to detect circulating antibodies will clinch the diagnosis.

Management

High doses of systemic corticosteroids (e.g. prednisolone 60 mg daily) may be required to control blistering in pemphigus and, more often than not, a lower maintenance dose is needed for the rest of the patient's life. Other immunosuppressive drugs (e.g. azathioprine) may be required. Pemphigoid surrenders to much lower doses of systemic corticosteroids and most patients can be weaned off this treatment eventually. Patients with dermatitis herpetiformis require full gastrointestinal investigation as they have a patchy gluten-sensitive enteropathy, demonstrable by jejunal biopsy. They should be encouraged to take a gluten-free diet as good compliance invariably leads to reduction in the dose of dapsone or sulphapyridine (Table 16.6) or cessation of such systemic treatment.

FURTHER READING

Fine J-D 1992 Bullous diseases. In: Moschella S L, Hurley H J (eds) Dermatology, 3rd edn. W B Saunders, Philadelphia
Priestley G C, Tidman M J, Weiss J C, Eady R A J 1990 Epidermolysis Bullosa: a Comprehensive Review of Classification, Management and Laboratory Studies. DEBRA, Crowthorne

Table 16.6 Some distinguishing features between pemphigus, pemphigoid and dermatitis herpetiformis

	Age	General health	Site of blisters	Nature of blisters	Blisters in mouth	Circulating antibodies	Fixed antibodies	Treatment
Pemphigus	Middle age	Poor	Trunk, flexures and scalp	Superficial and flaccid	Common	IgG to epidermal intercellular substance	IgG in epidermal intercellular substance	Corticosteroids Immunosuppressives
Pemphigoid	Old	Good	Often flexural	Tense and blood-filled	Rare	IgG to basement membrane region	IgG at basement membrane	Corticosteroids Immunosuppressives
Dermatitis herpetiformis	Primarily adults	Itchy	Elbows, knees, upper back, buttocks	Small, excoriated and grouped	Rare	IgG to the endomysium of muscle	IgA granular deposits in papillary dermis	Gluten-free diet Dapsone Sulphapyridine

SKIN REACTIONS TO LIGHT

Exposure to the sun is, in a number of respects, beneficial. It is essential for Vitamin D synthesis (p. 572) and it improves a number of common skin conditions such as psoriasis and atopic eczema. Many find a tan attractive and feel generally better after a period in the sun. On the other hand the drawbacks of excessive sun exposure are considerable. They include sunburn and the acceleration of skin ageing. There is also no doubt that ultraviolet irradiation is one very important factor in the cause of skin cancer and that certain skin eruptions are photosensitive. The photodermatoses can be divided into those rashes in which ultraviolet radiation (UVR) has a primary role and those where UVR is a triggering factor.

PRIMARY PHOTODERMATOSES

POLYMORPHIC LIGHT ERUPTION

The cause of this primary photodermatosis is unknown. As the name implies, a constellation of lesions, including erythema, papules, vesicles and plaques, appear on exposed skin about 24 hours after UVR exposure. Women are affected twice as often as men and the disorder usually starts in the spring and lasts for most of the summer. Sunscreens and protective measures are the cornerstone of treatment, but 'desensitisation' to UVR with carefully monitored and increasing doses of UVB or a short PUVA course (p. 952) at the beginning of the spring allows many patients to endure the summer months. Topical corticosteroids are also of some help.

CHRONIC ACTINIC DERMATITIS

This is a condition of unknown cause which primarily affects middle-aged and old men. Chronic and lichenified plaques of eczema are seen on the exposed skin, especially the face. Many patients have had eczema previously and a large proportion are allergic to plant oleoresins or to ingredients of cosmetics. Protective clothing, sun block preparations and the careful use of azathioprine provide the most effective therapy but sometimes the patient may be so exquisitely photosensitive that a darkened room provides the only significant relief during acute flare-ups of the condition.

SECONDARY PHOTODERMATOSES

PRE-EXISTING DISEASE

Herpes simplex infections, lupus erythematosus, cutaneous porphyrias, rosacea and vitiligo may all be triggered or exacerbated by UVR.

DRUG OR CHEMICAL-INDUCED PHOTOSENSITIVITY

Several drugs may cause a light-sensitive eruption by absorbing UVR. The reaction may be like an exaggerated sunburn, eczematous, bullous or pigmented. Common culprits are listed in the information box. Usually, specialised phototesting is not necessary. The incriminating drug is withdrawn or substituted with an unrelated compound.

TOPICAL AGENTS

Psoralens are found in many plants, especially umbelliferae (including wild parsley and giant hogweed) and some cosmetics. They absorb longwave ultraviolet irradiation and if UV exposure is sufficient, may cause a sunburn-like reaction with post-inflammatory pigmentation. Some local medications such as coal tar products may also photosensitise.

FURTHER READING

Norris P G 1993 Advances in understanding the pathogenesis of photodermatosis. Current Opinion in Dermatology 185–190

DISORDERS OF PIGMENTATION

DECREASED PIGMENTATION

OCULOCUTANEOUS ALBINISM

Little or no melanin is made in the skin and eyes in this disorder. There are two main types, tyrosinase negative and tyrosinase positive, distinguished by the hair bulb test. Both are inherited as autosomal recessive traits, the abnormal gene for each type being found on different chromosomes.

Clinical features

At birth the whole skin is white and pigment is also deficient in the hair, iris and retina. Albinos have poor vision, photophobia and rotatory nystagmus. Sunburn is common. As tyrosinase positive albinos grow older they gain a little pigment so that their hair becomes straw-coloured, their irides less translucent and their skin slightly freckled. As melanocytes are present, albinos have non-pigmented melanocytic naevi and may develop amelanotic malignant melanomas. Other skin tumours are also common in albinos living in the tropics.

Management

Avoidance of sun exposure, the use of sun blocks and protective clothing is essential, especially in the tropics. Termination of affected pregnancies, diagnosed by fetal biopsy at 20 weeks' gestation, may also be considered, especially for those living in sunny climates.

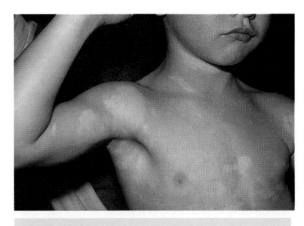

Fig. 16.15 Vitiligo: widespread patches in a youngster with a strong family history of autoimmune diseases.

VITILIGO

Vitiligo is an acquired condition, affecting 1% of all races, in which circumscribed depigmented patches develop.

Aetiology

There is complete loss of melanocytes from affected patches. There is a positive family history of the disorder in those with generalised vitiligo and this type is associated with autoimmune diseases such as diabetes, thyroid, adrenal disorders and pernicious anaemia. Trauma and sunburn may precipitate the appearance of vitiligo.

Clinical features

Segmental vitiligo is restricted to one part of the body, but not necessarily a dermatome. Generalised vitiligo (Fig. 16.15) is often symmetrical and frequently involves the hands, wrists, knees and neck as well as around the body orifices. The hair of the scalp and beard may also depigment. The patches of depigmentation are sharply defined and, in Caucasians, may be surrounded by 'white coffee'-coloured hyperpigmentation. Some spotty perifollicular pigment may be seen within the depigmented patches and is sometimes the first sign of repigmentation. Sensation in the depigmented patches is normal (cf. tuberculoid leprosy, p. 131). The course is unpredictable but most patches remain static or enlarge; a few repigment spontaneously.

Management

This is unsatisfactory. It is important to protect the patches from excessive sun exposure by clothing or sunscreen preparations. Camouflage cosmetics may be helpful especially in Blacks. Photochemotherapy with PUVA (p. 952) is rarely helpful.

PHENYLKETONURIA (p. 764)

This rare metabolic cause of hypopigmentation has a prevalence of about 1:25 000.

HYPOPITUITARISM

The hypopigmentation is due to a decreased production of pituitary melanotrophic hormones (p. 677). The complexion has a pale, yellow tinge; there is skin atrophy and thinning or loss of the sexual hair.

INCREASED PIGMENTATION

This is mostly due to hypermelanosis but other pigments may occasionally be deposited in the skin so that orange discolouration may suggest carotenaemia, a bronze colour haemochromatosis (p. 528) and other hues suggest drug eruptions (see information box).

LOCALISED HYPERMELANOSIS

Freckles (ephelides)
These are sharply demarcated light brown-ginger macules of up to 5 mm in diameter. They are most prominent on exposed sites; they multiply and become darker with sun exposure. The melanin in the basal cell layer of the epidermis is increased without melanocytic proliferation.

Lentigines
These are dark brown macules ranging from 1 mm to 1 cm across. Although discrete their outline may be irregular. Lentigines occur in childhood but are most common after middle age on the backs of the hands ('liver spots') and on the face. Lentigines have an increased number of melanocytes which produce excessive melanin.

Multiple lentigines are seen on and around the lips, buccal mucosa and fingers in the Peutz–Jeghers syndrome (associated with small intestinal polyposis and intussusception).

DIFFUSE HYPERMELANOSIS

Endocrine pigmentation
Chloasma describes discrete patches of facial pigmentation which occur in pregnancy and in some women taking oral contraceptives. Diffuse pigmentation, sometimes worse in the skin creases, may be a feature of Addison's disease (p. 715), Cushing's syndrome (p. 707), Nelson's syndrome, and chronic renal failure (p. 631). In all of these cases it is due to an increase in the levels of pituitary melanotrophic peptides (p. 677).

Drug-induced pigmentation
The information box lists some drugs which may cause hyperpigmentation, not invariably due to hypermelanosis alone but sometimes due to deposition of the drug or its metabolite, either of which may be complexed with melanin.

DRUG-INDUCED PIGMENTATION

Drug	Appearance
• Amiodarone	Slate-grey, exposed sites
• Arsenic	Diffuse bronze pigmentation with superimposed 'raindrop' depigmentation
• Bleomycin	Often flexural, brown
• Busulphan	Diffuse brown
• Chloroquine	Blue-grey, exposed sites
• Clofazamine	Red
• Mepacrine	Yellow
• Minocycline	Slate-grey, scars temples and shins
• Phenothiazines	Slate-grey, exposed sites
• Psoralens	Brown, exposed sites

FURTHER READING

Bologna J, Pawelek J M 1988 Biology of hypopigmentation. Journal of the American Academy of Dermatology 19: 217–255
Orlow S J 1993 Recent advances in oculocutaneous albinism. Current Opinion in Dermatology 73–77

DISORDERS OF THE HAIR AND NAILS

The condition of the hair and nails may reflect both local and systemic disease and omission of this part of the general examination could result in some important diagnostic clues being overlooked.

HAIR DISORDERS

The scalp hair should be inspected and its lustre, calibre, structure, kinks, breaks and frayed ends and density assessed. A search for nits and lice (p. 181) is essential when faced with an itchy scalp and adenopathy of the

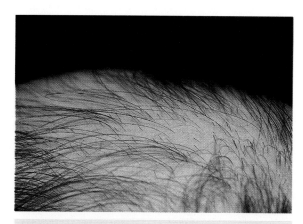

Fig. 16.16 Alopecia areata. Marked hair loss with diagnostic exclamation mark hairs.

posterior cervical chain. When assessing alopecia it is helpful to distinguish whether the hair loss is due to an abnormality of the hair shaft (as in some inherited diseases of scalp hair) or of the scalp and, in the latter, whether there is scarring or not.

ALOPECIA AREATA

This non-scarring condition appears as sharply defined non-inflamed bald patches, usually on the scalp. During the active stage of hair loss pathognomonic 'exclamation-mark' hairs are seen (broken off hairs of 3–4 mm long which taper off towards the scalp, Fig. 16.16). An uncommon diffuse pattern on the scalp is recognised. The condition may affect the eyebrows, eyelashes and beard. The hair usually regrows spontaneously in small bald patches, but the outlook is less good with larger patches and when the alopecia appears early in life or is associated with atopy. Alopecia totalis describes complete loss of scalp hair and alopecia universalis complete loss of all hair.

Aetiology

Aetiology is unknown but there is an association with autoimmune disorders, atopy and Down syndrome.

Management

Intralesional corticosteroid injections may hasten spontaneous regrowth of hair. Contact sensitisers (e.g. local diphencyprone) produce dramatic results in about a quarter of patients with alopecia totalis. Wigs may be the only answer in some women with extensive involvement.

ANDROGENETIC ALOPECIA

Male-pattern baldness is physiological in men over 20 years old though rarely it may be extensive and develop at an alarming pace in the late teens. It also occurs in females, but most obviously after the menopause. The well-known distribution (bitemporal recession and then crown involvement) is described as 'male-pattern' but this type of hair loss in females is often diffuse.

Aetiology

Androgenetic alopecia is often familial though the precise mode of inheritance is not clear. As the name implies the hair loss is androgen-dependent though those afflicted usually have normal levels of circulating androgens. When this type of alopecia is associated with other signs of virilisation in the female, especially if there is menstrual irregularity or cessation, full endocrinological assessment is required to exclude an androgen-secreting tumour of the adrenal or ovary.

Management

There is no medical cure for androgenetic alopecia. Topical minoxidil may slow hair loss or stimulate fine hair regrowth in the minority. Scalp surgery, hair transplants and wigs are welcomed by some.

HIRSUTISM

Hirsutism is the growth of terminal hair in a male pattern in a female. It should be distinguished from hypertrichosis which describes the growth of terminal hair in either sex in a non-androgenic distribution.

Hirsutism is often racial (e.g. Mediterranean Caucasians and Asians) and familial. Some degree of hirsutism is common after the menopause. The cause of most cases of hirsutism is unknown and only a small minority have a demonstrable hormonal abnormality.

Investigations

Full endocrinological investigations are required if hirsutism:

- occurs in childhood
- is of sudden onset
- is accompanied by signs of virilisation
- is associated with menstrual irregularity or cessation.

Tests will include diurnal cortisol levels, dexamethasone suppression test, ACTH, testosterone, sex-hormone-binding globulin, dehydroepiandrosterone sulphate, androstanedione, 17-OH progesterone, luteinising:follicular stimulating hormone ratio and ovarian ultrasound examination (when polycystic ovaries are suspected).

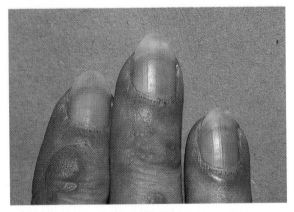

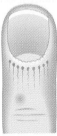

Fig. 16.17 Dermatomyositis. The erythema, dilated and tortuous capillaries in the proximal nail fold and the Gottron's papules on the digits are important diagnostic features.

Management

Any remediable endocrinological cause should be corrected. Oral anti-androgens (e.g. cyproterone acetate) are useful in idiopathic hirsutism. Electrolysis, shaving, waxing and depilatory creams are all helpful.

NAIL DISORDERS

The nail plate arises from the nail matrix and lies on the nail bed. The keratinous plate is produced by cells of the matrix and, to a much lesser extent, the bed. Finger nails grow about 1 cm every 3 months and toe nails at about a third of this rate.

NAIL FOLD DISORDERS

Examination of the nail folds should accompany examination of the nails. Paronychia describes inflamed and swollen nail folds. Chronic paronychia is seen most commonly in those with a poor peripheral circulation, in those involved in wet work, in diabetics and those who are over-enthusiastic when manicuring their cuticles. Ragged cuticles and dilated or thrombosed capillaries in the proximal nail folds are important pointers to connective tissue disease (Fig. 16.17).

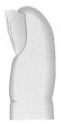

Fig. 16.18 The nail in pachyonychia congenita.

NAIL PLATE DISORDERS

These may be isolated abnormalities due to congenital disease or trauma or reflect other diseases, either systemic or those just involving the skin. Longitudinal ridging and beading of the nail plate is not abnormal and increases with age. Similarly, occasional white transverse flecks (striate leukonychia) are seen frequently in normal nails and are due to air spaces within the plate and not, contrary to popular belief, to insufficient calcium.

CONGENITAL DISEASE

Pachyonychia congenita is rare and inherited as autosomal dominant. The nails are grossly thickened, especially at the free edge (Fig. 16.18), and discoloured from birth.

TRAUMA

Splinter haemorrhages are fine linear dark brown flecks running longitudinally in the plate (Fig. 16.19). They are most commonly due to trauma but may be seen in nail psoriasis. They are also a sign of subacute bacterial endocarditis.

Subungual haematomas (Fig. 16.20) may appear as a crimson, purple or grey-brown discolouration of the nail plate, most frequently that of the big toe. Some-

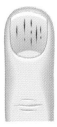

Fig. 16.19 Splinter haemorrhage running longitudinally in the nail plate.

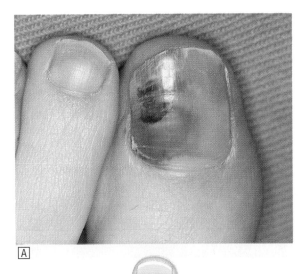

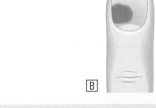

Fig. 16.20 Subungual haematoma A. A normally-coloured band would develop as shown in B, as the nail grows out.

times, but not always, there is a history of trauma. The abnormality appears suddenly and the nail folds remain uninvolved (cf. subungual malignant melanoma, p. 969). As the nail grows out, a normally coloured band develops proximally.

Habit-tic dystrophy is common. It is due to the habit of picking or fiddling with the cuticle of the thumb nail. This produces a ladder pattern of transverse ridges and furrows up the centre of the nail (Fig. 16.21).

Chronic trauma from ill-fitting shoes and from sport may cause malalignment and thickening of the nails,

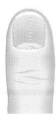

Fig. 16.21 Ridge and furrow pattern in the thumb nail in habit-tic dystrophy.

known as onychogryphosis, and lead to ingrowing toe nails.

THE NAIL IN SYSTEMIC DISEASE

Koilonychia (Fig. 16.22A) is a concave or spoon-shaped deformity of the plate which is a sign of iron deficiency. It is seen most often in countries where malnutrition is prevalent.

Beau's lines (Fig. 16.22B) are transverse grooves which appear at the same time on all nails, a few weeks after an acute illness, and which move out to the free margins as the nails grow.

Digital clubbing in its most gross form is seen as a bulbous swelling of the tip of the finger (Fig. 16.22C, D) or toe. The normal angle between the proximal part of the nail and the skin is lost. Causes include:

- **Respiratory**—bronchogenic carcinoma, asbestosis (especially with mesothelioma), suppurative lung dis-

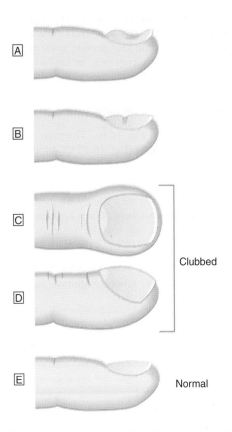

Clubbed

Normal

Fig. 16.22 The nail in systemic disease: A Koilonychia; B Beau's lines; C and D digital clubbing and E normal nail.

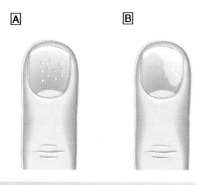

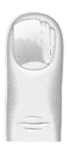

Fig. 16.24 Dermatophyte infection causes discolouration and crumbliness of the nail plate.

Fig. 16.23 The nail in psoriasis.

ease (empyema, bronchiectasis, cystic fibrosis), fibrosing alveolitis

- **Cardiac**—cyanotic congenital heart disease, sub-acute bacterial endocarditis
- **Other**—inflammatory bowel disease, biliary cirrhosis, thyrotoxicosis, familial.

Whitening of the nails is a rare sign of hypoalbuminaemia. 'Half and half' nails (white proximally and red-brown distally) are seen in some patients with renal failure. Rarely, drugs (e.g. antimalarials) may discolour nails.

THE NAIL IN SOME COMMON SKIN DISEASES

Psoriasis (see also Fig. 16.6). This may cause coarse pitting of the nail plate (Fig. 16.23A), onycholysis (separation of the nail plate from the nail bed, 16.23B), and subungual hyperkeratosis.

Eczema. Shiny nails may signify frequent rubbing of eczematous skin elsewhere. When eczema involves the distal phalanges the nail may be deformed with transverse ridging and thickening of the plate.

Lichen planus and severe alopecia areata may cause trachyonychia, a fine roughness and white discolouration of the nail plate.

Dermatophyte infection causes yellow-brown discolouration and crumbling of the plate which starts at the free margins and spreads proximally (Fig. 16.24). Usually only a few nails are infected and frequently only on one foot or hand.

FURTHER READING

Sawaya M E, Hordinsky M K 1992 Advances in alopecia areata and androgenetic alopecia. Advances in Dermatology 7: 211–227
Tosti A, Baran R 1993 Treatment of nail disorders. Current Opinion in Dermatology 96–100

SKIN TUMOURS

The increasing number of patients over 70 years old is paralleled by an increasing incidence of skin cancer. Only the most common benign tumours and a few malignant ones will be described in this section.

BENIGN TUMOURS

MELANOCYTIC NAEVI

Melanocytic naevi (moles) are localised benign proliferations of melanocytes. Their cause is unknown but they are often familial. They are very common, the average number on the skin in different populations ranging from 15 to 40. They are more profuse in Caucasians living in sunny climates. With the exception of congenital melanocytic naevi (which are present at birth or appear shortly after birth), most melanocytic naevi appear in early childhood, at adolescence and during pregnancy or oestrogen therapy. New lesions appear less often after the age of 20.

Clinical features

Acquired melanocytic naevi are classified according to the microscopic location of the clumps of melanocytes in the skin (Fig. 16.25). The *junctional* type shows these clumps at the epidermal–dermal junction, the *intradermal* type within the dermis and the *compound* type at both of the above sites. There is a reasonable correlation between their clinical and histological appearance. Junctional naevi are usually circular and macular; their colour ranges from mid to dark brown and may vary within a single lesion. Compound and intradermal naevi are similar to one another in appearance; both are nodules of up to 1 cm in diameter though intradermal naevi are usually less pigmented than compound naevi. Their surface may

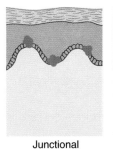 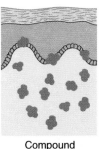 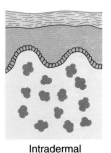

Junctional   Compound   Intradermal

Fig. 16.25 Classification of melanocytic naevi, based on microscopic location of the clumps of naevus cells.

be smooth, cerebriform or even hyperkeratotic and papillomatous and they are often hairy.

Clinically and histologically atypical melanocytic naevi (syn. dysplastic naevi) may run in some families in which cases of malignant melanoma are seen. These profuse, large and irregularly pigmented naevi are most obvious on the trunk. Their edges are irregular and they vary greatly in size, often being over 1 cm in diameter. Some are pinkish and an inflamed halo may surround them.

Whereas about 30–50% of malignant melanomas develop from melanocytic naevi the converse is far from true and only a minute percentage of melanocytic naevi become malignant. Malignant change is most likely in large congenital melanocytic naevi (risk estimated around 6%) and in atypical (dysplastic) melanocytic naevi (precise risk still unclear). However, as the skin can be so easily seen, there is an unrivalled opportunity to observe and report change which might signify early and curable malignancy. Any change (see information box below) in a mole deserves attention even though the reason for it is often not sinister.

SIGNIFICANT CHANGES IN MELANOCYTIC NAEVI

- Itch
- Enlargement
- Increased or decreased pigmentation
- Alteration in shape
- Irregularity of surface or edge
- Inflammation
- Ulceration
- Bleeding

Such changing lesions should be examined carefully remembering the 'ABCDE' features of malignant melanoma listed in the information box (p. 969).

Management

Excision and histological examination is needed when malignancy is suspected or is a significant risk, for example in a large congenital melanocytic naevus, when a naevus becomes repeatedly inflamed or traumatised and when a naevus is deemed ugly.

SEBORRHOEIC KERATOSIS (BASAL CELL PAPILLOMA)

These common benign epidermal tumours are unrelated to sebaceous glands. Their appearance is usually unexplained but multiple lesions may be inherited as an autosomal dominant. Occasionally they appear in the wake of an inflammatory dermatosis and, very rarely, a sudden eruption of multiple itchy lesions may be associated with an internal tumour.

Clinical features

These appear usually after the age of 50 years but flat inconspicuous lesions may be visible earlier. They are most commonly found on the trunk and face. The sexes are equally affected. The lesions vary in colour from yellow to dark brown and have a distinctive, raised and 'stuck-on' appearance. They are sometimes pedunculated. Their surface may have greasy scaling and scattered pinpoint keratin plugs. They become more profuse with age but remain benign.

Investigation

Biopsy is necessary only in dubious cases.

Management

They may be left alone but unsightly or easily traumatised lesions are simply removed by curettage under local anaesthetic or by cryotherapy.

PREMALIGNANT TUMOURS

ACTINIC KERATOSIS

These discrete, rough-surfaced lesions occur on light-exposed areas. They are caused by cumulative sun exposure. Caucasians living near the equator are most at risk and invariably develop them though they also affect the middle-aged and elderly in temperate climates. Actinic keratoses are not seen in Blacks. They are premalignant though only a few turn into squamous cell carcinomas.

Clinical features

The multiple pink or grey hyperkeratotic lesions seldom exceed 1 cm in diameter and are most common on the backs of the hands, the face and bald scalp. Many resolve spontaneously. Transition to squamous cell carcinoma, although rare, should be suspected if a lesion enlarges, ulcerates or bleeds.

Management

Cryotherapy with liquid nitrogen is effective, though multiple lesions may be treated with 5% 5-fluorouracil cream under specialist guidance. Lesions which do not respond to treatment should be regarded with suspicion and biopsied.

MALIGNANT TUMOURS

BASAL CELL CARCINOMA

This is the most common form of skin cancer and is usually found on the face of the middle-aged or elderly. The tumour invades locally but rarely metastasises. 'Rodent ulcer' is a term commonly used for slowly expanding ulcerative basal cell carcinoma. The malignant cells resemble basal keratinocytes.

Aetiology

Cumulative sun exposure is the most important factor in their development and these tumours are more common in Caucasians living near the equator. They may also occur in scars following vaccination and trauma or appear on skin previously treated with X-rays.

Clinical features

The most common type is the nodulo-ulcerative form. The earliest lesion is a small, glistening, skin-coloured papule, often with fine telangiectatic vessels on the surface, which slowly enlarges (Fig. 16.26). Central necrosis may occur which leaves an ulcer surrounded by a rolled pearly edge. Without treatment lesions may reach 1–2 cm in diameter over 5 to 10 years. Slow but relentless growth causes local tissue destruction. Sometimes this type of tumour becomes cystic or pigmented. The cicatricial variant of basal cell carcinoma is a slowly expanding yellow or grey, waxy plaque with an ill-defined edge. Fibrosis often follows ulceration and crusting and the lesion may appear as an enlarging scar. The superficial (multifocal) variant is seen most often on the trunk; it appears as a slowly enlarging pink or brown scaly plaque with a fine 'whipcord' edge. If left it may grow to 10 cm in diameter.

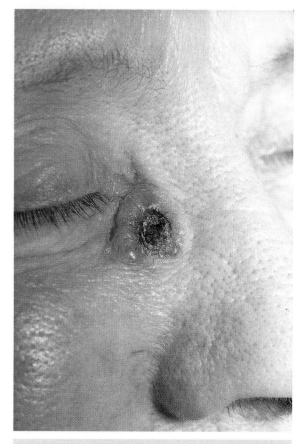

Fig. 16.26 Basal cell carcinoma. A slowly growing pearly nodule just below the inner canthus. The central crust overlies an ulcerated area.

Management

Excision, with a half centimetre of normal skin, is the treatment of choice for most patients. Lesions with an ill-defined edge are best excised by specialist surgeons, who might take advantage of microscopic examination of clearance *during* the operation (Mohs' technique). Radiotherapy is effective and should be reserved for biopsy-proven lesions when surgery is contraindicated. The cure rate for all types of basal cell carcinoma is over 95% but regular follow-up for at least three years is required to detect local recurrence.

SQUAMOUS CELL CARCINOMA

Aetiology

These malignant tumours of keratinocytes often arise in skin damaged by long-term ultraviolet radiation but also by X-rays and infra-red rays. Patients with certain rare genetic disorders, with defective DNA repair mechanisms, such as xeroderma pigmentosum, also develop multiple basal and squamous cell carcinomas. The integration of human papilloma virus DNA detected in some squamous cell carcinomas suggests an oncogenic potential for certain types of this group of viruses; immunosuppression and ultraviolet radiation appear to be important contributory factors.

Clinical features

Squamous cell carcinoma usually presents as a keratotic nodule, though anaplastic lesions may be seen as an ulcer with a granulating base and indurated edge. The tumour is common on the lip and in the mouth where it may be preceded by leukoplakia. Those arising in actinic keratoses seldom metastasise but all tumours should be treated promptly to prevent nodal spread.

Management

Treatment is similar to that for basal cell carcinoma.

MALIGNANT MELANOMA

Malignant melanoma attracts a disproportionate amount of attention because it is so lethal and prevention, early diagnosis and treatment are by far the best ways of combating its dangers. It is rarely seen in Blacks but its incidence in Caucasians in the UK and USA is doubling, approximately every 10 years. Sunlight is the most important cause. There is a higher incidence in Caucasians living near the equator (over 40 per 100 000 per annum) than those living in temperate zones (5–10 per 100 000 per annum). The tumour is rare before puberty and in areas of low incidence (including the UK) the tumour is twice as common in females. Those with blond or red hair, fair skin which tans poorly, many freckles and melanocytic naevi, dysplastic melanocytic naevi and a family or personal history of a previous melanoma have an increased risk of developing the tumour.

ABCDE FEATURES OF MALIGNANT MELANOMA

Asymmetry
Border irregular
Colour irregular
Diameter often greater than 0.5 cm
Elevation irregular

CLINICAL STAGES OF MALIGNANT MELANOMA

- Stage I: primary lesion only
- Stage II: regional nodal disease
- Stage III: distant disease (nodal or visceral)

Clinical features

The classification of invasive malignant melanomas is seen in the information box.

CLASSIFICATION OF CUTANEOUS MALIGNANT MELANOMA

Type of invasive melanoma	Presence of preceding in situ/radial growth phase
• Superficial spreading	+
• Lentigo maligna	+
• Nodular	−
• Acral lentiginous	+

Two-thirds of invasive melanomas are preceded by a superficial and radial growth phase characterised by an expanding, irregularly pigmented macule or plaque. Its margin is usually irregular with reniform projections. Lentigo maligna (in situ changes of malignancy only) and lentigo maligna melanoma occur most often on the exposed skin of the elderly. A speckled macular lentigo maligna may have been present for many years before a nodule of invasive melanoma appears within it (Fig. 16.27). The in-situ phase of superficial spreading melanoma, the most common type in Caucasians, seldom lasts for longer than two years, usually shows much colour variation and is often palpable. Acral lentiginous melanoma occurs on the palms and soles and is the most common type in the Chinese and Japanese. Nodular melanoma develops as a pigmented nodule with no preceding in-situ phase. All changing pigmented lesions deserve careful examination remembering the 'ABCDE' features of malignant melanoma. About 30–50% of melanomas appear to develop in a preceding melanocytic naevus (p. 966). A change in any naevus should raise suspicion of malignant transformation.

True amelanotic melanomas occur but are rare; flecks of pigmentation can usually be seen with a lens. Subungual melanomas present as painless, expanding areas of pigmentation under a nail and usually involve the nail fold.

The clinical stages of malignant melanoma are shown in the information box below.

The diagnosis should be established by local excision biopsy of the suspected lesion with 2 mm lateral clearance and with a cuff of subcutaneous fat deep to the tumour. Incisional biopsies are not recommended as a routine but may be unavoidable with some large and doubtful lesions and at certain sites.

Management

Only surgical excision is effective. A 3-cm clearance is recommended for tumours greater than 1 mm thick. Direct closure, without grafting, may be possible.

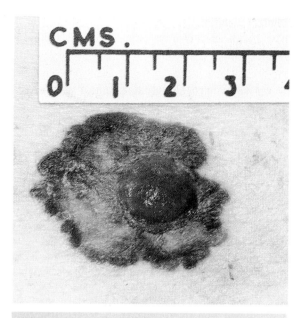

Fig. 16.27 Superficial spreading melanoma. The radial growth phase was present for about 3 years before the invasive amelanotic nodule developed within it. Note irregular outline, asymmetrical shape and different hues, including depigmented areas signifying spontaneous regression.

Tumours less than 1 mm thick are removed with a 1 cm clearance; direct closure is nearly always possible. Elective (prophylactic) local node dissection may benefit some patients with tumours of intermediate depth (2.0–3.5 mm). Palpable local nodes in Stage II patients should always be removed by radical block dissection. Chemotherapy, rarely curative, is palliative in 25% of patients with Stage III melanoma.

Prevention and early diagnosis are best achieved by education of those at highest risk who live or holiday in sunny climates. Successful campaigns have focused on regular self-examination and the ways in which sun exposure can be reduced by avoidance, clothing and sunscreen preparations. Public awareness and compliance has been encouraged by imaginative and gimmicky slogans like the Australian 'Slip, Slap and Slop' advice (slip on the shirt, slap on the hat and slop on the sunscreen).

Prognosis

The prognosis of patients with a malignant melanoma can be determined with reasonable accuracy. Those with clinical Stage III disease fare least well (less than 10% survive 2 years), patients with Stage II disease have a 20–30% chance and those with Stage I disease a 70% chance of surviving 5 years. The thickness of the tumour (measured microscopically by Breslow's method which gives the distance between the granular cell layer and the deepest part of the tumour) is a reliable predictor of the prognosis for patients with Stage I disease. The prognosis is excellent for those with tumours less than 1 mm thick (over 90% survive 5 years), but becomes less good with thicker tumours. The 5-year survival of patients with tumours greater than 3.5 mm thick is about 50%. In general, females fare better than males and tumours at certain sites (e.g. lower leg) are less aggressive.

FURTHER READING

Emmett A J J, O'Rourke M G E 1991 Malignant Skin Tumours, 2nd edn. Churchill Livingstone, Edinburgh
NIH Consensus Development Panel on Early Melanoma 1992 Diagnosis and treatment of early melanoma. Journal of the American Medical Association 268: 1314–1319
Veronesi U, Cascinelli N 1991 Narrow excision (1 cm margin): a safe procedure for thin cutaneous melanoma. Archives of Surgery 126: 438–441

THE SKIN AND SYSTEMIC DISEASE

Skin reactions can be linked with an underlying systemic disease in a number of ways as shown below in Table 16.7.

Only common or important associations will be discussed below.

NEUROFIBROMATOSIS

The skin markers of Von Recklinghausen's type of neurofibromatosis include scattered and discrete light brown (café au lait) macules, axillary freckling and a variable number of cutaneous neurofibromata (see page 1112). The tumours may be small and superficial or large and deep. Small circular pigmented hamartomas of the iris (Lisch nodules) appear in early childhood.

TUBEROUS SCLEROSIS

This is an autosomal dominant condition with hamartomas affecting many systems.

The classic triad of clinical features is mental retardation, epilepsy and skin lesions but not all are invariably present. The skin signs include small white oval (ash leaf) macules, pink or yellowish papules on the centre of the face (adenoma sebaceum), peri- and subungual fibromata and connective tissue naevi (cobblestone-like plaques at the base of the spine, sometimes called shagreen patches).

Table 16.7 Skin reactions in systemic disease
Part of a multisystem disease
Genetically determined (e.g. neurofibromatosis and tuberous sclerosis)
Xanthomas
Amyloidosis
Porphyria
Sarcoidosis
A non-specific and not invariable reaction pattern to a systemic disease
Urticaria
Erythema multiforme
Annular erythemas
Erythema nodosum
Pyoderma gangrenosum
Sweet's syndrome
Generalised pruritus
A sign of internal malignancy
Dermatomyositis
Generalised pruritus
Acanthosis nigricans
Superficial thrombophlebitis
A sign of internal organ failure
Liver: Generalised pruritus, pigmentation, spider naevi and palmar erythema
Kidney: Generalised pruritus and pigmentation
Pancreas (diabetes mellitus): Necrobiosis lipoidica
A result of a common genetic link with the systemic disorder
Dermatitis herpetiformis and gluten-sensitive enteropathy
Psoriasis and some types of arthropathy
The cause of the systemic disease
Exfoliative dermatitis causing high output cardiac failure
A result of treatment of the systemic disease
Drug eruptions

XANTHOMAS

These deposits of fatty material in the skin, subcutaneous fat and tendons may be the first clue to primary or secondary hyperlipidaemia (p. 766).

Various clinical patterns are seen which correlate well with the underlying cause. They include eruptive yellow papules on the buttocks (eruptive xanthomas), yellowish macules or plaques (plane xanthomas), small yellow-grey plaques around the eyes (xanthelasma palpebrarum), nodules over the elbows and knees (tuberous xanthomas) and subcutaneous nodules attached to tendons, especially those on the dorsal aspect of the fingers and the Achilles tendons (tendinous xanthomas). When xanthomas are detected the fasting blood lipids and the electrophoretic pattern of plasma lipoproteins must be measured though abnormalities will not always be detected.

AMYLOIDOSIS (p. 912)

Skin lesions are uncommon in systemic amyloidosis secondary to rheumatoid arthritis or other chronic inflammatory diseases.

Deposits of amyloid in the skin, appearing often as waxy plaques around the eyes, are prominent in primary systemic amyloidosis and in amyloid associated with multiple myeloma. 'Pinch purpura', appearing where the skin is traumatised, is due to amyloid infiltration of blood vessels and may also be a striking feature.

PORPHYRIA

Skin lesions do not occur in acute intermittent porphyria.

This is characterised by attacks of abdominal pain, neuropsychiatric symptoms and the passage of dark urine. Attacks may be triggered by drugs, especially barbiturates, oestrogens, griseofulvin and sulphonamides (see p. 773, Ch. 12).

Fragility, blistering (Fig. 16.28), hypertrichosis and scarring of exposed skin are features of cutaneous hepatic porphyria. The condition is most common in patients with alcoholic liver damage and previous viral hepatitis.

The autosomal dominantly inherited variegate porphyria is common in South Africa. The features include the systemic symptoms and drug provocation of acute intermittent porphyria and the skin signs of hepatic cutaneous porphyria.

SARCOIDOSIS (p. 381)

Skin lesions are seen in about one-third of patients with systemic sarcoidosis.

The clinical features include erythema nodosum, granulomatous deposits in long-standing scars, dusky infiltrated plaques on the nose and fingers (lupus pernio) and scattered brownish-red, violaceous or hypopigmented papules or nodules which vary in number, size and distribution.

URTICARIA

This common reaction pattern may be due to a particular food or food additive, a drug or, more rarely, an underlying systemic disease.

Aetiology

The final common pathway for all types of urticaria is the release of mediators which cause increased capillary permeability and the accumulation of fluid in the surrounding tissue. Histamine released from mast cells is important in most cases but kinins or serotonin may play a part in the deeper, more persistent, types of physical urticaria.

Many types of urticaria do not have an immunological or allergic basis. Amongst these are the physical urticarias which may be induced by heat, sweating, cold,

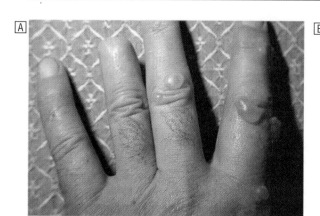

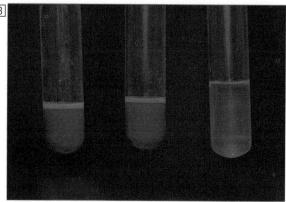

Fig. 16.28 **Cutaneous hepatic porphyria.** Ⓐ Recent skin fragility and blistering on the backs of the fingers. The signs, although trivial, are highly suggestive of cutaneous hepatic porphyria. The urine of this patient with alcoholic liver damage contained excessive uroporphyrins fluorescing coral pink under longwave ultraviolet when extracted. Normal control specimen seen on right Ⓑ.

pressure, sun exposure and even contact with water; their pathogenesis is diverse. Urticaria of sudden onset, widespread distribution and lasting only for a few days may be a manifestation of a type I allergic reaction, even associated with a serum sickness-like reaction (p. 43) and the history often reveals a clear-cut cause such as a particular food or drug.

Clinical features

Urticaria describes an eruption of itchy wheals (Fig. 16.29), sometimes accompanied by deeper and more diffuse swelling (angioedema) which is seldom itchy. By definition the wheals are evanescent and individual lesions are seldom present for longer than 12 hours; but the urticaria tendency may last for a few days, weeks or even years.

The most serious complications of acute urticaria are: anaphylactic shock—pallor, sweating, hypotension and collapse which may be preceded by headache, bronchospasm, nausea and vomiting; and angioedema, causing obstruction of the upper airway.

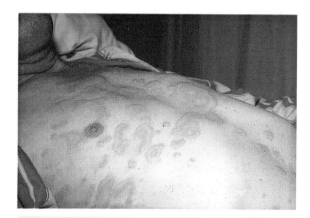

Fig. 16.29 **Widespread acute urticaria** due to penicillin allergy.

Investigation

A good history and examination will usually be more helpful than laboratory tests. First a physical cause should be excluded. If none is obvious an underlying systemic condition should be considered, including viral infections such as early viral hepatitis, infectious mononucleosis and primary HIV infection, but also systemic lupus erythematosus and thyrotoxicosis. Drugs, especially salicylates which are histamine releasers, should then come under suspicion. Occasionally, exacerbations may coincide with ingestion of a particular food and specially kept food diaries may help to identify causative items. Additives such as tartrazine, salicylates

and yeasts have received much attention. Finally, laboratory tests should be performed to confirm underlying systemic disease, to check the complement system in suspected familial angioedema and to look for an eosinophilia which might be a clue to parasitosis.

Management

Any obvious cause should be avoided and underlying systemic conditions should be treated. The majority of acute and subacute cases respond well to the new generation of non-sedative antihistamines, e.g. terfenadine 60–120 mg daily, but different antihistamine combinations may have to be tried in chronic cases. Calamine lotion is as good as any local treatment. Potential airway obstruction is an emergency and is treated with adrenaline (1 in 1000), 0.5 ml given slowly subcutaneously or intramuscularly followed by intravenous chlorpheniramine (10 mg) and intravenous hydro-cortisone (100 mg). If treatment is given early enough tracheostomy should be avoidable. The management of anaphylactic shock is similar and described on page 43.

HEREDITARY ANGIOEDEMA

Hereditary angioedema is a rare but important condition, inherited as an autosomal dominant. It usually presents in childhood with swellings of the skin and mucous membranes sometimes associated with bouts of upper gastrointestinal and upper respiratory tract obstruction. Trauma, for example during dental treatment, may precipitate attacks. It is due to a functional or quantitative deficiency of the inhibitor of the activated first component of the complement system which allows complement activation to go unchecked and mast cell degranulation, with liberation of vasoactive mediators, to occur. Intravenous infusion of fresh frozen plasma is the best treatment for acute attacks and anabolic steroids (e.g. danazol), which promote hepatic synthesis of the inhibitor, are used for maintenance treatment.

ERYTHEMA MULTIFORME

As its name implies this is a reaction pattern of multiform erythematous lesions. The precipitating factor may not be found in some cases but attacks are provoked by the factors listed in the information box below.

PRECIPITATING FACTORS FOR ERYTHEMA MULTIFORME

- Herpes simplex infections
- Other viral infections, e.g. orf, and mycoplasma
- Bacterial infections
- Drugs, especially sulphonamides, penicillins and barbiturates
- Internal malignancy or its treatment with radiotherapy

Clinical features

The multiform erythematous lesions may be urticaria-like and some have obvious 'bull's eye' or 'target' lesions. Blisters may be seen in the centre or around the edges of the lesions. In some cases blisters dominate the picture; the Stevens–Johnson syndrome is severe bullous erythema multiforme with emphasis on mucosal involvement including the mouth, eyes and genitals with accompanying constitutional disturbance.

Management

Severe cases are usually managed with tapering courses of systemic corticosteroids after treatment, if possible, of the primary cause.

ERYTHEMA NODOSUM

This characteristic reaction pattern is due to a vasculitis in the deep dermis and subcutaneous fat.

Erythema nodosum may be provoked by factors listed in the information box below.

PROVOKING FACTORS IN ERYTHEMA NODOSUM

- **Infections**
  Bacteria (streptococci, tuberculosis, brucellosis and leprosy), viruses, mycoplasma, rickettsia, chlamydia and fungi
- **Drugs**
  e.g. sulphonamides and oral contraceptives
- **Systemic disease**
  e.g. sarcoidosis, ulcerative colitis and Crohn's disease

Clinical features

Painful, palpable, dusky blue-red nodules are most commonly seen on the lower legs. Malaise, fever and joint pains are common. The lesions resolve slowly over a month leaving bruise-like marks in their wake.

Management

The underlying cause should be determined and treated. Bed rest and oral, non-steroidal anti-inflammatory drugs may hasten resolution. Tapering systemic corticosteroid courses may be required in stubborn cases.

PYODERMA GANGRENOSUM

This starts as an inflamed nodule or pustule which breaks down centrally and rapidly progresses to an ulcer with an indurated or undermined purplish or even pustular edge. Lesions may be single or multiple (Fig. 16.30). The condition is not bacterial in origin. Although it may arise in the absence of any underlying disease, it is usually associated with one of the following conditions: ulcerative colitis (found in about half of patients with pyoderma gangrenosum), Crohn's disease, rheumatoid arthritis, monoclonal gammopathies, leukaemia. Treatment is by control of the underlying disease and with systemic corticosteroids.

ACANTHOSIS NIGRICANS

This is a velvety thickening and pigmentation of the major flexures. It may be associated with obesity or insulin resistant diabetes but, if not, the chances are high of an underlying carcinoma, usually within the abdomen.

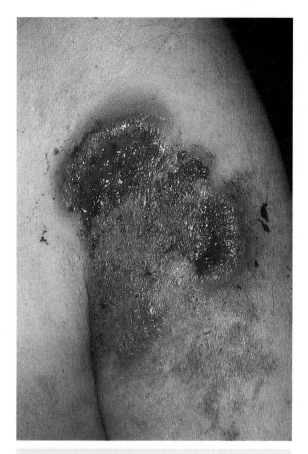

Fig. 16.30 Pyoderma gangrenosum: rapidly extending ulcer with purplish indurated edge.

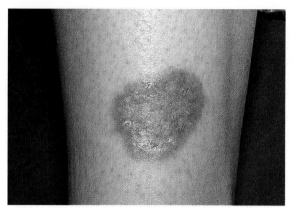

Fig. 16.31 Necrobiosis lipoidica: atrophic yellowish plaque on the skin of a diabetic.

NECROBIOSIS LIPOIDICA

This condition is important to recognise because of its association with diabetes mellitus. Less than 1% of diabetics have necrobiosis, but more than 85% of patients with necrobiosis will have or will develop diabetes.

Typically the lesions appear as shiny, atrophic and slightly yellow plaques on the shins (Fig. 16.31). Underlying telangiectasia is easily seen. Minor knocks may precipitate slow-healing ulcers. No treatment is effective.

DRUG ERUPTIONS

Cutaneous drug reactions are common and almost any drug can cause them. Drug reactions may reasonably be included in the differential diagnosis of most skin diseases. Although the mechanisms are poorly understood, drug eruptions may be classified as shown in Table 16.8.

Clinical features

The most common types of drug eruptions and their cause are listed in Table 16.9. It is important not to

GENERALISED PRURITUS

This is a symptom with many causes, rather than a disease in its own right. It may be due to a skin disorder (e.g. eczema, scabies, lichen planus) or to an internal cause such as those listed in the information box below.

INTERNAL CAUSES OF PRURITUS

- Liver disease, itching signals biliary obstruction
- Chronic renal failure
- Iron deficiency
- Polycythaemia. The itching is often triggered by a hot bath
- Thyroid disease, both hypo- and hyperthyroidism
- Internal malignancy, especially Hodgkin's disease and other lymphomas

---

DIAGNOSTIC CLUES TO DRUG ERUPTIONS

- Past history of reaction to suspected drug
- Introduction of suspected drug a few days before onset of rash
- Recent prescription of a drug commonly associated with rashes (e.g. penicillin sulphonamide, thiazide, allopurinol, phenylbutazone)
- A symmetrical eruption which may fit with a well-recognised pattern caused by one of the current drugs (Fig. 16.33)

Table 16.8   Drug eruptions and their mechanisms

Mechanism	Example
Non-immunological (non allergic)	
Unwarranted pharmacological effect	Striae due to corticosteroids, mouth ulcers due to methotrexate
Drug overdosage or failure to metabolise or excrete the drug	Morphine rashes in patients with liver disease
Drug interaction	Warfarin toxicity when co-administered with aspirin or phenylbutazone
Idiosyncratic reaction (odd reactions which may be genetically determined and are peculiar to an individual)	Drug-induced variegate porphyria
Phototoxic reaction	Chlorpromazine-induced light reactions
Altered skin ecology	Tetracyclines causing vaginal candidiasis
Exacerbation of pre-existing skin condition	Lithium and beta-adrenoceptor antagonist worsening of psoriasis
Immunological (allergic)	
Immediate hypersensitivity	Penicillin-induced urticaria
Immune complex reaction	Drug-induced vasculitis or erythema multiforme
Delayed hypersensitivity	Drug-induced exfoliative dermatitis or photoallergic reactions

Table 16.9   Drug eruptions and some drugs which may cause them

Name of reaction pattern	Clinical features	Drugs which commonly cause reaction
Toxic erythema	Erythematous plaques Morbilliform, sometimes with urticarial or erythema multiforme-like elements	Antibiotics (especially ampicillin) Sulphonamides, thiazide diuretics, phenylbutazone, para-aminosalicylic acid (PAS)
Urticaria	Itchy wheals, sometimes accompanied by angioedema	Salicylates and antibiotics
Allergic vasculitis	Painful, palpable purpura followed by necrotic ulcers	Sulphonamides, phenylbutazone, indomethacin, phenytoin and oral contraceptives
Erythema multiforme	Target-like lesions and bullae on the extensor aspects of the limbs	Sulphonamides, phenylbutazone and barbiturates
Purpura	Widespread purpura not due to thrombocytopenia or a coagulation defect	Thiazides, sulphonamides, phenylbutazone, sulphonylurea, barbiturates and quinine
Bullous eruptions	May be associated with above eruptions. May occur at pressure sites in drug-induced coma	Barbiturates, penicillamine, nalidixic acid
Exfoliative dermatitis	Universal redness and scaling, shivering	Phenylbutazone, para-aminosalicylic acid (PAS), isoniazid and gold
Fixed drug eruptions	Round, erythematous, and sometimes bullous, plaques develop at the same site every time the drug is given. Pigmentation left in wake	Tetracyclines, quinine, sulphonamides and barbiturates
Acneiform eruptions	Rash resembles acne (see text)	Lithium, oral contraceptive, androgenic or glucocorticoid steroids. Antituberculosis and anti-convulsant drugs
Toxic epidermal necrolysis	Rash resembles that of scaled skin (Fig. 16.32)	Barbiturates, phenytoin, phenylbutazone and penicillin
Hair loss	Diffuse	Cytotoxic agents, etretinate, anticoagulants, antithyroid drugs and oral contraceptives
Hypertrichosis		Diazoxide, minoxidil and cyclosporin A
Photosensitivity	Rash limited to exposed skin	Thiazides, tetracyclines, phenothioazines, sulphonamides, nalidixic acid and psoralens
Pigmentation	Irregular melanin pigmentation on face Slate-grey colour of exposed skin Diffuse yellow colouration of skin Streaky depigmentation of hair	Oral contraceptives Phenothiazines Mepacrine Chloroquine

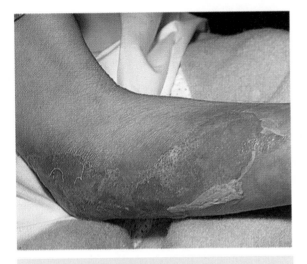

Fig. 16.32 Toxic epidermal necrolysis. In this case it was due to a barbiturate.

forget the possibility of a drug eruption when faced with a rash which is atypical of a known skin disease (Figs. 16.32, 16.33). Further clues to make the diagnosis are included in the information box.

Investigations

There are no specific investigations which help. Prick tests and in vitro tests for allergy are too unreliable for routine use. Readministration, as a diagnostic test, is usually unwise unless the reaction is mild and there is no suitable alternative drug.

Management

The first step is to withdraw the suspected drug(s). This may not be easy, or even possible, if there is no alternative available. The decision will depend on many factors including the severity and nature of the drug reaction, its potential reversibility and the probability that the drug caused the reaction. Supportive treatment with antihistamines or a tailored course of systemic cort-

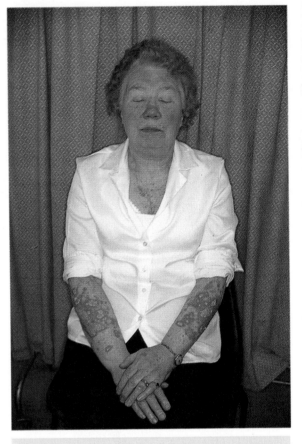

Fig. 16.33 Drug eruption: a weird but symmetrical erythematous scaly rash with a distribution suggesting a degree of photosensitivity. The rash persisted until the recently prescribed sulphonylurea was withdrawn.

icosteroids may be indicated depending on the type of skin reaction. The emergency treatment of anaphylactic shock is described on page 973.

FURTHER READING

Weissman K, Graham R M 1992 Systemic disease of the skin. In: Champion R H, Burton J L, Ebling F J G (eds) Textbook of Dermatology, 5th edn. Blackwell Scientific Publications, Oxford

Psychiatry

Diagnosis in psychiatry is mainly based on recognised patterns of subjective symptoms which are volunteered by the patient or elicited during a clinical interview. With the exception of the organic psychiatric disorders there are no objective markers of disease, such as radiological or laboratory abnormalities, by which diagnosis can be confirmed. In this context psychiatry differs from other branches of medicine where diseases have come to be classified in terms of their aetiology, such as an infective agent, biochemical abnormality or structural lesion. The symptoms of mental disorders involve abnormalities of behaviour, mood, perception, thinking and intellectual function. Some of these abnormalities impair judgement or contact with reality so that patients become a danger to themselves or other people. This is recognised in law and the Mental Health Act gives doctors the authority to treat patients against their will in exceptional cases. However, the great majority of patients with psychiatric disorders are managed in general practitioners' surgeries or hospital outpatient clinics in much the same way as patients with any other medical condition.

The number of inpatients in psychiatric hospitals has decreased sharply during the last three decades. In part this has been due to improved methods of treatment but it is also a result of government policy in many countries to treat patients in the community and to avoid hospital admission whenever possible. Long-stay patients have been moved out of hospital into community facilities such as hostels or group homes although the development of these facilities has not kept pace with plans for hospital closure. The overall result is that psychiatrists spend more time working in the community and have had opportunities to work more closely with their colleagues in general practice and other hospital specialties.

EPIDEMIOLOGY

Epidemiology is concerned with the study of disease in relation to the population in which it occurs, particularly its variation between subgroups and its association with environmental factors. Prevalence rates provide an estimate of how common a particular disease is in a given population; these rates can be expressed for a particular time (point prevalence) or for a given period (period prevalence). One-month and life-time prevalence figures for psychiatric disorders from a large American study are shown in Table 17.1.

These figures are probably representative of other Western countries. In the United Kingdom the preva-

Table 17.1 Prevalence rates of psychiatric disorders (%)*

	1-month	Life-time
Any psychiatric disorder	15.4	32.2
Affective disorders	5.1	8.3
Mania	0.4	0.8
Major depression	2.2	5.8
Dysthymia	3.3	3.3
Anxiety disorders	7.3	14.6
Phobia	6.2	12.5
Panic	0.5	1.6
Obsessive compulsive	1.3	2.5
Schizophrenia	0.7	1.5
Substance use disorder	3.8	16.4
Alcohol abuse	2.8	13.3
Drug abuse	1.3	5.9
Somatisation disorder	0.1	0.1
Antisocial personality disorder	0.5	2.5
Severe cognitive impairment	1.3	1.3

* From Regier D A, Boyd J H, Burke J D et al 1988 One-month prevalence of mental disorders in the United States. Archives of General Psychiatry 45: 977–986

lence of psychiatric illness in different populations can be summarised as shown below.

PREVALENCE OF PSYCHIATRIC ILLNESS IN DIFFERENT POPULATIONS, IN PERCENTAGES

• Community	15–20%
• General practice attenders	30%
• General hospital outpatients	20–30%
• General hospital inpatients	25–40%

The average general practitioner can expect to be consulted by one in seven of his patients because of psychiatric disorder during one year. The spectrum of illness treated in primary care differs from that treated by psychiatrists in outpatient clinics. General practitioners see a greater proportion of patients with neurotic illnesses and relatively few with psychotic illnesses; their patients are less severely ill than those attending a psychiatrist. There is considerable variation between general practitioners in their ability to identify psychiatric illness. Cases are likely to be missed especially if psychiatric illness is associated with physical illness or presents with somatic complaints.

Psychiatric disorders are commoner in inner city areas than in rural communities, and among women than men although the sex distribution becomes more even if personality disorders and alcohol abuse are taken into account.

CLASSIFICATION OF PSYCHIATRIC DISORDERS

Psychiatric disorders have traditionally been classified into two main groups, **organic** and **functional**. In the **organic** disorders a known physical aetiology can be established, the symptoms resulting from overt brain disease, as in dementia, or from metabolic upset or circulating toxins, as in acute delirium. In the **functional** disorders, such as schizophrenia, affective disorders and anxiety disorders, which constitute the large majority of psychiatric illnesses, it was implied that no such physical factors were present. The theoretical basis of this distinction is becoming weaker as evidence accumulates to demonstrate the presence of cerebral pathology and neurotransmitter disturbance at synaptic level in schizophrenia and the affective disorders. However, the term organic still has some use in clinical practice and will be retained here to describe certain disorders.

Another traditional distinction which has become eroded is the separation of the functional disorders into psychotic or neurotic, depending on the presence of certain 'psychotic' symptoms. These are abnormal beliefs (delusions), abnormal perceptions (hallucinations and illusions) and certain disturbances in the pattern of thinking. Neurotic symptoms, in contrast, are mainly exaggerations of emotions such as anxiety and depression which are universally experienced. Psychotic illnesses were often regarded as being associated with lack of insight while patients with neurotic disorders were considered to have insight into their condition. Although this is true as a generalisation there are important caveats. Many psychotic patients recognise the nature of their symptoms while some neurotic patients are strikingly lacking in understanding. Insight varies from time to time and its presence is not an all-or-none phenomenon, rather a matter of degree. Nor is it true to say that all psychotic illnesses are severe while neurotic illnesses are mild.

The two main classification systems currently used in clinical practice are the American Psychiatric Association's Diagnostic and Statistical Manual (4th edition), usually abbreviated to DSM-IV, and the World Health Organization's International Classification of Disease (10th edition), known as ICD-10.

The two systems are very similar but ICD-10 is the more widely accepted outside the United States. The classification of clinical syndromes used in this chapter will be based on ICD-10, an outline of which is shown in the information box.

CLASSIFICATION OF PSYCHIATRIC DISORDERS

- **Organic**
  Acute, e.g. delirium
  Chronic, e.g. dementia
- **Substance misuse**
- **Schizophrenia and delusional disorders**
- **Affective (mood) disorders**
  Depression
  Mania
  Recurrent affective disorders
- **Neurotic, stress-related and somatoform disorders**
  Anxiety disorders:
    Generalised anxiety
    Phobic anxiety
    Panic disorder
  Obsessive compulsive disorder
  Reaction to severe stress:
    Acute stress disorder
    Post traumatic stress disorder
    Adjustment disorder
  Dissociative (conversion) disorder
  Somatoform disorder
  Neurasthenia
- **Behavioural syndromes associated with physiological disturbance**
  Eating disorders
  Sleep disorders
  Sexual dysfunction
  Puerperal mental disorders
- **Personality Disorders**

AETIOLOGICAL FACTORS

The causes of most psychiatric disorders are unknown, yet there is considerable information concerning the range of factors which are regarded as important aetiologically. Causation is nearly always multifactorial and the aetiological factors should be regarded as having *predisposing*, *precipitating* or *maintaining effects*. The classification of these factors is shown in the information box (p. 980).

Genetic factors

There is a genetic contribution to several psychiatric disorders, including schizophrenia and affective illness. The evidence is derived from various observations: a higher prevalence of the disorder among first degree relatives than in the general population; a higher concordance rate in monozygotic than in dizygotic twins, even if the monozygotic twins have been reared apart; a higher prevalence rate for children of mentally ill parents who are brought up by healthy adoptive parents. Some disorders are due to single gene transmission. These include Huntington's chorea (autosomal dominant) and

Social network

Many psychiatrically ill patients are socially isolated. The lack of a network of people with whom they can interact socially often appears to be a contributory factor in their illness. Particularly important is the lack of a close, confiding relationship.

FURTHER READING

American Psychiatric Association 1994 Diagnostic and statistical manual of mental disorders, 4th edn. American Psychiatric Association, Washington
Regier D A, Boyd J H, Burke J D et al 1988 One-month prevalence of mental disorders in the United States. Archives of General Psychiatry 45: 977–986
World Health Organization 1992 The ICD-10 classification of Mental and Behavioural disorders. WHO, Geneva

some uncommon causes of mental retardation (see fragile X syndrome, p. 20). However, for the majority of psychiatric disorders in which heredity undoubtedly plays a role, no single gene has been isolated and it is assumed that several genes have an influence on the development of the condition.

Family background

Many patients with psychiatric disorders report an unhappy childhood background and it seems likely that a traumatic upbringing predisposes to future mental illness. Important factors are loss of a parent in childhood, either due to death or separation, parental disharmony and physical, especially sexual, abuse. In later life the family environment can adversely influence the course of an illness if parents are emotionally over-involved and express critical or hostile attitudes towards the patient.

Physical illness

Chronic physical ill-health predisposes to psychiatric disorder. There is an especially well-established link between brain injury and subsequent schizophrenic and depressive illness. Physical illness of acute onset can give rise to psychiatric disorder due either to its effect on cerebral anatomy and physiology or to its emotional significance and implications for the patient's future well-being.

Stressful life events

A wide range of stressful life events can precipitate episodes of illness in vulnerable people. These events usually involve a sense of loss and include death of a close relative, marital breakdown, redundancy, retirement and major financial crisis.

THE CLINICAL INTERVIEW

When a patient is referred to a psychiatrist the clinical interview obviously concentrates on evaluating psychological symptoms, exploring the patient's background and personality and assessing the patient's current mental state. However, many of the areas explored by a psychiatrist need to be included in an assessment conducted by a general practitioner or hospital specialist, particularly if the patient presents emotional complaints or has somatic symptoms which do not appear to have a physical basis. A physical examination, with particular attention to the neurological system, is an essential component of any psychiatric assessment.

Wherever the interview is conducted, interviewers should introduce themselves to a newly referred patient and explain the purpose of the interview. Patients should be allowed to describe their problems in their own words but the doctor must be in charge and guide the course of the interview by appropriate prompting and interjections. If possible the doctor should ask to see a reliable informant who should be interviewed separately. There are several aims to be borne in mind during the interview.

- **Reason for referral**
  Why the patient has been referred and by whom
- **Presenting complaints**
  The patient should be asked to describe briefly the symptoms for which help is requested
- **History of present illness**
  The patient should then be asked to describe the course of the illness from the time when symptoms were first noticed. The interviewer needs to ask direct questions to determine the nature, duration and severity of symptoms and factors associated with them
- **Family history**
  Description of parents and siblings, the patient's relationship with them and a record of mental illness in relatives
- **Personal history**
  Birth history, major events in childhood, developmental milestones, schooling, higher education, occupational history, sexual development, relationships, marriage, children, current social circumstances and forensic problems
- **Previous medical and psychiatric history**
  An enquiry into previous health, accidents and operations; use of alcohol, tobacco and other drugs. Direct questions may be needed concerning previous psychiatric history since this may not be volunteered, for example, 'Have you ever been treated for depression or nerves?' or 'Have you ever suffered a nervous breakdown?'
- **Previous personality**
  This refers to the characteristic patterns of behaviour and thinking which determine a person's adjustment to the environment—including attitudes, moral values, interests, quality of relationships with other people and reactions to stress. Personality attributes are usually developed by adolescence and are then stable throughout the person's life, and should be assessed independently of symptoms of psychiatric illness. However, certain personality types predispose to illness; an individual's personality will also influence the nature of the symptoms if psychiatric illness develops, and the emotional reaction if physical illness occurs. Several questionnaires are available for quantifying personality, the best known in Britain being the Eysenck Personality Questionnaire which measures extraversion, neuroticism and psychoticism as dimensions. For clinical purposes the most useful information can be obtained from a personality description given by one or more reliable informants who have known the patient well for many years.

MENTAL STATE EXAMINATION

Several aspects of the patient's current mental state will have become apparent while the history is being recorded. However, it is always necessary to proceed to ask about current symptoms. The sequence of questions should be flexible depending on which aspects of the mental state seem most important. These aspects are listed in the information box.

ASPECTS OF MENTAL STATE TO BE EXAMINED

- General appearance and behaviour
- Speech
- Mood
- Thought content
- Abnormal beliefs
- Abnormal perceptions
- Cognitive function

GENERAL APPEARANCE AND BEHAVIOUR

Describe succinctly the patient's appearance, dress and general tidiness. Is there a normal relationship with the examiner or is there avoidance of eye contact or uncooperative behaviour? Note any abnormalities of alertness and motor behaviour. For example is there restlessness or retardation? Does the patient pace repeatedly up and down the interview room?

SPEECH

Speed and fluency of speech should be noted. Is there retardation of speech or difficulty finding words? Does the patient speak excessively rapidly so that it appears speech is generated under pressure and it is difficult to interrupt the flow? Are there rapid changes in the topic of the conversation? Is it difficult to follow the patient's train of thought?

MOOD

Does the patient appear agitated, depressed or elated? These can be judged by facial expression, mannerisms, posture and other motor movements. The patient's subjective mood should be elicited by asking for a description of current spirits. Some patients find it difficult to describe their mood in terms of anxiety or depression; questions which help elicit their mood include inquiries as to whether they have lost the ability to enjoy themselves or derive pleasure from life (anhedonia) or whether they have lost interest in themselves and those around them. People who are depressed should be asked about feelings of low self esteem, guilt and worthlessness. It is also important to determine how they see their future. They should be asked about suicidal ideation, for example 'Do you ever feel that life is not worth living?'. Patients who reply positively need to be asked whether they have suicidal thoughts and active plans for putting an end to their lives.

Elated patients should be asked about feelings of grandiosity and general well-being. Manic patients may be irritable with the examiner who does not share their view of themselves. However, irritability is seen in other disorders of mood, not only mania.

THOUGHT CONTENT

Patients should be asked about their main preoccupations. This is best done simply by asking them to describe what is on their mind at present or what are their main worries. It can then be elicited whether the preoccupations are appropriate to the circumstances or whether they are indicative of psychological disorder. Is there evidence of phobic symptoms? A phobia is defined as an abnormal fear of an object or situation, the fear being sufficiently intense to lead to avoidance of the particular stimulus. Are there any obsessional symptoms? These are defined as thoughts, impulses or actions which enter the patient's mind repeatedly against his/her resistance but which nevertheless are recognised as his/her own thoughts. They are often associated with behavioural rituals such as repeated hand washing or checking.

ABNORMAL BELIEFS

It is necessary to establish whether the patient has any delusional beliefs. These are abnormal beliefs which are held with conviction and which cannot be argued away but which are out of keeping with the patient's social, cultural and educational background. They may be paranoid, grandiose or depressive in nature. Leading questions are often necessary to elicit delusional beliefs, for example, whether the patient believes anything unusual is going on or, if paranoid delusions are suspected, whether there are beliefs that people have malevolent intent. Primary delusions arise suddenly, often on the basis of a normal perception which is interpreted by the patient in a morbid manner. Thus the patient may see special significance in a particular arrangement of furniture in the room and conclude that there is a conspiracy organised by a secret political agency. Primary delusions of this type are characteristic of schizophrenia. Secondary delusions are those which occur due to some other psychological disorder such as a mood disturbance and they are commonly encountered in severe depression when they tend to involve gloomy themes of guilt, wickedness and punishment. When the mood is abnormally elated, as in mania, the delusions are typically grandiose.

ABNORMAL PERCEPTIONS

The patient may report unusual sensory experiences but more often these have to be elicited by direct questions such as 'Have you had any strange experiences recently'? or 'Do you ever hear people talking about you even though there is no one near you at the time'? The main abnormalities of perception are depersonalisation, illusions and hallucinations. Depersonalisation refers to an unpleasant subjective feeling in which the patient's body is perceived as if it is changed, lifeless or unreal. It is often accompanied by a sensation that the external world seems changed in that it appears grey, unreal or two-dimensional; this phenomenon is known as derealisation.

Illusions are abnormal perceptions of normal external stimuli. They occur most commonly in the auditory and visual modalities. Sounds appear distorted, muffled or louder than usual. Objects may be seen as larger (macropsia) or smaller (micropsia) than normal, distorted in shape or more vividly coloured. Hallucinations are sensory perceptions which occur in the absence of external stimuli. They can also occur in any sensory modality. It is important to establish whether the patient perceives the sensation as emanating from within the mind or from the outside world. It is also important to establish the degree of insight into the experience. Hallucinations which arise from within the patient's mind and whose origins the patient recognises are known as pseudohallucinations. Auditory hallucinations are characteristic of schizophrenia and affective psychoses. Visual, olfactory, gustatory and tactile hallucinations usually indicate organic mental disorder.

COGNITIVE FUNCTION

Intellectual abilities need to be assessed, particularly with regard to the possibility of mental handicap or dementia. They can be gauged from the history of the patient's educational background and attainments but can also be assessed during the interview from the patient's fluency, vocabulary and grasp of the interviewer's questions.

The level of consciousness should be noted. Does the patient remain alert throughout the interview or is there a tendency to drift off and lose the ability to concentrate on what is being asked? Concentration can be assessed more thoroughly by asking the patient to perform a simple repetitive task, such as subtracting 7 from 100 serially or repeating the months of the year backwards. Memory should be assessed under several headings. Recall of recent and distant events is determined by the patient's ability to describe details of personal history, dating back to childhood. It is also important to determine the ability to recall events occurring during the last few days and weeks. Registration is determined by presenting the patient with simple new information such as a name and address and then asking for this to be repeated immediately. The ability to consolidate and recall the information is checked by asking for the information to be repeated five minutes later, during which time the patient's attention should be diverted to other tasks. Memory is also assessed by checking on orientation. Does the patient know his/her exact location (orientation in place) and what day, date, month and year it is now (orientation in time)? Orientation in person refers to the patient's ability to describe details of personal identity, that is name, date of birth, marital state, address and other intimate details. Loss of personal orientation does not usually occur in organic brain disorders but is a feature of psychogenic amnesia. The patient should be asked to describe recent current affairs; this gives an indication of general intelligence and interest in external events.

It is useful to record patients' understanding of their problems, particularly whether they regard themselves as being ill or not. Finally doctors should note their own response to the patient. Did they feel sympathetic or warm towards the patient or were they made to feel irritable, frustrated or angry?

FURTHER READING

Institute of Psychiatry, London 1987 Notes on eliciting and recording clinical information, 2nd edn. Oxford University Press, Oxford
Leff J P, Isaacs A D 1990 Psychiatric examination in clinical practice, 3rd edn. Blackwell, Oxford

TREATMENTS USED IN PSYCHIATRY

Some of the treatment approaches in psychiatry are unfamiliar in other branches of medicine so they will be reviewed here before the clinical syndromes are discussed. The doctor is often the coordinating member of a multi-disciplinary team and needs to liaise closely with other professionals such as nurses, occupational therapists, social workers and psychologists, any one of whom may be responsible for a particular aspect of treatment.

PSYCHOLOGICAL TREATMENTS

PSYCHOTHERAPY

This is based on a continuing relationship between patient and doctor in which the patient confides his or her symptoms and the doctor uses his or her understanding of the patient in a therapeutic manner. There are two main types, supportive and interpretive. Supportive psychotherapy underlies all other treatments in psychiatry. Indeed it is a crucial element in treatment throughout clinical medicine, much more so than many doctors realise. It involves a process of empathic listening during which the doctor encourages patients to describe their symptoms, express their feelings and reflect on associated problems in their lives. A single interview conducted sympathetically often has a healthy cathartic effect, but usually the doctor has to see patients at regular intervals over a long period and be prepared for them to become dependent. The doctor should give an explanation of symptoms, advice, practical guidance and reassurance when indicated. Supportive psychotherapy does not aim at any fundamental psychological change but when successful it fosters a therapeutic alliance and improves compliance with other forms of treatment. In patients with incurable and chronic conditions it forms a vital source of emotional support over many years.

Interpretive psychotherapy, in contrast, attempts a radical restructuring of the patient's psychological conflicts and behaviour. It is based on one of the several schools of psychoanalytic theory and should only be conducted by professionals with special training. At the basis of all types of interpretive psychotherapy lies the assumption that the presenting symptoms result from unacceptable memories or conflicts which have been repressed so that they exist only in the patient's unconscious mind. Treatment aims at bringing these memories or conflicts into patients' consciousness by allowing them to associate freely or to describe the content of dreams which the therapist can interpret, and help them understand and modify their behaviour as a result. An important element in treatment is an analysis of the transference, a term which refers to the patients' attitudes and feelings towards the doctor. The transference is thought to reflect the patients' feelings towards other people during their development, particularly their parents. Patients suitable for this type of treatment have to be highly motivated and are usually suffering from anxiety, depression or certain types of personality disorders especially when these conditions are associated with disturbed interpersonal relationships. Treatment is contraindicated for those who have psychotic symptoms, paranoid traits, alcohol or drug abuse or who act in an antisocial manner. Interpretive psychotherapy is conducted during regular sessions of an hour's duration at least once a week and lasts for several months or even years. It can be conducted on an individual or group basis; its principles are also applied in marital and family therapy.

BEHAVIOUR THERAPY

Behaviour therapy is derived from the psychological principles of learning theory which state that many psychiatric disorders result from maladaptive patterns of learned behaviour. Treatment is aimed specifically at relief of symptoms. It is not thought necessary to modify or even understand aetiological factors from the patients' previous experiences. A behavioural analysis is essential before treatment is planned. This involves a detailed account of the symptoms, their severity, frequency and duration, together with an assessment of factors which trigger and maintain them. Several types of behaviour therapy have been evolved:

Systematic desensitisation

This is used in the treatment of phobias and other anxiety-related disorders. Its key elements are listed in the information box below.

KEY ELEMENTS OF SYSTEMATIC DESENSITISATION

- Training the patient to relax
- Constructing a hierarchy of anxiety-provoking situations
- Introducing the patient, while fully relaxed, to anxiety-provoking stimuli from the hierarchy, working from the least to the most distressing. This can be done in imagination or in real life

---

Flooding

This is also used in the treatment of phobias. It involves introducing the patient to the most stressful stimulus from the start and maintaining contact with the stimulus until anxiety subsides to normal levels. It stems from observations that anxiety eventually diminishes if avoidance of the anxiety-provoking stimulus is prevented. To allow this to occur, each session should last at least one hour and sometimes considerably longer.

Response prevention

This is used to treat the compulsive rituals which are characteristic of obsessional neurosis. The patient is exposed to stimuli which induce compulsive behaviour (e.g. checking or hand washing) but is prevented from carrying out the rituals.

Modelling

In this technique a therapist demonstrates normal behaviour in the presence of the stimulus. It is a useful supplement to response prevention. It is also used as a basis for social skills training.

Operant conditioning

This uses a system of positive and negative reinforcements to alter particular aspects of behaviour. Positive reinforcements (or rewards) are given following desired behaviour while negative reinforcements (or punishments) are used following undesired behaviour. Operant conditioning forms the basis of token economy systems used to reduce behavioural problems in chronic schizophrenia and mental handicap.

Bell and pad training

This is used in the treatment of enuresis. A special pad is placed under the patient's bed sheet. It contains an electrical circuit which is completed when wetted by urine, thereby sounding an alarm bell which wakes the patient. Micturition is interrupted and the patient gets up to complete emptying his or her bladder. After repeated training the patient learns to respond to sensations of bladder distension and wakens before micturition occurs.

COGNITIVE THERAPY

This approach is based on the assumption that some psychiatric disorders are due to a negative pattern of thinking which is an enduring characteristic. In depression a negative triad has been described, the three components of which are:

1. devaluation of the self
2. negative view of current life experiences
3. negative view of the future.

Cognitive therapy is a problem-orientated approach which aims at modifying patterns of thinking in a positive way; it is assumed that improvements in mood and behaviour will follow. The treatment has been used for depression, anxiety and eating disorders. The therapist has to identify the negative thoughts and help the patient see the connection between them and his mood or behaviour. The patient is encouraged to monitor the negative thoughts and to analyse them logically by examining the evidence on which they are based. The final step is to substitute positive patterns of thinking which are more in keeping with reality.

PHYSICAL TREATMENTS

DRUGS

Drugs used to treat psychiatric disorders are known collectively as psychotropics. They are classified according to their main mode of action (Table 17.2).

Table 17.2 Classification of psychotropic drugs

Action	Main groups	Clinical use
Antipsychotic	Phenothiazines Butyrophenones Thioxanthenes Substituted benzamides Dibenzodiazepine Benzisoxazole	Schizophrenia, mania, acute confusion
Antidepressant	Tricyclics and related drugs	Depressive illness, obsessive compulsive disorder
	Tetracyclics	Depressive illness
	Monoamine oxidase inhibitors	Depressive illness, phobic disorders
Mood stabilising	Lithium	Prophylaxis of manic depression, acute mania
	Carbamazepine	Prophylaxis of manic depression
Anti-anxiety	Benzodiazepines	Anxiety disorders, insomnia, alcohol withdrawal
	Beta-adrenoceptor antagonists	Anxiety (somatic symptoms)
	Azapirone	Anxiety disorders

Table 17.3 Antipsychotic drugs

Group	Drug	Usual dose
Phenothiazines	Chlorpromazine Thioridazine Trifluoperazine Fluphenazine	100–1500 mg daily 50–800 mg daily 5–30 mg daily 20–100 mg fortnightly
Butyrophenones	Haloperidol	5–30 mg daily
Thioxanthenes	Flupenthixol	40–200 mg fortnightly
Diphenylbutyl-piperidines	Pimozide	4–30 mg daily
Substituted benzamides	Sulpiride Remoxipride	600–1800 mg daily 150–450 mg daily
Dibenzodiazepine	Clozapine	25–900 mg daily
Benzisoxazole	Risperidone	2–16 mg daily

Antipsychotics

The essential mechanism of many of these drugs, which are also known as neuroleptics, is their ability to block central dopamine receptors. This has been thought to explain their antipsychotic effect. Antipsychotics are used to treat acute schizophrenia and mania and to prevent relapse in chronic schizophrenia. They are also useful in the management of disturbed behaviour due to acute confusional states. In low doses they are used to treat anxiety. The drugs have many unwanted side-effects so the indications for their use should be reviewed regularly. Weight gain due to increased appetite is common and may cause the patient to refuse further treatment. Side-effects related to dopamine blockade include parkinsonism, akathisia (an unpleasant, irresistible motor restlessness), acute dystonia (muscular spasm), tardive dyskinesia (persistent movements predominantly affecting the tongue and other facial muscles), gynaecomastia and galactorrhoea. The drugs also possess anticholinergic properties which cause dry mouth, blurred vision, constipation, urinary retention and impotence. In the elderly postural hypotension and hypothermia can occur. Hypersensitivity reactions include cholestatic jaundice, blood dyscrasias and photosensitive dermatitis. Ocular complications which can occur in long-term treatment are opacities in the cornea and lens; retinitis pigmentosa has been described with thioridazine.

Clozapine and risperidone have a much lower incidence of extrapyramidal side-effects, probably because of their strong blocking effect on serotonin (S_2) receptors and relatively weaker dopamine (D_2) blockade. Neutropenia occurs in 3% of patients treated with clozapine and several fatalities have occurred from agranulocytosis. Its use is currently restricted for schizophrenic patients who have not responded to other antipsychotic drugs and who are specially registered with a monitoring service. Blood counts have to be monitored weekly for the first 18 weeks of treatment and fortnightly thereafter. The drug must be stopped if neutropenia develops; the neutrophil count then reverts to normal levels. Other troublesome side-effects of clozapine include hypersalivation, weight gain and seizures. Commonly used antipsychotics are shown in Table 17.3.

Antidepressants

Commonly used antidepressants are shown in Table 17.4.

Tricyclic antidepressants

These are the drugs of first choice in the treatment of depressive illness. They inhibit the re-uptake of amines (noradrenaline and 5-hydroxytryptamine) at synaptic clefts and this action has been used to support the hypothesis that affective disorders result from a deficiency of these amines which serve as neurotransmitters in the central nervous system. There is a delay of 2 to 3 weeks between the start of treatment and the onset of therapeutic effect. Side-effects can be particularly troublesome during this period; they include anticholinergic effects, postural hypotension and cardiotoxicity. The recently introduced drugs, fluoxetine, fluvoxamine, paroxetine and sertraline are selective inhibitors of 5-hydroxytryptamine re-uptake. They are less cardiotoxic, less sedative and have fewer anticholinergic effects than tricyclics but can cause headache, nausea and anorexia. Their antidepressant effects are equivalent to those of tricyclics but they are generally

Table 17.4   Antidepressant drugs

Group	Drug	Usual dose
Tricyclics	Amitriptyline	75–150 mg daily
	Imipramine	75–150 mg daily
	Dothiepin	75–150 mg daily
	Clomipramine	75–150 mg daily
5-HT re-uptake inhibitors	Fluoxetine	20–80 mg daily
	Fluvoxamine	100–200 mg daily
	Sertraline	50–100 mg daily
	Paroxetine	20–50 mg daily
Tetracyclics	Mianserin	30–90 mg daily
Monoamine oxidase inhibitors	Phenelzine	60–90 mg daily
	Tranylcypromine	20–40 mg daily
	Moclobemide	300–600 mg daily

better tolerated. At present their high cost limits their use to patients for whom tricyclics are not effective or contraindicated because of side-effects.

The tetracyclic drug mianserin is an alpha$_2$-adreno-ceptor antagonist but has no effect on amine uptake. It has fewer side-effects than the tricyclics but can cause intolerable sedation and rarely leucopenia.

Monoamine oxidase inhibitors (MAOIs)

These increase the availability of neurotransmitters at synaptic clefts by inhibiting metabolism of noradrenaline and 5-HT. They are less effective than tricyclics for severe depressive illness but are equally effective for milder illness, particularly when depression is associated with anxiety and phobic symptoms. They also have a place in the management of primary phobic disorders. Monoamine oxidase inhibitors have acquired notoriety because of their interaction with various drugs such as amphetamines and opiates, and foods rich in tyramine such as cheese, pickled herrings, degraded protein and red wine. Amines accumulate in the systemic circulation causing a hypertensive crisis and fatalities have occurred from cerebral haemorrhage. These interactions have resulted in considerable anxiety about prescribing the drugs. However, they are relatively safe if the offending foods are avoided, and MAOIs are not used as often as they should be. Patients taking MAOIs should be given a card listing all the substances to be avoided. A newly introduced MAOI, moclobemide, is a reversible and selective inhibitor of monoamine oxidase, subtype A. It causes minimal potentiation of the pressor response to dietary tyramine so the need for dietary precautions is considerably reduced.

Mood stabilising drugs

Lithium carbonate

This drug, which inhibits neurotransmitter-stimulated phosphoinositide hydrolysis, is the main drug used in the prophylaxis of affective disorders. It should be given to patients who have had two or more episodes of illness requiring drug therapy within two years. It is more effective in bipolar illness (mania and depression) than in unipolar illness. Lithium is also used for acute mania and in combination with a tricyclic or MAOI for resistant depression. It has a narrow therapeutic range so regular blood monitoring is required to maintain a serum level of 0.5–1.0 mmol/l. This is usually achieved with a daily dose of 800–1200 mg. Toxic effects include nausea, vomiting, tremor and convulsions. With long-term treatment, weight gain, hypothyroidism, nephrogenic diabetes insipidus and renal failure can occur. Thyroid and renal function should be checked before treatment is started and every 6 months thereafter. Lithium has a significant teratogenic effect and should never be prescribed during the first trimester of pregnancy.

Carbamazepine

Recently carbamazepine, an established anticonvulsant drug, has been used successfully as prophylaxis in manic depression for patients who have not responded to lithium. The dose is 400–1200 mg daily although it is usual to start with a lower dose and increase it gradually. Common side-effects are drowsiness, ataxia, headache, rashes, nausea and vomiting.

Anti-anxiety drugs

Examples of commonly used anti-anxiety drugs are shown in Table 17.5.

Benzodiazepines

These agents have been used widely for the treatment of insomnia and anxiety-related disorders but they have been shown to cause dependence and withdrawal symptoms in many patients who have taken them for 6 weeks or more. These symptoms occur especially with short-acting benzodiazepines and if medication is stopped abruptly. They are listed in the information box below.

BENZODIAZEPINE WITHDRAWAL SYMPTOMS

- Anxiety
- Heightened sensory perception
- Hallucinations
- Epileptic seizures
- Ataxia
- Paranoid delusions

In view of problems of dependence, psychological methods of anxiety management should be considered first in the treatment of anxiety but if benzodiazepines are prescribed they should be given in short courses, no more than 3 weeks, to help with limited periods of stress, and the dose should be tailed off gradually thereafter.

Table 17.5   Anti-anxiety drugs

Group	Drug	Usual dose
Benzodiazepines	Diazepam	2–30 mg daily
	Chlordiazepoxide	5–30 mg daily
	Nitrazepam	5–10 mg daily
	Temazepam	10–20 mg at night
Beta-adrenoceptor antagonists	Propranolol	20–80 mg daily
Azapirone	Buspirone	10–45 mg daily

They have superseded chlormethiazole in the management of alcohol withdrawal. Buspirone, which is unrelated to any other psychotropic drug, is claimed not to have withdrawal effects nor does it have sedative or muscle relaxant properties. Its mode of action is slow, over 3 or 4 weeks, and this is obviously a disadvantage when a quick response is required.

Beta-adrenoceptor antagonists such as propranolol have a limited role in the treatment of anxiety where somatic symptoms are prominent.

ELECTROCONVULSIVE THERAPY (ECT)

Electroconvulsive therapy has been used in psychiatry for 50 years. It involves the administration of high voltage, brief, direct current impulses to the head while the patient is anaesthetised and paralysed by muscle relaxants. Electrodes can be placed either bilaterally, or unilaterally over the non-dominant hemisphere. Bilateral ECT is more effective but unilateral ECT causes less short-term memory impairment. The main use of ECT is for depressive illness but it is sometimes used in mania and acute schizophrenia. Indications are listed in the information box below.

INDICATIONS FOR ECT IN DEPRESSIVE ILLNESS

- Severe depression with paranoid or nihilistic delusions
- High suicidal risk where quick response is needed
- Failure to respond to a tricyclic and an alternative antidepressant
- Depressive stupor when food and fluid intake is inadequate
- Elderly or physically ill when tricyclic antidepressants may be unsafe
- Inability to tolerate side-effects of antidepressants

Up to 12 applications may be needed to produce optimal results. There has been a decline in its use following the introduction of psychotropic drugs but it remains the most effective treatment for severe depression with psychotic symptoms. ECT is safe and side-effects are few. Headache and a brief period of confusion often occur during the immediate post-ictal period. There may be amnesia for events occurring a few hours before (retrograde) and after (anterograde) ECT. Permanent anterograde amnesia has been claimed to occur but is infrequent. The contraindications to ECT are few; they are shown in the information box below.

CONTRAINDICATIONS TO ECT

- Recent myocardial infarction (within 3 months)
- Instability of cervical spine
- Raised intracranial pressure
- Cerebral haemorrhage
- Aortic aneurysm
- Acute respiratory infection

PSYCHOSURGERY

This treatment has been rendered virtually obsolete by modern drug therapy. It is now carried out for a small number of patients with severe, resistant depression or obsessional disorder and should only be undertaken at specialised centres. The operation involves a stereotactic technique to interrupt the frontolimbic pathways bilaterally.

FURTHER READING

Andrews G 1993 The essential psychotherapies. British Journal of Psychiatry 161: 447–451
Henry J A 1992 The safety of antidepressants. British Journal of Psychiatry 160: 439–441
Silverstone T, Turner P 1988 Drug treatment in psychiatry, 4th edn. Routledge, London

---

CLINICAL SYNDROMES

ORGANIC PSYCHIATRIC DISORDERS

This group of disorders results from pathological lesions within the brain or acting on the brain from a focus elsewhere in the body. According to their extent and rapidity of onset they can be classified as generalised or focal, acute or chronic.

DELIRIUM

Delirium, which is also known as acute confusional state, involves a global impairment of mental functions of acute onset. Its characteristic features are:

Impairment of consciousness

This sign, often overlooked, is fundamentally important. It covers a spectrum of impairment from a barely detectable dulling of alertness to deep coma. The patient appears drowsy and lethargic; the level of consciousness often fluctuates so that lucid periods alternate with drowsy spells. Consciousness is characteristically most impaired during the evening when there is decreased environmental stimulation. Clinical testing reveals impaired attention and concentration.

Memory disturbance

All aspects of memory-registration, retention and recall are affected. One of the earliest manifestations is disorientation in time and place, resulting from an inability to register the sequence of events and to learn new surroundings. Disorientation in place is particularly evident if the patient has recently been moved to unfamiliar surroundings, e.g. from home to hospital. Learning of other new information is impaired and there is faulty recall of past events, this being most marked for events in the previous few weeks.

Perceptual disturbance

In mild forms normal perceptions are distorted. Objects may be seen as larger (macropsia) or smaller (micropsia) than they are. They may be perceived as distorted in shape or be misinterpreted (illusions). Hallucinations are the most striking perceptual disturbance. Generalised organic reactions are characteristically associated with visual and tactile perceptual disturbances. Focal lesions in the temporal lobe can cause disturbances in taste and smell.

Difficulty in thinking

There is subjective difficulty in thinking clearly. Speed of thought is slowed, mental fatigue soon occurs and the pattern of thinking becomes muddled. The patient has difficulty grasping the essential features of the environment so that events are misinterpreted and secondary delusional ideas develop, often of paranoid nature.

Psychomotor changes

Mental and motor activity is retarded. There is little spontaneity, speech is sparse and responses to questions are slow in forthcoming. However, in some cases the reverse is true. The patient appears agitated and restless and there may be extensive hyperactivity to a dangerous degree. This clinical picture is often associated with toxic reactions to alcohol and other drugs.

Emotional changes

Anxiety, irritability and depression may accompany the other features. In severe cases the emotional response becomes apathetic.

Causes of an acute confusional state

The aetiology has to be determined from the history, physical examination and special investigations. The main causes can be grouped and are listed in the information box.

CAUSES OF ACUTE CONFUSIONAL STATES

Intra-cranial
- Trauma
- Vascular
  Transient ischaemic attack
  Cerebral haemorrhage
  Cerebral thrombosis
  Subarachnoid haemorrhage
  Subdural haemorrhage
- Epilepsy
  Post-ictal state
- Infection
  Encephalitis
  Cerebral abscess
  Meningitis
  AIDS
- Tumour
  Primary or secondary lesion

Extra-cranial
- Infections
  Exanthemata
  Septicaemia
  Pneumonia
  Urinary infection
- Toxic
  Alcohol
  Many therapeutic drugs (e.g. anticholinergics, beta blockers, L-dopa, isoniazid, corticosteroids)
- Endocrine
  Hyperthyroidism
  Hypothyroidism
  Hypoglycaemia
- Metabolic
  Uraemia
  Liver failure
  Electrolyte imbalances
  Remote effects of carcinoma
- Hypoxia
  Respiratory failure
  Cardiac failure
  Acute heart block
  Carbon monoxide poisoning

Rare causes
SLE, porphyria, Addison's disease, hypopituitarism, hypo/hyperparathyroidism, heavy metal poisoning, Wilson's disease, Vitamin B_{12} or folate deficiency

Management

The underlying cause must be determined; this usually involves admission to hospital where appropriate investigations are available. Once the cause is established specific treatment is given for the underlying lesion. Supportive measures are also necessary. The patient should be nursed in a well-lit room; frequent changes of nurses should be avoided so that rapport can be built up. Intravenous therapy may be required to correct fluid and electrolyte imbalance. Sedative drugs should not be given unless the patient's behaviour is disruptive; chlorpromazine (50–100 mg 8-hourly) or haloperidol (5–10 mg 8-hourly) are the drugs of choice except in delirium tremens when benzodiazepines (e.g. diazepam 10–20 mg 6-hourly) are preferred.

DEMENTIA

Dementia is defined as a clinical syndrome characterised by a loss of previously acquired intellectual function in the absence of impairment of consciousness. The syndrome results from a variety of pathological conditions which primarily or secondarily affect the brain. The commonest causes are Alzheimer's disease and cerebrovascular disease. Dementia is predominantly associated with the elderly but in some disorders, notably Alzheimer's disease, Pick's disease and Huntington's chorea, the onset of symptoms occurs in middle life. These conditions, known collectively as presenile dementias, have a strong familial disposition, Huntington's chorea being transmitted by an autosomal dominant gene. The key features of dementia are:

Loss of general intelligence

There is impairment of abstract thinking, judgement and problem solving ability. Thinking is slow and inflexible and the ability to reason logically is reduced.

Memory impairment

Minor degrees of forgetfulness are often the first signs of dementia and are noticed initially by relatives. Events of the recent past cannot be recalled so patients forget where they have left personal possessions and where they have been. Gas taps, electric lights and switches may be left on. People's names are forgotten, especially those who are newly introduced, and appointments are missed. Patients cannot learn to find their way around in new situations. Consequently they readily lose their way and eventually this applies even in familiar surroundings. Declining memory may lead to secondary delusions. For example, patients who forget where they have left important personal possessions may believe people are breaking into their homes and robbing them.

Personality change

There is a decline in personal manners and social awareness. Behaviour becomes rude, tactless and generally insensitive to the feelings of other people. Disinhibited behaviour may lead to episodes of aggression, sexual indiscretions or infringements of the law such as theft. These personality changes are often described as 'coarsening' in that they reflect exaggerations of the less desirable aspects of the patient's character which have previously been kept under restraint. Eventually there is a deterioration in personal appearance and hygiene. Urinary and faecal incontinence are common but appear to cause the patient little embarrassment. There is also a loss of volition and a general decline in interest. Patients may sit for hours without initiating any form of purposeful activity.

Emotional changes

Mood changes may be prominent during the early stages and cause some difficulty in differentiating dementia from affective disorders. Depression, anxiety or irritability may dominate the clinical picture. They appear to depend on some degree of insight into failing intellectual powers. Rapid changes of mood, emotional lability, are also common. In advanced dementia the emotional reaction becomes blunted and patients appear incapable of responding to emotionally charged events in their environment.

Aetiology

The main causes of dementia are shown in the information box.

ALZHEIMER'S DISEASE

Alzheimer's disease is a primary degenerative cerebral disorder with a characteristic neuropathology. Its onset is insidious, often in middle life (Alzheimer's disease of presenile onset) but the incidence is higher in later life (Alzheimer's disease of senile onset). Genetic factors are more important in the presenile variety which has a more rapid course and prominent focal cortical signs such as aphasia or apraxia. In cases with a senile onset the course is slower and there is a more general impairment of higher intellectual functions. Patients with Down syndrome appear to be at high risk of developing Alzheimer's disease.

The pathological changes result in widespread cerebral atrophy, particularly involving the cortex and hippocampus. Microscopy shows a marked reduction of neurons, neurofibrillary tangles and neuritic plaques with an amyloid core; aluminium silicate is present in the cores of mature plaques. Several neurochemical changes

CAUSES OF DEMENTIA

- **Degenerative**
  Alzheimer's disease
  Pick's disease
  Huntington's chorea
  Creutzfeldt–Jakob disease
  Parkinson's disease
- **Vascular**
  Cerebrovascular disease
  Cerebral emboli
- **Normal pressure hydrocephalus**
  Primary
  Secondary to head injury, subarachnoid
  haemorrhage or meningitis
- **Trauma**
  Post-traumatic dementia; boxer's
  encephalopathy
- **Space-occupying lesions**
  Cerebral tumour
  Subdural haematoma
- **Infections**
  AIDS
  Cerebral syphilis
  Viral encephalitis
- **Endocrine**
  Hypothyroidism
  Hypoglycaemia
  Hypopituitarism
- **Metabolic**
  Liver failure
  Renal failure
  Remote effects of carcinoma
- **Toxic**
  Alcohol
  Chronic barbiturate ingestion
  Heavy metals
- **Anoxia**
  Cardiac failure
  Heart block
  Cardiac arrest
  Respiratory failure
  Carbon monoxide poisoning
- **Vitamin deficiency**
  B_{12}, folic acid

CASE HISTORY

A 64-year-old man had been involved in three minor car accidents within a period of 2 months. His family had noticed he had become more forgetful following his early retirement 2 years previously and they arranged for him to be seen by his general practitioner. Clinical assessment showed him to be fully conscious; his mood was not depressed but he was overtly anxious when his intellectual functions were assessed. He had difficulty finding the correct words to describe common objects; he was incorrectly orientated in time and place; his recall of recent events was poor and the ability to learn new information was markedly impaired. The rest of the physical examination was normal. He was referred to a psychiatrist who made a diagnosis of Alzheimer's disease. Psychometric assessment confirmed the clinical impression of intellectual decline. A CT brain scan showed diffuse cortical atrophy and symmetrical enlargement of the lateral ventricles (Fig. 17.1). No focal lesions were seen. He was able to be supported at home by his family for another three years but his condition slowly deteriorated until he had to be transferred to a residential nursing home where he died 2 years later.

an accumulation of cerebral infarcts (multi-infarct dementia).

TRANSMISSIBLE DEMENTIAS

There has been increased interest recently in a rare group of dementias which are caused by a proteinaceous infectious agent, or prion, which can be transmitted from one individual to another. The most common human form of transmissible dementia is Creutzfeldt–Jakob disease which usually takes a rapidly fatal course, most patients dying within 2 years of the onset of symptoms. In addition to the rapid intellectual deterioration there are several neurological signs including myoclonus, cerebellar ataxia, rigidity and muscle wasting. In advanced stages of the disease there is a characteristic EEG pattern of bilateral, slow spike-and-wave discharges. Histologically the cerebral cortex shows neuronal degeneration, astrocytic proliferation and a vacuolated or 'spongiform' appearance.

Assessment and management

Diagnostic assessment is directed at confirming the diagnosis of dementia, determining its severity by assessing the degree of disability, and establishing the underlying cause. The history should be provided by a reliable informant who has known the patient for many years. Careful enquiry should be made concerning any family history of presenile dementia. Physical examination should be undertaken especially with the reversible causes of dementia in mind and particular attention

occur, including a reduction in acetylcholine and choline acetyltransferase.

CEREBROVASCULAR DEMENTIA

This usually follows a series of acute strokes or, less commonly, a single major stroke. In the former case there is a stepwise deterioration of intellectual function. Emotional lability is common; there are focal neurological signs and often evidence of vascular insufficiency elsewhere, including ischaemic heart disease and peripheral vascular disease. A more gradual onset occurs following a series of ischaemic episodes which produce

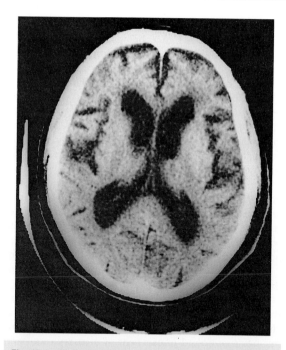

Fig. 17.1 Alzheimer's disease: CT brain scan showing cortical atrophy, widened sulci and enlarged lateral ventricles.

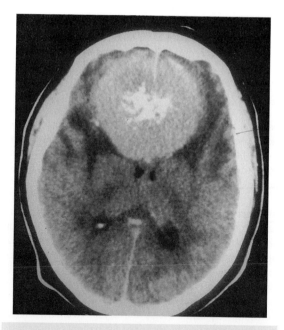

Fig. 17.2 Large frontal meningioma with a calcified centre—shown by contrast enhanced CT brain scan. The patient presented with a 5-year history of personality change, depression and incontinence.

needs to be given to detecting focal neurological signs. Several laboratory and radiological investigations (Figs 17.1 and 17.2) are required and are listed in the information box below. Newer techniques can diagnose more subtle abnormalities (Fig. 17.3).

INVESTIGATIONS FOR DEMENTIA

- Full blood count
- Urea and electrolytes
- Liver function tests
- Thyroid function tests
- Syphilitic serology
- HIV antibodies
- Chest radiograph
- CT brain scan

Detailed assessment of intelligence should be carried out by a clinical psychologist. There are several available tests, the most widely used being the Wechsler Adult Intelligence Scale (WAIS). This provides an intelligence quotient (IQ) which expresses an individual's test score as a percentage of the mean scores obtained by samples of the population on whom the tests were standardised. The WAIS comprises 11 subtests, 6 of which are concerned with words or numbers and whose scores are combined to give a Verbal IQ; 5 other subtests are concerned with spatial ability, such as recognising patterns, and are combined to give a Performance IQ. The Verbal and Performance IQs are combined to give a Full Scale IQ. Psychometric testing has several functions; it is use-

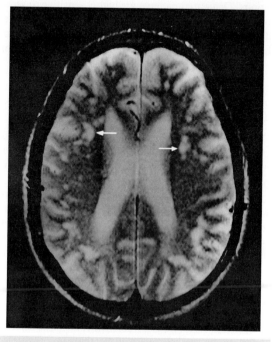

Fig. 17.3 Cerebrovascular dementia: MRI brain scan showing multiple, diffuse areas of vascular disease (arrowed).

ful when the diagnosis of dementia is in doubt, it gives a quantified assessment of deterioration, and repeat tests after an interval of at least 6 months allow the rapidity of change to be determined. Other specific psychological tests can be employed when localised lesions are suspected.

A behavioural assessment, conducted by an occupational therapist, indicates whether the patient has lost skills such as cooking, dressing, spatial orientation and the ability to handle money. These are important factors when considering whether independent living is still possible.

Any reversible cause should be treated appropriately, in which case a varying degree of functional recovery can be expected. In the majority of cases, where no remediable condition can be found, management should be directed at providing the best possible support for the patients and their families. Approximately half of Britain's elderly demented are maintained at home by their families. Local authority social services can provide domestic help and a meals delivery service. Attendance at a day centre can be arranged for patients whose relatives cannot cope with full-time supervision. For the more severely demented and for those without family support admission to residential homes for the elderly is necessary, while for those with heavy nursing requirements hospital admission becomes inevitable.

Drugs should be avoided unless there are specific indications. Demented patients are highly sensitive to sedative drugs; if medication is needed to treat episodes of confusion or excitement a small dose of a phenothiazine can be given, for example thioridazine 25 mg 8-hourly.

FOCAL ORGANIC DISORDERS

These arise from discrete cerebral lesions which affect specific cerebral functions, although in practice it is common for there to be some evidence of damage elsewhere in the brain.

In psychiatry the most significant disorder is the amnesic syndrome caused by thiamine deficiency. When this has an abrupt onset the patient becomes acutely confused; mental state examination reveals drowsiness, disorientation in time and place and an impaired ability to recall recent events or to register new information. Physical examination reveals a horizontal nystagmus, evidence of external ocular palsies, ataxia and peripheral neuropathy. This syndrome, known as Wernicke's encephalopathy, results from damage to the mammillary bodies, dorso-medial nuclei of the thalamus and adjacent areas of grey matter. In those who die in the acute stage microscopic examination of the brain shows hyperaemia, petechial haemorrhages and astrocytic proliferation. Wernicke's encephalopathy in Western countries is nearly always due to poor nutrition associated with chronic alcoholism; other causes are prolonged vomiting, diarrhoea and severe starvation.

Immediate treatment with thiamine 50 mg intravenously is essential to minimise permanent damage. Fluid replacement may also be required and intramuscular thiamine should be given daily until an adequate diet can be resumed. It is usual to give this with other vitamins in the form of parentrovite which is available as paired ampoules for injection, either as intravenous high potency, intramuscular high potency or intramuscular maintenance. One of the ampoules contains thiamine, riboflavin and pyridoxine and the other nicotinamide and ascorbic acid. 2–4 pairs of high potency intravenous ampoules are given 4–8-hourly for 2 days followed by high potency intramuscular injections daily for 5–7 days.

When recovery is incomplete a chronic amnesic syndrome develops, this being known as Korsakoff's psychosis. Characteristically the patient is fully conscious but has a profound impairment of memory recall and new learning ability. A striking feature is a tendency to confabulate, which has been defined as a falsification of memory in clear consciousness. For example if the patient is asked to describe his activities during the previous week he or she will reply by reporting events which have taken place many years previously. Confabulation probably results from an inability to distinguish the temporal sequence of past events. Other cognitive functions remain intact in the Korsakoff syndrome but the memory disturbance is often so profound that the patient is incapable of living independently and institutional care is required.

Amnesia also occurs in bilateral lesions of the hippocampus and hippocampal gyrus, which are situated on the inferomedial aspect of the temporal lobe. The conditions chiefly responsible are herpes simplex encephalitis and cerebrovascular disease localised to the posterior cerebral arteries. The clinical picture is similar to that of Korsakoff's psychosis except that confabulation does not occur.

Other deficits associated with focal brain lesions include expressive and receptive aphasias, apraxias and agnosias. These are described in detail in the Neurology chapter, page 1028 etc.

SUBSTANCE MISUSE

ALCOHOLISM

Alcohol consumption in the United Kingdom has risen greatly since the Second World War and this has been accompanied by increases in the social, psychological and physical problems due to alcohol. The term alcoholism is now used in a broad sense to describe a pattern of drinking which is harmful to the individual or to his or her family. The more restricted term, alcohol dependence, has the criteria listed in the information box.

CRITERIA OF ALCOHOL DEPENDENCE

- Narrowing of the drinking repertoire
- Priority of drinking over other activities
- Tolerance of effects of alcohol
- Repeated withdrawal symptoms
- Relief of withdrawal symptoms by further drinking
- Subjective compulsion to drink
- Reinstatement of drinking behaviour after abstinence

National statistics indicate that morbidity related to alcohol closely correlates with mean per capita consumption. Men are more likely to have alcohol-related problems than women, although the gap is closing. Approximately *one-quarter* of male patients in general hospital medical wards have a current or previous alcohol problem.

Aetiology

Although genetic factors make a small contribution to the development of alcohol abuse, cultural factors are much more important. Alcohol problems are rare among Muslims and Jews and common in countries which have large alcohol-producing industries, for example France, Italy and Portugal. In the United Kingdom problems are commoner among Scots and Irish. Availability of alcohol is important, as shown by high rates among those employed in the drink trade. Doctors previously held a high position in the occupational league table but are now only just above the average. There is a close correlation between consumption and the price of alcohol relative to average earnings. The cheaper the relative price the higher the consumption, with the effect that a larger proportion of the population will develop alcohol-related problems.

No consistent predisposing personality profile has been identified. Most people with alcohol problems are distinguished from the rest of the community simply by the fact that they drink more. The majority of alcoholics do not have an underlying psychiatric illness but in a few it appears that heavy drinking has developed in an attempt to relieve the unpleasant symptoms of an anxiety state, depression or schizophrenia.

Problems caused by alcohol

Many patients' alcohol problems are not detected by their doctors. A high index of suspicion is important,

particularly in cases where there are repeated consultations for vague symptoms or minor accidents. If in doubt a drinking history should be taken in which the patient is asked to describe a typical week's drinking. Consumption should be quantified in terms of units of alcohol; one unit contains approximately 9 g alcohol and is the equivalent of half a pint of beer, a single measure of spirits or a glass of table wine. Current opinion suggests that drinking becomes hazardous at levels above 21 units weekly for men and 14 units weekly for women. Conversely, there is some evidence which suggests that regular, modest consumption of alcohol may have a protective effect against the development of coronary artery disease. Laboratory tests are useful in confirming alcohol abuse. Mean corpuscular volume (MCV) or gamma-glutamyl transpeptidase (gamma GT) are raised in approximately 50% of problem drinkers. Although the low sensitivity of these tests makes them unsuitable for population screening, they are useful for monitoring treatment response in individual cases where their values were elevated originally.

Social problems

These include absenteeism from work, unemployment, marital tensions, child abuse, financial difficulties and problems with the law, including violence and traffic offences.

Psychological problems

Depression

This is common and is usually reactive to the numerous social problems which heavy drinking creates. Alcohol also has a direct depressant effect. Attempted suicide and completed suicide are much commoner in alcoholics than in the rest of society.

Morbid jealousy

This is a syndrome characterised by delusions of sexual infidelity. It is usually seen in alcoholics of sensitive or paranoid disposition whose sexual relationship has deteriorated because of impotence or rejection by the partner. The alcoholic suspects and accuses his or her partner of having a relationship with another person and goes to extreme lengths to obtain corroborative evidence, such as repeatedly searching the partner's personal possessions or employing a private detective to follow them. Accusations lead to violence and sometimes murder. Morbid jealousy can also occur in schizophrenia, depressive illness and paranoid personality disorder.

Withdrawal symptoms

These indicate physical dependence. The earliest manifestation is a subjective sensation of tension on waking in the morning. This may be accompanied by a tremor which makes it difficult to shave or hold a cup of tea. Another alcoholic drink relieves these symptoms, thus establishing a pattern of morning drinking. Less common but more serious withdrawal symptoms are epilepsy and delirium tremens, the latter having the features of a severe confusional state characterised by impaired consciousness, visual hallucinations, memory disturbance and seizures. Alcoholic hallucinosis also occurs following relative or absolute withdrawal. Its essential features are auditory hallucinations occurring in clear consciousness; the hallucinations take the form of derogatory or persecutory voices which discuss the individual in the third person or comment directly to him or her. They are similar to the auditory hallucinations reported by schizophrenics.

Vitamin deficiencies
These occur in alcoholics who have a severely impoverished diet. The most important is thiamine (B_1) deficiency which leads to the acute phenomena of Wernicke's encephalopathy or the chronic features of Korsakoff's syndrome (p. 992).

Direct toxic effects on the brain
These cause the familiar features of drunkenness. In very heavy drinkers there are periods of amnesia (alcoholic blackouts) for events which occurred during bouts of intoxication. When alcoholism has been established for several years, cortical atrophy can occur and the clinical picture of dementia develops.

Indirect effects on behaviour
These can result from head injury, hypoglycaemia and portasystemic encephalopathy.

Physical problems
These are protean and can affect virtually any organ in the body, giving rise to the comment that alcohol has replaced syphilis as the great mimic of disease. The diseases are grouped together in Figure 17.4 and are discussed in detail in their respective sections.

Management
Straightforward advice about the harmful effects of alcohol and safe levels of consumption is often all that is needed. In more serious cases patients may have to be advised to alter leisure activities or change jobs if these are contributing to the problem. Supportive psychotherapy is often crucial in helping the patient effect the necessary changes in lifestyle. Interpretive psychotherapy, either individual or group, can help patients who have recurrent relapses. Treatment of this type is available at specialised centres and is also provided by voluntary organisations such as Alcoholics Anonymous (AA).

Drug therapy also has a valuable role in treatment. Benzodiazepines are the drugs of choice for withdrawal symptoms and can be given safely in large doses (e.g. diazepam 20 mg 6-hourly) provided they are tailed off over a period of 5–7 days as symptoms subside. It is usual to give high dose vitamins during withdrawal treatment because of the possibility of thiamine deficiency. These are given in the form of 2–4 pairs of high potency intravenous ampoules of parentrovite (R) 4–8-hourly for 2 days followed by high potency intramuscular injections for 5–7 days. Only rarely are antidepressants required; the depressive symptoms, if present, usually resolve with abstinence. Phenothiazines (e.g. chlorpromazine 100 mg 8-hourly) are required for alcoholic hallucinosis. Disulfiram (200–400 mg daily) can be given as a deterrent to patients who have difficulty resisting sudden impulses to drink after becoming abstinent. The drug blocks the metabolism of alcohol, causing acetaldehyde to accumulate in the body. When alcohol is consumed by someone taking the drug there follows an unpleasant reaction consisting of headache, flushing, nausea and laboured breathing. Knowledge that this reaction will occur can provide an insurance against drinking and even remove craving. Disulfiram should always be seen as an adjunct to other treatments, especially supportive psychotherapy.

DRUG MISUSE

Dependence on illegal and prescribed drugs has become a major problem in Western countries during the last two decades. In the United Kingdom there are now 50 000–100 000 opiate addicts and 2% of the population regularly take benzodiazepines. Many of the aetiological factors which apply to alcohol abuse are also relevant to drug dependence. The main factors are cultural pressures, particularly within a peer group, and availability of a drug. In the case of some drugs availability has been increased by medical over-prescribing but there has also been a relative decline in price.

Benzodiazepines
More people are dependent on benzodiazepines than on any other group of drugs. They are effective anti-anxiety drugs if given in short courses but tolerance occurs after 6 weeks of daily consumption. Withdrawal symptoms can then occur if the drug is stopped abruptly. These include anxiety, increased sensory perception, epileptic fits and psychotic experiences. Withdrawal symptoms are particularly likely to occur with short-acting drugs such as lorazepam. Benzodiazepine dependence nearly always occurs because the drugs have been prescribed

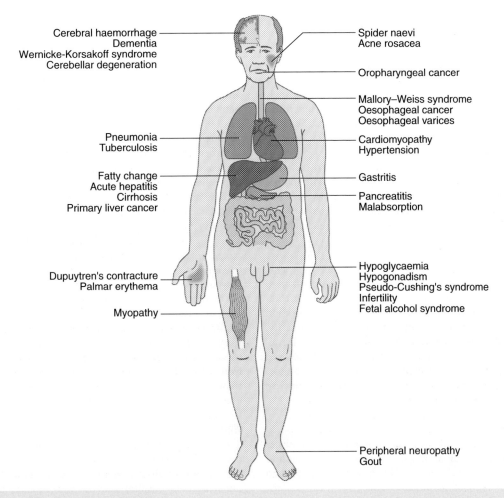

Cerebral haemorrhage
Dementia
Wernicke-Korsakoff syndrome
Cerebellar degeneration

Spider naevi
Acne rosacea

Oropharyngeal cancer

Mallory–Weiss syndrome
Oesophageal cancer
Oesophageal varices

Pneumonia
Tuberculosis

Cardiomyopathy
Hypertension

Fatty change
Acute hepatitis
Cirrhosis
Primary liver cancer

Gastritis

Pancreatitis
Malabsorption

Dupuytren's contracture
Palmar erythema

Hypoglycaemia
Hypogonadism
Pseudo-Cushing's syndrome
Infertility
Fetal alcohol syndrome

Myopathy

Peripheral neuropathy
Gout

Fig. 17.4 Physical effects of alcohol abuse.

for the wrong reasons or because repeat prescriptions have been issued for several months. However, there is also a vogue for intravenous benzodiazepines, notably temazepam, among some adolescent groups who have never been given medical prescriptions for the drug.

Cannabis

Cannabis, derived from the plant *Cannabis sativa*, is usually smoked mixed with tobacco. It quickly produces a sensation of relaxation and well-being; psychological dependence is common but tolerance and withdrawal symptoms are unusual. It is probably the commonest illegal drug taken in the United Kingdom and is often the only drug with which young people experiment. The extent of its use cannot be estimated reliably.

A toxic confusional state occurs after heavy consumption and acute psychotic episodes are well recognised. Long-term consequences of regular consumption

are also being appreciated. One of the first effects to be described was the 'amotivational syndrome', characterised by apathy and slothfulness. Cerebral atrophy has also been described and recent reports suggest that chronic consumption can lead to a schizophrenia-like illness.

Barbiturates

These are now rarely prescribed, having been replaced as hypnotics by benzodiazepines. However, they are still taken by some people who manage to obtain them indirectly from doctors. They soon cause dependence, and sudden withdrawal is very likely to cause epileptic fits. Barbiturates are dangerous in overdose because of their depressant effect on respiration.

Opiates

Morphine, heroin and codeine are the main drugs in this group, with heroin having become especially prominent recently. Heroin, which is taken orally, intravenously or by inhalation, gives a rapid, intensely pleasurable experience, often accompanied by heightened sexual arousal. Physical dependence occurs within a few weeks of regular high-dose injection, with the result that the dose is escalated and the addict's life becomes increasingly centred around obtaining and taking the drug. Intravenous users are prone to bacterial infections, hepatitis B and human immunodeficiency virus (HIV) infection through needle contamination. Accidental overdose is common. The withdrawal syndrome, which can start within 12 hours in some people, can present with intense craving, rhinorrhoea, lacrimation, yawning, perspiration, shivering, piloerection, vomiting, diarrhoea and abdominal cramps. Examination shows a tachycardia, hypertension, mydriasis and facial flushing.

Amphetamines

These have a stimulating central effect and are taken to produce increased energy, elevated mood and greater capacity for concentration. There is also a suppression of appetite which accounts for their use in obesity. Amphetamines are taken orally or intravenously. Physical dependence is unusual but withdrawal of the drug results in rebound depression, anxiety and fatigue. Chronic ingestion can cause a syndrome identical to paranoid schizophrenia.

Cocaine

Cocaine is becoming increasingly popular, taken either intravenously or by sniffing or 'snorting' the powder into the nostrils through a tube. Absorption occurs through the nasal mucous membranes and gives a rapid stimulating effect similar to amphetamine. Cocaine hydrochloride may be converted by a simple chemical process into freebase or 'crack' cocaine which can be smoked, giving a rapid onset of effect similar to intravenous use. A toxic psychosis occurs with high levels of consumption, and tactile hallucinations (formication) may be prominent. Chronic cocaine sniffing can cause ulceration of the nasal mucosa.

Hallucinogenic drugs

Lysergic acid diethylamide (LSD) and psilocybin (magic mushroom) are currently the most commonly used hallucinogens. Perceptual changes occur within 40 minutes of oral ingestion. Vision is affected most often; the subject experiences heightened visual awareness of objects, especially colours. Images may be distorted in shape or size and true hallucinations occur. These can be terrifying in nature, the experience then being referred to as a 'bad trip'. There may also be distorted perception of time, sounds and tactile sensations. Flashback experiences can occur several months after the last dose;

during these the psychotic experiences of LSD are experienced again with their original intensity. A chronic psychotic illness has also been reported after regular LSD use.

Ecstasy, the popular name for a synthetic amphetamine analogue, has become fashionable among young people for recreational use at dance parties or 'raves'. It has both stimulant and hallucinogenic properties, thus producing feelings of euphoria and emotional intimacy together with distorted sensory perceptions. There is no evidence that it is addictive but there are several reports of physical complications. Fatalities have occurred from cardiac arrhythmias, hyperthermia, disseminated intravascular coagulation and cerebral haemorrhage. Paranoid psychoses have also been reported.

Organic solvents

The inhalation of organic solvents (glue sniffing) has become popular in some adolescent groups. These substances produce acute intoxication characterised by euphoria, excitement, dizziness and a floating sensation. Further inhalation leads to loss of consciousness; death can occur from the direct toxic effect of the solvent or from asphyxiation if the substance is inhaled from a plastic bag.

Management of drug abuse

The first step in management is usually aimed at helping the patient withdraw from the drug. When there are signs of severe physical dependence withdrawal is best undertaken in hospital and this also enables physical complications, such as infections, to be treated. Decreasing doses of the relevant drug are given over a period of 1–3 weeks, the dose being titrated against objective withdrawal symptoms. Oral methadone is used for opiate dependence. In some cases complete withdrawal is not successful and the patient functions better if maintained on regular doses of oral methadone as an outpatient. This decision should only be undertaken by a specialist and the long-term supervision requires the patient to attend a specially designated drug treatment centre. The withdrawal period may need to be extended to several months for some drugs, for example benzodiazepines. A regime for managing benzodiazepine withdrawal is shown in the information box below.

Long-term support is necessary if patients are to remain drug free. Many doctors can achieve good results if they strike up a rapport with the patient. Complicated or relapsing patients should be referred to specialist centres. Support can also be provided by self-help groups and voluntary bodies such as Narcotics Anonymous.

MANAGING BENZODIAZEPINE WITHDRAWAL

1. Reduce daily dose by 1/8 every fortnight
2. For patients taking a drug other than diazepam and who cannot reduce it, switch to equivalent dose of diazepam preferably taken at night
3. Reduce diazepam by 2 or 2.5 mg every fortnight
4. If withdrawal symptoms occur maintain the dose until symptoms improve
5. Reduce dose further in fortnightly steps until drug stopped completely
6. Provide regular counselling
7. Avoid other drugs (e.g. beta antagonists, antidepressants) unless specifically indicated
8. It is better to reduce too slowly than too quickly. Successful withdrawal may take a year or more

SCHIZOPHRENIA

In terms of its disabilities and chronicity, schizophrenia is the most serious of all psychiatric illnesses. It affects 1% of the adult population at some time in their lives and, when uniform diagnostic criteria are used, the prevalence is similar throughout the world. Descriptions of schizophrenia in medical literature are sparse until the nineteenth century. Then the German psychiatrist Emil Kraepelin distinguished two major groups of insanity, manic depression which nearly always had a favourable outcome and dementia praecox which usually ran a chronic course. The term schizophrenia replaced dementia praecox after its introduction by Eugen Bleuler in 1911.

Aetiology

Genetic factors

There is no doubt that schizophrenia can be transmitted genetically. Relatives of a schizophrenic have a risk of developing schizophrenia much higher than the general population life-time risk of 1%, and this increases with the degree of genetic proximity. Siblings of a schizophrenic have an 8% risk of developing the illness, children have a 12% chance but when both parents are affected this increases to 35% or more. Twin studies have provided further support. The risk for dizygotic twins is approximately the same as for non-twin siblings whereas for monozygotic twins it is of the order of 45–60%. This high risk for identical twins prevails even if the twins have been reared apart. Similarly adoption studies have shown that the increased risk for children of a schizophrenic parent continues in those cases where the children have been adopted at birth and brought up by healthy parents.

Psychological factors

No convincing evidence has been found to support the various hypotheses that abnormal family relationships have a causal influence on schizophrenia. However, it is established that the family environment can influence the course of the illness. An atmosphere in which there are high levels of emotional expression appears harmful to schizophrenics and contributes to relapses of the illness. It is therefore advisable for patients to avoid returning to a family who are critical or who are emotionally over-involved and they do better in an emotionally neutral atmosphere which can be provided in a hostel or group home.

Psychological stress plays a part in precipitating episodes of the illness. It has been shown that schizophrenics are likely to have been exposed to a variety of adverse life events in the three weeks leading up to the onset of acute symptoms.

Viral infections

Epidemiological studies have consistently shown that schizophrenics are more likely to have been born in the winter months. This suggests the influence of some environmental factor on the development of schizophrenia and there is accumulating evidence to implicate viral infections, especially influenza, in intrauterine life or during the immediate post-natal period.

Cerebral disease

The introduction of the computed tomography (CT) scan has shown that up to one-third of chronically ill schizophrenic patients have evidence of brain damage, particularly ventricular enlargement. This brain damage may have been acquired in utero, at birth or in early childhood. Viral infections and obstetric complications have been implicated as causal factors, probably resulting in a neurodevelopmental disorder. The schizophrenia syndrome can also be associated with a wide range of cerebral pathology which becomes evident in adult life, including temporal lobe epilepsy, Huntington's chorea, cerebral tumor and demyelinating diseases. This is known as symptomatic schizophrenia.

Neurotransmitter disturbance

The final pathway by which the various aetiological factors cause schizophrenia may be by interfering with neurotransmitter substances in the brain. The most convincing hypothesis suggests that there is a functional overactivity in the dopaminergic neuronal systems in the mesolimbic and mesocortical areas. Drugs which stimulate central dopamine receptors, such as amphetamines and L-dopa, are known to induce symptoms identical to those seen in paranoid schizophrenia. On the other hand drugs which are effective in the treatment of schizophrenia are known to block dopamine receptors. There is also evidence from postmortem studies that the brains of schizophrenics have an increased number of dopamine receptors.

Immigration

Recent reports of exceptionally high hospital admission rates due to schizophrenia among the Afro-Caribbean population in Britain have renewed interest in the role of immigration and its associated stress in the development of the illness. This remains a controversial topic and it is not clear whether the incidence of schizophrenia among Afro-Caribbeans resident in Britain is higher than in their countries of origin. The influence of cannabis may be a contributory factor if the high rates are confirmed.

Clinical features

The term schizophrenia describes a clinical syndrome based on abnormalities reported in the patient's history and observed during mental state examination. The concept of schizophrenia varies slightly from one country to another and some psychiatrists attach particular diagnostic importance to the chronic duration of symptoms and onset before the age of 45. However, there is less debate about the characteristic mental state abnormalities. These appear to result from a breakdown in the normal ability to distinguish between experiences arising from the inner self and those coming from the outside world. This phenomenon is aptly described as a dissolution of ego boundaries. The most striking features are the **first rank symptoms** delineated by Kurt Schneider. He believed that a diagnosis of schizophrenia should be made if one or more of these symptoms is present and if the patient is not suffering from structural brain disease or a confusional state. The symptoms of first-rank importance are given in the information box.

In the **acute** stages of schizophrenia approximately **two-thirds** of patients have at least one first-rank symptom. The patient may have other symptoms which are of lower diagnostic significance but which in combination give rise to the diagnosis. These other symptoms are listed in the information box below.

The features described in the information boxes are known as the **positive symptoms** of schizophrenia and some of them are usually present during the acute illness. If there are recurrent episodes, or if recovery is incomplete, the clinical picture can change so that it becomes dominated by **negative symptoms**. These symptoms are listed in the information box below.

Course and prognosis

The four patterns of outcome which have been distinguished are listed in the information box below.

FIRST-RANK SYMPTOMS OF SCHIZOPHRENIA

- **Thought insertion**
  The experience of having thoughts put into one's mind by another person, or of thinking someone else's thoughts
- **Thought withdrawal**
  The experience of one's own thoughts being taken away
- **Thought broadcasting**
  The sensation that one's thoughts are known to other people, sometimes described as a feeling that thoughts are being transmitted by telepathy or radio waves
- **Passivity feelings**
  Emotions, bodily movements or specific sensations which are perceived as being caused and controlled by an external object or another person
- **Auditory hallucinations**
  Voices discussing the patient in the third person. One or more voices keeping up a running commentary on the patient's thoughts or actions. The experience of hearing one's own thoughts being spoken out loud; this is also known as 'thought echoing'
- **Delusional perceptions**
  A primary delusion which arises from a normal perception which is given delusional significance: e.g. a man who saw a woman lighting a cigarette immediately realised this meant he was to be the next king of England.

OTHER SYMPTOMS OF SCHIZOPHRENIA

- **Catatonia**
  Motor abnormalities of two extreme types, excitable overactivity on the one hand and bizarre posturing with abnormal muscle tone (waxy flexibility) on the other
- **Thought disorder**
  A loosening of association between concepts so that thinking lacks a logical flow and appears incoherent to other people
- **Neologisms**
  Newly made-up words
- **Delusions**
  Of a grandiose, paranoid, sexual or religious nature
- **Hallucinations**
  Visual, tactile, olfactory or gustatory
- **Affective change**
  The patient may appear bewildered or perplexed by his or her various strange experiences. There may also be incongruity of affect in which the patient laughs without appropriate stimulus or in response to events which would not be expected to elicit a jocular reaction

---

Several factors have been identified which influence the prognosis and these are listed in the information box.

Management

Hospital admission is necessary for a first episode of acute schizophrenia to permit a full physical and psy-

CASE HISTORY

A 24-year-old man was brought to hospital by the police after being involved in a fight with a neighbour whom he accused of inserting an electronic transmitter into his brain. One year previously he dropped out of university in his final year because of declining interest in his subject and difficulty concentrating on the relevant reading material. He believed that the electronic device had been inserted to transmit his thoughts to the police who he believed held him responsible for a political assassination. He also reported hearing the voices of his neighbour and local police officers talking about him in a derogatory and accusatory manner. His parents reported that a paternal grandmother had developed schizophrenia in middle age and had spent the last 20 years of her life in a psychiatric hospital. His symptoms responded well to treatment with chlorpromazine but he refused to take medication once he left hospital and he had to be readmitted 1 year later with a recurrence of similar symptoms.

PROGNOSTIC FACTORS IN SCHIZOPHRENIA

Good prognosis
- Acute onset of symptoms
- Obvious precipitating factor
- Prominent affective symptoms
- Catatonic symptoms
- No family history of schizophrenia
- Normal personality
- Stable work record
- Calm family environment

Poor prognosis
- Insidious onset of symptoms
- No precipitating factor
- Flattened affect
- No catatonic symptoms
- Family history of schizophrenia
- Schizoid personality
- Poor work record
- Highly emotional family environment

NEGATIVE SYMPTOMS OF SCHIZOPHRENIA

- **Social withdrawal**
  The patient avoids interacting with other people, appears unable to motivate himself or herself to work and cannot cope with daily living activities. He/she loses interest in himself/herself and other people. The patient's manner is generally apathetic
- **Poverty of speech**
  Speech is sparse, conversation is not initiated and answers to questions are monosyllabic or empty. The poverty of speech reflects the poverty of thinking
- **Flatness of affect**
  The patient's mood has a dull, monotonous quality. There is a loss of the normal day-to-day variation in mood and there is little or no response to emotionally charged external events.

OUTCOME IN SCHIZOPHRENIA

- 20% make a full recovery from the acute illness and have no relapses
- 35% recover completely but have repeated relapses with full recovery each time
- 35% have recurrent acute episodes with incomplete recovery each time. They are left with negative symptoms which become more disabling after each relapse
- 10% have a rapid downhill course from the outset and have persistent positive and negative symptoms

chiatric assessment and to allow medication to be increased quickly to suppress symptoms.

Neuroleptic drugs (Table 17.3, p. 985)
These are the mainstay of treatment and the choice is often governed by individual preference and familiarity with a particular drug. However, there are significant differences between the drugs. Thioridazine has fewer extrapyramidal side-effects, chlorpromazine can be given intramuscularly as well as orally, while trifluoperazine is less sedative than the other two. Haloperidol has fewer cardiotoxic effects. A conventional regime would be to start with chlorpromazine 100 mg 8-hourly building up gradually to a maximum of 1500 mg daily or until symptoms are abolished. Higher doses are required initially if the patient is aggressive or agitated, for example chlorpromazine 150 mg orally or intramuscularly 6-hourly. In patients who do not respond well to one drug, improvement can occur after switching to an equivalent dose of another preparation. When symptoms have improved it is usual to reduce the dose or to change to one of the long-acting intramuscular neuroleptics which need only be given once every two weeks (e.g. fluphenazine 20–100 mg fortnightly or flupenthixol 40–200 mg fortnightly). Depot injections improve compliance with treatment as many patients forget or cannot be bothered to take oral drugs every day once they are better. Dosage should be kept as low as possible to avoid recurrent psychotic symptoms. Parkinsonism is a troublesome side-effect and many patients require anti-Parkinsonian drugs as well (e.g. procyclidine 5 mg 8-hourly). Other extrapyramidal side-effects include akathisia, dystonias and tardive dyski-

nesia. The newer drugs, sulpiride, remoxipride and risperidone, can be used as alternatives if extrapyramidal symptoms develop. Clozapine, recently reintroduced after having been abandoned in the 1970s because of agranulocytosis, also has a low incidence of extrapyramidal side-effects and appears to be more effective than conventional neuroleptics in treating resistant schizophrenia. It has to be given under close haematological monitoring and this makes it relatively expensive.

The duration of drug treatment is controversial. When the features of the illness and the patient's premorbid adjustment suggest a favourable prognosis it is common practice to tail off medication gradually after 12 months and to stop it completely unless there are signs of relapse. When the prognosis is poor most psychiatrists continue maintenance medication indefinitely.

Social measures

These become increasingly important as the patient recovers. Schizophrenics do best in an environment which has a regular, predictable routine. Positive symptoms are exacerbated in highly-charged emotional situations while negative symptoms are induced in environments which are understimulating, such as was often the case in mental hospital wards for the chronically ill. Considerable efforts are now made to discharge the patient from hospital after a brief admission lasting only a few weeks. If the home environment is not suitable, accommodation can be provided in a hostel or group home. Alternatively if these facilities are unavailable family therapy conducted along behavioural lines can be arranged to help modify the family's behaviour towards the patient. The specific aims are to reduce the level of emotional expression and face-to-face contact thereby creating a more neutral atmosphere which is less harmful to the patient.

Those who are unable to return to their previous employment can regain occupational skills at special rehabilitation centres. Preparation for this facility can be made by regular occupational therapy during the hospital admission.

AFFECTIVE DISORDERS

The fundamental abnormality of an affective disorder is a disturbance of mood, either depression or mania. Depression is by far the commoner; most patients who have manic symptoms are also prone to depressive episodes but the reverse does not apply. In a few cases depressive and manic symptoms occur simultaneously or in rapid succession (mixed affective state).

There are many ways of classifying affective illnesses, none of which is entirely satisfactory. The simplest classification divides them into **primary** and **secondary** disorders.

Primary affective disorders

These are not secondary to any other psychiatric or physical illness but may be precipitated by a wide range of environmental factors. They are often recurrent; if recurrences always take a depressive form the term **unipolar** disorder is used; if the recurrences are both manic and depressive the term **bipolar** is used.

Secondary affective disorders

These follow another psychiatric (alcoholism, schizophrenia) or physical illness. In the latter case the mood change is usually due to the emotional impact of the illness but in some patients it is due to anatomical or physiological changes in the brain and may be the presenting feature of the underlying physical illness. These are described as organic or symptomatic affective disorders.

Epidemiology

Community studies have shown that the prevalence rate for depression, defined by strict operational criteria, is approximately 6–8% for women and 3–5% for men. Depression is commoner in the lower social classes and among inner city dwellers. Women in their child-bearing years are especially vulnerable.

Bipolar disorder is less common, having a prevalence rate of 1%. There is no difference in prevalence between the sexes nor between social classes.

Aetiological factors

Genetics

There is convincing evidence from adoption and twin studies of a genetic contribution to bipolar disorders although the mode of inheritance is not clear. The genetic basis of unipolar depression has not been established with such certainty.

Environment

Many environmental factors have been implicated but the three most consistently involved are loss of a parent in childhood, lack of social support and recent adverse life events. For women a profile of vulnerability factors has been defined and is given in the information box below.

While these factors do not in themselves necessarily cause depression, they increase the likelihood that depression will follow major life events involving a loss of some kind.

VULNERABILITY FACTORS FOR AFFECTIVE DISORDERS

- Loss of mother before age of 11
- Three or more children under 14 living at home
- Lack of confiding relationship
- Lack of full-time or part-time employment

Physical illness

All physical illnesses can be followed by depression, especially those like cancer and heart disease which carry serious implications. There is considerable interest in the role of viral illnesses in causing depression. Prolonged mood change can follow infectious mononucleosis or influenza. Some doctors believe a chronic fatigue syndrome (myalgic encephalomyelitis—ME) can be caused by coxsackie or other viral infections.

Depression, or less often mania, can be the presenting feature of cerebrovascular disease, neurological disorders such as multiple sclerosis and Parkinsonism and endocrine diseases such as Cushing's syndrome, Addison's disease and hypothyroidism. Mood change can also be associated with drug therapy, for example corticosteroids, beta-adrenoceptor antagonists and other anti-hypertensive drugs (e.g. alpha-methyl dopa). When mood disorders result directly from physical causes such as these they are known as organic affective disorders.

Personality

Some depressives have personality characteristics which are thought to predispose to the illness. These involve a negative attitude to oneself, the outside world and the future; the term 'cognitive triad' has been applied to these attitudes. The personality most typically associated with bipolar illness is a cyclothymic one.

Clinical features of depression

The most fundamental symptom, although not always the most prominent, is **depression of mood**. This varies considerably in severity from one patient to another and even within the individual from time to time. There is no clear separation between the mood change of a clinically depressed patient and everyday unhappiness. Mood varies on a continuum and the diagnosis of depressive illness is made depending on the presence of associated features. There may be a diurnal variation of mood, depression being most distressing early in the morning or at the end of the day. Accompanying psychological symptoms are loss of pleasure in life (anhedonia), loss of interest in oneself and others, low self-esteem, self-blame and hopelessness. Suicidal thinking is common. In mild depression this consists of a passive wish to be dead but in more severe cases there are active

thoughts of suicide and patients may have made detailed plans as to how they will end their lives. Severe depression may also be accompanied by feelings of guilt and worthlessness which are delusional in nature.

Somatic symptoms may dominate the clinical picture and are the symptoms with which depressed patients usually present to a general practitioner or physician. These symptoms are listed in the information box.

SOMATIC SYMPTOMS OF DEPRESSION

- Sleep disturbance (initial insomnia, early morning wakening or hypersomnia)
- Fatigue
- Headache
- Other pains (e.g. chest pain, abdominal pain)
- Anorexia
- Weight change
- Constipation
- Reduced libido
- Poor concentration
- Psychomotor retardation

The diagnosis of a depressive illness is based on the presence of mood disturbance together with some of the associated features. The criteria in the information box below are those currently proposed by the American Psychiatric Association for the diagnosis of a major depressive episode.

At least five of the symptoms listed in the information box below, including at least one of the first two, must be present nearly every day over a 2-week period. To justify the diagnosis of a major depressive episode it is also necessary to establish that the symptoms are not associated with a bereavement reaction, organic lesion or other psychotic disorder. The terms minor depressive episode or dysthymic disorder are applied to depressive symptoms which are not sufficiently severe to warrant the diagnosis of major depression.

DIAGNOSTIC CRITERIA FOR DEPRESSION

- Depressed mood most of the day
- Markedly diminished interest in almost all activities most of the day
- Significant weight loss or weight gain (at least 5% in one month)
- Insomnia or hypersomnia
- Psychomotor retardation or agitation
- Fatigue or loss of energy
- Feelings of worthlessness or excessive guilt
- Diminished ability to think or concentrate, or indecisiveness
- Recurrent thoughts of death or suicide; a suicide attempt or a specific plan for suicide

CASE HISTORY

A 44-year-old woman employed as a bank clerk complained of headaches, dizziness and poor concentration which prevented her working effectively. She was convinced she had a brain tumour and insisted that her general practitioner refer her to a neurologist. Physical examination was normal, as was a CT brain scan. At the follow-up interview the patient kept bursting into tears; she told the neurologist her father had died 9 months previously and her 16-year-old son had been treated for leukaemia, which was currently in remission. She reported weight loss of 6 kg, early morning waking and a recent complete loss of sexual desire. She was prescribed antidepressant medication and referred to a clinical psychologist for bereavement counselling. Within 3 months she had made a complete recovery and the medication was tailed off after a further 3 months.

Management

Outpatient management is appropriate in most cases. Admission is necessary when there is a strong risk of suicide or when social supports are inadequate. Compulsory admission under the Mental Health Act is required for suicidal patients who do not accept voluntary treatment.

Antidepressant drugs (Table 17.4, p. 986)

These relieve depressive symptoms in approximately two-thirds of patients. A tricyclic drug is the first choice of treatment. It needs to be given in adequate doses for at least 6 weeks (e.g. amitriptyline 75–150 mg at night) and then, if symptoms have responded it should be continued at a lower dose for at least 6 months to prevent relapse. Patients should be advised that there may be a delay of 2 to 3 weeks between starting treatment and therapeutic improvement. If response to a tricyclic is poor one of the other drugs such as a selective serotonin reuptake inhibitor (e.g. fluoxetine 20–80 mg daily) or monoamine oxidase inhibitor (MAOI) (e.g. phenelzine 15 mg 4 times daily) or mianserin (30–90 mg at night) should be tried. Some psychiatrists use an MAOI as a first choice drug when depression is accompanied by prominent anxiety or phobic symptoms or if there is hypersomnia or hyperphagia.

Cognitive therapy

This has been used successfully in combination with antidepressants and is indicated especially for patients whose depression seems to be perpetuated by a negative pattern of thinking.

Electroconvulsive therapy (ECT)

This is indicated when the risk of suicide is so great that one cannot wait for the delayed therapeutic effect of antidepressant drugs. ECT should also be given to patients in depressive stupor, when there are psychotic symptoms or when medication has been ineffective. In approximately 10% of cases depression does not respond to drugs used singly or to ECT. These patients should be treated with **combined antidepressants**, the most popular combination being lithium and a tricyclic or MAOI.

Clinical features of mania

The psychological features of mania are the exact opposite of those of depression. There is a sense of well-being which may be evident as elation or even ecstasy. Confidence and self-esteem are high; patients may have grandiose ideas which have little substance but upon which they may act. Thus they may embark on ruinous business ventures or put themselves at risk through reckless behaviour. The grandiose beliefs may involve delusions of being especially gifted or connected to well-known people such as royalty or entertainers. They feel highly energetic, thoughts come rapidly and speech is so fast that it appears to be generated under pressure. Thoughts jump from one topic to another with only chance connections between them (flight of ideas). There may be rhyming speech.

Motor activity is increased. Appetite is enhanced at first although in established mania the patient has no time to eat so weight falls and physical health suffers. The hours of sleep are reduced; typically patients wake after a few hours feeling full of energy and wanting to get on with work or leisure activities. Promiscuity may occur with consequent risk of exposure to sexually transmitted diseases.

CASE HISTORY

Increasing interpersonal problems at work led a 32-year-old journalist to be referred to an occupational health physician and thence to a psychiatrist. The patient had become grandiose in his manner during the previous 2 months, challenging the decisions of senior editorial staff and voicing his intention to take over the editorial chair. The quality of his writing had declined and he often failed to meet publishing deadlines. When seen he was elated in mood; he had an inflated opinion of his abilities, pressure of speech and constantly jumped from one topic to another. His manner was overfamiliar and he paced repeatedly up and down the interview room. He had twice previously been treated for depression and his father had committed suicide 3 years previously. He was considered to be in a manic phase of a bipolar affective illness and he was prescribed chlorpromazine as an outpatient with gradual recovery during the next 4 weeks. In view of the recurrent nature of his illness he agreed to take long-term prophylactic lithium.

Management

Neuroleptic drugs, either haloperidol (10–30 mg daily) or a phenothiazine (chlorpromazine 100–1500 mg daily) suppress the features of mania in nearly all cases. ECT is useful when symptoms are resistant to medication.

Lithium carbonate is indicated as prophylactic treatment for patients who have had two or more episodes of affective illness, either depression or mania, requiring medical treatment within the previous 2 years. Before starting lithium patients should be screened for thyroid (serum thyroxine, TSH and thyroid antibodies) and renal (plasma urea and creatinine) disease. Serum lithium should be kept within the therapeutic range of 0.5–1.0 mmol/l. This is usually achieved with a daily dose of lithium carbonate of 800–1200 mg. Lithium levels should be measured every 3 or 4 months and thyroid and renal function should be assessed 6-monthly.

It is not known how long lithium should be continued but, given that recurrent affective illnesses are largely constitutional, there is much to be said for continuing lithium indefinitely if relapses are prevented or attenuated. Recently carbamazepine (400–1200 mg daily) has been used as an alternative prophylaxis for patients who do not respond to lithium.

NEUROTIC, STRESS-RELATED AND SOMATOFORM DISORDERS

ANXIETY DISORDERS

Generalised anxiety

Anxiety is a universal experience which has an important protective function in the face of danger. It becomes morbid when symptoms are out of proportion to external circumstances or if they persist long after a threatening situation has been averted. However, there is no clear distinction between the features of normal and pathological anxiety. Symptoms of anxiety are prominent in other psychiatric disorders, such as depressive illness and schizophrenia, so it is important to look for features of these conditions before making a diagnosis of anxiety disorder. Several physical illnesses can present with anxiety and are listed in the information box.

These need to be considered in the differential diagnosis but special investigations are necessary only when there are suggestive features in the history or clinical examination.

If operational criteria are used, generalised anxiety disorder has a prevalence of between 2 and 5% with women being more susceptible than men.

PHYSICAL ILLNESSES WHICH MIMIC ANXIETY DISORDER

- Hyperthyroidism
- Phaeochromocytoma
- Hypoglycaemia
- Paroxysmal atrial arrhythmias
- Alcohol withdrawal
- Temporal lobe epilepsy

With regard to aetiology, genetic studies indicate there is a small genetic contribution. Many patients appear to have personality traits of high anxiety and poor tolerance of stress but perhaps the most important factors are unexpected life events which the patient cannot handle. Sometimes these are relatively minor events, within the range of everyday experience.

The clinical features of generalised anxiety are conveniently divided into two groups, psychological and somatic, and are shown in the information box below.

SYMPTOMS OF ANXIETY DISORDER

- **Psychological**
  Apprehension
  Fears of impending disaster
  Irritability
  Depersonalisation

- **Somatic**
  Tremor
  Sweating
  Palpitations
  Chest pain
  Breathlessness
  Headache
  Dizziness
  Diarrhoea
  Frequency of micturition
  Initial insomnia
  Poor concentration

Any of these can form the main presenting symptom; if somatic symptoms predominate, the patient is likely to regard himself or herself as physically ill, a view which is often shared initially by his or her doctor.

Phobic anxiety

A phobia is an abnormal fear which is brought on by a particular object or situation and which leads to avoidance of the provoking stimulus. Community surveys of phobic disorders have shown a prevalence of 6–8% but only a small proportion of these are sufficiently distressing to need treatment. Phobias have been classified as shown in the information box below.

Few clear aetiological factors have been identified. Most phobias are commoner in women and a genetic contribution is probably important. Psychologists have explained phobias in terms of learning theory as being due to conditioning following exposure to a traumatic event in childhood. However, it is unusual to uncover specific traumas when taking a history from a phobic patient.

The clinical features vary according to the type of phobia but the key elements are the psychological and somatic symptoms of anxiety together with avoidance. Agoraphobia is the most disabling because of the extensive range of provoking situations. Agoraphobic symptoms can be brought on in open spaces, crowded shopping centres, supermarkets, cinemas, churches and public transport. Symptoms become progressively more severe when the patient ventures further away from home, particularly when unaccompanied. Thus there is an increasing restriction in life style so that in extreme cases the patient is virtually house-bound. Social phobias are triggered by situations which involve personal interaction in public, such as eating or speaking in front of others. This type of phobia is particularly disruptive to social life and to the careers of people whose work involves public engagements. Animal and other specific phobias are less disruptive. The patient is often able to modify his or her behaviour without much difficulty so that daily activities are hardly affected. However, some specific phobias, such as of flying, may be sufficiently handicapping to require treatment.

Panic disorder

This consists of recurrent attacks of severe anxiety which are sudden and unpredictable. Although they are not related to particular situations they may lead to secondary agoraphobic symptoms. Panic disorder has a prevalence of less than 1%. Little is known about its aetiology; some psychiatrists regard it as a variant of depressive illness.

The key feature is a sudden attack of intense anxiety. Physical symptoms are prominent, especially palpitations, chest pain and breathlessness, and the patient often fears he or she is about to die. The attack lasts from a few minutes to as long as 2 hours. Between attacks the patient is free of anxiety although secondary avoidance behaviour may be prominent.

Management of the anxiety disorders

Psychological approach

Explanation and reassurance are essential in the management of all forms of anxiety. The nature of the symptoms should be explained and the patients reassured that they form part of a recognised illness. Reassurance is also needed to allay fears of physical illness if this can be done after appropriate examination and investigation. Specific relaxation techniques should be taught to those who do not respond to reassurance, and are always required for patients with panic attacks. For phobic disorders relaxation should be accompanied by graded exposure (desensitisation) or flooding.

Drugs

Drugs have a limited role. Benzodiazepines are prescribed less often than previously because of the risk of dependence but they are useful in treating anxiety when symptoms can be expected to last no more than a few weeks. Diazepam can be given in doses of 2–10 mg 8-hourly but should be reduced and tailed off after 3 weeks or dependence may occur. A beta-adrenoceptor blocking drug, such as propranolol 20–80 mg daily, can help when the peripheral somatic symptoms of anxiety are prominent. Antidepressant drugs, either a tricyclic (amitriptyline 50–150 mg at night) or MAOI (phenelzine 15 mg 6-hourly), are the most effective drugs in managing anxiety and should be used for generalised anxiety when symptoms do not respond to psychological approaches. They can be given in conjunction with behaviour therapy for phobic disorders and appear to be very effective for panic attacks.

OBSESSIVE COMPULSIVE DISORDER

An obsessional symptom is an unwanted thought or impulse which enters the subject's mind repeatedly despite his or her conscious resistance. These symptoms can occur in schizophrenia and depression but when they are primary phenomena a diagnosis of obsessive compulsive disorder is made. This has a prevalence of approximately 1–3%, but many people with the condition do not request treatment.

Aetiology

Genetic factors are important, as is the previous personality, which is usually characterised by traits of perfectionism, rigidity and conscientiousness. Organic brain disease has been implicated in the light of the occurrence of obsessional symptoms after outbreaks of encephalitis lethargica. However, in the great majority of cases seen in current practice there is no evidence of cerebral disease.

Clinical features

Obsessional symptoms are recognised as coming from the subject's own mind. Common themes include repeated thoughts of becoming aggressive or fears of contamination with dirt or chemical substances. These thoughts are often followed by rituals which are patterns of behaviour developed to relieve the anxiety generated by the original obsession. The rituals involve repeated checking, handwashing or changing of clothes. The condition tends to follow a relapsing course so patients may experience distress over many years.

CASE HISTORY

A 29-year-old woman was referred to a psychiatric department by her general practitioner because of a 14-year history of obsessional handwashing. During her adolescence she feared her hands might be contaminated with bodily excretory products such as urine, faeces or menstrual blood, either her own or other people's. She developed cleaning and hand washing rituals which took up to 3 hours to complete each morning and longer while she was menstruating. She avoided touching door knobs or other objects which she feared might have been contaminated by other people. If she did inadvertently touch such an object she would have to repeat her washing rituals and change into clean clothes. She had not worked for 2 years because her rituals prevented her getting to her office on time. A course of behaviour therapy involving exposure, response prevention and self-monitoring was devised and supervised by a specially trained nurse therapist. Within 6 months her washing rituals were reduced to 10 minutes each morning and she was able to limit subsequent washing to acceptable duration after going to the lavatory and before preparing food.

Management

Behaviour therapy is the preferred treatment. This should be carried out under specialist supervision and is most effective when the obsessional rituals are prominent. It consists of repeated exposure to the contaminated objects followed by prevention of the ritualistic behaviour (response prevention). Some patients are helped further if they can observe a therapist modelling normal behaviour in the presence of contamination. Treatment should be given over several sessions and relatives need to be enlisted as cotherapists to prevent recurrence of symptoms in the home environment. Obsessional thoughts not accompanied by rituals are more difficult to treat but some success has been claimed for various psychological techniques designed to interrupt the patient's pattern of thinking (thought stopping).

Additional benefit can be derived if medication is combined with behaviour therapy; clomipramine (50–150 mg daily) or one of the selective serotonin reuptake inhibitors are the drugs of choice in this condition.

REACTION TO SEVERE STRESS

Acute stress reaction

Following an exceptionally stressful event some people with no previous psychiatric history develop a characteristic pattern of symptoms which include a sense of bewilderment, anxiety, anger, depression, overactivity and withdrawal. The symptoms are transient; they start to subside within a few hours and have usually completely resolved within 3 days of their onset. Precipitating events include major accidents, military action, criminal assault and rape.

Post traumatic stress disorder

This is a delayed and protracted response to a stressful event of an exceptionally threatening or catastrophic nature, outside the range of everyday human experience, which would be likely to cause distress in almost everyone. The events include natural disasters, terrorist activity, serious accidents and witnessing violent deaths. There is usually a delay ranging from a few weeks to several months between the traumatic event and the onset of symptoms. Typical symptoms are recurrent intrusive memories (flashbacks) of the traumatic event, sleep disturbance, nightmares, autonomic arousal, emotional blunting and avoidance of any situation which evokes memories of the trauma. Anxiety and depression are associated features and excessive use of alcohol or drugs may complicate the clinical picture. The condition runs a fluctuating course, and most people recover within two years although in a small proportion the symptoms become chronic.

Management

Current opinion favours a preventive approach in the management of this disorder by arranging immediate counselling for those who have survived a major catastrophe with the aim of preventing the development of symptoms of post traumatic stress disorder (PTSD). Counselling can be of various types but the essentials are to provide support, direct advice and the opportunity for catharsis by reliving the trauma. In established PTSD structured psychological approaches, particularly cognitive therapy, are used, often in conjunction with antidepressant medication.

Adjustment disorder

This is a reaction to a stressful life event such as bereavement, separation, redundancy or the onset of a physical illness. The predominant symptoms are depression or anxiety, or a mixture of the two, but these are not sufficiently intense to justify the diagnosis of an affective or anxiety disorder. These symptoms develop within a month after the stressful event and do not last longer than 6 months. If they persist longer the diagnosis has to be revised according to the prevailing clinical picture.

Grief reactions are a particular type of adjustment disorder. A bereaved person usually experiences a brief period of emotional numbing followed by a period of distress lasting several weeks during which sorrow, tearfulness, sleep disturbance, loss of interest and a sense of futility are common. Perceptual distortions may occur including misinterpreting sounds as the dead person's voice or sensing the deceased's presence. The distinction between normal and abnormal grief is an arbitrary one. Considerable importance is given to the intensity and duration of symptoms and associated social dysfunction. Symptoms which are considered to indicate abnormal grief are suicidal ideas, denial of the loss, guilt and identification with the dead person by adopting some of his/her symptoms. An abnormal grief reaction which lasts longer than 6 months should be classified as a prolonged depressive reaction.

Adjustment disorders in general do not usually require psychotropic medication; patients can be helped by supportive measures, particularly reassurance, explanation and advice. Skilled psychotherapy is however required for patients with abnormal grief reactions.

DISSOCIATIVE (CONVERSION) DISORDER

This is one of the most controversial concepts in psychiatry. It has, at least temporarily, replaced the previously used term hysteria in the ICD-10 classification but many clinicians still prefer to retain 'hysteria' as a diagnostic category. Controversy has occurred because of the high rate of organic disease in patients previously diagnosed as having hysteria and also because of the multiple uses of the term which has been used to describe symptoms, a personality type, an epidemic phenomenon and clinical syndromes.

'Dissociative disorder' is best used to define a syndrome characterised by a loss or distortion of neurological function not fully explained by organic disease.

Aetiology

The condition is considered to result from unconscious psychological processes, implying that the patient lacks insight into the nature of the symptoms. In psychoanalytic terms dissociative disorder has been seen as a maladaptive way of coping with an unresolved psychological conflict, that is by becoming ill. The patient thus derives primary gain by relieving the conflict and secondary gain by obtaining sympathy and attention from others or by avoiding everyday responsibilities. It is certainly the case that dissociative disorder is more commonly diagnosed in women and children, groups who often lack an effective means of verbal communication because of an inferior social position.

The role of organic neurological disease is unclear. Although, by definition, the symptoms of hysteria are not themselves caused by organic disease, there is coexisting disease of the nervous system in up to 50% of cases. Organic disease may facilitate dissociative mechanisms and provide a model for symptoms, thus, for example, explaining the occurrence of pseudoseizures in patients with epilepsy.

Clinical features

The commonest symptoms of dissociative disorder mimic lesions in the motor or sensory nervous system and in classic cases there is apparent unconcern (belle indifférence) even in the face of gross physical disability. However, this is not always present and it should not be relied upon for diagnostic purposes. The presentations of dissociative disorder are given in the information box below.

COMMON PRESENTATIONS OF DISSOCIATIVE DISORDER

- Gait disturbance
- Loss of function in limbs
- Aphonia
- Pseudoseizures
- Sensory loss
- Blindness

Dissociative disorder can also involve higher mental functions, especially memory and general intelligence.

Dissociative amnesia usually develops acutely. The memory loss is patchy and inconsistent; a characteristic feature is a loss of personal identity so that the patient is unable to recall his or her name, address or other personal and family details. Memory loss of this degree does not occur in organic disease unless there is gross dementia. Dissociative amnesia is occasionally accompanied by a tendency to travel aimlessly many miles from familiar surroundings; this is known as a hysterical fugue. When global intelligence is affected the cognitive deficits are variable and the patient's behaviour is not in keeping with the apparent degree of dementia.

Management

A full physical and psychiatric assessment should be completed to determine whether other disorders are present. Once the doctor is satisfied that relevant organic disease has been excluded no further investigations should be undertaken and therapeutic effort should be directed towards restoring optimal function. Many patients resist the idea that their symptoms are not entirely somatic. Confrontation is best avoided and initial management should concentrate on simple explanation and reassurance that the symptoms conform to a recognised pattern and will get better with treatment. This involves identifying those factors which appear to have precipitated the symptoms and helping the patient to cope with them more adaptively. Secondary reinforcing factors in the patient's social network must be corrected and physical treatment, for example physiotherapy, should be arranged to provide an acceptable framework for recovery. Little is to be gained by debating how much insight the patient really has into his or her condition. Acute symptoms respond well to treatment. In resistant cases recovery can be helped by abreaction under the influence of hypnosis or small intravenous doses of amylobarbitone (250–500 mg given over 5–10 minutes). During abreaction the patient is encouraged to describe, in a cathartic manner, the emotional trauma which provoked the symptoms while the doctor makes use of the patient's enhanced suggestibility to predict symptom relief.

SOMATOFORM DISORDERS

The essential feature of this group of disorders is repeated medical consultation for physical symptoms which have no adequate physical basis. In most cases a psychiatric assessment will show that the physical symptoms bear a close relationship with stressful life events or emotional conflicts. Unfortunately the degree of psychological understanding which the patient achieves is often minimal and a physician's attempts to discuss the possibility of psychological causation are firmly resisted.

Several syndromes are described within this group; there is considerable overlap between them, both in aetiology and clinical presentation, and they also have similarities with dissociative disorder.

Somatisation disorder

This syndrome runs a chronic and fluctuating course over many years. Symptoms start in early adult life, are more frequent in women and may be referred to any part of the body. Common complaints include pain, vomiting, nausea, headache, dizziness, menstrual irregularities and sexual dysfunction. By the time the patient is referred to a psychiatrist there is usually a multitude of negative investigations and unhelpful operations, particularly hysterectomy and cholecystectomy.

Hypochondriacal disorder

This refers to a morbid preoccupation with the possibility of having a serious physical illness. Hypochondriacal symptoms commonly occur in anxiety and depressive disorders but occasionally they are primary and persist for many years. In a small proportion of cases conviction of disease reaches delusional intensity, the best known example being the conviction of parasitic infestation ('delusional parasitosis') which leads patients to consult dermatologists. Pimozide (2–12 mg daily) has been claimed to be effective for this syndrome. A preoccupation with bodily disfigurement (dysmorphophobia) leads to inappropriate requests for cosmetic surgery.

Somatoform autonomic dysfunction

Symptoms are referred to organs which are largely under autonomic control. The commonest examples involve the cardiovascular system (cardiac neurosis), respiratory system (psychogenic hyperventilation) and gut (psychogenic vomiting and irritable bowel syndrome).

Somatoform pain disorder

The cardinal feature is severe, persistent pain which cannot be explained by a physical illness or physiological disturbance. Sufficient emotional conflicts or psychosocial problems are evident to conclude that these are the main causal influences on the pain. Patients with this disorder usually make great demands for emotional support from their families and for treatment from the medical profession.

Management of somatoform disorders

Similar principles apply as in the management of dissociative disorders. Physical examination and investigations should be arranged according to the pattern of symptoms and once organic disease has been excluded requests for further investigations should be resisted if there is sufficient positive evidence to make a psychiatric diagnosis. Most of the somatoform disorders are chronic so complete recovery must not be expected. Treatment involves a multidisciplinary team approach and aims to minimise the rewards of the sick role and to encourage healthy behaviour. The attitudes of close relatives may need to be modified to effect these changes because they may have adopted an overprotective role, unwittingly reinforcing the patient's disability.

Antidepressant drugs have a limited role in treating depressive episodes when they arise; they are also useful in some cases of psychogenic pain.

NEURASTHENIA

Also known as chronic fatigue syndrome, this condition is characterised by excessive fatigue after minimal physical or mental exertion, poor concentration, dizziness and muscular aches. There may be various autonomic symptoms affecting the cardiovascular or gastrointestinal systems. The sleep pattern is altered, with frequent waking or hypersomnia.

This pattern of symptoms may follow a viral infection such as infectious mononucleosis, influenza or hepatitis; the term myalgic encephalomyelitis is used by those who favour a viral aetiology. However, in most cases there is no convincing evidence of viral infection, either from the history or antibody titres. There is a considerable overlap with the symptoms of an affective disorder and many psychiatrists regard neurasthenia as a variant of depression.

Current approaches to treatment favour an active programme of rehabilitation combined with cognitive therapy and antidepressant medication without sedative effects.

EATING DISORDERS

ANOREXIA NERVOSA

This disorder, which sometimes causes extreme emaciation, typically develops during adolescence and predominantly affects girls. Only 5–10% of cases occur in males; occasionally the condition develops in older women. There is a higher prevalence in the upper social classes and the patients are often hard-working, perfectionist and ambitious. One survey found a prevalence of 1% in girls at an independent school with another 5% showing some features of the condition. Theories about aetiology are speculative. Current social pressures to maintain a slim figure are thought to have caused a recent increased incidence. Some girls have a history of

obesity and embark on an extreme course of dieting after being teased about their fatness. Anorexia has also been regarded as an attempt to remain pre-pubertal by girls who have fears of sexual maturation. In other cases anorexia appears a nonspecific response to family crises which often involve the parental relationship. Hormonal changes have been suggested as aetiologically important. However, the endocrine abnormalities nearly always revert to normal following restoration of weight and are probably secondary to the effects of weight loss.

Clinical features

These are listed in the information box below.

> **ESSENTIAL DIAGNOSTIC CRITERIA FOR ANOREXIA NERVOSA**
>
> - Weight loss of at least 25% of original body weight (or weight 25% below norm for age and height)
> - Avoidance of high calorie foods
> - Distortion of body image so that the patient regards herself as fat even when grossly underweight
> - Amenorrhoea for at least 3 months

In boys, loss of sexual interest replaces amenorrhoea as a diagnostic criterion. Other features include a striking indifference to the weight loss and a denial of problems. Emaciation may be disguised by wearing loosely fitting clothes and hiding heavy objects in the clothing when weight is checked on scales. Subjects are often physically overactive; they may use laxatives or induce vomiting secretly after meals. Although they avoid carbohydrates and fats they are often preoccupied with food and enjoy making elaborate meals for their families. Other physical signs include a downy, lanugo hair on the trunk and limbs, hypotension, bradycardia and peripheral cyanosis. Psychosexual immaturity is often prominent.

Management

The first objective is to restore normal body weight, which is most likely to be achieved if a trusting relationship can be established with the patient from the first interview. Treatment can be conducted on an outpatient or day patient basis unless there is a risk of suicide or serious physical complications. Inpatient treatment should then be arranged. By educating the patient about the dangers of starvation it should be possible to establish the need for weight gain and to agree on a target weight which should be reached slowly in a controlled manner. If inpatient treatment becomes necessary the patient should be supervised during meals and for 1 hour subsequently to ensure vomiting does not occur. A series of target weights should be set and the patient is allowed increasing privileges and independence as each target is achieved. The final target should be within the normal range for the patient's age and height. Psychotherapy is an essential part of management. Individual therapy allows the patient to acquire insight into her condition and associated problems. Family therapy is also necessary to help resolve tensions which are nearly always evident by the time the patient presents for treatment.

The short-term prognosis is good if this programme is followed but the long-term outlook is less favourable. Approximately 20% make a full recovery, 20% remain chronically ill and 60% have recurring episodes of anorexia. Death occurs from suicide or physical complications in 5% of cases.

BULIMIA NERVOSA

This disorder was described in the late 1970s and may be related to anorexia nervosa. It is almost exclusively confined to women and the age of onset is slightly older than for anorexia. Prevalence has been estimated at 1% of women in their early twenties.

Clinical features
These are listed in the information box below.

DIAGNOSTIC CRITERIA FOR BULIMIA NERVOSA

- Recurrent bouts of binge-eating
- Lack of self-control over eating during binges
- Self-induced vomiting, purgation or dieting after binges
- Weight maintained within normal limits

The binges occur at least twice weekly and involve rich foods such as cakes, chocolates and dairy products; over 20 000 calories may be consumed during the day of a binge. Despite this intake weight is usually maintained within the normal range and menstruation is often regular. Physical complications from vomiting and purgation include erosion of dental enamel, hypokalaemia and metabolic alkalosis. Electrolyte and fluid disturbances can be sufficiently severe to cause cardiac arrhythmias or renal damage. A bilateral enlargement of the parotid glands is seen in some patients.

Management
Most treatment can be undertaken on an outpatient basis. Cognitive behaviour therapy is the currently preferred approach, the central component being self-monitoring of eating behaviour. The patient is asked to keep a full eating diary, together with a record of emotions and circumstances associated with binges. A series of tasks is set which are directed at helping the patient

cope more appropriately with provoking stimuli, thereby reducing the frequency and severity of binges. Treatment may need to be continued for several months; short-term results are encouraging but the long-term prognosis of the condition is not known.

OBESITY

This is the commonest form of eating disorder but it is rarely seen as a presenting problem in psychiatric practice. It is defined in terms of a high body mass index (BMI), i.e. weight in kilograms divided by the square of height in metres. The normal range of BMI is 20–25 (see p. 580) and on these figures one–third of the British population is obese. Obesity results from excessive intake of food and insufficient exercise, but constitutional and cultural factors are important in its aetiology and maintenance. There is no consistent association between obesity and psychiatric illness or personality traits but many obese people find the condition highly embarrassing. The management of patients with mild–moderate (BMI 25–40) and gross (BMI over 40) obesity is discussed on page 581.

SLEEP DISORDERS

This section discusses those sleep disorders in which psychological factors are considered to be the main aetiological influences. Sleep has a restorative function and is important for conservation of energy and growth. It comprises two distinct physiological states: rapid eye movement (REM) sleep and non-REM sleep. Non-REM sleep consists of four stages, two of which are known as 'slow wave' or deep sleep because they are associated with low frequency, synchronised waves on the electroencephalogram. REM sleep develops after progression through the various stages of non-REM sleep, usually within 90 minutes. It is the stage in which most dreaming occurs. During a night's sleep there is a cycle of non-REM and REM sleep with the episodes of REM becoming relatively longer.

Insomnia
Insomnia is a condition of inadequate quantity or quality of sleep. Difficulty falling asleep is the commonest complaint, followed by difficulty staying asleep and early wakening.

Insomnia may be a symptom of a depressive illness, anxiety disorder or other psychiatric condition. More commonly it arises at a time of increased life stress; some people then become preoccupied with lack of sleep and fear trying to get to sleep. This establishes a vicious circle which perpetuates the problem.

When insomnia results from a definite psychiatric illness treatment should be directed towards the underlying condition. Counselling, cognitive therapy, psychotherapy and medication all have their place. Sleep disturbance is a particularly distressing symptom of depressive illness, in which case an antidepressant drug with marked sedative properties (e.g. amitriptyline, dothiepin) should be prescribed to be taken at night.

Hypnotic drugs are useful for short-term treatment of insomnia which is due to acute stress which is likely to resolve, for example bereavement or separation. They should not be taken for longer than 3 weeks. Benzodiazepines such as temazepam (10–20 mg) are most commonly used. It is claimed that tolerance and dependence are less likely to develop with some of the newer hypnotics, for example zopiclone.

Drugs are not appropriate when insomnia is a chronic condition. In such cases much can be achieved by educating the patient about healthy sleep and by giving advice about regular exercise and avoiding heavy meals, alcohol and caffeine-containing drinks during the evening. Behavioural techniques such as relaxation exercises and various cognitive strategies to cope with intrusive thoughts are generally helpful.

Parasomnias

The two most important are sleep-walking and night terrors, both of which occur during slow-wave sleep. During sleep-walking vision and coordination remain intact but serious accidents can occur. It is important that these patients sleep in a protected environment so that it is impossible for them to fall from windows or down stairs.

Night terrors start with a frightening scream which is associated with sweating, increased heart and respiratory rates and a scared expression. The patient is usually unable to recall the episodes (unlike nightmares). It is claimed that parasomnias resolve with improved sleep hygiene, particularly reduced consumption of alcohol and caffeine.

SEXUAL DYSFUNCTIONS

These are the commonest sexual complaints which doctors see in practice. They include low sexual interest and various difficulties experienced during intercourse which reduce mutual satisfaction. Many sexual problems stem from ignorance and fear, often dating back to an excessively prudish upbringing which has caused inhibition in relation to sexual topics. Sexual dysfunction can occur transiently as a symptom of an anxiety disorder or depressive illness or it may be a manifestation of a relationship problem. Physical health has an important influence and needs careful assessment. Sexual interest and performance are impaired during any debilitating illness. Endocrine, cardiovascular and neurological disorders should be especially considered; for example, impotence may be a presenting feature of hypogonadism, diabetes, peripheral vascular disease or multiple sclerosis. Finally an alcohol and drug history should be taken. Any drug which has a depressant effect on the central nervous system can impair sexual function, as also can drugs which act on the peripheral autonomic system (e.g. alpha-methyldopa, phenothiazines, tricyclic antidepressants).

Impotence

This is the commonest sexual dysfunction among men. It involves complete or partial erectile failure with normal sexual desire. It is often transient and improves with reassurance. If persistent it can be helped by a behavioural programme in which the partner's cooperation is essential. The couple are instructed to carry out a graded series of mutually pleasurable sexual activities but intercourse is completely banned until an erection can be confidently maintained. Successful results have also been obtained by injecting papaverine into the corpora cavernosa and this treatment is now preferred in many clinics.

Premature ejaculation

This is defined as ejaculation prior to penetration or, if penetration occurs, before the partner can achieve orgasm. It is often associated with high levels of anxiety which appear to perpetuate the condition. Successful treatment is based on behavioural techniques derived from the work of Masters and Johnson.

Vaginismus

Vaginismus is due to spasm of the pelvic muscles which prevents full penetration. It results from intense fear of penetration on the part of the woman, and a conditioned reflex is established resulting in pelvic spasm even at the thought of intercourse. Treatment consists of instructing the patient in relaxation exercises followed by insertion of vaginal dilators of increasing size, initially by the doctor, then the patient and finally the partner.

Female orgasmic dysfunction

Most cases result from ignorance of sexual technique on the part of the patient or her partner. Counselling is usually effective in overcoming the problem. Approximately 10% of women appear physiologically incapable of orgasm due to absence of the bulbo-cavernosus reflex.

SEXUAL DEVIATIONS

Sexual deviations involve obtaining sexual arousal from inanimate objects or unwilling partners. Examples include exhibitionism (genital exposure in public), fetishism (arousal from female clothing), transvestism (arousal by dressing in clothes of opposite sex) and paedophilia (sexual arousal with children).

TRANSSEXUALISM

This rare condition results from a disturbance of gender identity. The patient, usually a man, is convinced he should have been born female and strongly identifies with feminine psychology. He wishes to live his life as a woman and may request medical help to do so. Transsexuals should be referred to special clinics where hormone therapy may be given to enable suitable patients to develop the secondary sexual characteristics of the opposite sex. Surgical treatment can be undertaken to reassign external genitalia if the patient can successfully adopt the lifestyle of the opposite sex for at least 12 months.

PUERPERAL MENTAL DISORDERS

There is a sharp increase in psychiatric illness following childbirth. Three different syndromes have been defined according to their severity and time of onset, although there is some overlap between them.

POSTNATAL BLUES

These occur in 50–60% of women following delivery. Symptoms are evident by the third postnatal day, reach a peak on the fifth day and subside rapidly during the next ten days. The predominant features are tearfulness, irritability, lability of mood, anxiety about the baby and poor concentration. These symptoms are unexpected and bewildering to a new mother and consequently cause considerable distress. Prompt recognition and reassurance by nursing staff nearly always succeed in alleviating this distress.

A hormonal basis has been suspected in view of the rapid changes in progesterone and oestrogen levels which follow childbirth. However, no consistent association has yet been found between hormonal changes and symptoms of the 'blues'.

POSTNATAL DEPRESSION

This is the most important psychiatric disorder following childbirth in terms of its frequency and disabilities.

Within 6 weeks of delivery 10–15% of mothers have developed a new episode of depressive illness. In addition to the usual features of depression there may be excessive concern about the baby's health, fears of harming the baby, guilt about maternal deficiencies and marital tensions including loss of sexual interest. Diagnosis may be missed at a routine postnatal examination because attention is concentrated on the baby's welfare and on possible gynaecological complications. Furthermore, women are embarrassed by admitting to feeling depressed after what is expected to be a joyful event in their lives.

Postnatal depression can last for several months if it is not treated. Once symptoms are recognised support and counselling should be arranged—counselling from a health visitor has been shown to have a significant effect in hastening recovery. Antidepressant drugs are required in severe cases.

Postnatal depression probably occurs as a result of various social and psychological changes following childbirth including giving up work, financial hardship, altered status, marital friction and the sheer exhaustion of broken nights.

PUERPERAL PSYCHOSES

These occur following approximately 0.2% of deliveries. Although they are infrequent they are severe and have a devastating effect on the mother's bonding with her child and on other family relationships.

The psychosis can take the form of affective (manic depressive) or schizophrenic illness. The former predominates, with lability of mood being a characteristic feature. Perplexity and disorientation are relatively more common than in psychoses unrelated to childbirth. In the majority of cases symptoms develop during the first fortnight after delivery. Transfer to a psychiatric ward is nearly always necessary and in some hospitals there are mother and baby units which allow the baby to be admitted with the mother. The theoretical advantage of this arrangement is that it enables mother-child bonding to develop without interruption. However, some mothers are so disturbed that they cannot relate adequately to their baby. Alternative arrangements should then be made for the baby's care until the mother's mental state has improved sufficiently for her to care for the child.

Neuroleptic or antidepressant drugs are prescribed depending on the nature of the psychosis. ECT is given for severe psychotic depression if it is accompanied by stupor, refusal to eat and drink, or suicidal risk.

The aetiology of puerperal psychosis is not understood. There is an increased risk of psychotic illness among first-degree relatives and an increased personal risk of psychosis not related to childbirth. Despite the intuitive appeal of a hormonal aetiology no distinct hormonal changes have been discovered. A psychological contribution is suggested by observations that puerperal psychoses are commoner in unmarried women, after a first child and following Caesarian section. These factors are probably important because of the increased stress associated with them.

The short-term outcome is nearly always good but there is at least a 20% risk of recurrent illness after a subsequent birth. If there have been previous episodes of affective illness unrelated to childbirth the risk of puerperal psychosis rises to 40%.

CASE HISTORY

Midwifery staff requested a psychiatric opinion on a 29-year-old woman who had given birth to her first child, a boy, by forceps delivery 6 days previously. There had been some concern about the child, who had developed neonatal jaundice, but this appeared to be resolving satisfactorily. The mother had become increasingly anxious about her son's health. She feared he was going to die and she refused to be reassured by a favourable report from the paediatrician. When interviewed by the psychiatrist she appeared retarded, very depressed and almost mute. Her few utterances indicated her to have a markedly low mood and nihilistic delusions about her son's health. It was learned that she had twice had hospital treatment for a bipolar affective illness. She was started on antidepressant medication but her condition deteriorated during the next few days until she was no longer eating or drinking adequately. Her condition improved dramatically after treatment with ECT and she was able to look after her baby under nursing supervision and then unsupervised. She was recommended to take long-term lithium therapy to prevent relapse, with the qualification that the drug should be discontinued if she wished to become pregnant again.

Psychotropic drugs in pregnancy and the puerperium

Certain precautions need to be observed when prescribing psychotropic drugs in pregnancy and the puerperium because of possible teratogenic effects during the first trimester, withdrawal symptoms following delivery and toxic effects on the baby of drugs excreted in breast milk. Lithium is the most dangerous drug concerned. It has definite teratogenic effects and should not be prescribed at all during the first trimester. If a woman taking prophylactic lithium wishes to become pregnant the drug should be stopped gradually beforehand and contraception continued until the drug is completely withdrawn. If pregnancy occurs while taking lithium the drug must be stopped immediately. Lithium is excreted in breast milk and can cause toxicity in the newborn baby. It should therefore be avoided in the puerperium if breastfeeding is practised.

Benzodiazepines also have a weak teratogenic effect. They can cause over-sedation (floppy baby syndrome) or withdrawal symptoms in the neonate immediately following delivery if taken beforehand, so they should be avoided in pregnancy and during lactation.

Tricyclic antidepressants, phenothiazines and butyrophenones do not appear to have teratogenic effects so they can be given during pregnancy if indicated clinically. They are excreted in breast milk in very small amounts; breast-feeding is therefore not contraindicated if the mother is taking these drugs.

PERSONALITY DISORDERS

Psychiatrists often disagree about this concept which refers to a pattern of enduring traits and behaviour which is maladaptive and which causes significant harm to the individual or those around him or her. The traits of personality disorder are exaggerations of those characteristics which are recognised in many normal members of society. They are usually well developed by late adolescence and persist relatively unchanged throughout life. The diagnosis of a particular type of personality disorder is made separately from a diagnosis of psychiatric illness. This recognises that an individual with a disordered personality may or may not experience discrete episodes of psychiatric illness.

Aetiological factors are not well understood. Many patients with personality disorders come from deprived families and have been subjected to physical and emotional abuse in childhood. Personality disorders tend to run in families but the relative influence of genetic and environmental factors is not clear.

Personality disorders are usually grouped according to particular traits which tend to go together.

Antisocial personality

Also known as psychopathic personality, this refers to recurrent delinquent behaviour with repeated offences against the law, aggression, impulsiveness and lack of feeling for other people. Antisocial personalities have an unstable record with regard to work, marriage and personal relationships. They often serve prison sentences but there is a high rate of re-offending.

Paranoid personality

These individuals are very sensitive to criticism and humiliations. They are excessively keen on establishing what they regard as their personal rights and defend them forcefully. They have an exaggerated sense of their own importance so they readily perceive a slight from others where none is intended. If things go wrong for them they blame other people. This is apparent if such people become medically ill, when they may accuse their doctor of negligence or bad practice. Relatives of paranoid personalities have a higher than average rate of paranoid psychoses.

Dependent personality

These people are indecisive and have difficulty coping with daily responsibilities. They demand constant support from other people and may enter into unsuitable relationships merely to avoid being left to fend for themselves. They tend to comply passively with the wishes of authority figures.

Histrionic personality

This term, sometimes called hysterical personality, is usually applied to women who display traits of egocentricity, emotional shallowness, vanity and dramatisation. Relationships are established quickly but do not last. Although they behave in a sexually provocative manner they are usually frigid and afraid of mature sexuality. The concept has been criticised as a caricature of femininity derived by male doctors. It does have some relationship with a tendency to develop hysterical conversion symptoms but most patients with hysteria have normal personalities.

Schizoid personality

People with this personality type are socially withdrawn, preferring solitary pursuits which are often of an eccentric nature. They appear aloof to other people but in fact are usually socially phobic. This personality type may contribute to the development of schizophrenia, in which case the prognosis is worse than for schizophrenics with normal personalities.

Obsessional personality

Minor obsessional traits of orderliness, cleanliness and punctuality are advantageous to most who possess them and essential for success in certain occupations, including medicine. They become handicapping when they lead to slowness, inflexibility and indecisiveness. Obsessional people are often insecure and like their lives to be as routine and predictable as possible. They may develop a florid obsessional neurosis under stress and are also prone to depressive illnesses during which their obsessional traits become more pronounced.

Management

See below under factitious disorders.

FACTITIOUS DISORDERS

This refers to individuals who, in the absence of a distinct psychiatric or physical disorder, repeatedly induce the signs or symptoms of disease. The behaviour is consistent and deliberate. It is often difficult to understand the underlying motives other than as an attempt to gain access to the role of patient and to fool doctors.

One pattern is seen predominantly in young women who usually work in nursing or one of the other professions allied to medicine. These patients surreptitiously fabricate the signs of disease, for example by regularly taking hormone preparations or by inducing anaemia by repeated bleeding. Other presentations include chronic ulcerating skin lesions (dermatitis artefacta), pyrexia of unknown origin, and hypoglycaemia.

Another form of factitious disorder, Munchausen's syndrome, is seen in patients who present with dramatic symptoms of a medical emergency such as myocardial infarction or intra-abdominal catastrophe. The patient fabricates a convincing history which persuades an unsuspecting doctor to undertake complicated investigations or exploratory surgery. If suspicions are aroused it may be possible to trace the patient's history showing that he or she has presented similarly at several other hospitals, often changing his or her name several times during the course of these travels. When confronted with the fraudulent nature of the symptoms the patients discharge themselves angrily, only to present again at another hospital shortly afterwards. This condition is named after the German Baron von Munchausen who was legendary for his inventive lying. Treatment is strikingly ineffective but it is important to recognise the syndrome to avoid unnecessary investigations.

Management

By their nature, personality disorders cannot be cured but some individuals can be helped to make necessary changes so that their behaviour is less distressing to themselves or other people. Various psychological treatments have been used and success has been claimed for behaviour therapy and interpretive psychotherapy. Some experts believe group therapy is especially helpful.

It is important to remember that people with personality disorders can develop other psychiatric illnesses, the features of which are coloured by underlying personality. These illnesses respond to conventional treatment but often remain undetected.

FURTHER READING

Bancroft J 1989 Human sexuality and its problems, 2nd edn. Churchill Livingstone, Edinburgh

Crow T J 1991 The search for the psychosis gene. British Journal of Psychiatry 158: 611–614

Huckle P L, Palia S S 1993 Managing resistant schizophrenia. British Journal of Hospital Medicine 50: 467–471

Lishman W A 1987 Organic psychiatry, 2nd edn. Blackwell, Oxford

Lishman W A 1990 Alcohol and the brain. British Journal of Psychiatry 156: 635–644

Ramana R, Paykel E S 1992 Classification of affective disorder. British Journal of Hospital Medicine 47: 831–835

Roberts G W 1991 Schizophrenia: a neuropathological perspective. British Journal of Psychiatry 158: 8–17

Shapiro C M 1992 ABC of sleep disorders. British Medical Journal, London

Sharp C W, Freeman C P L 1993 The medical complications of anorexia nervosa. British Journal of Psychiatry 162: 452–462

Strang J, Johns A, Caan W 1993 Cocaine in the UK — 1991. British Journal of Psychiatry 162: 1–13

Taylor D, Lewis S 1993 Delirium. Journal of Neurology, Neurosurgery and Psychiatry 56: 742–751

Thomas H 1993 Psychiatric symptoms in cannabis users. British Journal of Psychiatry 163: 141–149

SPECIAL ASPECTS OF PSYCHIATRY

PSYCHIATRIC PROBLEMS IN THE GENERAL HOSPITAL

There are several reasons why psychiatric illness is commoner in patients attending general hospitals than in the community.

PSYCHOLOGICAL REACTIONS TO PHYSICAL ILLNESS

Most physical illnesses cause some psychological upset, which is usually minor in degree and brief in duration. Sick people modify their lifestyle according to the severity of their illness; mood changes are common but are not distressing, nor do they interfere with adjustment to the illness. More pronounced mood changes can cause significant distress. They usually resolve with recovery from the physical illness and they are best regarded as adjustment disorders. Anxiety is the commonest reaction within the first few days following the onset of physical symptoms; depression is a later development. Explanation and reassurance help allay the emotional distress; specific psychiatric intervention is not necessary.

In a minority of patients a depressed mood persists for weeks or months after physical recovery and is accompanied by the characteristic symptoms of loss of interest, low self-esteem, sleep disturbance and weight change. The diagnosis of a secondary depressive illness is then warranted and treatment with antidepressant medication is required. Physically ill patients tolerate antidepressant drugs poorly. Lower doses than usual should be used initially and if side-effects to tricyclics are troublesome one of the newer drugs like fluoxetine (20–80 mg daily) can be given. Close collaboration between physician and psychiatrist is essential for optimal management. Nowhere is this more important than in the care of the elderly who are prone to multiple problems, physical, psychological and social.

Depression can prolong functional disability following physical illness, thereby delaying return to work and resumption of leisure activities. In other cases recovery is delayed even though there is no evidence of depression. These patients remain incapacitated and adopt a lifestyle of invalidism or abnormal illness behaviour. The explanation can be found by examining the patient's social environment, when various factors prolonging the disability may be uncovered. The patient may be avoiding returning to an unsatisfactory job, may be gaining attention from an otherwise unsympathetic partner or may be exaggerating symptoms for financial gain if compensation is involved.

Anxiety, depression or mania may be the presenting symptoms of various underlying physical illnesses. In these cases the psychological symptoms result from disturbances of neurotransmitter function or interruption of anatomical pathways in the brain. Physical examination is essential in patients presenting with a new episode of psychiatric illness and suspicion of underlying physical pathology should be aroused particularly in the circumstances listed in the information box.

POINTERS TO AN ORGANIC CAUSE FOR PSYCHIATRIC DISORDER

- Late age of onset of psychiatric illness
- No previous history of psychiatric illness
- No family history of psychiatric illness
- No apparent psychological precipitant

These symptomatic psychiatric disorders can occur in the conditions listed in the information box below.

SOMATIC PRESENTATION OF PSYCHIATRIC ILLNESS

Somatic symptoms such as fatigue, dizziness, headache and other pains are commonly experienced during periods of emotional stress. This becomes a medical problem when the symptoms are attributed to physical illness for which the patient requests medical attention. Many

ORGANIC CAUSES OF AFFECTIVE DISORDERS

- **Neurological**
  Cerebrovascular disease
  Cerebral tumour
  Multiple sclerosis
  Parkinson's disease
  Huntington's chorea
  Alzheimer's disease
  Epilepsy

- **Endocrine**
  Hypothyroidism
  Hyperthyroidism
  Cushing's syndrome
  Addison's disease
  Hyperparathyroidism

- **Infections**
  Glandular fever
  Herpes simplex
  Brucellosis
  Typhoid
  Toxoplasmosis

- **Collagen disease**
  Systemic lupus
  erythematosus

- **Malignant disease**

- **Drugs**
  Reserpine, phenothiazines
  Methyldopa, oral
  contraceptives
  Corticosteroids,
  phenylbutazone

patients with psychiatric illness present in this manner to their general practitioner or hospital specialist. This phenomenon, known as somatisation, results in considerable misdiagnosis because the somatic presentation misleads the doctor into suspecting physical illness and distracts attention from underlying psychiatric problems. Not only does the patient have somatic symptoms but sometimes there is also a concern about a specific physical illness such as cancer, heart disease, AIDS or myalgic encephalomyelitis.

Among patients attending general hospital medical clinics at least one-fifth have no significant organic disease to account for their symptoms but have a psychiatric illness which is only detected when specific questions are asked.

Most have a depressive illness or one of the anxiety disorders (generalised anxiety, panic attacks or phobic disorder). The symptoms may have an abrupt onset in which case the history is short and a good response can be expected to conventional treatment. In a small proportion there is a longer history of complaints and disability; these patients are often diagnosed as having hypochondriasis, Briquet's syndrome (somatisation disorder) or hysteria and are less easy to treat.

Aetiology

The presenting somatic complaints are often amplifications of normal physiological sensations or muscular aches which everyone experiences. During episodes of depression or anxiety these sensations are exaggerated, and interpreted in a morbid manner, thus becoming the focus for medical complaint. A family history or previous personal history of a particular physical illness may influence the location of symptoms as well as their

interpretation. Although somatisation is a universal phenomenon it is commoner in Third World cultures and in immigrants from those countries into Britain. The social stigma of being psychiatrically ill probably accounts for the higher prevalence of somatisation in these immigrant groups. Many patients selectively emphasise somatic symptoms when they visit their doctor because they believe there is more medical interest in physical illness. Their pattern of somatisation is subsequently reinforced if special investigations are arranged, particularly if these yield equivocal results.

GYNAECOLOGICAL DISORDERS

Several gynaecological disorders have been associated with psychiatric morbidity but there are few definite conclusions. A specific menstrual mood disorder has been described. This condition, also known as the premenstrual syndrome, is characterised by depression, irritability, tension, poor concentration and a general bloated sensation; it occurs a few days before the onset of menstruation and subsides rapidly once menstruation begins. In women with affective disorders symptoms are accentuated premenstrually but never clear completely so they continue throughout the cycle. No consistent hormonal abnormalities have been found to account for menstrual mood disorder. Symptomatic improvement may be achieved by giving progesterone or diuretics.

Therapeutic abortion, hysterectomy and the menopause may be followed by psychiatric illness in some women but for the majority there are no significant psychological complications.

ATTEMPTED SUICIDE

There was a steady increase in hospital admissions for suicide attempts from the early 1960s so that by the end of the 1970s there were over 100 000 admissions annually in Britain. Since then there has been a slight decrease but attempted suicide is still one of the commonest reasons for acute medical admission. The term attempted suicide is potentially misleading in that the majority of patients are not unequivocally trying to kill themselves. However, alternative terms such as parasuicide and deliberate, non-fatal self-harm have not been widely accepted and attempted suicide can be retained provided it is realised that it does not inevitably involve fatal intent.

Most suicide attempts involve overdose, either of prescribed or non-prescribed drugs. Less common methods include wrist slashing, asphyxiation, drowning, hanging, jumping from a height or in front of a moving vehicle, and using firearms. Methods which carry a high chance of being fatal are more likely to be associated with serious psychiatric illness.

Suicide attempts are commoner in women than in men and in young adults than in the elderly. In contrast completed suicide is commoner in men and in the elderly although there has recently been an increased rate of suicide in young adults. There is a higher incidence of suicide attempts among the lower socioeconomic groups, particularly those living in crowded, socially deprived urban areas. They often have a deprived family background due to early loss of a parent through death or separation. There are also links with alcohol abuse, child abuse, unemployment and recently broken relationships.

A thorough psychiatric and social assessment must be carried out in all cases. In most hospitals this involves an interview with a psychiatrist. This need not always be the case because it is now recognised that junior physicians, nurses and social workers can assess these patients competently if properly trained and supervised. The assessment should be undertaken after emergency medical treatment has been completed. In patients who have taken drug overdoses it is important that sufficient time has elapsed to allow the toxic effects of the drug to wear off. Topics to be covered when assessing a patient are listed in the information box below.

ASSESSMENT OF PATIENTS AFTER ATTEMPTED SUICIDE

- Explanation of attempt
- Degree of suicide intent
- Presence of psychiatric illness
- Current suicidal risk
- Previous suicide attempts
- Family and personal history
- Social support available to patient
- Patient's usual ability to cope with stress
- Further management

The patient should be asked about events occurring immediately before the act and whether the attempt had been planned beforehand. In some cases there will be clear evidence that suicide was intended; the patient may have recently made a will, disposed of treasured possessions, gone to considerable effort to avoid discovery or have left an explicit suicide note. All these help explain the motivation behind the attempt. The interviewer needs to assess the severity of any current symptoms of psychiatric illness and to assess what personal and social supports are available if the patient were to leave hospital.

The majority of patients have depressive and anxiety symptoms which are reactive to an acute life crisis super-

imposed on a background of chronic social and personal difficulties. They do not require psychotropic medication or specialised psychiatric treatment. They need emotional support and practical advice to help them cope with the crisis which has precipitated the attempt. A social worker may be the most appropriate person to provide this help. Admission to a psychiatric ward is necessary for patients who have a major psychiatric illness, who remain intent on suicide or who require temporary respite from intolerable domestic circumstances. Admission should also be arranged when further information is needed to clarify the patient's mental state.

Approximately 20% make a repeat attempt during the following twelve months and 1% succeed in killing themselves. Factors which are known to be associated with a increased risk of suicide after a suicide attempt are listed in the information box below.

RISK FACTORS FOR SUICIDE AFTER A SUICIDE ATTEMPT

- Psychiatric illness (depressive illness, alcoholism, schizophrenia)
- Age over 45
- Male sex
- Living alone
- Unemployed
- Recently bereaved, divorced or separated
- Chronic physical ill-health
- Drug or alcohol abuse
- Violent method used (e.g. hanging, jumping)
- Suicide note written
- History of previous attempts

PSYCHIATRIC EMERGENCIES

These can occur in the community or in hospital wards but one of the commonest locations where doctors encounter psychiatric emergencies is in the accident and emergency department of a general hospital. They require urgent action because the patient's behaviour is potentially dangerous to him or herself or other people; the behaviour disturbance may be aggression, extreme overactivity or suicidal activity.

Rapid assessment is required. Two main decisions need to be taken. First, is the behaviour disturbance due to psychiatric illness? If not, the patient may have to be dealt with by the police. If the patient is psychiatrically ill, the second decision is whether it is an organic or functional illness. A full history and mental state examination will be out of the question. As much information as possible should be obtained from informants. This should include enquiries about recent mood change, paranoid ideas or other psychiatric symptoms. There may be a history of previous psychiatric illness, recent physical illness, head injury or drug abuse. When assessing the patient's mental state the key elements are evidence of cognitive impairment, paranoid delusions, and aggressive or suicidal intent. It is also important to understand any triggering events which have precipitated the emergency.

Many aggressive and overactive patients are frightened because their behaviour is determined by paranoid experiences. They can be calmed by a confident, nonthreatening approach. It is helpful if they feel the doctor understands what has brought on their distress. If there is a high risk of violence, the patient must be restrained. This should not be attempted until sufficient staff are present to overpower the patient safely. The police need to be involved if the patient is armed or causing actual physical harm. Once restraints have been imposed it is likely that sedation will be required. Haloperidol is the drug of choice. It can be given intramuscularly at an initial dose of 10–20 mg; this can be repeated if necessary until the patient is calmed. A decision can then be taken about the next stage in management depending on the nature of the underlying psychiatric disorder.

COMMUNITY PSYCHIATRY

There has been a steady shift towards treating psychiatrically ill patients in the community during the last 30 years. To a large extent this has been made possible by the development of effective psychotropic drugs but it has also been facilitated by changing attitudes which have favoured the closure of large psychiatric hospitals and replacing them with smaller units closer to the populations which they serve. There has been a progressive decline in the number of patients resident in psychiatric hospitals but paradoxically an increase in the number of admissions, most of which are re-admissions.

The closure of hospital beds has mainly affected the care of the chronically ill but there has also been a trend to treat acutely ill patients in their homes. In some areas multidisciplinary community care teams have been established to provide home treatment with 24-hour availability of staff. It has been possible to treat even severely ill patients in this manner. Results have been shown to be as effective as those obtained by hospital based services. The community service does not appear to increase the burden on relatives, possibly because they receive more support from professional staff, and it is claimed to be more effective in keeping patients in long-term contact with psychiatrists.

Treatment of chronically ill patients, usually suffering from schizophrenia, in a community setting is generally successful if careful plans are made to discharge patients to appropriate residential facilities such as community hostels and if they continue to receive treatment after leaving hospital. Medication can be administered by a community psychiatric nurse at the patient's home or hostel or in a community mental health centre. Additional support can be provided by attendance at a day hospital or local authority day centre. The Community Care Act, which became law in England and Wales in 1993, gave responsibility to local authorities for the social aspects of community care for the mentally ill. For patients resident in hospital social requirements should be identified as soon as possible during their admission and discharge should not be implemented until their needs have been met. However, there are fears that this Act, desirable in principle, will lead to delayed discharge and a shortage of beds, thus making it more difficult to admit acutely ill patients.

Problems arise when chronically ill patients discharged into the community do not comply with treatment and lose contact with psychiatric services. Some of these people become homeless and lead a vagrant existence, contributing to the high prevalence of psychiatric illness among those in reception centres, in prisons or sleeping rough. Lack of adequate treatment eventually leads to an acute relapse during which the patients may be a risk to themselves or other people. At present little can be done to treat those who refuse to accept medication and nursing support in the community, but in response to some well publicised cases new legislation is now being introduced to ensure the delivery of community care and strengthen the safety net through which too many patients fall.

LEGAL ASPECTS OF PSYCHIATRY

Psychiatry has closer links with the law than most other branches of medicine because psychiatric illness sometimes impairs judgement to the extent that the patients are not considered fully responsible for their actions. A doctor may therefore be required to prepare a report if one of his patients is considered psychiatrically ill and has been charged with committing an offence. This may need to concentrate on whether the patient is able to understand the charge brought against him or her, fit to plead, able to instruct a lawyer, able to follow proceedings in court and able to understand the verdict. The report should describe the patient's background and mental state at the time of the assessment and give an opinion of the patient's mental state at the time the offence was committed. A summary should comment on the patient's criminal responsibility and make recommendations for future management if it is thought

Table 17.6 Important provisions of the Mental Health Act, 1983 (England and Wales)

Purpose	Section	Duration	Signatures required	Appeal
Emergency admission	4	72 hours	One doctor plus relative or social worker	None
Assessment and treatment	2	28 days	Two doctors (one approved) plus nearest relative or social worker	To Tribunal within 14 days of admission
Treatment	3	6 months	Two doctors (one approved) plus nearest relative or social worker	To Tribunal within first 6 months and once during each subsequent period for which detention renewed
Emergency detention of patient in hospital	5(2)	72 hours	Doctor in charge	None
Emergency detention of patient in hospital	5(4)	6 hours	Nurse (RMN status)	None
Assessment of persons in public places thought to be mentally ill and in need of safety	136	72 hours	Police officer	None

more appropriate for the patient to be treated in a medical context rather than to be sent to prison. This may involve a probation order conditional on regular psychiatric outpatient attendance.

All doctors in clinical practice need to be familiar with the legal aspects of admitting psychiatrically ill patients to hospital against their will or detaining them in hospital after admission. It should be reiterated here that these regulations apply only to a small minority, less than 10% of psychiatric inpatients.

The law in England and Wales is governed by the Mental Health Act, 1983. This is principally concerned with the grounds for detaining patients in hospital or placing them under guardianship. Application for compulsory admission to hospital can only be made when the patient, who is suffering from mental disorder, is not willing to be admitted voluntarily and ought to be detained in the interests of his or her own health or safety or with a view to the protection of other persons. The definition of mental disorder includes mental illness, mental impairment and psychopathic disorder, the latter resulting in abnormally aggressive or seriously irresponsible conduct. The Act introduced significant changes to improve patients' rights by allowing appeal against detention under certain sections of the Act. Appeals are heard by a Mental Health Review Tribunal. This consists of three members, a Circuit Judge or equivalent who acts as President of the Tribunal, a medical representative and a lay representative. Table 17.6 summarises the most important sections of the Act with which doctors need to be familiar.

Similar legislation for Scotland was passed by the Mental Health (Scotland) Act, 1984. Reasons for hospital admission and detention are similar to those for

Table 17.7 Important provisions of the Mental Health (Scotland) Act, 1984

Purpose	Section	Duration	Signatures required	Appeal
Emergency admission	24	72 hours	One doctor; consent of relative or mental health officer if practicable	None
Short term detention and treatment	26	28 days (further to Section 24 or 25(i))	Approved doctor in addition to recommendation under Section 24 or 25(i); consent of nearest relative or mental health officer if practicable	To Sheriff or Mental Welfare Commission
Non-urgent admission	18	6 months	Two doctors (one approved); nearest relative or mental health officer; Sheriff's approval	To Mental Welfare Commission; to Sheriff if detention extended after 6 months
Emergency detention of patient in hospital	25(i)	72 hours	Doctor in charge	None
Emergency detention of patient in hospital	25(ii)	2 hours	Nurse (RMN status)	None
Detention of person in public place thought to be mentally ill and in need of safety	118	72 hours	Police officer	None

England and Wales except that psychopathic disorder is not included. Appeals in Scotland can be made to the Mental Welfare Commission or to the Sheriff. The most important sections of this Act are summarised in Table 17.7.

FURTHER READING

Appleby L 1992 Suicide in psychiatric patients: risk and prevention. British Journal of Psychiatry 161: 749–758

Bass C, Benjamin S 1993 The management of chronic somatisation. British Journal of Psychiatry 162: 472–480

Goldberg D, Benjamin S, Creed F 1987 Psychiatry in medical practice. Tavistock, London

Hawton K, Fagg J, Platt S, Hawkins M 1993 Factors associated with suicide after parasuicide in young people. British Medical Journal 306: 1641–1644

Kendell R E, Zealley A K (eds) 1993 Companion to psychiatric studies, 5th edn. Churchill Livingstone, Edinburgh

Lloyd G G 1993 Acute behaviour disturbances. Journal of Neurology, Neurosurgery and Psychiatry 56: 1149–1156

R. E. Cull, R. G. Will

18

Diseases of the nervous system

ANATOMY, PHYSIOLOGY AND INVESTIGATION

Neurological disease accounts for about 20% of admissions to medical wards and is the underlying cause in a significant proportion of the long term disabled in the community: see Table 18.1.

Table 18.1   Incidence and prevalence of some neurological diseases

	Incidence/100 000	Prevalence/100 000
Migraine	250	2000*
Stroke	200	800
Carpal tunnel syndrome	100	—
Epilepsy	50	520**
Transient ischaemic attack	35	—
Essential tremor	25	300
Parkinson's disease	20	150
Cerebral metastasis	15	10
Benign intracranial tumour	10	50
Multiple sclerosis	5	100
Guillain-Barré syndrome	2	—
Motor neurone disease	1.5	6
Myasthenia gravis	0.4	5
Syringomyelia	0.4	7

* Severe
** Epilepsy on treatment

Neurological disorders comprise those affecting the brain, spinal cord, peripheral roots and nerves and the muscles. Although the nervous system may at first sight appear complex, because of its precise anatomy it is probably the most logical and predictable of the body's systems. A knowledge of basic anatomy and physiology of the nervous system is essential, for it can be applied to clinical examination and lead to often precise localisation of the lesions causing clinical problems. Diagnosis of the nature of such lesions is seldom possible from examination alone—few clinical signs are due only to one disease—and must be made by analysis of the history, clinical signs and results of investigation.

The history is all-important and in some disorders (e.g. migraine) is the only method of diagnosis. The time-course of symptoms may give valuable clues (Table 18.2).

THE MOTOR SYSTEM

Movements are achieved by contraction and relaxation of skeletal muscles. The motor unit (Fig. 18.1) is the final common pathway through which spinal, cerebral and cerebellar control systems act to coordinate movement. The motor unit comprises a spinal anterior horn

Table 18.2   Typical time-course of neurological symptoms

Disorder	Onset	Typical course
Epilepsy	Acute (seconds)	Recurrent attacks (minutes)
Vascular	Acute (seconds–minutes)	Recovery in hours–days
Migraine	Acute (minutes)	Recurrent attacks (hours)
Infective	Sub-acute (hours–days)	Worsening–recovering
Demyelination	Sub-acute (days–weeks)	Varying severity, site
Tumour	Slow (weeks–months)	Gradual worsening
Degenerative	Slow (months–years)	Gradual worsening

cell (or cranial nerve motor neurone), its motor axon and the muscle fibres it supplies. The number of muscle fibres innervated by one axon varies from 10 to 1000 or more in different muscles. The motor axons terminate in specialised end-plates on the muscle surface. Activity in the nerve releases acetylcholine at the end-plate, causing depolarisation of the fibre and activation of the contractile process. Muscle fibres may have different biochemical and contractile characteristics (Table 18.3); most muscles contain a mixture, though one type may predominate.

The activity of motor units is governed by both local spinal reflex activity and by descending pathways from the cerebrum and cerebellum. Spinal reflexes may be monosynaptic as in the stretch reflex or polysynaptic as with flexor withdrawal and extensor plantar responses. The important supraspinal mechanisms involved in movement control are the pyramidal, the extrapyramidal and the cerebellar systems. These descending pathways interact via excitation and inhibition of the motor neurones and also with one another within the brain (Fig. 18.2). Signs of damage to the motor unit (lower motor neurone) are listed in the information box (p. 1023).

Table 18.3   Main types of muscle fibre

Type	Contraction	Fatigue	Enzymes	Nerve activity
I	Slow	Resistant	Oxidative	Tonic
IIa	Fast	Resistant	Glycolytic Oxidative	Phasic
IIb	Fast	Prone	Glycolytic	Phasic

THE PYRAMIDAL SYSTEM

The neurones of origin of the pyramidal tracts lie in the cerebral cortex just anterior to the central sulcus in the pre-central gyrus or 'motor strip'. Fibres from the pyramidal cells come close together in the internal capsule which passes close to the thalamus and basal ganglia deep in the cerebral hemisphere. As it descends the brain stem, the pyramidal tract innervates contralateral cranial

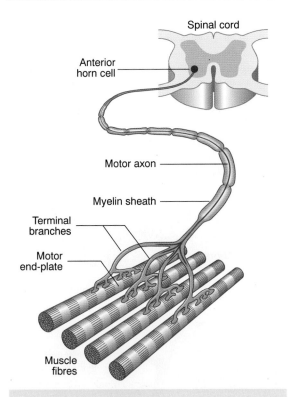

Spinal cord

Anterior horn cell

Motor axon

Myelin sheath

Terminal branches

Motor end-plate

Muscle fibres

Fig. 18.1   The motor unit.

SIGNS OF LESIONS AFFECTING MOTOR UNITS (LOWER MOTOR NEURONE)

- Weakness or paralysis of muscles supplied by affected motor neurone or axons
- Hypotonia
- Reduced or absent tendon reflexes
- Flexor (or absent) plantar response
- Wasting and fasciculation of affected muscle

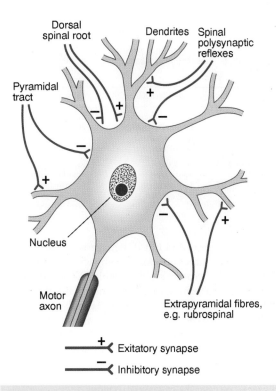

Dorsal spinal root

Dendrites   Spinal polysynaptic reflexes

Pyramidal tract

Nucleus

Motor axon

Extrapyramidal fibres, e.g. rubrospinal

+ Exitatory synapse

− Inhibitory synapse

Fig. 18.2   Synaptic influences on the activity of motor neurones.

nerve motor nuclei and sends fibres to the cerebellum via the middle cerebellar peduncle. At the lower medulla, the tract decussates, most of its fibres crossing over and descending the contralateral side of the spinal cord. As is seen in Figure 18.2 pyramidal fibres have both excitatory and inhibitory effects on the anterior horn cell. A strict topographical arrangement exists (Fig. 18.3) whereby specific areas of the precentral gyrus control movements of different parts of the contralateral side of the body. The larynx and pharynx are represented at the most inferior end of the gyrus, followed by relatively large contiguous areas for movements of the face, mouth and hand. The trunk is represented by a smaller area near the midline, and the foot on the medial aspect of the hemisphere.

In addition to causing weakness and impairment of fine movements, pyramidal tract lesions also cause increased muscle tone of spastic type ('clasp knife'), hyperactivity of stretch (tendon) reflexes and release of polysynaptic spinal reflexes, of which the extensor plantar response is the best example. These changes occur because of removal of the inhibitory effects of the pyramidal system on spinal neurones (see box on p. 1024).

The distribution of the weakness and the presence or

absence of cranial nerve deficits are of help in locating the site of a lesion involving the pyramidal tract (Table 18.4). The signs are listed in the information box below.

The motor cortex may be thought of as a store of basic instructions for eliciting movements. Activation of the motor strip causes several muscles to interact to produce movements. By contrast, motor unit activation at the spinal or peripheral nerve level causes only single muscles to contract. Damage to the pyramidal system above the decussation causes weakness or paralysis of voluntary movements on the contralateral side of the body. If the lesion is in the cortex, weakness may be limited to

SIGNS OF A PYRAMIDAL TRACT LESION

- Loss of voluntary movements
- Impaired fine movements
- Increased muscle tone
  Spasticity
  Clasp knife rigidity
- Exaggerated tendon reflexes and clonus
- Extensor plantar response
- Little or no muscular wasting
- Absent abdominal reflexes

Table 18.4 Distribution of weakness in pyramidal tract lesions

	Most affected	Least affected
Upper limb	Shoulder abduction Elbow extension Finger extension Finger abduction	Shoulder adduction Elbow flexion Wrist flexion Finger flexion
Lower limb	Hip flexion Knee flexion Foot dorsiflexion Foot eversion	Hip extension Knee extension Foot plantar flexion Foot inversion

one limb or part of it; but if damage is at a site where the pyramidal fibres are closely compacted (e.g. internal capsule) then weakness of the whole of one side of the body (hemiparesis) results. Lesions to the pyramidal tract below the medulla cause ipsilateral weakness. A characteristic pattern of weakness occurs with pyramidal tract lesions, especially if partial (Table 18.4). Signs of the level of lesions are listed in the information box.

SIGNS OF LEVEL OF PYRAMIDAL LESIONS

- **Cortex**
  Localised weakness (e.g. hand)
- **Internal capsule**
  Hemiplegia or hemiparesis
- **Brain stem**
  Cranial nerve deficit(s) with contralateral hemiparesis
- **Spinal cord**
  Weakness below lesion often bilateral

THE EXTRAPYRAMIDAL SYSTEM

This is a complex system of neurones and fibres which has reciprocal connections with the cerebral cortex, thalamus, cerebellar and brain-stem nuclei and spinal cord. The main collections of neurones involved are the

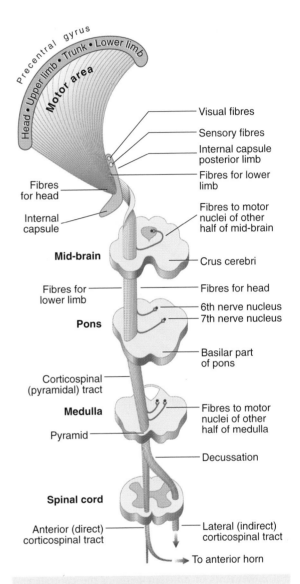

Fig. 18.3 The motor pathways.

caudate nucleus, putamen, globus pallidus, substantia nigra, and the subthalamic and red nuclei. The precise role of the extrapyramidal system is not well understood. It seems to be important in the activation of voluntary movements programmed in the motor cortex, and also in the involuntary adjustments of posture and muscle tone which enable willed movements to take place.

Lesions of the extrapyramidal system may cause various problems, depending on their site (Table 18.5).

Slowness in initiating movements (hypokinesis) and

Table 18.5 Clinical features of extrapyramidal lesions	
Signs	**Usual site of lesion**
Resting tremor	Substantia nigra, red nucleus
Muscular rigidity	Substantia nigra, putamen
Hypokinesis	Substantia nigra, putamen, globus pallidus
Chorea	Caudate nucleus
Hemiballismus	Subthalamic nucleus
Dystonia, athetosis	Putamen

CLINICAL FEATURES OF CEREBELLAR LESIONS

- **Incoordination of ipsilateral limbs**
  Past pointing (dysmetria)
  Intention tremor
  Decomposition of movements
  Impaired alternating movements
- **Loss of balance**
  Ataxic, broad based gait
  Leaning towards side of lesion
- **Dysarthria**
  Slurred indistinct speech
  Loss of normal rhythm
- **Nystagmus**
  Phasic usually horizontal nystagmus
  Maximal on looking to side of lesion
- **Hypotonia of limbs**
- **Decreased tendon reflexes**
- **Head tremor**
- **Head tilt**

difficulty with fine tasks are common, but muscular weakness is absent. Tendon reflexes are usually normal and plantar responses are flexor. Muscular tone may be either decreased (as in chorea) or increased in either a smooth fashion ('lead pipe') or have a phasic component as in the cog-wheel rigidity of parkinsonism.

THE CEREBELLUM

The cerebellum is concerned with the control of voluntary movements and the maintenance of posture and balance. It is closely connected to the vestibular system, and receives further proprioceptive input from the spinocerebellar tracts of the spinal cord which send fibres through the inferior cerebellar peduncle. Information about cortical motor instructions is relayed from the pyramidal tracts via the middle cerebellar peduncle to the cerebellum. The chief outputs are through the superior cerebellar peduncle to the ventrolateral thalamus and thence to the cerebral cortex, and also to the spinal motor neurones via the reticular formation, red nucleus and the vestibular nuclei. The midline (vermis) and the anterior lobe are concerned chiefly with maintenance and posture and balance, while the posterolateral lobes are responsible for coordination of the limbs (Fig. 18.4).

The cerebellum may be seen as a feedback computer which compares the intended actions of the motor cortex with the resultant movements of the body, and makes adjustments to the impulses relayed to the spinal motor neurones in order to achieve smooth control of movement and balance. The lateral parts of the cerebellum interconnect with the contralateral thalamus and cerebral cortex, thus controlling movements of the ipsilateral limbs. Clinical features of cerebellar lesions are listed in the information box (right).

THE SENSORY SYSTEM

The sensory system is responsible for transmitting information about the internal and external environment of the body to the brain. Not all sensory information is perceived consciously; much proprioceptive data is processed automatically by the cerebellum and basal ganglia. There are also mechanisms of variable gating at the spinal and cerebral levels whereby the amount of sensory information (especially relating to pain) which reaches consciousness is controlled. Superficial sensations of touch, warmth, cold and pain, and deep sensations of position, pressure and pain all begin peripherally in specialised receptor organs which transduce physical modalities into sensory nerve impulses. Sensory nerve fibres are elongated processes of the bipolar neurones of the dorsal root ganglia; their central processes pass in the dorsal root to the spinal cord and either synapse there or pass directly towards the brain. Two main relay systems for sensory information are important clinically: the *lemniscal* and the *spinothalamic*.

The lemniscal system is concerned with transmission of proprioceptive and well-localised touch information. Modalities such as joint position, two-point discrimination, and vibration sense use this pathway. The peripheral fibres are large, myelinated and fast conducting. They enter the dorsal horn of the spinal cord and without synapsing pass up the dorsal (posterior) columns to the gracile and cuneate nuclei in the lower medulla. Here they synapse, and second order fibres cross the midline and ascend the brain stem in the medial lemniscus, and thence to the thalamus (Fig. 18.5).

The spinothalamic system is the pathway for pain, temperature and poorly localised touch. The peripheral fibres for these modalities are smaller, slower conducting and sometimes unmyelinated axons. They enter the spinal cord in the dorsal root, and synapse in the dorsal horn. Most of the second order fibres cross the midline

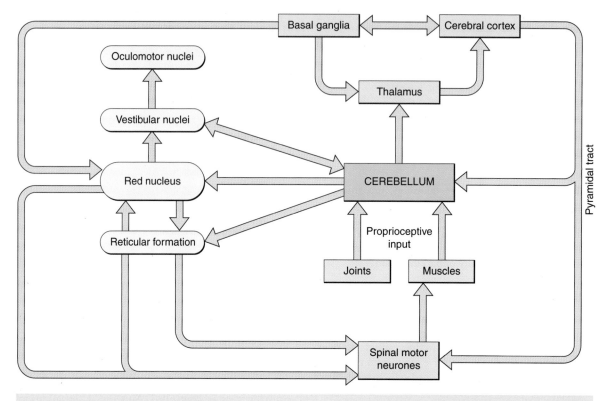

Fig. 18.4   Main connections of the cerebellum.

of the cord over the distance of several segments and ascend in the contralateral spinothalamic tracts, joining the medial lemniscus fibre to synapse in the thalamus. A topographical arrangement exists in the spinothalamic tract, such that fibres from the lower limb come to lie outermost and those from the upper limb innermost.

Both the main sensory pathways synapse in the ventro-postero-lateral nucleus of the thalamus. The post-synaptic fibres lie closely packed together in the internal capsule, immediately posterior to the pyramidal tract fibres. They project up to the post-central gyrus (primary sensory cortex) in a topographical arrangement, similar to that on the motor strip. Although some appreciation of sensation and pain probably occurs at the thalamus, the sensory cortex is necessary for localisation of sensations from different parts of the body and provides the accuracy needed for two-point discrimination and joint position sense. Further analysis goes on in the adjoining parietal lobe which is responsible for perception of pattern, shape, size, texture and weight.

Collateral fibres from the ascending sensory pathways also make contact with the reticular formation. This is a chain of interconnecting short fibre neurones which lies in the centre of the brain stem and projects up to the

midline thalamic nuclei, which in turn send fibres widely over the cortex. These non-specific projections (the reticular activating system) are important for maintaining awareness.

Lesions of the sensory system may cause negative and positive symptoms and signs. Negative symptoms of decreased sensation may be described as 'numbness', but also altered temperature perception may provoke descriptions of 'coldness'. Positive sensory symptoms may be paraesthesiae ('pins and needles'), warmth, burning, or tightness. The symptoms and signs caused by lesions at different levels are summarised in Table 18.6. Partial lesions of peripheral nerves or roots tend to cause altered sensation rather than anaesthesia. Because of disturbance of the normal gating of painful stimuli, these lesions often cause hypersensitivity to painful stimuli, but with reduced sensitivity to well localised touch (hyperpathia).

REFLEX ACTIVITY

Reflexes represent the simplest forms of integrated activity in the nervous system. The functional com-

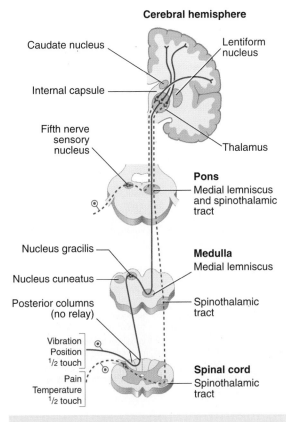

Cerebral hemisphere

Caudate nucleus

Lentiform nucleus

Internal capsule

Fifth nerve sensory nucleus

Thalamus

Pons
Medial lemniscus and spinothalamic tract

Nucleus gracilis

Medulla
Medial lemniscus

Nucleus cuneatus

Posterior columns (no relay)

Spinothalamic tract

Vibration
Position
1/2 touch

Spinal cord
Spinothalamic tract

Pain
Temperature
1/2 touch

Fig. 18.5 The sensory pathways.

ponents of a reflex are listed in the information box below.

FUNCTIONAL COMPONENTS OF A REFLEX

- A peripheral receptor organ
- A sensory nerve (or autonomic afferent)
- A central neurone or chain of neurones (spinal, cranial, or autonomic)
- A motor nerve (or autonomic efferent)
- An effector organ (skeletal/smooth muscle, gland)

The activity of a given reflex may be altered by local or descending neural influences acting on the central neurones. For example, tendon reflexes become exaggerated when there is damage to the pyramidal tract, or depressed when there is a cerebellar lesion.

Many reflexes involve not only activation of an effector muscle but also relaxation of antagonists. A simple way to consider reflexes is to divide them into monosynaptic (or oligosynaptic) and polysynaptic types.

MONOSYNAPTIC AND OLIGOSYNAPTIC REFLEXES

The best-known example of a monosynaptic reflex is the tendon stretch reflex. This serves to maintain muscle tone and to adjust it during movement. Clinically, the reflex can be tested by applying a sharp stretching force (hammer tap) to a muscle tendon. This activates stretch receptors in the muscle spindle organs which send a synchronised volley of sensory activity up the rapidly conducting large afferent fibres which enter the spinal cord at the dorsal root. The sensory fibres synapse directly on the anterior horn cell, promoting depolarisation by excitatory transmission. The motor-fibre volley passes to the same muscle, causing contraction which is observed as a brief jerk (see Fig. 18.6). The intrafusal fibres of the muscle spindle control the sensitivity of its stretch receptors, and are in turn adjusted by gamma efferent fibres whose activity is controlled by descending influences from the cerebellum, and pyramidal and extrapyramidal systems (Table 18.7) The tendon reflexes serve as a convenient way for the clinician to test the integrity of the reflex arc components at different spinal levels (Table 18.8) and also to judge changes in the descending (especially pyramidal) systems.

Other monosynaptic or oligosynaptic reflexes can be elicited in the cranial nerves. The **jaw jerk** is mediated by stretching the muscles of mastication, the reflex loop passing to and from the pons in the trigeminal nerves.

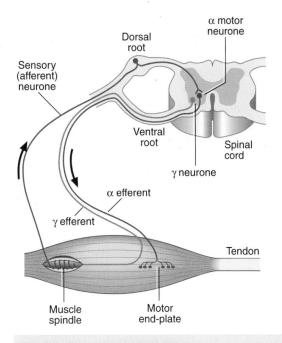

α motor neurone

Dorsal root

Sensory (afferent) neurone

Ventral root

Spinal cord

γ neurone

α efferent

γ efferent

Tendon

Muscle spindle

Motor end-plate

Fig. 18.6 The tendon stretch reflex.

Table 18.6   Symptoms and signs of sensory lesions

Site	Symptoms	Signs	Associated features
Peripheral nerve (partial)	Numbness, paraesthesiae (discomfort)	Reduced sensation in territory of nerve (hyperpathia)	Weakness of muscles supplied by nerve
Many peripheral nerves (polyneuropathy)	Numbness and paraesthesiae hands and feet	'Glove and stocking' reduced sensation, impaired vibration at extremities	Weakness of distal muscles, loss of tendon reflexes
Spinal root (radiculopathy)	Numbness, paraesthesiae, hypersenstivity, 'tightness'	Reduced sensation ± hyperpathia in dermatomal pattern	Weakness of muscles and reduced tendon reflexes of that segment
Posterior column	Numbness, 'band-like' sensation, unsteadiness, clumsiness	Reduced joint position sense, vibration and 2-point discrim and touch ipsilaterally; normal pain and temp	Sensory ataxia; loss of balance worse with closed eyes (Romberg's Test)
Spinothalamic tract	Numbness, warmth/coldness diffuse distribution contralaterally below lesion	Reduced pain and temp sensation below and contralateral to lesion; normal proprioception and vibration	Area of altered sensation begins several spinal segments below lesion
Brain stem (pons or lower)	Numbness and paraesthesiae face with coldness/warmth opposite limbs and trunk	Ipsilateral facial anaesthesia, with contralateral loss of pain/temperature limbs and trunk	May be lower cranial nerve lesions ipsilateral (V, VI, VII, IX, X, XI, XII)
(above pons)	Contralateral numbness or coldness/ warmth face, limbs, trunk	Contralateral reduced pain/temperature on face, limbs, trunk	Ipsilateral upper cranial nerve lesion (III, IV)
Thalamus	Diffuse deep pain on opposite side of body	Reduced touch, pain and temp + hyperpathia contralaterally to lesion	Pain threshold raised, but more unpleasant
Internal capsule	Contralateral numbness of face, limbs, trunk	Reduced touch, pain, temperature on face, limbs and trunk contralateral side	Hemiparesis or hemianopia if other parts of capsule involved
Sensory cortex	Numbness localised to limb or part of	Loss of position sense, 2-point discrimination and sterognosis	Weakness of affected part if motor cortex involved
Parietal lobe	Difficulty in identifying shape, size, texture; spatial disorientation	Impaired recognition of shapes, sizes; denial of limbs on affected side	Apraxia for purposeful movements/ speech, dressing apraxia, spatial problems

Table 18.7   Lesions affecting tendon reflex activity

Site of lesion	Effect on reflexes
Sensory fibres/roots	Diminished/absent
Motor neurone	Diminished/absent
Motor roots/nerves	Diminished/absent
Cerebellum	Diminished/pendular
Pyramidal tract	Increased ± clonus

Table 18.8   Segmental supply of tendon reflexes

Reflex	Spinal segment
Biceps	Cervical 5/6
Brachioradialis	Cervical 5/6
Triceps	Cervical 7
Finger flexors	Cervical 7/8
	Thoracic 1
Quadriceps (knee)	Lumbar 3/4
Hamstrings	Lumbar 5/sacral 1
Gastrocnemius (ankle)	Sacral 1

Lesions of the pyramidal tracts above the pons exaggerate the reflex. The **corneal reflex** is oligosynaptic, involving mainly the first division of the trigeminal sensory root as the afferent limb. Fibres enter the pons, descend in the tract of the fifth nerve and synapse in its nucleus from where second-order fibres pass to both facial nuclei to cause bilateral eye closure from contraction of orbicularis oculi. The reflex is diminished by lesions of the first trigeminal sensory division, by damage to the facial nerve and in lesions of the lateral pons and medulla.

POLYSYNAPTIC REFLEXES

These more complex reflexes involve chains of interconnected neurones within the spinal cord which activate several muscle groups to produce coordinated movements in response to usually noxious stimuli. The presence and sometimes nature of the reflexes is modified by descending fibre systems, particularly the pyramidal tracts. The **plantar reflex** is an example of polysynaptic activity. After the first year of life, the normal plantar response is flexion of the great toe, with adduction of the other toes. If the pyramidal tract is damaged or rendered temporarily non-functional (e.g. during an epileptic seizure), the same stimulus causes extension of the great toe and abduction of the other toes—the extensor plantar response. The **flexion withdrawal reflex** may be seen in conjunction with an extensor plantar response. Here a noxious stimulus will cause reflex flexion of the hip and knee to withdraw the foot from the stimulus. Sometimes when the pyramidal tract damage is severe, the ipsilateral flexion reflex is accompanied by extension of the opposite leg—the crossed extensor reflex.

The **abdominal reflexes** are also examples of polysynaptic activity which has protective function. Damage to the pyramidal tract on one side will abolish the reflex on that side, this phenomenon being particularly common in multiple sclerosis. Damage to the peripheral elements of the reflexes (T 8–12 spinal nerves) also abolishes the response, as do obesity, pregnancy, abdominal surgery and muscle laxity.

CONTROL OF THE BLADDER AND SPHINCTERS

BLADDER

The nerve supply to the bladder derives from three sources (Fig. 18.7):

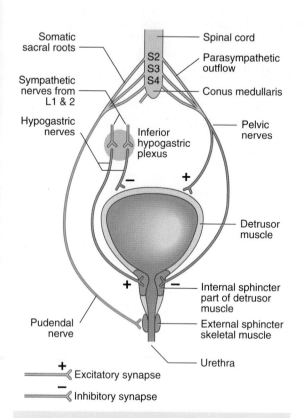

Excitatory synapse
Inhibitory synapse

Fig. 18.7　Nerve supply to the bladder and sphincters.

Sympathetic fibres

Coming from spinal segments L1 and 2 these pass via the inferior hypogastric plexus and the hypogastric nerves to the bladder wall and internal sphincteric part of the detrusor muscle. When activated they cause relaxation of the bladder wall but closure of the internal sphincter. These effects are inhibited by alpha-adrenergic blocking drugs such as phenoxybenzamine.

Parasympathetic fibres

These derive from the sacral outflow (S2–4) and pass to the bladder via the pelvic nerves. They effect contraction of the detrusor muscle and opening of the internal sphincter. These cholinergic effects are inhibited by drugs such as atropine and probanthine.

Somatic fibres

These also emerge from spinal segments S2–4 and pass to the skeletal muscle of the external sphincter. The same nerves supply the anal sphincter muscles.

Bladder function

Afferent fibres from the bladder wall pass via the pelvic and hypogastric nerves, and from the sphincters in the pudendal nerves. Distension of the bladder evokes reflex activation of parasympathetic neurones in the sacral 2–4 segments which causes detrusor contraction and sphincter opening to effect automatic bladder emptying. Reciprocal changes in the sympathetic outflow from L1 and 2 aid this process. Awareness of bladder fullness reaches consciousness via the lateral spinothalamic tracts of the spinal cord, eventually reaching the parasagittal part of the post-central gyrus. Voluntary inhibition of the bladder reflex and its release which permits micturition are controlled by the parasagittal part of the frontal cortex, the efferent fibres descending the spinal cord close to the pyramidal tracts. Several patterns of neurogenic bladder dysfunction may occur and these are listed in the information box overleaf.

RECTUM

The rectum has an excitatory cholinergic input from the parasympathetic sacral outflow, and inhibitory sympathetic supply similar to the bladder. Continence depends largely on skeletal muscle contraction in the puborectalis and pelvic floor muscles supplied by the pudendal nerves which influence the angle of the anorectum as well as the internal and external anal sphincters. Damage to the autonomic components causes constipation. Lesions affecting the conus medullaris, the somatic sacral 2–4 roots and the pudendal nerves cause faecal incontinence.

PATTERNS OF NEUROGENIC BLADDER DYSFUNCTION

Atonic Bladder
- Cause
  Damage to sacral segments of conus medullaris
  Damage to sacral roots/nerves and pelvic nerves
- Results
  Loss of detrusor contraction
  Difficulty initiating micturition
  Distension of bladder, overflow incontinence

Hypertonic Bladder
- Cause
  Spinal-cord damage involving pyramidal tracts above
  conus medullaris
  Frontal lobe lesions
- Results
  Urgency and urge incontinence
  Bladder/sphincter incoordination
  Incomplete bladder emptying

Cortical Lesions
- Post-central
  Loss of awareness of bladder fullness, incontinence
- Pre-central
  Difficulty initiating micturition
- Frontal
  Inappropriate micturition, loss of social control

PENILE ERECTION AND EJACULATION

These related functions are under autonomic control via the pelvic nerves (parasympathetic S2–4) and the hypogastric nerves (sympathetic L1 and 2). Descending influences from the cerebrum are important for psychogenic erection, but this can occur as a purely reflex phenomenon in response to genital stimulation. Erection is largely parasympathetic in control, and is impaired by drugs which have anticholinergic effects and also some anti-hypertensive and anti-depressant agents. Sympathetic activity is important for ejaculation, and may be inhibited by alpha-adrenoceptor antagonists.

SPEECH

Speech enables the communication of ideas from person to person by the use of verbal symbols produced by the larynx, pharynx, lips and tongue. A schematic representation of the mechanisms involved in speech and language is shown in Figure. 18.8. The important cortical area for language lies in the dominant hemisphere. This is on the left side for right-handed people; left-handers may have language functions mostly on the right, mostly on the left or shared between both sides. The cortical language areas are shown in Figure 18.9.

The posterior language (Wernicke's) area in the dominant temporo-parietal region is important in the comprehension of received speech and in the selection of words to express ideas. In simple terms, this area acts like a dictionary. A bundle of subcortical fibres, the arcuate fasciculus, connects it with the anterior speech (Broca's) area in the inferior third frontal convolution. Broca's area is important for the fluency and rhythm of speech and for the maintenance of grammar and syntax.

DYSPHASIA

Dysfunction of the language areas results in dysphasia, where there is disordered use of language with or without

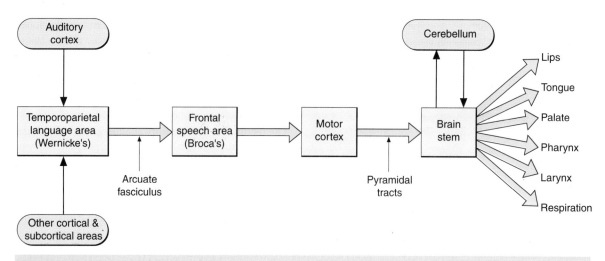

Fig. 18.8 Mechanisms of speech and language.

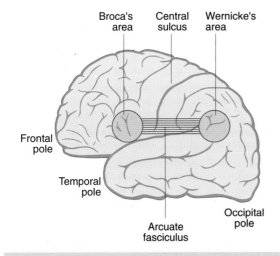

Broca's area   Central sulcus   Wernicke's area

Frontal pole

Temporal pole

Occipital pole

Arcuate fasciculus

Fig. 18.9 Cortical language areas in the left cerebral hemisphere.

impaired comprehension of received speech. Lesions of the anterior speech area cause **expressive dysphasia**, characterised by poor fluency, with reduced output of words, but usually preserved comprehension. By contrast, with damage to the temporo-parietal region, fluency, grammar and articulation are preserved, but the speech lacks correct meaning, with inappropriate letters or words (paraphasias) or entirely new words (neologisms). In addition there is a degree of difficulty with comprehension of heard speech (receptive dysphasia). Lesions in the perisylvian region, damaging the arcuate fasciculus, may have elements of both expressive and receptive difficulty, but are characterised particularly by impaired ability to repeat heard speech; this picture is known as **conduction dysphasia.** The features of lesions in the different language areas are shown in Table 18.9.

In clinical practice, analysis of speech is carried out not only to localise the lesion, but, in the case of a vascular or traumatic insult, to give some idea of prognosis. Global dysphasia carries a poor chance of recovery, while pure forms of anterior or posterior dysphasia

are more likely to recover, especially if repetition is preserved.

DYSARTHRIA

When the motor control systems for the muscles of speech, or the muscles themselves are impaired, dysarthria results. The dysarthric patient uses language normally with correct grammar, appropriate words, and retained comprehension; but speech is indistinct or even unintelligible because of weakness, slowness or incoordination of the muscles responsible (Table 18.10). The lesion causing dysarthria may be peripheral in the muscles of the face, tongue or pharynx; at their neuromuscular junctions; in the brain stem or the cerebellum, the pyramidal tracts or motor cortex, or in the extrapyramidal system.

DYSPHONIA

When there is impaired air flow, damage or dysfunction of the vocal cords or soft palate, the generation of notes is impaired. Speech may be softer, hoarse or husky. The generation of hard consonants (G or B) is impaired if the soft palate cannot close off the nasopharynx; this gives speech a 'nasal' quality (e.g. 'frog' becomes 'frong'). Severe damage to both vocal cords causes total lack of phonation—aphonia.

VISION

The visual system is frequently involved by intracranial disease because, starting in the eyes and terminating in the occipital cortex, its fibres traverse a wide area of the cerebrum. Light rays are refracted by the media and lens of the eye and an inverted image of the external world is focused on to the retina. Fine adjustment of focus is carried out by the ciliary muscle, under control of the third nerve parasympathetic outflow. The light-sensitive retinal rods and cones convert photic energy into nerve impulses which undergo preliminary integration at the

Table 18.9 Characteristics of dysphasias

Site	Output	Fluency	Paraphasias	Comprehension	Repetition
Anterior (Broca)	Reduced	Poor	Absent	Retained	Variable
Posterior (Wernicke)	Normal/increased	Good	Present	Impaired	Variable
Arcuate fasciculus (conduction)	Variable	Variable	Mild	Variable	Impaired
Fronto-parietal (global)	Very reduced	Poor	Jargon	Impaired	Impaired

Table 18.10   Causes of dysarthria

Site	Type	Characteristics	Associated features
Muscles of speech	**Myopathic**	Indistinct, poor articulation	Weakness of face, tongue and neck
Motor end-plate	**Myasthenic**	Indistinct with fatigue and dysphonia Fluctuating severity	Ptosis, diplopia facial and neck weakness
Brain stem	**Bulbar**	Indistinct, slurred, often nasal	Dysphagia, diplopia ataxia
Cerebellum	**'Scanning'**	Slurring, impaired timing and cadence, 'sing-song' quality	Ataxia of limbs and gait tremor head/limbs
Pyramidal tracts	**Spastic**	Indistinct, breathy, mumbling	Poor rapid tongue movements; increased reflexes and jaw jerk
Basal ganglia	**Parkinsonian**	Indistinct, rapid stammering, quiet	Tremor, rigidity, slow shuffling gait
Basal ganglia	**Dystonic**	Strained, slow	Dystonia, athetosis

retinal ganglion cells. Fibres from these cells make up the optic nerves which pass back through the optic foraminae towards the optic chiasm. Each optic nerve carries a covering of meninges which may transmit cerebrospinal fluid (CSF) pressure changes to the nerve head in the eye, causing optic disc swelling (papilloedema) if the pressure is elevated. Pathophysiologically, the optic nerve behaves more like cerebral white matter than peripheral nerve.

Because of the image inversion produced by the eye's optics, the temporal visual field is represented on the nasal retina, and the upper field on the lower retina. At the optic chiasm, fibres from the nasal retinae (temporal fields) cross over to the contralateral optic tract, while the temporal retinal fibres (nasal fields) remain uncrossed. The optic tract fibres pass mostly to the lateral geniculate bodies where some synaptic integration takes place. A few fibres leave before the geniculate and pass to the mid-brain to supply the afferent limb of the pupil light reflex. After the geniculate bodies, the optic radiation fibres sweep posteriorly through the temporal and parietal lobes towards the calcarine cortex in the occipital lobe. The vertical arrangement is maintained so that fibres in the parietal lobe come from the upper retinae

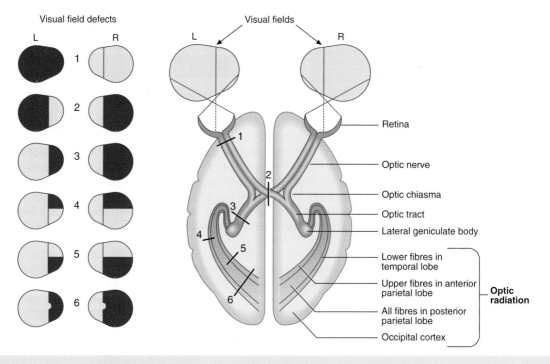

Fig. 18.10   Visual pathways and field defects.

Table 18.11   Clinical manifestations of lesions of the visual pathway

Site	Clinical features
Retina	Partial lesions—patches of visual loss (scotomas). Damage to macula causes severe loss of acuity. Large lesions diminish pupil light reflex
Optic nerve	Partial—scotomas, esp. central or between fixation and blind spot (centrocaecal). Vascular lesions tend to affect upper or lower field of one eye (altitudinal defects). Severe lesions cause blindness and loss of pupil light reflex
Optic chiasm	Midline lesions (e.g. pituitary tumour) damage crossing nasal fibres, causing bitemporal defects. Compression from below affects upper fields first. Lateral compression rare but causes loss in nasal fields of vision. Large chiasmatic lesions impair pupil light reflex bilaterally
Optic tract	Impairment of same side of vision in each eye often asymmetrically (incongruous homonymous hemianopia). Affected fields opposite side to lesion
Optic radiation	Homonymous hemianopia contralateral to lesion. Upper fibres (parietal)—lower quadrantic defects; lower fibres (temporal)—upper quadrantic
Occipital lobe	Contralateral homonymous hemianopia. Small lesions may cause homonymous scotomas, sectorial or altitudinal defects

(lower visual fields) and those in the temporal lobe from the lower retinae (upper fields) (Fig. 18.10). In the occipital lobe further analysis of visual information from the contralateral side of the visual field takes place. Cells in the calcarine cortex are synaptically connected so that they detect rectangular shapes, moving edges, and bars or lines in different orientations. Stereoscopic vision is also served in this area by cells activated by corresponding retinal points.

A variety of visual defects are associated with lesions of the visual pathway which help to localise the site of the disease (Table 18.11).

Clinical features of localised cerebral lesions

Although the brain functions in an integrated fashion, certain cortical areas are allied to specific functions. The effects of lesions at different sites are summarised in Figure 18.11.

INVESTIGATION OF THE NERVOUS SYSTEM

While clinical examination often will lead to accurate localisation of lesions within the nervous system, the precise diagnosis of the nature of such lesions relies firstly on analysis of the history and secondly on methods of investigation. The tests which offer the best diagnostic accuracy are frequently the most invasive and hazardous; as a general rule it is wise to begin investigation with

non-invasive screening tests and to select only the most appropriate invasive methods for each case.

IMAGING

Plain radiology

Plain radiographs are frequently normal even in the presence of quite advanced cerebral or spinal disease. Skull films are nevertheless useful for demonstrating sinus disease, fractures, pituitary tumours, bony metastatic deposits and calcified intracranial lesions. Abnormalities most likely to calcify include meningiomas, tuberculomas, oligodendrogliomas, giant aneurysms and arteriovenous malformations. Chronically raised intracranial pressure may sometimes be inferred from erosion of the clinoid processes of the pituitary fossa. Lateral shift of the calcified normally mid-line pineal gland can provide evidence of a mass lesion.

Plain spine radiographs may show evidence of degenerative bony changes, with reduction of the disc spaces and misalignment, and are particularly helpful after trauma. Oblique views of the cervical spine help delineate narrowing of the intervertebral neural exit foramina. Plain films also aid detection of metastatic or infective lesions affecting the spine, where erosion of the vertebral body, laminae or disc may be evident.

Contrast radiology

If a contrast medium (usually iodine based) is introduced into the cerebral blood vessels or the cerebrospinal fluid surrounding the brain or spinal cord, then normal and abnormal structures can be demonstrated.

Angiography

In conventional cerebral angiography contrast is injected into the carotid or vertebral arteries. Selective catheterisation of the relevant vessel is usually performed via a catheter inserted into the femoral artery in the groin. A series of radiograph films is taken usually in two planes during contrast injection so that arterial, capillary and venous phases can be studied (Fig. 18.12). In modern practice angiography is used mainly to study the extracranial and intracranial vessels, to outline regions of arterial disease, aneurysms and arteriovenous malformations. Conventional angiography carries a small but significant risk of stroke or death, particularly in the elderly and patients with vascular disease, and should be undertaken only if management is likely to be altered by the result.

Digital subtraction angiography (DSA)

This offers a less invasive way of demonstrating cerebral vasculature by computer enhancing techniques. Con-

1 Parietal lobe

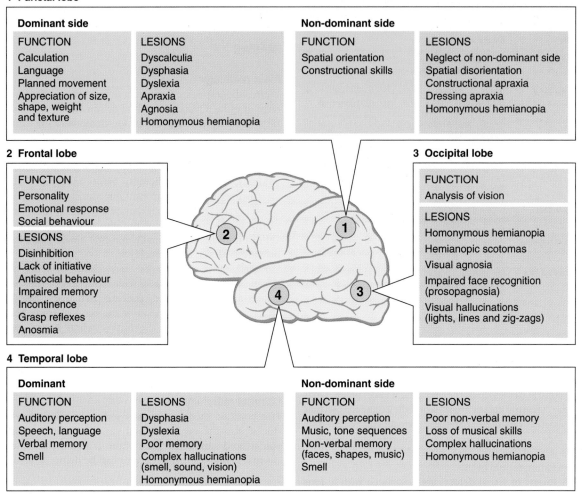

Dominant side

FUNCTION	LESIONS
Calculation	Dyscalculia
Language	Dysphasia
Planned movement	Dyslexia
Appreciation of size, shape, weight and texture	Apraxia
	Agnosia
	Homonymous hemianopia

Non-dominant side

FUNCTION	LESIONS
Spatial orientation	Neglect of non-dominant side
Constructional skills	Spatial disorientation
	Constructional apraxia
	Dressing apraxia
	Homonymous hemianopia

2 Frontal lobe

FUNCTION
Personality
Emotional response
Social behaviour

LESIONS
Disinhibition
Lack of initiative
Antisocial behaviour
Impaired memory
Incontinence
Grasp reflexes
Anosmia

3 Occipital lobe

FUNCTION
Analysis of vision

LESIONS
Homonymous hemianopia
Hemianopic scotomas
Visual agnosia
Impaired face recognition (prosopagnosia)
Visual hallucinations (lights, lines and zig-zags)

4 Temporal lobe

Dominant

FUNCTION	LESIONS
Auditory perception	Dysphasia
Speech, language	Dyslexia
Verbal memory	Poor memory
Smell	Complex hallucinations (smell, sound, vision)
	Homonymous hemianopia

Non-dominant side

FUNCTION	LESIONS
Auditory perception	Poor non-verbal memory
Music, tone sequences	Loss of musical skills
Non-verbal memory (faces, shapes, music)	Complex hallucinations
Smell	Homonymous hemianopia

Fig. 18.11   Features of localised cerebral lesions.

trast is injected either by a central venous bolus or a low dose arterial injection. With the venous route (DVI), there is less risk than with conventional angiography, but the image quality, especially of intracranial vessels, is inferior. Studies of sufficient quality may however be obtained to exclude a major stenosis of the cervical carotid and vertebral arteries.

Myelography and radiculography

It is usually necessary to introduce contrast liquid into the subarachnoid space by lumbar, cervical or cisternal puncture to investigate disorders of the spinal cord or roots. Water-soluble non-ionic contrast media are in routine use. The patient is tilted on a table so that contrast can be manipulated up or down the spinal sub-arachnoid space, permitting visualisation of the spinal cord (myelography—Fig. 18.14, top row) and lumbo-sacral roots (radiculography). Headache is a common sequel, and occasionally seizures, meningitis and muscle spasms occur. It is likely that Magnetic Resonance Imaging (MRI) will replace many myelographic examinations.

Pneumoencephalography

The injection of air into the lumbar subarachnoid space to outline the cerebral ventricles and CSF spaces is rarely performed. Air-CT meatography is a modern refinement in which small volumes of air are manoeuvred into the cerebello-pontine angle and CT images taken to outline the internal auditory meatus and the seventh and

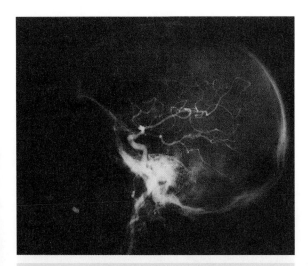

Fig. 18.12 Normal carotid angiogram (lateral view). It shows cervical carotid artery, its bifurcation and internal carotid circulation within the head.

eighth cranial nerves within it. The technique is used for the detection of small acoustic neuromas.

Computed tomography (CT)

This non-invasive technique has revolutionised investigation of the central nervous system. The method is very sensitive and will show the normal outlines of the brain, cerebral ventricles and CSF spaces (Fig. 18.13), and after intravenous contrast injection, some of the larger blood vessels. CT will demonstrate the vast majority of cerebral haemorrhages, tumours, cysts and abscesses and will readily demonstrate hydrocephalus and cerebral atrophy. Although many cerebral infarcts and subdural haematomas will also be seen, small early lesions may be undetected. Because of interference from bony structures CT is less useful for visualisation of the brain stem, cerebellum and spinal cord, but with modifications of technique, these structures can be demonstrated.

CT is largely non-invasive and carries little risk. Spinal CT scanning is used increasingly to outline disc protrusions, spinal canal stenosis and intramedullary lesions.

Magnetic resonance imaging (MRI)

This technique is a powerful, non-invasive tool for imaging the brain and spinal cord; but machines are as yet very expensive, and MRI is not yet widely available. MRI is particularly sensitive to differences between grey and white matter, and shows areas of demyelination (e.g. in multiple sclerosis) much more readily than CT. MRI is insensitive to compact bone and therefore renders

excellent images of the posterior fossa and cranio-vertebral region (Figs 18.14, lower row; 18.15). The technique is the investigation of choice for demonstrating lesions in suspected multiple sclerosis, brain-stem tumours and infarcts, and intrinsic lesions in the spinal cord, especially syringomyelia (Figs 18.39, 18.45). It is likely that MR images of the lower spinal cord will replace many myelographic examinations as more sophisticated equipment becomes available.

Radionuclide cerebral scanning

This method is reasonably efficient in the detection of meningiomas and arteriovenous malformations because they have increased blood supply and take up isotope more avidly than surrounding brain. However, it is considerably inferior to CT in detecting infarction, haemorrhage, gliomas and subdural collections, and gives no information about the cerebral ventricles unless isotope is injected into the CSF. The dynamics of isotope uptake can be studied by linking the gamma camera to a computer. Images of regional cerebral blood flow can be thus obtained.

Emission computed tomography

This is a further modification whereby the distribution of radio-labelled compounds is mapped by a moving array of scintillation detectors and the data reformatted into a two-dimensional image. Spacial resolution is inferior to X-ray CT, but functional changes such as oxygen and glucose uptake and neurotransmitter turnover can be studied. Such systems are costly and are used primarily for research.

CLINICAL NEUROPHYSIOLOGY

Electroencephalography (EEG)

Spontaneous electrical signals arising from the cerebral cortex can be recorded with electrodes placed on the scalp. Rhythmical waveforms (Fig. 18.16) can be detected, slower frequencies tending to predominate in the very young, during sleep and in disease states. Frequency bands are annotated as:

alpha:	7–13/s
beta:	>13/s
theta:	4–6/s
delta:	<4/s.

In alert adults alpha activity predominates, especially when the eyes are shut, and is found best over the posterior quadrants. In disease states (see Table 18.12), slow activity (theta and delta) may be focal or generalised.

The EEG is used mainly for detection and charac-

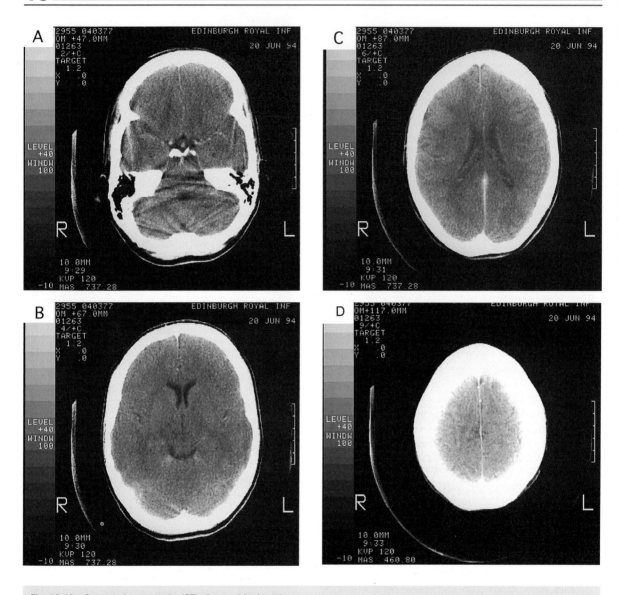

Fig. 18.13   Computed tomography (CT) of normal brain. [A] at level of cerebellum, temporal lobes and pituitary fossa; [B] section through cerebral hemispheres and upper brain stem; [C] section through cerebral hemispheres showing lateral ventricles; [D] upper part of cerebral hemispheres.

terisation of epileptic disturbances (Fig. 18.17), but also has a role in other states of altered brain function (e.g. encephalitis) where imaging techniques may be unhelpful. In epilepsy, focal or generalised high voltage fast transients (spikes and sharp waves) are recorded during seizures and sometimes interictally. The chance of detecting such phenomena is improved by hyperventilation, photic flicker, sleep and some drugs. In selected cases of diagnostic difficulty it is possible to record EEG from ambulant patients for 24 hours or longer using a light-weight tape recorder, or to use prolonged video-monitoring of the patient and his EEG simultaneously. It is important to recognise that up to 40% of patients with clinical epilepsy may have a normal routine EEG, and that an abnormal EEG record does not establish a diagnosis of epilepsy in the absence of appropriate history. In patients with severe epilepsy, intracranial electrodes placed through the foramen ovale or surgical burrholes may be used to identify an epileptic focus which may be subsequently resected.

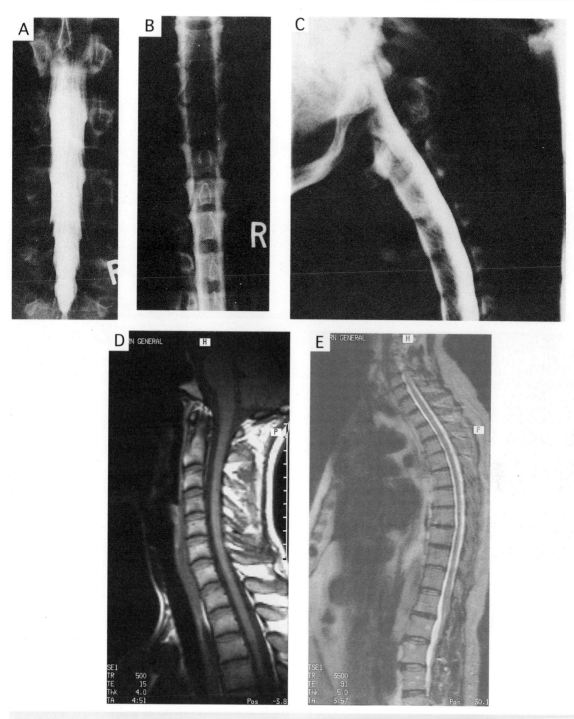

Fig. 18.14   Top row: Normal myelogram. Water soluble contrast (iopamidol) introduced by lumbar puncture at L2/3 level. A Anteroposterior view demonstrating the lumbo-sacral roots. B The cervical spinal roots can be identified in the posteroanterior view. C The cervical spinal cord is seen against the positive contrast as a central shadow.
Lower row: Magnetic resonance imaging (MRI) of normal spine. D Proton density image showing normal cervical spine and cord. The cerebellum and lower brain stem are seen at the top of the picture. E T2 weighted image of dorsal spine and cord.

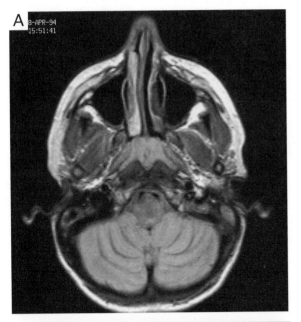

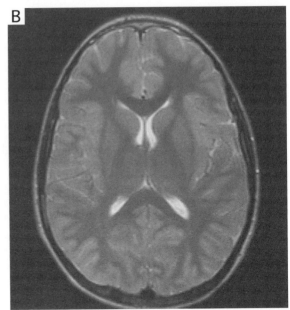

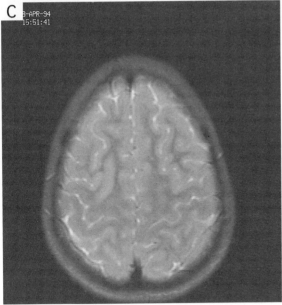

Fig. 18.15 Magnetic resonance images (MRIs) of normal brain: axial sections. [A] At level of lower brain stem, cerebellum and paranasal sinuses; [B] Mid cerebral hemisphere level showing cerebral ventricles, corpus callosum, deep cerebral white matter and basal ganglia. [C] Level of upper cerebral hemisphere, showing CSF spaces around cerebral sulci.

Evoked potential recording

The development of electronic signal averaging by computer techniques permits recording of very small cerebral or spinal event-related potentials. Stimulation by visual, sensory nerve or auditory routes is time-locked to the averager so that a processed signal, relatively free from interference, can be made up from 100–1000 evoked responses. Visually evoked potentials (VEP) are the most useful clinically, and are recorded with an array of scalp electrodes over the occipital region. The dominant response wave from a normal eye is a positive wave peaking at about 100 ms (Fig. 18.18). Lesions of the retina, optic nerve, chiasma, tract, radiation of cortex may all disrupt or delay the response, but demyelinating lesions of the optic nerve often cause marked delay with relatively good preservation of the wave form. A delayed VEP in a patient with clinically normal vision can therefore be of much diagnostic help in multiple sclerosis.

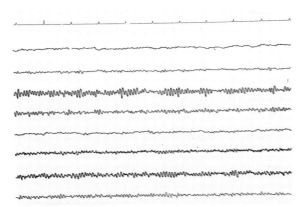

Fig. 18.16 Portion of an 8-channel EEG record taken from a normal adolescent. Four channels running anterior to posterior over the parietal regions are displayed from each side. Top four traces—right side; lower four—left side. Uppermost trace is a 1 second time marker. Note the posteriorly dominant 10/s waves—the alpha rhythm.

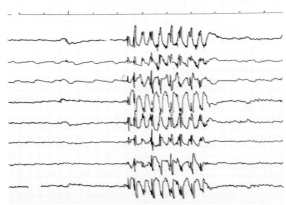

Fig. 18.17 Abnormal EEG from a patient suffering from generalised tonic-clonic seizures. This inter-ictal record shows a paroxysm of generalised spike and slow wave activity lasting about 3 seconds, during which the patient showed no clinical abnormality.

Electromyography (EMG)

Muscle or nerve action potentials can be detected by surface or needle electrodes. After electrical stimulation of a peripheral nerve trunk, compound action potentials can be recorded over the nerve's course, their normal amplitude varying from 5–30 microvolts. Compound muscle action potentials elicited by motor nerve stimulation are much larger (1–20 millivolts) and more readily recorded because the muscle amplifies the response. Many peripheral nerves can be stimulated and conduction velocities of motor and sensory fibres can be measured separately. Velocity and amplitude measurements help gauge the type and severity of polyneuropathies and may define the site of localised nerve compression, as in the carpal tunnel syndrome.

Demyelination of peripheral nerve causes marked reduction in conduction velocity, whereas primary axonal degeneration is associated with reduction of motor and sensory action potential amplitude with little or no reduction in velocity. Concentric needle EMG is used to sample motor units in muscle at rest and during voluntary activity. Primary myopathy is associated with reduction in motor unit amplitude and duration with normal numbers of units activated during effort. Denervation causes spontaneous fibrillation and fasciculation at rest, and a reduced number of normal or enlarged units during activity (Fig. 18.20). Repetitive stimulation of a motor nerve with trains of impulses at 3–15/s may detect a characteristic decremental response in myasthenia gravis, although false negative results are common. In Lambert–Eaton myasthenic syndrome (LEMS) higher frequency stimulation (20–50/s) nearly always produces striking incrementation of the motor response.

Table 18.12 EEG changes in disease states

Disorder	EEG pattern
Cerebral tumour	Focal theta/delta
Cerebral abscess	Focal delta
Cerebral infarct	Focal theta/delta
Encephalitis	Theta/delta/sharp waves usually generalised
Metabolic coma (e.g. hypoglycaemia)	Diffuse theta/delta
Sub-dural haematoma	Reduced amplitude over side of lesion
Epilepsy	Focal or generalised spikes, sharp waves, spike-wave complexes

Somato-sensory evoked potentials (SSEP) recorded from the brachial plexus, cervical spine and contralateral parietal area when the median or ulnar nerve is stimulated electrically may similarly help detect lesions in the sensory pathways. Similar responses may be produced over the lumbar and dorsal spine and vertex by posterior tibial nerve stimulation in the leg (Fig. 18.19). SSEP are less useful than VEP for detecting subclinical demyelination, but can be of help in delineating lesions of the brachial plexus, spinal roots and cord.

Auditory evoked potentials (AEP) in response to click stimuli arise largely from the brain stem, and may give evidence of cochlear, acoustic nerve or brain stem disorders.

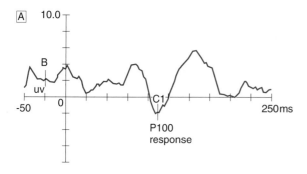

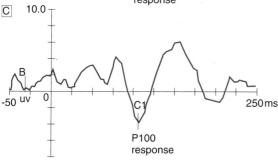

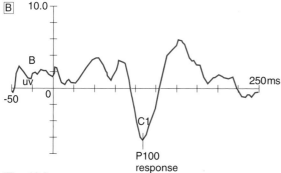

Fig. 18.18   Normal visual evoked responses elicited by reversing chequer-board pattern stimulus to right eye. [A] trace—right occipital; [B] trace—mid occipital; [C] trace—left occipital recording electrons. 100 individual responses are computer averaged to produce these traces. The major positive (downward) deflection occurs about 110 ms after the stimulus and is called the P100 response.

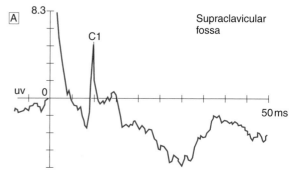

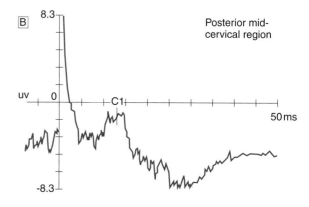

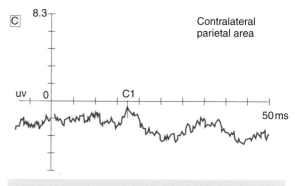

Fig. 18.19   Normal somato-sensory evoked response elicited by electrical stimulation of the median nerve at the wrist. Each trace is a computer average of 500 responses. [A] trace, recorded at supraclavicular fossa, shows a negative (upward) potential at 10 ms. [B] trace, recorded from posterior mid-cervical region, shows at C1 a negative response with a latency of 12–13 ms. [C] trace, recorded from contralateral parietal area, shows at C1 a smaller negative response of 17–18 ms latency.

BIOCHEMICAL TESTS

Tests of muscle breakdown

Enzymes released from muscle increase in concentration in peripheral blood in muscle disease. The highest enzyme levels are seen in active polymyositis and the more severe forms of muscular dystrophy. Widespread denervation may cause modest enzyme elevations. The enzymes most commonly measured are: creatinine phosphokinase (CPK), aldolase and lactate dehydrogenase (LDH).

Tests for specific disorders

Rare disorders of muscle and nerve metabolism can sometimes be diagnosed by measuring specific enzymes in blood or muscle. Some examples are listed in the information box on page 1042.

Compound muscle action potential responses: recordings over thenar eminence

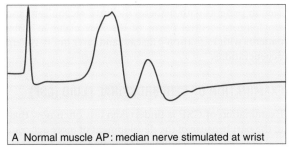

A Normal muscle AP: median nerve stimulated at wrist

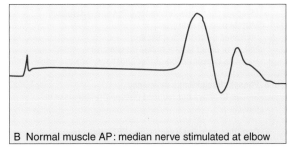

B Normal muscle AP: median nerve stimulated at elbow

Concentric needle electrode recordings

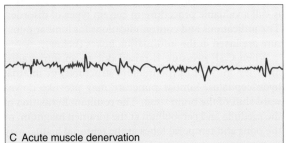

C Acute muscle denervation

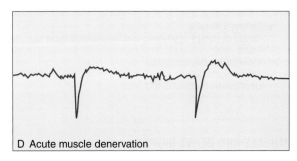

D Acute muscle denervation

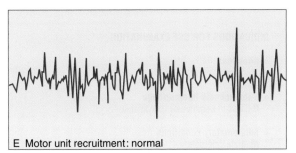

E Motor unit recruitment: normal

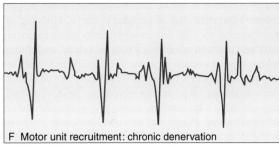

F Motor unit recruitment: chronic denervation

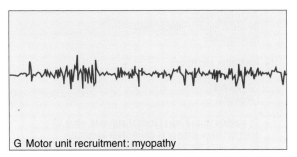

G Motor unit recruitment: myopathy

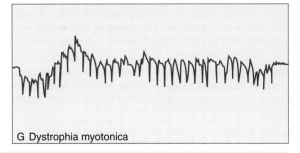

G Dystrophia myotonica

Fig. 18.20 Normal and abnormal electromyographic recordings. A and **B** show compound muscle action potential responses recorded with surface electrodes on the thenar eminence when the median nerve is stimulated at the wrist A and elbow B. Note the difference in latency; this is used to calculate conduction velocity—usually 50–60 m/s.
C–H show EMG recordings made with a concentric needle electrode. C shows small short duration fibrillation potentials, and D positive sharp waves, both features seen in acute muscle denervation. E shows a normal pattern of motor unit recruitment when a subject makes a strong voluntary muscle contraction. Impaired recruitment of enlarged motor units is seen in chronic denervation F. In myopathy G recruitment is full but the motor units are reduced in amplitude and duration. H shows an example of a high frequency burst of muscle activity recorded from a patient with dystrophia myotonica.

MUSCLE AND NERVE BIOPSY

Biopsy of skeletal muscle usually provides more helpful information than that of peripheral nerve. Histological examination with light microscopy, enzyme histo-chemistry and electron microscopy may be helpful in defining which type of muscle or nerve fibre is affected, whether any inflammation is present, and whether any abnormal accumulations (e.g. excess glycogen, lipid, amyloid, mitochondria) are present to suggest a specific defect of metabolism. Peripheral nerve is less easily biopsied without causing deficit. The distal sural nerve at the ankle or the superficial radial nerve at the wrist are the most suitable since the resultant sensory deficit is mild and localised. Partial thickness biopsy causes less sensory deficit. The pathological process, whether primarily affecting axons or myelin, may be evident, and abnormal infiltration (e.g. amyloid) is occasionally seen. The presence of perineural vasculitis is the most therapeutically useful finding, since corticosteroid therapy may be indicated.

Blood tests and other procedures used in the elucidation of nerve and muscle disorders are listed in Table 18.13.

TESTS OF THE AUTONOMIC NERVOUS SYSTEM

These are based mostly on measuring cardiovascular responses to the Valsalva manoeuvre, deep breathing, sustained hand grip and changing from lying to standing posture. Pupil cycle time is also relatively easily meas-ured with a slit lamp and stop watch, and gives an indication of parasympathetic function in the oculo-motor nerve. Peripheral autonomic abnormalities are seen in patients with diabetes mellitus, alcoholism, and amyloidosis; central forms of disorder occur in some patients with Parkinson's disease and rarer multi-system degenerations.

EXAMINATION OF CEREBROSPINAL FLUID (CSF)

Examination of CSF is undertaken less often now than in the past because of the development of more accurate and non-invasive techniques for demonstrating cerebral and spinal lesions. Nevertheless, examination of CSF obtained by lumbar (or occasionally cisternal) puncture is still a valuable procedure in certain types of disorder. The indications and contraindications for lumbar puncture are listed in the information boxes (below).

When CSF pressure is raised due to an intracranial mass lesion, shift of the midline structures, or internal hydrocephalus, lumbar puncture may provoke downward shift of the brain stem. The resultant herniation of the medulla and cerebellum at the foramen magnum, or the pons and temporal lobes at the tentorial hiatus, may

Table 18.13   Screening tests for nerve and muscle disorders

Neuropathy	Myopathy
Full blood count, ESR	Full blood count, ESR
Urea, electrolytes, calcium, creatinine	Urea, electrolytes, calcium, phosphate
Serum lipoproteins	Urinary calcium
Liver function tests	Liver function tests
Blood glucose ± tolerance test	Plasma and urinary corticosteroids
Thyroxine and TSH	Thyroxine and TSH
Plasma protein electrophoresis	Creatine phosphokinase
Urinary Bence–Jones protein	Lactate dehydrogenase
Urinary porphyrins	
Blood vitamin assays:	Tests of energy metabolism
B_{12} folic acid	(e.g. lactate production)
(thiamine, pyridoxine)	Tissue enzyme assays:
(nicotinamide, vitamin E)	myophosphorylase phosphofructokinase
Toxic metals (e.g. Pb, Hg) in urine, blood, hair, nails	acid maltase, carnitine,
Exclude drug intoxication	carnitine-palmitoyl transferase
Serum autoantibodies:	Serum autoantibodies:
Antinuclear	Antinuclear
Double-stranded DNA	Double-stranded DNA
Rheumatoid factor	Rheumatoid factor
	Acetylcholine receptor (myasthenia)
Nerve conduction/EMG	Nerve conduction/EMG
Nerve biopsy	Muscle biopsy
Exclusion of malignancy and systemic disorders:	Exclusion of malignancy and systemic disorders:
Chest radiograph	Chest radiograph
Faecal occult blood	Faecal occult blood
Abdominal ultrasound scan	Abdominal ultrasound scan
Prostate specific antigen	

be fatal. A sample of venous blood should be taken at the same time as CSF so that blood glucose and immunoglobulin levels can be compared with those in CSF. Normally CSF glucose concentration is about 2/3 that of blood. Small vessels are often damaged at lumbar puncture rendering the initial CSF sample blood-stained (traumatic tap). Usually the staining clears in subsequent collection tubes, and a mildly traumatic tap will not affect protein or IgG analysis especially if the sample is centrifuged. A clear supernatant distinguishes a traumatic sample from blood staining due to subarachnoid haemorrhage, where the fluid is yellow tinged (xanthochromic) due to the presence of bile pigments. Xanthochromia may be absent initially and take several hours to develop.

CONDITIONS UNDER WHICH LUMBAR PUNCTURE IS NOT PERFORMED

- Depressed consciousness especially if focal neurological signs present
- Papilloedema

Proceed to CT scan initially

CSF parameters in health and common disorders are shown in Table 18.14.

FURTHER READING

Cull R E, Whittle I R 1995 Examination of the nervous system. In: Munro J (ed) Macleod's Clinical Examination, 9th edn. Churchill Livingstone, Edinburgh
Perkin G D 1988 Diagnostic Tests in Neurology. Chapman & Hall Medical, London

DISORDERS AFFECTING THE CRANIAL NERVES

Cranial nerves are often involved singly or in groups by intracranial disease and occasionally by generalised neuropathies or myopathies. Intracranial disease such as cerebral tumour may involve a cranial nerve directly (e.g. acoustic neurinoma) or may cause secondary dysfunction of the nerve by stretching it or compressing it against other structures (e.g. sixth nerve palsy secondary to tentorial herniation of medial temporal lobe due to raised intracranial pressure).

Table 18.14 CSF parameters in health and some common disorders

	Normal	Subarachnoid haemorrhage	Pyogenic meningitis	Tuberculous meningitis	Viral meningitis	Multiple sclerosis
Pressure	50–180 mm CSF	Increased	Normal/ increased	Normal/ increased	Normal	Normal
Colour	Crystal clear	Blood-stained xanthochromic	Cloudy	Clear/cloudy	Clear	Clear
Cell count	0–4/mm^3	Increased red blood cells	Polymorphs 1000–50 000	Lymphocytes 50–5000	Lympho. 10–2000	Lympho. 0–100
Glucose	2/3 blood level	Normal	Decreased	Decreased	Normal	Normal
Protein	<500 mg/l	Increased	Increased	Increased	Normal/increased	Normal/increased
IgG/total protein %	<13%	—	(Not routinely measured)	—	—	Increased
IgG index	<0.45	—	(Not routinely measured)	—	—	Increased
Oligoclonal IgG bands	Absent	—	(Not routinely measured)	—	—	Present
Microbiology	Sterile	Sterile	Organisms on Gram stain and culture	Organisms on ZN stain and culture	Sometimes viruses	Sterile

I OLFACTORY NERVE

Nasal chemoreceptor fibres pass through the cribriform plate in the floor of the anterior cranial fossa and synapse in the olfactory bulb. Second order fibres pass along the olfactory tract, which lies on the floor of the anterior fossa under the frontal lobe, to the olfactory cortex in the anteromedial temporal lobe. Damage to the olfactory system may be bilateral (e.g. trauma and infection) or unilateral (e.g. frontal lobe tumour) (Table 18.15).

Table 18.15 Sites of damage to the olfactory pathway

Site	Example
Nasal mucosa	Upper respiratory infection
Cribriform plate	Head trauma
Olfactory tract	Frontal meningioma
Temporal lobe	Tumour or trauma

II OPTIC NERVE

The components of the visual system and the effects of lesions at various sites have been described above (pp. 1031–1033). Clinical testing of vision is summarised in the information box below.

Alterations in the appearance or reaction of the pupils occur for a variety of reasons (Table 18.16).

TESTS OF VISION

- **Visual acuity**
  Distance (6 m chart)
  Near (reading types)
- **Fields of vision**
  Confrontation
  Perimetry
- **Colour vision**
  Ishihara plates
- **Pupil reflexes**
  Light
  Accommodation
- **Ophthalmoscopy**

OPTIC DISC OEDEMA (PAPILLOEDEMA)

Optic disc oedema is recognised by swelling of the disc with blurring of its margins, often hyperaemia of the disc with loss of the normal central cup, and when acute, haemorrhages at the disc margins. The vessels on the disc become curved over its edges, the veins are engorged and cease to pulsate. The unifying mechanism for all forms of optic disc oedema is blockage of axonal transport in the optic nerve with swelling of its axons due to accumulation of subcellular organelles, which in turn results in capillary and venous congestion and further swelling of the disc (Fig. 18.21). Common causes of disc oedema are shown in the information box (p. 1045).

OPTIC NEURITIS

Aetiology

This is usually an acute inflammatory disorder causing demyelination in the optic nerve near the disc (optic neuritis) or more posteriorly (retrobulbar neuritis).

Table 18.16 Types of pupil abnormality

Defect	Example	Appearance	Direct light response	Consensual response in other eye	Near response
Afferent	Optic neuritis	Normal/large	Impaired	Impaired	Normal
III Nerve palsy	Cerebral aneurysm	Large	Impaired	Normal	Impaired
Myotonic (Adie's) pupil	Holmes–Adie syndrome	Small or large	Impaired	Normal	Normal with slow relaxation
Argyll–Robertson	Neurosyphilis	Small irregular	Impaired	Impaired (usually bilateral)	Normal
Horner's syndrome	Cervical sympathetic chain lesion	Small (+ptosis)	Normal	Normal	Normal

COMMON CAUSES OF OPTIC DISC OEDEMA (PAPILLOEDEMA)

- **Raised intracranial pressure**
  Cerebral tumour, abscess
  Hydrocephalus, oedema
  Haemorrhage, haematoma
- **Obstruction of ocular venous drainage**
  Central retinal vein occlusion
  Cavernous sinus thrombosis
- **Systemic disorders affecting retinal vessels**
  Hypertension
  Vasculitis
  Hypercapnia
- **Optic nerve damage**
  Demyelination (optic neuritis)
  Ischaemia
  Toxins (e.g. methanol)
- **Infiltration of optic disc**
  Sarcoidosis
  Glioma
  Lymphoma

Some cases follow an acute viral infection, this form being seen especially in children when the disorder may be bilateral. In adults it is usually part of the spectrum of multiple sclerosis (MS), and more than 50% of patients who have had optic neuritis eventually develop MS.

Clinical features

The onset of symptoms is acute or sub-acute, often with pain in the eye especially on movement, and blurring of central vision. A central scotoma is frequently present, causing marked reduction in visual acuity; the direct pupil light reflex is impaired. If the inflammatory process is close to the optic nerve head, optic disc oedema (papillitis) is seen in the acute phase. The visual evoked potential is diminished and delayed or absent early on, but may return later with a delayed latency or altered waveform. Recovery is usual within a few weeks, but some patients are left with impaired vision, especially

for colour, and occasionally vision fails to improve. Ophthalmoscopy after recovery may show pallor of the optic disc, particularly on its temporal side. Other causes of optic nerve damage are given in the information box below.

CAUSES OF OPTIC NERVE DAMAGE

- Optic neuritis
- Compression in or behind orbit, e.g. tumour, aneurysm
- Toxins, e.g. Methyl alcohol, cyanide, chloroquine
- Direct trauma
  Head injury
- Increased intraocular pressure
  Glaucoma
- Ischaemia
  Atherosclerosis, giant cell arteritis
- Raised intracranial pressure
  Disc oedema, secondary ischaemia

OPTIC ATROPHY

This is the end result of many processes which damage the optic nerve. There is loss of axons with glial proliferation and decreased vascularity of the nerve head. The disc appears pale white or grey and has clear margins (Fig. 18.22, p. 1048). The causes are listed in the information box below.

COMMON CAUSES OF OPTIC ATROPHY

- Previous optic neuritis, ischaemic or toxic damage
- Previous disc oedema from raised intracranial pressure
- Chronic optic nerve compression
- Chronic glaucoma
- Previous trauma
- Degenerative conditions e.g. Friedreich's ataxia

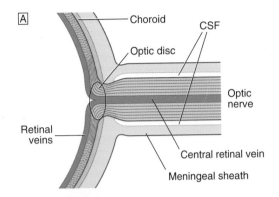

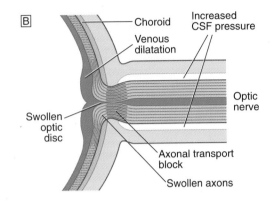

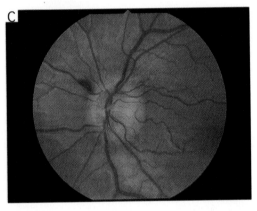

Fig. 18.21 Mechanism of optic disc oedema (papilloedema). Ⓐ Normal. Ⓑ Disc oedema (e.g. due to cerebral tumour). Ⓒ Fundus photograph of the left eye showing optic disc oedema with a small haemorrhage on the nasal side of the disc.

III OCULOMOTOR NERVE, IV TROCHLEAR NERVE, VI ABDUCENT NERVE

Together these three pairs of nerves are responsible for the control of the external ocular muscles. Their functions and the clinical abnormalities are summarised in Table 18.17 and Figure 18.23.

All three nerves can be damaged at various sites between nuclei in the brain stem and their end-plates on the external ocular muscles. Some common types of lesion are outlined in Table 18.18. The III and VI nerves are sometimes involved indirectly by mass lesions, hydrocephalus or cerebral oedema which stretch or compress the nerves against other structures; the cranial nerve palsies are then referred to as 'false-localising signs'.

SQUINT (STRABISMUS)

Squint occurs when the two eyes fail to move in a co-ordinated fashion. Diplopia results unless one eye has

Table 18.17 Cranial nerves III, IV and VI — clinical aspects

Nerve	Name	Muscles	Eye movements	Other functions	Signs of lesion
III	Oculomotor	Superior rectus Inferior rectus Medial rectus Inferior oblique	Elevation Depression Adduction Up/adduction	Levator upper eyelid Pupil constrictor Ciliary muscle	Ptosis Dilated pupil Abducted eye Divergent squint
IV	Trochlear	Superior oblique	Down/adduction	—	Oblique diplopia on down/in gaze
VI	Abducent	Lateral rectus	Abduction	—	Horizontal diplopia on lateral gaze Convergent squint

Table 18.18 Common lesions affecting cranial nerves III, IV and VI

Nerve	Site	Pathology	Clinical associations
III	Midbrain	Infarction Haemorrhage Demyelination	May or may not affect pupil; may be bilateral lesions; contralateral pyramidal signs
	Circle of Willis	Aneurysm at origin of posterior communicating artery	Pupil involved early, headache over affected eye
	Cavernous sinus	Int. carotid aneurysm Sinus thrombosis	VI and IV also often involved ± pain and proptosis of eye
	Orbit	Infarction of nerve e.g. in diabetes; giant cell arteritis	Pupil often spared, may be painful or painless
IV	Cavernous sinus	Carotid aneurysm Thrombosis	Seldom involved alone, usually VI and III lesions also
	Orbit	Trauma	Dislocation from trochlea
	Orbital fissure	Tumour Granuloma	Pain in eye, III and VI likely to be involved ± ophthalmic branch of V
VI	Pons	Infarction Haemorrhage Demyelination	± associated facial weakness, contralateral pyramidal signs
	Tentorial orifice	Compression Meningioma	May be secondary to raised intracranial pressure as false localising sign
	Cavernous sinus	Carotid aneurysm Thrombosis	± III and IV involvement
	Orbit	Infarction Tumour	May be secondary to diabetes or giant cell arteritis

very poor vision or the defect has been of long standing since childhood, when information from one eye becomes suppressed at cortical level (amblyopic eye). Squint may be paralytic or non-paralytic (concomitant).

Paralytic squint

This is due to weakness of one or more of the external ocular muscles because of lesions of the III, IV or VI nerves or of muscle disease (e.g. myasthenia gravis).

Non-paralytic or concomitant squint

This usually has onset in childhood, and is due to failure of development of normal fixation reflexes. This is commonly due to refractive error or some other ocular defect, and provision of appropriate correcting lenses may prevent the squint from becoming permanent.

NYSTAGMUS

Nystagmus describes a series of rhythmical oscillations of one or both eyes. The movements may be horizontal, vertical or rotatory, and the oscillations may be equal in velocity and amplitude to either side (pendular) or may have a slow phase and a fast phase in opposite directions (phasic or jerk nystagmus) (Fig. 18.24). By convention, the direction of phasic nystagmus is denoted by its fast phase, and the movement is usually exaggerated on gaze

to that side. The degree of phasic nystagmus can be graded from 1 to 3 and the causes are shown in Table 18.19.

Internuclear ophthalmoplegia

This curious disorder of eye movement is caused by lesions of the medial longitudinal fasciculus which links the sixth nerve nucleus in the pons with the third nerve nucleus in the midbrain. It causes disconjugation of lateral eye movements, especially during rapid changes of gaze, so that one eye is slow to adduct while the abducting eye shows coarse horizontal nystagmus ('ataxic nystagmus'). The disorder is frequently bilateral. Occasionally failure of full abduction with nystagmus in the adducting eye is seen. Often up-beating vertical nystagmus is present on up-gaze. The commonest cause is multiple sclerosis, but vascular disease, tumour, sarcoidosis and Wernicke's encephalopathy may be responsible.

Ocular nystagmus

Ocular fixation is poor when there is a defect of central vision, and may result in nystagmus. The defect is often congenital and sometimes associated with head tilt and titubation. The nystagmus is pendular in type to central gaze but may become phasic on lateral gaze, and tends to diminish with convergence. Pendular nystagmus may

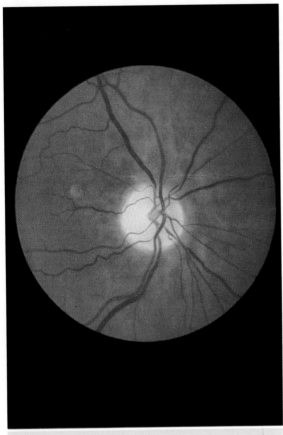

Fig. 18.22 Fundus photograph of the left eye of a patient with familial optic atrophy: note marked pallor of optic disc.

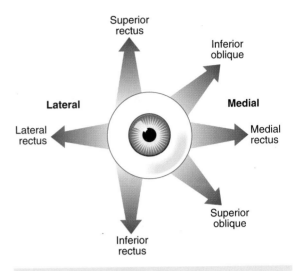

Fig. 18.23 External ocular muscle function.

Table 18.20 Motor and sensory functions of the trigeminal nerve

MOTOR
Masseter and temporalis muscles	Jaw closure
Medial and lateral pterygoid muscles	Jaw opening, side-side movement

SENSORY
Division I (Ophthalmic)
Division II (Maxillary)
Division III (Mandibular)
Areas of sensory supply:
Skin of face, cornea, mucosa of sinuses, mucosa of cheek, teeth, gums, tympanic membrane, anterior 2/3 of tongue

---

occur also in diffuse brain-stem disease due to multiple sclerosis or tumours.

Positional nystagmus
Nystagmus and usually vertigo may occur only in certain head positions. Two types of positional nystagmus are recognised.

Peripheral type
In benign positional vertigo, calcific degeneration in the utricle and saccule of the inner ear causes small particles to fall on to the cupola of the semicircular canals when the head is tilted back below the horizontal and turned with the affected ear lowermost. If the patient is put into

---

Table 18.19 Causes of phasic nystagmus

Site of lesion	Clinical features
Cerebellum	Horizontal nystagmus maximal on gaze to side of lesion
Vestibular apparatus or nerve	Horizontal or rotatory nystagmus maximal on gaze opposite to side of lesion (unless irritative lesion in labyrinth)
Midbrain, superior colliculus	Vertical up-beating nystagmus evoked by upward gaze
Pons-midbrain, medial longitudinal fasciculus	'Ataxic' nystagmus most marked in abducting eye, associated with internuclear ophthalmoplegia, vertical up-beating nystagmus on up-gaze
Lower medulla	Down-beating nystagmus on downward or lateral gaze

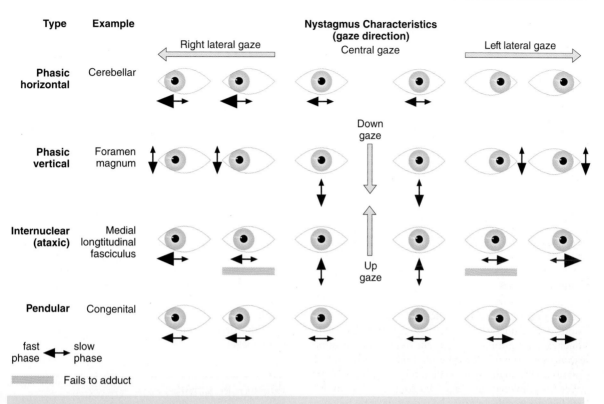

Type **Example**

Right lateral gaze

**Nystagmus Characteristics
(gaze direction)**
Central gaze

Left lateral gaze

**Phasic
horizontal** Cerebellar

Down
gaze

**Phasic
vertical** Foramen
magnum

**Internuclear
(ataxic)** Medial
longtitudinal
fasciculus

Up
gaze

Pendular Congenital

fast
phase ⟷ slow
phase

Fails to adduct

Fig. 18.24 **Common types of nystagmus**.

this position, after a latent period of a few seconds, vertigo is experienced and rotational nystagmus can be observed. If the position is maintained, the vertigo and nystagmus abate—usually within a minute. The condition may follow head injury, ear infection, and viral or vascular damage to the inner ear. Vestibular sedatives such as cinnarzine 15–30 mg 8-hourly or pro-chlorperazine 5–10 mg 8-hourly help suppress the symptoms which are troublesome when the patient lies down or turns over in bed.

Usually the disorder is self-limiting and settles after a few months.

Central type
Lesions of the cerebellum or brain-stem vestibular connections may cause positional nystagmus.

V TRIGEMINAL NERVE

The trigeminal nerve has motor and sensory roots. The motor root supplies the muscles of mastication (Table 18.20).

Lesions of the trigeminal system
The cranial motor neurones of the motor root lie in the pons. The principal trigeminal sensory nucleus lies close by and relays common touch and position sense to the contralateral medial lemniscus and thence to the thalamus. Fibres serving pain and temperature descend in the tract of the trigeminal nerve to the medulla and upper cervical region, where they synapse and cross the midline to join the spinothalamic tract. Lesions affecting the trigeminal sensory system may thus lie between the pons and the upper cervical spinal cord. Examples of lesions affecting the V nerve are listed in Table 18.21.

TRIGEMINAL NEURALGIA

Aetiology
This condition affects mainly middle-aged and elderly people. Occasionally younger patients suffering from multiple sclerosis develop similar symptoms. It was for many years regarded as idiopathic, but recent evidence suggests that in many patients an aberrant loop of artery

Table 18.21 Lesions affecting the trigeminal system

Site	Example	Clinical features
Pons	Infarction, demyelination	Motor and sensory function impaired, corneal and jaw flexes diminished
Medulla	Infarction, syrinx	Loss of pain and temperature sensation on face
Semi-lunar ganglion	Meningioma Aneurysm	All 3 sensory divisions may be involved
Cavernous sinus	Aneurysm Thrombosis	Ophthalmic division affected, corneal reflex impaired
Maxillary sinus	Antral carcinoma	Maxillary division affected
Infratemporal fossa	Nasopharyngeal carcinoma	Mostly mandibular division, sensory and motor involvement

is pressing on the trigeminal rootlets as they emerge from the pons.

Clinical features

Paroxysms of sharp lancinating pain radiating into the territory of one or more of the trigeminal sensory divisions are characteristic. The pain is often set off by touching or washing the face, shaving, tooth cleaning, eating, talking and exposure to cold. The II and III divisions are usually affected first, but the condition may spread to involve all three. Paroxysms of pain last only a few seconds, but may be repetitive or be followed by a dull ache. In its early course the disorder may show spontaneous remissions lasting weeks or months.

There are no abnormal motor or sensory signs of trigeminal nerve dysfunction, with the exception of localised trigger spots which set off pain when touched. If clinical abnormalities are present, the diagnosis is more likely to be of structural disease such as multiple sclerosis, meningioma, aneurysm or neurinoma.

Management

Membrane-stabilising drugs such as carbamazepine or phenytoin should be tried first. With carbamazepine sedative side-effects should be avoided by starting with a small dose (100 mg once daily or 12-hourly) and increasing gradually to 200–400 mg 8-hourly over the course of 2–3 weeks, aiming for a plasma level of 30–50 μmol/l. Slow introduction is not needed with phenytoin, but patients have differing tolerance within the range 150–500 mg/daily, an average dose being 300 mg/daily. Plasma level monitoring should be used to achieve about 40–80 μmol/l. Clonazepam 0.5–2 mg 8-hourly is sometimes effective.

Various surgical procedures can be considered if drug treatment proves ineffective, or its side-effects intolerable. These range from injection of the trigeminal ganglion with phenol or alcohol, radiofrequency thermo-coagulation of a branch of the ganglion, intracranial section of the trigeminal sensory root, and microvascular decompression procedures. The latter are theoretically the most attractive, but may be too hazardous in an elderly patient. Phenol injection or thermocoagulation can be carried out percutaneously and at low risk, but have the disadvantage of giving only temporary relief lasting weeks or months.

VII FACIAL NERVE

The chief function of the facial nerve is the supply of motor fibres to the muscles of facial expression. The facial motor neurones lie in the ventral part of the pontine tegmentum, their fibres looping around the sixth nerve nucleus before emerging from the lateral aspect of the pons. This portion of the nerve enters the internal auditory meatus at the cerebello-pontine angle, along with the acoustic nerve (VIII) and the nervus intermedius. The latter contains parasympathetic fibres concerned with salivation and lacrimation; at the geniculate ganglion it receives sensory fibres for taste on the anterior 2/3 of the tongue from the chorda tympani. A small sensory component serves cutaneous sensation on the external ear. As it passes through the petrous temporal bone, the facial nerve sends a small motor branch to the stapedius muscle (Tables 18.22 and 18.23).

IDIOPATHIC (BELL'S) PALSY

Bell's palsy is a common condition affecting patients of all ages and both sexes. The cause is unknown; viral infection, vascular damage, trauma, and cold exposure have all been implicated. The site of damage is probably the labyrinthine portion of the facial nerve within the facial canal. Swelling of the nerve at this site has been observed, and may be responsible for the initial loss of nerve impulse conduction leading to facial paralysis.

Table 18.22   Functional components of the facial nerve

Component	Connections	Function/supply
Somatic motor	VII nucleus in pons: facial nerve	Muscles of facial expression / stapedius
Visceral efferent parasympathetic	Superior salivary nucleus: nervus intermedius	Lacrimal gland, submandibular and sublingual salivary glands
Special afferent (taste)	Lingual nerve, chorda tympani, geniculate ganglion, nervus intermedius, tractus solitarius	Taste sensation on anterior 2/3 of tongue
Somatic afferent	Geniculate ganglion	Cutaneous sensation to external ear

Table 18.23   Causes of facial weakness

Site	Examples	Clinical features
Cortex	Cerebral infarction Haemorrhage Tumour	Contralateral facial weakness mainly of lower face often associated hemiparesis
Pons (nuclear)	Infarction Demyelination Haemorrhage Tumour	All parts of ipsilateral face weak; often VI nerve affected $\pm$ contralateral hemiparesis
Cerebello-pontine angle	Acoustic neurinoma Meningioma	All parts of face affected + deafness and tinnitus $\pm$ trigeminal nerve
Facial canal (petrous bone)	Bell's palsy Mastoiditis Herpes zoster	All parts of face affected $\pm$ loss of taste, salivation and lacrimation, hyperacusis if stapedius weak
Parotid gland	Tumour Sarcoidosis	Selective weakness of parts of face due to branch involvement
Neuromuscular junction	Myasthenia gravis	Associated ptosis and external opthalmoplegia, dysphagia, dysarthria, $\pm$ limb weakness
Muscles	Muscular dystrophy Myositis	Limb muscles also weak

Clinical features

The onset is subacute with symptoms coming on over a few hours or overnight. There may be pain in the face and around the ear before the patient or their family notice loss of movement on one side of the face. Sometimes patients describe the face as being numb, but objective evidence of loss of sensation (except taste) is lacking. The chorda tympani fibres are often affected so that taste is impaired on the anterior 2/3 of the tongue, and occasionally the tongue tingles on the affected side. Hyperacusis occurs if the nerve to stapedius is involved. More severe lesions cause loss of salivation and tear secretion.

Examination reveals weakness or paralysis of the facial muscles on one side, with failure of eye closure and visible upward deviation of the eye as this is attempted (Bell's sign, Fig. 18.25). The mouth is drawn over to the normal side and saliva may drool from it. The tongue may appear to deviate to the normal side, but this is usually due to distortion of the mouth and not hypoglossal weakness. A degree of dysarthria often accompanies the facial weakness. The facial appearance in an upper motor neurone lesion is shown in Figure 18.26.

Management

About 70–80% of patients with Bell's palsy recover spontaneously within 2–12 weeks. A short course of dexamethasone 2 mg 8-hourly for 5 days is worthwhile if the patient is seen within 48 hours of the onset. There is some evidence that this reduces oedema of the facial nerve, and may limit damage and speed recovery. The patient should wear a pad over the eye if eye closure is affected, especially during sleep, to protect the cornea.

Surgical decompression of the nerve in the facial canal is advocated by some but since most patients recover well without interference, and there is no good way of predicting poor outcome during the first few days of the condition (when surgery might be most helpful), the indications for operation are unclear.

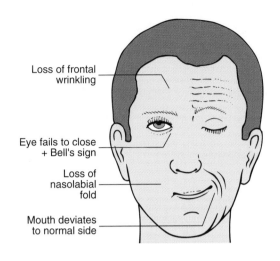

Loss of frontal wrinkling

Eye fails to close + Bell's sign

Loss of nasolabial fold

Mouth deviates to normal side

Fig. 18.25   Lesion of facial nerve or nucleus (lower motor neurone).

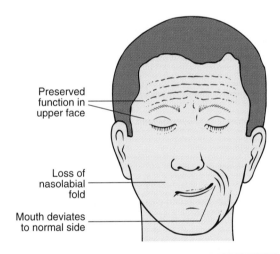

Preserved function in upper face

Loss of nasolabial fold

Mouth deviates to normal side

Fig. 18.26   Facial weakness due to lesion of precentral area or pyramidal tract (upper motor neurone).

Prognosis

Elderly patients with complete facial paralysis tend to have the worst prognosis. Slower or incomplete recovery can be predicted if facial EMG studies show marked reduction in the amplitude of evoked facial muscle action potentials after the first week. Preservation of the response and a measurable blink reflex are good prognostic signs. With a severe palsy, axonal degeneration occurs and recovery is slower and less complete. Aberrant reinnervation may take place, so that unwanted facial movements occur (e.g. the eye may close when the mouth is moved), sometimes adding to the disfigure-

ment. This problem can sometimes be alleviated by local injection of Botulinum toxin into the affected overacting muscles.

CLONIC FACIAL (HEMIFACIAL) SPASM

This disorder usually presents after middle age.

Clinical features

Symptoms usually start with intermittent twitching around one eye. Over the course of months or years, clonic twitches increase in frequency and severity so that the eye may close for a few seconds at a time, and gradually the movements begin to affect the lower face. The spasms are intermittent, sometimes being more prominent during talking and eating or when the patient is under stress. Occasionally sufferers report transient dulling of hearing on the affected side during a facial spasm—presumably due to stapedius contraction. Examination reveals, in addition to the spasms, mild weakness of the affected musculature.

Investigations

Facial nerve conduction studies are usually normal or show only minor defects of distal conduction and the blink reflex. EMG recording shows bursts of rapid motor unit firing during the spasms, with periods of silence interposed. The pathophysiology is believed to be due to an aberrant loop of artery irritating the facial nerve as it emerges from the pons—similar to the mechanism postulated for trigeminal neuralgia (see above).

Management

Treatment with carbamazepine or phenytoin as for trigeminal neuralgia may help reduce the frequency and severity of the spasms, but is often disappointing. If the disorder is severe and disfiguring, posterior fossa exploration and microvascular decompression may be justifiable, but the risks of this in an elderly patient must be balanced against the benign nature of the condition. Injections of Botulinum toxin into the affected muscles may control symptoms for several months, and is becoming an established treatment.

VIII VESTIBULO-COCHLEAR NERVE

The eighth cranial nerve transmits special sensory information from the vestibular system (head position and movement) and the cochlea (hearing). From the sensors in the inner ear the VIII nerve fibres pass through the internal auditory meatus, emerge at the cerebello-pontine angle and enter the brain stem at the ponto-med-

Table 18.24 Components, symptoms and signs of lesions affecting the VIII cranial nerve

Component	Sensors	Parameter	Symptoms of lesion	Signs of lesion
Vestibular	Utricle, saccule	Head position	Vertigo, loss of balance, oscillopsia, nausea, vomiting faintness	Poor balance, nystagmus, positional vertigo and nystagmus
	Semi-circular canals	Head movement		
Cochlear	Spiral hair cells	Hearing	Deafness, tinnitus	Sensorineural deafness

Table 18.25 Types of lesion causing vertigo

Site of lesion	Example	Clinical features
Labyrinth	Ménière's disease	Vertigo, deafness, tinnitus
VIII nerve	Acoustic neuroma	Deafness, tinnitus, vertigo, trigeminal and cerebellar signs
Vestibular neurones	Vertebral artery ischaemia	Vertigo, ataxia, diplopia, syncope, dysarthria
Cerebellum	Tumour, infarct	Vertigo, ataxia, dysarthria
Temporal lobe	Epilepsy, tumour	Vertigo accompanying seizures

ullary junction where they synapse in the vestibular and cochlear nuclei. Vestibular information is passed to the cerebellum, reticular formation, spinal motor neurones and oculomotor nuclei. Much of this information is involved with reflex control of head, eye and body posture but some of it reaches consciousness by a pathway to the superior temporal lobe. Auditory signals are relayed to the temporal lobe via the lateral lemniscus (Table 18.24).

VERTIGO

This is an hallucination of movement of either the body (or part of it) or the surroundings. The perceived movement may be of falling or rotating or a sensation that the outside world is spinning; sometimes the vertigo is so intense that the sufferer falls to the gound. Vertigo of labyrinthine origin is often marked, and accompanied by nausea, vomiting, oscillopsia, pallor and occasionally syncope. It is important to establish whether the patient is describing true vertigo, or less precise feelings of imbalance or light-headedness; the latter are less likely to be of vestibular origin. Table 18.25 lists the main causes of vertigo together with the site of lesion and relevant clinical features.

DEAFNESS

Deafness is often accompanied by tinnitus, especially when the lesion lies in the cochlea or auditory nerve. Blockage of the external auditory meatus or damage to the ear drum ossicular chain cause **conductive deafness**. Normally hearing through air transmission via the drum and ossicles is more efficient than conduction of

vibration by bone; this difference is reversed in conductive deafness. **Sensorineural deafness** is due either to disease of the cochlea or the auditory fibres in the VIII nerve and its connections in the brain stem. Both air and bone conduction hearing are affected, and tinnitus is often present. Common causes of deafness and tinnitus are listed in Table 18.26.

MÉNIÈRE'S DISEASE

This is a disorder of the inner ear in which there is excessive pressure and dilatation of the endolymphatic system. This results in damage to both the vestibular and cochlear sense organs. The cause is unknown, although there is some overlap with other functional vasospastic disorders such as migraine.

Clinical features

Symptoms rarely start before middle age; the patient suffers from recurrent bouts of profound vertigo, nausea and vomiting associated with deafness (especially for middle and low frequencies) and tinnitus. Acute attacks may be preceded by discomfort in one ear, and increasing tinnitus and deafness. The attack usually lasts several hours or a day, and is accompanied by prostration, pallor, vomiting, nystagmus and occasionally by syncope. Deafness and tinnitus tend to persist between attacks and sensorineural mid-low frequency hearing loss with loudness recruitment may be found on audiometry. Caloric tests show impaired vestibular function on the affected side.

Management

Bed rest and administration of vestibular sedatives are required during acute attacks. Cinnarizine (15–30 mg

Table 18.26 Common causes of deafness and their features

Type of deafness	Site of lesion	Example	Clinical features
Conductive	External meatus	Wax	Air conduction < bone conduction Weber's test → deaf ear
	Ear drum	Otitis media	Pain in ear, fever
	Ossicular chain	Otosclerosis	Progressive deafness; tinnitus
Sensorineural	Cochlea	Ménière's disease	Mid-low tone deafness, loudness recruitment, tinnitus, vertigo
	Cochlea	Noise induced	'Notch' pattern deafness for specific frequencies
	Cochlea	Senile	Deaf mainly for higher frequencies
	VIII nerve	Acoustic neuroma	Deafness, tinnitus, air conduction > bone conduction, Weber's test → normal ear

8-hourly) or prochlorperazine (5–10 mg 8-hourly) help suppress vertigo and vomiting. In more severe attacks, intramuscular injection of prochlorperazine 12.5 mg or cyclizine 50 mg may be required. Some authorities also give intravenous diuretics (frusemide 40 mg intravenously) to try to reduce the endolymphatic pressure. Prophylaxis from recurrent episodes is sometimes effective with vasodilators such as betahistine (8 mg 8-hourly), but if disabling attacks continue or hearing deteriorates progressively, surgical endolymph drainage may be necessary.

VESTIBULAR NEURONITIS

This a common disorder affecting mainly young adults. The aetiology is presumed to be due to viral infection, and it occasionally occurs in small epidemics.

Clinical features

There is usually a degree of systemic illness with fever, malaise, myalgia and gastrointestinal upset, suggesting that enteric viruses may be implicated. Vertigo, often with a marked positional element, accompanies the acute illness and may persist for days or several weeks, and sometimes relapses occur. Nystagmus is present in the acute phase, but there is no disturbance of hearing. Caloric tests may show impaired vestibular function on one or both sides.

Management

Treatment is with bed rest and vestibular sedatives as for Ménière's disease (see above). Recovery in a few weeks is usual, but sometimes symptoms persist with positional vertigo for several months, and there is some overlap with the post-viral fatigue syndrome (myalgic encephalomyelitis).

ACOUSTIC NEUROMA (NEURILEMMOMA)

This is a benign tumour arising from the covering tissues of the VIII nerve. The tumour usually starts in the internal auditory meatus and expands towards the cerebello-pontine angle, where it may involve the V and VII nerves, the cerebellum and the brain stem. Bilateral acoustic neuromas may occur in neurofibromatosis type II.

Clinical features

Early symptoms are unilateral deafness and tinnitus and insidious vertigo. Larger lesions cause facial numbness and weakness, ataxia and features of raised intracranial pressure. Examination reveals unilateral sensorineural deafness, and sometimes phasic nystagmus intially on looking away from the lesion. Later, as the tumour invades the cerebello-pontine angle, the nystagmus is of cerebellar origin and most marked on gaze towards the lesion. Facial numbness, and weakness, loss of the corneal reflex and onset of cerebellar and pyramidal tract sign are late features.

Investigations

Diagnosis at an early stage rests on demonstration of unilateral sensorineural deafness and impaired caloric vestibular function on the same side. A delayed or absent auditory evoked potential may be helpful at this stage. Plain radiographs or tomograms of the internal auditory meati may show enlargement or erosion of the canal. Larger tumours may be demonstrated by contrast enhanced CT scanning, but for small lesions air-CT meatography or high quality MRI scanning are more reliable.

Management

The results of surgical treatment are optimal when the tumour is still within the internal auditory meatus. Deaf-

Table 18.27 Components of the lower cranial nerves IX, X and XI

Nerve	Component	Nucleus	Functional supply
IX	Motor	Nucleus ambiguus	Stylopharyngeus
	Secretory	Inferior salivary nucleus	Parotid gland
	Sensory	Tractus solitarius	Common touch and taste for posterior 1//3 tongue, soft palate, tonsil, eardrum
X	Motor	Nucleus ambiguus	Palate, pharynx and larynx, heart, lungs, abdominal viscera dura,
	Parasympathetic	Dorsal vagal nucleus	ear, pharynx, soft palate
	Sensory	Spinal tract of V	
XI	Motor	Nucleus ambiguus (medullary portion)	Pharynx and larynx via X
		C1–5 anterior horn cells (spinal portion)	Trapezius, sternomastoid

ness and facial weakness may result, but long-term prognosis is good if complete removal of the lesion is achieved.

IX GLOSSOPHARYNGEAL NERVE, X VAGUS NERVE, XI SPINAL ACCESSORY NERVE

These nerves are grouped together because they all pass through the jugular foramen at the skull base, and tend to be affected as a group. Their cells of origin lie in the medulla oblongata (IX, X) and the upper cervical cord (XI), their roots emerging adjacent to one another. Their main functional components are shown in Table 18.27.

Isolated lesions of IX and X are very rare; usually they are affected together. Lesions at the jugular foramen tend to affect IX, X and XI simultaneously. Common examples of disorders of these nerves are listed in Table 18.28. Tumours of the jugular bulb (glomus) are rare; they present with involvement of all three nerves.

XII HYPOGLOSSAL NERVE

The hypoglossal nerve supplies motor fibres to the intrinsic and extrinsic muscles of the tongue. The hypoglossal nuclei lie in the medulla near to the midline beneath the floor of the IV ventricle. The nerves leave the medulla on its ventral aspect and pass through the

Table 18.28 Causes and features of lesions to cranial nerves IX, X and XI

Site	Causes	Clinical features
IX/X nuclei (medulla)	Infarction Syringobulbia Tumour Demyelination	Nasal voice, palatal weakness, absent gag reflex, impaired sensation posterior 1/3 tongue and pharyngeal wall, laryngeal stridor, bovine cough
Jugular foramen	Glomus tumour Metastatic tumour Meningioma	As above + spinal accessory nerve affected: weakness trapezius and sternomastoid
Diffuse lesions	Polyneuritis Guillain–Barré syndrome	Usually bilateral involvement
	Motor neurone disease Myasthenia gravis	No sensory deficit
Supra-nuclear (cortex, pyramidal tract)	Stroke Cerebral tumour Demyelination Motor neurone disease	Unilateral lesions do not cause persisting deficit (bilateral supply); bilateral lesions cause loss of coordination of pharynx and palate, brisk gag reflex (pseudobulbar palsy)
XI nucleus	As for IX, X	Same functions as IX and X
XI jugular foramen	Glomus tumour, etc.	Weakness of sternomastoid and trapezius
Supranuclear XI	Stroke etc., as for IX, X	Slowness and weakness of contralateral trapezius, but ipsilateral sternomastoid

Table 18.29   Causes of lesions of the hypoglossal nerve

Site	Causes
XII nucleus	Infarction
	Syringobulbia
	Tumour
	Motor neurone disease
Skull base	Metastatic tumour
	Meningioma
	Vertebral aneurysm
	Cranio-vertebral anomalies (e.g. basilar impression)
Neck	Trauma
	Surgery (e.g. carotid endarterectomy)

Table 18.30   Glasgow Coma Scale

Assessment	Score
Eye-opening (E)	
spontaneous	4
to speech	3
to pain	2
nil	1
Best motor response (M)	
obeys	6
localises	5
withdraws	4
abnormal flexion	3
extensor response	2
nil	1
Verbal response (V)	
orientated	5
confused conversation	4
inappropriate words	3
incomprehensible sounds	2
nil	1
Coma score = E + M + V	
Minimum	3
Maximum	15

hypoglossal canal at the skull base and cross the carotid vessels on their way to the tongue.

BULBAR AND PSEUDOBULBAR PALSY

Lesions of cranial nerves IX, X, XI, and XII often occur together, frequently because of vascular disease affecting the medulla. The resultant palatal, pharyngeal and tongue weakness causing dysphonia, dysphagia and dysarthria is known as 'bulbar palsy'. Bilateral supranuclear lesions affecting the pyramidal tracts (e.g. due to diffuse vascular disease, motor neurone disease, multiple sclerosis) cause loss of voluntary palatal and pharyngeal movements, but the gag reflex is preserved. The tongue is small (spastic) and shows poor rapid movement, this resulting in indistinct speech (spastic dysarthria). The jaw jerk is brisk. This state is known as 'pseudobulbar palsy'.

FURTHER READING

Cull R E, Whittle I R 1995 The nervous system. In: Munro J (ed) Macleod's Clinical Examination. Churchill Livingstone, Edinburgh
Patten J 1977 Neurological differential diagnosis. Harold Starke, London

COMA AND BRAIN DEATH

COMA

Assessment of conscious level is an essential component of neurological examination. Terms such as stuporose, semi-conscious and obtunded are ill-defined and have been superseded by a systematic assessment of the unconscious patient by the application of the Glasgow Coma Scale (Table 18.30).

This scale provides a grading of coma by the use of a numerical scale which allows serial comparisons and may provide prognostic information, particularly in traumatic coma.

There are a wide range of causes of coma (Table 18.31). The history of the mode of onset of coma and any precipitating event is crucial to establishing the cause. The first priority on examination is an assessment of cardiac and respiratory function. Neurological examination may reveal important findings, for example evidence of head injury, papilloedema, meningism or eye movement disorder. In the majority of cases, however, there are no focal neurological signs as drug overdosage or metabolic disturbance are the commonest causes of unexplained coma requiring hospital admission.

BRAIN DEATH

The widespread availability of mechanical ventilators has resulted in the survival of some patients with severe and irreversible brain damage, who would otherwise have died. Diagnostic criteria for brain death have been established in order that those patients with no possible chance of recovery may be identified and artificial ventilation discontinued.

The diagnosis of brain death depends on meeting a set of preconditions *all* of which must coexist (Table 18.32) and then applying a series of clinical tests (Table 18.33) *all* of which must be fulfilled.

Table 18.31   Causes of coma

Metabolic disturbance
Drug overdose
Diabetes mellitus—hypoglycaemia
                      ketoacidosis
                      hyperosmolar coma
Hyponatraemia
Uraemia
Hepatic failure
Respiratory failure
Hypothermia

Trauma
Cerebral contusion
Extradural haematoma
Subdural haematoma

Cerebrovascular disease
Subarachnoid haemorrhage
Intracerebral haemorrhage
Brain stem infarction/haemorrhage
Cerebral venous sinus thrombosis

Infections
Meningitis
Encephalitis
Cerebral abscess

Others
Epilepsy
Tumour
Thiamine deficiency

Table 18.32   Preconditions for considering a diagnosis of brain death

1. The patient is deeply comatose.
   a) There must be no suspicion that coma is due to depressant drugs, e.g. narcotics, hypnotics and tranquillisers.
   b) Hypothermia has been excluded—rectal temperature must exceed 35°C.
   c) There is no profound abnormality of serum electrolytes, acid base balance, or blood glucose concentrations, and any metabolic or endocrine cause of coma has been excluded.

2. The patient is maintained on a ventilator because spontaneous respiration had been inadequate or had ceased. Drugs including neuromuscular blocking agents must have been excluded as a cause of the respiratory failure.

3. The diagnosis of the disorder leading to brain death has been firmly established. There must be no doubt that the patient is suffering from irremediable structural brain damage.

FURTHER READING

Critchley E M R 1988 Neurological emergencies. W. B. Saunders, London. See pp. 21–95
Jennet B, Teasdale G, Braakman R, Minderhoud J, Heiden J et al 1979 Prognosis of patients with severe head injury. Neurosurgery 4: 283–289
Medical Royal Colleges 1979 Diagnosis of brain death. British Medical Journal 1: 332

Table 18.33   Tests for confirming brain death

ALL BRAIN STEM REFLEXES ARE ABSENT.

1. The pupils are fixed and unreactive to light.

2. The corneal reflexes are absent.

3. The vestibulo-ocular reflexes are absent—there is no eye movement following the injection of 20 ml of ice-cold water into each external auditory meatus in turn.

4. There are no motor responses to adequate stimulation within the cranial nerve distribution.

5. There is no gag reflex and no reflex response to a suction catheter in the trachea.

6. No respiratory movement occurs when the patient is disconnected from the ventilator long enough to allow the carbon dioxide tension to rise above the threshold for stimulating respiration ($PaCO_2$ must reach 6.7 kPa or 50 mm mercury).

The diagnosis of brain death should be made by two experienced doctors, one of whom should be a consultant and the other a consultant or senior registrar. The tests are usually repeated after an interval of 6–24 hours, depending on the clinical circumstances, before brain death is finally confirmed.

CEREBRAL TUMOURS

Cerebral tumours account for 2% of deaths at all ages. The majority are benign or malignant neoplasms arising from cellular components within the central nervous system, with metastatic tumours from systemic malignancies largely accounting for the remainder. Malignant brain tumours rarely give rise to extracerebral metastases and the clinical features and prognosis depend on the anatomical localisation and histological characteristics of the lesion.

Pathology

Primary intracerebral tumours are classified by their cell of origin and degree of malignancy, and vary in incidence by age and localisation (Tables 18.34, 18.35). Cerebral metastases usually occur in the white matter of the cerebral or cerebellar hemispheres and common primary sites are bronchus, breast, and gastrointestinal tract.

Benign intracranial tumours are slow growing but may cause disability and death by impinging on and displacing the intracranial contents. The commoner histological types are listed in Table 18.35. Cerebral lesions resembling tumours also occur in sarcoidosis, cysticercosis, echinococcosis (as hydatid cysts), and schistosomiasis. Tuberculoma is common in developing countries.

Meningiomas account for about a fifth of intracranial tumours. Intraventricular tumours, including colloid cysts of the third ventricle and choroid plexus papilloma,

Table 18.34 Malignant intracranial tumours

Histological type	Common site	Age
Glioma (astrocytoma)	Cerebral hemisphere Cerebellum Brain stem	Adult Childhood/Adult Childhood/Young adult
Oligodendroglioma	Cerebral hemisphere	Adult
Medulloblastoma	Posterior fossa	Childhood
Ependymoma	Posterior fossa	Childhood/adolescence
Microglioma (cerebral lymphoma)	Cerebral hemisphere	Adult

Table 18.35 Benign intracranial tumours

Histological type	Common site	Age
Meningioma	Cortical dura Parasagittal Sphenoid ridge Suprasellar Olfactory groove	Adult
Neurofibroma	Acoustic neuroma	Adult
Craniopharyngioma	Suprasellar	Childhood/adolescence
Pituitary adenoma	Pituitary fossa	Adult
Colloid cyst	Third ventricle	Any age

are rare but can cause an acute rise in intracranial pressure and sudden death.

Clinical features

The clinical features of an intracranial tumour relate to the site of the tumour and its rate of expansion. Symptoms and signs are produced by a number of mechanisms which are listed in the information box below.

CLINICAL FEATURES OF CEREBRAL TUMOURS

- Local effects on adjacent cerebral tissue
- Raised intracranial pressure
- Epilepsy
- False localising signs

Local effects

In general the focal disabilities produced by a cerebral tumour are of slow onset and progressive. Tumours may present at an early stage in areas of the brain such as the brain stem, where structural disturbance quickly results in a neurological deficit. In other regions, including the frontal lobe, the tumour may attain a large size before clinical evidence of a structural lesion is evident. The

clinical features of dysfunction in the various lobes of the brain are outlined on page 1034 (Fig. 18.11).

Occasionally localised oedema in the brain tissue surrounding a tumour will cause a rapid progression of symptoms and, rarely, haemorrhage into a tumour causes an acute presentation resembling a stroke.

Raised intracranial pressure

This may be caused by the tumour mass, reactive cerebral oedema or obstruction of cerebrospinal fluid pathways. The major features are:

1. *Headache.* This is a common but not invariable manifestation of cerebral tumour. Pain may be caused by distortion of or traction on nearby arteries, venous sinuses or meninges which are pain sensitive structures. The localisation of the headache does not generally correlate with the site of the tumour although posterior fossa tumours often cause pain in the occiput or nuchal area.

Headache due to raised intracranial pressure is felt diffusely over the cranium and may be aggravated by manoeuvres which further increase the intracranial pressure, including coughing, bending and straining. Typically the headache is most severe in the morning and may disturb sleep, although as intracranial pressure rises the pain becomes more constant.

2. *Impairment of conscious level.* This ranges from listlessness and drowsiness to coma and is related to the level of intracranial pressure. Cerebral tumours occupy space within the rigid skull but compensatory mechanisms involving alteration in the volume of fluid in cerebrospinal fluid spaces and venous sinuses may delay the development of raised pressure. Benign tumours may thereby attain a large size before causing a rise in intracranial pressure, but raised pressure develops early in rapidly expanding tumours or even acutely if the cerebrospinal circulation is obstructed by, for example, posterior fossa masses or intraventricular tumours. Raised intracranial pressure may also cause personality change including apathy, irritability, withdrawal and inattention.

3. *Papilloedema.* This is a significant but not invariable sign of raised intracranial pressure and may develop acutely or insidiously. Swelling of the optic nerve head may be accompanied by haemorrhages in the optic disc but often causes little subjective visual disturbance. Perimetry may reveal peripheral constriction of the visual field or enlargement of the blind spot but visual acuity is usually preserved. Rarely acute blurring of vision or transient blindness precipitated by postural change (visual obscurations) is a feature and indicates severely raised intracranial pressure. Papilloedema progresses in parallel to the level of intracranial pressure and eventu-

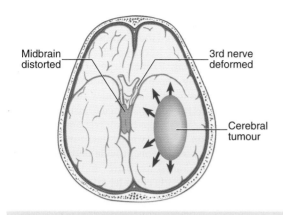

Fig. 18.27. **Cerebral tumour of the medial part of the temporal lobe** causing distortion of the midbrain and third nerve.

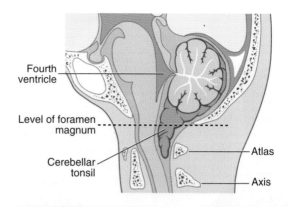

Fig. 18.28. **Downward displacement of the cerebellar tonsils below the level of the foramen magnum.**

ally results in visual failure due to extensive retinal haemorrhage or secondary optic atrophy. Rarely, but significantly, papilloedema may not develop in raised intracranial pressure, particularly if this is of acute onset as may occur in obstruction of cerebrospinal fluid pathways.

4. *Vomiting, bradycardia, arterial hypertension.* These develop as the intracranial pressure continues to rise and usually parallel the other clinical signs; but sudden vomiting may be an early feature of tumours of the cerebellar hemisphere.

Epilepsy

Infiltration by tumour cells of an area of cerebral cortex often invokes excitatory responses in neighbouring neurones and may result in an epileptic focus. The resulting seizures may be generalised or focal in nature, and the development of focal motor or sensory seizures in adult life should always suggest the possibility of a tumour.

False localising signs

The rise in intracranial pressure may not be uniform within the cerebral substance and sudden alterations in pressure relationships within the skull may lead to displacement of parts of the brain. Downward displacement of the temporal lobes due to a large hemisphere mass may result in stretching of the third and sixth cranial nerves, or pressure on the contralateral cerebral peduncle may result in ipsilateral upper motor neurone signs (Fig. 18.27). Another form of displacement is the downward movement of the cerebellar tonsils so that they impact within the foramen magnum thus compressing the medulla (Fig. 18.28). This 'coning' may result in brain-stem haemorrhage or acute obstruction of the cerebrospinal fluid pathways and is

often associated with loss of consciousness and paresis of the sixth and third cranial nerves, with dilatation of the pupil on the side of the lesion. The patient may adopt a decerebrate posture and death almost invariably ensues. This type of brain displacement may occur spontaneously in relation to critical levels of intracranial pressure, but is particularly likely to develop if the pressure dynamics are disturbed by lumbar puncture.

Investigations

Investigation for cerebral tumour should be considered in any patient presenting with the recent onset of progressive neurological dysfunction, symptoms or signs suggestive of raised intracranial pressure, or who develops epilepsy over the age of eighteen. Coma as a presenting feature is rare with the exception of intraventricular tumours which may suddenly obstruct cerebrospinal fluid pathways.

CT head scan is the definitive investigation for cerebral tumour, allowing accurate localisation of the lesion and providing some guidance as to the likely histological type (Fig. 18.29). Distortion of intracranial structures and the size of the ventricular system may also be assessed and high definition views or computerised reconstruction of the images may provide accurate evaluation of the extent of the tumour. Plain skull radiographs are rarely of diagnostic value with the exception of pituitary tumours and neoplasms which calcify, such as oligodendroglioma and craniopharyngioma. Chest radiography is an important investigation and may provide evidence of a pulmonary tumour or other systemic malignancy. Cerebral angiography provides information on the vascularity of the tumour and may be important if surgery is planned. Magnetic resonance imaging is of particular value in the investigation of tumours of the

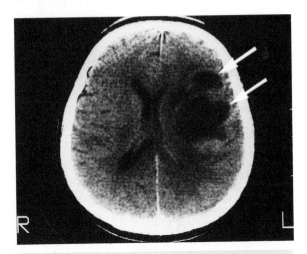

Fig. 18.29 CT scan of cerebral glioma. There is an irregular area of low density in the left cerebral hemisphere with surrounding oedema and shift of midline structures to the right (arrowed).

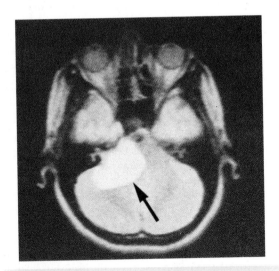

Fig. 18.30 MRI scan showing a large right acoustic neuroma distorting the cerebellum and brain stem.

posterior fossa and brain stem, areas in which the CT scan has a relatively poor resolution (Fig. 18.30).

Management

Medical

The medical management of cerebral tumours can never be anything more than temporary or palliative. Relief of raised intracranial pressure is often required when surgery is not possible or when life is threatened before investigation has revealed the diagnosis. The main therapeutic agent used to lower intracranial pressure is dexamethasone, 4 mg 4 times daily either orally or by injection. A striking improvement in conscious level is often produced and focal disabilities may regress. In severe and acutely raised intracranial pressure 16–20 mg of dexamethasone may be given intravenously or 200 ml of a 20% solution of the osmotic agent mannitol may be infused. These treatments provide only a temporary decrease in intracranial pressure and neurosurgical advice should be urgently considered.

Surgical

Surgery is the mainstay of treatment, although only partial excision may be possible if the tumour is inaccessible or if its exposure is likely to cause unacceptable brain damage. Tumours may invade areas of the brain where excision of small amounts of tissue is likely to cause major disability. The accurate diagnosis of an intracranial lesion does however have important implications for management and prognosis, and biopsy by direct or stereotactic technique should be considered even if the tumour cannot be removed.

Meningiomas and acoustic neuromas offer the best prospects for complete removal without unacceptable damage to surrounding structures. Meningiomas of the olfactory groove, suprasellar area and the convexity of the cerebral hemisphere only rarely recur, while those of the sphenoid ridge can often only be partially excised although recurrence is commonly delayed for many years. Craniopharyngiomas and colloid cysts are technically more difficult to remove in their entirety and, in common with other benign tumours, the possibility of complete excision depends on early diagnosis. Pituitary adenomas can be extirpated and surgery can often be performed by a trans-sphenoidal route, thus avoiding the necessity for a craniotomy. Prolactin or growth hormone secreting tumours may respond to medical treatment with bromocriptine.

Radiotherapy and chemotherapy

Radiotherapy and chemotherapy have only a marginal effect on survival in cerebral metastases and malignant gliomas in adults. Ependymomas and low grade gliomas in children and young adults are often radiosensitive and a combination of radiotherapy and chemotherapy has greatly improved the prognosis in medulloblastoma. Radiotherapy also reduces the risk of recurrence of pituitary adenoma after surgery and is often used as an adjunct to operative treatment in meningiomas in which the anatomical site precludes complete excision (e.g. sagittal sinus, skull base).

Table 18.36 Causes of hydrocephalus

Communicating	Obstructive
Infection e.g. bacterial or tuberculous meningitis	**Congenital** e.g. Arnold–Chiari malformation, aqueduct stenosis
Head injury	**Tumours** e.g. metastasis, glioma, ependymoma, colloid cyst
Subarachnoid haemorrhage	**Cerebral haemorrhage** e.g. brain stem or cerebellum
Idiopathic e.g. 'normal pressure' hydrocephalus	**Infection** e.g. cerebellar abscess

Prognosis

Gliomas can rarely be completely excised and infiltration may spread beyond the radiologically evident boundaries of the tumour. Recurrence is common even if the mass of the tumour is apparently removed, although survival in some cases may be prolonged for several years. Partial excision may be useful in alleviating raised intracranial pressure, but survival in highly malignant gliomas (glioblastoma multiforme) is measured in months even if such a decompressive procedure is attempted.

Ependymomas and medulloblastomas may be excised with minimal residual disability, but often recur with seeding of the tumour via the cerebrospinal fluid. Oligodendrogliomas are often slowly growing and relatively benign in the early stages, but may transform to a more malignant form and behave as gliomas.

The prognosis in benign tumours is good provided complete surgical excision can be achieved.

HYDROCEPHALUS

Hydrocephalus (dilatation of the ventricular system) may be due to obstruction of the cerebrospinal fluid circulation or failure of absorption of cerebrospinal fluid by the arachnoid villi, which lie in the parasagittal region (Fig. 18.31). Obstruction may occur anywhere within the ventricular system, but is most common in the narrow channels in the third ventricle, aqueduct and fourth ventricle and may be caused by tumour or a congenital anomaly such as aqueduct stenosis. Impairment of cerebrospinal fluid absorption may follow meningitis, head injury, subarachnoid haemorrhage or sagittal sinus thrombosis (Table 18.36).

In 'normal pressure' hydrocephalus the dilatation of the ventricular system is caused by intermittent rises in cerebrospinal fluid pressure, which occur particularly at night. The condition occurs predominantly in old age and the characteristic clinical features are dementia, ataxia of gait and incontinence.

Diversion of the cerebrospinal fluid by means of a shunt procedure between the ventricular system and the peritoneal cavity or right atrium may result in a prompt relief of symptoms in obstructive or communicating hydrocephalus, but the result is less predictable in 'normal pressure' hydrocephalus.

FURTHER READING

Shapiro W R 1986 Therapy of adult malignant brain tumours: what have the clinical trials taught us? Seminars in Oncology 13(1): 38–45

Vecht C J, Avezaat C J J, van Putten W L J et al 1990 The influence of the extent of surgery on the neurological function and survival in malignant glioma. A retrospective analysis in 243 patients. Journal of Neurology, Neurosurgery and Psychiatry 53: 466–471

Whittle I R 1992 Origins and management of peritumoural brain dysfunction. Neurosurgery Quarterly 2(3): 174–198

HEADACHE AND FACIAL PAIN

Custom usually restricts the term headache to describe pains in the region of the cranial vault, while pain in the maxillary and mandibular regions may be classified as facial pain. Although the lines of demarcation are often vague, headache and facial pain are considered separately.

HEADACHE

Headache is one of the most common and difficult clinical problems in medicine. In the majority of patients, the cause is trivial and reversible and a careful clinical history and examination often allows a specific diagnosis thereby avoiding unnecessary investigation. Headache may presage serious intracranial disease, but the clinical features of raised intracranial pressure or meningitis can usually be distinguished from those of the more common forms of headache.

Pain in the head may be due to lesions in nearby structures such as the eye and ear causing referred headache, it may be due to meningeal irritation, vascular disturbance, traction and distortion of intracranial structures, or to psychogenic causes. The clinical features of the commoner causes of headaches are listed in Table 18.37. Headache of raised intracranial pressure due to a mass lesion is described on page 1058.

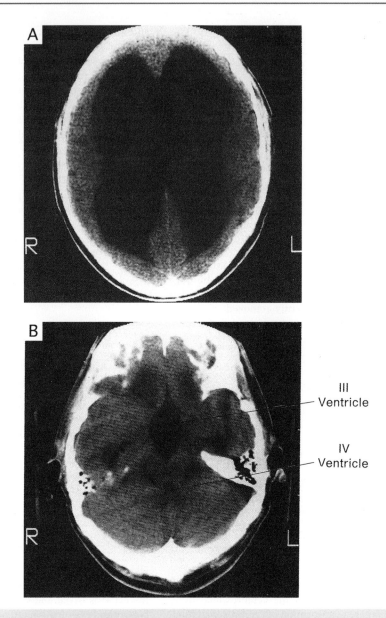

Fig. 18.31 CT scan in hydrocephalus. [A] There is a marked enlargement of the lateral ventricles. [B] The lower cut shows enlargement of the third ventricle and a normal fourth ventricle consistent with a diagnosis of aqueduct stenosis.

Investigations for headache

The extent and nature of investigations are determined by the history and clinical examination. In the great majority of patients no specific investigation is necessary, other than perhaps an ESR and serology for syphilis. Plain skull radiograph is of little diagnostic value but may provide reassurance in some patients. CT head scan is rarely necessary, but should be considered if raised intracranial pressure is suspected, if there are focal neurological signs or if there is diagnostic doubt.

TENSION HEADACHE

Clinical features

This is the commonest form of headache. The pain is usually constant and may be generalised or predominantly nuchal. It is characterised as dull, tight, or like a pressure, and there may be a sensation of a band round the head or pressure at the vertex. In contrast to migraine, the pain may continue for weeks or months without interruption although the severity may vary, and there is no associated vomiting or photophobia. The patient can usually continue normal activities and the pain may be less noticeable when the patient is occupied. Local tenderness may be present over the skull vault or in the occiput but this should be distinguished from the acute pain precipitated by skin contact in trigeminal neuralgia.

Stress or anxiety are common precipitants to tension headache and there is sometimes an underlying depressive illness. Anxiety about the headache itself may lead to continued propagation of symptoms, and patients often become convinced of a serious underlying condition. A detailed history followed by a meticulous examination helps not only to clarify the diagnosis but may provide reassurance to the patient. A careful explanation of the symptoms and likely precipitants of tension headache are more likely to be beneficial than analgesics.

Management
Treatment of underlying anxiety or depression may be helpful, but many forms of stress are not amenable to medical intervention.

MIGRAINE

Migraine is characterised by episodic headache, which is typically unilateral and often associated with vomiting and visual disturbance. In many patients, however, the headache is bitemporal and generalised and there may be no associated focal visual or neurological disturbance. The single most characteristic feature is the episodic nature of the headache.

Pathogenesis
In migraine with aura, there is a decrease in cerebral blood flow at the onset of an attack and relative oligaemia may result in focal disturbance of cortical function, particularly in the occipital and parietal lobes. During the phase of headache, there is dilatation of the extracranial arteries, which may be related to fluctuations in blood 5-hydroxytryptamine levels.

Approximately half of patients who suffer from migraine have an affected relative, suggesting a genetic predisposition. Dietary factors, including chocolate, cheese and alcohol, may precipitate attacks, and episodes may occur more frequently perimenstrually, at weekends or in patients taking oral contraceptives. Stress and anxiety may initiate attacks or lead to perpetuation of headache,

and stress and migraine headache not uncommonly co-exist.

Clinical features
The condition usually starts after puberty and continues until late middle life. Attacks occur at intervals which vary from a few days to several months, and last for hours to days. Premonitory symptoms occur in some patients in the form of zig-zag lines, flashing coloured lights, or defects in the visual field, and in others dysphasia, hemiparesis or hemianaesthesias may develop in association with the headache. The headache is usually localised to the frontal region and spreads to affect the whole of one side of the head, but may become generalised. The pain is severe and throbbing and may be associated with vomiting, photophobia, pallor, and prostration, which may necessitate the patient taking to bed in a darkened room. Variants are shown in the information box overleaf.

Management
Dietary or other precipitants to attacks should be avoided, and may sometimes be identified by advising the patient to keep a diary of attacks. The oral contraceptive pill should be stopped if the attacks are frequent or if there is associated focal neurological disturbance.

Acute attacks of common migraine usually respond to soluble aspirin (600–900 mg) or paracetamol (1 g) with or without an antiemetic such as metaclopramide or prochlorperazine. In classical migraine, ergotamine tartrate, 0.5–1.0 mg sublingually, rectally or by inhaler, may abort the headache phase if taken as soon as visual or sensory symptoms are felt. Ergotamine itself causes nausea and vomiting and many patients cannot tolerate it. Excessive use may lead to vasospasm and, paradoxically, headache. No more than 12 mg should be given in a week, and it is contraindicated in pregnancy, ischaemic heart disease and peripheral vascular disorders. The serotonin agonist sumatriptan is a newly introduced agent for acute migraine attacks, 100 mg tablets, no more than 300 mg per 24 hours. It is also available in an injection, 6 mg subcutaneously, no more than 2 injections per 24 hours. This preparation is highly effective, but costly.

If migraine attacks occur frequently enough to disrupt work and social life (e.g. weekly), then drug prophylaxis is justified. Useful agents are propranolol (40–80 mg 8-hourly), and pizotifen (1.5–3 mg at night). Antidepressants such as amitriptyline (25–100 mg at night) may be helpful. All these agents have some blocking activity on 5-HT receptors, and in resistant cases methysergide (1–2 mg 8-hourly) is often effective. This is a potent 5-HT antagonist and can cause retroperitoneal

Table 18.37 Clinical features in headache

Cause	Site	Duration	Character	Associations
Tension	Generalised/nuchal	Constant	Dull, tight pressure	Local tenderness, anxiety/depression
Migraine	Unilaterla/bitemporal	Episodic	Aching, throbbing	Prostration, nausea, vomiting, photophobia, visual features
Temporal arteritis	Temporal	Constant (nocturnal)	Burning	Scalp tenderness, jaw claudication, malaise
Meningitis	Generalised/nuchal	Acute progressive	Throbbing	Meningism, pyrexia
Raised pressure	Generalised	Progressive	Throbbing	Papilloedema, drowsiness, vomiting

CLASSIFICATION OF PRINCIPAL FORMS OF MIGRAINE

- **Classical migraine (migraine with aura)**
  Visual or sensory symptoms precede or accompany the headache

- **Common migraine (migraine without aura)**
  No visual or sensory features
  Headaches, nausea, vomiting, photophobia

- **Hemiplegic migraine**
  Prolonged headache lasting hours or days, followed by hemiparesis which recovers slowly over days

- **Basilar migraine**
  Occipital headache preceded by vertigo, diplopia, dysarthria ± visual and sensory symptoms

- **Cluster headache (migrainous neuralgia)**
  Affects mostly males. Bouts of severe pain around one eye with associated epiphora and nasal congestion

fibrosis with prolonged use; it should be given for courses of only 3 months and renal function should be carefully monitored.

BENIGN INTRACRANIAL HYPERTENSION

This is a rare condition, usually occurring in obese young women, in which raised intracranial pressure develops without a space-occupying lesion. The aetiology is uncertain, although the condition can be precipitated by drugs including tetracycline, steroids, and the oral contraceptive pill.

Management
Treatment involves withdrawal of any precipitating medication and diet; in patients in whom chronic papilloedema threatens vision, lumboperitoneal shunt may be necessary.

FACIAL PAIN

Common causes of facial pain are listed in Table 18.38. The differentiation between the causes of facial pain depends primarily on the clinical history. The treatment of trigeminal neuralgia is discussed on page 1049. Migrainous neuralgia may respond to ergotamine tartrate (see above), sumatriptan, or oxygen inhalation, but in many patients prophylactic therapy with lithium carbonate 0.25–2 g daily, methysergide 1–2 mg 8-hourly, or steroids may be necessary. Atypical facial pain often responds to antidepressant medication, while a prosthetic device to correct malocclusion and sometimes surgery are indicated in temporo-mandibular arthritis.

FURTHER READING

Diamond S, Dalessio D J 1991 The Practicing Physician's Approach to Headache, 5th edn. Williams and Wilkins, Baltimore

EPILEPSY

Epilepsy is defined as a group of disorders in which there are recurrent episodes of altered cerebral function associated with paroxysmal excessive and hypersynchronous discharge of cerebral neurones. The clinical accompaniments of these episodes—seizures—vary in manifestation from brief lapses of awareness to prolonged bouts of unconsciousness, limb jerking and incontinence.

Pathophysiology
In health the widely interconnected neurones of the cerebral cortex are held in a state of relative quiescence by inhibitory synaptic influences. Synchronous discharge amongst neighbouring groups of neurones is limited by

Table 18.38 Common causes of facial pain

Cause	Site	Duration	Character	Associations
Trigeminal neuralgia	Unilateral, maxillary/mandibular	Occurs in bouts	Lancinating	Triggering by touch, chewing, speaking, etc.
Migrainous neuralgia	Unilateral, ocular/cheek/forehead	Occurs in bouts	Severe throbbing (nocturnal)	Lacrimation, nasal blockage
Atypical facial pain	Bilateral/unilateral	Constant	Aching, boring	
Temporomandibular arthritis	Unilateral, angle of jaw, cheek	On chewing	Aching	Malocclusion

recurrent and collateral inhibitory circuits. The inhibitory transmitter gamma-aminobutyric acid (GABA) is thought to be particularly important in this role; drugs which block GABA receptors provoke seizures. There is also a large number of excitatory neurotransmitters, of which acetylcholine and the amino acids glutamate and aspartate are examples. Epileptic cerebral cortex exhibits hypersynchronous repetitive discharges involving large groups of neurones; intracellular recordings show bursts of rapid action potential firing, with reduction of the transmembrane potential (paroxysmal depolarisation shift). It is likely that both reduction in inhibitory systems and excessive excitation play a part in the genesis of seizure activity.

Classification

The chief division of seizure types is between **partial (focal) seizures** in which paroxysmal neuronal activity is limited to one part of the cerebrum, and **generalised seizures** where the electrophysiological abnormality involves large areas of both hemispheres simultaneously and synchronously (Table 18.39). If partial seizures remain localised, the symptomatology is elementary and depends on the cortical area affected; awareness is preserved, and the attack is termed 'simple'. If, however, the activity spreads to involve the reticular activating system at the thalamic level, awareness is lost and a 'complex partial seizure' results. Further spread may lead to a secondarily generalised seizure. Some generalised seizures arise without any clear focal onset, such patients appearing to have diffusely impaired cortical inhibitory mechanisms.

PARTIAL SEIZURES

Motor

Epileptic activity arising in the precentral gyrus causes partial motor seizures affecting the contralateral face, arm, trunk and leg. Seizures are characterised by rhythmical jerking or sustained spasm of the affected parts. They may remain localised to one part, or may spread to involve the whole side. Some attacks begin in one part (e.g. mouth, thumb, great toe) and spread gradually, this form being called Jacksonian epilepsy. Attacks vary in duration from a few seconds to several hours. More prolonged episodes may leave paresis of the involved limb for several hours after the seizure ceases (Todd's palsy).

Sensory

Seizures arising in the postcentral gyrus cause tingling or 'electric' sensations in the contralateral face and limbs. A spreading pattern like a Jacksonian seizure may occur.

Versive

A frontal epileptic focus may involve the frontal eye field, causing forced deviation of the eyes to the opposite side. This type of attack often rapidly becomes generalised to a tonic-clonic seizure.

Visual

Occipital epileptic foci cause simple visual hallucination such as balls of light or patterns of colour. Formed visual hallucinations of faces or scenes arise more anteriorly in the temporal lobes.

Psychomotor

Seizures which cause alterations of mood, memory and perception usually arise from the medial temporal lobe. This is a common form of epilepsy, causing both partial and secondary generalised seizures. Occasionally, a similar clinical picture arises from inferior frontal foci. Simple partial temporal lobe attacks may cause disordered perception such as undue familiarity (déjà vu) or unreality (jamais vu); complex hallucinations of sound, smell, taste, vision; emotional changes (fear, sexual arousal); visceral sensations (nausea, epigastric discomfort). Complex partial seizures may be preceded by an aura of these phenomena, lasting seconds or minutes, and then awareness is diminished or lost for typically several minutes. During this phase of a complex partial seizure, the sufferer may stare and be unresponsive to

Table 18.39   Clinical classification of epilepsy

Partial seizures	Generalised seizures (generalised from onset or secondary generalisation of partial seizure)
Simple (awareness preserved) Motor Sensory Psychomotor Visual Versive	Tonic-clonic (grand mal) Absence (petit mal) Akinetic Myoclonic
Complex (awareness lost) Temporal Frontal	

Table 18.40   Common causes of epilepsy

Generalised seizures (tonic-clonic, absences, myoclonus)	
Primary (idiopathic)	Genetic—family history
Diffuse cerebral insults	Encephalitis, anoxia, storage disorders
Metabolic disorders	Hypocalcaemia, hyponatraemia, hypoglycaemia, porphyria, hypoxia, renal and hepatic failure
Drugs and toxins	Alcohol, antidepressants, phenothiazines, amphetamines, local anaesthetics, metronidazole drug and alcohol withdrawal
Partial seizures	
Cerebral trauma	Birth injury, head injury, infarction and haemorrhage
Structural lesions	Vascular malformations, aneurysms, cerebral tumours, cysts, hydrocephalus
Infections	Meningitis, encephalitis, abscess, empyema, syphilis, tuberculosis, HIV, toxoplasmosis
Inflammation	Sarcoidosis, multiple sclerosis, systemic lupus erythematosus

PHASES OF A TONIC-CLONIC SEIZURE

- **Prodromal phase**
  Hours or days before attack, unease, irritability

- **Aura**
  Due to partial onset of seizure lasts seconds or minutes: e.g. olfactory hallucination, epigastric discomfort, déjà vu, jerking of one limb

- **Tonic phase**
  Rapid discharging of motor cortex cells causes tonic contractions of muscles; arms flexed and adducted, legs extended; respiratory muscle spasm causes 'cry' as air expelled; cyanosis; loss of consciousness. Lasts 10–30 s

- **Clonic phase**
  Less rapid, gradually slowing discharge of cortical cells; violent jerking of face and limbs; tongue biting, incontinence. Lasts 1–5 min

- **Post-ictal phase**
  Deep unconsciousness, flaccid limbs and jaw, loss of corneal reflexes, extensor plantar responses. Lasts a few minutes to several hours. Headache, confusion, aching muscles and sometimes automatic behaviour, occasional violence

Classical absences (petit mal)

This is a relatively uncommon form of generalised epilepsy, seen mostly in children. Typical absences are always due to primary generalised (idiopathic) epilepsy; the symptoms start in childhood or adolescence. During an absence attack the child stops activity, stares, may blink or roll up the eyes, and fails to respond to commands. Each attack lasts only a matter of seconds but many hundred absences may occur in a day. Occasionally, loss of posture occurs and the child falls but is able to get up again quickly (akinetic attack). The EEG recorded during attacks shows generalised bilaterally synchronous spike and wave complexes at a frequency of 3/s (see Fig. 18.17, p. 1039). Attacks may go unnoticed by the patient, and sometimes by their family.

Causes of epilepsy

Investigation of patients with epilepsy reveals no clear cause in many cases. Primary generalised (idiopathic) epilepsy usually causes tonic-clonic seizures without an aura, or less often, classical absences. In up to 40% of patients there is a family history of epilepsy in a close relative, heredity being particularly important in primary epilepsies. Generalised epilepsy is occasionally secondary to a definable cause (e.g. anoxia, hypocalcaemia), but it is partial seizures which have the highest incidence of a detectable cortical lesion. Partial seizures therefore warrant more intensive investigation, especially if they arise for the first time in adult life. Common causes of epilepsy are listed in Table 18.40.

Factors precipitating seizures

Sometimes specific trigger factors which set off seizures can be identified. Some are listed in the information box below.

questions. Automatic movements (e.g. lip smacking, swallowing, fidgeting with clothes) may occur at this stage, and some patients fall down. If the attack proceeds further, a tonic-clonic seizure may ensue.

GENERALISED SEIZURES

Tonic-clonic (grand mal)

This is a common type of seizure. If epileptic activity has spread from a focus by secondary generalisation, the patient may recall an aura of the elementary symptoms. The aura often lasts only a few seconds before consciousness is lost. Several phases can be identified, although they do not always occur on every occasion; they are summarised in the information box above.

Clinical features

The most important steps in making a diagnosis of epilepsy are listed in the information box above. In many patients these two steps are sufficient to establish the diagnosis, or may suggest an alternative (e.g. syncope).

Clinical examination is often unhelpful. Rarely, clinical features may suggest a specific diagnosis such as tuberous sclerosis or pseudohypoparathyroidism. A good general examination with emphasis on the nervous and cardiovascular systems should be performed. Particular points of note are listed in the information boxes above.

Investigations

The investigations which may be undertaken in a patient with suspected epilepsy are shown in the information box below.

Electroencephalography (EEG)

The EEG may help establish and characterise the type of epilepsy; interictal records are abnormal in about 60% of patients. Details of EEG recording methods and examples of abnormalities are given on pages 1035–1039. The yield of diagnostic abnormalities can be increased by prolonging recording time, and including a period of natural or drug induced sleep. In cases of diagnostic difficulty with frequent symptoms, ambulatory EEG recording or video/EEG monitoring may provide helpful information, but are costly and time-consuming. It is important to remember that a normal interictal EEG does not negate a good clinical diagnosis of epilepsy; but nor does an abnormal record establish a diagnosis in the absence of an appropriate history.

Computed tomography (CT)

CT brain scanning does not help establish a diagnosis of epilepsy but is often useful in defining or excluding a structural cause for seizures. As a general rule a CT scan should be performed if:

1. epilepsy starts after the age of 20 years
2. at any age if seizures have focal features clinically
3. the EEG shows a focal seizure source
4. control of seizures is difficult or deteriorates.

CT scanning is not required if a confident diagnosis of primary generalised epilepsy can be made clinically. Examples:

1. tonic-clonic seizures without aura, on waking in morning, in a teenager with a positive family history, EEG shows generalised paroxysms
2. typical absences in a child of 10, with 3/s spike and wave bursts on EEG.

Management

The nature of epilepsy should be explained to patients and their relatives. Many people with epilepsy feel stigmatised by society and may become unnecessarily isolated from work and social life. It should be emphasised that epilepsy is a common disorder which affects just under 1% of the population, and that good or complete control of seizures can be expected in more than 80% of patients.

Immediate care of seizures

Little can or need be done for a person having a major seizure. Some simple guidelines are listed in the information box above.

Restrictions

Until good control of seizures has been established, work or recreation above ground level, with dangerous machinery or near open fires should be avoided. Patients should take a shallow bath, only when a relative is in the house, and should not lock the bathroom door. Cycling and swimming should be discouraged until at least 6 months' freedom from seizures has been achieved, and swimming should always be in the company of someone who is aware of the slight chance of a seizure occurring. Any activity where loss of awareness might be very dangerous (e.g. mountaineering) should be discouraged.

Driving

Legal restrictions apply in the United Kingdom to vehicle driving. Patients with epilepsy must be free from all types of seizure for 1 year (on or off medication), or seizures must have been exclusively during sleep for a period of three years, before driving may be resumed. The patient should inform the licensing authorities about the onset of seizures, and it is also wise for them to notify their motor insurance company. Vocational drivers are not permitted a heavy goods or public service vehicle licence if any seizure occurs after the age of 5 years.

Anticonvulsant drug therapy

Traditionally, a single seizure has been regarded as an indication for investigation and assessment, but not for drug treatment unless a second attack follows closely. Prospective studies have shown that the recurrence rate after a first seizure approaches 70% during the first year, most recurrent attacks occurring within a month or two of the first. Further seizures are less likely if a trigger factor is definable (e.g. sleep deprivation, exhaustion). Drug treatment should certainly be considered after two seizures have occurred, and in some cases (very abnormal EEG, strong family history) a single unprovoked seizure is sufficient indication. There is some evidence to uphold the notion that the earlier seizures are brought under control, the more easily they will remain quiescent.

Use of anticonvulsant drugs

Several effective agents are available. Their mode of action is not well understood, but they probably affect both the stability of neuronal membranes and neurotransmitter systems by promoting inhibitory activity. Good or total control of seizures can be expected in about 80% of epileptic patients using a single drug in adequate dosage. Dose regimens should be kept as simple as is necessary to maintain therapeutic plasma levels of the drug; the simpler the regimen, the more likely the patient is to comply with it. Some useful guidelines are listed in the information box below.

Measuring plasma anticonvulsant drug levels

Levels of all the major antiepileptic drugs can be measured in blood routinely. Agents which have a long plasma half-life (e.g. phenytoin: 24–36 hours) can adequately be given once a day. Plateau levels taken 4–6 hours after the last dose are preferable to peak samples when measuring drugs with shorter half-lives (carbamazepine and sodium valproate). Plasma level monitoring is particularly useful for phenytoin, because of the marked variation in dose requirements between individuals and the saturation kinetics of the drug which give rise to an exponential dose/blood level relationship. The measurement of plasma levels for carbamazepine and the barbiturates are helpful but not essential; valproate levels are rarely a useful guide to adequate dosage, and serve often only to confirm patient compliance. It is important to recognise that quoted 'therapeutic' ranges are approximations from experience, and need not be adhered to rigidly if the patient is otherwise well.

Efficacy and choice of drug

Overall, generalised tonic-clonic seizures are more readily controlled than partial epilepsy. Although some agents seem more effective in certain types of seizure, with the exception of absence attacks there are no hard and fast rules as to which drug is superior. The choice may lie more in the suitability of a particular drug for a specific patient. For example, phenytoin and carbamazepine are not ideal agents for a young woman wishing to use oral contraception, because the drugs induce liver enzymes which render the contraceptive less effective. Sodium valproate should be avoided in children with progressive cerebral disorders because the risk of fatal hepatic damage is much higher in this group; it is also unsuitable for obese patients since it tends to cause weight gain.

The commonly used drugs, dose ranges, therapeutic levels and side-effects are shown in Table 18.41. A guide to the choice of appropriate drugs is given in Table 18.42.

Withdrawal of anticonvulsant therapy

After a period of complete control of seizures, withdrawal of medication may be considered. How long complete control should be achieved before considering withdrawal is debatable; periods of 2–4 years are usually required. Childhood onset epilepsy, particularly classical absence seizures, carries the best prognosis for successful drug withdrawal. Seizures which begin in adult life, particularly those with partial features, are the most likely to recur. Overall, the recurrence rate of seizures after drug withdrawal is about 40%; some adult patients tend to opt for continuation of therapy for they feel the threat of further attacks greater than continuing with medication. The EEG does not seem to be a good predictor of seizure recurrence but if the record is still very

abnormal, drug withdrawal is unwise. Withdrawal should be undertaken slowly, reducing the drug dose gradually over 6–12 months.

STATUS EPILEPTICUS

Status epilepticus exists when a series of seizures occurs without the patient regaining awareness between attacks. Most commonly this refers to recurrent tonic-clonic seizures (major status), this condition being a life-threatening state and therefore a medical emergency. Partial motor status is obvious clinically, but complex partial status and absence status may be difficult to diagnose, because the patient may merely present with a dazed, confused state. Status may be precipitated by abrupt withdrawal of anticonvulsant drugs, or major intracranial disasters (e.g. cerebral haemorrhage), and tends to be more common with frontal epileptic foci. Management is summarised in the information box.

MANAGEMENT OF STATUS EPILEPTICUS

- Maintain airway with oropharyngeal tube; give high-flow oxygen
- Give diazepam i.v. 10–20 mg over 1–3 min. This may cause hypotension and impair respiration; use i.v. only if resuscitation facilities available, otherwise rectal route safer
- Transfer patient to intensive care area; monitor BP, ECG, EEG and blood gases
- Set up i.v. infusion of diazepam 10–50 mg/h. Adjust dose to control seizures
- Give loading dose of phenytoin i.v. 18 mg/kg body weight at a rate no faster than 50 mg/min (omit if patient already taking phenytoin)
- Try chlormethiazole i.v. 0.5–1.2 g/hour by infusion if diazepam fails to control seizures
- If seizures still uncontrolled set up i.v. infusion of thiopentone. This usually necessitates assisted ventilation
- When seizures controlled, determine cause. Check electrolytes, calcium, glucose, urea. Consider urgent CT scan if patient not previously known to have epilepsy. In established epileptic, check plasma anticonvulsant levels

---

Epilepsy and pregnancy

Reference has already been made to the hepatic enzyme induction caused by carbamazepine, phenytoin and the barbiturates which accelerate metabolism of the oral contraceptives, causing breakthrough bleeding and contraceptive failure. The safest policy is for women taking these drugs to use an alternative contraceptive method,

Table 18.41 Major anticonvulsant drugs, doses, therapeutic ranges, side-effects

Drug	Seizure types	Dose range mg/day	Doses per day	Therap. range μmol/l	Side-effects dose related	Side-effects idiosyncratic	Side-effects long term
Phenytoin	Tonic-clonic Partial	150–600	1–2	40–80	Ataxia Nystagmus Lethargy Tremor Dystonia Confusion	Rashes Lymphadenopathy Blood dyscrasia Liver damage SLE[2]	Gum hypertrophy Hirsutism Folate deficiency Osteomalacia Neuropathy
Carbamazepine	Partial Tonic-clonic	200–2000	2–3	20–50	Drowsiness Ataxia Nystagmus Diplopia Headache Hyponatraemia	Rashes Dyspepsia Blood dyscrasia	Not recognised
Sodium valproate	Tonic-clonic Absences Myoclonus	400–3000	2–3	200–700 Poorly defined	Nausea Anorexia Tremor Drowsiness	Alopecia Thrombocytopenia Hepatic necrosis	Weight gain
Primidone	Tonic-clonic Partial	250–1000	2–3	50–150[1]	Nausea Drowsiness Ataxia Nystagmus	SLE[2]	Folate deficiency Osteomalacia Neuropathy
Phenobarbitone	Tonic-clonic Partial	60–180	1–2	50–150	Drowsiness Lethargy Ataxia Nystagmus	Rashes SLE[2]	As primidone
Ethosuximide	Absences (petit mal)	500–1500	2	200–700	Dizziness Insomnia	Nausea Rashes Blood dyscrasia	
Clonazepam	Partial (adjunctive)	1–6	2–3	50–300	Drowsiness Irritability		Useful effects decline after a period of weeks
Lamotrigine	Complex Partial (+ absences)	200–400	2		Dizziness Diplopia	Blood dyscrasia Skin rash	
Gabapentin	Complex Partial	600–1200	3		Drowsiness Ataxia		

[1] Measured phenobarbitone.
[2] SLE: Systemic lupus erythematosus.

but it is sometimes possible to overcome the problem by giving a higher oestrogen dose (50–80 μg) preparation.

Epilepsy may worsen during pregnancy, particularly during the third trimester when plasma anticonvulsant levels tend to fall. More frequent monitoring of blood levels during pregnancy is therefore advisable. All the major anticonvulsant drugs have been associated with an increased incidence of fetal congenital abnormalities (cleft lip, spina bifida, cardiac defects). The risk is greatest during the first trimester. It is seldom possible to withdraw or change therapy before conception, but carbamazepine may be less teratogenic than the other agents. Occasionally in a well-controlled patient anticonvulsants can be withdrawn before conception, but if seizures have occurred in the preceding year this is unwise as the risk to the fetus from uncontrolled maternal seizures is probably greater than the teratogenic effects.

FURTHER READING

Laidlaw J, Richens A, Chadwick D (eds) 1993 A Textbook of Epilepsy, 4th edn. Churchill Livingstone, Edinburgh
Trimble, M R (ed) 1989 Chronic Epilepsy, its Prognosis and Management. John Wiley & Sons, Chichester

Table 18.42	Guidelines for selection of anticonvulsant drugs	
Seizure	**Types**	**Drug preference order**
Tonic-clonic	Primary generalised	Valproate Phenytoin Carbamazepine Barbiturates
	Secondary generalised	Phenytoin Carbamazepine Valproate Barbiturates
Partial		Carbamazepine Phenytoin Valproate Lamotrigine Gabapentin Barbiturates Benzodiazepines
Classical absences (petit mal)		Valproate Ethosuximide Lamotrigine

Table 18.43	Vascular disorders causing stroke	
Causing infarction		
Atherosclerosis		Extracranial Intracranial
Arteriolar sclerosis		Hypertensive Degenerative Inherited
Embolism		From heart From vessels
Arteritis		Infective Giant cell SLE, polyarteritis Granulomatous
Dissection		Traumatic Spontaneous
Vasospasm		Migraine Subarachnoid haemorrhage Angiography
Causing haemorrhage		
Aneurysms of major arteries (berry) **Small arteriolar aneurysms** (hypertensive) **Arteriovenous malformations** **Atheromatous aneurysms** **Infective aneurysms** (mycotic) **Head trauma**		

CEREBRAL VASCULAR DISORDERS

STROKE

Damage to brain tissue due either to cerebral infarction or haemorrhage ('stroke') is the third commonest cause of death in developed countries. Stroke is uncommon below the age of 50 and affects males 1.5 times more often than females. Younger people occasionally sustain a stroke because of trauma to cerebral vessels, inflammatory disorders of arteries, or congenital vascular anomalies. In an average population, the annual incidence of new strokes is 2 per 1000 people. Stroke is therefore a prominent cause of disability, particularly in the elderly. Pathological studies indicate that 80–85% of strokes are due to cerebral infarction; 15–20% are caused by haemorrhage. The most common vascular disorder underlying stroke is atherosclerosis affecting intracranial and extracranial arteries; less common mechanisms are listed in Table 18.43. Strokes are common in patients with other cardiovascular disorders, particularly ischaemic heart and peripheral vascular disease. The major risk factors for stroke are listed in Table 18.44.

Table 18.44	Risk factors for stroke	
Major risks		**Other risks**
Arterial hypertension Cigarette smoking Diabetes mellitus Hyperlipidaemia Polycythaemia Thrombocythaemia		High alcohol intake Positive family history Oral contraceptives Trauma

CEREBRAL INFARCTION

Occlusion of a major cerebral artery usually leads to infarction unless, as in some young people, a collateral circulation is well developed. Thrombosis at the site of atheromatous degeneration in a major cerebral vessel is probably the commonest mechanism, but embolism of thrombotic or atheromatous material from the heart or an extracranial artery is also frequent (see Fig. 18.32). Thromboemboli of cardiac origin may arise from mural thrombus after myocardial infarction, and are often associated with atrial fibrillation, especially when it is secondary to valvular disease. Cardiac emboli tend to be large and cause occlusion of one of the principal cerebral arteries or a major branch, thereby causing usually major strokes. By contrast, emboli arising from the carotid bifurcation are more often particulate, due to deposition of platelets, and often cause minor or transient cerebral or ocular symptoms.

Once deprived of blood supply cerebral tissue undergoes infarction within a few minutes. Released excitatory amino acids may exacerbate the neuronal damage by promoting calcium influx. The damaged neurones and glia become oedematous after some hours, the resultant cerebral oedema causing more damage by further impairing cerebral blood flow.

CEREBRAL HAEMORRHAGE

About half the strokes caused by cerebral haemorrhage are due to subarachnoid bleeding from rupture of an aneurysm at the circle of Willis or less commonly from an arteriovenous malformation. In other patients, haemorrhage is mainly into the cerebral substance and is due to rupture of small perforating arteries or arterioles weakened by hypertension or atheromatous degeneration (Fig. 18.33). Intracerebral haemorrhage of this type tends to occur at three distinct sites:

1. The internal capsule—from lenticulo-striate arteries
2. The pons—from perforating branches of the basilar artery
3. The cerebellum.

Subarachnoid haemorrhage may induce secondary arteial spasm and thereby cerebral infarction. Although large cerebral haemorrhages cause severe disability, small bleeds in the deep cerebral white matter may cause only mild and transient defects. Cerebellar haemorrhage can be fatal if secondary compression of the brain stem occurs.

Classification of stroke
The clinical classification of a stroke is given in the information box below.

CLINICAL CLASSIFICATION OF STROKE

- Completed stroke
  Major
  Minor
- Evolving stroke
- Transient ischaemic attack (TIA)

Completed stroke
This is an episode of focal cerebral dysfunction, due either to cerebral infarction or haemorrhage, with symptoms lasting longer than 24 hours. Strokes usually evolve rapidly over a few minutes, and reach maximum disability within an hour or two. Sometimes a slower course occurs, the disability advancing gradually over several hours or days. This is known as an evolving stroke, or 'stroke in evolution'. Headache is a common accompaniment to acute stroke and does not help distinguish infarction from haemorrhage. Epileptic seizures, vomiting and depressed consciousness may also occur, the latter usually indicating a severe lesion. The precise features of a stroke depend on the vascular territory involved. Figure 18.34 shows the territories of the three main cerebral arteries; Table 18.45 sets out the features of stroke lesions at different sites.

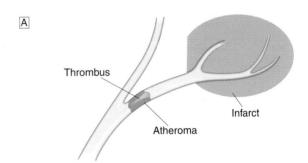

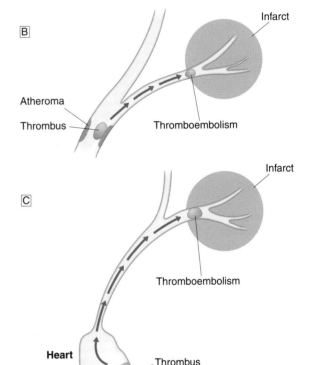

Fig. 18.32   Mechanism of stroke—cerebral infarction.
A Thrombosis at site of atheroma. B Embolism from major artery.
C Thromboembolism from cardiac source.

Evolving stroke
In some patients the symptoms worsen gradually or in a step-wise fashion over a matter of hours or days. This clinical picture can be due to cerebral tumour or subdural haematoma, but is more often due to slow occlusion of a major cerebral vessel such as the internal carotid or the middle cerebral artery.

Minor stroke
Some patients with a completed stroke improve rapidly, with recovery from disability over the course of the first

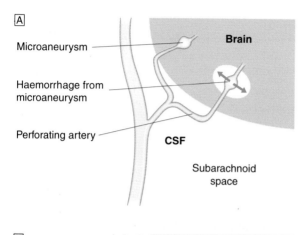

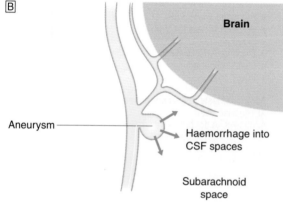

Fig. 18.33 Mechanism of stroke—cerebral haemorrhage.
Ⓐ Intracerebral (hypertensive). Ⓑ Subarachnoid (aneurysmal).

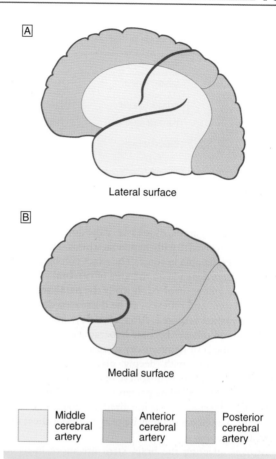

Fig. 18.34 Supply territories of cerebral arteries. Ⓐ Lateral view of left hemisphere. Ⓑ Medial view of right hemisphere.

week or two. The rather arbitrary definition of minor strokes is useful because such patients can be managed in much the same way as cases of transient ischaemia (see below).

Transient ischaemic attack (TIA)

This is an episode of focal neurological dysfunction due to cerebral ischaemia in which symptoms last less than 24 hours. In many TIAs symptoms last only a few minutes; it is likely that a minor degree of infarction takes place when symptoms last longer than an hour, and indeed many patients with TIAs have minor neurological signs. The most frequent mechanism of TIA is embolism of thrombus or platelet material from the extracerebral arteries, especially the internal carotid artery at its origin in the neck. Less often a cardiac source of emboli is responsible. In some patients a severe stenosis of a major artery causes focal cerebral ischaemia by interference with haemodynamics so that changes in overall perfusion pressure (e.g. due to standing up or

exertion) provoke TIA symptoms. This type of attack is more commonly encountered in the vertebro-basilar circulation where symptoms of vertigo, diplopia, ataxia and syncope are triggered by postural changes or neck movements. Patients with carotid TIAs often experience retinal embolic events, causing transient monocular blindness (amaurosis fugax).

TIAs are important because they may herald a completed stroke. This is particularly relevant for carotid territory TIAs which carry an annual risk of completed stroke of about 5%; vertebrobasilar TIAs are less sinister, but still carry an increased risk. About 25% of patients who have suffered a completed stroke report symptoms of one or more TIA before the onset of the major event. A TIA is therefore an important warning symptom, which should alert the doctor to investigate and attempt to prevent more serious events.

Clinical features

The clinical diagnosis of a stroke is usually straightforward. The majority of patients exhibit greater or lesser

Table 18.45   Features of stroke in different arterial territories

Main artery	Branch	Clinical features	Side
Internal carotid	Middle cerebral	Hemiparesis (face and arm > leg), hemianaesthesia Dysphasia, dysarthria, dyspraxia, hemianopia	Opposite side to lesion
	Anterior cerebral	Hemiparesis (leg > arm and face), incontinence	
Vertebral	Posterior cerebral	Hemianopia, cortical blindness, amnesia Thalamic pain	Nuclear symptoms ipsilateral to lesion: contralateral sensory and pyramidal signs
	Cerebellar basilar	Ataxia, diplopia, nystagmus, dysarthria, dysphagia, facial weakness/numbness, bilateral sensory symptoms, loss of consciousness	

degrees of hemiparesis, dysphasia (if the dominant hemisphere is involved), with hemianaesthesia and homonomous hemianopia in some. The exact combination of these features depends on the area of cerebral cortex or deep white matter involved. Initially the paralysed limbs may be flaccid and reflexes can be decreased despite an extensor plantar response. After a few days, tone usually increases and reflexes become hyperactive on the affected side. Ataxia or hemisensory disturbance may dominate the picture with deeply placed small lacunar infarcts. With severe hemisphere damage, flaccid hemiplegia is accompanied by paresis of gaze to the affected side, and consciousness is impaired as cerebral oedema develops. Papilloedema may be present under these circumstances.

Strokes affecting the brain stem are more likely to cause loss of consciousness because of damage to the reticular activating system. The cardinal features of brain-stem stroke are a combination of nuclear signs on the side of the lesion (e.g. oculomotor palsy, palatal weakness) and pyramidal and spinothalamic signs in the contralateral limbs. A characteristic syndrome occurs with infarction of the lateral medulla, due to occlusion of either the posterior-inferior cerebellar artery or the vertebral artery itself; there is ipsilateral ataxia, nystagmus, facial numbness and palatal palsy and sometimes ipsilateral Horner's syndrome; damage to the spinothalamic tract causes impairment of pain and temperature sensation contralateral to the lesion.

In addition to careful assessment of the neurological lesions, general examination should pay special attention to the cardiovascular system, noting blood pressure, cardiac rhythm, peripheral vasculature, arterial bruits and any cardiac murmurs.

Further details regarding the assessment of impairment following stroke are given on page 1122.

Investigations

The more routine tests are given in the information box below.

ROUTINE TESTS IN STROKE PATIENTS

- Full blood count, ESR
- Serological tests for syphilis
- Blood glucose
- Blood urea, electrolytes, proteins
- Chest radiograph
- ECG

Additional tests in younger patients
Antinuclear factor
Antibodies to double-stranded DNA
Anti-cardiolipin antibodies
Lupus anticoagulant
Cholesterol

CT scanning

With the exception of MRI, CT scanning provides the only reliable method of distinguishing cerebral infarction from haemorrhage. Clinical assessment has been shown to be very unreliable, and if any treatment with anticoagulants or even antiplatelet drugs is planned, CT scanning is essential to exclude cerebral haemorrhage. Occasionally a cerebral tumour presents as a stroke, usually because of haemorrhage into the lesion. Early or very small infarcts may not be detected by CT, but the vast majority of haemorrhages will be. Examples of typical lesions are shown in Figures 18.35 and 18.36. Infarcts appear as areas of low density usually with little or no mass effect unless they are very large. Some contrast enhancement may be present within infarcts especially after a few weeks when they exhibit increased vascularity.

Angiography

This is not usually indicated during the acute phase of a stroke unless a specific cause such as arterial dissection is suspected and intervention is likely to result. Angiography may exacerbate the stroke symptoms.

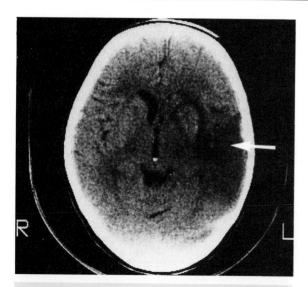

Fig. 18.35 CT scan of cerebral infarction. A large wedge-shaped low density lesion is seen in the left temporoparietal area (arrow), due to infarction in the territory of the middle cerebral artery. The left lateral ventricle is compressed, indicating that there is oedema associated with recent infarction.

MANAGEMENT OF ACUTE STROKE—GENERAL MEASURES

Careful nursing
- Regular turning of patient to avoid pressure sores; skin kept dry and clean

Care of airway
- Oropharyngeal tube with regular suction of secretions if patient unconscious

Fluid balance
- Nasogastric feeding if patient cannot swallow; bladder catheterisation if incontinent

Physiotherapy
- Start immediately to prevent joint contractures; to clear chest secretions; to promote recovery of strength and coordination

Speech and occupational therapy
- Start once acute stage over to assess functional problems and to encourage recovery of skills

Echocardiography

This is sometimes performed if there is a suggestion of a cardiac source of embolism causing a stroke and anticoagulation is being considered. In a young patient with an unexplained stroke, echocardiography may demonstrate cardiac thrombus, vegetations or myxoma.

Management

General measures for managing patients with an acute stroke are listed in the information box.

Specific management

Blood pressure

Many patients show a reactive rise in blood pressure in the acute phase of a stroke. This is a compensatory change attempting to maintain cerebral blood flow; hypotensive agents should not be used at this stage unless there are features of accelerated hypertension or signs of end-organ involvement. If treatment is necessary, this should be gentle to avoid a sudden lowering of cerebral perfusion pressure, which can exacerbate infarction.

Anticoagulation

There is usually no indication for the use of anticoagulants in acute stroke. The only positive indications are: if there is a clear persisting embolic source (e.g. atrial fibrillation; dissection of carotid artery) or if the features of stroke are evolving over hours or days.

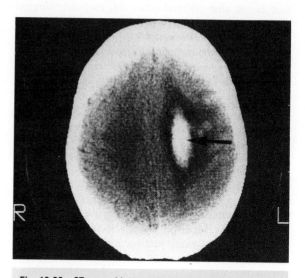

Fig. 18.36 CT scan of intracerebral haemorrhage. A large high-density lesion typical of recent haemorrhage is seen deep in the left hemisphere (arrow). The likely site of bleeding is in the internal capsule, in which region hypertensive microaneurysms often rupture.

In both instances, cerebral haemorrhage or tumour must be ruled out by urgent CT scanning before anticoagulation is started. Initial treatment should be with an intravenous infusion of heparin; oral warfarin may be instituted at the same time, and the heparin withdrawn after 3–4 days. When there is an established cerebral infarct, anticoagulation carries a risk of causing bleeding into the lesion. This risk has to be weighed against the risk of further progression of the stroke due to further emboli or extension of thrombus.

Oedema-reducing agents

Osmotic agents (i.v. mannitol 20%, 200 ml) and potent steroids (dexamethasone 4 mg i.v. 6-hourly) may help reduce mortality in patients with severe strokes and secondary cerebral oedema by limiting brain swelling and brain-stem compression. They are not indicated for an uncomplicated stroke, and their use in severe stroke is debatable because they have not been shown to prevent disability.

Vasodilating agents

There is no good evidence to support the use of vasodilators in acute stroke. Inhibitors of the excitatory amino acids are currently under evaluation.

Surgery

Carotid arterial surgery carries a high risk during the first month after cerebral infarction, and early surgical treatment of carotid occlusion has not been shown to be of benefit. Neurosurgical evacuation of a cerebral haematoma is sometimes indicated if, for example, the patient continues to deteriorate and the lesion is easily accessible. In cerebellar haemorrhage with secondary brain-stem compression, urgent surgical drainage of the haematoma may be life-saving.

Continuing management

Rehabilitation

About 30% of stroke patients will die as a direct result of the acute lesion. Of the survivors, most will recover some useful function over periods ranging from 1 to 12 months. At this stage, active help from enthusiastic physiotherapists, speech and occupational therapists is invaluable. (See page 1122, Chapter 19, for further details on stroke rehabilitation.) The risk of further strokes is 5–10% per annum and if risk factors can be identified they should be corrected as far as possible. Aspirin 300 mg/day reduces the risk of further stroke and death by about 25% but carries a small increase in the risk of cerebral haemorrhage. Patients who make a good functional recovery should be managed along the lines described for TIA in the information box (right).

Management of TIA

Risk factors

These should be identified and corrected. Hypertension, smoking and diabetes mellitus are the most important.

CLINICAL ASSESSMENT OF TIA AND MINOR STROKE

History
- Vascular territory involved
- Duration of symptoms
- Associated cardiac, peripheral vascular or retinal symptoms
- Other possible diagnoses (epilepsy, migraine, hypoglycaemia)

Examination
- Hypertension
- Diabetes mellitus
- Hyperlipidaemia
- Arterial disease (peripheral pulses, carotid or subclavian bruits)
- Cardiac disease (arrhythmias, murmurs)
- Previous CNS damage (weakness, sensory loss, incoordination, reflex, changes)
- Ocular involvement (retinal emboli, arterial disease)

Investigation
- Routine tests as for stroke (p. 1074)
- Special tests
  - **Vertebral/basilar TIA**
    - Lying/standing blood pressure
    - 24-hour ECG monitoring
    - X-rays of cervical spine
  - **Carotid TIA**
    - CT brain scan
    - Carotid Doppler ultrasound scanning
    - Arteriography (DVI or formal angiography)*

*Only if carotid surgery is contemplated

Hyperlipidaemia and polycythaemia are also worth treatment in younger patients.

Antiplatelet agents

Aspirin 300 mg/day reduces the risk of stroke by 25% and of death by 30%. If patients are intolerant of 300 mg of aspirin, lower doses (75–150 mg/d) may be tried instead. A new agent, Ticlopidine, is also likely to be useful in such cases, but is not yet available in the UK.

Anticoagulants

The use of oral anticoagulants in TIA has not been subjected to randomised clinical trials. These drugs carry more risk than aspirin, and are usually given only if there is a definable cardiac source of thromboemboli. They are occasionally useful when TIAs fail to come under control with antiplatelet agents, and arterial surgery is not possible.

Arterial surgery

Carotid endarterectomy by an experienced surgeon lowers the risk of further TIA and stroke. In order to be effective there must be a suitable stenosis at the origin of the internal carotid artery on the symptomatic side and the patient must be fit for operation. Large trials have shown surgery to give definite benefit to patients with a symptomatic carotid stenosis of greater than 70%. There is still uncertainty regarding patients with moderate stenosis, but surgery is not indicated when stenosis is less than 30%. Totally occluded vessels cannot be treated in this way, and by-pass procedures have not been shown to improve outlook. Carotid endarterectomy carries an operative risk of stroke or death in up to 10% of cases, and this has to be weighed against that of spontaneous stroke (5% per annum).

SUBARACHNOID HAEMORRHAGE

Subarachnoid haemorrhage (SAH) accounts for about 8% of all strokes. In more than 50% of patients, SAH is due to rupture of an aneurysm of one of the major cerebral arteries or their branches at the circle of Willis. Figure 18.37 shows the common sites of aneurysm formation, usually at the branch points of the arteries. Other causes of SAH are listed in the information box below.

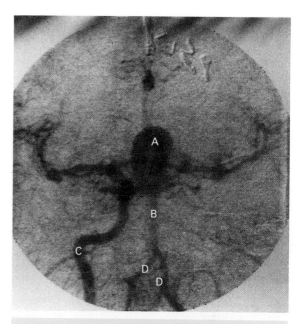

Fig. 18.37 Digital venous imaging (DVI)—intracranial view demonstrating a large saccular aneurysm arising from the basilar artery. Smaller aneurysms are also seen on the middle cerebral arteries. [A] Basilar aneurysm. [B] Basilar artery. [C] Internal carotid artery. [D] Vertebral artery.

CAUSES OF SAH

- Ruptured aneurysm
- Arteriovenous malformations
- Extension of intracerebral haemorrhage
- Haemorrhage into cerebral infarct
- Haemorrhage into cerebral tumour
- Rupture of atheromatous vessel
- Rupture of mycotic aneurysm
- Clotting disorders, anticoagulation

Clinical features

SAH often occurs during exertion (e.g. straining, sexual intercourse) when blood pressure is increased. There is usually sudden severe headache which radiates occipitally; neck pain and stiffness often follow. Consciousness may be lost and sometimes a tonic-clonic seizure is provoked. Some patients experience small warning headaches a few days before a major SAH. Examination reveals a variable degree of unconsciousness, photophobia and irritability. Neck stiffness is usually present, but may be absent in the earliest stages. Kernig's sign tends to develop later. Fundoscopy may show subhyaloid haemorrhages and sometimes optic disc oedema. Focal neurological signs may be present because of bleeding into the brain substance or from cerebral ischaemia consequent on arterial spasm. In severe cases, signs of decerebration with extensor posturing and extensor plantar responses are seen. A bruit may be audible over the head or eyes if bleeding is from an arteriovenous malformation.

Investigations

CT scanning

This is the investigation of choice; it will demonstrate the presence of subarachnoid blood in about 90% of cases (Fig. 18.38).

Lumbar puncture

This should be undertaken if SAH is suspected and if the scan fails to show bleeding. This will show uniformly blood-stained CSF; after 3–4 hours the supernatant becomes xanthochromic. A lumbar puncture is unnecessary and hazardous if CT scan shows definite subarachnoid blood.

Management

If SAH is proven, urgent transfer to a neurological unit for cerebral angiography is usually indicated unless the patient is deeply comatose. Surgical clipping of the

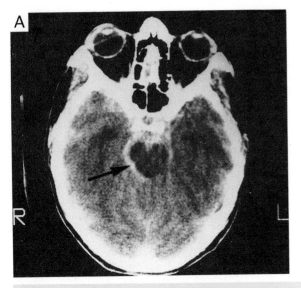 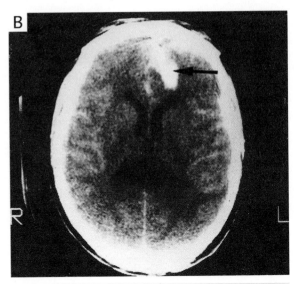

Fig. 18.38   CT scan of subarachnoid haemorrhage. Ⓐ Extensive blood (high density) in the basal cisterns, outlining the brain stem. Ⓑ There is a small intracerebral component to the haemorrhage in the left frontal lobe making it likely that the source of bleeding is from a ruptured aneurysm at the junction of the anterior cerebral and the anterior communicating arteries.

aneurysm is usually feasible. The majority of second haemorrhages occur about 14 days after the initial SAH and surgery should ideally be performed before this time. If the patient is alert and fit, operation within the first few days is successful, but in some patients surgery is delayed to allow arterial spasm to settle.

Other features of cerebral aneurysms and arteriovenous malformations

Cerebral aneurysms may present in ways other than SAH and some of these are listed in Table 18.46. For features of arteriovenous malformations see the information box below.

OTHER VASCULAR DISORDERS

GIANT CELL ARTERITIS—see page 924.

Cerebral venous thrombosis

Thrombosis of cerebral veins and venous sinuses is uncommon. The causes are listed in the information box below.

Cortical vein thrombosis

This causes local cerebral dysfunction (epilepsy, hemiparesis, dysphasia) though the area involved may enlarge if spreading thrombophlebitis occurs.

ARTERIOVENOUS MALFORMATIONS

Clinical features
- Subarachnoid haemorrhage
- Epilepsy
- Headache
- Vascular steal episodes (like TIAs)
- Tinnitus, vascular noises in head

Investigations
- CT scan with contrast enhancement
- Cerebral arteriography

Management
- Surgical resection (not always possible)
- Stereotactic radiotherapy (reduces risk of haemorrhage)
- Therapeutic embolisation
- Anticonvulsants if epilepsy present

CAUSES OF CEREBRAL VENOUS THROMBOSIS

Predisposing causes
- Polycythaemia
- Dehydration
- Hypotension
- Pregnancy
- Oral contraceptives

Local causes
- Paranasal sinusitis
- Facial skin infection
- Otitis media, mastoiditis
- Meningitis, subdural empyema
- Skull fracture
- Penetrating head and eye wounds

Table 18.46   Other presentations of cerebral arterial aneurysms

Mechanism	Vessel	Lesion
Compression of cranial nerves	Carotid aneurysm in cavernous sinus Internal carotid/posterior communicating aneurysm Anterior communicating artery aneurysm	IV, III, VI palsies III nerve palsy Optic nerve/chiasm lesions
Compression of cerebral tissue	Middle cerebral artery Basilar artery	Epilepsy, hemiparesis Diplopia, ataxia, tetraparesis

Cerebral venous sinus thrombosis

The clinical features of cerebral venous sinus thrombosis depend on the sinus involved. They are listed in the information box below. CT scanning may show evi-

---

CLINICAL FEATURES OF CEREBRAL VENOUS SINUS THROMBOSIS

Cavernous sinus
- Proptosis, ptosis, headache, external and internal ophthalmoplegia, papilloedema, reduced sensation in trigeminal first division
- Often bilateral, patient ill and febrile

Superior sagittal sinus
- Headache, papilloedema, seizures
- May involve veins of both hemispheres causing advancing motor and sensory deficits

Transverse sinus
- Hemiparesis, seizures, papilloedema
- May spread to jugular foramen to involve cranial nerves IX, X, XI

---

dence of sinus occlusion but is often normal. There may be evidence of cerebral oedema with small ventricles, and low density changes at sites of cortical infarction. Angiography or MRI scanning show impaired filling of veins and sinuses. CSF is under increased pressure, may be xanthochromic with excess of red and white blood cells and have an increased protein content. Appropriate broad spectrum antibiotics should be given intravenously, and any infected site (paranasal sinus, middle ear, facial abscess) must be drained. Cerebral oedema may respond to dexamethasone 4 mg 8-hourly. The use of anticoagulants is controversial but may be helpful in limiting the spread of thrombosis early in the disorder.

FURTHER READING

Humphrey P 1994 Stroke and transient ischaemic attacks. Journal of Neurology, Neurosurgery and Psychiatry 57: 534–543

Kopitnik T A, Samson D S 1993 Management of subarachnoid haemorrhage. Journal of Neurology, Neurosurgery and Psychiatry 56: 947–959

MOVEMENT DISORDERS

This is a varied group of conditions in which there are abnormal involuntary movements, and in some cases impaired voluntary movements, without loss of muscle strength. The extrapyramidal system (p. 1024) and particularly the basal ganglia are believed to be the main sites of dysfunction although the pathophysiology is often poorly understood. The main types of disorder and their likely site of damage are listed in Table 18.47.

PARKINSONISM

In his essay on 'The Shaking Palsy', James Parkinson described the three main components of the syndrome that bears his name: tremor, muscular rigidity and hypokinesis.

Hypokinesis or bradykinesis describes slowness in initiating and repeating voluntary movements, despite normal muscular strength. These features are described in more detail below. The pathophysiological mechanism which links the various forms of parkinsonism is either defective release or impaired postsynaptic response to the neurotransmitter dopamine in the cor-

Table 18.47   Movement disorders and putative sites of causative lesions

Movement disorder		Sites of lesion
Tremor Hypokinesis Rigidity	} Parkinsonism	Substantia nigra Corpus striatum
Chorea		Caudate nucleus
Athetosis Dystonia	}	Putamen Corpus striatum
Hemiballismus		Sub-thalamic nucleus

pus striatum. The causes of parkinsonism are listed in Table 18.48.

IDIOPATHIC PARKINSONISM (PARKINSON'S DISEASE)

Parkinson's disease has an overall prevalence of about 1/1000 of the general population but it is more common in the elderly, the prevalence rising to 1% of those over 60 years.

Aetiology

The cause of the disease is unknown. Genetic factors are not important in typical cases, and there is no good evidence for a viral mechanism. The discovery that methyl-phenyl-tetrahydropyridine (MPTP) caused severe parkinsonism in drug addicts has provoked the theory that the idiopathic disease might be due to an environmental toxin. There is some evidence to suggest that parkinsonism is more common in country areas frequently sprayed with herbicides, some of which (e.g. paraquat) have chemical similarity to MPTP.

Pathology

There is depletion of pigmented neurones in substantia nigra, hyaline material (Lewy bodies) in nigral cells, atrophic changes in the substantia nigra and depletion of neurones in locus caeruleus.

Clinical features

Both sexes are affected equally. The onset of the disease is usually after the age of 50 years, the incidence increasing with advancing age. Occasionally symptoms start in the third or fourth decades. Classical features of tremor, rigidity and hypokinesis may be absent initially, when non-specific symptoms of tiredness, aching limbs, mental slowness, depression and small handwriting (micrographia) may be noticed.

Tremor

Tremor at rest, affecting one or both hands, is often the reason for referral. Tremor may also affect the legs, mouth and tongue; head tremor is rare. Tremor may remain the predominant symptom for some years.

Hypokinesis

This may develop gradually. Many patients have difficulty in initiating rapid fine movements, and slowness of gait and difficulty with tasks such as fastening buttons or writing.

PHYSICAL ABNORMALITIES IN PARKINSONISM

General
- Expressionless face
- Greasy skin
- Soft, rapid, indistinct speech
- Flexed posture

Gait
- Slow to start walking
- Shortened stride
- Rapid small steps, tendency to run (festination)
- Reduced arm swinging
- Impaired balance on turning

Tremor
Resting 4–6 Hz
- Usually first in fingers/thumb
- Coarse, complex movements, flexion/extension of fingers
- Abduction/adduction of thumb
- Supination/pronation of forearm
- May affect arms, legs, feet, jaw, tongue
- Intermittent, present at rest and when distracted
- Diminishes on action
Postural 8–10 Hz
- Less obvious, faster, finer amplitude
- Present on action or posture, persists with movement

Rigidity
Limbs
- Cogwheel type, mostly upper limbs, phasic element to stiffness in all directions of movement
- Plastic (lead pipe) type, mostly legs and trunk
Trunk
- Flexed, stooped posture

Hypokinesis
- Slowness initiating movements
- Impaired fine movements, especially of fingers
- Poor precision of repetitive movements

Rigidity of muscular tone

This causes stiffness and flexed posture. As the disease advances, speech becomes softer and indistinct; postural balance reflexes tend to decline so that falls occur.

There are a number of abnormalities on neurological examination and these are listed in the information box (above).

The features of parkinsonism may be unilateral initially, but gradually bilateral involvement is the rule. Muscle strength and reflexes remain normal; plantar responses are flexor. Facial reflexes may be enhanced despite paucity of facial expression, thus tapping the forehead causes repetitive blinking (glabellar tap sign). Eye movements may show impaired upgaze and convergence. Sensation is normal and intellectual faculties are not markedly affected although many patients

Table 18.48 Causes of parkinsonism

Mechanism	Example
Impaired release of dopamine	
Idiopathic	Parkinson's disease
Drugs depleting dopamine stores	Reserpine, tetrabenazine
Toxins damaging dopaminergic neurones	Methyl-phenyl-tetrahydropyridine
	Manganese
Viral infection	Encephalitis lethargica
	Japanese 'B' encephalitis
Trauma	Repeated head injury—'punch drunk' syndrome
Blockade of striatal dopamine receptors	Phenothiazines
	Butyrophenones
Damage to striatal neurones	Viral infection
	Multisystem atrophy
Miscellaneous	Wilson's disease
	Huntington's disease
	Cerebral tumour
	Neurosyphilis

become depressed, and some show mild cognitive impairment as the disease advances.

Investigations

Usually a diagnosis of Parkinson's disease can be made on clinical grounds; detailed investigation is not required in a typical patient. Some exceptions are listed in the information box below.

TESTS IN PARKINSONISM

- **Serological tests for syphilis**
  All patients
- **CT brain scanning**
  Patients under age 50
  Signs entirely unilateral
  Atypical clinical signs (e.g. pyramidal)
- **Tests to exclude Wilson's disease**
  Young patients (2nd to 4th decade): serum caeruloplasmin, serum copper, urine copper, and liver function

---

Management

Any identifiable cause should be treated. Drug induced parkinsonism may respond to withdrawal of the causative drug but the features may persist for many months and in some patients are permanent. It is possible that such patients have idiopathic disease that has been unmasked by the drug.

Drug therapy

- *Anticholinergic agents.* These have a useful effect on tremor and rigidity, but do not help hypokinesis. They can be prescribed early in the disease before hypokinesis is a problem, but should be avoided in patients over 65

because they cause confusion and hallucinations. Other side-effects include dry mouth, blurred vision, difficulty with micturition and constipation. Many anticholinergics are available; benzhexol (1–5 mg 8-hourly) and orphenadrine (50–100 mg 8-hourly) are in common use.

- *Amantidine.* This has a mild, usually short-lived effect on hypokinesis, but may be used early in the disease before more potent treatment is needed. It acts by potentiating the action of endogenous dopamine. A dose of 100 mg 8-hourly or 12-hourly is adequate. Side-effects include livedo reticularis and oedema due to vasodilatation, confusion and seizures.

- *Selegiline.* This is an inhibitor of monoamine oxidase type B. Its action is to reduce the rate of removal of dopamine at central synapses and thereby potentiate and prolong its action. Although used mainly as an adjunctive agent to L-dopa (see below), it has a mild therapeutic effect in its own right and may delay the need for more potent agents if used in patients with mild early disease. The usual dose is 10 mg in the morning.

- *L-dopa containing agents.* The rationale for this treatment relies on the fact that the enzyme converting the precursor DOPA to dopamine is dependent on the concentration of available substrate. Thus, although the number of dopamine-releasing terminals in the striatum is diminished in Parkinson's disease, it is possible to overdrive the remaining neurons to produce more dopamine by administering DOPA. More than 90% of orally administered L-dopa is decarboxylated peripherally in the gastrointestinal tract and blood vessels to dopamine and only a small proportion reaches the brain. This peripheral conversion is responsible for the high incidence of side-effects (nausea, vomiting, vasodilatation) encountered when L-dopa was used alone. The problem is largely overcome by giving along with the L-dopa a peripherally acting decarboxylase inhibitor. This combination therapy permits a much lower dose of L-dopa to be used and markedly reduces the incidence of side-effects. Two combination preparations are available:

L-dopa + carbidopa (4:1 and 10:1 ratios available)
L-dopa + benserazide (4:1 combination).

Each preparation is formulated in doses of 50, 100 and 250 mg of L-dopa. Initial treatment should be with the 50 mg strength 8-hourly or 12-hourly, increasing gradually over 2–4 weeks to 100 mg 8-hourly. The therapeutic effect increases gradually over the first 4–8 weeks even when the dose is held steady. Tremor, rigidity and especially hypokinesis are improved. Nausea and vomiting are uncommon and can be offset with a peripheral dopamine antagonist such as domperidone 10 mg. Dose-related side-effects are mainly involuntary movements, particularly orofacial dyskinesias, limb and axial dystonias, and occasionally depression, hallucinations and delusions. The L-dopa dose may be increased gradually up to 800–1000 mg/day, but higher doses often induce troublesome involuntary movements.

Late deterioration in response to L-dopa therapy occurs after 3–5 years in one-third to one-half of patients. Usually this manifests as fluctuations in response at different times of the day (the 'on-off' effect). In simplest form this is end of dose deterioration due to progression of the disease and loss of capacity to store dopamine. More complex fluctuations are unpredictable changes in response hour to hour with periods of hypokinesis, tremor and dystonia alternating with dyskinesia and agitation. End of dose deterioration can often be improved by dividing the L-dopa into smaller but more frequent doses (e.g. 50–100 mg every 1.5–3 hours) or by converting to a slow-release preparation. Individual doses may be potentiated and prolonged by the addition of the selective type B monoamine oxidase inhibitor selegiline, 10 mg daily. In more difficult cases the combination of low doses of a dopamine receptor agonist like bromocriptine to frequent small doses of L-dopa can be beneficial.

• *Dopamine receptor agonists.* Although a number of drugs which stimulate striatal postsynaptic dopamine receptors have been tried clinically, only bromocriptine, pergolide and lisuride are freely available. The drugs are very costly, and when used alone, less well tolerated and less impressive in controlling parkinsonism than L-dopa. Dyskinesias and fluctuations in response are less likely, but the incidence of side-effects (nausea, vomiting, mental changes) is higher. Initially 1–2.5 mg bromocriptine is given with food, and the dose increased slowly to 2.5 mg 8-hourly over the first week. Nausea can be suppressed with domperidone 10 mg with each dose if necessary. The dose can then be built up slowly over

several months to 60 mg daily or more, depending on response and tolerance. There may be a case for using bromocriptine alone or in low dose combination with L-dopa in young patients who will require treatment for many years. In a minority of patients with severe fluctuations in response, subcutaneous injections of apomorphine can be useful in providing rapid dopamine receptor stimulation.

The management of parkinsonism depends on the stage of the disease: see Table 18.49.

Surgery
Stereotactic thalamotomy is rare, because of good response to medication, but is worth considering when severe unilateral tremor fails to respond to drugs. It is too early to judge whether implantation of fetal midbrain or adrenal cells into the basal ganglia of parkinsonian patients will prove of long-term value. Pallidotomy has shown promising benefit recently, and is currently under evaluation.

Physiotherapy and speech therapy
Patients at all stages of Parkinson's disease benefit from physiotherapy which helps reduce rigidity and corrects abnormal posture. Speech therapy is indicated for more severe cases where dysarthria and dysphonia interfere with communication.

Prognosis
The outlook for patients with idiopathic parkinsonism is variable, and depends partly on the age of onset. If symptoms start in middle life, the disease is usually slowly progressive and likely to shorten life-span because of the complications of immobility and tendency to falling. Onset after the age of 70 is unlikely to shorten life or to become severe. L-dopa itself may accelerate the loss of nigral neurones, so treatment should probably be withheld until symptoms are significant and the dose kept low enough to relieve major symptoms without inducing dyskinesias.

MULTI-SYSTEM ATROPHY (SHY-DRAGER SYNDROME)

This is a relatively rare sporadic condition seen in middle-aged and elderly patients. Features of parkinsonism often without tremor are combined with varying degrees of autonomic failure, cerebellar involvement and pyramidal tract degeneration. The parkinsonism is usually of an akinetic rigid form and often accompanied by marked neck flexion. The response to L-dopa and direct dopamine agonist drugs is disappointing, probably because of degeneration of post-synaptic neurones in the basal ganglia. Autonomic features can be very

Table 18.49 Therapeutic strategy in Parkinson's disease

Stage	Features	Drugs
Early	Tremor, rigidity	Under age 65: Anticholinergics Amantidine Selegiline Over age 65: Avoid anticholinergics; Amantidine Selegiline
Moderate	Tremor, rigidity, hypokinesis	L-dopa combinations Anticholinergics In younger patients consider low dose bromocriptine + L-dopa combination
Severe	Tremor, rigidity, hypokinesis, dyskinesias, fluctuations	Frequent small doses of L-dopa combination (1.5–3 hourly) ± selegiline 10 mg/d ± low dose bromocriptine 15–30 mg/d Other dopaminergic agonists (pergolide, lisuride) Subcutaneous apomorphine

disabling with severe postural hypotension, sphincter disturbances and sometimes respiratory stridor. The severe parkinsonism is often accompanied by postural instability and frequent falls, and many patients die from the complications of progressive disability within a few years of disease onset. Management of the autonomic failure includes measures to combat postural hypotension (head-up sleeping position, compressive stockings, oral fludrocortisone).

OTHER MOVEMENT DISORDERS

Chorea

The term chorea is used to describe jerky semi-purposive movements which may affect the limbs, face or trunk. They are variable in manifestation even in the same patient at different times. The patient is not able to control them, although they may get worse with anxiety and always disappear during sleep. The causative lesion is usually in the caudate nuclei of the basal ganglia.

In adult life the most common cause of chorea is the inherited disorder Huntington's disease (see below) but other causes include drugs, particularly L-dopa and phenothiazines, viral encephalitis and acute rheumatism, metabolic disturbances, particularly hyperthyroidism, and occasionally pregnancy or oral contraceptives. Rare causes include vascular disease due to systemic lupus erythematosus and polycythaemia rubra vera. Management depends on the underlying cause but chorea may respond to dopamine receptor antagonists such as phenothiazines or butyrophenones, e.g. haloperidol 0.5–1.5 mg 8-hourly. Dopamine depleting agents such as tetrabenazine 25–50 mg 8-hourly may also

be useful, as may sodium valproate 200–1000 mg 8-hourly.

Hemiballismus

This term describes wild flailing proximal movement of the arm and leg on one side of the body. A causative lesion is usually a small area of vascular infarction in the contralateral subthalamic nucleus. The disorder is seen typically in elderly hypertensive patients. Management with either dopamine receptor antagonists or tetrabenazine as described for chorea may be helpful, but if the movements fail to respond then stereotactic thalamotomy is sometimes necessary. In typical cases, due to small vascular lesions, the abnormal movements usually cease within a few weeks of onset, although the patient may become exhausted if they are not controlled in the earlier stages.

Athetosis and dystonia

Athetosis describes slow writhing distal movements usually affecting fingers, hands, toes or feet. Dystonia describes more sustained abnormal posture usually affecting the limbs, neck or trunk. The causative lesions usually lie within the basal ganglia, particularly the putamen. Sometimes well defined causes such as kernicterus, birth injury, hypoxia encephalitis or vascular lesions may be defined. In other cases of late onset dystonia the cause may be obscure but is sometimes familial. Management is often very difficult, although some patients respond to progressively increased doses of anticholinergic agents such as benzhexol where doses building up from 6 mg to 100 mg a day may be tried. Baclofen 5–20 mg 8-hourly and benzodiazepines, e.g. diazepam 2–10 mg 8-hourly, may be tried. A minority of patients with dystonia respond to L-dopa as outlined for Parkinson's disease. If the dystonia is strictly uni-lateral then stereotactic surgery may be considered. Focal dystonias may be treated by local injections of Botulinum toxin (see Spasmodic Torticollis below).

HUNTINGTON'S DISEASE

This is an inherited disorder with autosomal dominant transmission affecting both males and females in adult life. The abnormal gene is located on chromosome 4 and has been found to be due to a base-triplet repeating sequence of variable length. Symptoms typically begin in middle adult life although occasionally juvenile onset occurs. Adult onset cases usually begin with chorea fol-lowed by progressive dementia and occasionally seiz-ures. In juvenile onset cases a parkinsonian syndrome is more common.

Investigations

Diagnosis is principally made on a positive family history and the finding of caudate nucleus atrophy on CT scan or MRI. Now that the causative gene has been defined, pre-symptomatic diagnosis is possible.

Management

Management at present is symptomatic only. The chorea may respond to tetrabenazine or dopamine antagonists as described above for chorea. Long-term psychological support and eventually institutional care is needed as dementia progresses. Genetic screening and counselling of potentially affected relatives should help reduce the incidence of the disease.

WILSON'S DISEASE (HEPATOLENTICULAR DEGENERATION)—see p. 529.

RHEUMATIC CHOREA (SYDENHAM'S CHOREA)

This disorder is seen less frequently now that strep-tococcal infections are effectively treated. It usually occurs as a sequel to streptococcal infection, frequently of the pharynx. It affects principally children and ado-lescents and is more common in females.

Clinical features

Clinically the disease is characterised by the onset of chorea, often accompanied by emotional lability. Serology demonstrates increased anti-streptolysin titres in blood.

Management

Sedation and a prescription of dopamine receptor antag-onists as for chorea (see above) are usually helpful and the underlying infection should be treated with phenoxy-methylpenicillin 250–500 mg 8-hourly. Prognosis is good and most cases recover within a few weeks, although relapses occasionally occur during pregnancy.

KERNICTERUS

This term describes damage to the basal ganglia and cerebral cortex by high levels of unconjugated bilirubin in premature infants with haemolytic disease. Early clini-cal features are convulsions, opisthotonos, rigidity and coma. If the child survives, later features are the devel-opment of athetosis, choreoathetosis, deafness, mental subnormality and spasticity. The disorder is preventable principally by the avoidance of rhesus incompatibility and by prompt exchange transfusion of severely jaun-diced neonates.

SPASMODIC TORTICOLLIS

This is a relatively common form of late onset segmental dystonia. The disorder is seen principally in middle-aged adults and there is usually no definable cause. The pathophysiology is not well understood but may involve the basal ganglia or possibly disordered vestibular input.

Clinical features

Dystonic movements involving the head turning to one side (torticollis) or extending (retrocollis) occur par-ticularly at times of stress. Aching pain in the affected muscles particularly the sternomastoid on one side is characteristic.

Management

Treatment with drugs such as anticholinergics or tetra-benazine is disappointing although benzodiazepines are occasionally effective. The treatment of choice is injec-tion of Botulinum toxin (5–20 ng) into the affected ster-nomastoid and posterior cervical muscles. The toxin binds to the motor nerve terminals and prevents acetylcholine release for several months. Side-effects are usually few but occasionally dysphagia and dysphonia occur. Surgical denervation of the affected sterno-mastoid muscle is sometimes necessary but rarely cura-tive.

TARDIVE DYSKINESIA

This term describes the onset of involuntary movements usually involving facial grimacing, chewing and tongue movements following the use of dopamine receptor drugs such as phenothiazines or butyrophenones. It is more common in elderly patients and usually begins some years after treatment has started. Management is difficult but sometimes withdrawal of the causative drug is helpful. Substituting a more selective agent (e.g. sulpiride 200–400 mg 12-hourly) or the use of tetrabenazine 25–50 mg 8-hourly may be beneficial.

TICS

This term describes repeated stereotyped brief movements usually involving the face and limbs. Occasionally vocalisation occurs (see below). The movements are to a certain extent under the control of the patient and get worse with anxiety and improve with relaxation. They are presumed to be due to a functional disorder of the basal ganglia and are more common in childhood. More complex tics accompanied by vocalisations, often with obscene utterances (coprolalia) and rude gestures (copropraxia), occur in the Gilles de la Tourette syndrome. This may start in childhood or adolescence and persist into adult life. Both types of disorder tend to respond to dopamine receptor antagonists such as sulpiride 200–400 mg 12-hourly, pimozide 1–4 mg 8-hourly or haloperidol 0.5–1.5 mg 8-hourly.

FURTHER READING

Marsden C D, Fahn S 1987 Movement disorders (1 and 2). International Medical Reviews. Butterworths, London

DEMYELINATING DISEASES

MULTIPLE SCLEROSIS

Multiple sclerosis affects 1 in 2000 of the population in Britain and is one of the commonest neurological causes of long-term disability.

Aetiology

The cause of the disease remains unknown. Epidemiological evidence suggests an environmental influence on causation: the prevalence varies in relationship to latitude with low prevalence in the tropics and high prevalence in the temperate zones of both northern and southern hemispheres. Migration before the age of 15 between areas of contrasting prevalence affects the risk of developing the disorder, and children born in Britain of immigrants from areas of low prevalence have the same risk of developing the condition as the indigenous population.

A genetic influence on susceptibility is suggested by a tenfold increase in risk in first degree relatives and the higher concordance for multiple sclerosis in monozygotic twins in comparison with dizygotic twins. HLA tissue-typing has demonstrated an increased prevalence of haplotypes A3, B7, Dw2 and DR2 in affected patients

Table 18.50   Common presentations in multiple sclerosis

Mode of onset	Frequency
Weakness or loss of control of one or more limbs	50%
Visual symptoms (including optic neuritis)	30%
Sensory symptoms	10%
Miscellaneous	10%

SYMPTOMS SUGGESTIVE OF MULTIPLE SCLEROSIS

- Optic neuritis
- Tingling in spine or limbs on neck flexion (Lhermitte's phenomenon)
- Exacerbation of symptoms by exercise or rise in body temperature
- Trigeminal neuralgia under the age of 50
- Recurrent facial palsy

in Britain, but different haplotypes have been associated with an increased risk for multiple sclerosis in other countries. An immune mechanism is suggested by increased levels of activated T lymphocytes in the CSF, and increased immunoglobulin synthesis within the central nervous system. There are increased levels of antibody to some viruses, including measles virus, in the CSF but this may be an epiphenomenon.

The relative importance of environmental, genetic and immunological factors is unresolved: multiple sclerosis is likely to be multifactorial in origin.

Pathology

The acute lesion is the plaque, a circumscribed area of demyelination with swelling of axis cylinders and patchy infiltration of inflammatory cells. Gliosis follows and the chronic lesion is a scar with a shrunken greyish appearance, most commonly occurring in the periventricular region, the optic nerves and the subpial regions of the spinal cord.

Clinical features

Characteristically the clinical course involves relapsing and remitting neurological dysfunction, mainly affecting the optic nerves, brain stem, cerebellum and spinal cord. The first manifestation may occur at any age, but onset before puberty or after the age of 60 is rare. There is no typical clinical history, but some types of presentation are more frequent and suggestive symptoms may develop in the course of the illness (see Table 18.50 and the information box above).

The symptoms and signs of the first attack usually recover within 1–3 months and after a variable interval there may be a recurrence, in many cases within 2 years.

Frequent relapses with incomplete recovery indicate a poor prognosis and in many patients a phase of progressive deterioration supersedes the phase of relapse and remission. In a minority of patients there may be an interval of years or even decades between attacks and in some, particularly if optic neuritis is the initial manifestation, there is no recurrence. In the middle-aged, multiple sclerosis may present with a spastic paraparesis, which may be only slowly progressive.

The physical signs depend on the localisation of areas of demyelination, and reflect the common pathological sites of plaques, with some physical signs occurring frequently and others rarely. Common physical signs are listed in the information box. No sign is specific to multiple sclerosis and diagnosis depends on the identification of combinations of signs, for example optic atrophy and paraparesis, or mixed cerebellar and pyramidal signs in the limbs. Sensory signs are almost invariable at some time in the course of the disease, but are usually less prominent than sensory symptoms. Some patients become euphoric and, although significant intellectual impairment is unusual, mild impairment of memory is common.

COMMON PHYSICAL SIGNS IN MULTIPLE SCLEROSIS

- Upper motor neurone signs
- Optic atrophy, afferent pupillary defect, impaired colour vision, internuclear ophthalmoplegia
- Nystagmus, dysarthria, ataxia
- Peripheral impairment of position sense and vibration sensation

---

INVESTIGATIONS IN MULTIPLE SCLEROSIS

- **Evoked potentials**
  Visual
  Auditory
  Somatosensory
- **CSF examination**
  Cell count
  Immunoglobulin content
  Protein electrophoresis
  (oligoclonal bands)
- **Myelogram**
- **CT/MRI scan**

Table 18.51   Treatment of complications of multiple sclerosis

Complication	Treatment
Spasticity	Baclofen 15–100 mg*
	Diazepam 2–15 mg*
	Dantrolene 25–400 mg*
	Chemical neuronectomy
	Physiotherapy
Ataxia	Isoniazid 600–1200 mg*
	Clonazepam 2–8 mg*
Dysaesthesia	Carbamazepine 200–1800 mg*
	Phenytoin 200–400 mg daily
	Tricyclic antidepressant
Urinary symptoms	Propantheline 30–90 mg*
Failure to store urine	Oxybutynin 10–20 mg*
	Imipramine 25 mg 8-hourly
Failure to empty bladder	Bethanecol 30–120 mg*
	Baclofen 15–100 mg*
	Intermittent self-catheterisation

* In divided dosage.

Investigations

The diagnosis of multiple sclerosis depends clinically on the demonstration of lesions occurring at different times and at different sites in the central nervous system. Investigation is aimed at providing evidence for an inflammatory disorder and for multiple sites of neurological involvement (see the information box).

There is no specific test for multiple sclerosis and, although abnormalities may be revealed by any of these investigations, interpretation depends on the rest of the clinical picture. Visual evoked potentials can detect clinically silent lesions in up to 70% of patients, but auditory and somatosensory evoked potentials are less frequently of diagnostic value. The CSF may show a lymphocytic pleocytosis in the acute phase and persistent elevation of gammaglobulin or oligoclonal bands of IgG in 70–90% of patients between attacks. CT scan may show plaques, but MRI scan is the most sensitive technique for imaging lesions in multiple sclerosis and is positive in over 95% of definite cases (Fig. 18.39). Oligoclonal bands occur in a range of other disorders, and the MRI appearances in multiple sclerosis cannot be distinguished from those of cerebrovascular disease or cerebral vasculitis. Diagnosis depends on the clinical history and examination, taken in combination with the investigative findings.

It is important to exclude potentially curable conditions such as syphilis, vitamin B_{12} deficiency and spinal cord compression.

Management

There is no curative treatment but much can be done to support the patient during the course of the illness. Management is aimed at specific therapy for the underlying condition and symptomatic treatment of complications.

Corticosteroids may promote more rapid and complete recovery in acute exacerbations. Drug regimes

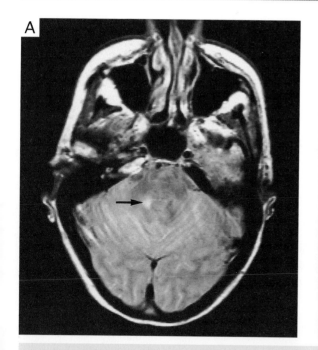 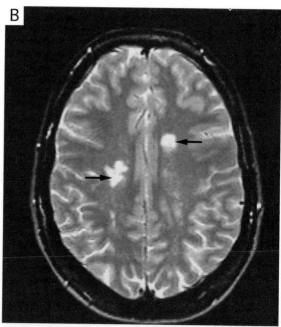

Fig. 18.39 MRI scan in multiple sclerosis. T2 weighted images showing areas of high signal in Ⓐ brain stem and Ⓑ deep cerebral white matter (arrow).

include oral dexamethasone 2 mg three times daily for 10 days or a course of oral prednisolone reducing in dosage over 2–3 weeks starting with an initial dosage of 30 mg daily. Intravenous methylprednisolone 500 mg daily for 5 days or 1 g daily for 3 days has been increasingly used in recent years for more severe relapses. Prolonged administration of steroids does not alter the long-term prognosis and immunosuppressive agents including azathioprine are of little benefit. Recent research suggests that beta interferon may significantly reduce the frequency of relapses in multiple sclerosis but, as with other therapies including cyclosporin, more evidence is needed before beta interferon can be regarded as an established treatment. Gluten-free diet, linoleic acid supplements or hyperbaric oxygen therapy are not of benefit.

The treatment of complications of multiple sclerosis is summarised in Table 18.51.

Of prime importance is the encouragement and support of patients and their relatives. A frank discussion of the diagnosis and prognosis is necessary and may dispel fears, which are often ill-founded. Periods of physiotherapy may improve functional capacity in those patients who become disabled and assessment by the occupational therapist will provide guidance in the provision of aids within the home and to improve mobility. The social worker can advise patients on financial allowances for the disabled and the provision of social services support.

The care of the bladder is particularly important. Infections should be treated with an appropriate antibiotic. Incontinence, urgency and frequency may be treated pharmacologically, by external drainage or by urinary catheter, which may be passed intermittently by the patient rather than left permanently indwelling. The choice of treatment is difficult to make clinically and urodynamic assessment may be necessary in patients with troublesome symptoms. Sexual dysfunction is a source of anxiety in many patients and may be relieved by skilled counselling.

Prognosis

The outlook cannot be predicted with confidence in any individual patient and, although approximately 5% of patients die within 5 years of onset, a rather larger proportion remain well and retain unlimited mobility for 20 years.

FURTHER READING

Compston D A S 1990 Risk factors for multiple sclerosis: race or place. Journal of Neurology, Neurosurgery and Psychiatry 53: 821–823
Compston D A S 1990 The dissemination of multiple sclerosis. Journal of the Royal College of Physicians of London 24: 207

INFECTIONS OF THE NERVOUS SYSTEM

The major infections of the nervous system are listed in the information box.

VIRAL INFECTIONS

VIRAL MENINGITIS

Viral infection is the commonest cause of meningitis, and usually results in a benign and self-limiting illness requiring no specific therapy. Viral (aseptic) meningitis is usually a much less serious illness than bacterial meningitis unless there is associated encephalitis, which is rare. The majority of patients suffering from this condition have a transient self-limiting illness and never reach medical attention. A number of viruses can cause meningitis, the commonest being echoviruses and the mumps virus. Causes of meningitis and encephalitis are listed in the information box above.

Clinical features

Viral meningitis usually occurs in isolation without clinical evidence of parenchymal involvement of the nervous system. Causative organisms include arena, echo, and coxsackie viruses, but in the majority of patients no specific virus is isolated. The condition occurs mainly in children or young adults, with the acute onset of headache and irritability and the rapid development of meningeal irritation. There may be a high pyrexia, but focal neurological signs are uncommon.

Meningeal irritation ('meningism') may occur in bacterial, viral, and fungal infections and in a range of non-infectious conditions including subarachnoid haemorrhage, malignant disease, and connective tissue disorders such as sarcoidosis and systemic lupus erythematosus. Careful interpretation of CSF indices is essential to accurate diagnosis (Table 18.52).

Investigations

The CSF contains an excess of lymphocytes, but normal glucose and protein levels.

Management

There is no specific treatment and the condition is usually benign and self-limiting. The patient should be treated symptomatically in a quiet environment. Recovery usually occurs within days, although a lymphocytic pleocytosis may persist in the CSF.

Meningitis may also occur as a complication of a viral

Table 18.52   Cerebrospinal fluid indices in meningitis

Condition	Cell type	Cell count	Glucose	Protein	Gram stain
Viral	Lymphocytes	10–2000	normal	normal	−
Bacterial	Polymorphs	1000–50 000	low	normal/elevated	+
Tuberculous	Polym/Lymph/mixed	50–5000	low	elevated	often −
Fungal	Lymphocytes	50–500	low	elevated	±
Malignant	Lymphocytes	0–100	low	normal/elevated	−

Table 18.53   Viruses causing encephalitis transmitted by mosquitoes and ticks

Infection	Vector	Endemic in
Yellow fever	Mosquito	Africa and South America
Japanese encephalitis		South-East Asia
Ross river fever		Australia
California encephalitis		North America
Omsk haemorrhagic fever	Tick	Russia
Louping-ill		North Britain

infection primarily involving other organs; for example in mumps, measles, infectious mononucleosis, herpes zoster and hepatitis. Complete recovery is the rule without specific therapy.

VIRAL ENCEPHALITIS

A range of viruses cause encephalitis but there is no recognisable combination of symptoms and signs specific to virus type. Only a minority of patients have a history of recent viral infection and viral isolation is often unrewarding. The development of effective therapy for some forms of encephalitis therefore enhances the importance of clinical diagnosis. The viruses which are transmitted by mosquitoes and ticks are shown in Table 18.53.

Pathology

Inflammation can occur in the cortex, white matter, basal ganglia and brain stem and the distribution of lesions varies with the type of virus. Inclusion bodies are often present in the neurones and glial cells and there is an infiltration of polymorphonuclear cells in the perivascular space. There is neuronal degeneration and diffuse glial proliferation, often associated with cerebral oedema.

Clinical features

Viral encephalitis presents with acute onset of headache, often accompanied by fever. Disturbance of consciousness ranging from drowsiness to deep coma supervenes early and may advance dramatically. Meningism

occurs in 75% of patients and there may be a variety of focal signs such as aphasia, hemiplegia, tetraplegia, or cranial nerve palsies. Epilepsy and raised intracranial pressure commonly develop as the condition progresses. Rabies presents a distinct clinical picture and is described on page 1091.

Acute encephalitic illness may occur in HIV infection, occasionally at the time of infection, but more commonly as a manifestation of AIDS.

Encephalitis lethargica occurred in epidemic form in the 1920s and was presumed to be of viral aetiology although this has never been established. Parkinsonism may be a late sequel of this disease.

In *herpes encephalitis* signs of temporal lobe dysfunction may be detected and confusional states, which may be misdiagnosed as a psychosis, develop.

Investigations

The differential diagnosis of viral encephalitis is summarised in the information box below.

DIFFERENTIAL DIAGNOSIS OF VIRAL ENCEPHALITIS

- Acute metabolic encephalopathy
- Cerebral tumour
- Stroke
- Bacterial meningitis/abscess
- Tuberculous meningitis

Approximately half of all patients suspected on admission as suffering from viral encephalitis have other diseases. The investigations listed in the information box below are indicated in suspected viral encephalitis.

INVESTIGATIONS IN VIRAL ENCEPHALITIS

- Full blood count
- Biochemical screen
- Viral studies
- CT scan (MRI scan)
- CSF examination
- Electroencephalogram

CSF examination may be hazardous and should be preceded by a CT scan, which will exclude a structural lesion and may provide evidence of reactive oedema. The cerebrospinal fluid usually contains excess lymphocytes, but polymorphonuclear cells may predominate in the early stages and occasionally the fluid is normal. The protein content may be elevated, but the glucose is normal. The electroencephalogram is usually abnormal with diffuse slow-wave activity, but is nonspecific unless there are periodic discharges to suggest herpes simplex encephalitis. Serological tests and culture may identify the causative virus, but are usually available too late to influence treatment.

Management

Patients suffering from viral encephalitis require skilled nursing care and careful monitoring of fluid balance and nutritional state. Anticonvulsant treatment is often necessary (p. 1068) and raised intracranial pressure is treated with dexamethasone 4 mg 6-hourly. Herpes simplex virus encephalitis may respond to acyclovir 10 mg/kg intravenously 3 times daily. This medication is relatively safe and should be given to all patients suspected of suffering from viral encephalitis as specific diagnosis is often impossible.

Even with optimum treatment mortality is 10–30% and a significant proportion of survivors have residual epilepsy or cognitive impairment.

BRAIN-STEM ENCEPHALITIS

This presents with dysarthria, diplopia or cranial nerve palsies. The CSF is lymphocytic with a normal glucose. The causative agent is presumed to be viral, although listeria meningitis may cause a similar syndrome and requires specific treatment with ampicillin 500 mg 6-hourly.

POLIOMYELITIS

Aetiology and pathology

The disease is caused by one of three related polio viruses which comprise a subdivision of the group of enteroviruses. It is much less common following the widespread use of oral vaccines but is still a major problem in developing countries. Infection usually occurs through the nasopharynx.

The virus is liable to affect the grey matter of the spinal cord, brain stem and cortex and has a particular propensity to damage anterior horn cells especially those within the lumbar segments. There is often accompanying infiltration of the meninges with lymphocytes.

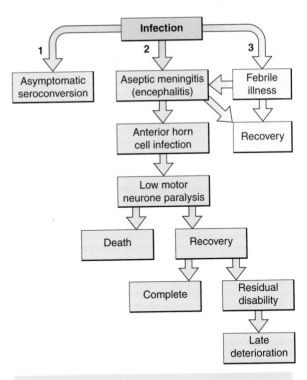

Fig. 18.40 Poliomyelitis—possible consequence of infection.

Clinical features

Figure 18.40 illustrates the various features of the infection. The incubation period is 7–14 days. At the onset there is usually mild fever and headache which improves after a few days. Many patients do not progress beyond this stage. In other instances, after a period of well-being lasting approximately a week, there is recurrence of pyrexia and headache accompanied by neck stiffness and signs of meningeal irritation. Paralysis may occur later and is of variable extent. Weakness of one muscle group may progress to widespread paresis. Respiratory failure may supervene if intercostal muscles are paralysed or the medullary motor nuclei are involved.

Investigations

The CSF shows a lymphocytic pleocytosis, a rise in protein and a normal sugar content. Poliomyelitis virus may be cultured from CSF and stool.

Management

In the early stages bed rest is imperative. At the onset of respiratory difficulties a tracheostomy and intermittent positive pressure ventilation are required. Subsequent treatment is by physiotherapy and orthopaedic measures.

Prognosis

Epidemics vary widely in their incidence of abortive and non-paralytic cases and in mortality rate. Death occurs from respiratory paralysis. Muscle weakness is maximal at the end of the first week and gradual recovery may then take place for several months. Any muscle showing no signs of recovery by the end of a month will not regain useful function. It is difficult to make a more definitive prediction about the extent of permanent disability until 3–6 months after the onset. Second attacks are very rare but occasional patients show late deterioration in muscle bulk and power many years after the initial infection.

Prevention

This is by immunisation.

HERPES ZOSTER (SHINGLES)

Herpes zoster is the result of reactivation of the varicella/zoster virus which has lain dormant in a posterior nerve root ganglion following chickenpox earlier in life. Reactivation may be apparently spontaneous (as usually occurs in the middle-aged or elderly) or be due to immunosuppression as in patients with malignant disease or AIDS. Chickenpox may be contracted from a patient with shingles but the reverse does not occur.

Clinical features

The first symptom is usually severe continuous pain in the distribution of the affected nerve root. After 3 or 4 days the skin in the affected area becomes reddened and vesicles appear which dry up over 5 or 6 days leaving small scars. The pain of zoster usually subsides as the eruption fades, but occasionally, especially in old people, it may be followed by a persistent and intractable neuralgia.

Any dorsal root ganglion may be infected, most commonly those supplying the trunk where two or three adjacent dermatomes on one side only are often involved. Infection of the trigeminal ganglion usually involves the ophthalmic division; the vesicles appear on the cornea and may lead to corneal ulceration with the danger of scarring and impairment of vision (ophthalmic herpes).

Segmental muscle wasting may occur sometimes from involvement of the motor root. The virus occasionally invades the spinal cord or the brain giving rise to myelitis or encephalitis.

Management

Idoxuridine may be applied to the skin in a 5% solution in the early stages of the evolution of the rash; 0.1% drops are used for corneal infections. Oral acyclovir 800 mg 5 times daily is useful if started early and sys-

Table 18.54 Sources of infection in rabies		
Area	**Source**	**Transmission**
World-wide	Dogs, other canines, cats	Bite, lick
	Cattle, etc. (to farmers)	Hand into mouth
	Other mammals	Bite, lick
	Man (undiagnosed)	Corneal graft
North America	Skunks and raccoons	Bite, lick
Central and South America	Vampire bats	Bite
	Cave-dwelling bats	Salivary aerosols

temic acyclovir in a dose of 5 mg/kg 8-hourly is indicated for immunocompromised patients or when infection is severe. The treatment of post-herpetic neuralgia is difficult. Analgesics are often unhelpful, but amitriptyline 25–100 mg daily and transcutaneous nerve stimulation are sometimes effective.

Ramsay–Hunt syndrome

Herpes zoster infection of the geniculate ganglion presents with vesicles in the auricle and less often on the palate. The facial nerve is usually involved, leading to ipsilateral facial paralysis and impairment of taste. Oral acyclovir 800 mg 5 times daily may be of benefit if started early.

RABIES

Rabies is caused by a rhabdovirus which infects the central nervous tissue and salivary glands of a wide range of mammals, and is usually conveyed by saliva through bites or licks on abrasions or on intact mucous membranes. Man is most frequently infected from dogs. In Europe the maintenance host is the fox and in recent years the zoonosis has spread from Poland westwards through Germany and France (Table 18.54).

The incubation period, during which the virus is spreading centripetally along axons to the brain, varies in man from a minimum of 9 days to many months but is usually between 4 and 8 weeks. Severe bites, especially if on the head or neck, are associated with short incubation periods.

Clinical features

Only a proportion of people bitten by a rabid animal develop the disease, but once manifest it is almost invariably fatal. At the onset there may be fever, and paraesthesia at the site of the bite. A prodromal period of from 1 to 10 days, during which the patient is increasingly anxious, leads to the characteristic fear of water, 'hydrophobia'. Although the patient is thirsty, attempts at drinking provoke violent contractions of the diaphragm and other inspiratory muscles and thereafter, even the sight or sound of water may precipitate distressing spasms and attacks of panic. Delusions and hallucination may develop accompanied by spitting, biting and mania, with lucid intervals in which the patient is acutely anxious. Cranial nerve lesions develop and terminal hyperpyrexia is common. Death ensues, within a week of the onset of symptoms.

In a small proportion of cases there is an ascending paralysis without mental excitement and these patients survive on average 12 days.

Investigations
During life the diagnosis is usually made on clinical grounds but rapid immunofluorescent techniques can detect antigen in corneal impression smears or skin biopsies.

Management
A few patients with rabies have survived. All received some post-exposure prophylaxis, and needed intensive care with facilities to control cardiac and respiratory failure. Otherwise, only palliative treatment is possible once symptoms have appeared. The patient should be heavily sedated with diazepam 10 mg 4–6 hourly, supplemented by chlorpromazine 50–100 mg if necessary. Nutrition and fluids should be given intravenously or through a gastrostomy.

Prevention
Pre-exposure prophylaxis is required by those who by profession handle potentially infected animals, those who work with rabies virus in laboratories and those who live at special risk in rabies endemic areas. Protection is afforded by two intradermal injections of 0.1 ml human diploid cell strain vaccine, or two intramuscular injections of 1 ml, given 4 weeks apart, followed by yearly boosters.

Post-exposure prophylaxis
The wounds should be thoroughly cleaned, preferably with a quaternary ammonium detergent or soap; damaged tissues should be excised and the wound left unsutured. Rabies can usually be prevented if treatment is started within a day or two of biting. Delayed treatment may still be of value. For maximum protection hyperimmune serum and vaccine are required.

The safest antirabies antiserum is human rabies immune globulin; the dose is 20 i.u./kg body weight. Half is infiltrated around the bite and half is given intramuscularly at a different site from the vaccine. The dose of hyperimmune animal serum is 40 i.u./kg; hypersensitivity reactions, including anaphylaxis, are common.

The safest vaccine, free of complications, is human diploid cell strain vaccine; 1.0 ml is given intramuscularly on days 0, 3, 7, 14, 30 and 90. In developing countries, where human rabies globulin may not be obtainable, 0.1 ml of vaccine should be given intradermally into 8 sites on day 1, with single boosters on days 7 and 28. Where human products are not available and when risk of rabies is slight (licks on the skin, or minor bites of covered arms or legs) it may be justifiable to delay starting treatment up to 5 days while observing the biting animal or awaiting examination of its brain rather than use the older vaccine.

The biting animal should be confined, if possible. If it is healthy after 5 days, it does not have rabies and treatment is stopped. If it dies, or is killed, the brain is examined by immunofluorescence for Negri bodies. If positive, treatment is continued.

Control of spread
Human rabies is an infrequent disease even in endemic areas. Its fearful manifestations, however, justify stringent attempts being made to limit its spread and prevent its importation into uninfected countries such as Britain. Measures to control rabies are listed in the information box below.

CONTROL OF RABIES

- License and vaccinate domestic dogs
- Kill stray dogs
- Monitor reservoir hosts
- Control and quarantine imported animals
- Vaccinate at-risk animals and man

JAPANESE ENCEPHALITIS

This arbovirus is transmitted to man by the bites of infected culicine mosquitoes which have fed on infected animals or birds, notably nestling herons. Pigs and other domestic animals are important sources of infection, acting chiefly as amplifiers of the virus brought to them by mosquitoes. The virus is widespread in the Pacific Islands from Japan to Guam in the Philippines, Taiwan, Borneo, Malaysia and Singapore and is spreading slowly west across the Indian subcontinent. Devastating epidemics, with a high mortality rate, have occurred. In endemic areas, serological surveys indicate a high incidence of subclinical infection and only sporadic cases may be encountered. Inflammatory and degenerative changes are found in the brain.

Clinical features
Many infections are subclinical. Overt disease may occur at any age, although children are particularly susceptible.

Typical clinical features of encephalitis (p. 1089) develop quickly and last from a few days to 2 weeks or longer and convalescence is prolonged. The CSF is under raised pressure and an increase of cells and protein appears within several days. Persistent neurological damage is common. The mortality in overt disease varies from 15 to 40%.

Investigations
The virus has only rarely been recovered from the blood or CSF but in fatal cases may sometimes be obtained from the brain. A rise in antibody titre is the usual basis for diagnosis.

Management
There is no specific treatment. Skilled nursing for the patient in coma may be life-saving.

Prevention
The elimination of breeding places of the vector mosquitoes, the control of piggeries, and the use of insecticides, where practicable, should be instituted. A vaccine, made in Japan and available in Britain, is safe and effective.

SUBACUTE SCLEROSING PANENCEPHALITIS

This is a rare, chronic, progressive and eventually fatal neurological disease caused by the measles virus, presumably as a result of an inability of the nervous system to eradicate the virus. It occurs in children and adolescents, usually many years after the primary virus infection. The onset is insidious with intellectual deterioration, apathy and clumsiness followed by myoclonic jerks, rigidity and dementia.

The CSF may show a mild lymphocytic pleocytosis and the electroencephalogram is distinctive with periodic bursts of triphasic waves. Although there is persistent measles specific IgG in serum and CSF, antiviral therapy is ineffective and death ensues within years.

PROGRESSIVE MULTIFOCAL LEUCO-ENCEPHALOPATHY

This is a rare condition which usually occurs as a complication of reticulosis, leukaemia, or carcinomatosis, but may also develop in previously fit individuals. A papovavirus, SV40, has been identified as the causative organism and pathologically there is widespread demyelination of the white matter within the cerebral hemispheres. CT scan shows areas of low density in the white matter and associated clinical signs include dementia, hemiparesis and dysphasia which progress rapidly, leading to death within weeks or months.

SLOW VIRUS INFECTIONS

A number of neurological diseases develop many months or even years after infection with transmissible agents which have properties distinct from conventional viruses.

KURU

This is a disease which occurs only in the members of a cannibalistic New Guinea tribe and is probably transmitted by eating the brains of dead tribal members. There is degeneration of grey matter, most marked in the cerebellum, causing a progressive ataxia.

CREUTZFELDT–JAKOB DISEASE

The typical features are rapidly progressive dementia, myoclonus and a characteristic EEG pattern. Creutzfeldt–Jakob disease is transmissible in the laboratory to chimpanzees and rarely from person to person, for example by human growth hormone, but the nature of the transmissible agent remains uncertain.

POST-VIRAL SYNDROMES

ACUTE DEMYELINATING ENCEPHALOMYELITIS

This occurs about a week after diseases such as measles and chickenpox or following vaccination, and is probably immunologically mediated. There are areas of perivenous demyelination widely disseminated throughout the brain and spinal cord.

Headache, vomiting, pyrexia, confusion and meningism are presenting features and fits or coma may develop. Flaccid paralysis and extensor plantar responses are common and cerebellar signs may be present, particularly when the disorder follows chickenpox. The CSF may be normal or show a small increase in mononuclear cells and protein.

POST-INFECTIVE POLYNEURITIS

This condition, commonly referred to as the Guillain–Barré syndrome, may rarely develop during or immediately after a virus infection, usually of the upper respiratory tract. (See pp. 1106–1107.)

Table 18.55   Bacterial meningitis

	Common	Less common
Neonate	Gram-negative bacilli (*E. coli*, Proteus, etc.) Group B streptococci	*Listeria monocytogenes*
Pre-school child	*Haemophilus influenzae* *Neisseria meningitidis* *Streptococcus pneumoniae*	*Mycobacterium tuberculosis*
Older child and adult	*Neisseria meningitidis* *Streptococcus pneumoniae*	*Listeria monocytogenes* *Mycobacterium tuberculosis* *Cryptococcus neoformans* (in immunosuppressed) *Staphylococcus aureus* (skull fracture) *Haemophilus influenzae*

MYALGIC ENCEPHALOMYELITIS (ME)

This is also known as the post-viral syndrome or chronic fatigue syndrome. Enteroviruses have been postulated as a possible cause. The syndrome not infrequently occurs following infectious mononucleosis. It is most commonly seen in teenagers and young adults, especially those with more demanding occupations or preparing for examinations.

ME is an ill-defined condition with a range of symptoms including malaise, fatigue, myalgia, headache and exhaustion. There are no abnormal physical signs and no specific test for the syndrome but serum antibodies to coxsackie-B or Epstein–Barr viruses may be present. Although a proportion of affected individuals respond to antidepressant medication, many patients become chronically disabled and all that can be offered currently is sympathy and moral support.

BACTERIAL INFECTIONS

BACTERIAL MENINGITIS

Bacterial meningitis is usually secondary to a bacteraemic illness although infection may result from direct spread from an adjacent focus of infection in the ear, skull fracture or sinus. Any bacterium can cause meningitis but some are more frequent causes than others (Table 18.55). Bacterial meningitis has become less common but the mortality and morbidity remain high despite the availability of an increasing range of antibiotics. An important factor in determining prognosis is early diagnosis and the prompt initiation of appropriate therapy.

Pathology

The pia-arachnoid is congested and infiltrated with inflammatory cells. A thin layer of pus forms and this may later organise to form adhesions. These may cause obstruction to the free flow of CSF leading to hydrocephalus, or may damage the cranial nerves at the base of the brain. The CSF pressure rises rapidly, the protein content increases and there is cellular reaction which varies in type and severity according to the nature of the inflammation and the causative organism. Pneumococcal meningitis is often associated with a very purulent CSF and a high mortality especially in older adults.

Clinical features

Headache, drowsiness, fever and neck stiffness are the usual presenting features of bacterial meningitis. Neck stiffness can be elicited by passive flexion of the neck which is resisted as a result of muscle spasm. In severe bacterial meningitis the patient is usually comatose and there may be focal neurological signs. In pneumococcal and haemophilus infections there may be otitis media. Pneumococcal meningitis is often associated with pneumonia, especially in older patients and alcoholics. It is common in patients without functioning spleens.

Neisseria meningitidis

The meningococcus is the commonest cause of bacterial meningitis in Britain where an increasing proportion of meningococci have become sulphonamide-resistant; fortunately, all strains remain sensitive to penicillin. Spread is by air-borne route and epidemics occur, particularly in cramped living conditions or when the climate is hot and dry, e.g. areas of Africa. The organism invades through the nasopharynx producing septicaemia which is usually associated with pyogenic meningitis. Complications of meningococcal septicaemia are listed in the information box below.

Chronic meningococcaemia is a rare condition in which the patient can be unwell for weeks or even months with recurrent fever, sweating, joint pains and transient rash. It usually occurs in the middle-aged and elderly.

Table 18.56   Chemotherapy of bacterial meningitis

	Drug of choice	Alternative agents
Meningococcal	Benzylpenicillin	Chloramphenicol Cefotaxime
Pneumococcal	Cefotaxime*	Chloramphenicol
H. influenzae	Cefotaxime	Chloramphenicol
Neonatal Gram-negative bacilli Group B streptococci	Cefotaxime Gentamicin + ampicillin	Gentamicin + ampicillin Chloramphenicol
L. monocytogenes	Gentamicin + ampicillin	Co-trimoxazole Rifampicin
C. neoformans	Amphotericin + flucytosine	Fluconazole
M. tuberculosis	see p. 361	

* Penicillin-resistant pneumococci now common worldwide.

Listeria monocytogenes

This has recently emerged as an increasing cause of meningitis in the immunosuppressed, diabetics, alcoholics and pregnant women. It can also cause meningitis in the neonatal period.

Investigations

In bacterial meningitis the CSF is cloudy (turbid) due to the presence of many neutrophils (often more than 1000 cells/mm³), the protein content is significantly elevated and the glucose reduced. Gram film may reveal the identity of the causative organism but this is by no means always so even after the results of culture are available. Blood cultures may be positive.

Management

The choice of antibiotic depends on the infecting organism. Tables 18.56 and 18.57 give guidance as to the preferred antibiotic:

1. if the organism has not been identified
2. if the organism is known.

The dose of the various antibiotics which must be given intravenously depends on the age and weight of the patient.

Prevention of meningococcal infection

Household and other close contacts of patients with meningococcal infections, especially children, should be given 2 days of rifampicin. The dose for adults is 600 mg twice a day. A single dose of 500 mg of ciprofloxacin is an alternative. Children under 1 year are given 5 mg/kg 12-hourly and those over 12 months 10 mg/kg 12-hourly. Vaccines are available for the prevention of disease caused by meningococci of Groups A and C, but not Group B which is the commonest serogroup isolated in many countries including Britain.

TUBERCULOUS MENINGITIS

Pathology

The condition occurs most commonly shortly after a primary infection in childhood or as part of miliary tuberculosis. The usual local source of infection is a caseous focus in the meninges or brain substance adjacent to the CSF pathway.

The brain is covered by a greenish, gelatinous exudate especially around the base, and numerous scattered tubercles are found on the meninges.

Clinical features

The clinical features are listed in the information box below.

Table 18.57   Treatment of pyogenic meningitis. Cause unknown

Neonate
Gentamicin + ampicillin
or
Third generation cephalosporin (e.g. Cefotaxime)

Pre-school child
Cefotaxime

Older child and adult
Cefotaxime

CLINICAL FEATURES OF TUBERCULOUS MENINGITIS

Children	**Adults**
- Lassitude	- Malaise
- Loss of interest in toys	- Headache
- Unwillingness to talk	- Vomiting
- Anorexia	- Low-grade fever
- Constipation	
- Headache	

Investigation

The CSF is under increased pressure. It is usually clear but, when allowed to stand, a fine clot ('spider web') may form. The fluid contains up to 400 cells/mm^3, predominantly lymphocytes. There is a rise in protein and a marked fall in glucose. Detection of the tubercle bacillus in a smear of the centrifuged deposit from the CSF may be difficult. The CSF should be cultured on appropriate media but as the result will not be known for up to 6 weeks, treatment must be started without waiting for confirmation.

Management

Chemotherapy should be started as soon as the diagnosis is made using one of the regimens including pyrazinamide described on page 362. All patients should also receive prednisolone, 10 mg 6-hourly. Surgical methods for ensuring ventricular drainage must be adopted if obstructive hydrocephalus develops. Skilled nursing is essential during the acute state of the illness and measures must be taken to maintain adequate hydration and nutrition.

The intensive regime of drug treatment should be continued for 8 weeks and followed by a continuation phase.

Prognosis

Untreated tuberculous meningitis is fatal in a few weeks but complete recovery is the rule with modern treatment if it is started before the appearance of focal signs or stupor. When treatment is started at a later stage the recovery rate is 60% or less and the survivors may be mentally deficient, epileptic, deaf, blind or show some other permanent neurological deficit.

TETANUS

This disease results from infection with *Clostridium tetani*, which exists as a commensal in the gut of man and domestic animals and is found in the soil. Infection enters the body through wounds, often trivial, such as those caused by a splinter, a nail in the boot or a garden fork or following septic infection such as a dirty abrasion. Tetanus is rare in Britain and occurs mostly in gardeners and farmers. By contrast the disease is common in many developing countries where dust contains spores derived from animal and human excreta. If childbirth takes place in an unhygienic environment *Tetanus neonatorum* may result from infection of the umbilical stump or the mother may develop the disease.

In circumstances unfavourable to the growth of the organism, spores are formed and these may remain dormant for years in the soil. Spores germinate and bacilli multiply only in the anaerobic conditions which occur in areas of tissue necrosis or if the oxygen tension is low as a result of the presence of other organisms, particularly aerobic ones. The bacilli remain localised but produce an exotoxin with an affinity for motor nerve endings and motor nerve cells. The anterior horn cells are affected after the exotoxin has passed into the blood stream and their involvement results in rigidity and convulsions. Symptoms first appear from 2 days to several weeks after injury—the shorter the incubation period, the more severe the attacks and the outcome may well be fatal with an incubation period of only a few days.

Clinical features

Much the most important early symptom is trismus—spasm of the masseter muscles which causes difficulty in opening the mouth and in masticating, hence the name 'lock-jaw'. This tonic rigidity spreads to involve the muscles of the face, neck and trunk. Contraction of the frontalis and the muscles at the angles of the mouth gives rise to the 'risus sardonicus'. There is rigidity of the muscles at the neck and trunk of varying degree. The back is usually slightly arched and there is a board-like abdominal wall.

In the more severe cases violent spasms lasting for a few seconds to 3 to 4 minutes occur spontaneously, or may be induced by stimuli such as moving the patient or making a noise. These convulsions are painful, exhausting and of very serious significance especially if they appear soon after the onset of symptoms. They gradually increasē in frequency and severity for about 1 week and the patient may die from exhaustion, asphyxia or aspiration pneumonia. In less severe illness convulsions may not commence for about a week after the first sign of rigidity and in very mild infections they may never appear. Autonomic involvement may cause cardiovascular complications such as hypertension.

Rarely the only manifestation of the disease may be 'local tetanus'—stiffness or spasm of the muscles near the infected wound—and the prognosis is good if treatment is commenced at this stage.

Investigations

The diagnosis is made on clinical grounds. It is rarely possible to isolate the infecting organism from the original locus of entry. Spasm of the masseters due to dental abscess, septic throat or other causes is painful, in contradistinction to tetanus. Conditions which can mimic tetanus include hysteria and phenothiazine overdosage.

Tetanus is still one of the major killers of adults, children and neonates in the tropics where the mortality rate can be nearly 100% in the newborn and around 40% in others.

Management

This should be begun as soon as possible. The essentials are shown in the information box.

TREATMENT OF TETANUS

- **Neutralise absorbed toxin**
  i.v. injection of 3000 IU of antitoxin
- **Prevent further toxin production**
  Debridement of wound
  Benzylpenicillin 600 mg 6-hrly i.v.
  (metronidazole if allergic to penicillin)
- **Control spasms**
  Nurse in a quiet room
  Avoid unnecessary stimuli
  i.v. diazepam—if spasms continue paralyse patient and ventilate
- **General measures**
  Maintain hydration and nutrition
  Treat secondary infections

Prevention

Active immunisation must be given. Contaminated injuries are treated by debridement. The immediate danger of tetanus can be greatly reduced by the injection of 1200 mg of penicillin followed by a 7-day course of oral penicillin. For those who are allergic to penicillin, erythromycin should be used. When the risk of tetanus is judged to be present, an injection of 250 units of human tetanus antitoxin should be given and an intramuscular injection of toxoid which should be repeated 1 month and 6 months later. For those already protected only a booster dose of toxoid is required.

LYME DISEASE — see p. 137.

NEUROSYPHILIS

Neurosyphilis may present as an acute or chronic process and may involve singly or in combination the meninges, blood vessels and parenchyma of the brain and spinal cord. The clinical manifestations are diverse and, although the condition is now rare, early diagnosis and treatment remain important.

Clinical features

The clinical and pathological features of the three most common presentations are summarised in Table 18.58.

Neurological examination reveals signs appropriate to the anatomical localisation of lesions. Pupillary abnormalities, described by Argyll Robertson, may accompany any neurosyphilitic syndrome. The pupils are small and irregular, and react to convergence but not directly to light. Delusions of grandeur suggest general paresis

of the insane, but more commonly there is simply progressive dementia. The combination of physical signs in tabes dorsalis are characteristic. Argyll Robertson pupils are found in 90% of patients and there is depression of tendon reflexes, hypotonia, distal impairment of deep pain sensation in the legs resulting in perforating painless ulcers and Charcot joints, and impairment of pin-prick sensation over the nose, perineum and distal lower limbs.

The clinical syndromes outlined above may occur in combination giving rise to mixed pictures, which may mimic many other neurological disorders.

Investigations

Routine screening for syphilis is warranted in the great majority of neurological patients. Serological tests (page 183) are positive in the serum in most patients, but CSF examination is essential if neurological involvement is suspected. Active disease is suggested by an elevated cell count, usually lymphocytic, and the protein content may be elevated to 0.5–1.0 g/l with an increased gamma-globulin fraction. Serological tests in the CSF are usually positive, but progressive disease can occur with negative CSF serology.

Management

The essential part of the treatment of neurosyphilis of all types is the injection of procaine penicillin 600 mg–1.2 g daily for 3 weeks (p. 184). Further courses of penicillin must be given if symptoms are not relieved, or the condition continues to advance, or the CSF continues to show signs of active disease. The cell count returns to normal within 3 months of completion of treatment, but the elevated protein takes longer to subside, and some serological tests may never revert to normal. Evidence of clinical progression at any time is an indication for renewed treatment.

OTHER FORMS OF MENINGITIS

Fungal meningitis (cryptococcosis)—see p. 147.

This usually occurs in patients who are immunosuppressed or have a focus of fungal infection. It is a recognised complication of HIV infection (p. 96). The CSF findings are similar to those of tuberculous meningitis, but the diagnosis can be confirmed by microscopy or specific serological tests.

Malignant meningitis

The cerebrospinal fluid may contain reactive lymphocytes with a low CSF glucose and the diagnosis depends on cytological examination, which may be enhanced by cytospin techniques.

Table 18.58   Clinical and pathological features of neurosyphilis

Type	Pathology	Clinical features
Meningovascular (5 years)*	Endarteritis obliterans Meningeal exudate Granuloma (gumma)	Stroke Cranial nerve palsies Seizures/mass lesion
General paralysis of the insane (5–15 years)*	Degeneration in cerebral cortex/cerebral atrophy Thickened meninges	Dementia Tremor Bilateral upper motor signs
Tabes dorsalis (5–20 years)*	Degeneration of sensory neurones Wasting of dorsal columns Optic atrophy	Lightning pains Sensory ataxia Visual failure Abdominal crises Incontinence Trophic changes

* Interval from primary infection.

Sarcoidosis or connective tissue disorder

The distinction between meningitis in these conditions and infectious conditions can be difficult and often rests on the recognition of the systemic features of these disorders.

In some areas meningitis may be caused by spirochaetes (leptospirosis p. 136), Lyme disease (p. 137), syphilis (p. 183), rickettsia (typhus fever p. 114) or protozoa (amoebiasis p. 153).

CEREBRAL ABSCESS

Bacteria may be introduced into the cerebral substance through penetrating injury, direct spread from sinuses or the middle ear, or through embolism from systemic infection, most commonly subacute bacterial endocarditis or pulmonary abscess. The site of abscess formation and likely causative organism are related to the source of infection (Table 18.59).

Initial infection leads to local suppuration followed by loculation of pus within a surrounding wall of gliosis, which in chronic abscess may form a tough capsule. Multiple abscesses occur particularly with metastatic spread.

Clinical features

Cerebral abscess may present acutely with fever, headache, meningism and drowsiness, but more commonly presents over days or weeks as a cerebral mass lesion with little or no evidence of infection. Epilepsy, raised intracranial pressure and focal hemisphere signs occur alone or in combination and distinction from a cerebral tumour may be impossible on clinical grounds.

Investigations

Lumbar puncture is potentially hazardous in raised intracranial pressure and CT scan should always precede lumbar puncture if focal neurological signs are present. The CT scan shows single or multiple low density areas which enhance peripherally with contrast to provide a ring appearance with central low density and surrounding cerebral oedema (Fig. 18.41). Plain skull radiograph may provide evidence of sinusitis and there may be an elevated blood white cell count and ESR in patients with active local infection.

Management

Antimicrobial therapy should be recommended once the diagnosis is made and the likely source of infection should guide the choice of antibiotic (Table 18.59). The presence of a capsule may lead to a persistent focus of infection despite antibiotics and in these patients surgical treatment by repeated burrhole aspiration or excision of abscess may be necessary. Anticonvulsants are often necessary as there is a high incidence of epilepsy which may develop acutely or in the recovery phase.

Table 18.59   Site, source and organism in cerebral abscess

Site of abscess	Source of infection	Likely organism
Frontal	Frontal sinusitis	Streptococcus
Temporal	Otitis media	Streptococcus Bacteroides Proteus
Cerebellar	Otitis media	Streptococcus Bacteroides Proteus
Parietal	Embolic	Streptococcus Bacteroides Proteus
Any site	Trauma	Staphylococcus

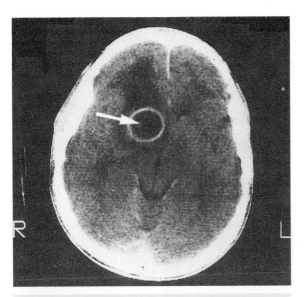

Fig. 18.41 CT scan in cerebral abscess (after contrast enhancement). There is ring enhancement of a lesion deep in the right cerebral hemisphere with surrounding cerebral oedema and shift of midline structures to the left.

Prognosis

The mortality rate remains at 10–20% despite an improvement in available surgical and medical treatments and in some patients this is related to delay in diagnosis and initiation of treatment.

SUBDURAL EMPYEMA

This is less common than cerebral abscess and occurs as a complication of frontal sinusitis, osteomyelitis of the skull vault, or middle ear disease. A collection of pus in the subdural space spreads over the surface of the hemisphere causing underlying cortical oedema or thrombophlebitis.

Clinical features

Epilepsy and progressive hemiparesis are common presentations.

Investigations

The diagnosis rests on plain skull radiograph, to provide evidence of a focus of infection, and CT head scan. This may show a subdural collection with underlying cerebral oedema but may be normal. The diagnosis is often dependent on suspicion of subdural empyema in patients with a local focus of infection.

Management

Pus is aspirated via a burrhole and appropriate parenteral antibiotic treatment commenced. Any local source of infection must be treated to prevent reinfection.

SPINAL EPIDURAL ABSCESS

Clinical features

The characteristic clinical features are pain in a root distribution and progressive transverse myelitis with paraparesis, sensory impairment and sphincter dysfunction. Infection is usually metastatic, but a primary source of infection is easily overlooked.

Investigations

Plain radiographs of the spine may show osteomyelitis, and urgent neurosurgical intervention, preceded by myelography or MRI, is essential to prevent complete and irreversible paraplegia.

Management

Decompressive laminectomy relieves the pressure on the dura and allows the abscess to be drained and organisms to be cultured. The patient must be given appropriate intravenous antibiotics.

FURTHER READING

Wood M, Anderson M (eds) 1988 Neurological Infections. W B. Saunders, London

DISEASES OF THE SPINAL CORD

COMPRESSION OF THE SPINAL CORD

Acute spinal cord compression is one of the commonest neurological emergencies encountered in clinical practice. Early diagnosis is essential to allow appropriate management and may prevent persistent and disabling neurological deficit. Pressure on the spinal cord may arise from lesions of the vertebral column, the spinal meninges, or the spinal cord and common causes are listed in Table 18.60.

A space-occupying lesion within the spinal canal may involve nerve tissue directly by pressure or indirectly by interfering with the blood supply. Oedema from venous obstruction impairs neuronal function, and ischaemia from arterial obstruction leads to necrosis of the spinal cord. The earlier stages are reversible, but severely dam-

Table 18.60	Causes of spinal cord compression	
Site	**Frequency**	**Causes**

Vertebral (extradural)	80%	Trauma
		Intervertebral disc
		Secondary carcinoma
		  Breast
		  Prostate
		  Bronchus
		Myeloma
		Tuberculosis

Meninges (Intradural extramedullary)	15%	Tumours
		  Meningioma
		  Neurofibroma
		  Ependymoma
		  Metastasis
		  Lymphoma
		  Leukaemia
		Epidural abscess

Spinal cord (Intradural intramedullary)	5%	Tumours
		  Glioma
		  Ependymoma
		  Metastasis

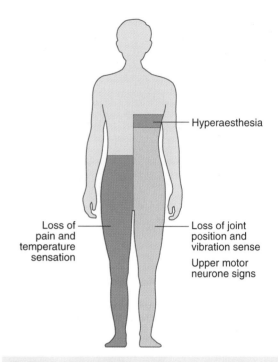

Hyperaesthesia

Loss of pain and temperature sensation

Loss of joint position and vibration sense

Upper motor neurone signs

Fig. 18.42   Physical signs in hemi-section of the cord (Brown–Sequard syndrome).

aged neurones do not recover, enhancing the importance of early diagnosis and treatment.

Clinical features

The onset of symptoms of spinal cord compression is usually slow but can be acute with trauma or metastases, especially if there is arterial occlusion. The symptoms are:

1. pain, localised over the spine or in a root distribution, which may be aggravated by coughing, sneezing or straining;
2. paraesthesia, numbness, or cold sensations, especially in the lower limbs, which spread proximally often to a level on the trunk;
3. heaviness, weakness or stiffness of the limbs, most commonly the legs;
4. urgency or hesitancy of micturition, leading eventually to urinary retention.

Pain and sensory symptoms occur early, while weakness and sphincter dysfunction are usually late manifestations.

The signs on examination vary according to the level of cord compression and the structures involved. There may be tenderness to percussion over the spine if there is vertebral disease, and this may be associated with a local kyphosis. Involvement of the roots at the level of compression may give dermatomal sensory impairment and lower motor signs at the corresponding level. Interruption of fibres in the spinal cord causes sensory loss and upper motor neurone signs below the level of the lesion, and there is often disturbance of sphincter function.

The distribution of these signs varies with the level of the lesion:

1. above the fifth cervical segment—upper motor neurone signs and sensory loss in all four limbs;
2. between fifth cervical and first thoracic—lower motor neurone signs and segmental sensory loss in the arms and upper motor neurone signs in the legs;
3. thoracic cord—spastic paraplegia with a sensory level on the trunk;
4. lumbosacral cord and cauda equina—lower motor neurone signs and segmental sensory loss in the legs. (The spinal cord ends at approximately the T12/L1 spinal level and spinal lesions below this level can only cause lower motor neurone signs.)

The **Brown–Sequard syndrome** results if damage is confined to one side of the cord. On the side of the lesion there is a band of hyperaesthesia with below it loss of proprioceptive sense and upper motor neurone signs. On the other side there is loss of spinothalamic sensation (pain, temperature) as fibres of that tract decussate soon after entering the cord (Fig. 18.42).

Investigations

Patients with a short history of progressive spinal cord compression should be investigated urgently. Investigations necessary are listed in the information box below.

Plain radiographs may show bony destruction and soft-tissue abnormalities and are an essential part of investigation (Fig. 18.43). Routine investigations, including chest radiograph, may provide evidence of systemic disease. Myelography localises the lesion and, with CT in suitable cases, defines the extent of compression and associated soft-tissue abnormality. The CSF should be taken for analysis at the time of myelography, and in cases of spinal block shows a normal cell count, very elevated protein and xanthochromia (Froin's syndrome). Acute deterioration may develop after myelography and it is preferable to alert neurosurgeons before such procedures are undertaken.

Management

The treatment and prognosis depend on the nature of the underlying lesion. Benign tumours should be surgically excised and a good functional recovery can be expected, unless a marked neurological deficit has developed before diagnosis. Extradural compression due to malignancy is the commonest cause of spinal cord compression and has a poor prognosis, although useful function can be regained if treatment is initiated within 24 hours of the onset of severe weakness or sphincter dysfunction. Surgical decompression may be appropriate in some patients, but has a similar prognosis to needle biopsy, to establish the histological nature of the tumour, followed by radiotherapy. Traumatic lesions of the vertebral column require specialised treatment in a neurosurgical centre.

PARAPLEGIA

This may result from many causes such as tumours, trauma and other forms of spinal compression, multiple sclerosis, subacute combined degeneration of the cord and, in India, lathyrism.

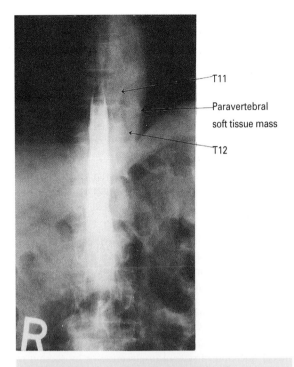

T11
Paravertebral soft tissue mass
T12

Fig. 18.43 Myelogram in malignant spinal cord compression. The column of contrast medium is obstructed at the level of T11/T12. There is partial collapse of the body of the T11 vertebra with loss of the pedicle and a paravertebral soft tissue mass at this level on the left side.

Management

This must be directed to the cause but management of the paraplegia itself is most important if complications, which may in themselves lead to death, are to be avoided. Pressure sores, urinary infections, renal calculi, faecal impaction and contractures can all be prevented.

Skin

Pressure sores are liable to develop because of the loss of sensation, diminished blood supply and immobility. The patient must be turned every 2–4 hours to a position which avoids pressure on bony prominences such as the sacrum and heels. The skin must be kept dry and clean and the patient nursed, if possible, on a specially designed mattress or bed.

If pressure sores develop, the patient must not lie on the affected side and scrupulous asepsis must be observed. Skin grafting may be necessary and it is important to maintain nutrition.

Bladder

Aseptic intermittent catheterisation must be performed if retention occurs. An indwelling catheter is not desirable as it predisposes to infection, reduces bladder capacity and promotes calculus formation. Many paraplegic patients are able to establish automatic bladder emptying, often assisted by manual compression of the lower abdomen; in others intermittent self-catheterisation or a urinary diversion procedure may be necessary. Urinary infection should be treated promptly and an adequate fluid intake encouraged.

Bowel

Constipation must be prevented by suitable diet and laxatives. Enemas or manual evacuation may be necessary if the faeces become hard and impacted.

Paralysis

Spasticity can lead to the development of flexor spasm and contractures in the limbs which may be prevented by regular passive movement of the limbs and by nursing the patient in postures that discourage flexion of the joints. A cradle to remove the weight of the bedclothes from the lower limbs may help prevent reflex stimulation and foot-drop deformity. In severe spasticity, without hope of recovery, flexor spasms can be relieved by intrathecal injection of phenol in glycerine or by section of the anterior nerve roots.

Rehabilitation

A great deal can be done by rehabilitation when the cause of paralysis is not progressive. Patients may learn to walk with calipers or to use a wheelchair. Many achieve independence, may follow suitable occupations, and take part in a variety of recreational activities.

CERVICAL SPONDYLOSIS

Degenerative change in the cervical spine is a common radiological finding in the middle-aged and elderly. Degeneration of the intervertebral discs and secondary osteoarthrosis (cervical spondylosis) is often asymptomatic, but may be associated with neurological dysfunction. The C5/6, C6/7, and C4/5 vertebral levels and C6, C7 and C5 roots respectively are most commonly affected (Fig. 18.44).

CERVICAL RADICULOPATHY

Compression of a nerve root occurs when a disc prolapses laterally and may develop acutely or more gradually due to osteophytic encroachment of the intervertebral foramina.

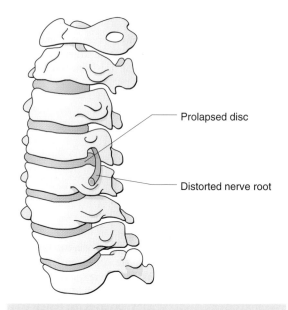

Fig. 18.44   C4/5 vertebral level. A lateral disc protrusion compressing the C5 root.

Table 18.61   Physical signs in cervical root compression

Root	Muscle weakness	Sensory loss	Reflex
C5	Biceps, deltoid, spinati	Upper lateral arm	Biceps
C6	Brachioradialis	Lower lateral arm, thumb, index finger	Supinator
C7	Triceps, finger and wrist extensors	Middle finger	Triceps

Clinical features

The patient complains of pain in the neck which may radiate in the distribution of the nerve root. The neck is held rigidly and neck movements may exacerbate pain. Paraesthesia and sensory loss may be found in the affected segment and there may be lower motor neurone signs, including weakness, wasting and reflex impairment (Table 18.61).

Investigations

Plain radiographs, including lateral and oblique views, should be obtained to confirm the presence of degenerative changes and to exclude other conditions, including destructive lesions. Electrophysiological studies rarely add to the clinical examination, but may be necessary if there is doubt about the diagnosis.

Management

Conservative treatment with analgesics and a cervical collar results in resolution of symptoms in the great majority of patients. In chronic nerve root compression cervical myelography or MRI scan may be indicated in the few patients who require surgery in the form of foraminotomy or disc excision.

CERVICAL MYELOPATHY

Dorsomedial herniation of a disc and the development of transverse bony bars or posterior osteophytes may result, alone or in combination, in pressure on the spinal cord or the anterior spinal artery, which supplies the anterior two-thirds of the cord.

Clinical features

The onset of symptoms is usually insidious and painless, although acute deterioration may occur after trauma, especially hyperextension injury. Upper motor neurone signs develop in the limbs, with spasticity of the legs usually appearing before the arms are involved. Dermatomal sensory loss is common in the upper limbs, while pain, temperature and joint position sense may be impaired in the legs. The neurological deficit usually progresses gradually and disturbance of control of micturition is a late feature.

Investigations

Plain radiographs confirm the presence of degenerative changes and myelography may be indicated if surgical treatment is being considered. MRI scan has the advantage of being non-invasive and is a sensitive technique for demonstrating disordered anatomy; it may also show areas of high signal within the spinal cord at the level of compression. Imaging of the cervical spine should be considered if there is diagnostic doubt or prior to surgery.

Management

Surgical procedures, including laminectomy and anterior discectomy, may arrest progression in disability but do not usually result in neurological improvement, and they carry a significant risk, particularly in the elderly. The judgement as to when surgery should be undertaken may be difficult. Manipulation of the cervical spine is of no proven benefit and may precipitate acute neurological deterioration.

Prognosis

The prognosis in cervical myelopathy is unpredictable. In many patients the condition stabilises or even improves without intervention, but if progressive disability does develop surgical decompression may be essential.

SYRINGOMYELIA

In this condition cavities filled with fluid and surrounded by glial cells develop near the centre of the spinal cord and may communicate with the central canal. The expanding cavity disrupts second-order spinothalamic neurones, may extend laterally to damage the anterior horn cells, and may compress the long fibre tracts.

Aetiology

The most frequent cause is blockage of the exit foramina of the fourth ventricle. Cerebrospinal fluid cannot escape into the subarachnoid space and the pressure rise within the closed ventricular system is communicated to the central canal of the cord, which expands along irregular paths of least resistance. In the majority of patients obstruction to the flow of CSF is due to congenital herniation of the cerebellar tonsils through the foramen magnum (Chiari Type I malformation) and in others to basal arachnoiditis or, rarely, following trauma. Following disturbed CSF dynamics hydrocephalus may occur in association and, rarely, extension of the cavities caudally produces brain-stem dysfunction (syringobulbia).

Clinical features

Patients usually present in the third or fouth decade and symptoms are of insidious onset and slowly progressive. Pain in the neck or shoulder is common and patients may seek advice because of sensory loss in the upper limbs. The most characteristic physical sign is dissociated sensory loss (loss or depression of pain and temperature sensation with preservation of other sensory modalities), which has an upper and lower level in a mantle or hemi-cape distribution. Loss of protective sensory function leads to trophic lesions such as painless burns or ulcers on the hands, and sometimes painless, deranged joints (Charcot joints) in the upper limbs. Wasting of the small hand muscles is a common early feature and loss of one or more reflexes in the arm almost invariable. Upper motor neurone signs develop in the legs as the condition progresses.

Kyphoscoliosis, pes cavus and spina bifida are common associations. Upward extension to involve the lower brain stem leads to dysarthria, palatal palsy, Horner's syndrome, nystagmus and sensory loss on the face.

Investigations

Plain radiographs may demonstrate congenital anomalies around the foramen magnum or expansion of the cervical canal. The most sensitive and least invasive investigation for syringomyelia is magnetic resonance imaging (Fig. 18.45), although myelography, often combined with CT scan, allows accurate diagnosis in the great majority of patients.

Management

Surgical decompression of the foramen magnum or the syrinx itself may arrest progression of the neurological deficit and often alleviates pain. The results of surgery are however often disappointing and in some patients the condition continues to progress and worsens if the brain stem is involved.

LUMBAR DISC HERNIATION

Low back pain, 'lumbago', is the commonest medical cause of inability to work, but in the great majority of patients is due to abnormalities of joints and ligaments in the lumbar spine rather than herniation of an intervertebral disc. Pain in the distribution of the lumbar or sacral roots is more often due to disc protrusion, but is also a feature of other rare but important disorders including spinal tumour, malignant disease in the pelvis and tuberculosis of the vertebral bodies.

Acute lumbar disc herniation is often precipitated by trauma, usually by lifting heavy weights while the spine is flexed. The nucleus pulposus may bulge or rupture the annulus fibrosus, giving rise to pressure on nerve endings in the spinal ligaments, changes in the vertebral joints, or pressure on the nerve roots.

Clinical features

The onset may be sudden, often following trauma to the back, or gradual and repeated episodes of low back pain may precede sciatica by months or years. Constant aching pain is felt in the lumbar region and may radiate to the buttock, thigh, calf and foot. Pain is exacerbated by coughing or straining and may be relieved by lying flat.

The altered mechanics of the lumbar spine results in loss of lumbar lordosis and there may be spasm of the paraspinal musculature. Root pressure is suggested by limitation of flexion of the thigh on the affected side if the straight leg is raised (Lasegue's sign). If the third or fourth lumbar roots are involved Lasegue's sign may be negative, but pain in the back may be induced by hyperextension of the hip (femoral nerve stretch test). The roots most frequently affected are S1, L5 and L4 and the signs of root pressure at these levels are summarised in Table 18.62.

Investigations

Plain radiographs of the lumbar spine

These may show no abnormality in acute disc herniation or there may be narrowing of the disc space. There may be degenerative changes including osteophyte formation at the margins of the vertebral bodies in chronic low back pain, and plain radiographs also exclude other conditions such as malignant infiltration of a vertebral body.

Myelography

This is required if there is diagnostic doubt or for purposes of localisation before operation. It is unlikely to be of diagnostic value unless there is clinical evidence of root compression and is rarely indicated if pain is the only clinical feature.

MRI scan

Using external coils, this has the potential to supersede myelography and has the great advantage of being non-invasive.

Management

The initial treatment in all patients is bed rest on a firm mattress, if necessary supported by wooden boards. Provided rest is absolute, with prohibition from sitting up or leaving the bed for toilet purposes, pain and neurological signs, if present, resolve in over 95% of patients. Bed rest should be continued for 2–4 weeks and on recovery the patients should be instructed in back-

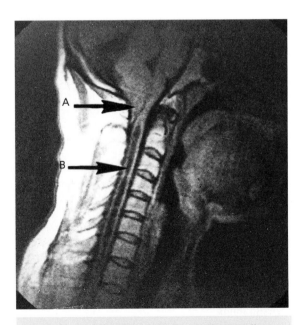

Fig. 18.45 Sagittal MRI scan showing a syrinx extending the length of the cervical cord. There is associated displacement of the cerebellar tonsils (Arnold–Chiari Type I) downward. A = cerebellar tonsil; B = syrinx.

Table 18.62 Physical signs in lumbar root compression

Disc level	Root	Sensory loss	Weakness	Reflex
L5/S1	S1	Sole and lateral foot	Eversion of foot	Ankle
L4/L5	L5	Outer calf and dorsum foot	Dorsiflexion of hallux/toes	Hamstring
L3/L4	L4	Inner calf	Inversion of foot	Knee

strengthening exercises and advised to avoid physical manoeuvres likely to strain the lumbar spine.

Injections of local anaesthetic or steroids may be a useful adjunct to bed rest if symptoms are due to ligamentous or joint dysfunction.

In a few patients with clinical evidence of nerve root compression, surgery may have to be considered if there is no response to conservative treatment or if progressive neurological deficits develop. Central disc prolapse with bilateral symptoms and signs and disturbance of sphincter function requires urgent surgical decompression.

LUMBAR CANAL STENOSIS (OR CAUDA EQUINA CLAUDICATION)

This is due to a congenital narrowing of the lumbar spinal canal, exacerbated by the degenerative changes which commonly occur with age.

Clinical features

Characteristically the patients, who are usually elderly, develop exercise-induced weakness and paraesthesia distally in the legs. These systems progress rapidly with continued exertion until the patient can no longer walk, but are quickly relieved by a short period of rest. Physical examination is usually normal at rest, with preservation of peripheral pulses, but weakness or reflex loss may be detected if the patient is examined immediately after exercise.

Investigations

Plain radiographs of the lumbar spine show narrowing of the lumbar canal, which may be confirmed by myelography, CT scan, or MRI.

Management

Extensive lumbar laminectomy results in an often complete relief of symptoms and recovery of normal exercise tolerance.

FURTHER READING

Braakman R 1994 Management of cervical spondylitic myelopathy and radiculopathy. Journal of Neurology, Neurosurgery and Psychiatry 57: 257–263

DISORDERS OF PERIPHERAL NERVES

Peripheral nerves are made up of axons, which represent elongated processes originating from neurones in the anterior horn cells of the spinal cord and dorsal root ganglia. These are enveloped in a series of Schwann cells which form the fatty myelin sheath. Pathological processes may affect cell bodies, the myelin sheath, or the connective tissue and blood vessels of peripheral nerves. Although these processes cannot be clinically distinguished, a knowledge of the pathological nature of a neuropathy is helpful in assessing prognosis and deciding on treatment. The clinical classification of peripheral nerve lesions comprises involvement of one or more individual peripheral nerves or a generalised polyneuropathy.

MONONEUROPATHY

The most frequent causes of damage to a single nerve are entrapment, particularly in fibro-osseous tunnels, trauma and diabetes mellitus.

ENTRAPMENT NEUROPATHIES

The diagnosis of these conditions rests on the often characteristic clinical history and a careful evaluation of the physical signs (Table 18.63).

Management

Lateral popliteal nerve palsies and radial nerve palsies are commonly due to local trauma, and complete recovery in 6–8 weeks can be expected without intervention. Meralgia paraesthetica often develops in relation to weight loss or gain and may respond to appropriate dietary advice and reassurance. Carpal tunnel syndrome and ulnar nerve palsy may remit if patients are advised to avoid activities involving repetitive wrist movement or pressure on the elbows. Precipitating causes including diabetes mellitus and hypothyroidism should be excluded. Persistent symptoms may respond to noc-

Table 18.63 Symptoms and signs in entrapment neuropathy

Nerve	Symptoms	Muscle weakness/wasting	Area of sensory loss
Median (at wrist) (carpal tunnel syndrome)	Pain and paraesthesia on palmar aspect of hands and fingers, waking the patient from sleep. Pain may extend to arm and shoulder	Abductor pollicis brevis	Lateral palm and thumb, index, middle and half ring finger
Ulnar (at elbow)	Paraesthesia on medial border of hand, wasting and weakness of hand muscles	All small hand muscles, excluding abductor pollicis brevis	Medial palm and little, and half ring finger
Radial	Weakness of extension of wrist and fingers, often precipitated by sleeping in abnormal posture, e.g. arm over back of chair	Wrist and finger extensors Supinator	Dorsum of thumb
Peroneal	Foot drop, trauma to head of fibula	Dorsiflexion and eversion of foot	Nil or dorsum of foot
Meralgia paraesthetica	Tingling and dysaesthesia on lateral border of the thigh (lateral cutaneous nerve of the thigh)	Nil	Lateral border of thigh

turnal splinting of joints, but in some patients decompression of the carpal tunnel or transposition of the ulnar nerve may be necessary. In these electrophysiological investigation is advisable pre-operatively in order to confirm the diagnosis and site of compression.

POLYNEUROPATHY

ACUTE POLYNEUROPATHY

Guillain–Barré syndrome (acute inflammatory or post-infective poly-neuropathy) develops 1–4 weeks after viral infection in 70% of patients and more rarely follows surgery or immunisation. Pathologically there is demyelination of spinal roots or peripheral nerves, which is almost certainly immunologically mediated.

Clinical features

The characteristic clinical feature is muscle weakness, which is more marked proximally than distally and progresses, often rapidly. Distal paraesthesia ascending proximally is common, and bilateral facial weakness develops in 50% of patients. The most striking findings on examination are diffuse weakness and widespread loss of reflexes. In the majority of patients muscle weakness progresses for 1–3 weeks, but occasionally rapid deterioration with respiratory failure develops within hours.

Investigations

The protein content of the CSF is raised at some stage of the illness but may be normal in the first 10 days. There is usually no rise in cells and a lymphocytosis of greater than 50/mm³ should raise the possibility of an alternative diagnosis. Electrophysiological studies are usually normal in the early stages of Guillain–Barré syndrome, but may be helpful if there is diagnostic doubt. Acute porphyria (p. 773) may cause a neuropathy similar to Guillain–Barré syndrome but may be excluded by urinary porphyrin estimation. Serum lead should be measured if there are only motor signs.

Management

During the phase of deterioration regular monitoring of respiratory function is essential. Respiratory failure may develop with little prior clinical warning and the development of dyspnoea or a drop in vital capacity below 1 litre may indicate the urgent necessity for intubation and positive pressure ventilation. Steroid therapy is ineffective, but plasma exchange and intravenous immunoglobulin therapy shorten the duration of ventilation and improve the prognosis provided treatment is started within 14 days of the onset of symptoms.

Prognosis

Overall 80% of patients recover completely within 3–6 months, 10% die, and 10% are left within residual neurological disability which can be severe.

MONONEURITIS MULTIPLEX

In this condition, multiple peripheral or spinal nerve lesions occur serially or concurrently. Pathologically there is ischaemia of the peripheral nerves due to vasculitis of the vasa nervorum, which renders the nerves susceptible to mechanical compression. Common causes are: polyarteritis nodosa, rheumatoid arthritis, diabetes mellitus, sarcoidosis and leprosy.

Table 18.64   Physical signs in brachial plexus lesions

Site	Root	Affected muscles	Sensory loss
Upper plexus (Erb–Duchenne)	C5 (C6)	Biceps, deltoid, spinati, rhomboids, brachioradialis (triceps, serratus ant.)	Patch over deltoid
Lower plexus (Dejerine–Klumpke)	T1 (C8)	All small hand muscles, claw hand (ulnar wrist flexors)	Ulnar border hand/forearm
Thoracic outlet syndrome	C8/T1	Small hand muscles, ulnar forearm	Ulnar border hand/forearm (upper arm)

BRACHIAL PLEXUS LESIONS

Trauma is the commonest cause of damage to the brachial plexus, and frequently involves forced separation of head and shoulder or excessive abduction of the arm. Other causes include neoplasia in the cervical lymph nodes or pulmonary apex, compression at the thoracic outlet, and damage due to radiotherapy of the axillary area.

Clinical features

The clinical signs depend on the anatomical site of damage (Table 18.64). There may be associated vascular symptoms in thoracic outlet syndrome including blanching and cyanosis of the fingers, and physical signs including asymmetry of radial pulses and a subclavian bruit.

Management

Regular passive movements of the affected limb prevent contractures while nerve fibres are regenerating. Splinting is ineffective, except in Erb's paralysis, and surgery is rarely indicated. Minor symptoms due to thoracic outlet syndrome often settle with rest and physiotherapy, but surgical treatment of underlying congenital anomalies such as cervical rib or fibrous band may be necessary if neurological signs progress.

The prognosis for recovery in traumatic lesions is dependent on the site and severity of neuronal damage and may be assessed electrophysiologically.

NEURALGIC AMYOTROPHY

Clinical features

This presents with severe pain over one shoulder and sometimes follows infection, inoculation or operation. Within days paralysis develops in the painful muscles, most commonly deltoid, spinati and serratus anterior and is rapidly followed by muscle wasting. There may be a patch of sensory loss over the deltoid and occasionally more extensive involvement of the muscles of the upper arm.

Table 18.65   Causes of peripheral neuropathy

Genetic
Hereditary motor and sensory neuropathy (Charcot–Marie–Tooth disease)
  Type I: demyelinating
  Type II: axonal
  Type III: congenital

Metabolic
Diabetes mellitus
Renal and hepatic failure
Paraproteinaemia
Amyloidosis
Acute intermittent porphyria
Hypothyroidism

Toxins
Alcohol
Heavy metals
Organic solvents
Drugs, e.g. amiodarone, vincristine, hydrallazine, phenytoin

Connective tissue disorders
Polyarteritis nodosa
Rheumatoid arthritis
Systemic lupus erythematosus

Deficiency states
Deficiency of vitamins A, B_2, B_6, B_{12} and E
Folate deficiency

Infections
Leprosy
Diphtheria
Typhoid
HIV

Malignant disease
Carcinoma of bronchus and other malignant tumours, including lymphoma and myeloma

Prognosis

Pain usually subsides within 1–2 weeks and complete recovery of paralysis and wasting can be expected in 3–6 months in the great majority of patients.

CHRONIC POLYNEUROPATHY

There are numerous causes of peripheral neuropathy (Table 18.65), but classification by clinical type (motor, sensory, or mixed) and by whether axons or myelin are predominantly affected (as judged by electrophysiological studies) allows a narrowing of diagnostic possibilities in the individual patient.

Clinical features

When the causal lesion lies in the nerve cell body, the first manifestations are at the distal end of the longest nerves. This gives rise to the typical picture of a generalised polyneuropathy with distal paraesthesia usually affecting the feet and then later the hands, which progresses proximally up the limbs. These sensory symptoms are associated with diminution of superficial sensation in a 'glove and stocking' distribution. There is distal weakness with diminished or absent tendon reflexes.

Investigations

The clinical features localise the lesion to the peripheral nerves. A careful clinical history, including details of family history, drug intake and potential exposure to toxins, is essential. Routine screening for a metabolic disorder should be undertaken and the possibility of diabetes mellitus must be excluded. Nerve conduction studies may be necessary if there is diagnostic doubt or if the condition is progressive. These studies confirm the presence of a neuropathy and provide an estimation of the nerve conduction velocity, which indicates whether the axons or myelin are primarily affected. In some cases, and in particular those in which a vasculitic aetiology is suspected, sural nerve biopsy may be indicated.

Management

No cause is found in the majority of patients with peripheral neuropathy and in many patients no treatment is necessary as the condition may stabilise or progress only slowly. Empirical treatment with steroids may be attempted if there is a progressive neurological deficit, but this is usually disappointing.

Exposure to drugs or toxins should be avoided if a causal link is suspected and in metabolic neuropathy appropriate treatment should be initiated without delay. Deficiency states require appropriate vitamin supplements and absolute abstention is essential in chronic alcoholism.

No specific therapy is available for hereditary neuropathies, but advice from physiotherapists and occupational therapists is important in helping patients to maintain their functional capacity and this also applies to other forms of chronic neuropathy.

FURTHER READING

Asbury A K, Gilliatt R N (eds) 1984 Peripheral Nerve Disorders. Butterworths, London
Hughes R A C 1990 Guillain–Barré Syndrome. Springer Verlag, London

DISEASES OF MUSCLE

The voluntary muscles are subject to a range of disorders, which result in a limited spectrum of symptoms and physical signs. These are listed in the information box below.

DISORDERS OF VOLUNTARY MUSCLES

- Muscular dystrophy
- Metabolic and endocrine myopathy
- Inflammatory myopathy
- Congenital myopathy
- Toxic myopathy
- Disorders of the neuromuscular junction

Diagnosis is largely clinical, depending on a recognition of the distribution of affected muscles, the identification of associated signs and symptoms, and, in many patients, a thorough family history. In some muscular dystrophies a specific genetic anomaly has been identified, for example in Duchenne dystrophy and dystrophia myotonica, and this may allow a specific diagnostic marker.

MUSCULAR DYSTROPHY

Progressive muscular dystrophy is a group of hereditary disorders characterised by progressive degeneration of a group of muscles without involvement of the nervous system.

Clinical features

The wasting and weakness are symmetrical, there is no fasciculation, tendon reflexes are preserved until a late stage and there is no sensory loss. Differential diagnosis depends on the age at onset, distribution of affected muscles, and type of inheritance (Table 18.66).

Investigations

The diagnosis of muscular dystrophy can be confirmed by electromyography and muscle biopsy. Creatinine kinase is markedly elevated in Duchenne muscular dystrophy, but is normal or only moderately elevated in the other types.

Dystrophia myotonica may be diagnosed by the distribution of muscle weakness and other features including myotonia (slow relaxation of muscle), cataract, ptosis, frontal baldness and gonadal atrophy.

Management

There is no specific therapy for these conditions, although advice from the physiotherapist and occu-

Table 18.66   Diagnostic features in muscular dystrophy

Dystrophy	Inheritance	Age at onset (yrs)	Muscles affected
Duchenne	X-linked recessive	3–10	Proximal legs and arms, then general
Limb girdle	Autosomal recessive	10–30	Pelvic girdle, shoulder girdle or both
Facio-scapulo-humoral	Autosomal dominant	10–40	Facial, shoulder girdle, serratus anterior
Dystrophia myotonica	Autosomal dominant	Any age (20–60)	Temporalis, facial, sternomastoid, distal limbs, myotonia

pational therapist may help the patient to cope with disability. Genetic counselling is an important component of management. Due to the recent mapping of the genetic disorders present in Duchenne dystrophy and dystrophia myotonica and in some other dystrophies, DNA analysis may allow early diagnosis and prenatal testing. Genetic counselling is an essential component of management.

Most patients with Duchenne dystrophy die within ten years of diagnosis, while the life-span in limb girdle and facio-scapulo-humeral dystrophies is unaffected. Premature death due to respiratory or cardiac failure is the usual outcome in dystrophia myotonica.

METABOLIC AND ENDOCRINE MYOPATHY

Muscle weakness may develop in a range of metabolic and endocrine disorders and is usually reversible. The causes are listed in the information box.

METABOLIC AND ENDOCRINE CAUSES OF MUSCLE WEAKNESS

Acute muscle weakness	Proximal myopathy
Hypokalaemia	Hyperthyroidism
Hyperkalaemia	Hypothyroidism
Hypocalcaemia	Cushing's syndrome
Hypercalcaemia	Addison's disease

Clinical features

The weakness is often acute and generalised in metabolic disorders, while a proximal myopathy predominantly affecting the pelvic girdle is a feature of some endocrine disorders, and may develop without other manifestations of hormonal disturbance. An awareness of the possibility of these conditions is the most important factor in diagnosis. Hypo- and hyperkalaemia may occur in familial periodic paralysis, which is a dominantly inherited condition characterised by attacks of profound weakness lasting for several hours and often precipitated by exertion.

Muscle pain on exercise is the characteristic feature

of myophosphorylase deficiency (McArdle's syndrome) and a number of other rare recessively inherited disorders of metabolism (p. 1042).

INFLAMMATORY MYOPATHY OR POLYMYOSITIS (see p. 918)

CONGENITAL MYOPATHY

This is rare and presents in infancy with muscular weakness and limpness. Serum enzymes may be normal or slightly elevated and the electromyogram is usually myopathic. The syndrome may be caused by a number of specific conditions which have a variable inheritance, and are defined by the type of structural abnormality present in skeletal muscle fibres. Most patients have a slowly progressive disease and there is no specific therapy.

TOXIC MYOPATHY

A wide variety of drugs may cause disorders of muscle, including carbenoxolone, thiazide diuretics and steroids. Alcohol may cause a spectrum of muscle disease varying from a mild, proximal weakness to severe muscle necrosis. Avoidance of the offending agent usually results in recovery of muscle function.

Penicillamine rarely causes a myasthenic syndrome, which may persist on drug withdrawal.

DISORDERS OF THE NEUROMUSCULAR JUNCTION

MYASTHENIA GRAVIS

This condition is characterised by progressive failure to sustain a maintained or repeated contraction of striated muscle.

Aetiology and pathology

Nicotinic receptors of acetylcholine in the post-junctional membrane of neuromuscular junctions are blocked or lysed by a complement mediated auto-immune reaction between receptor protein and anti-etylcholine-receptor antibody. The antibody is produced by B lymphocytes defectively controlled by T lymphocytes because of a disorder of the thymus gland. About 15% of patients, mainly of late onset, have an encapsulated or locally invasive thymoma. The majority, including all young individuals, have one of a number of thymic abnormalities, the most characteristic being germinal centres in the medulla of the gland. The latter group has a marked personal and familial relationship with other autoimmune diseases (p. 44), and many have inherited an immunoreactive gene which is linked to some of the HLA haplotypes; in a North European population these are HLA-B8 and DRw3. Inheritance of this gene is not obligatory for myasthenia and nothing is known about possible triggering factors for the spontaneous disease. Penicillamine may be one such breaker of immunological tolerance.

Clinical features

The disease usually appears between the ages of 15 and 50 years and females are more often affected than males. It tends to run a remitting course especially during the early years. Relapses may be precipitated by emotional disturbances, infections, pregnancy and severe muscular effort.

The cardinal symptom is abnormal fatigue of the muscles; movement although initially strong rapidly weakens. Intensification of symptoms towards the end of the day or following vigorous exercise is characteristic.

The first symptoms are usually intermittent ptosis or diplopia but weakness of chewing, swallowing, speaking or of moving the limbs also occurs. Any muscle of a limb may be affected, most commonly those of the shoulder girdle, so that the patient is unable to undertake work above the level of the shoulder, such as combing the hair, without frequent rests. Respiratory muscles may be involved and respiratory failure is a not uncommon cause of death. Asphyxia occurs readily as the cough may be too weak to clear foreign bodies from the airways. Muscle atrophy may occur in long-standing cases. There are no signs of involvement of the central nervous system.

Investigations

Recommended investigations are listed in the information box.

The intravenous injection of a short-acting anticholinesterase, edrophonium hydrochloride, is a valuable diag-

---

INVESTIGATION OF MYASTHENIA GRAVIS

- Tension test
- Autoantibody screen (including skeletal muscle antibody)
- Thyroid function tests
- Anti-acetylcholine receptor antibody titre
- PA and lateral chest radiograph/CT scan of thorax
- EMG

---

nostic aid (the Tensilon test). An initial dose of 2 mg is injected and a further 8 mg given half a minute later if there are no undesirable side-effects. Improvement in muscle power occurs within 30 seconds and usually persists for 2 or 3 minutes.

Screening for other autoimmune disorders, particularly thyroid disease, is necessary and elevated acetylcholine receptor antibody is found in 80% of cases, although much less frequently in ocular myasthenia. Positive skeletal muscle antibodies suggest the presence of thymoma and all patients should undergo radiological investigation to exclude this condition. EMG with repetitive stimulation may show a characteristic decremental response.

Management

The principles of treatment are:

1. to maximise the activity of acetylcholine at the remaining receptors in the neuromuscular junctions
2. to limit or abolish the immunological attack on motor endplates.

The duration of action of acetylcholine is greatly prolonged by inhibiting its hydrolysing enzyme, acetylcholinesterase. The most commonly used anticholinesterase drug is pyridostigmine, which is given orally in a dosage of 60–120 mg at intervals determined by supervised trial (2–8 hours). Side-effects, including diarrhoea, colic and other autonomic symptoms, may be controlled by propantheline (15 mg as required).

Overdosage of anticholinesterase drugs may cause a cholinergic crisis due to depolarisation block of motor endplates, with muscular fasciculation, paralysis, pallor, sweating, excessive salivation and persistently small pupils. This may be distinguished from severe weakness due to exacerbation of myasthenia (myasthenic crisis) by the clinical features and if necessary by the injection of a small dose of edrophonium hydrochloride. Sudden weakness from either cause may require intermittent positive pressure ventilation to save life, and early intubation before a crisis has developed will normally remove the need for tracheostomy.

The immunological disorder is treated by various procedures which are listed in the information box below.

IMMUNOLOGICAL TREATMENT OF MYASTHENIA

- **Thymectomy**
  Should be performed as soon as feasible in any patient with myasthenia not confined to extraocular muscles, unless the disease has been established for more than seven years; the indication for surgery is the stage of myasthenia gravis, not the presence of thymoma

- **Plasma exchange**
  Removing antibody from the blood may give marked improvement but, as this is usually brief, such therapy is normally reserved for myasthenic crisis or for preoperative preparation

- **Intravenous immunoglobulin**
  An alternative to plasma exchange in the treatment of severe myasthenia gravis

- **Corticosterold treatment**
  May cause improvement but this is commonly preceded by marked exacerbation of myasthenic symptoms and should be initiated in hospital. It is usually necessary to continue treatment for months or years, with the possibility of adverse effects, and steroids are not recommended for first-line management

- **Other immunosuppressant treatment**
  e.g. azathioprine 2.5 mg/kg daily, may be of value in reducing the dosage of steroids necessary to control symptoms and in some cases may allow steroids to be withdrawn

---

Prognosis

Prognosis is variable. Remissions sometimes occur spontaneously. When myasthenic affection is confined to the eye muscles, prognosis for life is normal and disability slight. Rapid progression of the disease more than 5 years after its onset is uncommon. Thymectomy, perhaps followed by high dosage steroid treatment, often leads to marked improvement so that disability is minimal and life expectancy normal. When the disease is associated with a thymoma, even if this is removed, the outlook is markedly worse.

FURTHER READING

Walton J (ed.) 1988 Disorders of Voluntary Muscle. Churchill Livingstone, Edinburgh

---

DEGENERATIVE DISORDERS

MOTOR NEURONE DISEASE

This is a progressive disorder of unknown cause, in which there is degeneration of spinal and cranial motor neurones and pyramidal neurones in the motor cortex. About 5% of cases are familial, the disorder having autosomal dominant in heritance to a gene defect on chromosome 21. A variety of possible causes including viral infection, trauma, exposure to toxins, and electric shock have been suggested, but no sound evidence exists to support any of these in typical cases. The prevalence of the disease is about 5 per 100 000; males are affected more often than females.

Clinical features

These are listed in the information boxes below and overleaf.

CLINICAL FEATURES OF MOTOR NEURONE DISEASE

- **Age of onset**
  Usually after age 50 years, occasionally in 30–50 years group
- **Course**
  Symptoms often begin focally in one part and spread gradually but relentlessly to become widespread
- **Signs**
  Wasting and fasciculation of muscles, weakness of muscles of limbs, tongue, face and palate (dysarthria, dysphagia)
  External ocular muscles and sphincters usually remain intact
  Pyramidal tract involvement causes spasticity, exaggerated tendon reflexes, extensor plantar responses
  No objective sensory deficits
  No intellectual impairment
- **Death**
  Usually within 3–5 years of onset from respiratory failure/infection, immobility and inability to swallow

---

Investigations

In many patients the clinical features are diagnostic. Electromyography helps confirm the presence of fasciculation and denervation, and is particularly helpful when pyramidal features predominate. Sensory nerve conduction is normal and motor studies show loss of axons with only modest reduction in conduction velocity. Myelography and CT brain scanning are sometimes necessary to exclude local spinal or cerebral disease when clinical abnormalities are localised. CSF examination is usually normal; a mild elevation of protein concentration may be found. Treatable disorders such as diabetes mellitus, syphilis, sarcoidosis, and spinal disorders should be excluded.

Management

No treatment alters the progress of this disease. Mental and physical support, with help from occupational and speech therapists and physiotherapists, is essential to keep the patient's quality of life as good as possible. Mechanical aids such as splints, walking aids, wheelchairs and communication devices all help to maintain morale of both the patient and their carers. Feeding by percutaneous gastrostomy or naso-gastric tube may be necessary if bulbar palsy is marked.

Prognosis

Motor neurone disease is progressive, most patients dying within 3–5 years of the onset of symptoms. Younger patients and those with early bulbar symptoms tend to show a more rapid course, whereas older patients and those with mainly peripheral involvement may survive 10 years. Death is usually from respiratory infection and failure, and the complications of immobility. Relief of distress in the terminal stages warrants the use of opiates and sedative drugs.

SPINAL MUSCULAR ATROPHIES

These are a group of genetically determined disorders affecting spinal motor and cranial motor neurones characterised by proximal and distal wasting, fasciculation and weakness of muscles. Involvement is usually symmetrical, but occasional localised forms occur. With the exception of the infantile form, progression is slow and the prognosis better than in motor neurone disease, from which they can usually be distinguished

by the age of onset and rate of progress. Examples are given in Table 18.67.

HEREDITARY ATAXIAS

This is a group of inherited disorders in which degenerative changes occur in the cerebellum, brain stem, pyramidal tracts, spinocerebellar tracts and optic nerves. Onset may be in childhood or in middle adult life. Most childhood forms are of recessive inheritance, while the late onset disorders are usually autosomal dominant. Clinically, combinations of cerebellar, pyramidal, sensory and extra-pyramidal features may occur. Recognition and classification of the disorders is important to give a prognosis and accurate genetic counselling. Patterns of involvement are listed in Table 18.68.

NEUROFIBROMATOSIS (VON RECKLINGHAUSEN'S DISEASE)

This is a genetic disorder of autosomal dominant inheritance probably due to an abnormal gene on chromosome

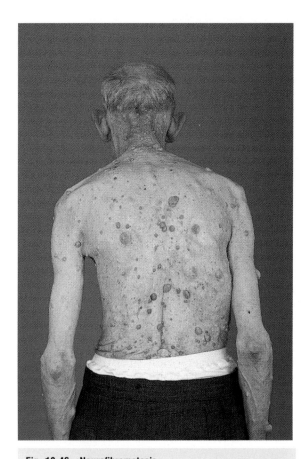

Fig. 18.46   Neurofibromatosis.

Table 18.67 Types of spinal muscular atrophy

Type	Onset	Inheritance	Features	Prognosis
Werdnig–Hoffman	Infancy	Autosomal recessive	Severe muscle wasting/weakness	Poor
Kugelberg–Welander	Childhood, adolescence	Autosomal recessive	Proximal weakness and wasting. EMG shows denervation	Slowly progressive disability
Distal forms	Early adult life	Autosomal dominant	Distal weakness and wasting of hands and feet	Good, seldom disabling
Bulbospinal	Adult life, males only	X-linked	Facial and bulbar weakness, proximal limb weakness	Good

Table 18.68 Types of hereditary ataxias

Type	Inheritance	Onset	Clinical features
Friedreich's ataxia	Autosomal recessive	8–16 years	Ataxia, nystagmus, dysarthria, spasticity, areflexia, proprioceptive impairment, diabetes mellitus, optic atrophy, cardiac abnormalities. Chairbound by age 20 usually
Ataxia telangiectasia	Autosomal recessive	Childhood	Progressive ataxia, athetosis, telangiectases on conjunctivae, impaired DNA repair, immunodeficiency, tendency to malignancies
Olivo-ponto-cerebellar atrophy	Autosomal dominant	Adult life	Slowly progressive ataxia, spasticity, dysarthria, extrapyramidal features, optic atrophy, deafness, pyramidal signs
Hereditary spastic paraplegia	Autosomal dominant	Adult life	Slowly progressive spasticity affecting legs > arms, extensor plantar responses, sensory signs minimal or absent

22. Multiple fibromatous tumours develop from the neurilemmal sheaths of peripheral and cranial nerves (Fig. 18.46). Most of the lesions are benign but sarcomatous change occasionally occurs. Cerebral gliomas, meningiomas, endocrine tumours (e.g. phaeochromocytoma), intellectual subnormality and epilepsy may be associated with the cutaneous manifestations.

Two genetically distinct forms of neurofibromatosis are now recognised (Table 18.69).

The peripheral form is readily recognised by the cutaneous lesions which gradually increase in number throughout life. Investigation and treatment is only indicated if there are symptoms of cerebral or spinal involvement, or if malignant change is suspected. Because the central form may have no cutaneous signs, a family history of cerebral or spinal lesions should be noted with care.

Table 18.69 Types of neurofibromatosis

Type 1 Peripheral form > 70% of cases	Multiple cutaneous neurofibromas, 'soft' papillomas, café-au-lait patches, axillary freckling, iris fibromas, plexiform neurofibromas, spinal neurofibromas, aqueduct stenosis, scoliosis, endocrine tumours
Type II Central form	Few or no cutaneous lesions, bilateral acoustic neuromas, cerebral and optic nerve gliomas, meningiomas, spinal neurofibromas

FURTHER READING

Critchley E, Eisen A (eds) 1992 Diseases of the Spinal Cord. Springer Verlag, Berlin

DISORDERS OF SLEEP

Normal sleep is thought to be under control of the reticular activating system in the upper brain stem and diencephalon. During overnight sleep, a series of repeated cycles of EEG patterns can be recorded. As drowsiness occurs, alpha rhythm disappears (stage I) and the EEG gradually becomes dominated by deepening slow activity which reaches delta frequencies in stages III and IV. After 60–80 minutes this slow-wave pattern is replaced by a short spell of low amplitude EEG background on which are superimposed rapid eye movements (REM). After a few minutes of REM sleep, another slow-wave spell starts and the cycle repeats several times throughout the night. The REM periods tend to become longer as the sleep period progresses. Dreaming takes place during REM sleep; it is accompanied by muscle relaxation, penile erection and loss of tendon reflexes. REM sleep seems to be the most important part of the sleep cycle for refreshing cognitive processes;

deprivation of REM sleep causes tiredness, irritability and impaired judgment.

DISORDERS OF SLOW-WAVE SLEEP

Sleep talking and sleep walking
Automatic behaviour not recalled by the sufferer may take place during light sleep. Such phenomena are common in normal children. Sleep walking is uncommon in adults.

Night terrors
These occur as sudden arousals from deep (stage III and IV) slow-wave sleep. They are more common in children, but may affect adults. The sufferer wakes in a state of agitation, screaming and fearful. Occasionally violent behaviour occurs. The agitation may last many minutes.

DISORDERS OF REM SLEEP

Nightmares
These are frightening dreams from which the sufferer wakes in a state of fear or agitation. Most normal people have experienced such phenomena.

Sleep paralysis
This may occur in otherwise normal people, but is more commonly reported by those with the narcoleptic tetrad (see below). The person wakes in the night or morning and is aware of their surroundings, but is unable to move or speak for seconds or minutes. This probably represents dissociation between the inhibitory part of the REM sleep system and the waking role of the reticular formation.

Hypnagogic hallucinations
These also sometimes affect normal people but are more common in narcolepsy/cataplexy. Frightening hallucinations are experienced soon after falling asleep, or just before waking.

Narcolepsy
This is abnormal. Sufferers experience recurrent bouts of irresistible sleep during which the EEG often shows direct entry into REM sleep. Sufferers tend to fall asleep when unstimulated or carrying out monotonous activity (bathing, eating, driving). The periods of sleep are usually short and the person can be woken relatively easily. They usually feel refreshed after waking. Paradoxically, overnight sleep is often fitful.

Cataplexy
This probably represents spontaneous activation of the REM sleep spinal inhibitory mechanism. Attacks are set off by surprise, emotion, laughter, fear and embarrassment. Muscle tone is lost in the limbs, face and trunk so that the sufferer sinks to the ground and is unable to move for seconds or minutes. Consciousness is not impaired and the EEG remains normal during attacks. Examination during an attack reveals loss of tendon reflexes and sometimes extensor plantar responses.

Narcolepsy, cataplexy, sleep paralysis and hypnagogic hallucinations may occur together in the same patient (Gélineau's tetrad); most often, narcolepsy and cataplexy occur together. The disorder has strong HLA association with DRw 2 and is sometimes familial.

Management
Narcoleptic attacks are treated by stimulant drugs such as dexamphetamine (5–10 mg 8-hourly). Cataplexy responds to tricyclic antidepressants, particularly clomipramine (25–50 mg 8-hourly).

SLEEP APNOEA/HYPOPNOEA SYNDROME
—see p. 328.

NUTRITIONAL NEUROLOGICAL DISEASES

Vitamin deficiency due to malabsorption or malnutrition can cause lesions in a number of sites in the nervous system (see pages 562–574).

Alcoholism—see pp. 992, 565
The commonest cause of vitamin deficiency in Britain is chronic alcoholism, in which the clinical effects of vitamin deficiency may be complicated by the neurotoxic effect of alcohol itself, including cerebellar degeneration, dementia, peripheral neuropathy and myopathy.

Central pontine myelinolysis occurs in alcoholics and following over-rapid correction of hyponatraemia. There is widespread destruction of myelin in the pons, resulting in tetraparesis, dysphagia and anarthria, and death.

Lathyrism
The consumption of pulses, a common constituent of many Indian diets, may produce an acute or slowly progressive spastic paraplegia if the pulses include *Lathyrus sativus* which contains a neurotoxin.

NEUROLOGICAL COMPLICATIONS OF ALCOHOLISM

- Wernicke's encephalopathy
- Korsakoff's syndrome
- Dementia
- Cerebellar degeneration
- Peripheral neuropathy
- Acute or chronic myopathy
- Toxic amblyopia
- Central pontine myelinolysis

Table 18.70 Paraneoplastic neurological syndromes

Disorder	Clinical features	Investigations
Peripheral neuropathy	Sensory-motor neuropathy	EMG Elevated CSF protein
Myopathy/myositis	Proximal muscle weakness	Myopathic EMG
Myasthenic syndrome	Generalised weakness Dry mouth Depression of tendon reflexes with post-contraction potentiation	Incremental EMG response
Cerebellar degeneration	Ataxia, nystagmus often rapidly progressive	CT scan
Encephalopathy	Progressive dementia Brain stem signs	CT scan
Myelitis	Motor neuropathy Spinal cord dysfunction	(Myelogram)

PARANEOPLASTIC NEUROLOGICAL SYNDROMES

These syndromes arise at a distance from a primary carcinoma in the absence of metastases. Although paraneoplastic syndromes may be associated with a variety of tumours, the most frequent primary sites are carcinoma of the lung, carcinoma of the breast, carcinoma of the ovary and lymphoma. Neural disturbance may occur at any stage during the development of the primary lesion and may antedate the symptoms directly attributable to the carcinoma by weeks or months. They may affect singly or in combination muscles and peripheral nerves as well as central neural structures and the brain (see Table 18.70).

Clinical features

The syndromes are most conveniently categorised anatomically, although over 50% of cases present with a mixed neuromyopathy.

Management

The treatment of the paraneoplastic syndrome is that of the primary lesion. Improvement and occasionally complete remission of a myasthenic-myopathic syndrome may occur with removal of the primary tumour but this is by no means invariable. In most instances the response of the neurological complications is unpredictable.

FURTHER READING

Posner J B, Furneaux H M 1990 Paraneoplastic syndromes. In: Wacksman B H (ed.) Immunological Mechanisms in Neurological and Psychiatric Disease. Raven, New York

W. J. MacLennan

19

Principles of geriatric medicine

DEMOGRAPHY OF AGEING

One of the most striking changes in the demography of developed countries has been the increased proportion of elderly individuals in the population. For example in Scotland between 1755 and 1990 the percentage of people over the age of 60 years has risen from 7.3 to 20.1 (Fig. 19.1). Much of the change has occurred over the last hundred years when there has been a dramatic reduction in perinatal and infant mortality, and a steady decline in the death rate from infectious disease throughout adult life. Over the last 20 years there has been a levelling off of the proportion aged 65 to 74 years, but a continuing increase in those aged 75 to 84 years, and a particularly steep increase in those aged 85 years and over (Fig. 19.2). The relevance of the latter to health and social services is that there is an exponential increase in disability, and mental and physical morbidity, in individuals over the age of 75 years.

Population projections suggest that demographic changes in many underdeveloped countries will be gradual, in contrast to developing countries where there will be at least a twofold increase in the proportion of the population over the age of 60 years (Fig. 19.3).

NORMAL OLD AGE

The practical value in defining the characteristics of normal ageing is that this provides a baseline against which the signs and symptoms of disease in elderly pat-

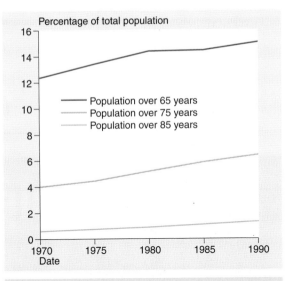

Fig. 19.2   Changes in the proportions of the population in Scotland over 65 years, over 75 years and over 85 years of age between 1970 and 1990.

ients can be assessed. It is an artificial concept, however, in that multiple pathology is so common in old age that individuals free from disease form a biological elite. There also is the problem that, with advancing age, there

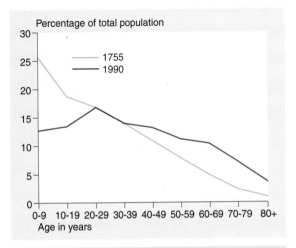

Fig. 19.1   The age structure of the population of Scotland in 1755 compared with that in 1990.

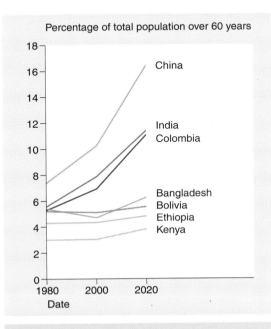

Fig. 19.3   Projected changes in the proportions of the population over 60 years of age between 1980 and 2020 in seven developing countries.

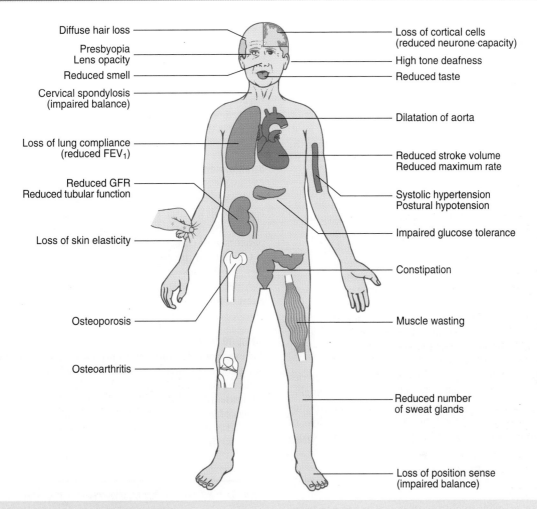

Diffuse hair loss

Presbyopia
Lens opacity

Reduced smell

Cervical spondylosis
(impaired balance)

Loss of lung compliance
(reduced FEV$_1$)

Reduced GFR
Reduced tubular function

Loss of skin elasticity

Osteoporosis

Osteoarthritis

Loss of cortical cells
(reduced neurone capacity)

High tone deafness

Reduced taste

Dilatation of aorta

Reduced stroke volume
Reduced maximum rate

Systolic hypertension
Postural hypotension

Impaired glucose tolerance

Constipation

Muscle wasting

Reduced number
of sweat glands

Loss of position sense
(impaired balance)

Fig. 19.4   Physiological effects of ageing.

is increase in variation, so that on average there may be a moderate decline in organ function; this remains unchanged in some elderly individuals, whereas in others it is so severe that it leaves them seriously incapacitated.

It also should be recognised that the effects of ageing are usually insufficient to interfere with the function of an organ under baseline conditions. The changes are sufficient, however, to reduce its reserve capacity, so that the stress of a mild illness or unaccustomed exercise may be sufficient to precipitate a crisis.

Though the effects of ageing are considered to be inevitable, the reality is that the rate of deterioration in organ function often can be reduced by factors such as regular exercise, or accelerated by bad habits such as cigarette smoking or heavy alcohol consumption.

Figure 19.4 outlines some of the more important organ and tissue changes associated with ageing.

Skin and integuments

Changes within the connective tissue result in the skin losing its elasticity and becoming wrinkled. The appearance is similar to that associated with dehydration, so that the condition is easily missed in elderly patients. Connective tissue damage is accentuated by excessive exposure to sunlight, and is particularly striking in fair-skinned individuals living in areas such as Australia or California.

A decline in the number of sweat glands means that elderly patients experience difficulty in regulating their temperature in warm weather. This manifests itself as a high incidence of cardiovascular disease during heat waves.

There is a diffuse loss of hair, and the hair also becomes finer. This is in contrast to the patchy changes associated with male pattern baldness. The stage at which depigmentation occurs is so variable that there is relatively little relationship between this and the age of an individual.

Cardiorespiratory system

There is a decline in the stroke volume of the heart, and in its maximum rate in response to exercise. A reduction in the elasticity of the lungs means that there is an increase in the physiological dead space, and that the rate of expiration measured as the forced vital capacity is reduced. The practical effect of these changes is that there is a decline in the maximal oxygen consumption. The rate of this decline is reduced in individuals who indulge in regular physical exercise, and is accentuated in cigarette smokers.

Vascular system

An increase in the rigidity of large arteries causes an increased systolic pressure. Although the condition is extremely common in old age, it is not 'normal' in that it is associated with an increased cardiovascular mortality and morbidity, which is reduced by effective control of the hypertension.

Impaired autonomic function and rigidity of arteries and veins result in a fall in blood pressure on changing from a supine to erect posture. This often is asymptomatic but may cause lightheadedness or even loss of consciousness. A wide range of diseases and drugs accentuate the process.

Homeostasis

There is a decline in glucose tolerance due to a reduced tissue sensitivity to insulin. Although common, it is not 'normal' in that it is associated with an increased risk of diabetic complications.

There is a decline in the glomerular filtration rate resulting in the delayed elimination of many drugs such as digoxin or chlorpropamide. Tubular damage reduces the ability of the kidney to concentrate urine, so that old people are particularly susceptible to drugs and disorders which cause dehydration.

Central nervous system

There is a decline in the number of neurones in the cerebral cortex, but this has only minor effects on mental function. Psychological differences between young and old people relate to cultural and environmental factors rather than ageing. Changes in the vestibular nuclei, the cerebellum and dorsal columns, damage to position sense receptors in the neck, and lower limb muscle weakness all contribute to a deterioration in balance.

Musculoskeletal system

A decline in the number of anterior horn cells results in muscle weakness and wasting. The process often is accentuated by the physical inactivity which may follow retirement, and can be minimised or reversed by taking regular physical exercise.

Physical exercise also is useful in reducing the rate of bone loss described in Chapter 15.

Special senses

Chemical changes in the lens result initially in rigidity of the structure associated with impaired close vision (presbyopia). Later on the lens becomes opaque with loss of vision (cataract). The process is accentuated in patients with diabetes mellitus.

Changes in the cochlea result in a high tone hearing loss (presbycousis).

A decline in taste and sense of smell affect appreciation of food.

Immune function

Ageing, poor nutrition and chronic ill health in many old people interact with each other to interfere with immune function. Results of this include an attenuated inflammatory response so that the local and systemic effects of infection are masked, and there is an impaired delayed cutaneous response to injected antigen.

ATYPICAL PRESENTATION OF DISEASE

The effects of age changes, impaired immunological function, poor nutrition, multiple pathology, sensory deficits, psychiatric disorders and intercurrent drug treatment interact to both modify and mask the typical symptoms and signs of disease in many elderly patients (Table 19.1).

GIANTS OF GERIATRIC MEDICINE

These refer to four of the most common causes of incapacity in elderly patients referred to a geriatric unit: acute confusion, urinary incontinence, immobility and falls. Resources of particular relevance to their management are the diagnostic skills of the geriatrician, and the team work of nurses, physiotherapists, occupational therapists, social workers and other professionals with skills supplementary to medicine.

Table 19.1 Disorders presenting with atypical features in elderly patients

Disorder	Atypical presentation in old age
Myocardial infarction or pulmonary embolism	Confusion, blackout, weakness, breathlessness and palpitations without chest pain
Bronchopneumonia	Confusion and rapid respiration, but no pyrexia and minimal chest signs
Appendicitis	Confusion and constipation or diarrhoea, but no pyrexia and few localising signs
Peptic ulcer	Anaemia, haematemesis or melaena without previous symptoms of dyspepsia
Urinary tract infection	Confusion and urinary incontinence, but no pyrexia or frequency and dysuria
Dehydration	No thirst, and skin changes indistinguishable from those of ageing
Hypothyroidism	Lethargy and general deterioration with no other characteristic symptoms and signs
Thyrotoxicosis	Apathy, weight loss and cardiac signs without anxiety, excess sweating or heat intolerance
Diabetes mellitus	Asymptomatic until onset of complications, e.g. nephropathy, neuropathy or retinopathy
Brain tumour	Confusion, drowsiness and focal neurological signs without headache or papilloedema

ACUTE CONFUSION

Since an acute confusional state usually is the result of organic disease, its investigation and treatment lie within the remit of geriatric or general medicine rather than psychiatry.

URINARY INCONTINENCE

Urinary incontinence is a symptom rather than a disease. A detailed clinical assessment and appropriate investigation often lead to the identification of a remediable cause.

Aetiology

Confusion and immobility associated with acute illness often result in urinary incontinence. This usually settles with resolution of the illness, but in a proportion of cases the incontinence persists.

A common neurological cause of chronic urinary incontinence is damage to the cerebral cortex with damage to normal bladder inhibition, so that the bladder has a small volume and increased tone, and empties frequently. Disorders responsible for this include cerebrovascular disease, Alzheimer's disease or Parkinson's disease. Cord damage due to multiple sclerosis, trauma or a tumour is less common in old age, but can result in complete loss of control over micturition

with a small volume bladder emptying automatically at regular intervals. Damage to afferent parasympathetic fibres in disorders such as a diabetic autonomic neuropathy gives rise to a large volume atonic bladder in which there is a continuous dribbling overflow incontinence.

Local causes of urinary incontinence include pressure on the bladder resulting from faecal impaction, stress incontinence due to a pelvic floor weakness in women, or disordered micturition associated with prostatic obstruction in men. After the menopause, atrophic changes in the vagina may be accompanied by similar abnormalities in the mucosa of the urethra and trigone giving rise to urinary frequency and urge incontinence.

Other causes of urinary incontinence include the use of drugs such as diuretics, or inability to reach the lavatory in time because of poor mobility. There also are instances in which incontinence is a manifestation of anxiety, or an attention-seeking device.

Assessment

The history should include details on the duration and timing of the incontinence, any associated urinary symptoms, and drug treatment. Particular attention should be given to examination of the abdomen, central nervous system, rectum, perineum, vulva and vagina. If the patient is in hospital, the nursing staff should keep an incontinence chart which records all episodes of both micturition and incontinence.

Further investigation is dependent upon the clinical features. A culture of the urine is normally taken, though infection and incontinence often are coincidental. Pelvic ultrasound examination may identify chronic urinary retention, while catheterisation followed by cystometrography provides details of dynamic filling pressures within the bladder. Cystoscopy and cinefluoroscopy also may be of value in cases of particular diagnostic difficulty.

Treatment

The mainstay of treatment is toilet training in which patients are encouraged to anticipate episodes of incontinence by regular emptying of their bladder. Practical measures such as modifying the dose of a diuretic or facilitating access to the lavatory also may be effective. Faecal impaction should be treated. More specific treatment with a bladder relaxant such as oxybutinin may be useful as an adjunct to toilet training in patients with a hypertonic bladder. An oestrogen cream should be used where there is atrophic vaginitis. If there is stress incontinence, exercises for the pelvic floor should be organised, and consideration given to reconstructive surgery. In men, prostatectomy may relieve overflow incontinence, but may make things worse if there is coincidental neurological damage.

As a last resort, intractable urinary incontinence should be managed by devices such as catheters, urinals, incontinence pads or marsupial pants.

IMMOBILITY

Age changes in the neurological and musculoskeletal system described already, and a high prevalence of disorders such as stroke, Parkinson's disease, osteoarthritis and osteoporosis, interact to make poor mobility one of the most common problems to afflict elderly patients.

Since there often is little reserve capacity in skeletal muscles, even a period in bed may be sufficient to render an elderly patient immobile. It is essential, therefore, that, after an acute illness, an active programme of rehabilitation is started as soon as possible. Any delay is likely to result in weeks of incapacity. It also is important to identify and treat any deterioration of mobility in an elderly individual living at home. The geriatric day hospital is a useful facility in this respect.

FALLS

There is an increased incidence of falls with advancing age. Environmental factors such as trailing flexes, poorly sited banisters or loose rugs can contribute to these, but there usually is an underlying disorder. Frequently more than one is identified in individual patients.

Although a careful history should be taken, this often is vague and misleading. Physical examination should include an assessment of standing balance and gait, and measurement of lying and standing blood pressures. Subsequent investigation depends upon the clinical findings, but may include a 24 hour ECG tape, electronystagmography and computerised tomography of the brain.

STROKE REHABILITATION

Stroke is one of the most devastating disorders to afflict elderly patients. The investigation and immediate management of stroke are described in Chapter 18, and this section concentrates on rehabilitation of the patient once the condition has been stabilised.

Assessment

The first stage in rehabilitation is to perform an assessment of impairment associated with the stroke (see information box). Muscle function is only one aspect of this and attention should also be directed to aspects such

---

CAUSES OF FALLS IN ELDERLY PATIENTS

Neurological
- Cerebrovascular disease
- Parkinson's disease
- Dementia
- Visual impairment
- Impaired position sense
- Vertebrobasilar insufficiency
- Transient ischaemic attacks
- Epilepsy

Cardiovascular
- Aortic stenosis
- Adams–Stokes attack
- Sick sinus syndrome
- Postural hypotension

Locomotor
- Osteoarthritis
- Other arthropathies
- Muscle weakness
- Cervical spondylosis

Otological
- Benign positional vertigo
- Ménière's disease
- Labyrinthine ischaemia
- Acoustic neuroma

Drugs
- Diuretics
- Psychotropic agents
- Antidepressants
- Tranquillisers and hypnotics
- Anticonvulsants

---

as sensation, parietal lobe function, speech and mental function.

ASSESSMENT OF IMPAIRMENT IN STROKE

- **Motor function** muscle power, muscle tone, contractures
- **Balance** sitting, standing, walking
- **Sensation** position sense is particularly important
- **Parietal lobe function** apraxia, agnosia, neglect, denial of disability
- **Vision** hemianopia, visual neglect
- **Cognitive ability** observe behaviour, administer a mental status questionnaire
- **Mood** depression (administer geriatric depression scale), emotional lability
- **Speech** dysphasia (motor, receptive, fluent), dysarthria
- **Swallowing** observation, cinefluoroscopy (if indicated)
- **Autonomic function** urinary incontinence, postural hypotension

This is followed by an evaluation of disability which involves an assessment of **mobility** (including ability to transfer), **activities of daily living (ADL)** (washing, bathing, dressing, feeding and toileting), **instrumental activities of daily living (IADL)** (cooking, performing housework, shopping). It also is important to record details of the home background, the level of support available from relatives, friends and neighbours.

With this information to hand, it is possible to organise a programme of rehabilitation. Dependent upon circumstances this may take place in hospital, at a day hospital, or in the patient's own home. A large number of professionals may be involved (Table 19.2). It is essential that their efforts are coordinated, and that there is effective communication. One way of facilitating this

Table 19.2   Composition and remit of rehabilitation team

Profession	Remit
Hospital doctor	Assessment of impairment, coordination of programme
Physiotherapist	Promotion of balance, mobility and upper limb function
Occupational therapist	Assessment and promotion of ADL and IADL, home assessment visit and organisation of appropriate aids
Speech therapist	Treatment of speech disorders, advice and management of dysphagia
Dietitian	Nutritional support of patients with dysphagia
Hospital nurse	Reinforcement of rehabilitation programme, continuous assessment, communication with other professionals and with relatives
Hospital social worker	Communication with patient and relatives, organisation of home support services or (where appropriate) institutional care, liaison with volunteers and stroke clubs
General practitioner	Initial referral for specialist services, organisation of continuing assessment and support at home
Care manager	Assessment of needs and organisation of services for continuing community care

is to hold regular case conferences at which all members of the team are represented.

DRUG TREATMENT

A number of physiological changes associated with ageing combine to modify the way in which elderly patients handle drugs and respond to them (Table 19.3). Added to these are the effects of both multiple pathology and polypharmacy. A practical consequence is that there is a high incidence of drug side-effects in elderly patients. The risk of these can be minimised by starting off treat-

MEASURES TO IMPROVE DRUG COMPLIANCE BY ELDERLY PATIENTS

- Prescribe the minimum of drugs necessary
- Provide patient with counselling on medication (doctor, nurse or pharmacist)
- Label containers with large letters giving times and doses
- Provide a card with names of drugs, their purposes, their dose and their times of administration
- Consider calendar packs or drug dispensers
- Carefully review all repeat prescriptions
- Discourage hoarding of drugs not in current use
- Where appropriate, involve carers in administration

ment with small doses and carefully monitoring the response, and only prescribing a drug if the chances of benefit are greater than the risk of side-effects. Attention should also be given to the likelihood of interaction with concurrent medication. Most elderly patients show a high level of compliance with instructions on medication, but those with physical or mental incapacity experience particular difficulty, as do those on complex regimes.

FURTHER READING

Cardozo L 1991 Urinary incontinence in women: have we anything new to offer? British Medical Journal 303: 1453–1457
Graham H J, Firth J 1992 Home accidents in older people: role of primary health care team. British Medical Journal 305: 30–32
Kelly J G, O'Malley K 1992 Principles of altered drug handling in the elderly. Reviews in Clinical Gerontology 2: 11–19
Lindeman R D 1992 Changes in renal function with age. Drugs and Aging 2: 423–431
Luxon L M 1993 Disorders of hearing and balance. Reviews in Clinical Gerontology 3: 347–358
Wade D T 1992 Stroke: rehabilitation and long-term care. Lancet 339: 791–795

Table 19.3   Effects of ageing on the pharmacokinetics and pharmacodynamics of drugs

Age change	Practical consequences	Example
Reduced first pass metabolism through liver	Increased initial level of drugs	Increased initial level of propranolol
Decreased lean body mass	Increased level of water soluble drugs	Increased level of digoxin
Increased percentage body fat	Decreased level of fat soluble drugs	Decreased level of phenothiazines
Reduced plasma binding	Increased activity of protein bound drugs	Increased activity of warfarin
Impaired renal excretion	Cumulation of slowly excreted drugs	Cumulation of digoxin
Impaired hepatic oxidation/hydroxylation	Increased level of drugs	Increased level of theophylline
Decrease in number of drug receptors in cells	Increased sensitivity to drugs	Increased sensitivity to benzodiazepines

NOTE: The importance of these changes is dependent upon the properties of a particular drug. One change occasionally cancels out the effect of another.

A. A. H. Lawson

20

Acute poisoning

Acute poisoning is a common and urgent medical problem in all developed, and many developing, countries of the world. In Britain it accounts for 15–20% of all acute medical emergency admissions to hospital. The different types of acute poisoning, and their relative frequency in patients above the age of 12, are shown in the information box. In young children, particularly below the age of five, they are virtually all accidental, whereas in older age groups the great majority are intentional and self-inflicted but not suicidal. For this reason, the terms self-poisoning, para-suicide and non-fatal deliberate self-harm are used to distinguish this major type. The preferred term is self-poisoning, which does not imply motive and is defined as a conscious impulsive action designed to secure redress of an intolerable situation with, often, strong manipulative motives. Criminal homicidal poisoning by comparison is rare.

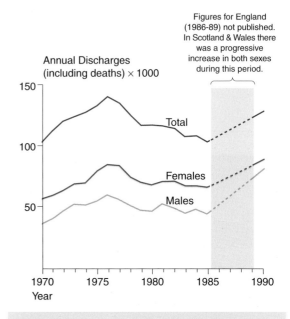

Fig. 20.1 Estimated total discharges and deaths due to the adverse effects of medicinal agents and chiefly non-medicinal substances. (Combined figures for Scotland, England and Wales 1970–90).

TYPES OF ACUTE POISONING AND THEIR RELATIVE IMPORTANCE AS CAUSES OF ADMISSION TO HOSPITAL IN PATIENTS ABOVE THE AGE OF 12

Type		Admissions to hospital (% of total)
Accidental		10
Intentional	True attempted suicide	10
	Self-poisoning (parasuicide)	80
	Homicide	rare

This chapter deals with the clinical features, diagnosis, treatment and prevention of acute poisoning. Food poisoning is discussed on page 123. Brief reference is made to industrial and agricultural poisons.

EPIDEMIOLOGY

The trends in total discharges and deaths due to acute poisoning in Scotland, England and Wales are shown in Figure 20.1. There was a dramatic and progressive increase in incidence until about 1976, since when there was a relative decline in the frequency of admission until 1985, but since then an increase. This variation may be partly due to changes in admission policy for acute poisoning across the country during recent years. As a result many symptomless children and up to 40% of adults reaching Accident and Emergency Departments are discharged and a further 30% are treated at home by their general practitioners. Many patients are thought not to seek medical advice and recover in their own homes. Despite this the number of patients admitted with acute poisoning remains well in excess of 100 000 each year and the true incidence of poisoning in the community is much higher.

Social patterns

Acute self-poisoning in societies of western origin is more common in females than in males in all age groups, the composite ratio of females to males being about 1.4:1.0. The major rise in incidence has been among patients in the second and third decades, reaching levels that are now many times higher than amongst the middle-aged and elderly. The main social factors resulting in this increase have been described (p. 1146).

In societies with different cultural and religious backgrounds the incidence of self-poisoning has also risen but different patterns occur. In India, for example, males are more commonly involved in self-poisoning than females and alcohol is much less involved.

Up to 50% of those who self-poison have done so before, and 20% will attempt it again within twelve months. These figures for repetition are remarkably consistent from year to year in different centres in the UK, as is the frequency with which suicide follows self-poisoning. This is the case particularly in socially high-risk groups, in whom the incidence of subsequent suicide is about 1% per annum. A broadly similar picture occurs

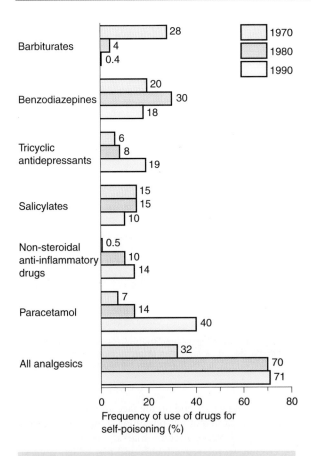

Barbiturates 28 / 4 / 0.4

1970
1980
1990

Benzodiazepines 20 / 30 / 18

Tricyclic antidepressants 6 / 8 / 19

Salicylates 15 / 15 / 10

Non-steroidal anti-inflammatory drugs 0.5 / 10 / 14

Paracetamol 7 / 14 / 40

All analgesics 32 / 70 / 71

0   20   40   60   80
Frequency of use of drugs for self-poisoning (%)

Fig. 20.2   Self-poisoning in Scotland (1970–90): the changing pattern of drugs involved. (Source: Scottish Hospital In-patient Statistics. Common Services Agency Information Services Division, Trinity House, Edinburgh.)

in other European countries, and in the United States there are 2.3 million acute poisonings every year.

Changing pattern of poisonings

Drugs have always been the most frequent agents taken by adults and, after household products, are the commonest substances ingested by children. At least 30% of self-poisoning episodes involve more than one drug, and alcohol will be taken together with the drug by 60% of males and 40% of females. In adults more than 60% ingest drugs that have been prescribed for themselves or a close relative and so the pattern of acute poisoning closely reflects prescribing habits. It is not surprising, therefore, that the major groups of drugs involved in acute poisoning at the present time are benzodiazepines, tricyclic and related antidepressant drugs and analgesics, which include paracetamol, non-steroidal anti-inflammatory drugs, salicylates and opiate analogues. The changing fashions are shown in Figure 20.2.

Mortality statistics

In all European countries and also in those with predominant populations from European sources, such as in North America and Australasia, completed suicide is commoner in the elderly over 60 years and more common in all age groups in males than in females. This is

---

SEX AND AGE DIFFERENCES IN SELF-POISONING COMPARED WITH COMPLETED SUICIDE DUE TO POISONING

Self-poisoning (non-fatal)	Completed suicide due to poisoning
Commoner in: Females than males (M:F 1:1.4) 2nd and 3rd decades	Commoner in: Males than females (M:F 4.7:1) 6th decade and above

---

in contrast to the patterns found in self-poisoning. There are large national differences which have persisted throughout this century with few changes in the rank order of countries for which statistics are available. In the United States and Australia studies of suicide rates in immigrant populations from different countries have demonstrated variations in the population similar to those of the country of origin, suggesting that these variations are true national characteristics.

Since 1960 the suicide rate due to poisoning for young adults has increased in both sexes in more countries than it has decreased, and among the elderly similar trends are appearing. In Britain more than 80% of deaths due to poisoning occur outside hospital and so it is important that hospital statistics should not be considered alone in an estimate of the physical consequences of poisoning in the community. In hospital, for example, there has been a dramatic fall in mortality due to this cause over the last 40 years. In 1945 up to 25% of patients admitted with acute barbiturate poisoning died. The mortality from that cause has now been reduced to 0.45%, and less than 1% for all poisonings. Even in severely ill patients less than 2% should die. Currently the main drugs causing death of self-poisoning patients admitted to the hospital are analgesics, antidepressant drugs and benzodiazepines. The major causes of death from poisoning outside hospital are carbon monoxide, benzodiazepines, tricyclic antidepressants, paracetamol and salicylate. Collectively, these account for almost 4000 deaths each year in the UK. Acute carbon monoxide poisoning usually occurs from deliberate inhalation of car exhaust fumes or accidentally as a result of incomplete combustion of natural gas by faulty domestic appliances. A similar pattern occurs in the United States but in Britain non-medicinal products, with perhaps the exception of inhaled solvents, cause few deaths, whereas in America a significant mortality results from cleaning and polishing agents, pesticides and petroleum distillates.

In other parts of the world, particularly India, East Asia and Africa, accidental poisoning due to snake bite is an important cause of mortality, accounting for over 30 000 deaths every year.

DIAGNOSIS

In Britain information can be obtained immediately, on a 24-hour basis, regarding the ingredients of a substance and the approximately fatal dose of a poison, from any one of the centres providing the National Poisons Information Services.

POISONS INFORMATION CENTRES—24 HOUR SERVICE (UK AND REPUBLIC OF IRELAND)

London	0171 635 9191	Birmingham	0121 554 3801
	0171 955 5095	Leeds	01132 430715
Edinburgh	0131 536 1000		01132 432799
Cardiff	01222 709901	Newcastle	0191 232 5131
Belfast	01232 240503	Dublin	003531 379964
			003531 379966

TOXBASE on-line poisons information service is available to users within the National Health Service throughout the UK.

Clinical features

The clinical features of most poisons are non-specific, but the diagnosis is seldom in doubt as the circumstantial evidence is often strong and many patients, or their relatives or friends, give a clear history of it. When this information is lacking difficulties arise, particularly when the patient is unconscious. The range of substances involved in acute poisoning is so great, with many patients taking mixtures, often with alcohol, that it is impossible to provide comprehensive clinical diagnostic guidelines. Many drugs in overdose produce complex neurological features of a non-specific type and so the state of the pupils, abnormalities of eye movements, nystagmus and changes in limb reflexes may not have the same significance as they would have in primary neurological disease. It is helpful, therefore, to remember that the commonest cause of unconsciousness in the age group 15–35 is acute drug overdosage. The clinical features of some drugs taken are listed in Table 20.1. Other useful clinical features are evidence of self-injury, either old or recent, especially on the flexor aspects of

Table 20.1   Clinical features of drugs or poisons

Clinical features	Possible drug or poison ingested/inhaled
Vomiting Depressed respiration Pinpoint pupils	Opiates and related analogues Cholinesterase inhibitors Dextropropoxyphene*
Widely dilated pupils Bladder distension Absent bowel sounds Cardiac arrhythmias Upper motor neurone signs	Tricyclic antidepressants
Sweating Tinnitus Deafness Hyperventilation	Salicylates
Buccal corrosive burns	Strong acids, alkalis, phenols, cresols, paraquat
Characteristic smell	Alcohol, volatile hydrocarbons, solvents
Hypothermia	Chlorpromazine Barbiturates
Skin blisters	Barbiturates Tricyclic antidepressants Carbon monoxide

* Especially likely to cause respiratory arrest, particularly if taken with alcohol or sedatives. Administration of specific opiate antagonist naloxone (0.4–2.0 mg i.v.) may be both therapeutic and diagnostic.

the arms and wrists and on the face and hands. Also, all patients suspected of self-poisoning should be examined carefully for venepuncture marks, abscesses or skin ulceration on the arms, hands and feet which suggests 'main-lining' by a drug addict. It is important to remember that with some serious poisonings, such as paraquat, clinical features may not become apparent for up to 36 hours after ingestion.

Identification

An increasing number of tablets and capsules are marked with a code letter and number and others can be recognised by their characteristic appearance. When in doubt, however, more precise identification may be obtained from hospital pharmacists and information services. The only conclusive identification is, however, toxicological analysis of urine, gastric aspirate or plasma and simple rapid screening methods are available for approximately 90% of common poisonings. It is important that the correct specimens are sent for analysis when the poison has been taken orally. Samples of vomitus or gastric aspirate, taken in the first few hours following ingestion, are ideal for diagnostic confirmation. Urine is a good alternative and often more appropriate than blood as the concentration of toxic substances or related metabolites is almost always much higher in urine than in serum or plasma. The appropriate samples are 50 ml gastric content or urine, with no added preservative, and 10 ml whole blood. Although these analyses can be carried out the results seldom influence treatment, but may be of value for medico-legal purposes. *Important common exceptions are salicylate or paracetamol overdoses in which rapid and accurate measurement of the blood levels is vital for the correct management of the poisoning.*

ASSESSMENT OF SEVERITY

The individual variation in response to drugs is very wide, depending on differences in tissue tolerance, drug interaction and the ability of an individual patient to metabolise the toxic substance. It is, therefore, dangerous to allow efforts to identify and quantify the poisoning by laboratory means to delay emergency supportive treatment. In general, therefore, the severity of any poisoning must be judged on the basis of clinical assessment. This initial evaluation is of paramount importance, not only for determining the patients' condition from which their progress may be appraised, but also for deciding upon the treatment required.

Poisonous substances may give rise to **primary toxic effects**, which may result in **organ damage** of a nonspecific or specific type (Fig. 20.3). The ensuing organ damage may then lead to respiratory or metabolic disturbance, or a combination of these, hence to a variety of clinical features. Initial physical examination, therefore, should be directed to determining the magnitude of disturbance of these vital functions and although it must be rapid, it must also be sufficiently comprehensive to detect any coincident disease which may influence the treatment given.

Neurological assessment

In overdoses of hypnotic, sedative and psychotropic drugs, estimation of the level of consciousness is the most important initial part of the neurological assessment. In acute poisoning, drug effects may produce such complex neurological abnormalities that this is most effectively done using a simple grading system such as the Edinburgh coma scale (Table 20.2). In addition, depression of respiratory, circulatory and metabolic function must be assessed.

Respiratory function

A practical and simple screening measurement of respiratory function is measurement of the respiratory minute volume using a Wright spirometer. If the minute volume is less than four litres, significant respiratory depression should be assumed and arterial blood gas analysis undertaken immediately. Accurate monitoring of the respiratory rate is a valuable part of the assessment

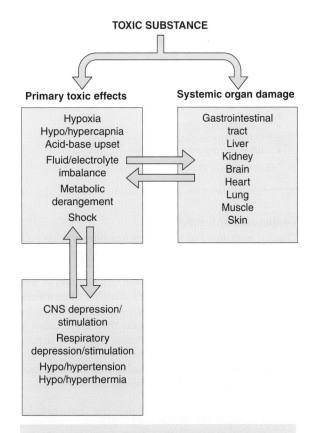

TOXIC SUBSTANCE

Primary toxic effects — Systemic organ damage

Hypoxia
Hypo/hypercapnia
Acid-base upset
Fluid/electrolyte imbalance
Metabolic derangement
Shock

Gastrointestinal tract
Liver
Kidney
Brain
Heart
Lung
Muscle
Skin

CNS depression/stimulation
Respiratory depression/stimulation
Hypo/hypertension
Hypo/hyperthermia

Fig. 20.3 Main ways in which a toxic substance may cause organ damage with resultant functional disturbance.

of respiratory efficiency in poisoned patients. A consistent very high respiratory rate may result in a high minute volume even if only the dead space is ventilated. Both the respiratory rate and the minute volume should be measured at the same time so that a rough measurement of alveolar ventilation may be made. Measurement of arterial blood gases should also be performed as soon as possible (p. 603). Note that, although the anatomical dead space is about 150 ml, this is almost halved by

Table 20.2 Edinburgh Coma Classification: impaired levels of consciousness in patients with acute poisoning

Grade of severity	Definition
0	Fully conscious
1	Drowsy but responsive to vocal command
2	Unconscious but responsive to minimal painful stimuli
3	Unconscious but just responsive to strong painful stimuli
4	Unconscious with no response to stimuli

insertion of an endotracheal tube. The information box below lists conditions to consider.

RESPIRATORY RATE > 20 PER MINUTE

Consider
- Acidosis
- Acute pulmonary oedema
- Pneumonia (inhalation/hypostatic)
- Adult respiratory distress syndrome *

* Develops 12–48 hours after initial poisoning

Cardiovascular function

Clinical assessment of circulatory function in acute poisoning is often difficult since the typical features of shock may not be apparent in the presence of central nervous depression and hypothermia. True shock occurs in less than 10% of all cases of acute poisoning but when it does occur it poses a severe threat to the patient's recovery. In practice it is reasonable to assume that shock exists if the systolic blood pressure falls below 90 mmHg in patients over the age of 50 and below 80 mmHg in younger patients. The procedures for dealing with shocked patients are listed in the information box below.

MONITORING OF ALL 'SHOCKED' PATIENTS

- Core/peripheral temperature deficit measured (low reading rectal thermometer) as guide to adequacy of tissue perfusion
- Fluid intake and urine output measured (indwelling urinary catheter attached to urimeter) as guide to renal perfusion
- Continuous ECG monitoring to detect cardiac arrhythmias

Depression of metabolism is a common feature of many types of overdosage. Moderate hypothermia is present when the rectal temperature is 30–36°C and below 30°C this is potentially life-threatening as the body temperature in these circumstances tends to fall progressively unless active reheating is given. Hypothermia is a significant finding as it contributes to shock, acidosis and hypoxia. In severely poisoned patients electrolyte balance should be monitored by appropriate biochemical testing.

GENERAL PRINCIPLES OF TREATMENT

Specific antidotes are available in only about 2% of acute poisonings (Table 20.3). Some of these cause significant

Table 20.3 Poisonings for which there are specific drug therapies

Poisoning	Antidote	
Benzodiazepines	Flumazenil	see p. 1137
Cholinesterase inhibitors (organophosphorus insecticides)	Pralidoxime mesylate Obidoxime Atropine	see p. 1143
Cyanide	Dicobalt edetate Sodium nitrite Sodium thiosulphate	see p. 1140
Gold, mercury, arsenic, copper, zinc	Dimercaprol 2.5–5 mg/kg body weight by deep i.m. injection every 4 hours for 2 days; 2.5 mg/kg body weight twice daily for 7–14 days	
	Penicillamine 250 mg–2 g daily orally in divided doses	
Iron	Desferrioxamine	see p. 1142
Lead (inorganic)	Sodium calcium edetate 50–75 mg/kg body weight by slow i.v. injection daily for 5 days (each 2 g being diluted with 250 ml isotonic saline)	
	Penicillamine	see above
Opiates and analogues	Naloxone	see p. 1136
Paracetamol	Methionine N-acetylcysteine	see p. 1133
Thallium	Prussian blue 10 g twice daily until urinary excretion of thallium < 0.5 mg per 24 hours	

side-effects and therefore they should be used only where the patient has serious and possibly life-threatening poisoning. Treatment in the great majority of cases, therefore, is dependent on the application of basic but good quality modern intensive therapy on a background of careful clinical assessment, coupled with a sound knowledge of the poison involved. Although the mortality in hospital is low, there are many 'near misses' in those who subsequently recover and so patients with significant poisoning should be regarded as genuine medical emergencies.

EMERGENCY MEASURES

These are listed in the information boxes.

Prevention of absorption of the poison

Patients with inhalant poisoning must be removed to fresh air as quickly as possible, but rescuers should under no circumstances expose themselves to toxic gases without care for their own safety and, if necessary, use appropriate breathing apparatus. When a liquid or solid poison capable of cutaneous absorption is in contact with the

ESTABLISHMENT AND MAINTENANCE OF A CLEAR AIRWAY

- Remove dentures, debris and secretions from the mouth and fauces
- If patient drowsy but has good cough and gag reflex, nurse semi-prone and if possible insert oropharyngeal airway. The neck should be extended
- If more deeply unconscious and gag reflex in doubt, insert cuffed endotracheal tube. In this case the neck should be slightly flexed
- Keep airway patent by regular aspiration of secretions
- Tracheostomy should be considered only if endotracheal intubation is required for longer than 7–10 days

MAINTENANCE OF RESPIRATION

- If PaO_2 is <10 but >8 kPa and the $PaCO_2$ is between 5.3 and 6.6 kPa, high-flow oxygen (6–8 l per minute) should be given. In patients with suspected or known chronic obstructive airways disease use initially 24% Ventimask with an oxygen flow rate of 4 litres per minute. Provided the $PaCO_2$ has not risen after 30 minutes, higher concentrations of oxygen may be given
- In the presence of more serious impairment of ventilation as indicated by a rising $PaCO_2$, administer high-flow oxygen using an Ambu bag as an emergency measure whilst arranging intubation and more formal mechanical ventilation (p. 331)

MAINTENANCE OF CIRCULATION

'Shocked' patients
Correct hypoxia
Correct acidosis
Elevate foot of bed
If no response, institute further measures (p. 215)

In serious cardiac arrhythmias
Correct hypoxia
Correct acidosis
Administer anti-arrhythmic drugs* (p. 234)

Intensive cardio-respiratory resuscitation may be required (p. 233 onwards)

*Particular attention must be given to the pharmacological actions of the poisoning to avoid adverse reactions to the anti-arrhythmic therapy.

patient's clothes these must be removed and any poison on the skin washed off carefully with soap and water. Care should also be taken during these procedures to avoid personal contamination. When the poison has been swallowed, measures to limit further absorption of ingested poisons include the following.

Oral adsorbents

Activated charcoal given with water can be usefully used when emesis and gastric aspiration and lavage are contraindicated, and also as an adjunct to these procedures. It can bind many poisons in the stomach and so reduce their absorption. It should be given as soon as possible after the poison is taken but can be effective up to 4 hours and longer with modified-release preparations. In the case of emesis, the vomiting should be over before the charcoal is given. The effective ratio of charcoal to estimated amount of poison to be adsorbed is of the order of 10:1. It is therefore most useful when the poison ingested is toxic in small doses. Repeated doses of activated charcoal by mouth can enhance the elimination of some drugs, as shown in the following information box. The usual dose is 50 g initially then 25 g 4-hourly.

INDICATIONS FOR USE OF REPEAT DOSES OF ACTIVATED CHARCOAL

After overdose of
- Salicylate
- Carbamazepine
- Dapsone
- Digoxin
- Barbiturates
- Phenytoin
- Quinine
- Theophylline

Induction of emesis

The oral administration of syrup of ipecacuanha paediatric BPC has gained popularity in the treatment of poisoned patients as a means of effective gastric emptying. The effective dosage regimen is 10 ml in children aged 6–18 months, 15 ml in older children and 30 ml in adults. This should be followed by a drink of 200 ml water. The dosage may be repeated after 20 minutes if emesis has not occurred. This is the treatment of choice in young children in whom gastric emptying is indicated, but its use should be reserved for hospital practice in view of the danger of aspiration pneumonia. The indications for this treatment and gastric lavage are listed in the following information box.

Gastric aspiration and lavage

The technique of gastric aspiration and lavage is described in the information box.

Other methods of elimination of poisons

If considerable absorption has occurred the patient may be gravely ill; hence more active measures to enhance elimination of the poison may be required. These can

INDICATIONS FOR INDUCED EMESIS AND GASTRIC LAVAGE

Induction of emesis
- Use only in conscious patients with good gag reflex and within 4 hours of ingestion of a potentially toxic dose of poison. In salicylate poisoning the interval is 24 hours and in tricyclic antidepressant overdose, 12 hours
- Contraindicated with petroleum distillates due to the danger of aspiration into the lungs
- Contraindicated following ingestion of corrosive substances

Gastric aspiration and lavage
- As for emesis except:
- Perform in all unconscious patients irrespective of time since ingestion, since the dose taken is clearly toxic and, therefore, gastric motility and emptying may be considerably impaired. This is provided the airway has been protected by insertion of an endotracheal tube. Take special care in chronic alcoholics and patients with chronic liver disease in view of the danger of rupture of oesophageal varices
- In a very few corrosive poisonings, e.g. paraquat, the danger of systemic toxicity is so high that cautious lavage may be considered

TECHNIQUE OF GASTRIC ASPIRATION AND LAVAGE

- Proceed only if there is a good cough reflex or if a cuffed endotracheal tube has been inserted
- Place the patient recumbent in the left lateral position (Fig. 20.4)
- Pass a lubricated large bore disposable plastic Jacques tube (36–40 French gauge). The position of the tube may be checked by aspiration of gastric content or by blowing a small amount of air down the tube and auscultating over the epigastrium
- Aspirate by lowering the free end of the tube, to which a large funnel is attached, below the level of the patient. If required for toxicological analysis, collect 50 ml of the fluid aspirated or of the first lavage cycle
- Lavage is carried out by pouring 300 ml portions of warm water slowly down the tube and syphoning as for aspiration until the recovered fluid is clear. Care should be taken to empty the stomach as far as possible after each lavage

be carried out only in hospital because of the technical skill and special apparatus required. They include forced diuresis (p. 1135), peritoneal dialysis, haemodialysis and haemoperfusion. In recent years attempts have been made to develop safer ways of increasing removal of toxic substances from the body. The most effective of these is haemoperfusion whereby heparinised blood from the patient is passed through a column containing granules of activated charcoal coated with synthetic acrylic hydrogel or, alternatively, ion exchange resins. This method may be life-saving for some severe poisonings, such as those due to medium- and short-acting barbiturates, glutethimide, methacholine and meprobamate, for which previous techniques of elimination were inadequate. It is indicated, however, only in seriously ill patients in whom intensive supportive therapy fails.

Additional supportive therapy

Hypothermia is common in severely poisoned patients. In moderate cases (p. 1130) the aim of treatment is to prevent further heat loss by nursing the patient covered in a space blanket in a humid but warm room between 26 and 29°C. In severe hypothermia, where the above treatment is ineffective, active heating is required. This may provoke serious cardiac arrhythmias and irreversible peripheral circulatory failure and so should be done with caution, especially in elderly patients. Reheating may be achieved by heating the inspired air by passing administered oxygen through a Water's canister, or by immersing one forearm in water at 43°C in addition to the above measures. Intravenous fluids should be brought to warm room temperature prior to infusion. Acid-base disturbances should be corrected and fluid and electrolyte balance achieved by appropriate replacement therapy. Epileptiform convulsions should be treated with intravenous diazepam (pp. 1070–1071).

PSYCHIATRIC ASSESSMENT

It is important to recognise that the management of poisoned patients, particularly the very large majority who are suffering from self-poisoning, is incomplete without early and adequate psychiatric assessment and management. It is established that the size and severity of the overdose bear little relation to the degree of the underlying psychological or sociological upset (Table 20.4)

Table 20.4 Psychiatric disposal of patients admitted with acute poisoning related to the depth of coma (Edinburgh classification) at the time of admission

Psychiatric disposal	Grade of coma		
	0–2 (%)	3 (%)	4 (%)
In-patient psychiatric care	20	31	28
Out-patient psychiatric care	36	38	34
Other (e.g. GP, social care)	44	31	38

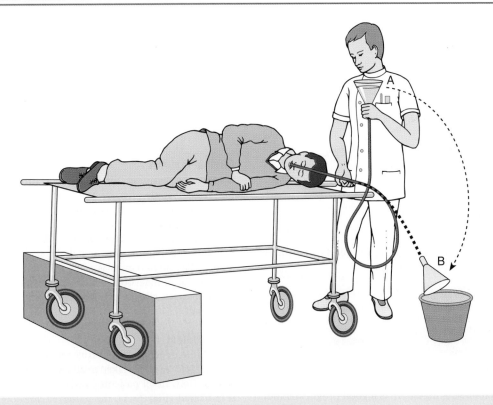

Fig. 20.4   Position of patient for gastric emesis and gastric aspiration and lavage.

Ideally the psychiatrist should become involved as quickly as possible before the circumstances of the poisoning are obscured or rationalised. In reality, however, the numbers of patients presenting with acute poisoning are now so great that it has become necessary to try to be more selective in the patients actually admitted to hospital for this reason.

The recognition of patients who have genuine suicidal tendencies, or may be in need of other help in association with their poisoning, is difficult in practice, particularly for young and inexperienced doctors in Accident and Emergency Departments. There is no problem if the patient is significantly poisoned as all of these require admission for physical as well as psychiatric assessment. The difficulty arises when the patient shows only minimal signs of acute poisoning and, from the history, there is little likelihood of any physical signs appearing later. The risk of repetition and possibly suicide remains and the decision for admission or not has to be made. Where there is any doubt, however, it is wise for the patient to be admitted to hospital.

CLINICAL FEATURES AND MANAGEMENT OF COMMON ACUTE POISONINGS

PARACETAMOL (ACETAMINOPHEN)

This drug is remarkably safe in therapeutic doses and most cases of poisoning are deliberate. Severe toxicity may occur after the single dose ingestion of as little as 10–15 g (20–30 tablets) in adults and 150 mg/kg in children. The most serious effects are acute liver failure and, less commonly, renal tubular necrosis. The cause of the liver damage is the formation of a highly reactive metabolite (N-acetyl-*p*-benzoquinonimine) which binds to vital cell membrane enzymes. Hepatic glutathione normally inactivates this metabolite but in paracetamol poisoning the glutathione becomes depleted. The administration of precursors such as acetylcysteine and methionine is highly effective in restoring the levels of glutathione and preventing or reducing liver damage. As a result of many studies it has been found that a single plasma paracetamol level, after 4 hours and up to

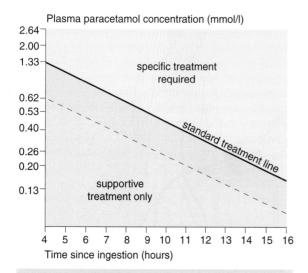

Plasma paracetamol concentration (mmol/l)

specific treatment required

standard treatment line

supportive treatment only

Time since ingestion (hours)

Fig. 20.5 **Graph for prediction of hepatic toxicity in acute paracetamol poisoning in relation to plasma paracetamol concentrations as an indication for the use of specific protective treatment.** Dotted line represents treatment line in patients on regular enzyme-inducing drugs including alcohol (see information box).

16 hours following ingestion, is a good prognostic indicator for the development of liver damage. The risk of this complication is increased 60% when levels are above the standard treatment line (Fig. 20.5). Emergency measurement of blood levels is essential, therefore, in the assessment of this poisoning.

INDICATIONS FOR ACETYLCYSTEINE THERAPY

- Antidote treatment is effective in protecting the liver when a single plasma paracetamol level is above the standard treatment line (Fig. 20.5)
- Patients taking regular enzyme inducing drugs (e.g. carbamazepine, phenytoin, rifampicin, phenobarbitone and alcohol) are at higher risk of liver damage and should be treated at plasma paracetamol levels half as great as the standard treatment line (Fig. 20.5)
- It is still worth giving antidote in all patients who have taken a potentially dangerous overdose (more than 150 mg/kg) and who present 16–24 hours later. Treatment may be stopped 24 hours after ingestion if the patient has escaped clear evidence of liver or renal damage

---

Despite this, paracetamol poisoning is the commonest cause of acute liver failure in the UK and is a major cause of death due to poisoning. The development of liver damage is best assessed by measurement of the prothrombin time, serum creatinine concentration and blood pH. More than 36 hours after overdose a poor prognosis is indicated as outlined in the information box.

PARACETAMOL POISONING: INDICATIONS OF POOR PROGNOSIS

- INR above 3.0, Prothrombin time >36 s
- Serum creatinine >200 μmol/l
- Blood pH below 7.3
- Clinical signs of encephalopathy

Clinical features

Nausea and vomiting, the only early features of poisoning, usually settle after 24 hours. If they persist longer and are accompanied by right hypochondrial pain, liver necrosis is likely. After about 36 hours in severe poisoning, more severe toxic effects may develop, including hypotension, hypothermia, metabolic acidosis and renal failure. The main danger is acute liver failure (maximal 3–5 days after ingestion) which may result in encephalopathy, haemorrhage, hypoglycaemia, cerebral oedema and death.

Management

In addition to general supportive measures, gastric emptying should be undertaken in all patients within 4 hours of ingestion. In all patients in whom specific treatment is indicated (Fig. 20.5), the preferred antidote is intravenous acetylcysteine. This is given in an initial dose of 150 mg/kg in 200 ml glucose 5% over 15 minutes, followed by serial infusions of 50 mg/kg in 500 ml glucose 5% in 4, 8 and 8 hours (total 300 mg/kg in 20 hours).

Oral methionine is an alternative. It is substantially cheaper than acetylcysteine, but its absorption is unreliable in patients who are vomiting. Its success as an antidote is, therefore, less certain and it has not been shown to be effective more than 12 hours following the overdose. The dosage regimen is 2.5 g orally every 4 hours for 4 doses.

If there is evidence of likely severe liver damage, full medical prophylaxis to combat liver failure must be started. These patients may be candidates for liver transplantation (p. 534) and advice should be sought from a specialist liver centre. Current indications for liver transplantation following paracetamol overdose are either (i) an arterial pH of <7.3 (or pH <7.25 if N-acetylcysteine has been given) or (ii) the combination of grade III/IV encephalopathy, serum creatinine >300 μmol/l and a prothrombin time of >100 s. Those who develop severe liver damage and recover do not suffer long-term sequelae.

SALICYLATES

Although the incidence of acute salicylate overdose has fallen in recent years (p. 1126) it continues to be an important cause of poisoning. The clinical features are usually unimpressive even in serious overdose and so emergency measurement of blood levels is essential in assessing the severity of the poisoning. Young children are more susceptible to the toxic effects than adults, mainly due to the complex and altering metabolic disturbances which occur. In all patients there is a mixed acid-base upset due to a combination of respiratory alkalosis and metabolic acidosis. In adults the former tends to predominate, whereas in children acidaemia is the main and persistent acid-base abnormality. The toxicity of salicylates is due to the amount of free salicylate in the body, and the urinary excretion of the free form of drug increases in relation to the alkalinity of the urine. This forms the rationale for the highly effective forced alkaline diuresis therapy described below.

Severe toxicity can be expected if the patient has taken 50 or more 300 mg tablets in a single dose and a plasma salicylate level of 50 mg/100 ml (3.6 mmol/1) in adults indicates moderate or severe toxicity. If, however, the salicylate has been ingested more than 12 hours previously a considerable quantity of active drug may have been taken up by the tissues and the plasma level may be misleadingly low. In these circumstances, the determination of arterial blood pH, blood gases and serum potassium are better indications of the severity of the poisoning.

Clinical features

This poisoning may result in formidable fluid, electrolyte and acid-base upsets. The main toxic effects are described in the following information box.

CLINICAL FEATURES OF ACUTE SALICYLATE OVERDOSE

- Coma is common in children, but in adults occurs only in severe poisoning
- Tinnitus, deafness and blurring of vision are common
- Vomiting, restlessness and sweating may result in severe dehydration
- Hyperventilation causes an initial respiratory alkalosis which is often followed by a metabolic acidosis which may be intense, especially in children
- Hypokalaemia is common due to acid-base shifts
- Marked acidosis should be regarded as a grave complication as it may herald the sudden development of acute pulmonary oedema and respiratory or cardiac arrest

---

Management

Management is mainly directed towards prevention of further absorption, and removal of the salicylate from the body. In addition to general supportive measures, gastric emptying should always be undertaken up to 24

hours after ingestion (p. 1132). Activated charcoal 100 g should be left in the stomach after lavage and, if tolerated, given orally (50 g) every 4 hours thereafter until recovery (p. 1131).

In mild cases (plasma level below 2.2 mmol/l), where there is usually little vomiting, patients should be simply encouraged to drink freely. In more serious poisoning (plasma salicylate above 2.2 mmol/l in children and above 3.6 mmol/l in adults) active measures to remove absorbed salicylate are required. The method of choice is forced alkaline diuresis, the regimen for which is shown as follows.

MANAGEMENT REGIMEN FOR FORCED ALKALINE DIURESIS

Intravenous infusion of:
saline 0.9%
dextrose 5% } 500 ml in rotation
sodium bicarbonate 1.26%

- In adults these solutions should be given at a rate of 2 l/hour for 3 hours and 500 ml/hour thereafter until the plasma salicylate is below 2.2 mmol/l; in young children the infusion rate is 30 ml/kg/hour and should continue until the blood level is below 1.0 mmol/l
- 1 g potassium chloride should be added to each 500 ml unit from the sixth unit in the infusion regimen
- Careful monitoring of fluid replacement, electrolyte and acid-base status is essential

---

If forced alkaline diuresis is not possible because of renal or cardiac impairment, haemodialysis is effective.

NON-STEROIDAL ANTI-INFLAMMATORY DRUGS

This is a varied group of compounds (p. 897). There are many preparations available and they are prescribed for a wide range of common conditions. The toxic effects are relatively similar. Mefenamic acid is the most significant one taken in overdose and is liable to cause convulsions.

Clinical features

These are listed in the information box.

Management

General supportive therapy and gastric emptying (p. 1132) if within 4 hours of ingestion. After gastric lavage, leave 100 g activated charcoal in the stomach and give oral activated charcoal 50 g every 4 hours until recovery. Convulsions can be controlled by intravenous diazepam.

OPIUM ALKALOIDS

The narcotic analgesics include codeine, dihydrocodeine, dextropropoxyphene, buprenorphine, dipipanone, pentazocine, pethidine, methadone, morphine and heroin. As they are drugs of addiction, they are often in the possession of individuals who are involved in the illicit drug scene and are prone to take overdoses. Drug tolerance, particularly in addicts, may be present to a marked degree and so assessment of the severity of the poisoning largely depends on the individual clinical response of the patient.

Clinical features

These are similar for the whole group of drugs, but the severity of the toxic effects depends on the potency of the preparation taken. Respiratory depression is the usual mode of death in fatal poisonings.

Management

Naloxone is a true antidote for narcotic overdose. It acts rapidly but its effects are short-lasting and so repeat doses may necessary. It is potent and so in patients dependent on narcotics it should be used with caution as it may precipitate acute withdrawal features. At the same time its use can be life-saving and it is also valuable as a diagnostic aid in unconscious patients when the cause of coma is in doubt.

TRICYCLIC ANTIDEPRESSANTS

Tricyclic and related antidepressant drugs in acute overdose have toxic effects as listed below. Many different preparations are available on the market but those in common use are listed (p. 985).

Clinical features

The main toxic effects, which usually appear 1–2 hours after ingestion, usually settle within 18–24 hours.

Management

In view of the complexity of the toxic effects, patients should always be admitted to hospital.

BENZODIAZEPINES

This group of drugs (p. 986) remains a significant cause of acute overdose and, outside hospital, of death due to poisoning (p. 1127). Despite this, in patients admitted to hospital the toxic effects are usually surprisingly mild. However, they often feature in poisoning due to multiple overdose and potentiate the effects of other central nervous system depressants, and may contribute to severe toxicity.

Clinical features

These include impairment of level of consciousness, ataxia, dizziness, hypotension and ventilatory depression, but recovery is usually rapid.

Management

Good general supportive measures are adequate in almost all cases.

An antidote has recently become available in the form of flumazenil given intravenously 200 μg over 15 seconds then 100 μg at 60-second intervals if required, to a maximum dose of 2 mg provided the patient is under intensive care. Alternatively it may be given by continuous intravenous infusion (100–400 μg/hour) according to response. In acute overdose patients, flumazenil should be used **only as an aid to differential diagnosis** and only with expert advice as its use may cause many serious toxic effects.

THEOPHYLLINE

This and related drugs are often prescribed as sustained release formulations and so toxic effects may be delayed. The clinical features and management of theophylline overdose are given in the information boxes.

CLINICAL FEATURES OF THEOPHYLLINE OVERDOSE

- Nausea and vomiting (often severe), abdominal pain, haematemesis and diarrhoea
- Thirst, polyuria, hypokalaemia, hyperventilation and agitation are common
- Cardiac arrhythmias, hypotension, metabolic acidosis and convulsions indicate severe poisoning with a poor prognosis, particularly in the elderly

---

PREVENTION OF ACUTE POISONING

An indication of the size and complexity of the problem has been given in the introduction to this chapter. The scope for preventive action is clear.

MANAGEMENT OF THEOPHYLLINE OVERDOSE

- Urgent gastric lavage and leave activated charcoal 100 g in stomach afterwards and give 50 g orally every 4 hours, if possible, until full recovery to enhance elimination of the drug
- Good intensive supportive care including cardiac monitoring
- Correction of hypokalaemia may require large doses of potassium chloride intravenously with ECG control
- Control agitation and convulsions with i.v. diazepam
- Provided the patient is **not asthmatic**, marked tachycardia and hypokalaemia may be reversed by i.v. propranolol
- In severe poisoning with a plasma level of theophylline above 60 mg/l, haemoperfusion should be considered

---

About 60% of patients consult their doctors in the month prior to taking the overdosage and many do so within a week of their action. Also a considerable number poison themselves again after discharge from hospital or during active treatment for psychiatric conditions such as depression. There can be no doubt, therefore, that doctors can make a very important contribution to the prevention of poisoning by learning to recognise the danger signs of imminent overdosage and take the appropriate preventive action. General practitioners are particularly well placed for this purpose as not only can they assess the personality concerned, but also the social and family circumstances which are often the main cause of the problem. For example, it has become apparent that some poisoning incidents in young children occur as an expression of abuse by their parents. Improvements are required in the social services in order that response to such difficulties should be more immediate and effective.

At all ages a major predisposing factor is the ready availability of medicaments and toxic household products. The major cause of acute poisoning incidents is intentional self-poisoning which, as has been stated, is usually of an impulsive and conscious type. The availability of drugs is particularly relevant in this group.

Another important factor in acute poisoning is that many tablets and capsules are supplied in a variety of attractive colours and shapes, often similar to popular sweets and therefore very appealing to children. The danger is increased by parents who, often with the best intentions, encourage their children to take medicines by suggesting that the tablets are in fact sweets. Also, many potent and dangerous drugs are dispensed as pleasant elixirs and syrups with an increased danger of overdosage in the unwitting youngster. Methods of preventing acute poisoning which have proved of value are listed in the following information box.

In Britain, poison information services answer questions only from members of the medical profession, but experience in other countries suggests that the scope of these services could be widened with benefit to the community. In the United States, for example, poison control centres have provided information and advice direct to the general public and fulfilled a valuable educational role whereby, for example, parents have become more aware of the importance of keeping drugs and household products out of the reach of toddlers. As a result, in many parts of the United States the incidence of childhood poisoning has fallen substantially.

In the recent past the numbers of prescriptions in Britain for sedative and psychotropic drugs has risen in a most dramatic way and there is no reason to suspect that serious psychiatric illness had undergone any major increase in the same time. This suggests that much prescribing of sedative and antidepressant drugs was inappropriate and was given often for psychosocial problems rather than significant psychiatric disorder.

Considering the large number of people involved and the vast range of possible toxic substances used in industry, accidental industrial poisoning is uncommon in Britain. This is largely due to the vigilance and initiative of industrial medical officers and to the effectiveness of legislation which regulates the safe storage, transport and use of potentially toxic substances. Also, many essential processes in industry involving the use of dangerous poisons have been made safer by the introduction of automated mechanical techniques which avoid exposure of workers to the risk.

Inevitably, the management of patients with acute poisoning rests with the medical profession and the social services, and it is easy to criticise their apparent inability to improve the situation. The basic problem, however, lies within the community. Until a more responsible attitude emerges with a willingness to be more supportive towards the emotional problems of individuals, there seems little doubt that acute self-poisoning will continue to be an expression of a plea for help to correct a situation which for the individual has become intolerable.

NOTES ON CLINICAL FEATURES AND TREATMENT OF POISONING AND ENVENOMATION BY SPECIFIC AGENTS

(including common insect stings and poisoning by marine animals, mushrooms, scorpions, snakes, spiders, ticks and vegetables)

The following descriptions are directed primarily towards adults. For children, appropriate adjustments in doses of drugs suggested in treatment regimens would require to be made.

Amphetamine group

Clinical features

Alertness, excitement, tremor and insomnia are common. Confusion, aggressiveness, hallucinations and even homicidal tendencies may occur. Initial excitement may give way to lethargy and depression. Brisk reflexes, tachycardia and hypertension occur and nausea, vomiting, diarrhoea and abdominal colic may be severe. In heavy overdosage convulsions and deep unconsciousness are characteristic.

Management

(1) General measures. (2) Droperidol (5–15 mg) or haloperidol (5–10 mg) by slow intravenous injection are the recommended treatments. Alternatively, chlorpromazine 100 mg intramuscularly. (3) In severe poisoning, forced diuresis using intravenous ammonium chloride to make the urine acid.

Barbiturates

Clinical features

Absorption is unpredictable but drowsiness and coma develop rapidly. The duration of cerebral depression varies greatly with the type of barbiturate taken, the dose and the tolerance of the patient. In general a large dose of short- or medium-acting barbiturate causes more severe poisoning than long-acting phenobarbitone. Changes in the pupils and limb reflexes are very variable and are unreliable guides to the severity of the poisoning. Withdrawal features such as restlessness, insomnia, delirium and convulsions may occur. Ventilatory depression and hypotension may be severe. Hypothermia is common and if severe may be associated with renal failure. Bullous lesions occur in 6% of patients with acute barbiturate overdosage, especially with short- or medium-acting drugs.

Management

(1) General measures with particular emphasis on respiratory and cardiovascular support. (2) Gastric lavage if within 4 hours of ingestion. Leave 5 g activated charcoal in stomach after lavage and, if conscious, 25 g orally every 4 hours. (3) When these measures fail, haemodialysis for phenobarbitone and barbitone, and charcoal haemoperfusion for short- and medium-acting barbiturates.

Beta-adrenoceptor antagonists

Clinical features

Bradycardia and hypotension with low output cardiac failure. Bronchospasm. Cardiorespiratory arrest may occur. Drowsiness, delirium, fits and hallucinations. Hypoglycaemia.

Management

(1) Gastric aspiration and lavage if appropriate and intensive supportive measures. (2) When bradycardia is severe, atropine 0.6–3 mg intravenously (50 μg/kg in children), followed if necessary by isoprenaline 2 mg diluted in 500 ml normal saline or 5% dextrose at a rate of 20–40 drops per minute depending on the response. A cardiac pacemaker should be inserted. (3) If significant hypotension occurs, the inotropic action of glucagon is beneficial—50–150 μg/kg intravenously over 1 minute, followed by an infusion of 1–5 mg/h. In severe cases dobutamine infusion 2.5–20 μg/kg per minute may be effective. (4) For bronchospasm, salbutamol by nebuliser. Intravenous salbutamol or aminophylline may be required. (5) Intravenous glucose for hypoglycaemia.

Carbon monoxide

This is a particularly dangerous poisoning and most deaths occur shortly after exposure due to hypoxia resulting from the formation in the blood of carboxyhaemoglobin. Carbon monoxide has an affinity for haemoglobin 300 times that of oxygen. Acute poisoning now usually results from the inhalation of smoke, car exhaust, incomplete combustion of fuel gases due to faulty heaters or flues, and is a major cause of completed suicide.

Clinical features

The most dangerous effects are on the central nervous system and myocardium. It is important to remember that tissue oedema due to capillary leakage may be delayed hours or days after initial exposure. Agitation, confusion, signs of raised intracranial pressure and deep coma all may occur. Central nervous system damage may become quickly permanent with loss of intellect, personality change, parkinsonism and cerebral infarction. Cardiac arrhythmias, hypotension and myocardial infarction are common. The pink colour of the skin and mucous membranes, so often described, is unusual unless in very severe poisoning. Pallor is more common and skin bullae may develop.

Management

This is very urgent and after emergency measures have been taken, patients should be admitted to hospital as soon as possible. (1) Remove the patient to fresh air and administer 100% oxygen as soon as available. (2) Immediate and efficient cardiorespiratory resuscitation (p. 233) should be given as required and continued until spontaneous respiration starts or there is clear evidence that recovery is impossible. (3) Cerebral oedema can be anticipated in all severe poisonings and is treated by intravenous infusion of mannitol 1 g/kg as a 20% solution over 15 minutes followed by 500 ml dextrose 5% over the next 4 hours. (4) If available, hyperbaric oxygen therapy, which is highly effective in seriously poisoned patients, should be considered if the patient is or has been unconscious or has a carboxyhaemoglobin concentration above 40%.

Cocaine

This is now a common drug of abuse. Acute toxicity may arise following inhalation, ingestion or injection.

Clinical features

Euphoria, excitement, restlessness, feeling of great power, vomiting, pyrexia, mydriasis, delirium, tremor, convulsions, hyperreflexia. Hypertension, hypotension, tachycardia, ventricular arrhythmias, cardiac failure. Hyperventilation and respiratory failure.

Management

Symptomatic and supportive measures. *Note*: Avoid beta-adrenoceptor antagonists to treat hypertension or sinus tachycardia as these cardiac effects tend to be transient and beta-blockade may cause cardiac failure.

Corrosives

Clinical features

Stains and burns of the mouth, lips and fauces. Abdominal pain, shock and hepatic or renal damage.

Management

(1) General measures. (2) Gastric lavage is contraindicated in severe poisoning. (3) Neutralise acid or alkali. Milk by mouth is often the most effective available treatment. (4) Analgesics, blood transfusion and correction of acid-base balance all may be required.

Cyanides and hydrocyanic acid

Clinical features

Odour of bitter almonds with shallow breathing; pink colour of skin and mucosa; widely dilated pupils and shock.

Management

This is very urgent. (1) General measures. (2) Cobalt edetate 600 mg in 20 ml intravenously over 1 minute. (3) If no recovery in the next minute, repeat 300 mg cobalt edetate. (4) If no response to cobalt edetate, give 10 ml i.v. of 3% sodium nitrite solution, followed by 25 ml i.v. of 50% sodium thiosulphate solution. (5) If ingested, gastric lavage with 50% sodium thiosulphate. (6) Correct acidosis with i.v. sodium bicarbonate.

Digoxin (p. 239)

Dinitro-ortho-cresol weedkillers

Clinical features

These may develop very rapidly. Yellow skin and burns of the lips and mouth. Anxiety, restlessness, fatigue, convulsions and coma. Tachypnoea, pulmonary oedema, hyperpyrexia and intense sweating are common. Acute renal and liver failure may result.

Management

(1) Wash exposed skin. (2) Sedation with chlorpromazine 100 mg intramuscularly. (3) General measures. (4) Tepid sponging to reduce temperature.

Domestic bleach

Clinical features

Local irritation if in contact with skin. If inhaled, cough and possible pulmonary oedema. If ingested, burning sensation of mouth and fauces, nausea and vomiting.

Management

(1) Gastric lavage with 2.5% sodium thiosulphate or alternatively with milk. If severely ill, sodium thiosulphate (1%) 250 ml intravenously.

Ethanol

See blood levels, page 1128.

Clinical features

Inebriation. Ataxia and blurred vision. Impaired level of consciousness. Especially in children, severe hypoglycaemia and convulsions, tachycardia and slow respiration.

Management

General supportive measures. Correct hypoglycaemia with i.v. dextrose.

Fish and other marine animals

Poisonous fish are numerous and widely distributed around the world. In some areas they are a common source of poisoning.

CIGUATERA POISONING. This is common, particularly in the Indo-Pacific and the Caribbean. It occurs sporadically after eating reef-dwelling fishes, which are popular items of diet. It is impossible to identify fish which are poisonous from others which are not and the toxins responsible are unaffected by all forms of preparation and cooking. Ciguatoxin is the cause of poisoning and the primary source is thought to be an alga (*Gambierdiscus toxicus*) eaten by herbivorous fish such as parrot fish and surgeon fish. Ultimately carnivorous fish such as barracuda also become poisonous.

Clinical features

The onset of symptoms is usually 1–6 hours after eating toxic fish, but may vary from a few minutes to 30 hours. Numbness and paraesthesiae of the lips, tongue and throat are common, followed by abdominal pain, diarrhoea, headache, arthralgia and myalgia. In 20% of patients, dyspnoea, hypotension and paresis occur.

Management

Principally symptomatic with bed-rest and analgesics. Most patients recover after about 3 days, but sometimes arthralgia and myalgia may be prolonged.

SCROMBOID FISH POISONING. The flesh of scromboid fish, such as mackerel, tuna, bonito and skipjack, has a high free histidine content. Many bacteria decarboxylate histidine to histamine, and if fish become contaminated by these organisms, large amounts of histamine accumulate in the flesh.

Clinical features

Flushing, headache, dizziness, abdominal cramps and symptoms of gastroenteritis occur. These usually develop 30 minutes after ingestion and the upset lasts for about 4 hours.

Management

Symptomatic.

SHELLFISH POISONING. Paralytic shellfish poisoning results from eating filter-feeding shellfish such as mussels, clams, oysters and scallops contaminated by the toxic protozoa, *Gonyaulax catanella* and *G. tamarensis*. The neurotoxin involved is called saxitoxin. These protozoa tend to colour the sea when present in numbers and fishing communities are well aware that it is dangerous to eat molluscs when the tide is red, blue or green. Food poisoning due to infected shellfish is described on pages 123–124.

Clinical features

Circumoral paraesthesiae, a 'floating' feeling, headache, nausea, vomiting and diarrhoea are common with, in severe cases, weakness, dysarthria and respiratory depression.

Management

(1) Gastric aspiration and lavage. (2) Symptomatic and supportive therapy. A less severe, but similar, poisoning results from eating shellfish contaminated by another dinoflagellate, *Gymnodinium breve*. The resultant illness is self-limiting, requiring only symptomatic treatment.

TETRODOTOXIC POISONING. This is generally known as 'puffer fish poisoning'. These fish are found in all warm and tropical seas. In Japan the detoxicated puffer fish ('fugu') is a popular delicacy. The mortality is as high as 50% because tetrodotoxin is one of the most powerful neurotoxins known.

Clinical features

Early symptoms are circumoral paraesthesiae, malaise, hypotension, dizziness and a feeling of 'floating in air'. In severe poisoning, ataxia, dysphagia and profound descending neuromuscular paralysis develop.

Management

Symptomatic, as there is no known antidote.

VENOMOUS MARINE ANIMALS. Serious illness from venomous marine creatures is rare in temperate waters. Poisoning by sea snakes is described under snake bites.

VENOMOUS FISH. Although many species occur, only two major groups are of real significance, the sting-rays

and scorpion fishes. All sting-rays inhabit warm or tropical coastal waters with the exception of one fresh water variety in South America. These fish will sting only if stood upon by mistake. Scorpion fish include the zebra fishes, the true scorpion fishes and the stone fishes. The spines of these fish are their offensive weapons and they are all capable of aggressive stinging. The stone fishes are particularly poisonous and zebra fishes are becoming popular for domestic aquaria.

Clinical features

Immediate intense pain and swelling at the site of the sting. Severe tissue necrosis may occur and systemic features include nausea, vomiting and diarrhoea. Cardiac arrhythmias may occur.

Management

(1) Analgesics and local anaesthesia if pain severe. (2) Careful cleansing of the wound and surgical removal of the sting sheath if it has been retained. (3) The venoms are heat-labile and if possible the wound should be immersed in water as hot as can be borne, for 1 hour. (4) In the case of stone fish, antivenoms are available.

VENOMOUS MOLLUSCS. Only two members of this very large species are venomous to man. These are the cone shells and the octopuses. The cone shells are not uncommon causes of poisoning as the colourful shells are eagerly collected. These predatory gastropods catch their prey by shooting out a dart-like tooth attached to a muscular venom gland. The only octopuses of importance are the small blue ringed octopuses of Australia which have toxic saliva and this may flow into wounds made by the beak of the octopus.

Clinical features

There is a local inflammatory response with generalised paraesthesiae. This is rapidly followed by muscular paresis which in severe poisoning may result in respiratory failure. Fatalities have occurred.

Management

Symptomatic and supportive therapy.

VENOMOUS COELENTERATA. These include the hydroids, jellyfish, sea anemones and corals. Although many of these animals may cause painful and at times disfiguring stings, few fatalities have resulted. The most important are the Portuguese man-of-war (*Physalia physalis*), sea wasps (*Cubomedusae*) and the true jellyfishes *Chironex fleckeri* and *Chiropsalmus quadrigatus*. Some authors suggest that only *Chironex* should be considered truly lethal. The precise toxins are not yet fully identified but haemolytic, dermatonecrotic and cardiotoxic substances have all been isolated.

Clinical features

All species cause intense pain at the site of envenomation and large wheals appear which may become necrotic, leading to extensive scar formation. Severe abdominal and generalised pains may result. In severe poisoning the patient rapidly loses consciousness with cyanosis and hypotension. Death may occur quickly or be delayed for some hours.

Management

(1) Analgesics and local anaesthesia if pain severe. (2) Any tentacles must be carefully removed with adhesive tape. The bare hand should not be used as the tentacles may still be capable of causing stings for many hours after removal from the water. Vinegar can be used to inactivate adhering tentacles, but alcohol solutions should not be used as this may stimulate further stinging. (3) Antivenom for sea-wasp stings is available.

At certain seasons 'Irukandji stings' affect bathers in the sea off N.E. Australia. They are caused by minute *Carybdeid* (simple sea-wasps). Acute poisoning develops in a few minutes characterised by violent abdominal and generalised pains, vomiting and prostration. After a few days of acute illness, full recovery always occurs.

Insect stings

Stings from ants, wasps, hornets and bees result only in local pain and swelling, unless the sting is on the mouth or tongue when local oedema may cause respiratory distress. Occasionally deaths may result from very extensive stings or more commonly due to severe anaphylaxis in individuals previously sensitised particularly to bee stings.

Clinical features

(1) Local pain and oedema. (2) Severe cases may become shocked; local tissue necrosis, acute haemolysis and acute nephritis may occur.

Management

Bee stings are acid and wasp, hornet and ant stings are alkaline. Local application is soothing, e.g. bicarbonate for bee, vinegar for wasp; systemic antihistamines may be helpful. The barbed bee stings should be removed as soon as possible as the gland attached continues to release venom. In severe sensitivity reactions, subcutaneous adrenaline (0.5 ml) and hydrocortisone (100 mg) intravenously may be life-saving. Allergic patients should carry adrenaline for immediate self-injection. In some, desensitisation has proved helpful.

See also scorpion, spider and tick.

Iron salts

Clinical features

These are more severe in children but this poisoning is potentially dangerous at all ages. It occurs in four stages. The predominant initial features are epigastric pain, nausea and vomiting. Haematemesis is frequent and may cause shock. Respiration and pulse are rapid. These symptoms may settle after a few hours and there may then be a quiescent period lasting for up to several days, suggesting that all is well, but then frequent black and offensive stools may be passed and acute encephalopathy and circulatory failure may follow. Most deaths occur in this second stage, but even if the patient survives, acute liver and renal failure may develop later and both carry a high mortality. Particularly in children, 2–6 weeks after ingestion, stricture formation may occur in the upper gastrointestinal tract, especially in the pyloric antrum, with vomiting and other features of high intestinal obstruction. A serum iron concentration > 90 μmol/l indicates the need for treatment.

Management

Speed is essential. (1) An intramuscular injection of 2 g desferrioxamine is given immediately (1 g in a child). (2) Gastric lavage is performed, following which 5 g desferrioxamine is left in the stomach. (3) This is followed by an intravenous infusion of desferrioxamine in saline, dextrose or blood. The amounts should not exceed 15 mg/kg body weight per hour up to a maximum of 80 mg/kg in 24 hours. (4) Full supportive treatment for convulsions, shock, acidosis, blood loss and electrolyte disturbance.

Lithium carbonate/citrate

Clinical features

Nausea, vomiting, apathy and sluggishness. Coarse tremor, hypertonicity, vertigo, dysarthria, muscular rigidity and twitching, ataxia, convulsions. Hepatic dysfunction. ECG changes including first degree AV block, prolongation of QRS and QT intervals.

Management

(1) Gastric emesis or lavage, if appropriate. (2) Supportive therapy. (3) Peritoneal or haemodialysis if plasma level > 5 mmol/l. Haemodialysis is the more effective. Continue dialysis till plasma lithium level is < 1 mmol/l. *Note*: Forced diuresis is ineffective.

Mushrooms

Serious poisoning is uncommon in Britain. Considering the many types of fungi, a relatively small number are poisonous. The difficulty is that identification of these harmful species is not easy and often dangerous mushrooms grow in the same places as edible varieties. The commonest types of mushroom poisoning result from eating species containing heat-labile toxins, many of which have not been identified. These cause acute and sometimes severe abdominal colic with diarrhoea, nausea and vomiting developing about 2 hours after ingestion. Occasionally the features are those of muscarine toxicity with parasympathetic stimulation which can be counteracted with atropine 0.6–2.0 mg i.v. in the adult. If the patient is excited or disorientated, atropine should not be given and chlorpromazine prescribed instead. The Common Ink Cap (*Coprinus atramentarius*) contains coprine which has a disulfiram-like action and, if taken with alcohol, provokes acute vomiting.

A trend amongst adolescents has been to ingest 'Magic' mushrooms (*Psilocybe semilanceate*) and *Panaeolus foenisecii* containing psilocybin and psilocin, which are hallucinogens. The amount required to obtain a 'trip' varies greatly from individual to individual and so some develop acute toxic effects. Acute gastroenteritis may result with visual hallucinations lasting up to 6 hours. Occasionally the symptoms last for several days and acute psychiatric upset has been reported continuing for weeks.

DEATH CAP (*AMANITA PHALLOIDES*). This mushroom accounts for 90% of all deaths due to mushroom poisoning in Britain. It contains two types of toxin; phallotoxins, which cause severe gastroenteritis within 6–12 hours of ingestion, and amatoxins, which also may cause gastric upset, but the major effect is delayed and results in liver and renal tubular damage. These toxins are heat-stable and may survive cooking.

Clinical features

After an initial delay of 6–12 hours and occasionally as long as 24 hours, acute and usually severe gastroenteritis with abdominal colic. The patient may then seem to improve before the onset of liver and renal damage.

Management

(1) If possible the mushrooms eaten should be identified, ideally by an expert in mushrooms. It is useful to remember that the later the onset of abdominal symptoms, the more likely it is to be a serious poisoning. (2) Gastric aspiration and lavage. (3) Careful medical care for liver and renal failure if these develop. Haemodialysis and haemoperfusion are ineffective in removing the toxins but the former may be required for renal failure and the latter for liver failure.

Other species of mushroom which produce similar toxic effects to *A. phalloides* are the North American

Deadly Agaric (*A. verna*), *A. virosa* and some types of *Galerina*.

Organophosphorus compounds

Clinical features

These insecticides are very toxic. Being cholinesterase inhibitors, the symptoms and rationale of treatment are explained by excess cholinergic activity. Clinical features include constricted pupils, cold perspiration, salivation, nausea, vomiting and diarrhoea; twitching, which may go on to convulsions, bradycardia, bronchospasm, intense bronchorrhoea and pulmonary oedema.

Management

(1) Remove contaminated clothing and wash skin, but take care to wear protective gloves. (2) General measures including meticulous care of the airway. (3) Atropine 2 mg intravenously, but if cyanosis is present this must first be corrected by oxygen therapy. The atropine is repeated at 5–10 minute intervals to achieve full atropinisation and this is maintained for at least 2–3 days. (4) Pralidoxime should be given in addition to atropine in a dose of 30 mg/kg intravenously at a rate not exceeding 500 mg per minute and repeated every 30 minutes as necessary. More recently obidoxime 3 mg/kg body weight by intramuscular injection has been reported to be more effective than pralidoxime as it has a faster action and crosses the blood-brain barrier. When these cholinesterase reactivators take effect the dosage of atropine should be reduced to avoid atropine toxicity.

Paraffin and petroleum distillates

Clinical features

Pallor, vomiting and diarrhoea, cough and breathlessness.

Management

(1) Do not wash out stomach (p. 1132). (2) Antibiotics if aspiration has occurred. (3) General measures.

Paraquat dichloride

This herbicide is very toxic in the concentrated liquid form supplied to farmers and horticulturalists. A granular preparation is available for domestic use.

Clinical features

These may be divided into local and systemic effects.

Local: contact with the eyes results in severe corneal and conjunctival inflammation. On the skin, acute irritation and even blistering may occur. If inhaled, epistaxis and severe pharyngitis/laryngitis. Following ingestion, burning sensation in the mouth, oesophagus, and abdomen. Ulceration of the lips, tongue and pharynx. These features may be absent at first but develop gradually over several hours and are usually at a peak within 24 hours.

Systemic: usually follow ingestion and involve multiple organ failure. Nausea, sweating and vomiting. Tremors and convulsions may occur. Some days after ingestion (even up to a week) dyspnoea with pulmonary oedema due to a relentless proliferative alveolitis and bronchitis. Myocardial and renal failure may accompany these changes but often resolve spontaneously or respond to supportive treatment. Methaemoglobinaemia occurs rarely. Death is usually from respiratory failure.

Management

(1) Immediate emesis and gastric lavage leaving 250 ml of a 30% solution of Fuller's Earth, or 7% Bentonite, in the stomach. Repeat doses of Fuller's Earth (or Bentonite) every 4 hours for the following 48 hours. This should be accompanied by regular doses of magnesium (or sodium) sulphate orally to prevent the above adsorbent material causing intestinal obstruction. (2) Supportive treatment with special emphasis on fluid and electrolyte balance. (3) Haemoperfusion or haemodialysis may be of value if started early, in mild or moderately severe poisoning, but do not prevent a fatal outcome in severe cases. (4) Methylene blue 1–2 mg/kg body weight (0.1 ml of a 1% solution/kg body weight) slowly intravenously if methaemoglobinaemia occurs.

Scorpion stings

Many genera of scorpions are found in the tropics and subtropics. Stings can cause dangerous poisoning. In Mexico, for example, 1000 deaths occur per year. Paired poison glands are situated in the terminal segment of the jointed tail.

Clinical features

(1) Intense local pain occurs immediately around the single puncture site, followed by erythema, swelling and sometimes ecchymosis. (2) Severe systemic features may follow, especially in children, such as sweating, salivation, nausea, vomiting and respiratory depression. Cardiac arrhythmias, myocarditis and acute pulmonary oedema may occur. Disseminated intravascular coagulation may occur, and in Trinidad, acute but usually reversible pancreatitis is a feature of stings from the scorpion, *Tityus trinitatis*.

Management

(1) A firm pressure bandage should be applied to limit the spread of the neurotoxic venom. As soon as possible dehydroemetine 1.0–1.5 mg/kg body weight should be given as single therapy by local infiltration at the site of sting, or by i.m. injection. Corticosteroids in addition in severe cases. (2) Analgesics and general supportive therapy. (3) In children, antivenom (5 ml i.m.) should be given if available. (4) Specific treatment of disseminated intravascular coagulation, if present.

Snake bite

In Britain there is only one indigenous poisonous snake, the adder (*Vipera berus*) which seldom causes significant poisoning. Serious snake bites may still occur as dangerous snakes are kept in zoos and by amateurs, often in less than ideal circumstances. There are three families of medically important venomous snakes. All have fangs at the front of their mouths whereby they inject venom from the parotid glands. The *Elapidae* (cobras, mambas, kraits, tiger snakes, and coral snakes) are found in all parts of the world except Europe. They are land snakes and have short fangs, the venom of which produces neurotoxic features. Local tissue necrosis may occur, a feature characteristic of venom of Asian cobras and the African spitting cobra. The *Hydrophidae* (sea snakes), which abound in the Asian-Pacific coastal waters, also have short fangs and characteristic flattened tails. The venom of these snakes is myotoxic. The *Viperidae*, which have long erectile fangs, are divided into *Viperinae* (true vipers) such as the European adder, Russell's viper and carpet viper. These occur in all parts of the world except America and the Asian-Pacific area. The second subgroup is the *Crotalidae* (pit vipers) such as rattlesnakes, Fer-de-lance and Malayan pit viper which have a small heat-sensitive pit between eye and nostrils. The venom of the *Viperidae* is vasculo-toxic.

At least 50% of people bitten by snakes suffer few or no toxic effects as little or no venom has been injected. By contrast if the dose of venom is high, mortality without effective treatment is 10% in *Elapidae* poisoning within 5–20 hours of the bites, 10% for sea snakes within 15 hours and 1–15% in *Viperidae* within 2 days. In the early stages snake bite is very unpredictable and all patients must be carefully monitored for at least 12 hours.

First aid measures

Firm pressure bandaging of the bite area and immobilisation of the part substantially delays spread of the venom. Patients are often very apprehensive and should be reassured and sedated if necessary.

Clinical features

Local pain and fang marks are very variable and of no help in diagnosis.

Viperidae

Local swelling starts almost immediately. This is also a feature of poisoning in bites by Asian cobras and the

African spitting cobra, but may not develop for up to 2 hours. Early signs of systemic poisoning, which may develop within 15 minutes of the bite, include vomiting, hypotension and signs of abnormal bleeding from or into any site. Later signs include increase in local swelling, which may become massive over 48–72 hours with associated bruising. Blister formation around the site of the bite is common and spreading blisters suggest a large dose of venom and may precede necrosis. Local tissue necrosis with an offensive putrid smell is typical of cobra bites. Shock may occur and haemorrhage into a vital organ which is often fatal may occur up to a week after the bite if antivenom has not been given.

Elapidae

There is seldom any local swelling. Vomiting, hypotension and a polymorph leucocytosis suggest systemic envenomation. More specific signs of muscle weakness such as ptosis, glossopharyngeal palsy and cough indicate severe poisoning and may be delayed for 10 hours after the bite. There is a danger of respiratory paralysis, and ECG changes and rises in cardiac enzymes occur.

Hydrophidae

The early features are similar to *Elapidae*. More specific signs are generalised myalgia, with the appearance of myoglobinuria 3–5 hours later. Paresis of the limbs may follow with respiratory paralysis within a few hours of the bite, although it may be delayed for up to 60 hours. Hyperkalaemia may result in cardiac arrest, and acute renal failure may occur.

Management

(1) The site of the bite should be cleansed and then left strictly alone; otherwise the risk of infection is increased. If skin necrosis occurs, sloughs should be excised with skin grafts applied as appropriate. (2) General measures, including intravenous fluids, should be given to support vital functions. (3) Sedatives are required if the patient is apprehensive. (4) Appropriate antitetanus prophylaxis should be given taking account of the patient's immune state. (5) Antivenoms should be given only if there is clear evidence of systemic poisoning. Some local effects, however, especially necrosis, may be avoided or minimised if antivenom is given within 4 hours of the bite. This is the case in bites by Asian cobras, African spitting cobras, puff adders and rattlesnakes. In *V. berus* bites, the only poisonous snake in Britain, adult patients may have prolonged and painful local swelling which can be effectively treated by Zagreb antivenom if given within the first few hours. All antivenoms may cause severe allergic reactions which may be fatal. Appropriate precautions, therefore, are mandatory. The potency of the antivenom should be checked by first making sure that

it is clear and has no opacities. Depending on the severity of poisoning, 20–100 ml antivenom is diluted in 2–3 volumes of isotonic saline. This is then given by slow intravenous infusion (15 drops per minute). Adrenaline (1:1000 solution) must be immediately available. If a reaction occurs the drip is stopped temporarily and 0.5 ml adrenaline injected intramuscularly. Provided the adrenaline is given at the first sign of anaphylaxis, it is rapidly effective and the drip can be restarted with care. Several injections of adrenaline may be indicated. There is marked variation in the requirements of different patients for antivenom. Therefore it is important to give sufficient antivenom to counteract the toxic effects of the poisoning and children require the same doses of antivenom as adults. This is especially important in neurotoxic poisoning.

Spider bite

Only a few genera of spiders are harmful to man. *Lactrodectus* species are found only in warm climates. The Black Widow Spider (*L. mactans*) is the most dangerous and occurs only in the tropics. The Funnel Web Spider (*Atrax robustus*) also quite often causes venomous bites. These spiders are shy, inhabiting dark corners of sheds, basements and foundations of houses and outside privies. Death may occur in up to 6% of cases, especially in young children.

Clinical features

(1) Burning of the bite site. (2) After about 1 hour, generalised muscular pain, which may simulate an acute abdomen, nausea and vomiting. (3) Pyrexia, sweating and shock.

Management

(1) 10–20 ml calcium gluconate (10%) by slow intravenous injection. (2) Analgesics. (3) If severe systemic toxicity give specific antivenom if available.

In the Southern States of America, Central and South America, the Brown Recluse Spider (*Loxosceles reclusa*) and related species may be found in houses and outbuildings. The spider often crawls into clothing and bedclothes. Poisoning is relatively uncommon but important as it results in necrosis at the site of the bite, which is slow to heal. Fever, vomiting and rashes may occur and occasionally haemolysis and thrombocytopenia. Analgesics should be given as required and antihistamines and corticosteroids are considered helpful.

Tick bite

Tick paralysis is due to venom in the saliva of certain hard ticks. Those most likely to cause trouble are the scrub tick, cattle tick and brown dog tick. If such a tick remains attached to the skin for some days there is increasing and spreading paralysis with a danger of respiratory failure, and mechanical ventilation may be required. If the tick is removed in time the patient recovers.

Vegetable toxins

The harmful effects of the ingestion of various bush teas (p. 519) are mentioned elsewhere.

EPIDEMIC DROPSY (ARGEMONE POISONING). This is seen mainly in India and in Indian communities elsewhere when curried dishes are prepared with mustard oil contaminated by extracts from the seeds of the poppy weed, *Argemone mexicana*, which contain the toxin, sanguinarine. This substance interferes with the oxidation of pyruvic acid, which accumulates and causes dilatation of capillaries and small arterioles. Haemangiomas may develop.

Clinical features

Nausea, vomiting, diarrhoea and fever occur followed by the development of peripheral oedema and cardiac failure. There is erythematous mottling of the skin and raised haemangiomas may appear. Severe glaucoma may result.

Management

All contaminated mustard oil must be identified and further exposure avoided. Supportive therapy for cardiac failure is effective, but the response may be slow.

VOMITING SICKNESS OF JAMAICA (ACKEE POISONING). The unripe fruit of the common West Indian and South American tree, *Blighia sapida*, contains a water-soluble toxin, capable of blocking gluconeogenesis in the liver. If eaten, especially by undernourished children, severe and prolonged hypoglycaemia may result. Vomiting, loss of consciousness and convulsions are common. Continuous intravenous infusion of glucose should be started as soon as possible. Without treatment the mortality is high.

Industrial and agricultural poisoning

Lead (p. 60), cyanide (p. 1140), mercury (p. 60), beryllium (p. 386) and cadmium are potential causes of industrial poisoning. In agriculture many highly toxic weedkillers, including paraquat and the dinitro-ortho-cresol group, and organophosphorus insecticides have been developed in recent years. They have been responsible for only a small number of cases of acute poisoning in Britain owing to effective legislation for controlling their use. In some countries, however, they have caused many deaths.

FURTHER READING

Beaumont G 1989 The toxicity of antidepressants. British Journal of Psychiatry 454–458

Diekstra R F 1989 Suicide and the attempted suicide: an international perspective. Acta Psychiatrica Scandinavica 354 Suppl. 1–24

Ferner R 1993 Paracetamol poisoning—an update. Prescriber's Journal 33(2): 45–50

Ilano A L, Raffin T A 1990 Management of carbon monoxide poisoning. Chest 97(1): 165–169

Meredith T J 1994 Epidemiology of poisoning. Pharmacology and Therapeutics 59: 251–256

Morgan H G, Vassilas C A, Owen J H 1990 Managing suicide risk in the general ward. British Journal of Hospital Medicine 44(1): 56–59

Nordentoft M, Breum L, Munck L K, Nordestgaard A G, Hunding A et al 1993 High mortality by natural and unnatural causes: a 10 year follow-up study of patients admitted to a poisoning treatment centre after suicide attempts. British Medical Journal 306: 1637–1640

Platt S, Bille-Brahe U, Kerkhof A, Schmidtke A, Bjerke T et al 1992 Parasuicide in Europe: the WHO/EURO multicentre study on parasuicide. I: Introduction and preliminary analysis for 1989. Acta Psychiatrica Scandinavica 85(2): 97–104

Vale J A, Meredith T J 1986 Acute poisoning due to non-steroidal anti-inflammatory drugs. Clinical features and management. Medical Toxicology 1(1): 12–31

21

Appendices

NOTES ON INTERNATIONAL SYSTEM OF UNITS (SI UNITS)

Examples of basic SI units

Length	metre (m)
Mass	kilogram (kg)
Amount of substance	mole (mol)
Energy	joule (J)
Pressure	pascal (pa)

Examples of decimal multiples and submultiples of SI units

Factor	*Name*	*Symbol*
10^6	mega-	M
10^3	kilo-	k
10^{-1}	deci-	d
10^{-2}	centi-	c
10^{-3}	milli-	m
10^{-6}	micro-	μ
10^{-9}	nano-	n
10^{-12}	pico-	p
10^{-15}	femto-	f

Volume. The basic SI unit of volume is the cubic metre (1000 litres). Because of its convenience the litre is used as the unit of volume in laboratory work.

Amount of substance ('molar') concentration (e.g. mol/l, μmol/l) is used for substances of defined chemical composition. It replaces equivalent concentrations (mEq/l), which is not part of the SI system. For univalent ions such as sodium, potassium, chloride and bicarbonate the numerical value is unchanged. For divalent ions such as calcium and magnesium the numerical value is halved.

Mass concentration (e.g. g/l, μg/l) is used for all protein measurements, for substances which do not have a sufficiently well defined composition and for serum vitamin B_{12} and folate measurements. The numerical value in SI units will change by a factor of 10 in those instances previously expressed in terms of 100 ml.

SI units are not employed for enzymes, nor usually for immunoglobulins.

BIOCHEMICAL VALUES

Reference ranges are largely those used in the Department of Clinical Biochemistry, the Royal Infirmary, University of Edinburgh. These can vary from laboratory to laboratory, depending on the assay method used and other factors; this is especially the case for the enzyme assays. Although the SI system of units is widely used in the UK, *units* of measurement can vary and lead to laboratory differences.

No details are given of the collection requirements which may be critical to obtaining a meaningful result.

Unless otherwise stated, reference ranges apply to adults; **values in children may be different.**

The values quoted for blood, except for Table 21.1, refer to plasma or serum. Serum is preferred for some analyses, especially certain hormones and electrophoretic studies.

Table 21.1   Arterial blood analysis

Analysis	Reference range	Units
Bicarbonate	21–27.5	mmol/l
Hydrogen ion	36–44	nmol/l
$PaCO_2$	4.4–6.1	kPa
PaO_2	12–15	kPa
Oxygen saturation	Normally >97	%

Table 21.2   Cerebrospinal fluid

Analysis	Reference range	Units
Cells	Up to 5 (all mononuclear)	cells/mm³
Chloride	120–170	mmol/l
Glucose	2.5–4.0	mmol/l
IgG index*	<0.65	
Total protein	100–400	mg/l

* A crude index of increase in IgG attributable to intrathecal synthesis

Table 21.3   Reference values in venous plasma for the more common analytes in adults

Analysis	Reference range	Units
α_1-Antitrypsin	1.7–3.2	g/l
Alanine aminotransferase (ALT)	10–40	U/l
Albumin	36–47	g/l
Alkaline phosphatase	40–125	U/l
Amylase	50–300	U/l
Aspartate aminotransferase (AST)	10–35	U/l
Bilirubin (total)	2–17	μmol/l
Calcium	2.12–2.62	mmol/l
Carboxyhaemoglobin	Not normally detectable Up to 1.5% in non-smokers	%
Caeruloplasmin	150–600	mg/l
Chloride	95–107	mmol/l
Cholesterol (total)	[See note 1]	
HDL-Cholesterol	0.5–1.6 (M) 0.6–1.9 (F)	mmol/l
Copper	13–24	μmol/l
Creatine kinase (MB isoenzyme)	Normally <6% of total CK	

Table 21.3 continued

Creatine kinase (total)	30–200 (M)	U/l
	30–150 (F)	
Ethanol	Not normally detectable	mmol/l
	65–87	
	(marked intoxication)	
	87–109	
	(stupor)	
	>109	
	(coma)	
Creatinine	55–150	μmol/l
Ferritin	15–350 (M)	μg/l
	8–300 (F)	
Gamma-glutamyl transferase (GGT)	10–55 (M)	U/l
	5–35 (F)	
Glucose (fasting)[2]	3.6–5.8	mmol/l
Glycated haemoglobin (HbA$_1$)	4.5–8	%
Immunoglobulin A	0.5–4.0	g/l
Immunoglobulin G	5.0–13.0	g/l
Immunoglobulin M	0.3–2.2 (M)	g/l
	0.4–2.5 (F)	
Iron	14–32 (M)	μmol/l
	10–28 (F)	
Iron binding capacity	45–72	μmol/l
Lactate	0.4–1.4	mmol/l
Lactate dehydrogenase (total)	230–460	U/l
Lactate dehydrogenase (urea-stable)	100–300	U/l
Lead[3]	<1.7	μmol/l
Magnesium	0.75–1.0	mmol/l
Osmolality	280–290	mmol/kg
Phosphate (fasting)	0.8–1.4	mmol/l
Potassium (plasma)	3.3–4.7	mmol/l
Potassium (serum)	3.6–5.1	mmol/l
Protein (total)	60–80	g/l
Sodium	132–144	mmol/l
Total CO$_2$	24–30	mmol/l
Transferrin	2.0–4.0	g/l
Triglycerides (fasting)	0.6–1.7	mmol/l
Urate	0.12–0.42 (M)	mmol/l
	0.12–0.36 (F)	
Urea	2.5–6.6	mmol/l
Zinc	11–22	μmol/l

Notes

1. Cholesterol (total) ideally   <5.2 mmol/l
            mild increase   5.2–6.5 mmol/l
            moderate increase   6.5–7.8 mmol/l
            severe increase   >7.8 mmol/l

(as defined by the European Atherosclerosis Society)

2. Values quoted for venous plasma or serum.
Diagnostic criteria for 75 g oral glucose tolerance test (venous plasma) are detailed in Table 12.18, p. 734.

3. Up to 1.2 μmol/l in children

Table 21.4 Reference values for the more common analytes in urine

Analysis	References range	Units
Albumin	[See note 1]	
Calcium	1.2–3.7	mmol/24 h
	(low calcium diet)	
	Up to 12	
	(normal diet)	
Copper	Up to 0.6	μmol/24 h
Cortisol	9–50	μmol/mol creatinine
Creatinine	10–20	mmol/24 h
5-Hydroxyindole-3-acetic acid (5-HIAA)	10–45	μmol/24 h
Metanephrines (conjugated)	Up to 3	μmol/24 h
Oxalate	80–490 (M)	mmol/24 h
	40–320 (F)	mmol/24 h
Phosphate	15–50	mmol/24 h
Porphyrins (total)	90–370	nmol/24 h
Potassium[2]	25–100	mmol/24 h
Protein	Up to 0.3	g/l
Sodium	100–200	mmol/24 h
Urate	1.2–3.0	mmol/24 h
Urea	170–600	mmol/24 h

Notes

1. Albumin/creatinine ratio (ACR) and urinary albumin excretion rate (AER) are used to detect microalbuminuria, i.e. excessive albumin excretion in patients with diabetes mellitus, which is of predictive value in identifying patients at risk of progression to diabetic nephropathy. The test should only be carried out in the absence of overt proteinuria (dipstix negative).

ACR
Reference range:	<3.5 mg albumin/mmol creatinine
'Borderline':	3.5–10 mg albumin/mmol creatinine
Positive test:	>10 mg albumin/mmol creatinine

AER
Reference range:	<20 μg albumin/min
Microalbuminuria:	20–200 μg albumin/min

2. The urinary output of electrolytes such as sodium and potassium is normally a reflection of intake. This can vary widely, especially on a cultural, worldwide basis. The values quoted are more appropriate to a 'Western' diet.

Table 21.5 Concentrations of therapeutic drugs in blood

Drug	Sample time	Therapeutic range	Units
Anticonvulsant drugs			
Carbamazepine	Just before next dose	17–51	μmol/l
Phenobarbitone	Not critical	65–170	μmol/l
Phenytoin	Not critical	40–80	μmol/l
Valproate	Just before next dose	300–600	μmol/l
Antibiotics			
Amikacin	Peak: 1 h after i.v. dose	15–30	mg/l
	Trough: pre-dose	5–10	
Gentamycin	Peak:1 h after i.v. dose	8–12	mg/l
Tobramycin	Trough: pre-dose	<2	
Netilmycin			
Streptomycin	Peak: 1 h after i.v. dose	15–40	mg/l
	Trough: pre-dose	<5	
Vancomycin	Peak: 1 h after i.v. dose	30–40	mg/l
	Trough: pre-dose	5–10	
Others			
Cyclosporin	Just before next dose	70–300	nmol/l
Digoxin	6–18 h after last dose	1.0–2.6	nmol/l
Lithium	12–18 h after last dose	0.6–1.0	mmol/l
Quinidine	Just before next dose	2–5	mg/l
Salicylate	Just before next dose	Up to 250	mg/l
Theophylline	Just before next dose	55–110	μmol/l

Notes
1. Care should be taken in comparing values between different laboratories. This is especially important since drug measurement units can be different. In the above table, both SI *and* non-SI units feature.
2. Drug pharmacokinetics are dependent on the *individual*. For within-individual comparison, it is advisable to sample at the same relative time(s) in relation to drug administration.

Table 21.6 Tumour markers

Tumour marker	Application
α_1-fetoprotein	Hepatoma, teratoma
Acid phosphatase (prostatic isoenzyme)	Prostate
Bence–Jones protein	Multiple myeloma
CA 15.3	Breast
CA 125	Ovary
Calcitonin	Medullary carcinoma of thyroid
Carcinoembryonic antigen (CEA)	Colon, GI
Human chorionic gonadotrophin	Choriocarcinoma, testicular tumours, hepatoma
Prostate-specific antigen	Prostate

Notes
1. Tumour markers have little place in diagnosis, the exceptions being HCG in the detection of choriocarcinoma and Bence–Jones protein (BJP) in the detection of multiple myeloma. For this reason, reference ranges have not been given.
2. Measurements are useful in monitoring disease progress and in the diagnosis of recurrence.

Table 21.7 Chemical investigations for gastrointestinal tract disease

Disease	Chemical investigation	Reference range (if applicable)	Units	Other comments
Peptic ulcer				
Zollinger–Ellison syndrome	Pentagastrin test, plasma [gastrin]	Basal acid secretion <5 Stimulated acid secretions <45 (male) Stimulated acid secretions <35 (female)	mmol/h	
Completeness of vagotomy	Insulin-hypoglycaemia test	[H$^+$] increases to no more than 20 in any sample	mmol/l	Usually samples taken at 15, 30, 45 and 60 mins after insulin. Glucose must fall to <2.2 mmol/l
Acute pancreatitis				
	Plasma amylase activity	50–300	U/l	Smaller and more transient increases found in almost any acute abdominal condition. Typically (but not always) high values in acute pancreatitis, but not specific for this condition
Chronic pancreatitis				
Direct (invasive) tests	Secretin/CCK-PZ test	Juice volume >2 HCO$_3^-$ output >10 HCO$_3^-$ concentration >80	ml/kg/h mmol/h mmol/l	
Indirect tests	BT-PABA/^{14}C-PABA test Fluorescein dilaurate test	— —	— —	Hydrolysis BT-PABA impaired in chronic pancreatitis Fluorescein dilaurate hydrolysis impaired
Wilson's disease				
	Liver copper	<50 >250 (Wilson's disease)	μg/g dry weight	
Haemochromatosis				
	Liver Iron	40–60 >1000 (Haemochromatosis)	μg/100 mg dry weight	
Intestinal malabsorption				
Fat malabsorption	Faecal fat excretion Triglyceride breath test	<18 —	mmol/24 h —	Average over 5-day collection Based on metabolism ^{14}C-triolein to ^{14}CO$_2$ and measurement of latter
Carbohydrate absorption	Xylose absorption test	>15% excreted at 2 h or >35% at 5 h (urine) >0.3 (blood concentration at 2 h)	% mmol/l	5 g test
Disaccharide absorption	Disaccharide tolerance tests	—	—	
Amino acid transport	Urine chromatography	—	—	
Bacterial colonisation	Urinary indican excretion	—	—	Tryptophan metabolised to indican by bacteria in gut
	[^{14}C]-xylose breath test	—	—	Bacteria increase degradation [^{14}C]-xylose to ^{14}CO$_2$
Intestinal permeability	Cellobiose/mannitol ratio	—	—	Cellobiose *permeability* increased and mannitol *absorption* decreased in e.g. coeliac disease

Table 21.8 Hormones

Hormone	References range	Units	Comments
Adrenocorticotrophic hormone (ACTH)	Up to 20 (07:00–09:00)	mU/l	Nycthemeral rhythm, so sampling time is critical. Avoid stress. Unstable
Cortisol	160–565 (at 08:00) <205 (at 22:00)	nmol/l	Nycthemeral rhythm, so sampling time is critical. Avoid stress
Follicle-stimulating hormone (FSH) (Male)	1.5–9.0	U/l	
Follicle-stimulating hormone (FSH) (Female)*	3.0–15 (early follicular) Up to 20 (mid-cycle) >30 (post-menopausal)	U/l	
Gastrin	Up to 120	ng/l	Collect after overnight fasting. Unstable.
Growth hormone (GH)	Very variable, usually less than 2, but may be up to 50 with stress	mU/l	Avoid stress. Stimulation and suppression tests required
Insulin	Highly variable	mU/l	Levels can only be interpreted in relation to plasma glucose and body habitus
Luteinising hormone (LH) (Female)*	2.5–9.0 (early follicular) Up to 90 (mid-cycle) >30 (post-menopausal)	U/l	
Luteinising hormone (LH) (Male)	1.5–9.0	U/l	
Oestradiol-17β (Female)	110–180 (early follicular) 550–1650 (mid-cycle) 370–770 (luteal) <150 (post-menopausal)	pmol/l	
Oestradiol-17β (Male)	<200	pmol/l	
Parathyroid hormone (PTH)	10–55	ng/l	
Progesterone (Male)	<2.0	nmol/l	
Progesterone (Female)	<2.0 (follicular) >15 (Mid luteal) <2.0 (post-menopausal)	nmol/l	
Prolactin (PRL)	60–390	mU/l	Avoid stress
Testosterone (Male)	10–30	nmol/l	
Testosterone (Female)	0.8–2.8	nmol/l	
Thyroid stimulating hormone (TSH)	0.15–3.15	mU/l	
Thyroxine (free) (free T$_4$)	10–27	pmol/l	Reference range may change in pregnancy
Tri-iodothyronine (T$_3$)	1.0–2.6	nmol/l	
TSH receptor antibodies (TRAb)	<7	U/l	

* Luteal phase values similar to follicular phase.

Notes
1. A number of hormones are unstable, and collection details are critical to obtaining a meaningful result. Refer to local hospital handbook.
2. Values in the table are only a guideline; hormone levels can often only be meaningfully understood in relation to factors such as sex (e.g. testosterone); age (e.g. FSH in women), time of day (e.g. cortisol), or regulatory factors (e.g. insulin and glucose, PTH and [Ca^{2+}]. Also, reference ranges may be critically method-dependent.

HAEMATOLOGICAL VALUES

Table 21.9 Haematological values

	SI units	Other units
Bleeding time (Ivy)	2–8 min	
Body fluid (total)		50% (obese)–70% (lean) of body weight
Intracellular		30–40% of body weight
Extracellular		20–30% of body weight
Blood volume		
Red cell mass, men	0.027–0.035 l/kg	
women	0.023–0.029 l/kg	
Plasma volume (both sexes)	0.04–0.05 l/kg	
Total blood volume, men	75 ± 10 ml/kg	
women	70 ± 10 ml/kg	
Erythrocyte sedimentation rate*		
Adult male	1–10 mm/h	
Adult female	3–15 mm/h	
Fibrinogen	1.5–4.0 g/l	
Folate—serum	2.2–18 μg/l	
—red cell	> 160 μg/l	
Haemoglobin—men	130–180 g/l	
—women	115–165 g/l	
Haptoglobin	0.3–2.0 g/l	
Leucocytes–adults	$4.0–11.0 \times 10^9$/l	
Differential white cell count		
Neutrophil granulocytes	$2.0–7.9 \times 10^9$/l	40–75%
Lymphocytes	$1.5–4.0 \times 10^9$/l	20–45%
Monocytes	$0.2–0.8 \times 10^9$/l	2–10%
Eosinophil granulocytes	$0.04–0.4 \times 10^9$/l	1–6%
Basophil granulocytes	$0.01–0.1 \times 10^9$/l	0–1%
Mean corpuscular haemoglobin (MCH)	27–32 pg	
Mean corpuscular haemoglobin concentration (MCHC)	30–35 g/dl	30–35%
Mean corpuscular volume (MCV)	76–100 fl	
Packed cell volume (PCV) or haematocrit–men	0.40–0.54	
–women	0.35–0.47	
Platelets	$150–350 \times 10^9$/l	
Prothrombin time	10.5–14.5 s	
Prothrombin ratio	2.0–4.5	
APTT (heparin control)	1.5–2.5	
Red cell count–men	$4.5–6.5 \times 10^{12}$/l	
–women	$3.8–5.8 \times 10^{12}$/l	
Red cell life span (mean)	120 days	
Red cell life span $T\frac{1}{2}$ (^{51}Cr)	25–35 days	
Reticulocytes (adults)	$25–85 \times 10^9$/l	0.2–2%
Vitamin B_{12}	170–1600 ng/l	

*Higher values in older patients not necessarily abnormal

DRUG NOMENCLATURE AND PRESCRIPTION

In this book, the names that have been given for drugs have almost invariably been those approved for use in Britain. Generic or non-proprietary titles are devised or selected by the British Pharmacopoeia Commission and published by the Health Ministers at regular intervals. It must be realised, however, that many countries have their own national non-proprietary names, and that the World Health Organization also has its own list. Usually these various names are similar, but there are significant differences; for example, paracetamol (BP) is listed as acetaminophen in the United States Pharmacopeia. Proprietary names are given in this book only in exceptional circumstances, but can usually be found in the British National Formulary (BNF), the Data Sheet Compendium and as an addendum to some textbooks. There may be many totally different names for the same substance, and this can cause confusion. Doctors must also be prepared to interpret the jargon used by addicts about drugs of dependence and their effects.

Abbreviations used in relation to the administration of drugs are i.m. (intramuscular injection), i.v. (intravenous injection) and s.c. (subcutaneous injection). The BNF recommends the use of English without abbreviations for prescriptions but recognises that certain Latin abbreviations are used. For instance, frequency of doses is given throughout this book as 12-hourly, 8-hourly, etc., but students may often meet, among others, b.d. (12-hourly), t.d.s. or t.i.d. (8-hourly) and q.i.d. (6-hourly), nocte (at night) and mane (in the morning). The dosage given is a guide for use in adults of average build and should be checked against that in a national formulary or in the manufacturer's instructions. It is particularly important to confirm that a dosage given in mg/kg body weight is indeed correct, and great care must be taken to ensure that no error occurs in the quantity of a drug prescribed for an infant or child. Important factors which will affect drug dose and frequency include use in the elderly and children, the presence of renal or hepatic dysfunction and concurrent medication. All drugs, whenever possible, should be avoided during pregnancy, especially the early months.

Some drugs, for example in the chemotherapy of malignant disease, are prescribed in weight of drug per square metre of body surface. With the use of a nomogram, the body surface area can be calculated from the height in centimetres and the weight in kilograms.

Patient compliance (i.e. the taking of medicines as prescribed) is improved if instructions are simple and specific, especially for the elderly. Polypharmacy should be avoided if possible, one reason being the danger of interaction between drugs. Pharmacodynamic and pharmacokinetic interactions can cause iatrogenic disease and increased hospital admissions, particularly in the elderly and those with impaired organ function. Basic information on these and other aspects of prescribing is available in the current issue of the BNF.

STANDARD REFERENCE BOOKS

APBI Data Sheet Compendium (updated yearly)
British Medical Association and The Pharmaceutical Society of Great Britain (updated 6-monthly). The British National Formulary
Martindale—The Extra Pharmacopoeia 1993, 30th edn. Pharmaceutical Press, London

FURTHER READING

Dollery C T (ed) 1992 Therapeutic Drugs, 2 vols plus supplements 1 (1992) and 2 (1994). Churchill Livingstone, Edinburgh

INCUBATION PERIODS, IMMUNISATION SCHEDULES AND NOTIFIABLE DISEASES

Table 21.10 Incubation periods of important infections

Infection	Incubation period	
	Maximum range	Normal range
Short incubation periods (<7 days)		
Anthrax	2–5 days	
Bacillary dysentery	1–7 days	
Cholera	Hours–5 days	2–3 hours
Diphtheria	2–5 days	
Gonorrhoea	2–5 days	
Meningococcaemia	2–10 days	3–4 days
Scarlet fever	1–3 days	
Intermediate incubation periods (7–21 days)		
Amoebiasis	14 days–months	21 days
Chickenpox	14–21 days	
Lassa fever	7–14 days	
Malaria	8 days–months	
Measles	7–14 days	10 days
Mumps	12–21 days	18 days
Poliomyelitis	3–21 days	7–10 days
Psittacosis	4–14 days	10 days
Rubella	14–21 days	18 days
Trypanosoma rhodesiense infection	14–21 days	
Typhoid fever	7–21 days	
Typhus fever	7–14 days	12 days
Whooping cough	7–10 days	7 days
Long incubation periods (>21 days)		
Brucellosis	Days–months	
Filariasis	3 months–years	
Hepatitis A	2–6 weeks	4 weeks
Hepatitis B	6 weeks–6 months	12 weeks
Leishmaniasis—cutaneous	1 week–months	
—visceral	2 weeks–2 years	2–4 months
Leprosy	Years	2–5 years
Rabies	Variable	2–8 weeks
Schistosomiasis	Weeks–years	
Tuberculosis	Months–years	
Trypanosoma gambiense infection	Weeks–years	

Table 21.11 Periods of infectivity in childhood infectious diseases

Chickenpox
5 days before rash to 6 days after last crop

Diphtheria
2–3 weeks (shorter with antibiotic therapy)

Measles
From onset of prodromal symptoms to 4 days after onset of rash

Mumps
3 days before salivary swelling to 7 days after

Rubella
7 days before onset of rash to 4 days after

Scarlet fever
10–21 days after onset of rash (shortened to 1 day by penicillin)

Whooping cough
7 days after exposure to 3 weeks after onset of symptoms (shortened to 7 days by antibiotics)

Table 21.12 Immunisation schedule recommended in Britain

Age	Visits	Vaccine	Intervals
3–12 months	3	Three administrations of DTP+ OPV and *Haemophilus influenzae* type B	6–8 weeks 4–6 months
12–24 months	1	MMR vaccination	
1st year at school	1	Booster DT+OPV	
10–13 years	1	BCG for the tuberculin negative	
Girls: 11–13 years	1	Rubella vaccination	
15–19 years or on leaving school	1	Td+OPV	

DTP = Diphtheria, tetanus, pertussis ('triple') vaccine
OPV = Oral poliomyelitis vaccine
DT = Diphtheria, tetanus vaccine
Td = Tetanus, low dose diphtheria toxoid
MMR = Measles, mumps and rubella vaccine

Table 21.13 Immunisation schedule recommended by WHO for developing countries

Age	Vaccine
Birth or first contact	BCG
6, 10, 14 weeks	DPT and OPV
9 months	Measles
12 months	Yellow fever (in endemic areas)
18–24 months	DPT and OPV
5 years	DT and OPV

MMR and Hepatitis B are being introduced to schedules in many areas, also meningococcal vaccine in epidemic seasons

DTP = Diphtheria, tetanus, pertussis ('triple') vaccine
OPV = Oral poliomyelitis vaccine
DT = Diphtheria, tetanus vaccine
MMR = Measles, mumps and rubella vaccine

Table 21.14 Indications for prophylactic immunoglobulins

Human normal immunoglobulin (Pooled immunoglobulin)
Virus A hepatitis (travellers* and debilitated children)
Measles (child with heart or lung disease)

Human specific immunoglobulin
Virus B hepatitis (needlestick injuries, sexual partner)
Tetanus (susceptible injured patients)
Rabies (post-exposure protection)
Chickenpox (immunosuppressed children)
Respiratory syncytial virus infection (high risk infants, e.g.
   premature—investigational use)

* If not protected by active immunisation

Table 21.16 Notifiable infectious diseases in Britain

Under the Public Health (Control of Diseases) Act 1984
Cholera
Food poisoning
Plague
Relapsing fever
Smallpox
Typhus

Under the Public Health (Infectious Diseases) Regulations 1988
Acute encephalitis
Acute poliomyelitis
Anthrax
Diphtheria
Dysentery (amoebic or bacillary)
Leprosy
Leptospirosis
Malaria
Measles
Meningitis
Meningococcal septicaemia (without meningitis)
Mumps
Ophthalmia neonatorum
Paratyphoid fever
Rabies
Rubella
Scarlet fever
Tetanus
Tuberculosis
Typhoid fever
Viral haemorrhagic fever

Table 21.15 Indications for chemoprophylaxis

Infection to be prevented	Indication for prophylaxis	Antimicrobial agent indicated	Adult dose
Diphtheria	Susceptible contacts	Erythromycin	500 mg 6-hourly for 5 days
Meningococcal infection	Susceptible contacts	Rifampicin Ciprofloxacin	600 mg 12-hourly for 2 days 500 mg as single dose
Whooping cough	Susceptible contacts	Erythromycin	500 mg 6-hourly for 7 days
Tuberculosis	Susceptible contacts	Isoniazid	300 mg daily for 6 months
Rheumatic fever	Following rheumatic fever	Penicillin	250 mg twice daily
Endocarditis	Heart valve lesion	Amoxycillin or Erythromycin	see p. 295
Tetanus	Wound or injury	Erythromycin	500 mg 6-hourly for 7 days
Gas gangrene	Wound or injury	Penicillin or Metronidazole	600 mg 6-hourly for 5 days 500 mg 8-hourly for 5 days
Abdominal/pelvic sepsis	Colonic or gynaecological surgery	Gentamicin or Cephalosporin+Metronidazole (single dose)	
Malaria	Travel to malarious countries	Depends on country (see page 148)	

Illustration acknowledgements

WE ARE GRATEFUL TO THE FOLLOWING INDIVIDUALS AND ORGANISATIONS FOR THE LOAN OF ILLUSTRATIONS:

Chapter 1
Fig. 1.18: Dr J. Tolmie

Chapter 4
Illustrative material supplied by Dr R Davidson and the EM and Histopathology Unit, London School of Hygiene and Tropical Medicine
Figs 4.7, 4.9, 4.13, 4.14: Audio-Visual Department, St. Mary's Hospital, London, W2
Figs 4.19, 4.49: Professor J A A Hunter
Fig. 4.20: Institute of Ophthalmology, Moorfields Eye Hospital, London
Fig. 4.24: Reproduced with permission of the World Health Organization
Fig. 4.35: Professor K Vickerman

Chapter 5
Fig. 5.73A, B: Dr B Cullen

Chapter 6
Figs 6.1, 6.10B: British Lung Foundation
Figs 6.6, 6.7: Dr J Reid
Fig. 6.9: Professor N J Douglas
Fig. 6.12B: Dr A Greening

Chapter 7
Figs 7.1, 7.2, 7.3, 7.6, 7.8, 7.13, 7.14, 7.17, 7.19: Dr G M Fraser
Fig. 7.5: Dr D H Cummack

Chapter 8
Figs 8.10, 8.13, 8.16: Dr P Hayes and Dr K Simpson

Chapter 9
Fig. 9.3: Dr R G Whitehead
Fig. 9.4: Professor W Gordon
Fig. 9.6: Institute of Ophthalmology

Chapter 11
Illustrative material supplied by Dr S Forbes, Dr I Beggs, Dr J Reid
Figs 11.3, 11.5, 11.6, 11.8, 11.34: Dr P Robinson, St. James' University Hospital, Leeds
Fig. 11.7: Dr D Fowler, Leeds General Infirmary

Fig. 11.13: Professor G B Fogazzi, Ospedale Maggiore, Milan

Chapter 12
Fig. 12.44: Dr I Campbell and Dr M Macdonald

Chapter 14
Figs 14.2, 14.3: Reproduced with permission from the Cancer Research Campaign

Chapter 15
Fig. 15.26: Reproduced with permission from the Arthritis and Rheumatism Council

Chapter 18
Figs 18.14A, B, C, 18.35, 18.36, 18.37, 18.38A: Dr D Kean
Figs 18.21C, 18.22: Dr B Cullen
Figs 18.29, 18.31A, B, 18.41, 18.43: Dr R J Sellar
Figs 18.30, 18.45: Dr R Grant

THE FOLLOWING FIGURES ARE REPRODUCED WITH PUBLISHERS' PERMISSION AS LISTED:

Chapter 1
Fig. 1.14: Dr M Mikkelsen, from Brock D J H, Rodeck C H, Ferguson-Smith M A 1992 Prenatal Diagnosis and Screening. Churchill Livingstone, Edinburgh

Chapter 3
Figs 3.3, 3.4: the Lung and Asthma Information Agency Factsheet 93/5, quoting the National Environment Technology Centre (Warren Spring Laboratory)

Chapter 4
Fig. 4.25: Bryceson A D M, Pfaltzgraff R E 1990 Leprosy, 3rd edn. Churchill Livingstone, Edinburgh
Figs 4.34, 4.36A: Knight R 1982 Parasitic Disease in Man. Churchill Livingstone, Edinburgh
Fig. 4.46: Gibbons L M 1986 SEM Guide to the Morphology of Nematode Parasites of Vertebrates. Commonwealth Agricultural Bureau International, Farnham Royal, Slough

Chapter 5

Fig. 5.10: Hampton J R 1994 The ECG Made Easy, 4th edn. Churchill Livingstone, Edinburgh

Figs 5.41, 5.42, 5.43: Copyright European Resuscitation Council: from Resuscitation 22 (1992): 111–121

Fig. 5.75: Hampton J R 1992 The ECG in Practice, 2nd edn. Churchill Livingstone, Edinburgh

Chapter 6

Fig. 6.12C: Reproduced with permission from Brewis R A L et al 1995 Respiratory Medicine, 2nd edn. Baillière Tindall, London

Fig. 6.18: Reprinted from Medicine International Spring 1991: 3711, by permission of Medicine International Ltd and Prof. A Tattersfield

Fig. 6.19: Geddes D 1993 Cystic fibrosis: gene therapy trials come to the UK. MRC News, Spring 1993. Medical Research Council/Smith Ward Studios

Fig. 6.27: The Lung and Asthma Information Agency Factsheet 93/1, quoting the Office of Population Censuses and Surveys

Fig. 6.29: Johnson N McL 1986 Respiratory Medicine. Blackwell Scientific Publications, Oxford

Chapter 7

Fig. 7.11A,B: Hayes P, Simpson K 1995 Gastroenterology and Liver Disease. Churchill Livingstone, Edinburgh

Chapter 8

Fig. 8.16: Hayes P, Simpson K 1995 Gastroenterology and Liver Disease. Churchill Livingstone, Edinburgh

Fig. 8.19: Shearman D J C, Finlayson N D C 1989 Diseases of the Gastrointestinal Tract and Liver, 2nd edn. Churchill Livingstone, Edinburgh

Chapter 9

Fig. 9.7: World Health Organization 1976 Report of a Joint WHO/USAID Meeting, Vitamin A Deficiency and Xerophthalmia (WHO Technical Report Series No. 5 W

Chapter 11

Table 11.9: Boulton Jones J M et al 1982 Diagnosis and Management of Renal and Urinary Diseases. Blackwell Scientific Publications Ltd., Oxford

Fig. 11.10: Whitworth J A, Lawrence J R (eds) 1987 Textbook of Renal Disease. Churchill Livingstone, Edinburgh

Chapter 12

Fig. 12.13: Toft A D et al 1978 New England Journal of Medicine 298: 643–647

Fig. 12.16: Nussbaum S R et al 1987 Clinical Chemistry 33/8: 1364–1367

Fig. 12.17: Broadus A E et al 1988 New England Journal of Medicine 319(9): 556–563

Fig. 12.49: Gaw A 1995 Clinical Biochemistry: 120. Churchill Livingstone, Edinburgh

Fig. 12.50: Hale P J, Nattrass M 1989 Clinical Endocrinology 30: 29–38. Blackwell Scientific Publications Ltd., Oxford

Chapter 13

Fig. 13.10: based on Hoffbrand A V, Pettit J E 1992 Essential Haematology, Fig. 6.3, by permission of Blackwell Scientific Publications Ltd., Oxford

Chapter 14

Table 14.1: Reproduced from Doll R, Peto R 1982 The Causes of Cancer, by permission of Professor Sir Richard Doll and Professor R Peto of Imperial Cancer Research Fund Cancer Studies Unit, and Oxford University Press

Chapter 15

Fig. 15.20: Maddison P J, Isenberg D A, Woo P, Glass D N 1993 Oxford Textbook of Rheumatology. Oxford University Press, Oxford

Fig. 15.29: Schumacher H R (ed) 1993 Primer on the Rheumatic Diseases, 10th edn: 99. Arthritis Foundation, Atlanta

Chapter 18

Figs 18.25, 18.26: Munro J, Edwards C R W 1995 Macleod's Clinical Examination, 9th edn. Churchill Livingstone, Edinburgh

Chapter 20

Fig. 20.2: Scottish Hospital In-patient Statistics, Common Services Agency, Edinburgh

Bold type indicates major entry.

D

J